Advanced Surgical Practice

Advanced Surgical Practice

Edited by

Aljafri Abdul Majid, MBBS (Monash), BMedSc (Hons), FRCSEd, FRCSEd (Cardiothoracics)

Consultant Cardiothoracic Surgeon
University Hospital, Kuala Lumpur, Malaysia
Professor, Department of Surgery, Faculty of Medicine, University of Malaya
Member, Panel of Examiners, Royal College of Surgeons of Edinburgh

Andrew Kingsnorth, BSc, MBBS, MS, FRCS, FACS

Honorary Consultant Surgeon
Derriford Hospital, Plymouth
Professor of Surgery, Plymouth Postgraduate Medical School
External Undergraduate Examiner, Oxford, London and Kuala Lumpur; Member, Court of
Examiners, Royal College of Surgeons of England

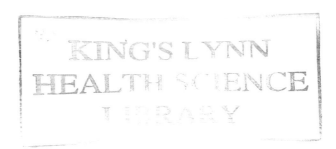

GMM

LONDON • SAN FRANCISCO

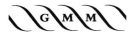

©2003
Greenwich Medical Media
4th Floor, 137 Euston Road,
London
NW1 2AA

870 Market Street, Ste 720
San Francisco
CA 94109, USA

ISBN 1 841100188

First Published 2003

www.greenwich-medical.co.uk

Distributed worldwide by Plymbridge Distributors Ltd and in the USA by Jamco Distribution

Typeset by Phoenix Photosetting, Chatham, Kent
Printed and bound in Great Britain by The Bath Press, Bath

Contents

Preface

This is the third in a series of books designed to meet the needs of the new generation of surgical trainees. The first two *Fundamentals of Surgical Practice* and *Principles of Surgical Practice* were prepared with the Basic Surgical Trainee in mind. This book *Advanced Surgical Practice* has been prepared for Specialist Registrars embarking on Higher Surgical Training in General Surgery.

Surgical training is now divided into two stages, the first being Basic Surgical Training leading to the award of the MRCS upon satisfactory completion of the stipulated requirements and examinations. This is followed by the second stage of Higher Surgical Training leading to the award of the FRCS on achieving success in one of the Intercollegiate examinations in a surgical specialty such as General Surgery, Orthopaedics, Surgical Neurology, Cardiothoracic Surgery or Urology. This two-tier system comprising the MRCS as an entrance requirement and an Intercollegiate Fellowship as an exit qualification, has, despite considerable initial debate, become firmly established, and the 'old style' Fellowship of 'Surgery in General' will soon cease to be awarded. Thus for doctors wishing to specialise in General Surgery the Intercollegiate Specialty Fellowship in General Surgery is now mandatory.

A very detailed curriculum, training requirements and syllabus in General Surgery has been drawn up by the SAC with input from the various subspecialty associations to produce the next generation of General Surgeon. The scope of General Surgery has widened considerably and it is now divided into eight subspecialties. Thus it is expected that a General Surgeon besides having a broad knowledge of the field of General Surgery may now subspecialise in one (or at most two) subspecialties.

The syllabus drawn up by the SAC consists of 10 schedules of knowledge and skills. The first two, emergency surgery and critical care are essential for all Higher Surgical Trainees in General Surgery. The remaining 8 schedules cover each of the subspecialties such as upper gastrointestinal surgery, breast surgery, endocrine surgery and vascular surgery. Each of these subspecialty schedules are further subdivided into three levels of training designated as Training in General Surgery (TIGS), Essential Subspecialty Training (EST) and Advanced Subspecialty Training (AST).

In this book we have concentrated on covering the topics listed as TIGS and EST in the 8 schedules dealing with the subspecialties since this essentially constitutes the core knowledge needed by Specialist Registrars in General Surgery. The topics in the first two schedules have been covered to some extent in the BST/MRCS programmes as well as in Fundamentals of Surgical Practice and Principles of Surgical Practice. Where appropriate they are also dealt with in the relevant subspecialty chapters.

Thus the book is divided into eight sections dealing with each of the subspecialties. In general, the beginning of the chapter deals with the theory whilst towards the end of each chapter we have incorporated a section on operative surgery which details operations which have been marked as 'index operations' in the syllabus. We hope that this combination of theory and practice will make it convenient for the busy trainee who when reading up on a particular topic will be able to have both theoretical and operative surgery aspects available, and thus save some time. At the end of each chapter we felt it appropriate to have a short list of Further reading consisting of studies which have been referred to in the text or recent reviews rather than a long list of references.

As mentioned in the preface to *Fundamentals of Surgical Practice*, the first book in our series, the process of training in surgery has undergone considerable revision over the last decade or so as a result of the change in philosophy in surgical training. This change in philosophy has arisen as a result of the rapid advances which have taken place in surgery as well as increased expectations and demands from patients and the public at large. It is hoped that this book and this series (with almost 100 chapters from about 100 surgical authorities) will contribute positively to the creation of *'Tomorrow's Surgeons'*.

AAM & ANK
Plymouth and Kuala Lumpur 2002

Foreword

The practice of surgery and surgical training are in the process of rapid change. Increasing specialisation and sub-division with demarcation lines and special examinations are confusing for both trainers and trainees. There is a danger that the broad education that used to be a traditional requirement for surgeons will change into a rigorous, technological syllabus, with progress and assessments similar to that required of an airline pilot (perhaps licensed to fly only one type of aircraft!), besides being required to put in sufficient – but not too many – hours as well as provide evidence of continuing education to keep up-to-date. The technological advances, particularly laparoscopic, endoscopic and radiological, represent the beginning of an even more rapid phase of change.

Thus, the surgeon who wishes to practise in the traditional way will need to spend most of his or her life training in the individual specialities in order to work in places such as developing countries, where the most modern and technologically advanced equipment will not be available!

The three volumes, *Fundamentals of Surgical Practice*, *Principles of Surgical Practice* and *Advanced Surgical Practice* should be of value to the surgeon who wishes to be an expert in a chosen speciality but nevertheless values a wider education. *Advanced Surgical Practice* is designed for the new Specialist Registrars in General Surgery. The short, well-written chapters cover the pathology, clinical aspects, and special investigations and describe the operative procedures most commonly performed in the subject of the chapter.

The text and illustrations are clear and, by combining the clinical and operative aspects in each chapter, the reader is provided with a broad and interesting view of the subject, which is unusual in surgical texts. I am sure that readers will enjoy this volume and find that their study for the specialist examination in general surgery will become a pleasant and instructive exercise.

Sir Roy Calne FRCS FRS
Emeritus Professor of Surgery,
University of Cambridge,
England
September 2002

Ackowledgements

The editors would like to thank all the contributors for the time and effort they have taken in the preparation of their chapters. Special thanks go to David Gardner for his drawings and to Nora Naughton and her team for their role in the production of this book. We would like to record that it has been a pleasure to work with Greenwich Medical Media, the publishers, and we are especially indebted to Geoff Nuttal, Gavin Smith and Gill Clarke for all their support.

AAM and ANK

Section 1

Upper gastrointestinal surgery

1

The oral cavity and salivary glands

William Ignace Wei, Po Wing Yuen

THE ORAL CAVITY

Surgical anatomy

The oral cavity is divided by the teeth into two parts: the outer smaller space is termed the vestibule and a larger inner portion, the oral cavity proper.

The vestibule is bounded externally by the lips and cheek and internally by the alveolus comprising the gum and teeth. The oral cavity proper is bounded anteriorly and laterally by the alveolus while posteriorly it communicates with the oropharynx through the oropharyngeal isthmus.

The roof of the oral cavity consists of the hard and soft palate, while the greater part of the floor is formed by the anterior two-thirds of the tongue. The lateral aspect of the floor is covered by reflection of the mucosa from the undersurface of the tongue to the inner surface of the mandible. This part is termed the floor of the mouth (Figure 1.1).

The wall of the oral cavity consists of mucosa, submucosa and muscle layers. The mucous membrane lining the mouth is continuous with skin at the free margins of the lips and with the mucous lining of the pharynx at the oropharyngeal isthmus. It is loosely draped over the submucosa and muscular layer at the buccal mucosa area while it is thick and adherent to the periosteum on the hard palate and alveolus.

The tongue

The tongue is a muscular organ with a tip, root, curved dorsum and an inferior surface and has an epithelial lining of squamous cells. The root is attached to the hyoid bone and the mandible and between these bones it is in contact with the geniohyoid and mylohyoid muscle.

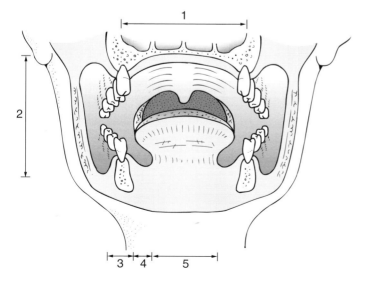

Figure 1.1 Schematic diagram of the regions in the oral cavity, 1 = palate; 2 = buccal mucosa; 3 = alveolus; 4 = floor of mouth; 5 = tongue.

The dorsum is convex in shape extending from anterior to posterior. The V-shaped groove that separates the anterior part from the posterior part of the tongue is named the sulcus terminalis. The limbs of the V run from a median pit, the foramen caecum, which marks the upper end of the thyroid diverticulum.

The anterior part (oral part) of the tongue has free margins whilst its tip rests against the incisor teeth. The oral tongue is covered with fungiform and filiform papillae. The mucous membrane on the undersurface forms a fold, the frenulum linguae, which reflects onto the floor of the mouth. Its nerve of sensation is the lingual nerve and the nerve of taste is the chorda tympani, a branch from the facial nerve.

The posterior part (pharyngeal part) of the tongue, also known as the base of the tongue, lies behind the palatoglossal arches and forms the anterior wall of the oropharynx. It is devoid of papillae but exhibits a number of low elevations, the lingual tonsils. The nerves of sensation and taste for this part of the tongue are derived from the glossopharyngeal nerve.

The lip

Skin on the outside and mucous membrane on the inside encloses the orbicularis oris muscle, labial vessels, nerves and minor salivary glands.

The floor of the mouth

This is a semilunar space over the mylohyoid and hyoglossus muscles, extending from the inner surface of the lower alveolar ridge to the undersurface of the tongue. Its posterior boundary is the base of the anterior pillar of the tonsil. Its medial boundary is the frenulum of the tongue and it contains the openings of the sublingual and submandibular glands. A thin layer of non-keratinised stratified squamous epithelium forms its lining.

The cheek

The cheek forms the side of the face and includes all the lining of the buccal mucosa. It is supported by the buccinator muscle which interdigitates with the orbicularis muscles anteriorly. The cheek is cushioned by the buccal fat pad anterior to the masseter muscle and is perforated by the parotid duct opposite the second upper molar. It is lined by non-keratinised stratified squamous epithelium.

Lymphatic drainage

Three groups of lymphatic vessels drain the tongue. They are the marginal, central and the dorsal vessels, which drain to the jugulodigastric and jugulo-omohyoid nodes.

The anterior part of the floor of the mouth has a bilateral lymphatic drainage to the submental nodes and then to the middle group of nodes of the deep cervical chain on both sides. The lateral and posterior parts of floor of mouth drain to the submandibular and deep jugular nodes on the same side.

The lymphatics of the cheek drain into the submental and submandibular nodes before reaching the deep jugular chains.

The lymph nodes located in the neck are arbitrarily divided into five levels or regions (Figure 1.2). The lymphatic drainage of various primary tumours in the head and neck region has been found to be associated with lymph nodes in different levels in the neck. The presence of a metastatic lymph node in a particular level may indicate the location of the primary tumour. In general, the primary stations of lymphatic drainage of the oral cavity are the cervical lymph nodes located at levels I, II and III in the neck.

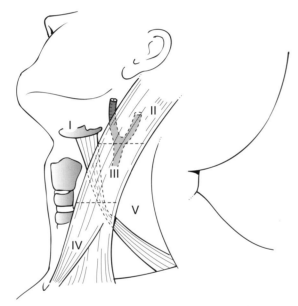

Figure 1.2 Schematic drawing of the distribution of cervical lymph nodes into five levels in the neck.

INTRAORAL CANCER

Aetiological factors

The association between tobacco and carcinoma of the oral cavity is well established. Smoking in any form is associated with a six-fold increased incidence of developing carcinoma in the oral cavity. In India and other parts of the world, the habit of chewing tobacco leaf, betel nut and slaked lime is associated with an increased incidence of intraoral carcinoma, especially that of the buccal mucosa.

Carcinoma of the oral cavity has been associated with heavy alcohol consumption in worldwide studies. Alcohol may exert its effect either directly as a carcinogen or indirectly as a co-

carcinogen. Vitamin deficiency associated with poor nutrition in alcoholics may contribute indirectly towards the development of carcinoma. The effects of alcohol and tobacco may have a synergistic effect. The risk of developing intraoral carcinoma in a smoker who is also a heavy drinker is 15 times that of a person who neither smokes nor drinks. The carcinogenic effects of tobacco and alcohol are also site specific. Smoking is more related to carcinoma of the lip and palate whilst alcohol is associated with carcinoma of the tongue and the floor of the mouth.

Other aetiological factors for the development of intraoral carcinoma include Plummer–Vinson syndrome, poor oral hygiene, mechanical irritation from sharp teeth or dentures, human papilloma virus infection and syphilis. Exposure to sunlight is associated with carcinoma of the lip. Ultraviolet rays are damaging to the lip mucosa since it lacks a protective pigmented layer.

Evaluation of intraoral cancer

The aim of assessment of intraoral cancer is to determine the extent of the primary tumour, involvement of the cervical lymph nodes and also the presence of distant metastases.

The extent of the primary tumour can be determined by clinical examination, endsocopic examination and, when indicated, examination under anaesthesia. When infiltration of the mandible is suspected, imaging studies such as plain radiographs or computed tomography may give additional clues (Figure 1.3).

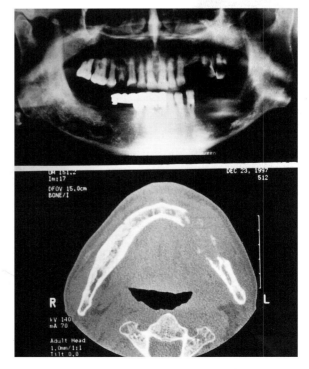

Figure 1.3 *Upper*: Orthopantomogram showing erosion of the mandible. *Lower*: Computed tomography showing erosion of the mandible

The status of cervical lymph node metastases is assessed with clinical examination. Fine needle aspiration biopsy of the enlarged lymph nodes is performed to confirm the status of the lymph nodes. Ultrasound-guided aspiration should be carried out whenever indicated (Figure 1.4).

The presence of distant metastasis is frequently evaluated with chest radiographs and liver function tests. In recent years, positron emission tomography has also been used to assess systemic metastasis (Figure 1.5).

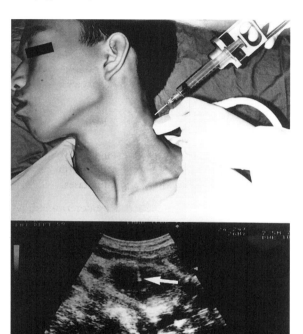

Figure 1.4 *Upper.* Fine needle aspiration biopsy of a cervical lymph node. *Lower.* Ultrasonography showing the needle (arrow) in the lymph node.

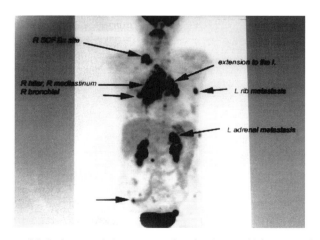

Figure 1.5 Positron emission tomography showing multiple metastasis in different parts of the body.

Staging of intraoral cancer

As with other malignancies, the clinical staging system allows the clinician to plan treatment strategies, compare therapeutic results and evaluate the prognosis of patients suffering from intraoral carcinoma. Tumour (T) staging is based on the size of the tumour and extent of local invasion. Nodal (N) staging is based on the size of the metastatic cervical lymph nodes as well as the number of nodes in the neck (Box 1.1).

Box 1.1   TNM staging system for intraoral carcinoma*

Primary tumour (T)
Tis	Carcinoma *in situ*
T1	The greatest dimension of the tumour is less than 2 cm
T2	The greatest dimension of the tumour is between 2 and 4 cm
T3	The greatest dimension of the tumour is more than 4 cm
T4	Tumour invades adjacent structure (tongue, mandible, skin)

Nodal involvement (N)
N0	No regional lymph node metastasis
N1	Single ipsilateral lymph node, greatest dimension less than 3 cm
N2a	Single ipsilateral lymph node, greatest dimension between 3 and 6 cm
N2b	Multiple ipsilateral lymph node, greatest dimension less than 6 cm
N2c	Multiple bilateral or contralateral lymph node, greatest dimension less than 3 cm
N3	Metastatic lymph node, greatest dimension more than 6 cm

Distant metastasis (M)
M0	No distant metastasis
M1	Distant metastasis

Stage grouping
Stage I	T1N0M0
Stage II	T2N0M0
Stage III	T3N0M0; T1,T2 or T3 N1M0
Stage IV	T4N0M0; T4N1M0; any T,N2 or N3 M0; any T any N, M1

---

* Modified from American Joint Committee for Cancer Staging and End Result Reporting (1988)

However, there are weaknesses with TNM staging.

- Whilst width and length are used for assessing the extent of tumour growth, depth of the tumour is not taken into account.

- In the evaluation of lymph node status, infiltration into surrounding structures and the location of the nodes are not taken into account.

Notwithstanding the above, the TNM staging system still remains popular for its simplicity. It has been suggested that the patient's performance status, nutritional condition and level of immunocompetence should also be built into future staging systems.

Second primary carcinoma

This is defined as a cancer that is geographically separate and not connected with the neoplastic epithelial change of the primary carcinoma. The incidence of second primary carcinoma following an initial intraoral carcinoma is 14% and most second carcinomas develop in the head and neck region. The concept of field carcinogenesis may be applicable here. Carcinogens such as tobacco and alcohol cause multiple genetic abnormalities in the epithelial cells. Alterations in the expression of certain genes such as Rb and p53 are critical events in the development of cancer.

The second primary cancer usually develops within two years of the initial treatment and is frequently the cause of treatment failure in those patients who present with early-stage primary carcinoma. The risk of developing multiple primaries in those patients who have stopped smoking after successful treatment of their primary carcinoma is one-sixth of those who continue to smoke.

CARCINOMA OF THE TONGUE

This is the second most common intraoral carcinoma following carcinoma of the lip in Western countries. In other races, it is the most frequently encountered intraoral carcinoma.

Leucoplakia is an important premalignant condition and presents clinically as a white keratotic plaque that cannot be rubbed off. Long-term studies have shown that 4%–18% of oral leucoplakia eventually transform into invasive carcinoma. Erythroplakia is a red mucosal plaque that does not arise from an obvious mechanical or inflammatory cause. The incidence of malignant transformation from erythroplakia is seven times that of leucoplakia; hence all erythematous areas in the oral cavity should be biopsied.

Clinical features

Carcinoma of the tongue usually occurs in males in their sixth and seventh decades of life. Carcinoma of the oral tongue arises from the lateral border over 50% of the time and occurs at the junction of the anterior and middle one-third. Early lesions take the form of a non-healing ulcer. The intrinsic muscle of the tongue offers no barrier to tumour growth and the tongue cancer may grow to significant size before it produces symptoms. The tumour may be exophytic or ulcerative in nature (Figure 1.6). When the sensory nerves supplying the tongue are affected, the patient may experience local pain and referred pain to the ear. Infiltration of the musculature of the floor of mouth will lead to ankyloglossia while involvement of the tonsillar pillars from carcinoma located in the posterior one-third of the tongue will lead to dysphagia and slurring of speech. When the carcinoma infiltrates deeper to involve vessels of significant size, spontaneous bleeding may occur.

About 30% of patients suffering from carcinoma of the tongue on presentation have cervical lymph nodes located in levels I, II or

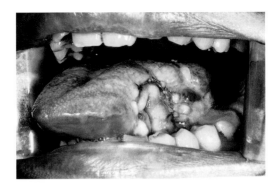

Figure 1.6 Exophytic carcinoma of the tongue over the lateral border of tongue.

III. When the carcinoma crosses the mid-line, bilateral neck lymph node metastasis may occur.

Investigations

Besides carrying out the investigations listed above to assess the status of metastasis to cervical lymph nodes and to distant sites, the local extent of carcinoma of tongue should be determined with an examination of the patient under anaesthesia. This eliminates the pain and apprehension associated with clinical examination and allows for a more accurate assessment, particularly regarding local extent of the carcinoma.

A biopsy of the suspected tongue carcinoma can also be taken when the patient is under general anaesthesia. The biopsy should be taken from the edge of the tongue ulcer. At this junctional region, the difference between normal and malignant cells is more obvious and adequate tissue can usually be obtained for histological examination. One of the complications of biopsy of the tongue is the associated bleeding. When the biopsy is taken from the edge of the ulcer, there is usually sufficient normal surrounding tissue around for haemostatic sutures to be inserted.

Treatment

This depends on the stage of the carcinoma. In general, for stage I and II carcinomas, radiotherapy and surgery produce similar results while for stage III or IV carcinomas, surgery followed by radiotherapy provides a greater chance of cure.

Early carcinoma

Radiotherapy, either by external beam radiation or brachytherapy, may be employed. The need for irradiation of the neck in early carcinoma of the tongue is debatable although in general, the neck is also included in the radiation field when external beam irradiation is administered.

Surgical resection of early carcinoma of the tongue is another therapeutic option and involves the transoral resection of the tumour with an adequate margin (1 cm of normal tissue measured from all sides of tumour). After resection, the defect can usually be closed primarily. The application of a split-thickness skin graft does not offer any additional advantage. The functional outcome after transoral resection of a part of the tongue is usually excellent and swallowing and speech functions return to normal after rehabilitation.

In view of the high incidence of metastases to cervical lymph nodes in carcinoma of the tongue, selective neck dissection with removal of the lymph nodes in level I, II and III on the side of the tumour is recommended. This is usually performed at the same time as the transoral resection.

Advanced carcinoma

For advanced carcinoma, surgical resection of the tumour followed by reconstruction and postoperative radiotherapy is the mainstay of treatment.

Resection

The primary tumour may be resected by a transoral hemi-glossectomy or partial glossectomy. When the tumour is extensive and crosses the mid-line, total glossectomy is indicated (Figure 1.7). When the carcinoma of the tongue extends laterally to involve surrounding structures, such as the floor of mouth, the mandible or posteriorly to affect the larynx, these structures will also need to be resected.

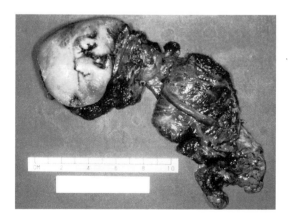

Figure 1.7 Specimen of total glossectomy with radical neck dissection.

Reconstruction

The aim of reconstruction is to fill the defect created after tumour resection and to provide maximum mobility of the tongue remnant. After a hemiglossectomy or partial glossectomy, the radial forearm free flap is a very good reconstructive option. The full-thickness skin does not contract and the mobility of the tongue remnant is retained. The donor defect can be covered

with a split-thickness skin graft or closed primarily if the skin island harvested is small. The resection and reconstruction can be performed simultaneously by two teams to reduce operating time. The skin island is sutured to the intraoral defect and the pedicle tunnelled through the floor of the mouth to be anastomosed to the vessels in the neck under magnification (Figure 1.8).

When total glossectomy or glossolaryngectomy is carried out for eradication of carcinoma of the tongue, the defect in the floor of the mouth is best closed with the pedicled pectoralis major myocutaneous flap. This flap is raised from the chest wall with the skin island lying on its surface. The pectoral branch of the acromiothoracic trunk, the main blood vessel of the muscle, lies on its undersurface. The pectoralis major muscle is then turned upwards to the neck together with its blood supply and the appropriately designed skin island. The skin island is used to line the defect in the floor of the oral cavity and the muscle bulk of the pectoralis major muscle is placed under the neck skin. This myocutaneous flap is easy to raise and has low associated morbidity. In addition, it provides tissue bulk for the whole floor of the mouth and this is essential for swallowing (Figure 1.9).

Postoperative radiotherapy

In view of the high recurrence rate locally and metastatic potential to the cervical nodes, full doses of external radiotherapy should be

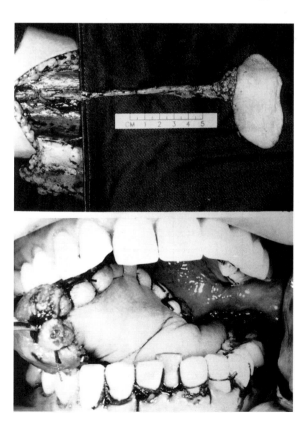

Figure 1.8 *Upper.* Radial forearm flap harvested. *Lower.* Skin island sutured in the mouth for reconstruction.

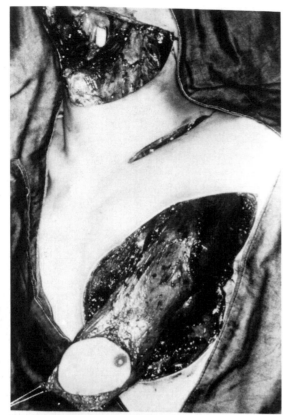

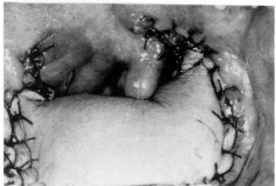

Figure 1.9 *Upper.* Pectoralis major myocutaneous flap raised. *Lower.* Skin island of pectoralis major myocutaneous flap sutured in mouth after total glossectomy.

delivered both to the primary site as well as to the neck. Irradiation is started once the wound has healed.

Treatment of cervical lymph nodes

N0 NECK

Carcinoma of the tongue is well known for its high propensity for subclinical nodal metastasis. Regional recurrence is the commonest site of recurrence for early-stage carcinoma. The regional recurrence rate of untreated N0 neck is around 30% for early T1 and T2 carcinoma and 90% appear within 20 months following surgery.

ASSESSMENT OF THE N0 NECK

More accurate nodal staging can be achieved nowadays with the help of CT scan, MRI and ultrasound screening of the N0 neck. Ultrasound-guided fine needle aspiration cytology carried out by experienced clinicians and cytopathologists is the most accurate diagnostic method (see Figure 1.4).

Although the above radiological investigations are recommended for the N0 neck, very small micrometastases within these non-palpable neck nodes continue to escape detection.

ELECTIVE NECK DISSECTION

In view of the high incidence of nodal recurrences in the neck, elective neck dissection of the N0 neck is increasingly practised. Elective neck dissection allows histopathological staging of the neck and for those node-positive necks this information may be used to guide subsequent postoperative radiotherapy. Elective selective neck dissection clearing the lymph nodes in levels I, II and III is the treatment strategy of choice for 'T' stage I and II carcinoma of the oral tongue.

N+ NECK

Radical neck dissection is the treatment of choice and should be performed together with resection of the primary carcinoma of the tongue. Resection of the sternomastoid muscle and other soft tissues in the neck provides space to accommodate the pectoralis major muscle used for reconstruction. Postoperative radiotherapy should also be administered.

Rehabilitation

After surgery, the patient is initially fed via a nasogastric tube and once the wounds have healed, oral feeding is started. Patients who receive postoperative irradiation often require a period of training before full functional recovery occurs.

CARCINOMA OF THE LIP

The incidence varies with geographical region and race. The incidence is high in southern Australia (13 per 100 000), northern Spain (11 per 100 000) and among fishermen of Newfoundland (50 per 100 000). It is, however, uncommon in Asia.

Besides tobacco and alcohol, other aetiological factors include thermal injury, mechanical irritation, trauma, poor oral hygiene, chemical exposure, immunosuppression, infection such as syphilis and prolonged exposure to harsh weather conditions such as wind, cold and dryness as well as cumulative exposure to ultra-violet light from the sun. This last factor may explain why over 90% of cancers of the lip occur on the lower lip, which is the part more exposed to direct sunlight.

Clinical features

Carcinoma of the lip usually presents as a non-healing ulcer and sometimes as a painless nodule. Any non-healing ulcer over the lip should thus be biopsied to achieve an early diagnosis. Metastasis to cervical lymph nodes is unusual.

Management

Radiotherapy, in the form of brachytherapy or external radiation for small tumours of less than 2 cm in diameter, results in a five-year survival of over 90%. The disadvantages of irradiation include cost of therapy, possibility of osteoradionecrosis and development of atrophy, fibrosis and telangiectasia.

Surgery is frequently employed as the definitive form of treatment as it offers the advantage of rapid and complete removal of the tumour.

For tumours involving a large portion of the lip but localised to the mucosa, mucosal resection is adequate. The defect can be covered by advancing intraoral mucosa from the inner aspect of the lip. For localised infiltrative carcinoma of the lip, surgical resection removing a V- or W-shaped piece of tissue with a margin of 4–6 mm is necessary to achieve tumour clearance. After adequate resection, the lip defect should be reconstructed to provide optimal preservation and restoration of anatomic and cosmetic function.

With full-thickness resections, the V-shaped defect may be closed primarily for defects up to one-third of the lip length. For larger defects, part of the normal lip may be switched around for optimal reconstruction. This cross-lip flap is transposed across the commissure as a one-stage procedure or across the mouth as a two-stage procedure (Figure 1.10).

As carcinoma of the lip rarely metastasises to the cervical lymph nodes, elective treatment of the neck is not necessary. Radical neck dissection is only carried out for clinically positive nodes.

CARCINOMA OF THE FLOOR OF THE MOUTH

Clinical features

Carcinoma of the floor of the mouth frequently presents as a non-healing ulcer with surrounding leucoplakia or erythroplakia. The majority of tumours are squamous cell carcinomas while the rest are malignant tumours arising from the sublingual glands or minor salivary glands. It may extend medially to the ventral surface of the oral tongue, laterally to the alveolar ridge and mandible, posteriorly to the posterior tongue, tonsillar region and retromolar trigone. Inferiorly, it may infiltrate the salivary glands and musculature of the floor of the mouth such as the mylohyoid. Cervical lymph nodes are palpable in around 50% of patients on

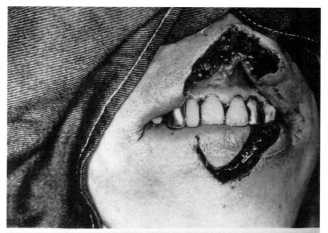
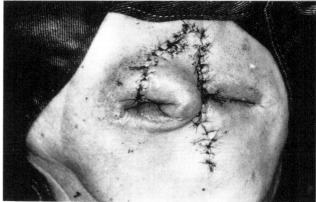
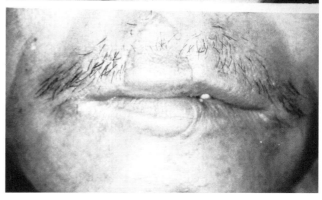

Figure 1.10 *Upper*: Defect created after resection of tumour over the upper lip and the lower lip flap is prepared for reconstruction. *Middle*: Lower lip flap switched up and insetted. *Lower*: Final result after dividing the soft tissue connection.

presentation. Distant metastasis is uncommon but must be excluded before radical curative treatment is instituted.

Investigations

A suspicious lesion in the floor of the mouth should be biopsied and, when indicated, examined under general anaesthesia. This should be carried out to determine the extent of the malignant growth before definitive treatment is planned.

In patients with teeth, the malignant growth rarely invades the mandible, as the periosteum is a good barrier to tumour infiltration. In the edentulous patient, the height of the mandible is reduced and the carcinoma of the floor of the mouth may extend laterally to involve the superior surface of the alveolus and invade the mandible through the empty tooth sockets. Computed tomography is a good means of detecting mandibular invasion (see Figure 1.3).

If metastasis to the cervical lymph nodes is suspected, fine needle aspiration cytology is indicated. For lymph nodes located deep in the neck, this can be performed under ultrasound guidance.

Endoscopic examination of the upper aerodigestive tract should be carried out to rule out a synchronous second primary tumour. Chest radiographs and other diagnostic tests to exclude metastases should also be performed before embarking on radical treatment.

Management

Primary tumour

For small lesions, surgery is the primary treatment modality, as it is simple and does not have many side effects. For patients who are not fit for operation because of underlying medical condition or other reasons, radiotherapy may be offered. This therapeutic modality may be delivered in the form of external beam irradiation or brachytherapy. The main complications are osteo-radionecrosis of the nearby mandible and xerostomia in the long term.

Resection and reconstruction

Small and superficial lesions are best treated by transoral excision with primary wound closure. When the defect cannot be closed primarily, a split-thickness skin graft can be used to cover the defect. The skin graft can be maintained in position with a tie-over dressing in the mouth for seven days. When a pedicle graft is required to cover a small area in the floor of the mouth, the nasolabial flap can be used. It is more applicable in edentulous patients (Figure 1.11).

When the carcinoma is more infiltrative and affects the musculature in the floor of the mouth, radical resection of the floor of the mouth is indicated. A combined oral and neck approach is used and the resultant defect is best closed with the radial forearm free flap. This fasciocutaneous flap is thin, pliable and can be sutured to fit the shape of the defect in the floor of the mouth. Its pedicle is joined to vessels in the neck. Tongue flaps should not be used for reconstruction of defects in the floor of the mouth as they reduce the mobility of the tongue and hence its function.

When carcinoma in the floor of mouth extends to involve the tongue, resection of the primary tumour together with partial glossectomy is indicated. The defect can again be reconstructed with the radial forearm free flap. Alternatively, when a large defect is created after tumour excision, the pectoralis major myocutaneous flap may be used for reconstruction although it is more bulky and may reduce the mobility of the tongue. It is, however, an easy flap to raise and very reliable.

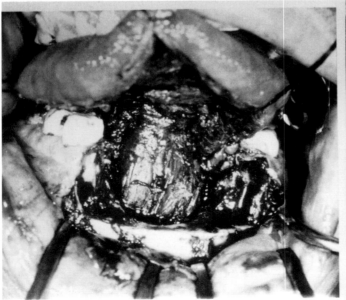 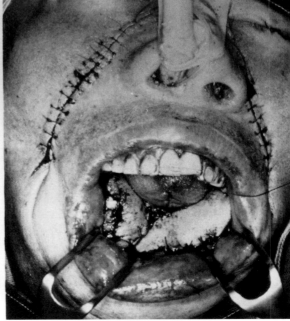

Figure 1.11 *Left*: Defect created after resection of carcinoma floor of mouth with partial mandibulectomy. *Right*: Bilateral nasolabial flaps insetted for reconstruction.

When the primary carcinoma involves the mandible, *en bloc* resection of the tumour with the mandible is indicated for tumour clearance. Either a partial mandibulectomy, removing the lingual cortex or upper half of the mandible (Figure 1.12), or, for more extensive tumours, segmental mandibulectomy may be needed to adequately excise the tumour.

After partial mandibulectomy, there is no need for mandibular reconstruction as long as the defect of the floor of the mouth is covered. After segmental mandibulectomy, the most appropriate method of reconstruction is microvascular free bone transfer, usually with a segment of fibula. Its overlying skin island (supplied by perforators of the peroneal vessel that supplies the fibula bone) can be used for reconstruction of the defect in the floor of mouth at the same time (Figure 1.13).

For advanced carcinoma, it is often the practice to provide a course of postoperative radiotherapy to the primary site as well as to the neck.

Treatment of cervical lymph nodes

This is similar to the management of lymph nodes in carcinoma of the tongue. For N+ lymph nodes, radical neck dissection should be carried out. For N0 necks, selective neck dissection of lymph nodes in levels I, II and III on the side of the lesion should be carried out electively.

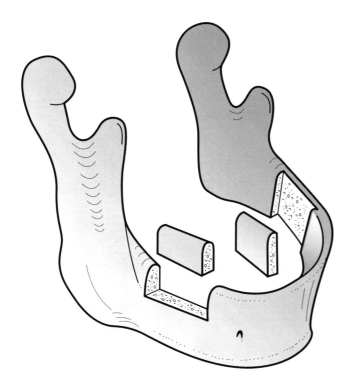

Figure 1.12 Schematic diagram showing partial resection of the mandible. Vertical resection of lingual aspect of mandible (*right*) and horizontal resection of upper part of mandible (*left*).

When the primary lesion crosses the mid-line, bilateral lymph node clearance should be performed.

CARCINOMA OF THE BUCCAL MUCOSA

Clinical features

About 10% of intraoral cancers, in Western countries are located in the buccal mucosa, whereas in India this site accounts for 40% of all intraoral cancers. This is related to the practice of chewing tobacco and betel nut. The macroscopic appearance commonly takes the form of an exophytic or verrucous growth arising from a preexisting leucoplakia. It may also appear to be an ulcer and infiltrate underlying musculature (Figure 1.14). Deeply invasive tumours can involve the skin and subcutaneous tissues. Medial extension of the carcinoma involves the upper alveolus and maxilla or inferiorly to the lower alveolus and mandible. When it extends posteriorly to infiltrate the pterygoid muscles the patient will have trismus, resulting in poor oral intake followed by wasting. Over 50% of patients on presentation have disease at an advanced stage.

Metastasis is usually to the submandibular group of lymph nodes although posteriorly situated tumours often metastasise to the jugulodigastric nodes. The incidence of occult cervical nodal metastasis is, however, not high (around 10%).

Management

Early malignancies in the buccal mucosa can be treated successfully with radiotherapy although it may lead to some degree of fibrosis and mild trismus.

When the growth has a distinct margin or when it infiltrates bone, surgical resection is indicated.

Resection and reconstruction

For small and superficial lesions, i.e. those less than 2 cm in diameter, transoral excision and primary closure of the defect is usually possible. The resection should be carried out together with frozen sections to ensure adequate tumour extirpation.

When the lesion is larger than 2 cm, transoral resection together with repair of the defect with a radial free forearm flap is the preferred method of treatment. The pedicle of the free flap is delivered to the neck and joined to the cervical vessels under magnification. The full-thickness skin of the flap does not contract and the complication of trismus is avoided. Although a split-thickness skin graft is easily applied, the graft may contract and result in trismus.

When the malignant growth extends deeply to involve subcutaneous tissue and skin, a through-and-through resection of

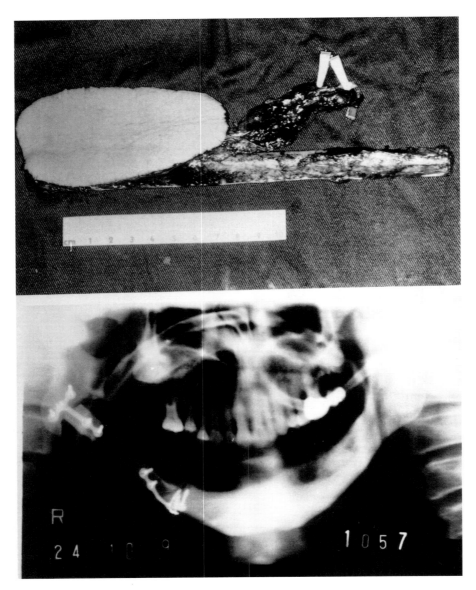

Figure 1.13 *Upper.* A segment of fibula bone harvested for reconstruction following a segmental mandibulectomy. The skin island is used for reconstruction of associated defect in the floor of the mouth. *Lower.* Postoperative X-ray showing the fibula bone.

the tumour is mandatory to achieve a curative resection. To reconstruct the resultant defect two linings, one for the skin exteriorly and one for intraoral resurfacing, are needed (Figure 1.15). The pectoralis major myocutaneous flap can be used to provide one lining and some bulk for the cheek while the delto-pectoral flap may be used for the other. Alternatively, the radial forearm flap can be used with the pectoralis major myocutaneous flap.

When the tumour extends to involve the maxilla, part of the involved maxillary bone has to be removed *en bloc* with the buccal mucosa tumour to effect a curative resection. The resultant defect under these circumstances has then to be reconstructed appropriately. A dental prosthesis may be used for reconstruction of the maxillary defect in addition to flaps used for reconstruction of the

intraoral defect. When the lesion involves the mandible, it can be removed together with the carcinoma of the buccal mucosa and the defect reconstructed.

For advanced buccal mucosa carcinoma, postoperative radiotherapy should be delivered to improve the chance of cure.

Treatment of cervical lymph nodes

For metastatic cervical lymph nodes, radical neck dissection is the treatment of choice. In view of the low incidence of occult metastasis, the benefit of elective treatment of the neck nodes is equivocal in carcinoma of the buccal mucosa. Close observation is usually adopted.

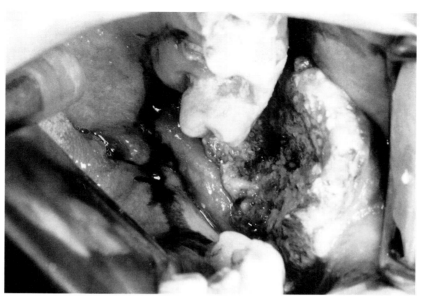

Figure 1.14 Ulcerative carcinoma of the buccal mucosa.

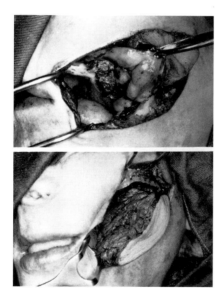

Figure 1.15 *Upper.* Defect created after through-and-through resection. *Lower.* Buccal mucosal defect reconstructed with pectoralis major myocutaneous flap for intraoral lining and deltopectoral flap for cutaneous resurfacing.

SALIVARY GLANDS

Parotid gland

Anatomy

The parotid gland lying on the lateral aspect of the face is situated between the ascending ramus of the mandible in front and the mastoid bone posteriorly. Superiorly is the zygomatic arch and posteroinferiorly it is limited by the sternomastoid muscle. Its lateral surface lies beneath the skin while its medial surface lies

over the styloid process and its associated muscles, stylohyoid, styloglossus and stylopharyngeus. Further medially is the carotid sheath with its contents and the superior portion of the lateral pharyngeal wall.

The gland is divided by the facial nerve into a larger superficial and a smaller deep lobe. The facial nerve emerges from the stylomastoid foramen to enter the posteromedial surface of the gland and it divides into two trunks, the temporofacial and the cervicofacial (Figure 1.16). It subsequently divides into five branches: temporal, zygomatic, buccal, mandibular and cervical. The facial nerve can be identified by one of the following methods.

- The main trunk of the facial nerve usually lies inferior and on a slightly deeper plane than the 'pointer'. Following the outer surface of the cartilaginous portion of the external auditory canal medially, the 'cartilaginous pointer' appears as the cartilage joins the bony portion of the canal.

- The vertical portion of the facial nerve can be identified within the mastoid cavity and traced through the stylomastoid foramen.

- The branches of the facial nerve can be identified peripherally and traced backwards to the main trunk.

The auriculotemporal nerve, the superficial temporal artery and vein leave the superior border of the parotid gland while the retromandibular vein enters at the inferior border. The greater auricular nerve bringing the cutaneous supply lies along the posterior border of the gland. The five branches of the facial nerve all leave the gland beneath its anterior border to enter the submuscular plane of the face.

The parotid duct formed by ductules among the parotid gland frequently originates from the superficial lobe, although it may

15

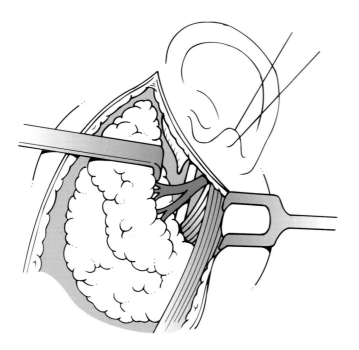

Figure 1.16 Schematic drawing of the two lobes of the parotid gland separated by the facial nerve which exits from the stylomastoid foramen behind the styloid process.

also exit from the deep lobe. It lies on the surface of the masseter muscle, 1 cm below and parallel to the lower border of the zygomatic arch. It turns medially at the anterior border of the masseter muscle, pierces the buccinator muscle, buccal fat pad and the oral mucosa opposite the upper second molar.

Infection and inflammation

Infection of the parotid gland is generally grouped into three categories.

- *Bacterial infections*: these are usually associated with mechanical blockage of the flow of saliva or associated with reduced production of saliva.
- *Viral infections*: some viruses tend to affect the salivary glands, in particular the parotid gland.
- *Granulomatous inflammation*.

Acute suppurative parotitis

This occurs as a result of retrograde ascending bacterial infection secondary to reduction in the production of saliva. This usually occurs in debilitated patients, both male and female, in their 60s or 70s. Patients in the postoperative period are particularly prone to develop this condition since there is less stimulation of salivation as a result of reduced oral intake. Saliva flow is reduced in dehydrated patients and when diuretics are given.

The patient usually experiences a tender swelling which rapidly appears in the affected gland (Figure 1.17); in 15% of patients, both parotid glands may be affected. Systemic manifestations may include fever, chills and malaise. Bimanual palpation of the gland may express purulent discharge from the opening of the parotid duct. The commonly cultured bacteria include *Staphylococcus aureus*, *Streptococcus pyogenes*, *Strep. viridans*, *Strep. pneumoniae* and *Haemophilus influenzae*.

Conservative treatment such as intravenous antibiotics, rehydration with electrolytes and fluids, improvement of oral hygiene and sialogogues should be instituted. Analgesics and local heat application help to lower the discomfort. Most acute suppurative parotitis subsides with conservative treatment. Occasionally, the infection may coalesce to form an abscess that may warrant external surgical drainage.

Recurrent suppurative parotitis in children

This presents as recurrent episodes of parotid gland swelling following a meal associated with malaise and pain in otherwise healthy children. Males are more frequently affected than females and the organism isolated is *Streptococcus viridans*. With appropriate antibiotic treatment, resolution of the parotid swelling and inflammation usually follows. Recurrent attacks of parotitis usually cease after adolescence. Rarely, the repeated attacks of parotitis progress to chronic sialadenitis.

Chronic parotitis

This is a localised condition of the parotid gland, characterised by repeated attacks of swelling and inflammation of the gland. The inflammation leads to parenchymal degeneration and fibrosis. The asymptomatic period may last a few weeks to a few months. Following repeated attacks of infection, the periductal fibrosis becomes irreversible and is the cause of obstruction of saliva flow.

The patient experiences repeated attacks of pain and swelling of the parotid gland. On examination, the gland is enlarged and indurated. Treatment is mainly conservative. When the symptoms become severe, surgical removal of the gland may be offered.

Viral inflammation of the salivary gland

Viral inflammation of the salivary gland mostly occurs through haematogenous dissemination.

Mumps

This acute non-suppurative parotitis is caused by the highly contagious paramyxovirus that is endemic in the community and spread by airborne droplets from salivary, nasal or urinary secretion.

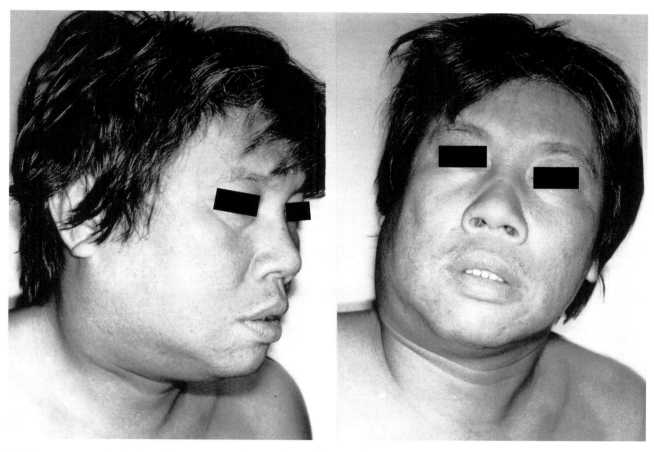

Figure 1.17 Immunocompromised patient with acute suppurative parotitis. Involvement of the surrounding muscle leads to the torticollis.

The patient usually is a child with initial symptoms of viral infection such as low-grade fever, malaise and headache. After an incubation period of 18 days, the patient experiences swelling and pain of one or both parotid glands. The pain is severe during eating as saliva is secreted from the inflamed salivary gland.

The diagnosis can be made from the typical clinical course and can be confirmed with haemagglutination inhibition and complement fixation tests. The treatment, as in all viral disease, is conservative, aiming at reducing complications. This includes adequate rest and hydration. More fulminant infection may progress to pancreatitis, nephritis, orchitis or even meningoencephalitis.

Acquired immunodeficiency syndrome (AIDS)

Human immunodeficiency virus is frequently associated with lymphoproliferative enlargement of the parotid gland together with reduced production of saliva.

The patient presents with gradual non-tender enlargement of one or more of the salivary glands with associated xerostomia. Biopsy of the gland shows inflammation similar to that of an autoimmune disease and the diagnosis can be confirmed by serological tests for the human immunodeficiency virus (HIV).

The treatment is usually conservative and surgical resection of the parotid gland is only indicated to rule out the possibility of lymphoma affecting the gland in these HIV-positive patients.

Sialolithiasis

Stones in the ductal system may occur as a result of stagnation of saliva or originate from a nidus of desquamated ductal epithelium. Stones are more common in the submandibular gland as the secretion of the gland is more mucoid in nature.

When stones form in the parotid gland, it is usually associated with chronic parotitis where the fibrosis causes narrowing of the ductal system. The patient frequently complains of swelling of the gland after food and this gradually subsides over a few hours. Occasionally, the stone can be detected with plain radiographs; otherwise, a sialogram may be necessary to confirm the nature and identify the location of the obstruction. When the stone is located at the orifice of the parotid duct, it may be removed by slitting the orifice under local anaesthesia. Meatoplasty of the ductal orifice is necessary following the removal of the stone. When stones are located in the proximal duct or within the gland, parotidectomy is necessary.

Neoplasms of the parotid gland

The parotid gland develops from ingrowths of the oral epithelium which develop into tubules which become the ductal system of the salivary gland. The acinar secretory cells empty into the intercalated duct that drains into the striated duct and then into the excretory duct. Every type of cell in the gland can undergo neoplastic transformation and this accounts for the variety of benign and malignant tumours arising from the parotid gland.

Benign tumours

CLINICAL FEATURES

Benign tumours of the parotid gland present as painless, mobile, slow-growing masses and do not change in size on eating. The facial nerve as a rule remains intact. A sudden increase in size of the mass may be caused by malignant change, cystic degeneration or bleeding into the tumour.

The location of the tumour may sometimes lead to other differential diagnoses. Those occurring at the tail of the parotid gland may be misdiagnosed as a lymph node (Figure 1.18). Benign tumours situated in the deep lobe of the parotid gland may only present externally as a vague parotid swelling. The tumour bulk may appear to push the tonsil or the soft palate into the oral cavity (Figure 1.19). The two most common benign tumours in the parotid gland are the pleomorphic adenoma and adenolymphoma.

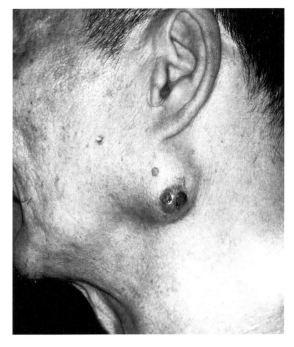

Figure 1.18 Tumour located in the lower part of the parotid gland may mimic an upper cervical lymph node.

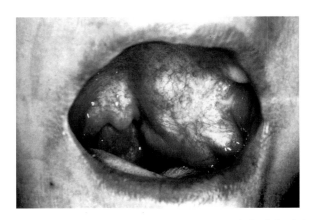

Figure 1.19 A deep lobe parotid tumour presenting as a bulge behind the soft palate.

DIAGNOSIS

Clinical course and examination contribute significantly to the diagnosis of benign parotid gland tumours. Imaging studies such as computed tomography or magnetic resonance imaging reveal the extent of the tumour but cannot differentiate between benign and malignant lesions.

Fine needle aspiration cytology is now commonly used for the evaluation of parotid neoplasms. With an experienced cytologist and good sampling of the neoplasm, its accuracy in differentiating benign from malignant conditions approaches 90%.

Pleomorphic adenoma

This is the most common benign tumour of the parotid gland. The term 'pleomorphic' refers to the origin of tumour, from both epithelial and connective tissue. This tumour usually presents in the fourth or fifth decade as a firm, painless and mobile mass in the parotid region. About 90% are in the superficial lobe while the remaining 10% are in the deep lobe. The macroscopic appearance of a pleomorphic adenoma is a solitary firm tumour with a thin and delicate capsule (Figure 1.20). Pseudopodia of tumour may actually extend beyond the capsule. The tumour must be removed with a thin rim of normal tissue to effect a curative resection. Enucleation of this tumour will result in local recurrence.

For tumours located in the superficial lobe, superficial parotidectomy has traditionally been the treatment of choice. In recent years, less extensive resection has been advocated. As long as the tumour is removed with a thin rim of tissue around the tumour, local recurrence is uncommon. When the main tumour is situated in the deep lobe, total parotidectomy with preservation of the facial nerve is indicated.

Adenolymphoma (Warthin's tumour)

This is the second most common benign tumour of the parotid gland which presents in the sixth decade as a mass over the angle of the mandible and has a male predominance (Figure 1.21). It is

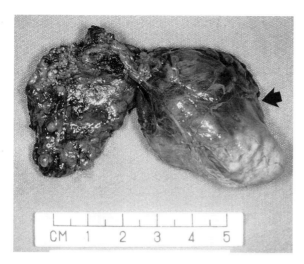

Figure 1.20 Resected specimen of a pleomorphic adenoma of the deep lobe of the parotid gland (arrow). The tumour was removed with superficial lobe.

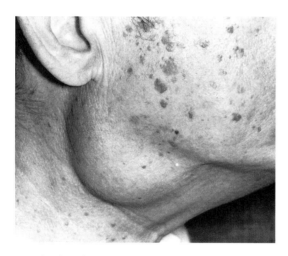

Figure 1.21 Adenolymphoma (Warthin's tumour) in an elderly man.

soft to firm in consistency, occurring at the angle of the mandible and is bilateral in 10% of patients. The tumour is usually encapsulated and contains lymphoid tissue on histological examination. Complete removal of the tumour via superficial parotidectomy with preservation of the facial nerve is the preferred treatment.

BENIGN LYMPHOEPITHELIAL LESIONS

This term covers a group of benign diseases which usually affect females in their fifth or sixth decades who present with unilateral, bilateral or even successive enlargement of the salivary gland and/or the lacrimal glands. The swellings are usually asymptomatic although there may be mild distending pain. The cause of the swelling is thought to be reactive and may be related to autoimmune disease. The clinical course of the pathology is benign although the development of lymphoma or anaplastic carcinoma is possible. The following group of diseases are considered to be benign lymphoepithelial lesions.

Mikulicz syndrome

This term is used to describe those patients with enlarged salivary gland and/or lacrimal gland as a result of systemic disease. The enlarged glands are asymptomatic. The treatment involves the management of underlying systemic disease.

Sjögren's syndrome

This is considered as a chronic autoimmune disease and characterised by the triad of keratoconjunctivitis, xerostomia and a collagen vascular disease such as rheumatoid arthritis. When the patient only has the former two syndromes, the term 'sicca complex' is used.

This is more commonly seen in females in their 50s and the enlargement of the glands is usually diffuse. The treatment aims to control symptoms.

Malignant tumours of the parotid gland

Malignancies of the parotid gland are challenging as the pathology is varied and complex, the biological course unpredictable and the anatomy of the facial nerve intricately related to the parotid gland. The incidence of malignancies of the salivary gland is 1–2 per 100 000. Around 85% of all neoplasms are in the parotid gland and of these, 20% are malignant lesions.

CLINICAL FEATURES

Patients usually present with a slow-growing mass in the parotid gland. Initially there is no pain but with increasing size, pain is present in about 20% of patients. Facial nerve involvement resulting in facial paralysis is seen in 10–15% of patients with malignancy of the parotid gland (Figure 1.22).

HISTOLOGICAL TYPES

Acinic cell carcinoma

This is regarded as a low-grade malignancy as it has a favourable biological behaviour. This carcinoma occurs in patients of all ages with a slight female preponderance. Patients usually present with an asymptomatic mass and the diagnosis is made after microscopic examination of the parotidectomy specimen. Where the surgical margins are clear, no further therapy is necessary. Otherwise, a completion total parotidectomy preserving the facial nerve is necessary. The best chance of cure lies in the complete surgical removal of the tumour. Five-year survival is over 85%.

Adenoid cystic carcinoma

The characteristic clinical features of this tumour are its slow growth over many years and the development of local recurrence or distant metastasis despite aggressive therapy. Despite this, even

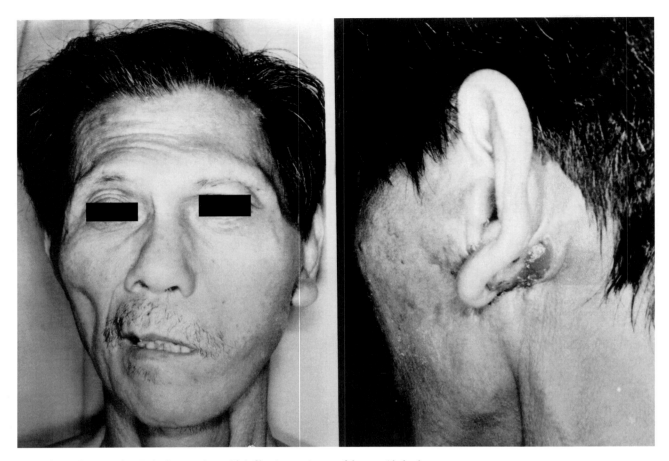

Figure 1.22 *Left*: Facial nerve palsy. *Right*: Same patient with infiltrative carcinoma of the parotid gland.

when patients have multiple pulmonary metastasis, they may survive several years.

Microscopically the tumour exhibits perineural spread and this may account for its high potential of local recurrence. Perineural spread and metastasis to cervical lymph nodes are associated with a worse prognosis. Three histological patterns have been recognised: tubular, cribriform and solid. The tubular pattern is associated with the best prognosis while the solid pattern is the worst. Most tumours present with a mixture of the three patterns.

Adequate surgical resection is the optimal treatment for this carcinoma and adjuvant radiotherapy helps to reduce local and regional recurrence. In view of the slow-growing nature of the carcinoma, an observation period of over 10 years is necessary. The five-year survival of 66% falls to 22% at 20 years.

Mucoepidermoid carcinoma

This is the commonest malignancy of the parotid gland. Patients usually present with a rapidly enlarging parotid mass which may be associated with facial nerve paralysis (Figure 1.23). Histologically, the tumour is composed of three types of cells present in variable amounts: the mucus-secreting, epidermoid and inter-

mediate cells. The prognosis depends on the degree of differentiation; the well-differentiated type (grade 1) has a low incidence of metastasis, the moderately differentiated type (grade 2) has a greater chance of local recurrence but rarely metastasises. The poorly differentiated type (grade 3) has the worst prognosis.

Poorly differentiated carcinoma has a high chance of metastasis to the cervical lymph node and elective neck dissection should be considered. Surgical resection remains the mainstay of treatment and the efficacy of postoperative radiotherapy depends on the proportion of epidermoid cells and the differentiation. The five-year survival for low-grade tumour is 70% and 40% for high-grade tumours.

Carcinoma ex-pleomorphic adenoma

This malignant tumour accounts for about 3–10% of all malignant parotid tumours and arises from 3–4% of all benign pleomorphic adenomas. The risk of developing malignancy increases with the duration of the benign tumour. The risk of malignancy is 1.5% up to five years but this increases to 9.5% after 15 years. The age at presentation is around 60 years, which is about 20 years after the occurrence of the pleomorphic adenoma.

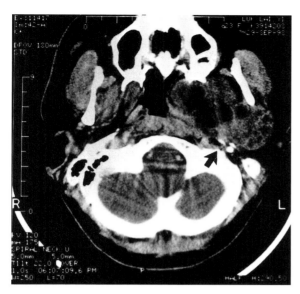

Figure 1.23 Computed tomography showing a mucoepidermoid carcinoma (arrow) involving the deep lobe of the parotid gland.

The clinical features include rapid increase in size of a long-standing benign tumour in the parotid gland. There may be associated pain, facial nerve palsy and infiltration of overlying skin. Tumours located in the deep lobe, larger than 2 cm in diameter and in a male patient over 40 years of age are more prone to the development of malignancy.

Histologically, three subtypes are recognised: carcinoma within the stroma of the benign lesion, invasive carcinoma and carcinosarcoma. The latter two types are associated with a poor prognosis especially if the tumour has invaded the surrounding tissue. Surgical resection with removal of all macroscopic tumour offers the best chance of cure. Postoperative radiotherapy is given to reduce the local recurrence rate.

This malignant tumour is classified as a high-grade malignancy, with 25% incidence of metastasis to cervical lymph nodes, and the prognosis is in general poor. The five-year survival is in the region of 30%.

Adenocarcinoma

This arises from the ductal epithelium of the parotid gland. It is more common in female patients at the sixth or seventh decade and is a glandular carcinoma. It resembles adenocarcinoma of other sites and is considered to be a high-grade tumour. It has a 50% incidence of metastasis to lymph nodes or to distant sites. Wide local excision with a clear margin gives the best chance of eradicating the disease. Radiotherapy does not seem to be effective for this tumour and the prognosis is poor.

Squamous cell carcinoma

This occurs in about 5% of all malignancies in the parotid gland and arises from the parenchyma of the gland and not from the involvement of a nearby lymph node with squamous cell carcinoma.

The patient usually presents with a rapidly enlarging parotid mass that is painful. Involvement of the facial nerve or the overlying skin is common. Surgery and radiotherapy are used for this condition. The incidence of distant metastasis is low but loco-regional recurrence has been reported to be in the region of 50% and the five-year survival is less than 10%.

Undifferentiated carcinoma

This tumour arises from the stem cell of the ductal system of the parotid gland and microscopically is similar to that of carcinoma arising from the nasopharynx. Endoscopic examination and biopsy of the nasopharynx should be performed to rule out the possibility that the lesion in the parotid is a metastasis.

Surgical resection followed by radiotherapy is the treatment of choice. Despite combined modality of treatment, the five-year survival rate is less than 10%.

Investigations

Radiological examinations are performed to detect distant metastasis. Computed tomography and magnetic resonance imaging are useful to delineate the extent of the primary tumour to facilitate planning of therapy. Fine needle aspiration cytology helps to confirm the clinical diagnosis of malignancy and in counselling the patient for the need for surgery or combined modality of treatment. However, it is not that useful in the determination of different pathological types of malignancy. It is of value in the detection of certain pathologies such as lymphoma or metastatic carcinoma so that surgical exploration can be avoided.

Treatment

The goal of therapy for malignant parotid gland neoplasms is to eliminate the disease with minimal morbidity and to reconstruct any residual functional defect. Surgery remains the mainstay of treatment and in extensive diseases, postoperative radiotherapy should be administered to improve the chance of eradicating the disease.

In general, when the tumour is small, located in the superficial lobe and of low malignancy, then superficial parotidectomy preserving the facial nerve is adequate. When the growth is in the deep lobe, total conservative parotidectomy should be performed. For more aggressive malignancies of the parotid gland without facial nerve paralysis, the current trend of surgical therapy is total conservative parotidectomy. Both superficial and deep lobes of the gland are removed while the facial nerve is preserved (Figure 1.24). There is no evidence to show that sacrificing the facial nerve under this circumstance improves local tumour control rate or survival.

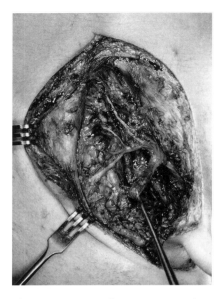

Figure 1.24 Total conservative parotidectomy was carried out, preserving the whole facial nerve.

When the malignant neoplasm of the parotid gland has affected the facial nerve, causing facial nerve paralysis, total radical parotidectomy, removing the whole gland together with the facial nerve, should be performed. The facial nerve defect should be grafted at the same session. Sural nerve obtained from the leg is used to bridge the gap between the facial nerve stump and the distal branches (Figure 1.25). Postoperative radiotherapy is usually administered for better tumour control. The functional recovery of the facial musculature is expected to be around 40–70% after two years.

Treatment of lymph nodes

Elective neck dissection is usually not carried out for malignancies of the parotid gland although there may be some grounds for performing it in the management of high-grade malignancies. Radical neck dissection is usually indicated as part of the management plan for patients with cervical lymph nodes on presentation.

Submandibular gland

Anatomy

The submandibular gland is triangular in shape and is composed of a larger superficial part and smaller deeper part separated by the mylohyoid muscle anteriorly. The two parts are continuous with each other. The lateral surface of the gland is covered by the deep cervical fascia, which also embraces the mandibular branch of the facial nerve. The body of the mandible covers part of the super-

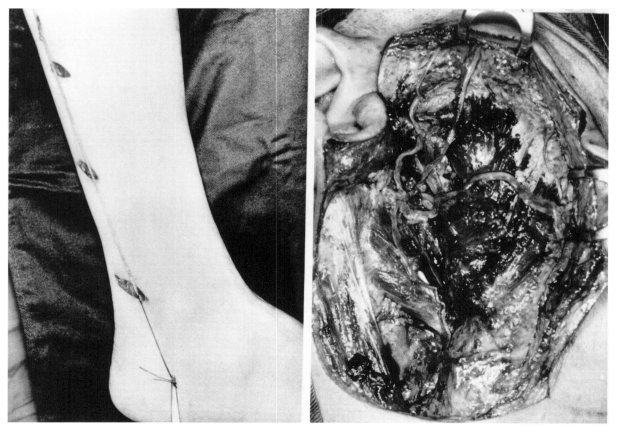

Figure 1.25 *Left*: Sural nerve prepared for grafting of the resected facial nerve. *Right*: Sural nerve used for grafting of the facial nerve.

ficial lobe. Its deep surface is related to the anterior belly of the digastric and the mylohyoid muscle.

The deep part of the submandibular gland lies under the mylohyoid muscle. The lingual nerve lies superior to the gland, attaching to it through the parasympathetic nerve fibres to the submandibular ganglion. The submandibular duct leaves the gland on its deep surface and travels superiorly to open into the floor of the mouth. The hypoglossal nerve and the lingual artery both lying deep to the duct also curve upwards and medially to enter the tongue base (Figure 1.26).

The parenchyma of the submandibular gland is composed of both serous and mucous glandular elements. Its parasympathetic innervation, which regulates the quality and quantity of secretion of saliva, reaches it through the chorda tympani via the lingual nerve.

Infection/inflammation

The causes of inflammation include acute suppurative sialadenitis, chronic sialadenitis and also viral infections related to human immunodeficiency virus.

Sialolithiasis

Stone formation is more frequently encountered in the submandibular gland than the parotid gland. The mucous secretions of the submandibular gland are more alkaline and viscous. The course of the submandibular duct is tortuous as it has to go upwards to empty into the floor of the mouth. Stagnation of saliva in the duct may lead to more stone formation.

The clinical features include painful postprandial enlargement of the submandibular gland that subsides over a few hours. For stones located near the opening of the submandibular duct, their presence can be confirmed with palpation or a plain radiograph (Figure 1.27). Stones located in the proximal part of the duct or within the gland can be detected by sialogram. This should be carried out to assess the status of the ductal system which may be damaged with repeated attacks of infection related to the obstructive nature of the stone.

Stones located near the orifice of the submandibular duct can be removed under local anaesthesia by splitting the opening (Figure 1.28). Meatoplasty of the orifice of the duct should be carried out to prevent future stenosis and stagnation of saliva. A sialogram should be performed subsequently to detect any stone in the gland and to assess the intraglandular ductal structure.

When the stone is located in the proximal part of the duct or within the gland or when there are multiple strictures in the ducts related to stone formation, removal of the gland through the neck is indicated.

Neoplasms of the submandibular gland

Clinical examination is carried out to differentiate a submandibular tumour from an enlarged submandibular lymph node. Bimanual palpation is sometimes helpful as the whole gland can be felt to be enlarged, in contrast to the oval shape of an enlarged, lymph node. When in doubt, fine needle aspiration should be performed to obtain further information on the nature of the swelling in the submandibular triangle.

Imaging studies such as computed tomography or magnetic

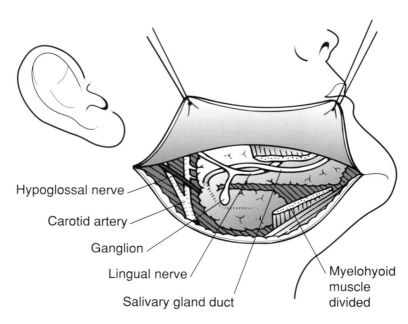

Hypoglossal nerve
Carotid artery
Ganglion
Lingual nerve
Salivary gland duct
Myelohyoid muscle divided

Figure 1.26 Schematic drawing of anatomy of the submandibular gland showing the structures on its deeper surface.

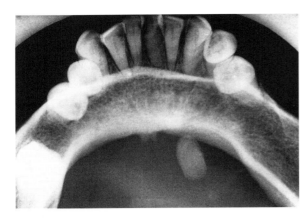

Figure 1.27 Plain radiograph of the floor of mouth showing a stone in the anterior part of the duct.

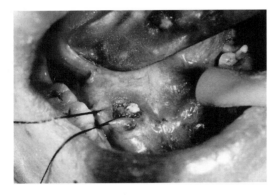

Figure 1.28 Stone in the anterior part of the duct removed by splitting the anterior portion of the duct and a meatoplasty is then carried out.

resonance imaging are useful to delineate the extent of the growth and involvement of the mandibular bone.

Benign tumours

Pleomorphic adenoma is the commonest benign lesion in the submandibular gland. It usually presents as a firm solitary swelling of the gland which enlarges only very slowly. The diagnosis can be confirmed with the clinical examination and fine needle aspiration biopsy of the mass.

Surgical resection of the whole submandibular gland with preservation of all nerves is the treatment of choice. Enucleation should not be performed, as it is associated with a high incidence of recurrence.

Malignant tumours

The commonest malignant tumour of the submandibular gland is adenoid cystic carcinoma. It accounts for 40% of malignant lesions

followed by mucoepidermoid carcinoma (17%) and adeno-carcinoma (11%).

The patient usually presents with a mass in the submandibular area and about 20% of them have associated pain in the mass related to the infiltration of nearby nerves such as the lingual nerve. The malignant growth may also affect the hypoglossal nerve, branches of trigeminal and facial nerves, depending on the extent of infiltration of the tumour.

Excision of the submandibular gland itself is not adequate. Besides the gland, other soft tissues in the submandibular triangle should be removed together with the lymph nodes in the region. The regional nerves should not be sacrificed unless they are grossly infiltrated by tumour. In view of the high incidence of adenoid cystic carcinoma occurring in the submandibular gland, frozen section of the nerves that go through the gland should be performed and any involved nerves resected in a retrograde fashion until the resection margins are clear of tumour. Metal clips should be applied to the nerve stump to aid in the planning of postoperative radiotherapy.

Postoperative adjuvant radiotherapy is usually recommended in cases of extensive disease with perineural spread and positive lymph node metastasis. The five-year survival of patients suffering from malignancy of the submandibular gland is around 40%. This is probably related to the high proportion of adenoid cystic carcinoma in the submandibular gland.

OPERATIVE SURGERY

Radical neck dissection

This operation aims to remove all the lymph nodes on one side of the neck. The sternomastoid muscle, internal jugular vein and the spinal accessory nerve are removed as part of the operation. This operation can be carried out alone or at the same session with resection of the primary tumour.

Patient preparation

The patient is prepared for general anaesthesia and the skin shaved from the mastoid to below the clavicle on the side of the operation. When the patient is scheduled for radical neck dissection, the operation is a clean one and no prophylactic antibiotic is required. However, when radical neck dissection is performed at the same time as resection of the primary tumour, prophylactic antibiotics are usually indicated. The choice of antibiotics depends on the nature of the operation for the primary malignancy. When the pharynx is expected to be opened, metronidazole together with a cephalosporin is selected. However, if the pharynx is not expected to be opened, only a cephalosporin is administered. All the antibiotics should be administered intravenously preoperatively and continued into the postoperative period for 5–7 days.

Anaesthesia and positioning

The operation is performed under general anaesthesia and venti-lation of the patient is maintained through an oral endotracheal tube. The ventilator/anaesthetic machine is usually located at the foot end of the patient to allow space for the surgeon and his or her assistants. The patient is placed in the supine position with a sandbag inserted beneath the shoulder to extend the neck. The head is tilted to the side opposite to the side of the planned radical neck dissection.

The surgeon stands on the right side of the head at around the shoulder level for a right-sided neck dissection. He or she may still stand on the right side for a left radical neck dissection or may elect to stand on the left side. The first assistant stands on the side opposite the surgeon and the second assistant stands at the head of the table.

Incision

A variety of incisions can be used for radical neck dissection. The most frequently used is the double Y incision that permits the exposure of all the structures in the neck. A disadvantage of this incision is that the two three-point junctions at the incisions may break down and expose the underlying vessels. This risk is increased with preoperative radiotherapy. The vertical limb of this incision also produces a cosmetically poor scar.

The two parallel incisions of MacFee avoid the three-point junction problem and the scars are hidden in the skin creases. When the two parallel incisions are more than 8 cm apart, the blood supply for the central skin flap is adequate even when a full dose of radiotherapy has been administered to the neck. When incisions of sufficient length are made, all the tissues in the neck can be exposed for dissection (Figure 1.29).

Surgical procedure

The skin flap (including the platysma) is raised.

The neck dissection should start from the angle furthest away from the suspected tumour-bearing lymph node and usually this is the inferior posterior angle. The angle between the anterior border of the trapezius muscle and the clavicle is first identified. The accessory nerve can be identified on the undersurface of the trapezius muscle and divided if necessary. The dissection extends along the superior border of the clavicle and the omohyoid muscle is divided (Figure 1.30).

When the dissection reaches the inferior anterior angle, the insertion of the sternomastoid muscle is divided to expose the internal jugular vein, vagus nerve and the common carotid artery. The phrenic nerve lying on the anterior scalene muscle is identi-fied behind the large vessels and protected. The internal jugular vein is divided between clamps while preserving the vagus nerve and common carotid artery. When the neck dissection is carried

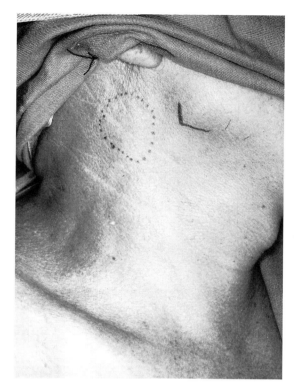

Figure 1.29 The patient is draped from the mastoid to below the clavicle and parallel incisions are used.

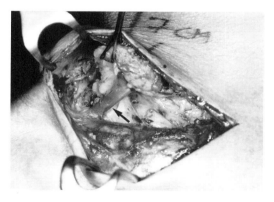

Figure 1.30 Dissection at the inferior posterior angle of the neck, showing the omohyoid muscle (arrow).

out on the left side, the thoracic duct coming up from the mediastinum behind the carotid artery entering into the junction between the subclavian vein and the internal jugular vein should be identified and ligated (Figure 1.31). The anaesthetist is requested to increase the intrathoracic pressure to allow the identification of any leakage of lymph. Any leaks found are sutured.

The soft tissue which includes all the lymph nodes together with the sternomastoid muscle is then lifted and turned upwards to reach the upper posterior angle while dividing the cervical plexus on the way. The sternomastoid muscle origin is detached from

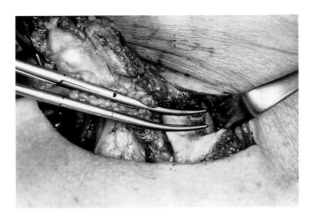

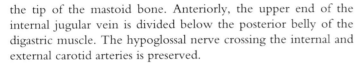

Figure 1.31 Dissection at the inferior anterior angle of the neck, showing clamps on the internal jugular vein.

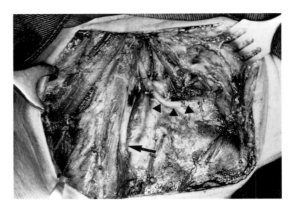

Figure 1.32 At completion of radical neck dissection, the carotid arteries, vagus nerve (arrow) and hypoglossal nerve (arrowheads) are preserved.

the tip of the mastoid bone. Anteriorly, the upper end of the internal jugular vein is divided below the posterior belly of the digastric muscle. The hypoglossal nerve crossing the internal and external carotid arteries is preserved.

The dissection of the superior anterior angle involves the dissection of the submental lymph nodes and submandibular gland. The anterior belly of the digastric muscle can be preserved or removed when indicated. The posterior edge of the mylohyoid muscle is identified and retracted to expose the deep part of the submandibular gland. The lingual nerve lying superior to the gland should be freed and displaced superiorly. The duct of the submandibular gland is freed and divided while preserving the hypoglossal nerve on its undersurface. (Figure 1.32).

When radical neck dissection is performed together with the removal of primary tumour and the pharynx is opened, there is a chance of leakage of the pharyngeal closure. The levator scapulae is lifted to cover the carotid vessels so that they will not be affected in case the patient develops a pharyngeal fistula.

Intraoperative hazards

Damage of the internal jugular vein will produce significant bleeding. Pressure should be applied to the bleeding site and the patient placed in the Trendelenburg position to prevent air embolism. Good exposure and suction are essential so that the damaged vessels can be identified and repaired. Damaged major

arteries are repaired after application of vascular clamps. Inadvertently divided major nerves should be repaired with interrupted sutures under magnification to achieve maximal apposition. The degree of recovery depends on the nature of the nerve divided; pure nerves recover much better than mixed nerves.

Postoperative management

The wound is closed in layers and suction drains are usually applied so that the neck skin flap will adhere to the deep tissue of the neck.

FURTHER READING

Gleeson M, Herbert A, Richards A. Management of lateral neck masses in adults. *BMJ* 2000; **320**(7248):1521–1524

Lee Rea J. Partial parotidectomies: morbidity and benign tumor recurrence rates in a series of 94 cases. *Laryngoscope* 2000; **110**(6):924–927

Robertson ML, Gleich LL, Barrett WL, Gluckman JL. Base-of-tongue cancer: survival, function, and quality of life after external-beam irradiation and brachytherapy. *Laryngoscope* 2001; **111**(8):1362–1365

Vokes EE, Weichselbaum RR, Lippman SM, Hong WK. Medical progress: head and neck cancer. *New England Journal of Medicine* 1993; **328**(3):184–194

Zenk J, Constantinidis J, Al-Kadah B, Iro H. Transoral removal of submandibular stones. *Archives of Otolaryngology – Head and Neck Surgery* 2001; **127**(4):432–436

Pharyngeal and oesophageal motility disorders

J.A.C. Thorpe

In 1883, Kronecker and Meltzer were the first to investigate the swallowing mechanism using oesophageal balloons. However, it was not until the 1950s that Ingelfinger and Code were able to provide more insight into oesophageal function using transducer probes. Today more reliable microtransducer and pH probe technology has revolutionised the assessment of normal and abnormal oesophageal function.

Before discussing the pathological aspects of pharyngeal and oesophageal motility disorders it is important to have a fundamental knowledge of normal physiology and the modern clinical techniques now adopted for the diagnosis of disorders of motility.

THE SWALLOWING MECHANISM

The swallowing mechanism is very complex. It involves an *oropharyngeal stage*, which lasts for one second and involves:

- elevation and retraction of the soft palate with nasopharyngeal closure

- upper oesophageal sphincter opening

- laryngeal closure

- tongue loading

- tongue pulsion

- pharyngeal clearance.

This is followed by an *oesophageal stage* where the bolus is transmitted to the stomach with orderly unidirectional peristalsis and coordinated relaxation of the lower oesophageal sphincter. The volume and consistency of the bolus affect the timing. The innervation, neuromuscular physiology and medullary control mechanisms are complex and still incompletely understood. The current model is described in Figure 2.1.

CLINICAL ASSESSMENT AND INVESTIGATIONS

A good clinical history and examination is invaluable in the assessment of pharyngeal and oesophageal motility disorders. The three clinical presentations are:

- heartburn

- dysphagia/odynophagia

- chest pain.

Gastro-oesophageal reflux disease (GORD) is often concomitant with oesophageal motility disorders and should also be considered. Dysphagia should not be confused with a globus sensation, i.e. a feeling of a lump in the throat.

There are many causes of pharyngo-oesophageal dysphagia including webs, strictures, carcinoma, extrinsic masses and denervation motility disturbance, e.g. scleroderma (failed peristalsis), or excessive/abnormal peristalsis (hypercontractile oesophagus), e.g. diffuse oesophageal spasm, nutcracker oesophagus.

Investigations

The following investigations will be necessary in most cases and their importance will be discussed in context with the individual motility disorder. Oropharyngeal and oesophageal disorders will be discussed separately.

- Record weight and dietary intake

- Haematological/biochemical profile

- Barium swallow/video barium

- Fibreoptic oesophagoscopy/endoscopic ultrasound

- Pharyngo-oesophageal manometry

- Twenty-four hour ambulatory pH monitoring

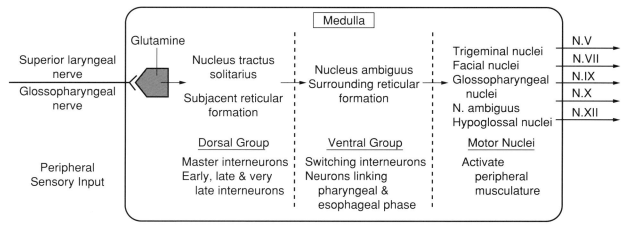

Figure 2.1 Current model of central control pathways of swallowing.

Oesophageal manometry

Manometric investigation is mandatory in most cases of dysphagia and essential prior to antireflux surgery or motility surgery. It is also a useful tool in evaluating the results of surgery.

Several recording techniques are used. The most accurate technique incorporates the use of multilumen catheters with small external diameter linked to a hydraulic capillary infusion system, e.g. the Arndorfer pump (Figure 2.2). This low-flow perfusion technique is very reliable and gives reproducible results. Technically the procedure requires some expertise and is used mainly for research. Modern microtransducer catheters are now very reliable although more expensive. They have the advantage of simplicity and ease of use and are well tolerated by patients because of their small diameter (Figure 2.3).

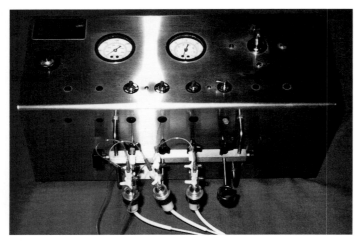

Figure 2.2 Andorfer hydraulic capillary infusion system for oesophageal manometry.

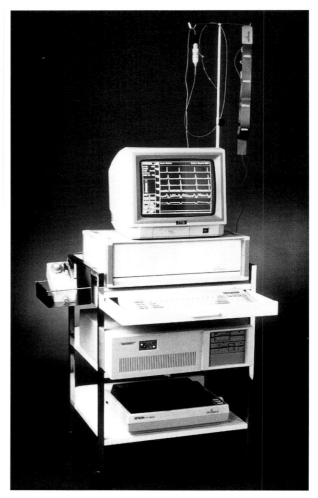

Figure 2.3 Modern mobile computerised system for oesophageal motility studies.

Technique

The catheter assembly is passed through the nose with topical anaesthesia and the patient encouraged to swallow small amounts of fluid through a straw. Once the transducers are in the stomach a positive pressure wave is obtained on inspiration or on palpation of the abdomen. A 1 cm station pull-through is then carried out. At the region of the hiatus a high-pressure zone (HPZ) is encountered which at its lower end represents the diaphragm and at its upper end the lower oesophageal sphincter (LOS) which on wet or dry swallow should relax completely to baseline pressure (0–5 mmHg) (Figure 2.4). Impaired relaxation is a feature of achalasia. The catheter bundle is then pulled back slowly at 1 cm intervals and peristaltic function assessed in the oesophageal body. The upper oesophageal sphincter is then located and resting pressure and the relaxation response assessed. With a transducer in the pharynx, pharyngo-oesophageal coordination can be assessed but interpretation of the responses in this area requires experience.

pH testing

This is an integral part of upper GI tract investigation and is usually combined with manometry. Once the HPZ is located at manometry or by X-ray localisation (usually unnecessary), the pH probe is placed 5 cm above the HPZ/LOS. The probe is usually calibrated to acid and alkaline pH and a reference electrode is placed on the skin. The probe is then connected to an ambulatory digital monitor and the patient sent home for 24 hours. The patient makes an accurate record/diary of eating habits, posture, medication and symptoms and a marker button can be pressed when the patient has significant symptoms. A computer analysis is then made and the 24-hour pH recording analysed. A standard computerised analysis and printout is then produced (Figure 2.5).

It is important to appreciate the computer criteria for the programme as these can differ. The pH recording is usually based on DeMeesters criteria and specific scores obtained. A reflux episode is defined as pH 4 or less. The normal pH in the oesophagus is pH 7. The computer analyses the total duration of pH <4, the total

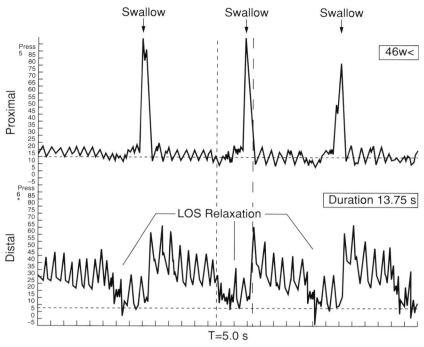

Figure 2.4 Manometric appearance of the lower oesophageal sphincter (LOS) with relaxation responses to swallow waves.

number of episodes and the duration of the longest episode. pH <4 for a period >4% of the 24-hour period studied is considered pathological.

Other types of pH probe can be used to assess bile reflux in special circumstances, e.g. post gastrectomy.

OROPHARYNGEAL DYSPHAGIA

Causes

High dysphagia can be caused by structural or propulsive abnormalities. Structural abnormalities may arise from trauma, radiation, surgery, tumours, caustic injury and congenital and acquired deformities. Propulsive abnormalities can result from dysfunction of intrinsic musculature, peripheral nerves or central nervous system.

Management

Fortunately, oropharyngeal dysphagia is relatively uncommon but poses a serious management problem. It is rarely amenable to

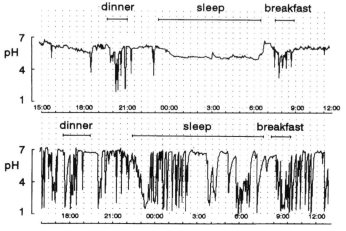

Figure 2.5 24 hour continuous ambulatory pH recording.

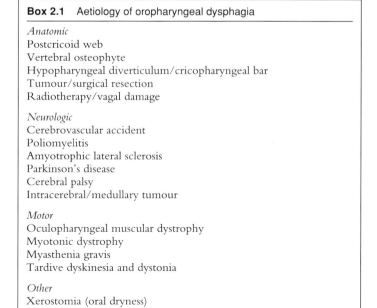

Box 2.1   Aetiology of oropharyngeal dysphagia

Anatomic
Postcricoid web
Vertebral osteophyte
Hypopharyngeal diverticulum/cricopharyngeal bar
Tumour/surgical resection
Radiotherapy/vagal damage

Neurologic
Cerebrovascular accident
Poliomyelitis
Amyotrophic lateral sclerosis
Parkinson's disease
Cerebral palsy
Intracerebral/medullary tumour

Motor
Oculopharyngeal muscular dystrophy
Myotonic dystrophy
Myasthenia gravis
Tardive dyskinesia and dystonia

Other
Xerostomia (oral dryness)

specific therapy. Dysphagia secondary to Parkinson's disease and myasthenia gravis often improves with medical therapy. However, therapy for most of these disorders is structured around the management of nutritional and aspiration complications.

Clinical evaluation should include a videocontrast swallow together with pharyngeal and upper oesophageal manometry if possible to assess which aspect of the swallow mechanism is abnormal. Technically, however, manometry may be difficult to perform and interpret accurately in these patients.

A nasal voice or nasal regurgitation suggests paresis of the soft palate. Inadequate bolus formation may be a consequence of tongue weakness; aspiration suggests impaired laryngeal elevation. Excess salivation may require cholinergic-type drugs and absence of salivation may necessitate lubricants or artificial saliva, which are now available.

Different feeding tactics, e.g. using a straw or infant feeder, and postural compensation can maintain oral intake of food. Physiotherapy and speech therapy are important in rehabilitating the stroke patient and a dietitian should monitor nutritional progress. Failure to maintain an adequate intake orally is an indication for fine-bore nasogastric feeding, a percutaneous endoscopic gastrostomy tube (PEG) or a fine-bore feeding jejunostomy.

Aspiration may require aggressive nasotracheal toilet, minitracheostomy or formal tracheostomy if severe.

Occasionally oesophageal dilatation or cricopharyngeal myotomy can be effective in some patients with a hypertensive or abnormally relaxing UOS and hypopharyngeal diverticulum.

OESOPHAGEAL MOTILITY DISORDERS

Presentation

Motility disorders affecting the body of the oesophagus usually present with symptoms of altered diet, dysphagia, odynophagia, chest pain and often heartburn and indigestion. Symptoms are usually chronic but may be acute. Chest pain can readily mimic an acute anginal attack or myocardial infarction. Up to 60% of patients with non-cardiac chest pain (NCCP) have an oesophageal disorder. The history is very important, with particular reference to diet, e.g. intolerance of fluids rather than solids would indicate achalasia.

Investigation

Dysphagia is a serious symptom and should always be investigated. Routine investigations should include:

- barium swallow/videobarium

- endoscopy

- manometry

- ambulatory pH monitoring.

Other investigations which may be of value include:

- ambulatory manometry

- Bernstein acid perfusion test

- edrophonium stimulation test for NCCP

- balloon dilatation sensitivity test

- endoscopic ultrasound

- oesophageal mucosal potential difference

- cerebral evoked response.

Table 2.1 provides a summary of the expected findings in various conditions.

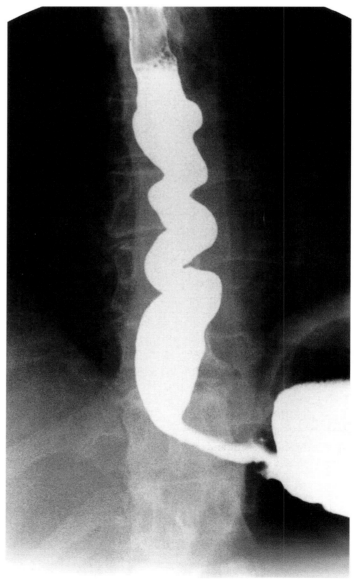

Figure 2.6 Contrast swallow of a 'corkscrew oesophagus' due to diffuse oesophageal spasm (DOS).

Table 2.1 Oesophageal motility disorders

Disorder	Radiology	Manometry	pH test / other
Achalasia	Bird's beak/rat-tail appearance at cardia	Normal–high LOS pressure, non-relaxing on swallow Synchronous spastic activity in oesophageal body	Not associated with reflux pH may be positive after myotomy
Diffuse oesophageal spasm	Spastic activity Reflux Corkscrew appearance Diverticulae	Normal–high spastic waves Occasional normal peristalsis Normal LOS	pH occasionally positive Muscle hypertrophy on EUS
Hypertensive LOS	Impaired oesophageal clearance	LOS pressure >45 mmHg May have impaired relaxation	Usually negative
Reflux/spasm	Reflux Spastic activity Hiatus hernia	Peristalsis normal Low-pressure LOS Occasional spastic wave forms	Positive pH test
Nutcracker	Spasm	Hypertensive peristalsis Normal–high pressure LOS May see impaired relaxation	Usually negative pH test Muscle hypertrophy on EUS
Scleroderma	Reflux Impaired oesophageal and gastric clearance	No peristalsis Flat trace Absence of LOS	pH positive

LOS, lower oesophageal sphincter; EUS, endoscopic ultrasound

Non-specific oesophageal motility disorders (NSOMD) – these are a distinct manometric group that do not fulfil the above criteria. They have impaired clearance with low-pressure swallow activity and occasional spastic activity. Non-transmitted swallows >30%

Management of oesophageal motility disorders

The majority of oesophageal motility disorders can largely be treated conservatively with reassurance, medication and occasional dilatation. The patient with persistent symptoms will need careful evaluation as inappropriate surgery to the oesophagus could result in lifelong problems with swallowing.

It is imperative prior to embarking on surgery that full investigations are carried out, especially to exclude carcinoma of the cardia, which may present as a pseudoachalasia.

Isosorbide dinitrate is of some use in DOS and anticholinergics, e.g. hyoscine or propantheline, may be used to reduce peristalsis (Figure 2.6). However, there have been no controlled trials of their efficacy. Calcium channel blockers, e.g. nifedipine and diltiazem, are occasionally effective in reducing spastic activity and non-cardiac chest pain. If there is evidence of gastro-oesophageal reflux, antacids/proton pump inhibitors are useful. Where there is evidence of low sphincter pressure and impaired oesophageal clearance, metoclopramide is a useful drug, which also improves gastric emptying.

Temporary subjective relief can be obtained by bouginage or balloon dilatation of the oesophagus in spastic disorders.

For patients with intractable symptoms and failed medication/dilatation, surgery may be indicated. This should be performed in a unit with expertise in the management of the oesophagus. It may be necessary to perform oesophagomyotomy (partial/complete) with the addition of an antireflux procedure, e.g. Belsey Mk IV repair, if there is documented gastro-oesophageal reflux.

It is important not to perform an overtight repair in the presence of impaired oesophageal motility, as dysphagia may well be worse postoperatively. Where diverticulae are present there is often an underlying motility disorder, e.g. DOS, and a myotomy should be added to the diverticulectomy (Figure 2.7).

In achalasia, balloon dilatation is preferred for the older patient but for the younger patient a Heller myotomy is recommended. This can be performed by a laparoscopic, thoracoscopic or minithoracotomy approach.

The results of surgery appear to be superior to balloon dilatation.

OPERATIVE SURGERY

Excision of a pharyngeal pouch (Zenker's diverticulum)

A pharyngeal pouch is a herniation of the pharyngeal mucosa through a muscular defect known as Killian's dehiscence in the posterior pharyngeal wall proximal to the cricopharyngeus. In 1874, the German pathologist Zenker was the first to describe the pulsion nature of the defect. This acquired defect is often associated with pharyngo-oesophageal incoordination. Clinically there is impairment of swallowing with dysphagia, regurgitation and often signs of aspiration to the lung. The patients are often elderly and have significant co-morbidity. The history is usually classic and there are few findings on clinical examination. Barium studies and manometry are essential to diagnose the disorder

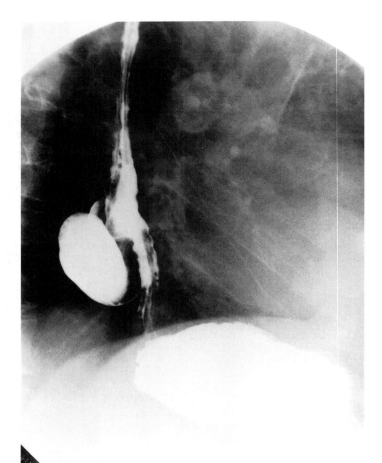

Figure 2.7 Contrast swallow showing a lower oesophageal diverticulum associated with oesophageal spasm.

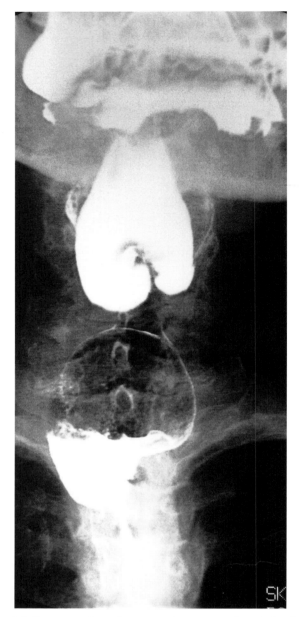

Figure 2.8 Contrast swallow of an upper pharyngo-oesophageal diverticulum (AP view).

(Figure 2.8). Manometry may not be easily tolerated but is useful to diagnose a hypertensive upper oesophageal sphincter, which may influence the surgeon on whether to add a cricopharyngeal myotomy. Endoscopy is also useful to exclude carcinoma but should be done with caution, as perforation is a well-known risk in this situation.

There are several surgical techniques to treat a pharyngeal pouch. The Dohlman procedure, which incorporates diathermy division of the septum by a peroral approach, has been superseded by a peroral division of the septum with an endoscopic stapler. The classical approach to the diverticulum is by a cervical incision and this operation is detailed below.

Patient preparation

In severe cases and in high-risk individuals the operation can be performed under local anaesthetic with sedation but it is preferable to perform the procedure under general anaesthesia. Adequate preparation is necessary with preoperative physiotherapy and antibiotics if there is significant aspiration and pneumonitis.

Technique (Figure 2.9)

- Supine position.
- Head extended and turned to right.
- 40–45 Fr Maloney bougie in oesophagus (place with care).
- Skin preparation and drape.
- Prophylactic antibiotic (24 hours).
- 5–8 cm oblique cervical incision.
- Incision along the anterior border of sternomastoid.

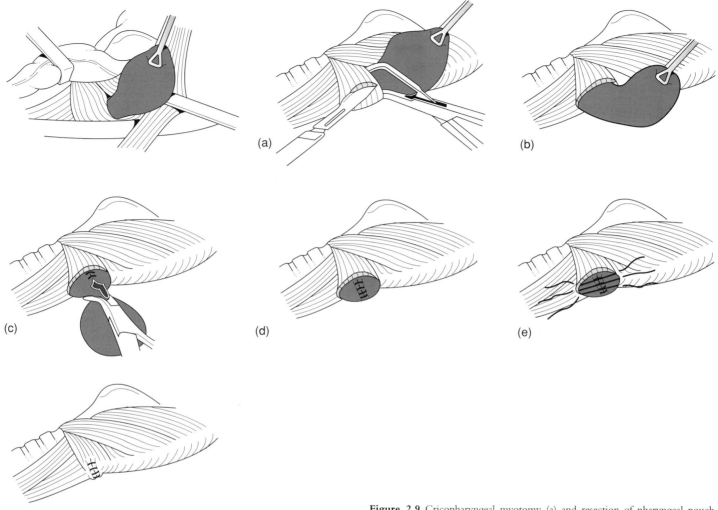

Figure 2.9 Cricopharyngeal myotomy (a) and resection of pharyngeal pouch (b–f).

- Retract sternomastoid laterally.

- Dissect retropharyngeal space cephalad to omohyoid.

- Diverticulum dissected and grasped with Allis forceps.

- Resect diverticulum above a Cooley or small Satinsky clamp.

- Oversew with 4 '0' polypropylene or staple with a 30 mm stapler.

- Divide cricopharyngeus if thickened with angle Potts' scissors.

- Close with a small Redivac or corrugated drain.

- Clips/subcuticular stitch to skin.

- Nil by mouth for 48 hours.

Postoperative management

After 48 hours and if the wound is dry fluid intake can commence cautiously with 30 ml of water per hour, building up rapidly to free fluids and soft diet. Clips are usually removed at 3–5 days.

Excessive wound drainage and inflammation may signify a cervical leak. This usually settles down with conservative management and intravenous feeding after one week. Occasionally patients may require an oesophageal dilatation if there is residual dysphagia. Recurrent laryngeal nerve injury has been reported but is usually transient.

Results

Good results have been reported in several series, with 85–95% success.

Modified Heller's oesophagomyotomy

Achalasia is a condition in which there is failure of the smooth muscle just above the cardia to relax on swallow (Figure 2.10). There is also a generalised disorder of peristalsis within the body of the oesophagus. Heller originally described a double myotomy

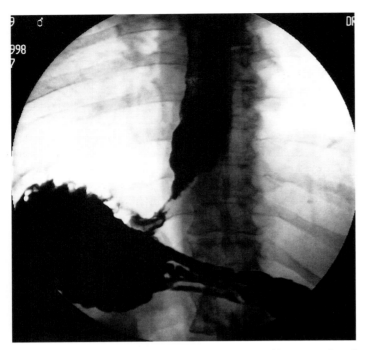

Figure 2.10 Contrast swallow of achalasia showing impaired lower oesophageal sphincter relaxation.

anteriorly and posteriorly but this has now been superseded by a single myotomy in the lower third of the oesophagus on its anterolateral aspect.

There are now several techniques for approaching the lower oesophagus: laparoscopy, thoracoscopy and open laparotomy and left anterolateral thoracotomy. All approaches have advantages and disadvantages, e.g. a higher incidence of recurrent achalasia with laparoscopic myotomy. Thoracotomy may be complicated with postthoracotomy wound pain but this is now less common with muscle-sparing minithoracotomy. The thoracoscopic approach is currently popular with good results.

In mega-oesophagus myotomy alone may be insufficient and oesophageal plication or even oesophagectomy may be required. A small carcinoma of the cardia may present with pseudoachalasia and the surgeon should be prepared and experienced enough to be able to explore and resect the stomach or oesophagus and reconstruct with small or large intestine.

In the presence of impaired oesophageal motility oesophageal emptying will continue to be impeded with continuation of symptoms.

In the following section the classic open approach via the thorax will be described.

Preoperative preparation

Patients appear to fall into two groups, the younger group aged 18–35 years and an elderly group aged 65–85 years, the latter having more co-morbidity. Stasis and regurgitation of food are

common and in a severely dilated oesophagus (mega-oesophagus/sigmoid oesophagus) (Figure 2.11), it may be necessary to perform preoperative endoscopy not only to empty the oesophagus to prevent aspiration pneumonia but also to exclude middle third squamous cell carcinoma of which there is an increased risk in chronic achalasia.

Operative technique

The patient is anaesthetised with a double-lumen tube and, if possible, a 45–50 Fr Maloney bougie is passed to the stomach. Antibiotic prophylaxis is given for 48 hours and subcutaneous heparin for thromboembolism prophylaxis.

The patient is positioned in a left thoracotomy position and the oesophagus is approached as follows:

- Left anterolateral thoracotomy sixth/seventh space. (Figure 2.12).

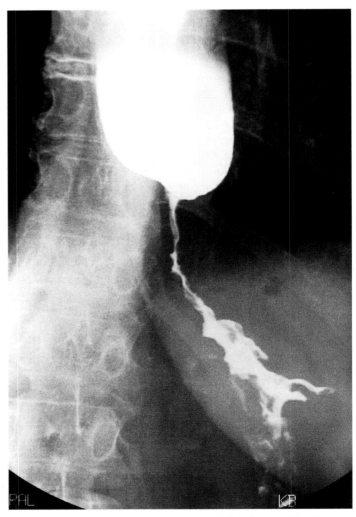

Figure 2.11 Close-up of lower oesophagus in achalasia showing dilated oesophagus and 'rat-tail' appearance.

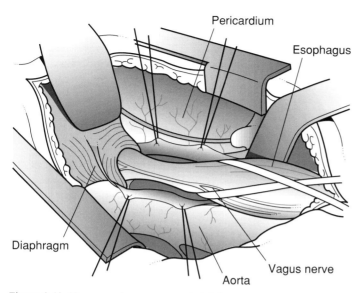

Figure 2.12 10 cm oesophagomyotomy via left thoracotomy.

- Ribs retracted and lung packed away.

- Oesophagus located and a tape passed around, dividing mediastinal pleura.

- 10 cm myotomy performed from the level of the inferior pulmonary vein to 1 cm onto the stomach, dividing some of the horseshoe-shaped fibres of the Collar of Helvetius. Angled Potts' scissors are useful. It is important not to disturb the anatomy of the hiatus as this will result in gastro-oesophageal reflux. If an adequate myotomy cannot be performed without doing this then it is advisable to add an antireflux procedure and a modified Belsey Mk IV is advocated. It is very important not to produce an overtight repair especially if a Nissen fundoplication is performed.

- Care with haemostasis.

- In the event of mucosal perforation close with a 4 '0' polypropylene suture.

- If hiatus disturbed perform modified Belsey Mk IV repair.

- Remove bougie.

- Pass a nasogastric tube.

- Close the chest with 25–28 gauge chest drain.

Postoperative management

The principal complication of myotomy is leakage. In view of this it is recommended to give nil by mouth for 3–5 days. The nasogastric tube should remain for 24 hours to prevent gastric distension and dilatation. Fluids are commenced cautiously at 30 ml/h from day 3 and built up rapidly to light diet initially. Chest radiographs on alternate days are recommended. If there is evidence of pleural effusion or pyrexia then a contrast swallow should be performed to exclude a leak.

Results

Good to excellent results in 80–90% patients have been reported in large series. Oesophagomyotomy either by the open or thoracoscopic technique appears to be the treatment of choice as results are superior to balloon dilatation.

FURTHER READING

Andreollo NA, Earlam RJ. Heller's myotomy for achalasia: is an added antireflux procedure necessary? *Br J Surg* 1987; **74**:765

Arndorfer RC, Stef JJ, Dodds WJ, Linehan JH. Improved infusion system for intraluminal manometry. *Gastroenterology* 1977; **73**:23

Castell JA, Dalton CB. *Esophageal Manometry*. Boston: Little, Brown, 1992

DeMeester TR, Wong CI, Wernley JA et al. Technique, indication and clinical use of 24-hr esophageal pH monitoring. *J Thorac Cardiovasc Surg* 1980: **79**:656

Ellis FH, Watkins E, Gibb SP, Heatley GJ. Ten-20 year clinical results after short oesophagomyotomy without an antireflux procedure (modified Heller operation) for esophageal achalasia. *Eur J Cardiovasc Surg* 1992; **6**:86

Payne WS, King RM. Pharyngoesophageal (Zenker's) diverticulum. *Surg Clin North Am* 1983; **63**:815

3

Neoplasms of the oesophagus

E.W.J. Cameron

BENIGN TUMOURS

Less than 2% of oesophageal tumours are benign and the majority are asymptomatic. Treatment, if needed, is by local excision rather than oesophageal resection.

Leiomyoma

Leiomyoma comprises about 60% of all benign tumours. They are intramural, usually larger than 5 cm diameter and are found in the distal third. Tumours larger than 5 cm may present with dysphagia and central chest discomfort. The differential diagnosis is made on the chest radiograph when a smooth mass is seen in the posterior mediastinum. Contrast swallow shows a typical smooth convexity bulging into the oesophageal lumen. CT scan and endoscopy confirm the diagnosis. If the lesion is greater than 5 cm diameter and/or is symptomatic it should be removed by enucleation from the oesophageal muscle layers, leaving the overlying mucosa and submucosa intact. This is done at open or video-assisted thoractomy. A local oesophagectomy with gastric replacement is needed when the leiomyoma erodes the mucosa or there is suspicion of leiomyosarcoma.

Polyp

These pedunculated lesions arise from mucosal cells and histologically are squamous epithelial, adenomatous, fibrovascular or lipomatous. Their peculiarity is the development of a long stalk attaching the polyp to the mucosa of the proximal third and they may literally present by regurgitation into the mouth. Polyps are seen on contrast swallow where they fill a segment of oesophageal lumen and resemble a foreign body or mobile food bolus. Polyp, stalk and mucosal base are removed by endoscopic snare and diathermy but if unmanageable at endoscopy then open oesophagostomy is used.

Haemangioma

A haemangioma is usually an incidental finding at endoscopy but occasionally presents as a source of minor upper gastrointestinal blood loss. When located in the distal third, it may be mistaken for a varix. Contrast CT scan shows a vascular tumour and haemangiomas are only removed if they are bleeding. Endoscopic ablation by diathermy, laser or sclerosing injection is also available.

Granular cell tumour

These tumours probably arise from Schwann cells and if large enough, cause mechanical obstruction. Frozen section biopsy may give a false-positive result for squamous carcinoma.

MALIGNANT TUMOURS

Pathology

Aspects of oesophageal malignant tumours have in the past been confused by failure in the literature to separate out squamous carcinoma, primary adenocarcinoma and adenocarcinoma of the gastric cardia. These lesions have and still are frequently combined together under the generic description 'oesophageal carcinoma' and although their pathological features are distinct, their clinical presentation, investigation and treatment are similar. Important uncertainties persist in determining the frequency of the cancers and their response to treatment.

Squamous carcinoma

In North America and Europe the tumour incidence increases with age, being uncommon under 40 years, is twice as frequent in males and occurs at a rate of around 3/100 000/annum. However, there are hyperendemic regions in North China, Iran and South Africa where rates exceed 100/100 000/annum. Because of this, local dietary factors such as nitrosamine-contaminated food have been implicated in the aetiology. Elsewhere, alcohol and tobacco are recognised as causative with a stepwise increase in risk with increasing consumption. Achalasia and Plummer–Vinson syndrome are alleged to be precancerous conditions but there is no clear evidence that gastro-oesophageal reflux is implicated.

Ninety percent of cancers occur in the middle or distal thirds of the oesophagus. Submucosal tumour may extend beyond the visible tumour margins and local invasion is into surrounding structures, notably central airway, lung, aortic adventitia, parietal pericardium and hiatus oesophagus. Haematogenous metastases are most frequent in lung and liver with lymphogenous spread to peri-oesophageal, scalene and coeliac nodes.

Adenosquamous carcinoma is a histological variant where glandular elements are found within a squamous pattern of malignancy. Carcinoma *in situ* is held to be precancerous and with time may extend to a more general field change in the oesophageal mucosa as well as the direct development of squamous carcinoma.

Adenocarcinoma

As mentioned above, there is continuing difficulty in clearly distinguishing between a primary adenocarcinoma of the distal third of the oesophagus and a gastric carcinoma at the oesophago-gastric junction and cardia which invades the oesophagus. Against this background it is thought that adenocarcinomas comprise between 10% and 20% of primary oesophageal malignancies. The majority of these develop where columnar cell metaplasia, the eponymous Barrett's mucosa, replaces the normal squamous mucosa. Other adenocarcinomas derive from submucosal mucous glands. Barrett's mucosa was thought to be a congenital anomaly but is now believed to develop as a response to chronic gastro-oesophageal reflux. With time the squamo-columnar junction can extend superiorly in the oesophagus and islands of columnar cells may be found in the more proximal squamous mucosa. Dysplasia can occur in the columnar cells and this change is pre-cancerous but not all dysplasias will go on to cancer. It is estimated that the presence of a Barrett's mucosa increases the risk of adenocarcinoma by a factor of 50. Local and metastatic spread of adenocarcinoma resembles that of squamous carcinoma.

Other malignant tumours

These together comprise 2% of all oesophageal malignancies. Small cell carcinoma presumably derives from APUD cells buried in the oesophageal mucosa and is both in embryological derivation, the primitive foregut, and subsequent behaviour analogous to small cell carcinoma of bronchus. It is a fast-metastasising tumour. At the other end of the biological spectrum is the quasi-benign and very rare oesophageal carcinoid. Malignant melanoma may be primary or secondary and the oesophagus is recognised as one of the non-cutaneous sites for primary melanoma.

Clinical features and diagnostic investigation

Symptoms

- Dysphagia for solids is the presenting symptom in over 90% of patients. This worsens to difficulty with fluids and saliva or sudden complete dysphagia due to bolus obstruction of the stenotic oesophageal segment.

- Regurgitation may succeed the onset of dysphagia and secondary aspiration causes cough and other symptoms of respiratory infection.

- Cough is incessant if there is a malignant oesophago-airway fistula.

- Odynophagia is more frequent with reflux disease than cancer.

- Constant pain in the back or epigastrium suggests tumour invasion into peripheral structures such as vertebral periosteum or the retroperitoneum.

- Usually dysphagia precedes any symptoms from a metastasis and severe weight loss and cachexia are signals of disseminated disease.

- A history of reflux symptoms is significant only for its association with columnar metaplasia in a Barrett's oesophagus.

- Vomiting is not a symptom of oesophageal carcinoma.

Signs

On general examination there is often no evidence of oesophageal carcinoma but a search should be made for signs of weight loss, scalene lymphadenopathy, chest infection and liver or epigastric mass.

Diagnostic investigation

Haematology and biochemistry

Anaemia and hypoproteinaemia reflect cachexia. It is unusual for oesophageal carcinoma to cause anaemia by direct blood loss from the primary. A leucocytosis is likely to follow from an associated respiratory infection. Uraemia is either due to dysphagic dehydration or, with abnormal liver function and hypercalcaemia, points to extensive secondary spread.

Imaging

PA and lateral chest radiographs are often normal but may show parenchymal lung infection, pulmonary metastases, a superior or posterior mediastinal mass or an air–fluid level lying in an obstructed oesophagus. The gastric air bubble may be missing.

Contrast swallow with *dilute* barium is ideally a precursor of endoscopy. It shows the level and longitudinal extent of the tumour, may prove aspiration with the appearance of contrast in the proximal airways or demonstrate an oesophago-airway (trachea, left or right main bronchus) fistula. If the patient is totally dysphagic it is unkind and wrong for a contrast swallow to be performed.

A CT scan of the thorax and abdomen is less good than a contrast swallow at delineating the lumenal anatomy of the primary but accurately shows the extralumenal bulk and lateral extent of the tumour. It is only a guide to possible T3 spread outwith the oesophageal muscle or T4 spread into adjacent structures. Lymph node size can be measured and nodes greater than 1 cm diameter are radiologically considered to be metastatic. However, N staging by CT scan is at best 60% accurate since lymph node enlargement is sometimes caused by infection, etc. and also because metastases are found in normally sized lymph nodes. Using lung settings, haematogenous pulmonary metastases will be seen more easily and at smaller size than on conventional chest X-ray. The abdominal CT scan is used to find metastases to the liver and to determine the presence of coeliac and para-aortic lymphadenopathy.

Liver ultrasound detects metastases and is valuable in conjunction with CT scan when there is diagnostic doubt between a metastasis and a simple cyst.

Endoscopy

Flexible oesophagoscopy under sedation and local anaesthetic is the standard invasive method to assess and biopsy oesophageal carcinoma. The proximal oesophagus is examined to confirm the normality of the squamous mucosa or to define the presence and level of the squamo-columnar junction in a Barrett's oesophagus or to search for radiographically invisible 'skip' lesions of metastatic carcinoma proximal to the primary. The proximal level of the primary is measured in centimetres from the upper alveolus and multiple biopsies are taken from the tumour. If possible, the endoscope is passed through the tumour and into the distal oesophagus, stomach and first part of duodenum to confirm absence of other lesions such as peptic ulceration or scarring and to check the suitability of the stomach for use as oesophageal replacement.

If resection is to follow quickly there is no point in exposing a patient to the risks of bouginage, intubation or stenting. However, these manoeuvres can be combined with diagnostic endoscopy when palliation of dysphagia or fistula is the only available treatment or is to be combined with radiotherapy or chemotherapy.

Endoscopic ultrasound is more accurate than CT scanning for staging tumour in the middle and distal thirds of the oesophagus. Tracheal air artefact is a limitation in the proximal third and ultrasound is baffled when the primary is stenotic and not safely dilatable. Ninety percent accuracy is claimed for the assessment of T staging by ultrasound and it also measures peri-oesophageal lymph node size but for N staging it has the same deficiencies as CT scan.

Rigid oesophagoscopy

Rigid oesophagoscopy is carried out with the patient under general anaesthetic, endotracheally intubated and paralysed. It is especially useful when the proximal oesophagus is filled with saliva, fluid and food debris which has to be cleaned out in order to see the primary lesion and is the best method for dealing with bolus obstruction. It also allows large size biopsy which is important when small flexible endoscopic biopsy provides inadequate material for the histological definition of dysplastic epithelium or necrotic tumour.

Laparoscopy

Laparoscopy is a recognised investigation for gastric carcinoma. Its value in oesophageal carcinoma is not known but it may have a place when the oesophageal primary involves the intraabdominal oesophagus or with laparoscopic ultrasound when liver metastases are suspected.

Bronchoscopy

Bronchoscopy is essential for all patients with proximal third lesions, oesophago-airway fistula or respiratory infection. It is imperative to recognise whether there is invasion of the tracheo-bronchial mucosa by the oesophageal carcinoma or airway narrowing by extrinsic compression. Occasionally an otherwise occult bronchial carcinoma with direct oesophageal invasion or

mediastinal lymphatic metastases which ulcerate into the oesophagus will mimic a primary oesophageal carcinoma.

Scalene lymph node biopsy

Open node biopsy or needle aspiration should be done if nodes are palpable on clinical examination. Routine biopsy of impalpable nodes is futile.

OPERATIVE SURGERY

Oesophagectomy

Patient preparation

Attempts to remedy weight loss immediately before resection are futile and meddlesome and operation should not be delayed because of weight loss. If a dysphagic patient faces combined modality treatment such as a prolonged course of chemotherapy before resection the simplest way of maintaining nutrition should be chosen from the possibilities: oral nutritional supplementation, nasogastric (Clinifeed) intubation, jejunostomy and total parenteral nutrition (TPN). A dietitian should see the patient before surgery to outline the postoperative dietary consequences and their palliation. However, dehydration has to be corrected with intravenous fluids and monitoring of urea, electrolytes and fluid balance. This scenario only occurs when patients present as an emergency with either total dysphagia or iatrogenic rupture of a carcinoma.

It is routine to give prophylactic broad-spectrum antibiotics at the induction of anaesthesia and for the first 24 hours thereafter. Metronidazole should also be given if the patient has dental infection. Preoperative instruction in chest physiotherapy is also routine.

Anaesthesia

General anaesthesia is induced by rapid sequence with cricoid pressure to prevent regurgitation into the pharynx.

Double-lumen intubation is used for all patients since it is the best means of preventing intraoperative aspiration of bronchial content into the dependent lung and because one-lung ventilation gives unimpeded access to the oesophagus through a thoracotomy.

Local analgesia by epidural, paravertebral or intercostal nerve block technique is set up in the immediate preoperative phase.

Minimum continuous haemodynamic and respiratory monitoring comprises systemic blood pressure (radial artery line), right atrial pressure (subclavian or internal jugular line), PaO_2 (pulse oximeter) and ECG.

Incisions

The surgical approaches to the oesophagus are listed in Table 3.1. There is no general agreement about which is best but there are theoretical factors which sway opinion.

- Management of anastomotic leak is thought to be easier with cervical anastomosis (three stage, transhiatal) and percutaneous local drainage than an intrathoracic anastomosis where rethoracotomy or covered stenting may be needed to gain control.

- Longitudinal cancer clearance is greatest with cervical anastomosis.

- Lateral cancer clearance with *en bloc* lymph node removal is best through a one-stage thoracolaparotomy which gives safest access to the descending thoracic aorta and the only access to all para-aortic lymph nodes. Two-stage transhiatal oesophagectomy clears only T1 and T2 tumours.

- There is debatable evidence that long-term postoperative reflux is lessened by creating a cervical rather than an intrathoracic anastomosis and by pyloric dilatation, myotomy or pyloroplasty to help gastric emptying.

Procedure

The steps (not given in order) of an oesophagectomy are summarised as follows:

- approach incision (Table 3.1)

- oesophageal mobilisation

- preparation of the stomach, jejunum or colon for oesophageal replacement

- oesophageal resection and anastomosis

- pleural drainage and closure.

However, important details of the procedure vary with the surgical approach, type and anatomy, the choice of oesophageal replacement and the anastomotic technique.

Approach

NECK

For right-handed surgeons the cervical oesophagus is approached through a skin and fascial incision along the anterior border of the left sternomastoid from hyoid to suprasternal notch. The carotid sheath is retracted laterally with division of the middle thyroid vein. Blunt dissection separates the oesophagus from trachea and prevertebral fascia and at transhiatal oesophagectomy the dissection is continued in the superior mediastinum to the level of the main carina.

RIGHT THORACOTOMY

The thoracotomy is made through the fifth interspace. The azygos arch is divided and the intrathoracic oesophagus separated from trachea, aorta, prevertebral fascia, parietal pericardium and hiatus oesophagus. The thoracic duct can be ligated close to the aortic hiatus to prevent chylothorax, a particular postoperative danger in removing T4 tumours.

LEFT THORACOLAPAROTOMY

The thoracotomy is made through the sixth or seventh interspace with division of the epigastric chondral margin. Division of the necks of the fourth or fifth ribs opens the wound to give an easy approach to the oesophagus in the superior mediastinum. If there is difficulty in access to this segment of the oesophagus, the left subclavian artery and arch of aorta are mobilised, the latter by division of the proximal intercostal arteries and the left superior intercostal vein. Otherwise the procedure in the distal oesophagus is similar in both left and right approaches.

Oesophageal replacement

Stomach is routinely used for oesophageal replacement. In two-stage operations the stomach is mobilised before the oesophagus. The short gastric and omental branches of the gastroepiploic artery are divided to free up the greater curvature and gain entry to the lesser sac. The lesser omentum is opened parallel to the lesser curvature, dividing the hepatic branch of the right gastric artery, if present. The intraabdominal oesophagus is separated from the right crus of the diaphragm.

The left gastric artery is divided at its origin from the coeliac. The stomach is transected across the cardia or more distally if a distal third carcinoma invades the cardia. The stomach is now pedicled on the first part of the duodenum and the right gastric and gastroepiploic vessels and is mobilised sufficiently to reach the neck. In transhiatal oesophagectomy the hand is passed up through the

Table 3.1 Approaches to the oesophagus		
Type	**Incision**	**Access**
One stage	Left thoracolaparotomy	Intrathoracic oesophagus, stomach, jejunum, colon
Two stage	Laparotomy before right thoracotomy (Ivor–Lewis)	As for left thoracolaparotomy
	Laparotomy before or simultaneous with left neck (transhiatal)	As for left thoracolaparotomy and cervical oesophagus
Three stage	Right thoracotomy before laparotomy and left neck	As for transhiatal

hiatus oesophageus to mobilise the distal two-thirds of the oesophagus. This manoeuvre severely compresses the left atrium and cardiac output can be dangerously compromised. In all techniques the stomach is pulled up through the hiatus into the chest or neck along the route of the resected oesophagus.

If stomach is not available, jejunum as a Roux-en-Y limb or colon pedicled on the middle or left colic arteries replaces the oesophagus.

Anastomosis

The oesophagus is transected at the selected level proximal to the tumour and the specimen removed. The vascularity of the oesophageal resection margin is protected by dissection of only a short segment proximal to the margin and by the avoidance of prolonged oesophageal cross-clamping. The highest part of the greater curvature is drawn up alongside the oesophagus and an oesophago-gastric anastomosis made either by suture or by circular stapler. Hand suturing varies from full-thickness continuous or interrupted single layer to more complicated two-layer techniques. In essence the squamous oesophageal mucosa and gastric serosa are the suture- and staple-holding tissues. Pedicled omentum can be wrapped around the intrathoracic anastomosis.

Postoperative management

Monitoring

Patients are returned to an intensive care or high-dependency unit where the intraoperative haemodynamic, respiratory and fluid balance monitoring is continued for several days.

Airway

Patients are extubated at the end of the operation and are nursed sitting up at 45° to reduce passive regurgitation and aspiration. Ten percent develop ventilatory failure and are supported by assisted ventilation. Chest physiotherapy is the initial treatment for retention of bronchial secretions supplemented by bronchoscopy and minitracheostomy.

GI tract

A nasogastric tube is left *in situ* and retained until gastric aspirate dries up. Some surgeons also place a feeding jejunostomy at operation. Most patients start oral fluids by the fifth postoperative day after a contrast swallow has confirmed an intact anastomosis and, with dietetic help, return to solid intake within a week. Evidence of gastric hold-up or anastomotic leak delays oral intake and nutrition is then maintained by total parenteral nutrition or jejunostomy. A small anastomotic leak is managed by neck or pleural drainage until it heals. Reoperation and preferably reanastomosis is needed to deal with a major leak.

Analgesia

Apart from the regional analgesic techniques set up at operation, opiate patient-controlled analgesia and intermittent IV opiate 'top-up' are used for pain control in response to pain scoring.

FURTHER READING

Baron TH. Current concepts: expandable metal stents for the treatment of cancerous obstruction of the gastrointestinal tract. *N Engl J Med* 2001; **344**(22):1681–1687

Geh JI, Crellin AM, Glynne-Jones R. Preoperative (neoadjuvant) chemoradiotherapy in oesophageal cancer. *Br J Surg* 2001; **88**(3):338–356

Lehnert T. Multimodal therapy for squamous carcinoma of the oesophagus. *Br J Surg* 1999; **86**(6):727–739

Whooley BP, Law S, Murthy SC, Alexandrou A, Wong J. Analysis of reduced death and complication rates after esophageal resection. *Ann Surg* 2001; **233**(3):338–344

Wijnhoven BPL, Tilanus HW, Dinjens WNM. Molecular biology of Barrett's adenocarcinoma. *Ann Surg* 2001; **233**(3):322–337

Surgical aspects of peptic ulcer disease

Frank J. Branicki

HAEMORRHAGE

Aetiology

More than 90% of patients with gastrointestinal haemorrhage (Box 4.1) have bled from a source proximal to the ligament of Treitz, i.e. upper gastrointestinal bleeding (UGIB).

Box 4.1   Sources of UGIB

Common
- Duodenal ulcer
- Gastric ulcer
- Gastric erosions
- Oesophageal varices

Less common
- Gastritis
- Duodenitis
- Mallory-Weiss tear
- Oesophagogastric cancer
- Reflux oesophagitis

Uncommon
- Dieulafoy's lesion
- Angiodysplasia
- Stromal tumour
- Gastric varices
- Portal hypertensive 'congestive' gastropathy
- Watermelon stomach
- Haemobilia
- Pancreatic cancer

Helicobacter pylori (Hp) infects approximately one half of the world's population and is a factor in the aetiology of 85–100% of duodenal ulcers and 70–90% of gastric ulcers. Ulceration can now generally be healed and recurrence prevented, without surgery, by eradication of Hp. Between 89% and 95% of peptic ulcer-related serious upper gastrointestinal events may be attributed to non-steroidal antiinflammatory drug (NSAID) use, Hp infection and cigarette smoking. Consumption of alcohol increases the risk of major gastric and duodenal haemorrhage in non-predisposed individuals (Box 4.2).

Approximately 20–25% of patients with peptic ulcer disease develop complications: bleeding, perforation or obstruction. Haemorrhage is the most common complication and carries the highest mortality rate. Approximately half the patients with bleeding peptic ulcer have no abdominal pain. In hospitalised patients, NSAIDs and anticoagulants, in association with stress and ageing, are frequently involved in peptic ulcer haemorrhage. Aspirin causes gastric mucosal erosions and enhances spontaneous microbleeding, chronic use being associated with uncomplicated gastric ulcer and with presentation with UGIB. Aspirin has an antihaemostatic as well as an ulcerogenic effect; a broken mucosa and inhibition of thromboxane synthesis both appear to be necessary for bleeding to occur. Thirty percent of patients with a history of aspirin-related UGIB have an exaggerated prolongation of skin bleeding time.

Box 4.2   Risk factors for UGIB
- Hp infection
- Advanced age
- Smoking
- History of peptic ulcer
- Oral corticosteroids/anticoagulants

Presentation

Despite improved endoscopic and surgical techniques, acute bleeding from peptic ulcer is a serious condition for which management is controversial. Optimal management is best facilitated by admission to a unit or team which has a special interest and members appropriately trained in resuscitation, therapeutic endoscopy and the expertise for surgical intervention. Often such a unit involves collaborative care by physicians and surgeons with clear lines of communication.

On presentation, it is important to establish as soon as possible whether there is active bleeding or overt evidence of hypovolaemia due to blood loss (Box 4.3). Shock, present in <15% of patients on admission, is recognised by imprecise signs and subjective symptoms. Critical reduction of blood flow to vital organs is described as shock. Shock has been defined in terms of systolic blood pressure <100 mmHg with or without an accompanying pulse rate of >100 beats/minute and peripheral circulatory failure. Loss of more than 30% of blood volume without therapy often results in death, maintenance of circulatory volume being more important than the actual red cell mass. Young patients can compensate for blood loss and only experience hypotension when in excess of 1 l of blood has been lost. Occasionally, patients may present having sustained head or other injuries secondary to a syncopal attack and the presence of melaena reveals the cause.

Box 4.3   Features of hypovolaemic shock indicating loss of 40% of blood volume
- Marked pallor
- Poor volume pulse
- Excessive sweating
- Rapid respiratory rate
- Cold extremities

Co-morbid illness

While the patient is being stabilised haemodynamically (see below), some elements of history can be obtained from family or friends, physical examination can be completed and investigations initiated. It is important to try and obtain from the stabilised patient an estimate of the volume of blood lost. A history of haematemesis confirms a UGIB site and 'coffee ground' vomitus indicates recent bleeding which is no longer active. Melaena, the passage of black, tarry pungent stool, may occur with as little as 100 ml of blood loss and, unless bowel actions are frequent and the colour of the stools assumes a maroon appearance, does not indicate continuing haemorrhage or rebleeding. Haematemesis following an episode of retching or vomiting suggests a Mallory Weiss tear at the gastro-oesophageal junction with bleeding occurring usually from the gastric mucosa.

It is obligatory to obtain a sound history of any co-existent disease, previous relevant abdominal medical disease, surgical procedures, drug ingestion and allergies. A history of chronic liver disease or identification of stigmata (gynaecomastia, spider naevi, palmar erythema, splenomegaly, testicular atrophy) are particularly relevant. The number of co-existent illnesses per patient is reported to be strongly related to mortality rate (Box 4.4). Peptic ulceration is the most common cause of UGIB in chronic renal failure whereas vascular ectasia, although less frequently encountered, is the most common cause of recurrent haemorrhage.

Box 4.4   Co-morbid illness related to mortality

- Diabetes mellitus
- Hypertension
- Ischaemic heart disease
- Previous cerebrovascular accident
- Previous pulmonary tuberculosis
- Chronic obstructive airways disease
- Cirrhosis
- Chronic renal failure
- Co-existent malignant disease

Mortality increases with the severity of the initial bleed, as indicated by hypotension, low haemoglobin level and large volume of blood transfusion, shock being the best clinical predictor of continued or recurrent bleeding. Elderly patients in shock admitted with their first peptic ulcer haemorrhage run the greatest risk of death. The presence of shock should help in the selection of patients for endoscopic therapy or surgery, as criteria based on the circulatory response to haemorrhage have proved to be of value in identifying patients at risk of exsanguination. Part of the problem is the potentially poor correlation between pressure and flow variables, which are difficult to assess but which are of overriding importance.

If bleeding is brisk and ongoing, endoscopy may be necessary during resuscitation. Oxygen is given via nasal specula to avoid hypoxia. Persistent and intractable bleeding occurs in 10% of patients with UGIB (Box 4.5).

Box 4.5   Upper gastrointestinal bleeding

- <20% of deaths related to uncontrolled rehaemorrhage
- Most fatalities attributed to co-morbid illness

Rebleeding

Rebleeding occurs in a further 10% and is associated with a 10-fold increase in mortality rate. Rebleeding is defined as:

- fresh haematemesis, or
- fall in systolic blood pressure to <100 mmHg or by 50 mmHg, or
- fall in haemoglobin concentration of 2 g/dl after correction of anaemia.

Risk assessment

It is essential to identify the high-risk patient with the high-risk lesion with endoscopic stigmata of recent haemorrhage (ESRH) (Table 4.1). Risk assessment and resuscitation proceed simultaneously as such assessment helps to rationalise decision making regarding management.

Table 4.1 Endoscopic stigmata of recent haemorrhage (ESRH) and rebleeding

	Rebleeding %
Active bleeding	100
Visible vessel and hypotension	80
Non-bleeding visible vessel	40
Oozing from adherent clot	35
Black or red spot	<10
Clean ulcer base	<2

Some studies have focused on outcome prediction based on clinical variables on presentation prior to endoscopy. Blood pressure response during the first hour of resuscitation strongly predicts outcome. Prediction of recurrent bleeding (Box 4.6) can be made with clinical scoring symptoms such as the Baylor Bleeding Score, which, although validated prospectively by the authors, has not been validated by others.

Consideration of both clinical and endoscopic findings is more likely to be of value with regard to management, particularly the identification of individuals considered to have a low risk of rebleeding not requiring prolonged hospitalisation and in whom discharge on the day of presentation with outpatient care is appropriate. The Rockall risk scoring system devised in the United Kingdom is based on a numerical score and includes no absolute exclusions and is intended to be applied to all aetiologies of UGIB, including varices (Box 4.7).

Patients identified by Rockall et al. as being at low risk had recurrent bleeding and mortality rates of 4% and 1% respectively, leading the authors to propose early hospital discharge of such patients. In a study in the United States which advocates early discharge of low-risk patients, one-third of those treated successfully as outpatients were classified by Rockall scoring as being at high risk. It is evident that models derived from multivariate analysis for predicting rebleeding and proactive guidelines to determine management strategies must include not only endoscopic findings but clinical variables such as severity of blood loss and the age and co-morbidity of the patient. There is, unfortunately, marked interobservation variability in identifying ESRH, other than spurting haemorrhage, and this may be due to differences in definition of terminology, lack of observer training or failure to wash target lesions. This implies that management strategies based too heavily on ESRH may result in inappropriate discharge of some patients who are at high risk.

Box 4.6 Risk factors for rebleeding and mortality	
High-risk patient	**High-risk lesion**
Co-morbid illness	High lesser curvature gastric ulcer
Shock on presentation	Posteroinferior duodenal ulcer
Severe anaemia	Large (>1 cm) ulcer size
	ESRH

Box 4.7 Rockall risk scoring system

- Age
- Shock
- Co-morbidity
- Diagnosis
- ESRH

Ulcer size

Ulcer size is known to be significantly associated with bleeding severity. Patients >60 years of age are more likely to have larger ulcers (>1 cm) and larger ulcers are associated with a higher prevalence of ESRH which are known to be associated with an increased risk of rebleeding, increased transfusion requirements and mortality (Figure 4.1). Octogenarians are particularly at risk when ulcer size exceeds 2 cm. Using logistic regression analysis, risk models for rebleeding and mortality have been constructed utilising the presence or absence of shock on presentation, ESRH, age >60 years and ulcer size >1 cm. In the absence of therapeutic endoscopy, there was a fivefold increase in predicted and actual rebleeding rates for patients with ulceration >1 cm in diameter with ESRH identifiable, one in three patients was documented to have a rebleeding episode. The rebleeding

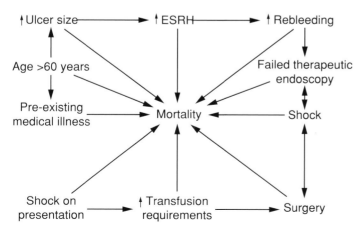

Figure 4.1 Risk factors for mortality.

model does not indicate which patients will succumb but helps to identify patients at risk. The rebleeding rate from gastric ulcers is higher than that for duodenal ulceration, gastric ulcers having at least double the mortality rate. More severe bleeding and poorer general condition are features of giant gastric ulcer and highlight the need for early diagnosis, rigorous resuscitation and early treatment. Giant (>3 cm) bleeding gastric ulcer has a poorer prognosis with high rates of mortality, need for surgery and operative mortality. While fixed management practices and guidelines are appealing, there is concern that treatment ought to be individualised according to evaluation of the patient (haemodynamic status, age, co-morbid illness, previous relevant history, Hp status) and the nature of the lesion (size, site, stigmata).

Management

Resuscitation

The cornerstones of management of UGIB are resuscitation followed by diagnostic endoscopy.
Resuscitation involves:

- airway protection
- oxygen (40–60%)
- vascular access (two 14 gauge cannulas)
- urinary catheter insertion
- correction of severe anaemia and coagulopathy
- non-invasive blood pressure measurement
- pulse oximetry
- central venous pressure measurement.

A central venous pressure line is helpful, particularly if there is any associated co-morbid cardiorespiratory disease.

The insertion of a urethral indwelling catheter will enable monitoring of the response to resuscitation and subsequent progress, a urine output of 0.5 ml/kg/h being desirable.

If bleeding is continuous and profuse then the source of bleeding needs to be identified and treated expeditiously to control haemorrhage as soon as possible.

Prompt and adequate intravascular volume replacement with isotonic crystallised solution (0.9N saline, Ringer's lactate) should commence immediately and, when available, packed cells should be transfused to maintain the haematocrit at about 30%. If there is intense vasoconstriction the haematocrit determination may be normal for the first few hours despite exsanguinating haemorrhage. Blood transfusion should not be withheld, despite a normal haematocrit, in the patient with brisk haemorrhage. Severe anaemia and coagulopathy must be corrected. Fresh frozen plasma (FFP) should be given (15 ml/kg) if the prothrombin time is at least 1.5 times higher than the mid range of the control value. If the prothrombin time is normal, then FFP is given after transfusion of six units of blood. Citrate toxicity after massive transfusion can be avoided by giving 10 ml 10% calcium gluconate after six units of blood, repeating this after every two further units.

Massive bleeding may contribute to myocardial hypoperfusion and infarction and cardiac arrest during severe haemorrhage is to be avoided by aggressive resuscitation at all costs. It is of interest, however, that research efforts in the pathophysiology of shock are now being channelled from normotensive to hypotensive, i.e. limited, fluid resuscitation with plasma substitutes. It is known that increasing mean arterial pressure may accelerate haemorrhage in experimental shock models.

Endoscopy

Endoscopy ought to be performed within 12–24 hours of presentation otherwise small superficial lesions such as erosions or bleeding from lesions such as Dieulafoy's disease (a prominent artery which reaches the mucosal surface) may be missed, making a definite diagnosis impossible. Some patients with brisk haemorrhage may have an overdistended stomach full of liquid, blood and clots, in which case there is a risk of pulmonary aspiration, especially if endoscopy is performed in a patient who already has an altered mental state or confusion. For this reason, experienced endoscopists often perform endoscopy in patients with UGIB without the use of intravenous sedation. Occasionally, it is advisable to perform endotracheal intubation to ensure airway protection in a patient considered to be at risk prior to endoscopic examination. Previously, gastric lavage with 500–1000 ml aliquots of fluid was advocated to remove clot and enable adequate visualisation at endoscopy. This is no longer recommended because of the risk of pulmonary aspiration in patients who may be hypoxic or have encephalopathy. Failure to clear a pool of blood in the gastric fundus at emergency endoscopy is, however, associated with significant morbidity and mortality, as small lesions may be missed.

A visible vessel is actually a fibrin clot plugging a side hole in an artery running parallel with the base of the ulcer. Visible vessels may be red, white or blue in colour and it has been suggested that the whitish pearl-like appearance of a protuberant vessel carries a greater risk of recurrent bleeding compared with dark coloured 'sentinel' clot. Different types of ESRH represent different stages in the healing process of a bleeding ulcer, a non-treated visible vessel taking about 4±2 days to disappear. The associated rebleeding risk diminishes as the vessel fades from the ulcer base. The optimal duration required for hospitalisation of patients with non-bleeding visible vessels at initial endoscopy is thus four days. Bleeding does not recur once ESRH are no longer seen and the time taken for stigmata to fade is not affected by age, gender, smoking, history of peptic ulcer, ulcer location, severity of bleeding, underlying systemic disease or endoscopic local therapy.

A clot is defined as adherent if it cannot be dislodged by irrigation with 200 ml of water. Most patients with a tightly adherent clot in an ulcer base have an uneventful course but 25% will rebleed within a month. Hence, there has been ongoing controversy as to whether adherent clot should be snared and removed, as it has been shown that identifying and treating the underlying visible vessel endoscopically results in lower rebleeding rates. Unfortunately, clot removal may provoke brisk haemorrhage and unless there is expertise and facilities are available for endoscopic treatment in the face of brisk bleeding, or a willingness to proceed to emergency surgery if so required, then it is perhaps prudent to leave adherent clot undisturbed.

Low-risk patients with stable low-volume bleeding, uncomplicated by co-morbid illness and issues such as anticoagulation and coagulopathy, and having a clean ulcer base can be discharged following endoscopy if there is a suitable home environment with family support. This may lead to reduced health expenditure but it is important to bear in mind that it is the elderly who run the greatest risk of rebleeding and death and some caution may need to be exercised in individual cases. The best prospects for a reduction in mortality from UGIB lie with prevention of rebleeding episodes. Age >60 years, haematemesis, shock and ESRH are each associated with a high risk of further haemorrhage.

Endoscopic therapy

Treatment is indicated for acute bleeding, the non-bleeding visible vessel and possibly, in experienced hands, the adherent clot (Table 4.2). It may prove beneficial in the subset of patients with independent predictors of rebleeding, i.e. co-morbid illness, shock and initial haemoglobin ≤10 g/dl.

Table 4.2 Endoscopic therapy for UGIB

Non-thermal	Thermal
Injection therapy	Electrocoagulation
● adrenaline	● monopolar
● sclerosant (polidocanol, ethanolamine)	● bipolar
	● multipolar
● fibrin glue	Heater probe
● thrombin	Argon laser coagulator
Mechanical	Nd:YAG laser
● haemoclips	
● band ligation	
● endoloops	

INJECTION THERAPY

The mechanism of action of injection therapy may include tamponade, vasoconstriction, tissue dehydration and thrombogenesis. Adrenaline (1:10 000) is injected submucosally around the periphery of the visible vessel or clot in all four quadrants, followed by injection centrally. Local gastric blood flow is reduced by tamponade, vasoconstriction and platelet aggregation. A disposable 23 or 25 gauge sclerotherapy needle is used which can pass through any endoscope with an instrument channel diameter of ≥1.8 mm, i.e. a paediatric endoscope. The needle is flushed free of air and the injection action double-checked before proceeding. Aliquots of 0.5–1.0 ml of adrenaline are given to a total of 10–20 ml and this rarely gives rise to complications, because most of the drug is metabolised in the first pass through the line, although tachycardia is sometimes precipitated. Local tamponade with distilled water has been reported to be as effective. Adrenaline injection alone reduces rebleeding, need for surgery and mortality and, in view of low cost, availability and simplicity of usage, is considered by many to be the endoscopic treatment of choice. Alternatively, injection of 0.1–0.3 ml aliquots of absolute alcohol for a total of 1–2 ml will lead to rapid dehydration and fixation of the tissues. There is no convincing evidence that a combination of injection treatments confers any advantage over single agent therapy, although adrenaline and thrombin is a combination favoured by some endoscopists who hold the view that addition of 600–1000 IU of human thrombin is optimal therapy. Sclerosants such as polidocanol and ethanolamine oleate hold no advantage over adrenaline but have been reported to cause extrahepatic biliary obstruction secondary to sclerosis of the distal common bile duct. Sclerosants must not be injected blindly because of the risk of perforation.

COMPLICATIONS OF ENDOSCOPIC INJECTION

These include:

- enlarged ulcer bed
- bleeding from exposed vessels
- perforation.

Such complications are not evident with haemoclipping. Adrenaline itself may cause gastric ischaemic necrosis and haemorrhage but this is less problematic; oesophageal perforation has been reported after endoscopic sclerotherapy with adrenaline and 1% polidocanol for bleeding Mallory-Weiss tears. By contrast, fibrin glue does not cause tissue damage but appears to be effective only if injected repeatedly. Application of haemoclips for bleeding peptic ulcer is easy and safe, even in patients in poor general health, and is now widely practised. The endoscopic injection of adrenaline or fibrin glue and application of heat coagulation can stop active bleeding in more than 90% of patients.

Electrocoagulation/heater probe

Monopolar electrocoagulation is not recommended as it is difficult to control the treatment depth and the risk of perforation is far greater than with the bipolar electrode (BICAP) where the circuit is completed by the patient or ground electrode. The heater probe develops a temperature of 100°C during treatment and coagulates the bleeding vessel; with the BICAP, heat is generated by radiofrequency energy with an electrical circuit completed between the pair of electrodes at the tip. Microwave coagulation occurs through dielectric heat similar to a microwave oven with heat generated by molecular excitation. Tissue adherence is common and requires application of a dissociation-current before safe removal. The argon plasma coagulator is a non-contact, multi-directional technique which shows promise, whereas the use of laser therapy (argon, Nd:YAG), although efficacious, is not favoured due to its non-portable nature, preventing bedside usage, and cost considerations.

Both the BICAP and heater probe recommended are 3.2 mm (10 Fr) in size, requiring a large endoscopic channel, and this enables forceful tamponade of the lesion. The BICAP is used at a low, 15–20 watt setting with 6–8 prolonged 10–14-second pulse periods of coagulation. Alternatively, short two-second bursts or a single burst totalling 10–20 seconds can be used before changing the position of the probe; when effective, the lesion appears charred. The heater probe delivers a fixed amount of energy and a setting of 25–30 joules is usually chosen. Four applications of 30 joule pulses, each delivered in eight seconds, is applied before changing the position of the probe. The preset energy level is delivered with each activation of the generator so, unlike the BICAP, it is not necessary to keep the foot switch depressed during treatment.

Twenty percent of patients with active bleeding or a non-bleeding visible vessel rebleed after endoscopic therapy with the BICAP, heater probe or injection therapy. Repeat endoscopic treatment results in haemostasis in half the group, i.e. 10%. Retreatment obviates the need for urgent surgical intervention but is associated with an increased risk of perforation. The addition of heater probe treatment after endoscopic injection of adrenaline, which is not thrombogenic, confers an advantage for control of spurting ulcer haemorrhage and has gained popularity in an attempt to avoid the need for retreatment of the high-risk lesion. The need for surgery to deal with spurting arterial haemorrhage is 30% following adrenaline alone, but the additional application of the heater probe reduces the surgical intervention rate to 7%. Contact thermocoagulation, in addition to injection of a thrombogenic agent, has been shown to improve outcome. Thermal contact methods can coapt, i.e. flatten and weld together, the endothelial surfaces of a blood vessel. Heater probe and BICAP may be superior to injection and laser therapy in deeply excavated duodenal ulcers which may be more accessible with wheeling to produce endoscopic coaptation so as to lie flat on the vessel. All thermocoagulation probes contain built-in irrigation devices for washing blood and clots. The technique is not difficult to learn. Junior endoscopists obtained similar initial haemostasis and rebleeding rates (92.6%, 26.4%) with heater probe therapy when compared with those achieved by more senior clinicians (96.2%, 22.7%). The morbidity rate is very acceptable – a metaanalysis of 30 randomised controlled trials of endoscopic haemostasis of non-variceal UGIB found treatment induced bleeding in only 0.4% of patients undergoing thermocoagulation, with perforation in 0.7%.

A tendency towards better results has been noted in patients receiving a second-look endoscopy 24 hours following endoscopic therapy. Scheduled repeat endoscopy cannot, however, be routinely recommended after successful endoscopic treatment when selection of patients for second look is based on endoscopic Forrest criteria at first presentation (Box 4.8). Follow-up endoscopy and biopsy, however, is recommended for all patients with gastric ulcer or complicated duodenal ulcer.

Box 4.8	Forrest classification of ESRH
Type 1A	Active spurting haemorrhage
Type 1B	Oozing haemorrhage
Type 11A	Non-bleeding visible vessel
Type 11B	Adherent clot
Type 11C	Flat pigmented spot
Type 111	Clean ulcer base

Endoscopic Doppler ultrasonography can detect movement of blood in vessels and act as a guide to endoscopic therapy. Pulsed Doppler, range gated ultrasonography avoids interference from unrelated arteries and is a better guide than continuous Doppler. It has been advocated to better direct endoscopic therapy in bleeding peptic ulcer but is not in routine use. It may well be helpful in the detection of Dieulafoy's disease, which accounts for up to 5% of UGIB disease, in patients with unexplained UGIB. A relatively large calibre (2–3 mm) vessel may be seen penetrating the muscularis mucosae for 2–4 cm. Injection therapy or haemoclipping, etc. can be performed at the same procedure but vascular ligation or wedge resection is required if endoscopic therapy for Dieulafoy's lesion fails.

In a metaanalysis of 25 randomised controlled trials, endoscopic therapy at initial endoscopy produced significant relative reductions:

- rebleeding (↓69%)
- the need for surgery (↓62%)
- mortality (↓30%).

Heavy bacterial counts of Hp are believed to precipitate bleeding episodes from duodenal ulcers. At endoscopy, if the patient's condition permits, it is helpful to identify Hp infection by taking antral/prepyloric biopsies for either rapid urease testing (RUT) (e.g. CLO test) or histological examination or both. Unfortunately, the RUT has a variable false-negative rate that can be as high as 40–50% in bleeding duodenal ulcer. Blood adversely affects the performance of the biopsy urease test. This is mediated by the buffering effect of serum albumin on the pH indicator, rather than by a direct effect on urease activity. Anti-Hp IgG antibody titres may document past infection.

Endoscopic haemostasis of bleeding upper gastrointestinal tumours is safe and initially effective and may provide time for further investigation and appropriate management.

Box 4.9	Failure of endoscopic therapy	
Gastric ulcer		*Duodenal ulcer*
Active arterial bleeding		Age
High lesser curvature ulcer		Shock
Ulcer size >2 cm		Haemoglobin level
		Ulcer size >2 cm
		Posteroinferior location

Pharmacotherapy

Octreotide is safe and may be beneficial in peptic ulcer haemorrhage. It can be used as first-line treatment to reduce splanchnic blood flow in a patient with brisk peptic ulcer haemorrhage, prior to transferral to hospital. It is known that blood clot in a peptic ulcer is unstable in a low pH environment. The use of proton pump inhibition may prevent rebleeding by elevating intragastric pH in patients in whom endoscopic haemostasis is successful. Profound acid suppression may prevent clot lysis. In patients with bleeding peptic ulcer and a non-bleeding visible vessel, infusion of omeprazole has been reported to decrease the rate of further bleeding, the need for endoscopic therapy and surgery. Treatment must be given by continuous infusion rather than bolus injection and optimal dosage is 8 mg/h of omeprazole after an initial loading dose of 40–80 mg, to aid the physiological cascade of haemostasis and improve overall outcome. On multivariate analyses, omeprazole has now been shown to be an independent factor for prevention of rebleeding after multipolar electrocoagulation for haemostasis of bleeding peptic ulcer.

Surgery

Proof that eradication of the *H. pylori* infection results in cure of peptic ulcer disease has led to a reappraisal of the indications for surgery and the nature of procedures performed.

Exsanguinating haemorrhage is often due to bleeding of a large-calibre artery >1 mm in diameter. Vessels of this size may be difficult to seal with therapeutic endoscopy. Therapeutic endoscopy for rebleeding may be successful in the patient considered to be at exceptional risk if surgery were to be performed. Endoscopic retreatment for rebleeding has been shown to reduce the need for surgery without increasing the risk of death and has fewer complications than surgery. Co-morbid illness increases the likelihood of postoperative morbidity and mortality. Surgery is, however, recommended after two or even three attempts at endoscopic therapy in the patient considered to be a high-risk surgical candidate. With effective endoscopic therapy and the belief that the ulcer diathesis can be cured by Hp eradication, there is a temptation to persist with endoscopic treatment, particularly in the elderly. This may be dangerous as repeated blood loss, hypovolaemia and multiple blood transfusions lead to poor outcome when surgery is delayed. The aggressive use of endoscopic therapy has led to fewer patients needing surgery but these patients often have serious co-morbid illness. Thus, mortality for surgery after unsuccessful endoscopic treatment is high.

Emergency surgery

Emergency surgery to control bleeding carries a mortality of 10–20%. Surgery is, however, advisable in patients in danger of exsanguination, but more than two-thirds of patients with major bleeding are poor surgical risks. The place of surgery therefore continues to be controversial, although it is accepted that surgical intervention in selected high-risk patients can lead to a reduction in overall mortality if performed early enough in the clinical course. The essence of good treatment is early diagnosis and timely operation but the problem remains as to how to make the right decision and operate on the right patient at the right time with the right procedure. Decisions about when to intervene surgically have become more difficult as there has been an atrophy of ulcer surgery all over the world. Understandably, there is some reluctance to advocate early surgery in the elderly who may tolerate even expeditiously performed procedures very poorly. In particular, poor results for emergency surgery are encountered in patients with congestive cardiac failure, chronic renal failure, cirrhosis or co-existing malignant disease. In patients with co-morbid illness, emergency surgical intervention was accompanied by disturbingly high mortality figures not influenced by whether the surgery was performed either early or as late as possible during the acute bleeding episode.

On multivariate analysis in patients <80 years of age, the risk of mortality following treatment was significantly associated with postoperative complications, highlighting the importance of technical considerations. Although avoidance of operation is attractive, it has to be borne in mind that such patients may weather a surgical procedure better than continued bleeding. Although trials often define the need for surgery as treatment failure, an alternative view is that endoscopic control may facilitate early elective operation in selected patients at high risk of rebleeding. A successful outcome may require a combination of endoscopic therapy and surgery.

Early elective surgery

Although early elective operation has been considered appropriate for elderly patients at high risk for further bleeding, it is salutary to recall that surgery carries inherent risks of its own with inevitable morbidity in such patients. For those at low risk of recurrent haemorrhage, early operation is associated with an unacceptable operation risk. False-positive predictions of the need for surgery can occur. Early elective surgery for gastric ulcer that is unlikely to rebleed is recommended only rarely: the long-term sequelae of gastric resection do not justify operation. However, reported 30-day mortality rates for gastric and duodenal ulceration of 6.2% vs 1.6% respectively suggest that, in the absence of definitive endoscopic treatment, early elective operation ought to have been performed more readily so as to obviate the high mortality rate of 24% for emergency surgery to control bleeding from gastric ulceration.

Endoscopic therapy for control of haemorrhage has thus become so successful that, for the management of even large ulcers, it is practised whenever possible, regardless of ulcer size, and surgical intervention is advocated only for continued uncontrolled rebleeding or when gross stenosis is also present, causing symptoms which fail to resolve on conservative management. Thus, despite enthusiasm in the recent past for proximal gastric vagotomy with duodenotomy ± ulcer excision/plication, the excellent results now being obtained with endoscopic retreatment of ulcers which rebleed suggests that surgery on an early elective basis, even in younger patients, may be inappropriate in most circumstances. Indeed, patients <70 years of age do not seem to benefit from early elective operation after endoscopic haemostasis of arterial bleeding.

Indications for surgery

Surgery must be seriously considered when:

- 1500 ml of whole blood are needed in any 24-hour period after initial stabilisation

- bleeding occurs continuously for more than 24 hours from onset (12–18 hours in patients >60 years)

- endoscopic retreatment fails in the patient with significant rebleeding.

Choice of procedure (Table 4.3)

For small ulcers, underrunning or ulcer excision may be considered adequate but for larger ulcers a technically difficult gastrectomy is often required. Unfortunately, the postoperative

Table 4.3 Operations for emergency treatment of bleeding peptic ulcer

	Duodenal ulcer	Gastric body and prepyloric ulcer
Ulcer plication or excision (P/E)	+	+
Truncal vagotomy and pyloroplasty (plus P/E)	+	+
Truncal vagotomy and antrectomy	+	+
Proximal gastric vagotomy	+	−
Billroth I gastrectomy	−	+
(Polya) Billroth II gastrectomy	+	−

rebleeding rate has been shown to be significantly higher in patients treated by simple underrunning or ulcer excision than by conventional definitive, i.e. more radical, surgery. Rebleeding in the postoperative period, which carries a 40% mortality rate, may arise from a suture or staple line, the initial ulcer treated or a second overlooked lesion.

Patients undergoing surgery for severe haemorrhage may be best served by a relatively aggressive approach. Truncal vagotomy and pyloroplasty (TVP), with ulcer underrunning or excision, is the best surgical approach at emergency operation in poor-risk patients with bleeding duodenal or gastric ulcer.

DUODENAL ULCERS

Proximal gastric vagotomy (PGV) with ulcer underrunning may be appropriate in selected good-risk patients with duodenal ulcer. Because of the risk of rebleeding following ulcer plication and TVP in large (>2 cm) posterior duodenal ulcers, it is recommended that a two-thirds Billroth II gastric resection be carried out in good-risk patients (Figure 4.2). The ulcer base, which is plicated, is left *in situ* and excluded from the gastrointestinal tract by suturing the inferior margin of the ulcer to the transected duodenal cuff, continuity being restored with a gastrojejunal anastomosis. Following Billroth II resection, it is essential to avoid obstruction of the afferent limb at the stoma. Should this arise, then duodenal stump leakage or pancreatitis may prove lethal. In peptic ulcer patients, the ulcer recurrence rate after Roux-en-Y gastrectomy without vagotomy is consistently higher than after Billroth II resection. Thus, gastrectomy with Roux-en-Y anastomosis without the addition of vagotomy cannot be recommended.

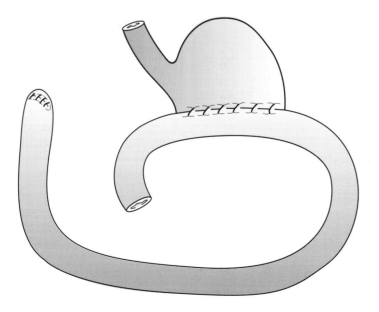

Figure 4.2 Billroth II gastrectomy with Polya anastomosis–proximal jejunum to greater curvature (Moynihan).

GASTRIC ULCERS

For gastric ulcers a more radical approach involving partial gastrectomy is often favoured since it reduces bleeding recurrence rates without increasing mortality. Mortality is minimal in patients with an APACHE II score <15 and partial gastrectomy can be performed with low risk. A gastric ulcer occurring at the incisura does not co-exist with duodenal or pyloric ulcers and is treated most frequently with a 50% distal gastrectomy and Billroth I (gastroduodenal) anastomosis but PGV with ulcerectomy for gastric ulcer is an alternative. A posterior gastric ulcer penetrating the pancreas is best treated by mobilising the surrounding stomach free from the ulcer bed which is then plicated and left *in situ*; the stomach containing the ulcer defect is then resected. Selective vagotomy – antrectomy has been advocated for patients with pyloric or prepyloric ulcer and pyloric obstruction, but occasionally patients develop disabling symptoms postoperatively which militate against its usage. More recently, pylorus-preserving, vagus-preserving gastrectomy for peptic ulcer disease (gastric, duodenal) was associated with better quality of life outcomes than Billroth procedures. Most stomal ulcers are single and are located at the mid-part on the jejunal side. A bleeding stomal ulcer may be managed solely by ulcer plication. Alternatively, truncal vagotomy and/or resection of the anastomosis can be performed with further gastric resection undertaken as deemed necessary.

LAPAROSCOPIC/LAPAROSCOPICALLY ASSISTED PROCEDURES

A small transverse incision in the right upper quadrant can be used to underrun the arterial bleeding point in the duodenum followed by pyloroplasty, the wound then being closed over a 10 mm trocar sheath. With the addition of three more ports, truncal vagotomy can be completed laparoscopically. A more minimalist laparoscopic approach has been advocated with duodenotomy and when excision/plication is planned on an early elective basis for duodenal ulcer without the addition of vagotomy, to be followed by Hp eradication therapy. The technique has been recommended to control bleeding from small duodenal ulcers related to Hp infection and NSAID-induced ulceration. Uncontrolled bleeding from gastric ulcer has also been dealt with laparoscopically, employing a transgastric approach with suture ligation performed via intragastric cannulae under endoscopic guidance.

TVP VS PGV

In a metaanalysis of 12 prospective randomised controlled trials comparing TVP and PGV for duodenal ulcer, the likelihood of adverse long-term sequelae (rapid gastric emptying, diarrhoea) was higher with TVP, whereas the likelihood of ulcer recurrence was higher with PGV. Alterations in biliary motility increase the risk of gallstone formation after most, but not all, definitive surgical procedures for ulcers. Gallstones are more likely after TVP than PGV which spares the hepatic branches of the vagus. Long-term follow-up after open proximal gastric vagotomy has shown that ulcer recurrence occurs in <10% of patients if the operation is performed by an experienced surgeon. Its success is due to a more complete division of preganglionic gastric vagal fibres ('extended' PGV) and the liberal use of pyloric reconstruction in patients with juxtapyloric ulceration; dumping, diarrhoea and gastric atony are quite rare. The section of all vagal fibres to the gastric fundus is essential for complete vagotomy. Many also advocate division of vagal branches running with the right gastroepiploic artery at the gastric antrum. It is the effect of vagotomy on stimulated rather than upon basal acid secretion that cures duodenal ulcer; the apparent basal hypersecretion of patients with duodenal ulcer is due to an increased parietal cell mass. Eighty percent of recurrences occur after 10 years of follow-up.

GASTRIC RESECTION VS VAGOTOMY

Compared with vagotomy, gastric resections are associated with an increased likelihood of emptying problems and nutritional disorders including iron deficiency anaemia and B12 deficiency, requiring lifelong supplementation. A significant reduction in bone mass density, especially of the lumbar spine, has been reported after partial gastrectomy in comparison with postvagotomy findings. Postgastrectomy bone disease may be the result of a calcium deficit which increases calcium release from bone and impairs calcification of newly formed bone matrix. Adequate supplementation of calcium and vitamin D is strongly recommended.

LAPAROSCOPIC VS OPEN SURGERY

Laparoscopic PGV is technically demanding but is feasible and safe, producing short-term results comparable to open surgery. Initial postoperative gastric acid secretion studies have shown similar results for laparoscopic and conventional open PGV. The main advantage of an elective laparoscopic procedure are reductions in hospital stay and overall recovery period of 70% and 50% respectively. Delayed gastric emptying may occur after open or laparoscopic PGV or highly selective anterior and posterior truncal vagotomy. The latter is a simplified vagotomy (Hill-Barker) which was proposed more than 15 years ago. Stapling modifications of the original Taylor procedure of posterior truncal vagotomy and anterior seromyotomy (conventional and laparoscopic) are said to be more rapid and technically easier with excellent long-term results. It can be performed safely laparoscopically with a reported recurrence rate of 4.2% after follow-up of 2–41 months.

H. pylori eradication and recurrence of bleeding

When conservative treatment or endoscopic therapy for bleeding duodenal ulcer has been successful, eradication of documented Hp infection significantly reduces the rate of ulcer recurrence and rebleeding is virtually abolished for at least four years. In populations of duodenal ulcer patients without predisposing risk factors for ulcer bleeding, Hp eradication prevented the occurrence of ulcer-related haemorrhage for up to a year after therapy.

Consistent 95% Hp eradication can be achieved with triple therapy employing a proton pump inhibitor twice daily together with any two of the following drugs: nitroimidazole, clarithromycin or amoxycillin in appropriate dosages taken two or three times daily and concurrently for a week. Compared with dual therapy, triple drug regimens are more likely to eradicate Hp and less likely to generate resistant strains among surviving organisms. Patients need to understand the vital importance of compliance. Dependent on geographical location, antibiotic resistance may lead to treatment failures requiring alternative drug regimens. Culture of the fastidious organism is not routinely performed, but may be considered when treatment repeatedly fails. Pretreatment with proton pump inhibitor does not significantly reduce the efficacy of triple therapy. Eradication of Hp is associated with more side effects and poor compliance but is more effective than acid suppression maintenance therapy in reducing the recurrence rate after duodenal ulcer.

For prevention of ulcer recurrence, testing after eradication therapy is important. Reinfection rates are as low as 3%. Testing after Hp eradication therapy can be carried out at one month following cessation of treatment. A simplified 13C urea breath test, without a test meal, is simple to perform and a single point breath evaluation after ingestion of 13C-labelled urea yields, with a chosen threshold, had a sensitivity and specificity for *H. pylori* infection of 92% and 95% respectively.

Maintenance treatment for acid suppression is not required after successful eradication. Cure of the Hp infection is more effective than long-term maintenance therapy, with H_2 receptor antagonists, in the prevention of recurrent peptic ulcer haemorrhage. Data showing a recurrence rate of 10%, operation rate less than 10% and a mortality rate of 5% represent the present standard of interdisciplinary treatment for bleeding peptic ulcer.

Acid suppression therapy nevertheless remains essential for treatment of Hp-negative ulceration, aspirin/NSAID-induced ulceration and hyperactity-related ulcer. Even when prolonged, acid suppression so far appears safe and generally well tolerated. High-risk patients, however, may warrant maintenance therapy with misoprostol, which has been shown to be effective in the prevention of NSAID-induced gastric and duodenal ulcers as well as for reducing the risk of haemorrhage and perforation. Routine misoprostol, often associated with diarrhoea, is not cost effective because of the low incidence of clinically significant bleeding in patients taking NSAIDs (Box 4.10).

Box 4.10 NSAID ingestion

- Hp and NSAID perforation are two distinct entities
- Increased risk of complicated peptic ulcer with multiple NSAIDs or high-dose single agent
- Risk for ulcer bleeding increased 3–5-fold
- Risk of ulcer perforation increased 5–8-fold
- NSAIDs account for 25% of peptic ulcer perforations
- Discontinue or reduce NSAID dosage in patients with ulceration
- Select NSAID with lowest risk
- Use cautiously in patients with risk factors for UGIB

Patients discharged after peptic ulcer haemorrhage have a substantially reduced life expectancy, perhaps related to co-morbid illness.

Implementation of trauma stress ulcer prophylaxis in guidelines limiting therapy to patients with risk factors for bleeding has led to an 80% decrease in drug costs and did not affect the frequency of major UGIB.

When endoscopy is unsuccessful in identifying or controlling gastrointestinal haemorrhage, arteriography with digital subtraction is useful for diagnosis of UGIB provided blood loss is occurring at a rate of >1 ml/min. Transcatheter arterial embolisation may induce haemostasis in 90% of patients with co-morbid disease who have endoscopically uncontrolled massive bleeding from duodenal ulcer. Superselective embolisation with the use of coaxial catheter systems using microcoils alone, microcoils and polyvinyl alcohol particles and microcoils with gelatin sponge particles is safe.

PYLORIC STENOSIS

Presentation and management

Patients may present with a long history of peptic ulcer disease, a succussion splash on examination with or without evidence of hypokalaemic alkalosis. Proton pump inhibition preceded by endoscopic gastric drainage is effective for relief of symptoms attributable to peptic pyloric stenosis, obviating the need for surgery or balloon dilatation. Nevertheless, gastric emptying studies for solids and liquids remain prolonged in almost half the patients. Balloon dilatation and sustained acid reduction therapy was recommended as first-line treatment of pyloroduodenal strictures, because the procedure is safe and is likely to be successful in half the patients in whom dilatation is technically possible. More than 25% of patients, however, require multiple sessions for dilatation and perforation is a well-recognised complication.

One of the surgical procedures proposed is laparoscopic truncal vagotomy with endoscopic pyloric balloon dilatation but the efficacy of such an approach has not been validated prospectively. Open truncal vagotomy (TVG) and gastrojejunostomy for chronic duodenal ulcer has been reported to be complicated by dumping in 12%, which is troublesome in 4% of patients, occasional episodes of postvagotomy diarrhoea in 6% and bile vomiting in 17%. Laparoscopic TVG is feasible treatment for pyloric stenosis. Alternatively, on completion of laparoscopic truncal vagotomy, a gastrojejunostomy may be fashioned expeditiously by minilaparotomy, 4–5 cm incision.

Fifty percent of patients with stenosis are infected with Hp and resolution of outlet obstruction after Hp eradication has been reported. Gastric outlet obstruction may be associated with a large inflammatory mass surrounding a contained microperforation.

> **Box 4.11** Procedures for pyloric stenosis
> - Balloon dilatation
> - Truncal vagotomy and pyloroplasty/gastrojejunostomy
> - Truncal vagotomy and antrectomy
> - Polya (Billroth II) gastrectomy

PERFORATION

Aetiology

The role of *Helicobacter pylori* infection in the aetiology of peptic ulcer perforation remains controversial.

A small clinical series of patients has been reported with duodenal ulcer perforation in whom, despite the presence of gastritis, *H. pylori* infection could not be confirmed on RUT, biopsy and histological examination of antral pouch biopsies and culture, implying that duodenal ulcer patients with Hp-negative status may have a greater predilection for perforation.

In contrast, persistence of ulceration six weeks following patch repair has been found to be associated with *H. pylori* infection, suggesting that eradication therapy should be given to all patients with ulcer perforation.

Whether eradication of Hp can alleviate the strong ulcer diathesis in patients with non-NSAID related peptic ulcer is unknown. In Istanbul, *H. pylori* was found in antral biopsies of 88% of patients with perforated duodenal ulcers, the organisms being present in the mucosa and also extending through the wall of the ulcer. Hp was present in antral biopsies of all patients with the organism in the wall of the ulcer. On immunohistochemical screening, Hp infection was more prevalent in perforated ulcer (92%) than in bleeding peptic ulcer (55%) or stenotic ulcer (45%), perforated ulcer being associated with significantly more Hp infection and changes of gastritis. A close relationship was observed between perforated ulcer and the density of the Hp infection determined semi-quantitatively using immunohistochemical stains. Patients with perforated ulcers are a heterogeneous group with recurrent ulcer disease, a majority having Hp infection. No significant difference in cytotoxin genes cagA and vacA was demonstrable between patients with ulcer perforation and age- and gender-matched patients with peptic ulcer in whom surgery was not required.

In Hong Kong 70% of 73 patients with perforated duodenal ulcer had evidence of *H. pylori* infection on intraoperative gastroscopy and antral biopsy, 80% if NSAID usage was excluded. Of interest, the Hp infection group was significantly younger, with a male preponderance, and had significantly less NSAID consumption and more prolonged dyspepsia than Hp-negative patients. Hp infection probably does play an important role in perforation of non-NSAID related duodenal ulcer.

Granulocytes, particularly eosinophils, have been reported in the granulation tissue of perforated gastric ulcers in Japan. The extracellular matrix of the stomach wall consists mainly of collagen types I and III which are selectively degenerated by matrix metalloproteinase-1 (MMP-1). MMP-1 RNA has been detected in the cytoplasm of the infiltrating eosinophils, raising the possibility that these may play an important role in ulcer recurrence after gastric perforation. The degree of eosinophil infiltration may be a marker for perforation risk. The control of MMP gene expression represents a potential strategy for the treatment of recurrent gastric ulcer.

Concomitant NSAID, smoking and alcohol usage is a pervasive association. Recent data have suggested that acid suppression therapy may be useful in prevention of ulceration in patients taking NSAIDs. Elderly patients using two or more NSAIDs should be considered at risk for ulcer development and treated prophylactically with ulcer-healing drugs. NSAID drug usage and ulcer complications may become epidemic. Selective COX II inhibitors or NO-NSAIDs that incorporate a nitroxybutyl moiety may prove to be efficacious at lower risk. Future introduction of new NSAIDs may not have a major effect on decreasing gastrointestinal complications because 'over the counter' purchase of aspirin is so widespread.

Box 4.12   Smoking decreases:

- gastric mucosal blood flow
- gastric mucus secretion
- gastric prostaglandin production
- salivary epidermal growth factor secretion
- duodenal mucosal bicarbonate secretion
- pancreatic bicarbonate secretion

Smokers are more likely to develop ulcers, ulcers in smokers are more difficult to heal as smoking impairs the therapeutic effects of H_2 receptor antagonists, and ulcer relapse is more likely in smokers. Smoking thus plays a significant facilitative role in the development and maintenance of peptic ulcer disease. It is a major cause of ulcer perforation in patients <75 years. Cigarette smoking did not increase the recurrence rate of peptic ulceration after eradication of Hp.

An ischaemic process has been postulated as the cause of a temporal association between crack cocaine use and duodenal ulcer perforation which is well documented. An acid-reducing procedure is therefore not recommended and omental patch repair alone is considered appropriate.

Spontaneous gastroduodenal perforation is a rare and lethal complication in cancer patients receiving chemotherapy. Unfortunately, the diagnosis is often delayed for 3–4 days, leading to a high mortality rate.

Presentation

Postbulbar duodenal ulcer complicated by intramural perforation and abscess formation has been described and this may carry a high mortality because of delay in diagnosis and treatment secondary to a lack of peritoneal signs. Liver and pancreatic penetration by peptic ulcer are well-recognised complications with gastrobronchial fistula a rarity. Occasionally, the patient presents with chest pain mimicking myocardial ischaemia. ECG findings include T wave inversion in leads V2–4 which return to normal after surgery.

Radiographic or sonographic air which can be detected in up to 92% of patients with perforated peptic ulcer lacks specificity. Small amounts of gas, <1 ml, can be detected by careful positioning of the patient and taking a chest radiograph when the patient has been upright for 15 minutes. Supine and lateral decubitus films are also of value. In the absence of free gas, air may be instilled via a nasogastric tube and the radiograph repeated. For some patients whose symptoms are settling on presentation and in whom conservative treatment is being considered, a water-soluble contrast gastroduodenogram is recommended to exclude free extravasation of contrast widely into the peritoneal cavity, in which case surgery is indicated. Barium usage is avoided as it may occasionally cause barium peritonitis if free leakage is present. Direct sonographic documentation of a perforation tract within the anterior wall of the gastric antrum has been described. Isolated thickening of the duodenal wall with an echogenic line within are considered features of duodenal ulcer; extension of the line beyond the duodenal wall and periduodenal fluid indicate perforation. In perforated peptic ulcer, contrast-enhanced thin-section spiral CT shows wall thickening and enhancement and inflammatory change in perigastroduodenal soft tissues or organs. Discontinuity of the gastroduodenal wall and/or tiny air bubbles in the proximity may indicate the site of perforation. Retroperitoneal perforation of duodenal ulcer is rare, diagnostic difficulties leading to an increased risk of a fatal outcome; presentation with scrotal sepsis also being reported.

As many as half the patients with perforated duodenal ulcer may have securely sealed spontaneously at the time of presentation. This has led to proposed management strategies which incorporate an initial period of conservative management and subsequent assessment in the expectation that surgery may be avoided in many patients. Conservative management without resorting to surgery has been shown in a randomised trial to carry a mortality rate comparable with simple closure, although the duration of hospital stay was greater in the non-operated group. If abdominal signs do not improve within six hours of first assessment or admission, surgery is recommended. Non-operative management is, however, controversial but is indicated for perforation that is believed to have sealed spontaneously at time of presentation. In a recent study of a non-operative approach, adherence to certain protocol guidelines was poor, notably those concerned with prevention of thromboembolism, use of antibiotics, use of contrast examination for diagnostic confirmation and referral for follow-up endoscopy. Perforation may be due to malignant gastric ulceration and the study highlighted the need for accurate diagnosis and the importance of follow-up endoscopy. Non-operative management is associated with a greater likelihood of intraabdominal abscess formation and a protracted hospital stay of about 14 days if drainage for five days is required. Drainage may prove to be inadequate, catheters rupture or become blocked, requiring multiple attempts at image-guided drainage or surgical intervention.

Risk factors for mortality

Attention to pre- and intraoperative resuscitation has been regarded as the single most effective therapy for reducing morbidity and mortality from perforation. The nature of surgery advocated for peptic ulcer perforation has evolved in recent years. Previous reports highlighted the superior results obtained when definitive acid-reducing procedures were performed at the time of omental patch repair when compared with patch repair alone. Emergency surgery with proximal gastric vagotomy as definitive treatment of perforated duodenal ulcer can be undertaken safely with minimal morbidity and without mortality in selected good-risk patients; ulcer recurrence rate in Hong Kong at three years follow-up after open PGV was 10.6%. Nevertheless, the knowledge that Hp infection may well have a significant aetiological role in peptic ulcer perforation has led to the view that omental patch repair alone is generally all that is required. Exceptions include the previously investigated patient who is known to be Hp negative on repeated testing and the repeated failure of eradication therapy due to poor compliance or antibiotic resistance. Acute gastric surgery carries high inpatient morbidity and a significant risk to life, particularly in the elderly. A minimalist approach as to the nature of the surgical procedure to be performed is now well supported.

Overall mortality for ulcer perforation is about 5%, being worse in patients >50 years and when the leukcocyte count is 9.5×10^6, when treatment is delayed more than 12 hours after perforation and when there is preoperative shock and renal failure, liver cirrhosis or immunosuppression. Tolerance to time delay is inversely proportional to age with fatality in patients <65 years being related to co-existent illness. Treatment delay of 24 hours for perforated peptic ulcer has been shown to be accompanied by a sevenfold increase in mortality rate, a threefold increase in morbidity and a doubling of the length of hospital stay when compared with treatment delay of <6 hours. Every effort needs to be made to perform surgery within 12 hours of perforation but this may not be achievable if a trial period of conservative therapy for spontaneous healing is advocated. Delay in diagnosis does result in increased mortality. Risk factors for mortality include concomitant illness, septicaemia and intraabdominal abscess. Reperforation after surgery for ulcer perforation carries a high mortality. Leakage from the same or another site is multifactorial in origin and reperforation is associated with co-existing malignancy, immunosuppression and preoperative shock.

Post-operative mortality is directly related to the number of risk factors present: 0%, 10%, 45% and 100% in patients with none, one, two and three of the risk factors (Box 4.13). Major medical illnesses and shock each conferred approximately three times the risk of mortality when compared with delay in surgery beyond 24 hours of perforation. Patients occasionally present in a moribund condition and pose a therapeutic dilemma; poor results may be anticipated regardless of non-operative management or operation intervention. Because the risk of serious ulcer recurrence with complicated disease is low (14%), it was concluded in a Swedish study that simple closure is adequate surgical treatment in the elderly.

Box 4.13 Risk factors for mortality after perforated peptic ulcer surgery

- Co-morbid illness
- Shock on presentation (<100 mmHg)
- Delay in operation >24 hours from time of perforation

Surgery (Table 4.4)

Taking abdominal complaints as the endpoint for future duodenal ulcer treatment, PGV performed on an elective or emergency basis is regarded as giving results superior to therapy with H_2 receptor antagonists and produces an almost identical level of complaints to that seen in the community. Definitive surgery at the time of perforation has been criticised in that some patients who might not develop recurrent ulcer are being placed at risk of adverse post-operative sequelae or death if acid-reducing surgery is performed.

Simple suturing of small ulcers has been recommended but, in an experimental study in rats, greater antiinflammatory and angiogenic activity and accelerated collagen synthesis were seen with patch repair when compared with simple suture closure. Basic fibroblast growth factor (bFGF) – mediated angiogenesis was noted, as well as transforming growth factor beta 1 (TGF-β1) activity within and around the omentum, resulting in abundant collagen production.

A variety of techniques have been described for closure of duodenal perforation, including ligamentum teres or omental patching/plugging and fibrin glue application. Sutureless repair with glue has been shown to be as safe as sutured patch repair and takes less

---

Table 4.4 Emergency procedures for perforated peptic ulcer	Duodenal ulcer	Gastric ulcer
Patch/plug repair		
omentum	+	+
ligamentum teres	+	+
Truncal vagotomy and pyloroplasty with or without ulcer excision	+	–
Truncal vagotomy and antrectomy	+	–
Proximal gastric vagotomy plus omental patch/plug	+	–
Billroth I gastrectomy	–	+
Polya (Billroth II) gastrectomy	+	–

time to perform. These may be accomplished in conventional open procedures or with a laparoscopic approach. Most popular is omental patch repair (omentopexy) and this is regarded as appropriate for perforations <2 cm in size (Figure 4.3). Larger perforations are believed to carry a risk of reperforation if patch repair is performed and some form of pyloroplasty or excisional surgery with gastric resection, with or without vagotomy, is preferred.

Peripatch leakage occurs in 5% of patients undergoing laparoscopic patch repair and poses a significant threat to life. Laparoscopic closure may be accomplished by an omental patch secured with sutures held by PDS clips or staples. Ligamentum teres repair with basket snare at upper endoscopy of the ligament pedicled at laparoscopy has been described. Similarly, endoscopic traction omental patch repair with duodenal suturing is also feasible. The duration of the laparoscopic procedure has now been reduced to <30 minutes with the aid of staples or fibrin glue plugging of the perforation site. Laparoscopic repair is associated with decreased postoperative pain but the procedure itself takes longer than open surgery and a number of studies have failed to show any significant difference between the two approaches in terms of hospital stay and return to normal activities. The major determinant of speed of recovery is likely to be the extent of peritoneal contamination and whether this gives rise to paralytic ileus.

Simple closure is safe even in relatively inexperienced hands but carries the disadvantage that, in the absence of anti-ulcer therapy, recurrence is a major cause of morbidity in patients with acute or chronic duodenal ulceration. Omentopexy alone is indicated for acute duodenal ulcer associated with drug ingestion or acute stress simple closure of stomal ulcer perforation is advisable in the high risk patient. A large perforation can be dealt with by suturing an intact seromuscular layer of jejunum to cover the defect or, in the good-risk patient, by resection of the stoma, part of the gastric remnant and refashioning of the gastrojejunostomy, with or without the addition of vagotomy.

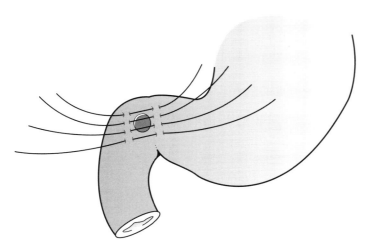

Figure 4.3 Suture placement prior to tying over an omental patch to close perforation.

Many surgeons previously held the view that definitive operation, with the prospect of lower ulcer recurrence rates, was the gold standard in the treatment of perforated duodenal ulcer but current opinion generally is that patch repair alone followed by detection and eradication of Hp infection is the preferred option for acute and chronic ulcers. If definitive surgery is believed to be advisable for duodenal ulcer, then a laparoscopic approach can also be employed for omental patch closure followed by laparoscopic proximal gastric vagotomy or posterior truncal vagotomy with anterior proximal gastric vagotomy (Hill-Barker) or seromyotomy (Taylor).

Perforated gastric ulcers may be excised or simply closed if the patient's condition does not favour Billroth I resection, closure being safe and effective in a majority. Frozen section of an excised ulcer or biopsy from the edge of the defect prior to closure is recommended. Gastrectomy has been advocated when there is a history of chronicity or when the nature of the ulcer, or associated ulcer haemorrhage, preclude safe, simple closure.

Laparoscopic surgery with CO_2 insufflation is not advocated in patients with delayed presentation and marked peritoneal contamination. The presence of peritonitis has previously been considered to be a contraindication to the laparoscopic approach because of the theoretical risk of malignant hypercapnia and toxic shock syndrome. Endotoxaemia is insignificant in most patients with perforated peptic ulcer. In patients with perforated peptic ulcer, laparoscopic patch repair does not reduce acute stress responses when compared with open surgery. Haemodynamic changes during laparoscopy are well recognised and may have an adverse effect in patients who have peritonitis, are hypovolaemic or even septic. Although postoperative septic shock occurs infrequently, it may prove lethal. Evidence from experimental work suggests that capnoperitoneum may aggravate peritonitis and induce septic shock due to increased intraabdominal pressure and distension of the peritoneum. Gasless laparoscopic treatment of perforated duodenal ulcer has been reported and may obviate such problems. The gasless technique enables continuous suction of fluid, blood, smoke and humidity without loss of camera view.

The use of abdominal drains at patch repair has now largely been abandoned. There was no difference in a randomised trial in the incidence or duration of postoperative pyrexia, return of bowel function or length of hospital stay, regardless of the presence or absence of drains. Routine use of drains was not effective in preventing postoperative fluid collections nor in decreasing the incidence of intraabdominal abscess. Migration of bacteria from the exterior via drains has been demonstrated as well as intestinal obstruction caused by drains.

H. pylori and recurrence of ulceration

H. pylori may not fully account for ulcer recurrence after peptic ulcer surgery. It has been suggested that *H. pylori* colonisation after vagotomy may promote the development of residual ulcer only in patients with incomplete vagotomy. *H. pylori* infection is frequently seen in the gastric remnant after operation for peptic ulcer disease but it does not appear to cause ulcer relapse in the gastric stump or at the anastomosis. In patients with ulcer recurrence after surgery, Hp infection was documented in only 42% who had undergone gastrectomy and 67% in whom vagotomy had been performed, the prevalence of Hp infection not differing between patients with or without ulcer recurrence. It is noteworthy, however, that the RUT is not sensitive for detecting *H. pylori* after acid reduction surgery. In a larger study, recurrent duodenal ulcer (18%) following surgery for perforated duodenal ulcer has been found to be correlated with positive Hp status. Following acid-reducing surgery, high-density Hp colonisation in the gastric antrum and corpus may only actually promote recurrence if vagotomy is incomplete. With constant aspirin abuse, recurrent ulceration is the rule and complications, especially stenosis, are common.

FURTHER READING

Branicki FJ. Perforated peptic ulcer. In: Jamieson G, Debas HT, eds. *Rob & Smith's Operative Surgery. Surgery of the Gastrointestinal Tract*, 5th edn. London: Chapman and Hall Medical: 530–536

Branicki FJ, Nathanson LK. Billroth II Gastrectomy. In: Nylus LM, Baker RJ, Fischer JE, eds. *Mastery of Surgery*, 3rd edn. 1997; 1:858–872. Boston: Little, Brown: 858–872

Branicki FJ, Ting ACW, Gertsch P et al. Bleeding peptic ulcer: an evolving role for surgical intervention. *J Gastroenterol Hepatol* 1998; 13(suppl):S227–S231

Chan VM, Reznick RK, O'Rourke K, Kitchens JM, Lossing AG, Detsky AS. Meta-analysis of highly selective vagotomy versus truncal vagotomy and pyloroplasty in the surgical treatment of uncomplicated duodenal ulcer. *Can J Surg* 1994; 37(6):457–464

Cook DJ, Guyatt GH, Salena BJ, Laine LA. Endoscopic therapy for acute non-variceal upper gastrointestinal haemorrhage: a meta-analysis. *Gastroenterology* 1992; 102(1):139–148

Dallemagne B, Weerts JM, Jehaes C, Markiewicz S, Lombard R. Laparoscopic highly selective vagotomy. *Br J Surg* 1994; 81(4):554–556

Forrest JAH, Finlayson Shearman DJC. Endoscopy in gastrointestinal bleeding. *Lancet* 1974; 2: 394–397

Hewitt PM, Krige JE, Funnell IC, Wilson C, Bornman PC. Endoscopic balloon dilatation of peptic pyloroduodenal strictures. *J Clin Gastroenterol* 1999; 28(1):33–35

Lau WY, Leung KL, Kwong KH et al. A randomized study comparing laparoscopic versus open repair of perforated peptic ulcer using suture or sutureless technique. *Ann Surg* 1996; 224(2):131–138

Leung JW, Lee JG. Non variceal upper gastrointestinal bleeding. *Gastrointest Endosc Clin North Am* 1997; 7(4):545–745

Longstreth GF, Feitelberg SP. Successful outpatient management of acute upper gastrointestinal haemorrhage: use of practice guidelines in a large patient series. *Gastrointest Endosc* 1998; 47(3):219–222

Poxon VA, Keighley MRB, Dykes PW, Heppinstall K, Jaderberg M. Comparison of minimal and conventional surgery in patients with bleeding peptic ulcer: a multicentre trial. *Br J Surg* 1991; 70:1344–1345

Rockall TA, Logan RFA, Devlin HB, Northfield TC. Selection of patients for early discharge or outpatient care after acute upper gastrointestinal haemorrhage. *Lancet* 1996; 347: 1138–1140

Rutgeerts P, Rauws E, Wara P et al. Randomized trial of single and repeated fibrin glue compared with injection of polidocanol in treatment of bleeding peptic ulcer. *Lancet* 1997; 350(9079):692–696

Saeed ZA, Ramirez FC, Hepps KS, Cole RA, Graham DY. Prospective validation of the Baylor Bleeding Score for predicting the likelihood of rebleeding after endoscopic hemostasis of peptic ulcers. *Gastrointest Endosc* 1995; 41(6):561–565

Sebastian M, Chandran VP, Elashaal YI, Sim AJ. Helicobacter pylori infection in perforated peptic ulcer disease. *Br J Surg* 1995; 82(3):360–362

Svanes C, Lie RT, Svanes K, Lie SA, Soreide O. Adverse effects of delayed treatment for perforated peptic ulcer. *Ann Surg* 1994; 220(2):168–175

Terdiman JP. Update on upper gastrointestinal bleeding. *Postgrad Med* 1998; 103(6):43–64

Wakayama T, Ishizaki Y, Mitsusada M et al. Risk factors influencing the short-term results of gastroduodenal perforation. *Surg Today* 1994; 24(8):681–687

Wyman A, Stuart RC, Ng EK, Chung SC, Li AK. Laparoscopic truncal vagotomy and gastroenterostomy for pyloric stenosis. *Am J Surg* 1996; 171(6):600–603

5

Gastric cancer

Mitsuru Sasako, Bruce Mann

Gastric cancer remains one of the most important malignancies throughout the world, with approximately 750 000 cases per year. Until the early part of the 20th century it was among the most common malignancies in Western countries. There has been a remarkable reduction in its incidence so that it has lost prominence in the West but it remains a major health issue in places including Japan, Korea and much of South and Central America.

Most gastric malignancies are adenocarcinomas. The next most common neoplasms are lymphomas, followed by gastrointestinal stromal tumours.

ADENOCARCINOMA

Epidemiology

The incidence of gastric cancer ranges from 6 cases/100 000 people/year in Caucasians in the USA to about 70 cases/100 000 people/year in North Eastern Japan. In all areas, the incidence in males is about twice that in females. It is more common in socio-economically deprived communities. Over the last 50 years, there has been a significant decline in the incidence worldwide, which has been confined to the intestinal type of carcinoma. The incidence of diffuse-type gastric cancer has remained constant or even increased. The net effect of this has been a shift in the type of gastric cancer from distal intestinal type to proximal diffuse type in many Western societies. The epidemiology of gastric cancer in Japanese communities in North America suggests strong environmental influences, as the frequency approaches that of white Americans in second-generation Japanese Americans.

Aetiology

The aetiology of gastric cancer has been partially elucidated. More is known about the cause of intestinal type cancer than is known about diffuse cancer.

- Infection with *Helicobacter pylori* is associated with gastric carcinoma. Populations at high risk of developing gastric cancer tend to have a high incidence of *H. pylori* infection and the infection tends to occur at a younger age. The risk of carcinoma is associated with infection with more virulent strains of *H. pylori* – cagA +ve strains. Inflammation and production of nitrosourea by this bacteria may induce cell proliferation, which might increase the chance of genetic changes.

- Smoking increases the risk, while alcohol does not have any effect.

- Dietary factors are also important. Diets high in salt and low in fresh fruit and vegetables have been linked to a high risk of gastric cancer.

- Gastric atrophy is common in areas with a high incidence of gastric cancer. Intestinal metaplasia, especially of the incomplete type, is also a high-risk lesion.

There is not yet an agreed unified theory to tie all these aetiological factors together. It is hypothesised that infection with *H. pylori* causes the chronic gastritis that eventually leads to gastric atrophy and a susceptibility to gastric cancer. High salt diets may promote the development of cancer, while diets high in fruit and vegetables may be protective. Such a theory is consistent with most of the current knowledge, but it is not proven. Little is known about the aetiology of proximal gastric cancer or the cause of the recent increase in the disease. *H. pylori* does not appear to be involved.

There are some premalignant conditions. Adenomatous gastric polyps, Menetriere's disease, pernicious anaemia and partial gastrectomy for benign disease more than 15 years ago are all associated with an increased risk of gastric adenocarcinoma.

Pathology

There are a number of classification systems for gastric adenocarcinomas. Borrmann's types 1–4 refer to macroscopic types polypoid/fungating, ulcerating with raised borders, ulcerating infiltrative and diffusely infiltrative types respectively. In the Japanese classification, Borrmann types 1–4 correspond to types 1–4 and those not classifiable are classified as type 5.

There are several classifications for histological types of gastric cancers: WHO classification, Lauren's classification, Ming's classification and Japanese classification. The most widely used system is the histological system of Lauren, with two broad categories of intestinal and diffuse. Some cancers show a mixed pattern. This classification is useful because it divides the disease into two groups with significantly different pathology, aetiology, epidemiology and prognosis. The male predominance is limited to the intestinal type of cancer and it is the main type in high-incidence countries such as Japan and Korea. There is a trend for distal tumours to be of the intestinal type and for proximal cancers to be diffuse. Intestinal cancers show glandular formation, while diffuse gastric cancer has a tendency to spread in the submucosal plane and malignant cells are often found many centimetres from the macroscopic edge of the tumour. In cases where this phenomenon is extreme, the whole stomach may be affected and take on a 'leather bottle' appearance – so called 'linitis plastica'. The other three classifications are similar to each other.

Gastric cancer is initially confined to the stomach. The duration of this phase is uncertain but Japanese data from screening programmes suggest that significant progression often occurs over 1–2 years. On the other hand, it is known that some well-differentiated intestinal-type cancers can remain localised for more than five years. It can spread directly into adjacent organs, including the oesophagus, duodenum, transverse colon, spleen, pancreas and liver. The other form of local spread is via the lymphatics (Table 5.1) to the perigastric lymph nodes and then to the para-aortic lymph nodes. Once the serosa is breached there is a high incidence of direct spread across the peritoneal cavity. It also spreads via the bloodstream, initially to the liver.

Table 5.1 Lymph node metastasis, spread according to the tumour depth (Data from 4485 pts surgically treated 1972–91 at NCCH (including incurable cases))

Depth		Number of pts	Lymph node (%)	Liver (%)	Peritoneum (%)
T1	M	1065	3.4	0	0
	SM	895	17.4	0.1	0
T2	MP	439	46.2	1.1	0.2
	SS	333	63.4	3.3	2.1
T3	SE	1187	79.5	5.5	14.7
T4	SI	566	89.8	11.7	33.7

Staging

The two main staging systems for gastric cancer are the TNM system (Table 5.2) and the Japanese Research Society for Gastric Cancer system. Recently the two staging systems have been revised to facilitate comparison between them. In the West, the TNM system is favoured. T staging relates to the depth of penetration of the gastric wall. T1 cancers are confined to the mucosa or submucosa, T2 tumours penetrate the muscularis, but do not breach the serosa. T3 means through the serosa, but not involving adjacent structures. T4 cancers are locally advanced, directly invading structures such as the liver or pancreas. The Japanese system is similar but subdivides T1 tumours into T1m (mucosal) and T1sm (submucosal) and divides T2 into T2mp (muscularis propria) and T2ss (subserosal).

'Early gastric cancer' (EGC) is the term given to T1 cancer, irrespective of the state of the lymph nodes. Early gastric cancers are subdivided according to the macroscopic appearance into protruded (type I), superficially elevated (IIa), flat (IIb), superficially depressed (IIc) and excavated (III). Many EGCs show a mixture of macroscopic types.

The N staging in the TNM system relates to the number of lymph nodes involved. It is important to note that in order to be accurately N-staged, at least 15 nodes must be examined. The Japanese system of N staging relates to the position of the involved lymph nodes. This is based on the belief that there are first-order and second-order nodes that are involved in gastric cancer sequentially. Involvement of second-order nodes is therefore much more prognostically significant. Recent analysis of results from large European and Japanese series have found that the TNM N staging provides more prognostic information. Japanese surgeons will continue to use the Japanese system because it ties in with the extent of lymph node dissection commonly practised there.

Clinical presentation

Early gastric cancer may be asymptomatic, but often presents with dyspepsia. It may be indistinguishable from benign causes of dyspepsia and the pain will usually respond at least initially to treatment with antacids or acid-suppressing medication. There may be accompanying anaemia from chronic blood loss. Loss of weight is not a feature of early gastric cancer. The main challenge is to identify those patients with dyspepsia who require investigation to exclude gastric cancer. Any patient over 45 years of age who develops new or different dyspepsia that lasts for more than two weeks should be investigated with a gastroscopy specifically searching for early gastric cancer. Japanese data show that many patients with EGC have symptoms. Out of 170 patients treated for EGC by surgery at NCCH in 1996, 75 (47%) had symptoms, such as epigastric discomfort (26 cases), pain (48 cases) and vomiting (one case); 36% of these patients were diagnosed outside a screening programme.

Table 5.2 TNM staging for gastric cancer

Definitions

Primary tumour
T1	Invades mucosa or submucosa
T2	Invades muscularis propria or subserosa
T3	Penetrates serosa without invasion of adjacent structures (excluding oesophagus or duodenum)
T4	Invades adjacent structures

Regional lymph nodes
N0	No regional nodal metastases
N1	Metastases in 1–6 regional nodes
N2	Metastases in 7–15 regional nodes
N3	Metastases in >15 regional nodes

Distant metastases
M0	No distant metastases
M1	Distant metastases

Stage Grouping

Stage	Criteria		
IA	T1	N0	M0
IB	T1	N1	M0
	T2	N0	M0
II	T1	N2	M0
	T2	N1	M0
	T3	N0	M0
IIIA	T2	N2	M0
	T3	N1	M0
	T4	N0	M0
IIIB	T3	N2	M0
IV	T4	N1, N2, N3	M0
	T1, T2, T3	N3	M0
	Any T	Any N	M1

With more advanced cancer, weight loss becomes a feature. Pain is often more severe and constant. It may be exacerbated by food and relieved by vomiting. The classic presentation of a patient with gastric cancer is that of a person with epigastric pain, nausea, anorexia and loss of weight. On examination the patient may be anaemic, with a palpable epigastric mass or an irregular enlarged liver. Troisier and Virchow described the finding of an enlarged left supraclavicular lymph node in metastatic gastric cancer. There may also be ascites and on rectal examination tumour may be present in the pelvis – Blumer's shelf. This picture is a description of a patient with advanced, incurable gastric cancer. Unfortunately many patients present with these features of metastatic disease.

Some distal gastric cancers present with acute complications of gastric outlet obstruction, while proximal cancers can lead to dysphagia. About 10–15% of gastric cancer patients have haematemesis and/or melaena.

Investigations

Blood tests

A full blood examination, serum electrolytes and liver function tests should be checked. The most common abnormalities are microcytic anaemia due to chronic blood loss, and abnormal liver function due to hepatic metastases. In some cases, the serum level of BUN is outside the normal range due to constant GI bleeding. In gastric outlet obstruction, there may be hypochloraemic alkalosis due to vomiting.

Upper GI endoscopy

Upper gastrointestinal endoscopy is the investigation of choice to diagnose or exclude gastric cancer. Some early gastric cancers are very subtle and so particular care needs to be taken to carefully examine the entire gastric mucosa, with biopsy of any suspicious areas. In addition, the mucosal abnormalities may be mild in extensive linitis plastica, where the tumour cells are primarily in the submucosal plane. Such a stomach does not distend normally. Barium contrast studies have been largely superseded in Western countries by endoscopy. They are still used routinely in Japan, both as part of mass screening and as part of preoperative assessment, especially to detect wall rigidity spreading over the area of a mucosal abnormality.

Endoscopic ultrasound (EUS)

EUS is complementary to upper GI endoscopy and CT scanning. The normal stomach wall has five distinct layers. EUS with a high-frequency (7.5–12 MHz) transducer is quite accurate at assessing the T stage. Its sensitivity for detecting nodal metastases is better than that of CT but it still cannot reliably exclude nodal disease, because more than 38% of lymph nodes containing metastatic gastric cancer are 5 mm or less in size. In gastric cancer the information available from EUS is most useful regarding the spread in submucosal or deeper layers. Thickening of the gastric wall implies tumour extension.

Computed tomography

CT scanning is important for excluding hepatic metastases and also in showing gross nodal involvement. CT scanning is poor at assessing the primary tumour and frequently fails to show small-volume peritoneal and hepatic disease.

Laparoscopy

Laparoscopy is becoming established as an essential part of the preoperative staging of gastric cancer. It is very sensitive for the detection of small-volume hepatic or peritoneal disease, especially if combined with laparoscopic ultrasound. As the survival of these patients is not improved by a palliative resection of the primary tumour, they can be spared the pain and potential morbidity and mortality of an open operation. Laparoscopic peritoneal lavage cytology may identify patients at high risk for peritoneal relapse. All of this may be important in the future in modifying treatment.

Serum markers

CEA and CA 19–9 are often elevated in patients with gastric carcinoma, but are of little importance in routine clinical use.

Screening

In Japan there are mass screening programmes for early gastric cancer. They use either double-contrast barium radiology or serum pepsinogen isoenzyme test to screen people over the age of 40. Approximately 15% of all Japanese over the age of 40 undergo this screening annually. This has resulted in a major increase in the proportion of EGC, such that almost 50% of all gastric cancers diagnosed in Japan are EGC, and a fall in the mortality rate. Screening is not cost effective in low-incidence countries.

Clinical management

Diagnosis and staging

Once a gastric cancer is suspected, the diagnosis must be confirmed via a gastroscopy and biopsy. The only potentially curative treatment is surgery and so preoperative investigations are directed at establishing whether or not the patient is potentially curable and on determining whether the patient's medical condition is optimised prior to surgery. CT scanning is used to identify liver metastases or gross nodal disease or ascites. Increasingly laparoscopy is used to identify small-volume hepatic or peritoneal disease. If the cancer has distant metastasis or bulky local lymph node metastasis there is no survival advantage in removing the stomach. Patients with such disease can be spared the morbidity and potential mortality of a laparotomy by accurate preoperative staging. Patients with bulky nodal but no distant metastasis may be candidates for trials of neoadjuvant chemotherapy. In patients with major bleeding from the primary tumour or where there is actual or impending intestinal obstruction, palliative surgery is indicated.

Surgery

The appropriate operation for gastric cancer depends on the site, histological subtype and extent of the tumour. In general there should be a 2–3 cm macroscopic margin around an intestinal-type tumour showing a clear tumour border, and a 5–7 cm margin around a diffuse-type tumour. If possible, a distal gastrectomy is used. If the tumour is either proximally located or so extensive

that an adequate margin cannot be achieved with a distal gastrectomy, then a total gastrectomy is the preferred option.

The extent of lymph node dissection is a controversial issue. Traditionally, most Western surgeons have removed the stomach and those lymph nodes located in the fatty tissues along the greater and lesser curves. In contrast, Japanese surgeons have long believed that better results are possible if an extensive lymph node dissection is performed. They have performed meticulous studies mapping the pattern of nodal metastases from tumours arising in various parts of the stomach. Analysis of these results has led to a classification of lymph nodes as N1, N2 and N3 lymph nodes for tumours arising from the various parts of the stomach. In general, the N1 nodes are those adjacent to the greater and lesser curves of the stomach and those at the origin of the right gastric and right gastroepiploic arteries. N2 nodes are those around the left gastric common and, proper hepatic and splenic arteries and the coeliac axis and those at the splenic hilum, while N3 nodes are located in

Table 5.3 Lymph node groups (compartments 1–3) by location of tumour (reproduced with permission from *Gastric Cancer* 1998; **1**: 3)

Lymph node station	Location	LMU/MUL MLU/UML	LD/L	LM/M/ML	MU/UM	U	E+
No.1	rt pracardial	1	2	1	1	1	
No. 2	lt paracardial	1	M	3	1	1	
No. 3	lesser curvature	1	1	1	1	1	
No. 4sa	short gastric	1	M	3	1	1	
No. 4sb	lt gastroepiploic	1	3	1	1	1	
No. 4d	rt gastroepiploic	1	1	1	1	2	
No. 5	suprapyloric	1	1	1	1	3	
No. 6	infrapyloric	1	1	1	1	3	
No. 7	lt gastric artery	2	2	2	2	2	
No. 8a	ant comm hepatic	2	2	2	2	2	
No. 8p	post comm hepatic	3	3	3	3	3	
No. 9	celiac artery	2	2	2	2	2	
No. 10	splenic hilum	2	M	3	2	2	
No. 11p	proximal splenic	2	2	2	2	2	
No. 11d	distal splenic	2	M	3	2	2	
No. 12a	lt hepatoduodenal	2	2	2	2	3	
No. 12b,p	post hepatoduod	3	3	3	3	3	
No. 13	retropancreatic	3	3	3	M	M	
No. 14v	sup mesenteric v.	2	2	3	3	M	
No. 14a	sup mesenteric a.	M	M	M	M	M	
No. 15	middle colic	M	M	M	M	M	
No. 16a1	aortic hiatus	M	M	M	M	M	
No. 16a2,bl	paraaortic, middle	3	3	3	3	3	
No. 16b2	paraaortic, caudal	M	M	M	M	M	
No. 17	ant pancreatic	M	M	M	M	M	
No. 18	inf pancreatic	M	M	M	M	M	
No. 19	infradiaphragmatic	3	M	M	3	3	2
No. 20	esophageal hiatus	3	M	M	3	3	1
No. 110	lower paraesophag	M	M	M	M	M	3
No. 111	supradiaphragmatic	M	M	M	M	M	3
No. 112	post mediastinal	M	M	M	M	M	3

M: lymph nodes regarded as distant metastasis   E+: lymph node stations re-classified in cases of esophageal invasion

the retropancreatic area and in the para-aortic position. Operations to completely remove the N1, N2 and N3 lymph nodes are referred to as D1, D2 and D3 lymph node dissections respectively. Results of thousands of these operations clearly demonstrate that there are significant numbers of long-term survivors among patients who have definite metastatic disease in lymph nodes not usually removed in 'standard' gastrectomy (Table 5.3) (Figure 5.1).

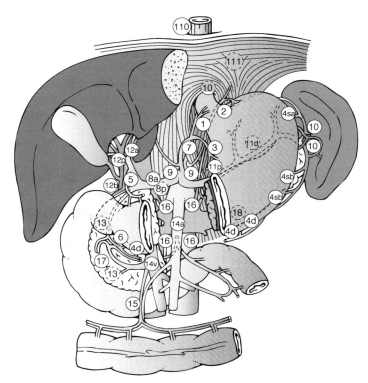

Figure 5.1 Lymph node station numbers.

Results of two randomised controlled trials comparing a D1 and D2 dissection in Western countries have not shown an overall advantage to the more extensive operation. Trials in the United Kingdom and the Netherlands found the D2 dissection to be associated with a higher operative morbidity and mortality. Overall there was no statistically significant survival advantage. In subset analysis, some groups of patients did appear to benefit from the bigger operation, but the conclusion is that a D2 dissection should not be the standard operation in the West. Most Japanese centres and many major Western centres will continue to perform D2 dissection, on the basis that they have shown they can do it safely, that there is certainly better prognostic information after a D2 and that some patients may gain a survival benefit.

In Japan, where EGC comprises up to half the gastric cancers diagnosed, a variety of conservative surgical options have been devised. For small intramucosal early gastric cancers that have virtually no chance of having lymph node metastases, endoscopic mucosal resection (EMR) is carried out using a wide-bore endoscope with operating channels. Saline is injected into the

submucosal plane and then the cancer is either snared, as for a polypectomy, or dissected from the submucosal plane. The specimen is carefully examined and if the margins are positive or if there is significant submucosal involvement (T1SM2), then open surgery is needed. Very good results have been reported but it is only suitable for very early differentiated intestinal cancers – unusual in the West. Laparoscopic wedge excision is also possible for the same type of early mucosal cancers of larger size.

Chemotherapy

Multiple drug chemotherapy is useful in the treatment of metastatic gastric cancer. The combination of 5-fluorouracil, adriamycin and mitomycin C or methotrexate has recently been replaced by the combination of epirubicin, cisplatin and 5-fluorouracil. The median survival of patients with irresectable gastric cancer is increased from about five months with supportive care to about nine months with chemotherapy.

There is no proven benefit from currently available chemotherapy given as an adjuvant, although metaanalysis of many trials has suggested a benefit. Available trials have tested a variety of combinations given after apparently curative surgery. As these have been negative, the next series of trials are investigating whether chemotherapy given before surgery will be more effective. There have been many examples of preoperative (induction) chemotherapy being effective in reducing the size of gastric cancers and making them more easily resectable, but there is no proof that this improves the long-term survival.

Intraperitoneal chemotherapy, either intraoperative or postoperative, is being investigated for its potential ability to reduce the incidence of intraperitoneal recurrences.

More recently there have been reports of a survival benefit from adjuvant chemoradiotherapy after 'curative' resection of gastric cancer. While this is a promising development, many questions remain to be answered before it becomes standard treatment.

Prognosis

Overall the survival rates from stomach cancer remain poor. In most countries, the reported five-year survival rate is between 10% and 20%. Japan is the striking exception, with reported five-year survival of around 70%.

The prognosis depends on the pathological type and stage. Diffuse gastric cancers and proximal cancers have a worse prognosis than intestinal-type and distal cancers. In particular, the number of lymph nodes involved and the depth of penetration of the gastric wall are critical. Once there are many nodes involved or the tumour penetrates the serosa (T3 tumours) the prognosis is poor. Interestingly, the prognosis of diffuse-type cancer is better than intestinal type if the tumour remains as T1 or T2.

Recurrence is common in gastric cancer and it usually occurs with 1–3 years of initial presentation. The common sites for recurrence are in the gastric bed (at the site of the surgery), in the liver and within the peritoneal cavity.

Treatment of recurrence is difficult and may not be effective. Surgical resection of metastases is rarely curative and surgery is largely reserved for management of bowel obstruction in a patient with a good performance status. Patients in whom metastatic disease is diagnosed should be considered for palliative chemotherapy.

LYMPHOMAS

Primary gastric lymphomas make up about 5% of gastric malignancies and most are non-Hodgkin's lymphomas. The symptoms are similar to those of gastric carcinoma, although bleeding and perforation are more common with lymphoma. Diagnosis is not usually suspected, but is found on biopsy of a mucosal lesion or ulcer.

Gastric mucosal associated lymphoid tissue (MALT) lymphomas are low-grade lymphomas that tend to remain localised to the stomach. The disease is associated with infection with *H. pylori* and the cells within gastric MALT lymphoma have been shown to proliferate in response to *H. pylori* antigens.

The appropriate treatment is controversial. Most high-grade lymphomas have been treated by surgery, followed by adjuvant chemotherapy. More and more they are treated with combination chemotherapy, either alone or with radiotherapy. Antibiotics to eradicate *H. pylori* are effective in treating MALT lymphoma and the first step of the treatment for this disease. Non-responders are treated either by radiotherapy or surgery. Surgery is sometimes required for life-threatening complications of haemorrhage or perforation during chemotherapy.

SOFT TISSUE TUMOURS

Benign and malignant soft tissue tumours are occasionally found in the stomach. They are known as gastrointestinal stromal tumours (GIST). Tumours less than 5 cm in size may have potential to metastasise but rarely have metastases at the time of initial treatment. Malignant tumours can spread and recur in the liver or the peritoneal cavity. Lymph node metastasis occurs in 10–20% of cases when the tumour is large. Tumours showing lymph node metastases have never been treated successfully, so lymph node dissection is abandoned for this disease. These tumours may present when small if the overlying mucosa ulcerates and causes haematemesis and/or melaena. At gastroscopy there is a characteristic appearance of a submucosal lesion protruding into the stomach, with ulceration of the overlying mucosa and so-called 'bridging folds'. Malignant lesions that do not bleed tend to be diagnosed late, with non-specific symptoms of vague abdominal pain and early satiety. Wedge excision is adequate for small tumours, while a gastrectomy may be needed for larger tumours. Lymph node dissection is not a part of the treatment. Recently Imatinib Mesilate has been proven effective to this disease.

OPERATIVE SURGERY

Principles of surgical resection for gastric neoplasms

For gastric carcinoma the definitive procedure is the complete removal of the primary tumour with sufficient surgical margins and an adequate lymph node dissection.

For interstitial tumours, such as leiomyosarcoma, a partial resection of the stomach ensuring histologically clear margins is adequate.

For gastric lymphoma, a 'routine' total gastrectomy ('*de principe*') with D1 or D2 dissection has been the treatment of choice. Combined chemoradiotherapy alone is being evaluated in phase II and III trials as an alternative to surgery followed by adjuvant chemotherapy.

Distal gastrectomy with D2 lymph node dissection

Indication

For a distally located carcinoma, a distal two-thirds gastrectomy or distal subtotal gastrectomy with D2 lymph node dissection is the procedure of choice in Japan and many Western centres.

Technique

The procedure begins with a laparoscopy or laparotomy to confirm that curative resection is possible. As part of the laparotomy, the duodenum is mobilised and the para-aortic area exposed and examined for nodal metastases. Suspicious nodes are submitted for frozen section. If there are hepatic or peritoneal metastases or grossly involved para-aortic lymph nodes, there is no survival benefit to extended lymph node dissection, although resection of the primary tumour may be necessary for palliation. If there are involved para-aortic lymph nodes without peritoneal or hepatic metastasis, neoadjuvant chemotherapy is recommended.

The gastrectomy starts with dissection of the greater omentum from right to left as far as the splenocolic ligament. For T3 or T4 tumours the omentectomy should be combined with dissection of the anterior leaf of the transverse mesocolon. This is because many T3 or T4 cancers have adhesions to or invade the anterior (but not the posterior) leaf of the mesocolon. In all cases it is essential to dissect deep to the anterior leaf of the mesocolon to identify the origin of the right gastroepiploic vessels.

The gastroepiploic vein can be identified by finding the accessory right colic vein, which joins the right gastroepiploic vein to form the gastrocolic trunk. The gastroepiploic vein is ligated and divided at its origin. The anterior leaf of the mesocolon continues as the capsule of the pancreas. This is dissected from the pancreas from the inferior to the superior border and the dissection continued towards the duodenum as far as the gastroduodenal artery. This artery is followed caudally to the root of the right gastroepiploic artery, which is ligated and divided. The gastroduodenal artery is then traced superiorly to its origin from the common hepatic artery. Visualisation of this junction is the last step of this phase of the dissection.

The lesser omentum is divided close to the left lateral segment of the liver. If present, an accessory left hepatic artery is ligated. The anterior surface of the hepatoduodenal ligament is incised a few centimetres below the hepatic hilum as far as the left edge of the common bile duct and then straight down to the duodenum. A few supraduodenal vessels are ligated and divided to clear the superior border of the duodenum. The tissue in the hepatoduodenal ligament is cleared from right to left. The origin of the right gastric artery can easily be found by following the gastroduodenal artery cephalad. It is ligated and divided. The duodenum is then divided with a linear cutting stapler and the staple line oversewn with interrupted or continuous sutures.

The next step is the dissection of the lymph nodes above the pancreas. The stomach is reflected upwards and to the left to expose the area along the superior border of the pancreas and the pancreas is gently retracted caudad. The dissection is carried out from right to left, starting by incising the connective tissue along the superior border of the pancreas from the gastroduodenal artery to the middle part of the splenic artery. As the left gastric vein often crosses the common hepatic artery, this procedure must be carried out carefully. The node dissection starts by removing the node-bearing connective tissue from the left side of the proper hepatic artery and portal vein. The dissection continues to the left, with skeletonisation of the proper and common hepatic arteries. The tissue on the right crus is dissected from the retroperitoneum, giving a view of the right side of the celiac axis. The origin of the left gastric artery is identified and doubly ligated and divided. The node dissection is continued along the proximal half of the splenic artery, as far as the origin of the posterior gastric artery. This artery is the first major branch of the splenic artery going cephalad. It is preserved when the tumour is located in the antrum but often ligated during a distal subtotal gastrectomy for a mid-stomach cancer. Stripping off all the retroperitoneal tissue on both crura behind the stomach is continued to the oesophageal hiatus.

The origins of the left gastroepiploic vessels are exposed close to the splenic hilum and ligated. Branches of the left gastroepiploic vessels are ligated and divided on the greater curve to prepare the site of gastric division and anastomosis. All the short gastric vessels should be preserved in a subtotal distal gastrectomy to preserve the blood supply of the gastric remnant. Splenectomy is not part of a D2 distal subtotal gastrectomy.

The node-bearing tissue along the lesser curve is cleared from the site of transection up to the gastro-oesophageal junction. This requires meticulous dissection and ligation of many small branches of left gastric vessels. The stomach is then transected using a linear cutting stapler. A gross margin of 3 cm for a well-circumscribed

type and 5 cm for invasive type is adequate, although a total gastrectomy with wider margin is always needed for Borrmann type 4 (linitis plastica type) tumours.

The major methods of reconstruction are a Billroth II gastrojejunostomy and a Roux-en-Y, end-to-side gastrojejunostomy. We recommend a retrocolic Roux-en-Y reconstruction as a safe procedure with minimal incidence of biliary reflux gastritis. Billroth I gastroduodenostomy should be reserved exclusively for young patients with minimum tension at the anastomosis.

Total gastrectomy with D2 lymph node dissection

There are three methods of total gastrectomy, depending on the approach to management of the spleen and pancreas.

- If the cancer involves the body or tail of the pancreas (T4 tumour) or if metastatic nodes on the splenic artery are adherent to the pancreas, this part of the organ should be resected *en bloc* with the stomach.

- Pancreas-preserving total gastrectomy with splenectomy is frequently used in Japan. This allows complete removal of the lymph nodes along the splenic artery, with much less pancreatic leakage and subsequent intraabdominal infection than occurs with distal pancreatectomy.

- In the West, both pancreas and spleen are usually preserved.

The procedure is the same as a distal gastrectomy until the division of the left gastric artery. The spleen and the body and tail of the pancreas are mobilised whether or not a splenectomy is planned.

If a splenectomy and distal pancreatectomy is part of the procedure, the splenic vein and artery are identified behind the body of the pancreas. These vessels are ligated and divided prior to transection of the pancreas. The standard approach to dividing the pancreas is to divide it with a knife and then to ligate the small vessels and pancreatic duct with non-absorbable sutures. The gastrectomy is completed as described below and a drain is placed close to the divided pancreas in case of a pancreatic fluid leak.

The standard Japanese approach to a total gastrectomy for a T2 or T3 tumour is the pancreas-preserving technique. In this procedure the splenic artery is divided distal to the origin of the pancreatico magna artery and the branches of the splenic artery to the pancreas are individually ligated. This results in an *en bloc* dissection of all the lymph nodes along the distal splenic artery and splenic hilum (Figure 5.2). It is critical to preserve the splenic vein and its pancreatic tributaries as far as the tail of the pancreas, to avoid venous congestion, resulting in the complication of pancreatic necrosis.

The spleen is not usually removed in a total gastrectomy in the West. In order to preserve the spleen yet still achieve an adequate node dissection, a meticulous dissection of all the nodes along

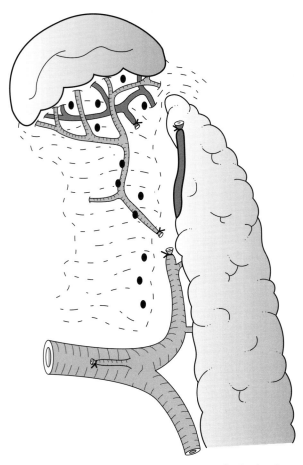

Figure 5.2 The first branch of the splenic artery is usually the dorsal pancreatic artery, which may be a direct branch of the celiac artery, and the second is the pancreatico magna artery. In this procedure, the splenic artery is divided distal to the pancreatico magna artery, while the splenic vein is preserved close to the tip of the tail of the pancreas.

splenic vessels is required. In this technique, the dissection of the splenic hilum nodes may often be incomplete. Short gastric vessels are ligated near the origin.

After dealing with the spleen and/or pancreas the dissection is continued up to the cardio-oesophageal junction. It is necessary to identify and divide the cardio-oesophageal branches from the left inferior phrenic vessels. The oesophagus is then encircled and the anterior and posterior vagal trunks are specifically divided to allow the lower end of the oesophagus to be mobilised.

Our standard approach to reconstruction after total gastrectomy is via an oesophago-jejunostomy with a Roux-en-Y. There is a range of alternatives, including jejunal interposition and jejunal pouches, but none of the variations has any proven advantage. The simplest and safest approach is the Roux-en-Y.

An oesophago-jejunostomy can be hand sewn or fashioned with a circular stapling device. We believe that a stapled anastomosis should be standard practice since experience at the National Cancer Centre Hospital in Tokyo has shown that hand-sewn anastomosis carries a significantly higher leakage rate despite the anastomoses being performed by highly experienced and dedicated gastric surgeons.

Postoperative care

The nasogastric tube placed across the anastomosis is removed on day 1 or 2, providing the drainage volume is small. There is no advantage to prolonged nasogastric tube drainage, unless the volume aspirated happens to be large.

Large-bore drains are placed close to the duodenal stump, the pancreas stump or the stripped pancreas tail and also close to the gastro-jejunostomy. These are connected to low suction until the patient is taking fluids. The most common complication after a D2 total gastrectomy is the leakage of pancreatic juice and subsequent intraabdominal infection. To predict this, it is useful to measure the amylase level in the drain fluid. If the amylase level is low, the drains close to the pancreas stump or stripped pancreatic tail can be removed early. If it is high, they should remain in place until the risk of these complications disappears.

After a distal or total gastrectomy, the patient may start taking fluids after about four days, provided there are no postoperative complications. We do not routinely perform a contrast study. After a total gastrectomy with high risk of leaking, we usually perform a contrast study after 4–7 days. If there is no extravasation, the patient commences fluids and the drainage tubes are removed.

FURTHER READING

Ajani AJ. Treatment of patients with upper gastrointestinal carcinomas. *Semin Oncol* 1997; **24**:S19–72–76

AJCC. *Cancer Staging Manual*, 5th edn. Philadelphia : Lippincott-Raven, 1997

Bonenkamp JJ, Hermans J, Sasako M, van de Vilde CJH. Extended lymph node dissection for gastric cancer. *N Engl J Med* 1999: **340**:908–914

Burke EC, Karpeh MS, Conlon KC, Brennan MF. Laparoscopy in the management of gastric adenocarcinoma. *Ann Surg* 1997; **225**:262–267

Cuschieri A, Weeden S, Fielding J et al. Patient survival after D1 and D2 resections for gastric cancer: long-term results of the MRC randomized surgical trial. *Br J Cancer* 1999: **79**:1522–1530

Earle CC, Maroun JA. Adjuvant chemotherapy after curative resection for gastric cancer in non-Asian patients: revisiting a meta-analysis of randomised trials. *Eur J Cancer* 1999; **35**:1059–1064

Japanese Gastric Cancer Association. *Japanese classification of gastric carcinoma*, 2nd English edition. *Gastric Cancer* 1998; **1**:10–24

Macdonald JS, Smalley S, Benedetti J et al. Postoperative combined radiation and chemotherapy improves disease-free survival (DFS) and overall survival (OS) in resected adenocarcinoma of the stomach and GE junction. *Proc ASCO* 2000; **19**:1a

Noda N, Sasako M, Yamaguchi N, Nakanishi Y. Ignoring small lymph nodes can be a major cause of staging error in gastric cancer. *Br J Surg*. 1998; **85**:831–834

Sasako M, Sano T, Katai H, Maruyama K. Radical surgery. In: Sugimura T, Sasako M, eds. *Gastric Cancer*. Oxford: Oxford University Press, 1997

6

The small bowel

Douglas M. G. Bowley, Andrew N. Kingsnorth

INVESTIGATIONS OF THE SMALL BOWEL

Small bowel diseases frequently behave insidiously and lack distinctive clinical features. Diagnostic delay and false-negative investigations are common. Complete assessment of the small bowel may require the expertise of a specialist GI radiologist (Figure 6.1). Luminal distension is a requirement for all small bowel imaging, as collapsed loops can hide even large lesions. Oral contrast gives suboptimal distension but may be more acceptable to the patient than intubation-infusion (enteroclysis), which can be poorly tolerated in the absence of sedation.

Diagnostic methods

Barium studies

Small bowel follow-through

This examination follows a column of barium as it moves through the gastrointestinal tract (GIT). The complete examination depends on transit time, but can take up to six hours. The false-negative rate for small bowel follow-through can be as high as 40% compared to a rate of under 10% for enteroclysis.

Small bowel enema (enteroclysis)

Placing a nasoduodenal catheter allows barium to be infused directly into the small bowel, allowing a quicker and more accurate assessment than small bowel follow-through. Enteroclysis is reliable, with a high negative predictive value. The principal advantage of enteroclysis is that the jejunum can be optimally distended. Information about function is obtained indirectly by defining distensibility or fixation of small bowel loops. However, overlapping loops of bowel can limit interpretation and enteroclysis only gives indirect information about the bowel wall and surrounding structures.

Ultrasound and CT

Ultrasound can detect intraluminal and extraluminal tumours, but is only accurate for tumours >6 cm. CT is highly successful in identifying small bowel tumours and can also help to stage tumour progression by identification of metastases. CT accurately demonstrates bowel wall and extraluminal structures but lacks ability to provide functional information. CT enteroclysis may also be used (Figure 6.2).

Magnetic resonance enteroclysis

Abdominal magnetic resonance (MR) imaging has improved in recent years, aided by availability of respiratory triggering, breath-hold sequences to suppress motion artefact and effective luminal contrast agents. MR is considered by some radiologists to be the optimal method of small bowel imaging because of the soft tissue

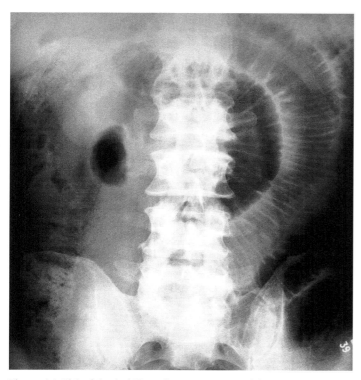

Figure 6.1 Plain abdominal X-ray demonstrating typical features of small bowel obstruction. Dilated small bowel loops in upper quadrant. Courtesy of Dr S.A. Jackson.

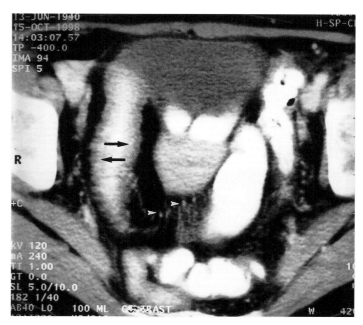

Figure 6.2 Intravenous contrast-enhanced CT scan of the pelvis in a patient with active Crohn's disease demonstrating a thick-walled terminal ileum (arrows) with engorged vasa recta (arrow heads). Courtesy of Dr S.A. Jackson.

contrast it can provide, the multiplanar imaging capabilities and the lack of ionising radiation. Real-time imaging of the small bowel during infusion can be obtained using breath-hold sequences; these images can provide functional information.

Radionuclide scans and angiography

Red blood cells labelled with technetium can be used to screen for occult GI bleeding. As little as 5 ml of luminal blood will give a positive scan. Delayed acquisition of images may be misleading as pooling of blood distal to a bleeding point may lead to incorrect localisation.

Selective visceral angiography can be used to localise GI haemorrhage and may be useful to delineate subserosal or actively bleeding tumours. Angiography can detect bleeding at a rate of 0.5 ml/min. A typical neoplasm may have multiple feeding arteries and draining veins, with irregular vessels and venous pooling.

Enteroscopy

Push-type enteroscopy

Specialised jejunoscopes or sterilised colonoscopes can be used to intubate the proximal jejunum, allowing targeted biopsy and polypectomy. Use of an overtube that limits looping of the endoscope allows deeper intubation of the jejunum. Retrograde examination of the terminal ileum may be performed during colonoscopy and, when combined with upper GI push enteroscopy, has been called 'two-way enteroscopy'. In expert hands two-way enteroscopy can provide a diagnosis in approximately 30% of patients with occult GI bleeding who had a previously normal barium follow-through.

Sonde-type enteroscopy

The word 'sonde' has a French origin and means 'bend'. Sonde instruments are introduced transnasally, a balloon at the tip is inflated and peristalsis propels the instruments distally. The bowel is examined as the instrument is withdrawn. Although a total small enteroscopy is possible, deflection of the tip is not possible, so the mucosa cannot be viewed totally and sonde endoscopes do not have instrumentation channels, so intervention is not possible. The role of sonde endoscopy is therefore somewhat limited.

Intraoperative enteroscopy

Intraoperative endoscopy requires cooperation between the surgeon and the endoscopist but allows a view of the entire mucosal surface of the small bowel for the endoscopist and a transilluminated and surface view of the vascular pattern of the bowel for the surgeon. A colonoscope or push enteroscope is passed into the duodenum and the surgeon helps to manipulate the scope into the proximal small bowel. Thereafter, the surgeon telescopes the bowel over the colonoscope, attempting to minimise the creation of artefact by scope trauma. The bowel is examined as the scope is withdrawn and any suspicious lesions can be marked by the surgeon and dealt with by excision or resection.

Laparoscopic-assisted enteroscopy is being evaluated in certain centres.

NEOPLASMS OF THE SMALL BOWEL

Despite its anatomical location between two regions of high cancer risk, the small bowel rarely develops neoplastic tumours. The inner surface area of the small bowel comprises about 80–90% of the entire GIT, but small bowel tumours comprise only 2% of all GI malignancies. Within the small intestine, the sites at the highest risk are the duodenum, for adenocarcinomas, and the ileum, for carcinoids and lymphomas. In industrialised countries, small bowel cancers are predominantly adenocarcinomas; in developing countries, lymphomas are much more common. The incidence of small bowel cancer rises with age and has generally been higher among males than among females. The risk factors for small bowel cancer include dietary factors similar to those implicated in large bowel cancer and other medical conditions, including Crohn's disease and polyposis syndromes. Protective factors may include rapid cell turnover, a general absence of bacteria, an alkaline environment, enzymatic detoxification of ingested carcinogens, rapid luminal transit, secretions containing immune protective factors and differences in the cellular biology of the epithelium compared to the stomach and colon.

Small bowel lymphoma is associated with infectious agents, such as human immunodeficiency virus (HIV) and Epstein–Barr virus (EBV).

Clinical presentation

- Small bowel neoplasms commonly present with iron deficiency anaemia; they are the second most common cause of obscure GI bleeding, accounting for 5–10% of all cases of chronic blood loss. Among patients with occult GI bleeding small bowel tumours are the most common lesions in patients below the age of 50 years.

- Presentation with obstruction may be caused by luminal blockage with tumour or intestinal kinking or the tumour may form the apex of an intussusception.

- Intussusception is rare in adult life, accounting for <5% of GI obstruction, roughly half of which are associated with neoplasms.

- Periampullary tumours of the duodenum may present with obstructive jaundice.

Pathology

Small bowel neoplasms may be classified as:

- adenomas and adenocarcinomas
- endocrine cell tumours
- lymphomas
- hamartomas
- other tumours.

Adenomas and carcinomas

Small bowel adenomas and carcinomas mimic their more common counterparts in the large intestine. They are similar in risk factors, geographic distribution, microscopic features and clinical significance. However, while colorectal cancer incidence rates in the United States have been falling since the mid-1980s, the incidence of small bowel carcinoma is rising. When multiple, small bowel adenomas principally in the duodenum are closely associated with familial adenomatous polyposis (FAP).

Adenomas may be:

- tubular
- villous
- tubulovillous.

Most adenomas occur in the duodenum and malignancy is more likely with large, multiple, villous and periampullary tumours. Small bowel carcinomas are unevenly distributed throughout the small bowel, with diminishing incidence proximal to distal. Most are annular and constricting but polypoid or fungating carcinomas occur. They may be multiple in 15–25% of patients and metastases are present in 50% at the time of presentation. The most common site is the periampullary region of the duodenum. Pancreaticoduodenectomy is the operation of choice for resectable lesions of the second part of the duodenum but palliative bypass may be necessary. Distal small bowel tumours should be resected when possible.

Association with inflammatory bowel disease

Patients with inflammatory bowel disease are at increased risk of developing intestinal carcinomas. There is an approximately 12-fold increased risk of small bowel cancer in Crohn's disease (Figure 6.3).

Association with hereditary polyposis syndromes

Familial adenomatous polyposis (FAP) is an autosomal dominant condition characterised by the development of multiple adenomas

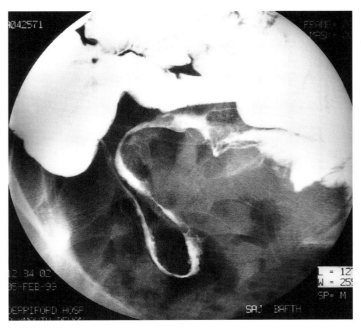

Figure 6.3 Small bowel meal study demonstrating terminal ileal involvement in a patient with Crohn's disease. Courtesy of Dr S.A. Jackson.

in the colon. Untreated, FAP invariably leads to colorectal cancer. Adenomas are present in the duodenum in 60–90% of patients with FAP but also occur in the small bowel distal to the duodenum, with the proximal jejunum having the highest prevalence. The incidence of duodenal polyposis increases with age and progression from adenomas to carcinoma may be rapid. The risk of duodenal cancer is about 100 times that of the general population. Duodenal carcinoma is now the most common cause of death in FAP and endoscopic surveillance of the upper GIT is recommended to identify high-risk patients and to diagnose cancer at an early stage. The St Mark's Hospital group recommend starting screening at the age of 20 years. Because of the high prevalence of adenomas in the periampullary region of the duodenum and proximal jejunum, side-viewing endoscopes and push enteroscopy are recommended for complete surveillance. The potential risk for adenocarcinoma is also increased in hereditary non-polyposis colorectal cancer (HPNCC). Although small bowel carcinoma is not considered a main tumour of the syndrome, HPNCC family members incur small bowel cancers at approximately 25 times the expected incidence.

Endocrine cell tumours

Carcinoid tumours

In 1907, Oberndorfer introduced the term 'carcinoid' to describe a mid-gut tumour that was morphologically distinct and less aggressive in behaviour than intestinal adenocarcinoma. Carcinoid tumours are often indolent, asymptomatic tumours but a small proportion are malignant and difficult to manage.

Carcinoid tumours are neuroendocrine tumours derived from enterochromaffin or Kulchinsky cells. Data from the US National Cancer Institute suggest an annual incidence of occurrence in up to 10% of postmortems. Approximately 74–90% of all carcinoid tumours occur in the GIT and most occur in the ileum. Some 35% of patients with ileal carcinoid will have more than one lesion; some may have >100. Macroscopically, carcinoids are solid tumours, yellow in appearance, reflecting a high lipid content. The cells stain with potassium chromate and are hence termed enterochromaffin; they also take up and reduce silver and are called argentaffin. Some take up silver but are unable to reduce it and are called argyrophil.

The ability of carcinoid cells to synthesise 5-hydroxytryptamine (5HT) from dietary tryptophan is a hallmark of the tumour. A breakdown product excreted in urine, 5-hydroxyindoleacetic acid (5HIAA), is classically associated with carcinoid tumours. However, many other hormones may be produced and released, including gastrin, kinins, prostaglandins and somatostatin.

Typical argyrophil carcinoids, which may secrete gastrin to give rise to the Zollinger–Ellison syndrome, may occur as part of the inherited multiple endocrine neoplasia syndrome type 1 (MEN-1).

Only 20–35% of small intestinal carcinoids are malignant and metastasise, the risk being related to the size of the tumour. Tumours larger than 2 cm in diameter are more likely to be symptomatic and also more likely to metastasise. The most common clinical presentation is periodic abdominal pain and intermittent bowel obstruction; bleeding is rare.

Most patients with mid-gut and metastatic carcinoid have abnormal metabolism of tryptophan. In health, 99% of typtophan is metabolised to produce nicotinic acid with only 1% being converted to 5HT. In carcinoid tumour, production of 5HT predominates and the breakdown product 5H1AA appears in the urine. A deficiency of nicotinic acid can arise leading to pellagra (dermatitis, diarrhoea and dementia). If 5HT is secreted into the systemic circulation carcinoid syndrome may appear.

Carcinoid syndrome

Most patients with carcinoid syndrome have metastatic carcinoid tumours. The syndrome is characterised by flushing and diarrhoea with, less commonly, heart valve dysfunction, wheezing and pellagra.

Investigation

Measurement of 24-hour urine 5H1AA is highly specific. Certain foods (avocado, banana) can cause false-positive readings and certain medication (aspirin, phenothiazines) can cause false-negative results.

Localisation of tumours can be difficult. Endoscopy with endoscopic ultrasound, barium studies, CT scanning, angiography and enteroscopy are all used. As most carcinoid tumours possess a somatostatin receptor, somatostatin-receptor scintigraphy is the best single imaging technique to identify the presence, location and extent of small bowel carcinoid tumours (Figure 6.4).

Treatment

Surgery is the only curative therapy for carcinoid tumours. Local resection and clearance of local lymph nodes is the treatment of choice for isolated primary carcinoids. Because tumours may secrete extensive amounts of hormones and manipulation of the tumour may induce vasomotor and metabolic instability, prophylactic infusion of somatostatin analogues has recently been adopted for patients undergoing embolotherapy or surgery as prophylaxis against carcinoid crisis. Liver transplantation has been used with some success for hepatic metastatic carcinoid.

Adjuvant therapy for carcinoid syndrome

- Lifestyle modification to avoid precipitating factors such as alcohol, spicy food and strenuous exercise.

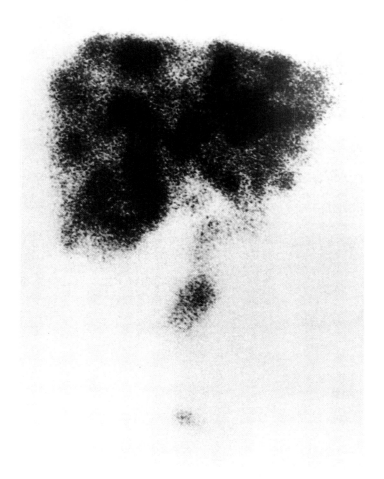

Figure 6.4 ^{111}In DTPA octreotide scinitigram demonstrating ileal carcinoid tumour with diffuse liver metastases. Courtesy of Dr E.A. van Royen.

- 5HT-release inhibitors such as octreotide or its long-acting analogues.

- Hepatic metastases may be treated with embolotherapy.

- Receptor-targeted therapy: carcinoid cells can be reduced in size and 5HT output by specifically targeting them with radioactive indium-labelled octreotide.

Lymphomas

Non-Hodgkin's lymphoma (NHL) of the GIT accounts for 4–20% of all NHLs and is the most common extranodal site of presentation.

Primary GI lymphoma accounts for 20–30% of malignant neoplasms of the small bowel but this represents <5% of all primary gut malignancies. The stomach is the major GI organ affected by lymphoma and in this site is associated with *Helicobacter pylori* infection. The small bowel may be affected by mucosa-associated lymphoid tissue (MALT) lymphoma, diffuse large cell lymphoma, mantle cell lymphoma, follicular lymphoma and immunoproliferative small intestinal disease (IPSID). A number of risk factors for GI lymphoma have been identified; infection with *Helicobacter pylori* and HIV, immunosuppression after solid transplantation, coeliac disease and inflammatory bowel disease. The predominant symptoms in small bowel lymphoma are abdominal pain, obstruction, malabsorption and weight loss.

Patients may present acutely with obstruction or perforation and diagnosis may be made at laparotomy. The prognosis of patients who have complete resection of disease is better than those with incomplete resection. When resection is not feasible treatment is usually with anthracycline-based chemotherapy, followed in some cases by radiotherapy. Five-year survival is approximately 75% for patients with indolent B cell lymphomas and only 25% for those with T cell tumours.

Box 6.1	Staging of gastrointestinal non-Hodgkin's lymphoma
Stage 1	Tumour confined to GI tract Single primary or multiple non-contiguous lesions
Stage 2	Tumour extending in abdomen from primary GI site Nodal involvement II1 local (paraintestinal) II2 distant (mesenteric, para-aortic, pelvic)
Stage 3	Penetration of serosa to involve adjacent organs/tissues
Stage 4	Disseminated extranodal involvement or GI lesions with supradiaphragmatic nodal involvement

Immunoproliferative disease of the small intestine (IPSID)

IPSID, alpha heavy-chain disease and Mediterranean lymphoma all refer to subgroups of B cell lymphoma affecting the small intestine. IPSID usually affects men and women of low socioeconomic status in Mediterranean and Middle Eastern regions with poor sanitation and hygiene. Males aged 10–30 years are most often affected. The lymphoma arises in association with diffuse plasma cell infiltration of the small intestine (IPSID). The plasma cells often synthesise an abnormal immunoglobin heavy chain, which is detectable in serum and urine.

The symptoms are usually diarrhoea, malabsorption, weight loss and abdominal pain. Small intestinal bacterial overgrowth and parasitosis are common features and treatment with tetracyclines can produce clinical, histological and immunological remission. The role of radiotherapy and surgery in IPSID is unclear. IPSID is a highly lethal condition with five-year survival of around 20–25%.

Multiple Lymphomatous Polyposis (MLP)

In patients with MLP, polypoid tumours are distributed through the GIT with the jejunum and terminal ileum being the most common sites. The cell type of this lymphoma resembles cells in the mantle zone of the lymph node follicle and at presentation there is frequently disseminated involvement of lymph nodes, blood and bone marrow as well as the intestine.

Primary intestinal T-cell lymphoma

Approximately 10–25% of primary small intestinal lymphomas arise from T cells. These lymphomas tend to appear as ulcerating plaques or strictures in the proximal small bowel in contrast to B cell lymphomas, which typically form annular or polypoid masses in the terminal ileum.

T cell lymphoma of the small intestine is often associated with long-standing coeliac disease when it is known as enteropathy-associated T cell lymphoma (EATCL). Patients with EATCL are often in their sixth or seventh decade and the diagnosis of malignancy should be suspected if patients develop a strict gluten-free diet. The prognosis is extremely poor with few patients surviving beyond one year.

Lymphoma in the immunosuppressed

Congenital and acquired immunodeficiency is associated with an increased incidence of NHL. Lymphoma arising in the setting of immunodeficiency is more likely to be extranodal and GI lymphoma is common. Epstein–Barr virus has been shown to be associated with virtually all lymphomas associated with immunosuppression. Lymphoma is commonly associated with AIDS and the introduction of antiviral chemotherapy that prolongs survival in AIDS patients has seen an increasing incidence of these lesions.

NHL represents about a quarter of all cancers in patients who have undergone solid-organ transplantation. Recipients of small bowel, heart/lung or heart transplants who require high degrees of immunosuppression have the highest incidence of NHL, up to 30%, while only about 5% of kidney transplant patients will develop lymphoma. Transplantation-associated lymphoma is strongly associated with cyclosporin therapy.

Treatment is difficult and involves surgery, when feasible, reduction of immunosuppression, antiviral therapy and chemotherapy. Outcome is poor with median survival of only six months.

Lymphoma in children

Lymphomas constitute approximately 10% of all childhood cancers in North America, of which about 60% are non-Hodgkin's type (NHL). According to a large series by the US Children's Cancer Group (CCG), 85% of NHL involves the bowel, including bowel infiltration from tumours arising in extraintestinal sites (kidney, spleen and ovary). Two-thirds of these involved the small bowel, with the overwhelming majority of primary lymphomas arising in the ileocaecal region.

With modern chemotherapeutic protocols the survival rate in patients undergoing complete resection approaches 100%. Complete resection eliminates the tumour burden and also eliminates the risk of perforation due to chemotherapy-induced mural necrosis where tumour has replaced the bowel wall. However, in the CCG series, over half of the paediatric abdominal lymphomas were too extensive to permit complete resection at laparotomy. If complete resection is not possible, then survival rates fall to around 50% and attempts at subtotal resection may result in complications that adversely affect outcome. Hence aggressive debulking of disease should be avoided.

Hamartomas

Peutz–Jeghers syndrome (PJS)

PJS is a polyposis syndrome characterised by mucocutaneous pigmentation and diffuse GI hamartomas. It is an autosomal dominant condition that occurs once in every 120 000 births. The PJS gene has recently been identified. PJS is recognised as a cancer predisposition syndrome and a hamartoma-adenoma-carcinoma sequence has been postulated. Polyps of varying size from a few millimetres to several centimetres may be found throughout the gut, most commonly in the small bowel. Clinical presentation is usually with intussusception, bleeding or obstruction. The relative risk of dying from GI malignancy in PJS has been estimated as 13-fold greater than the general population. Up to 75% of PJS-associated GI cancers occur in those less than 50 years old. Surveillance of the upper and lower GIT is achieved with upper GI endoscopy and colonoscopy with terminal ileoscopy but the middle small bowel is more challenging to screen. Push enteroscopy allows limited exploration and polypectomy in the jejunum, but surgery with intraoperative enteroscopy, either open or laparoscopically assisted, may be necessary.

PJS is also associated with extraintestinal manifestations, particularly genital tract tumours.

Juvenile polyposis

Juvenile polyps are also hamartomas and were first described in 1957. Solitary juvenile polyps occur in 1% of children but juvenile polyposis (JP) is much more rare. JP can be classified into three groups:

- JP of infancy
- generalised JP
- JP of the colon.

JP of infancy is a rare form of the disease and presents with diarrhoea, haemorrhage, intussusception, rectal prolapse and a protein-losing enteropathy. The entire GIT is affected and prognosis is related to the extent of the disease with death occurring before the age of two years in severe cases.

The generalised form of JP, with hamartomas in the stomach, small bowel and colon, presents with rectal bleeding and anaemia. The condition usually presents in childhood; only 15% of patients present as adults. About 9% of polyps in JP occur in the small bowel and the usual presentation is with bleeding, intussusception or obstruction. A family history of the condition is found in 20–50% of patients with an apparently autosomal dominant trait. Epithelial dysplasia may be observed and JP is recognised as a premalignant condition with a cumulative risk of colorectal cancer of >50%.

Myoepithelial hamartomas

Myoepithelial hamartomas are rare tumours thought to arise as a result of displacement of pancreatic cells along the gastrointestinal tract during embryogenesis, which differentiate into various pancreatic elements; the most highly differentiated form is heterotopic pancreas. An alternative theory is pancreatic metaplasia of endodermal tissues.

Haemangiomas

Haemangiomas are considered to be hamartomas by some authorities and represent <10% of small bowel tumours. They may be cavernous, capillary or mixed forms and present with GI bleeding. Small bowel haemangiomas may be associated with cutaneous lesions, such as cavernous skin haemangiomas in the blue rubber bleb naevus syndrome or with cutaneous haemangiomas and soft tissue hypertrophy in the Klippel–Trenaunay–Weber syndrome.

Lymphangiomas

These are rare neoplasms that account for around 3% of small bowel benign tumours.

Brunner's gland adenomas

Brunner's gland adenomas are rare duodenal neoplasms thought to be duodenal hamartomas with a predominance of Brunner's gland elements. They may achieve a large size and usually present with obstruction or bleeding but are usually amenable to endoscopic removal.

Other tumours

Gastrointestinal stromal tumours (GIST)

GISTs are mesenchymal neoplasms originating in the muscular wall of hollow viscera (Figure 6.5). They are rare compared to neoplasms arising from the epithelium. GISTs are divided into three groups.

- Well-defined or fully realised lines of differentiation such as leiomyomas or schwannomas.

- Poorly differentiated features or only partial or incomplete features of differentiation but with no histological signs of malignancy.

- Those showing malignant characteristics that are defined as gastrointestinal stromal sarcoma (GISS). GISSs are uncommon malignant tumours, which represent 2–5% of all soft tissue sarcomas; 35% will originate in the small bowel and symptoms are those of pain, obstruction, bleeding or a mass. Unlike retroperitoneal sarcomas, GISSs tend to be symptomatic at an early stage and tumours are therefore more amenable to complete resection.

Secondary malignancies

The small bowel serosa is often involved with cacinomatosis peritonei, but metastatic lesions may also be seen in malignant

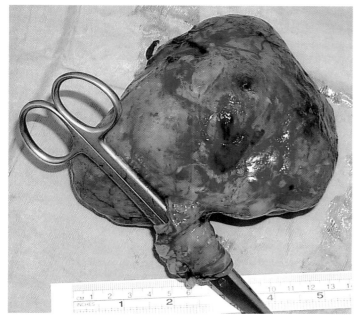

Figure 6.5 Gastrointestinal stromal tumour (GIST) arising from a section of terminal ileum.

melanoma or carcinoma of the lung or breast. Malignant melanoma is the most common tumour to metastasise to the gastrointestinal tract. Up to 60% of patients with malignant melanoma are found to have metastases at postmortem and roughly half will be in the small bowel. Between 1% and 4% of patients with melanoma will have clinically apparent gastrointestinal metastases antemortem. Symptoms are usually bleeding (either overt or occult), obstruction, intussusception, weight loss, malabsorption or protein-losing enteropathy. Radiologically, the lesions may appear as mural nodules, target lesions or large masses or with diffuse small bowel involvement. Endoscopy may be of limited value as the melanoma typically metastasises to small bowel serosa and mesentery. Surgery may be beneficial, with palliation of symptoms in >70% of patients who undergo resection or bypass. However, long-term survival is poor. Cutaneous melanoma precedes the onset of gastrointestinal symptoms by an average of four years but metastatic lesions have been reported 21 years after apparently definite treatment of the primary tumour. At postmortem in patients with non-small cell lung cancer small bowel metastases can be identified in 5% of cases, but these patients usually have multiple metastases at other sites.

AIDS-associated tumours

Malignant neoplasia complicates AIDS in approximately 12% of cases. The most common malignant neoplasm is Kaposi's sarcoma (KS) (60%), followed by lymphoma (35%) and miscellaneous tumours (6.5%). The GIT is involved in around 30% of patients with AIDS and neoplasia. Gastrointestinal KS is one of the most frequent neoplastic diseases seen in AIDS and the small bowel is one of the most frequently involved areas. Cutaneous KS usually precedes intestinal involvement and visceral involvement is usually silent but associated with shorter survival as compared to cutaneous KS.

Endoscopically the lesions are macules or nodules of red or violet colour and are frequently ulcerated. The yield of biopsy may be low as the tumour is situated in the submucosa. GI bleeding is the most common presenting feature.

Malignant lymphoma is the second most common malignancy seen in individuals with HIV infection. GI involvement is found in 10–25% of AIDS-related lymphoma but in contrast to GI lymphoma in immunocompetent individuals, more than 90% of AIDS patients will have lymphoma disseminated beyond the GIT at presentation. AIDS-related lymphomas are of predominantly intermediate and high-grade B cell non-Hodgkin's type. There is evidence that EBV plays a role in the pathogenesis of AIDS-related lymphoma.

Lipomas

Lipomas comprise 15–25% of small bowel tumours and are usually asymptomatic but may bleed or cause obstruction because of intussusception.

Neurogenic tumours

Neurofibromas may occur alone or in association with von Recklinghausen neurofibromatosis (VRNM). The gut is involved in 15–25% of patients with VRNM and 10–15% of neurofibromas will show sarcomatous change.

SMALL BOWEL OBSTRUCTION

Before the advent of modern surgical practice, most intestinal obstructions were caused by hernia. However, the aetiology of small bowel obstruction (SBO) has changed with the increase in intraabdominal surgery and elective abdominal wall hernia surgery and currently 60% of SBO is caused by adhesions.

The causes of SBO are:

- adhesions – 60%
- hernia – 15%
- neoplasms – 6%
- inflammatory causes (e.g. Crohn's) – 5%
- ischaemic bowel – 5%
- intussusception – 4%
- miscellaneous – 5%

Adhesions

Adhesions are the consequence of injury that may be traumatic, thermal, ischaemic, inflammatory or due to a foreign body reaction. By far the most common cause of adhesional obstruction is previous abdominal surgery. Approximately 4–5% of patients with a previous laparotomy will develop SBO. This figure varies depending on the type of surgery, with surgery in the infracolic compartment appearing to predispose to SBO. Some operations, such as restorative proctocolectomy, are associated with a very high incidence of subsequent SBO, perhaps up to 20%.

Hernia

Abdominal wall hernias carry a risk of strangulation and bowel obstruction if left unoperated. In one study, the cumulative probability after three months of strangulation for inguinal hernias was 2.8%, rising to 4.5% after two years. For femoral hernias the cumulative probability of strangulation was 22% at three months and 45% at 21 months. Mortality is increased for strangulated hernia due to late diagnosis and referral and increased co-morbidity in the elderly. For these reasons, elective repair of abdominal hernias is advocated and a reduction in the incidence of bowel obstruction secondary to hernia has been observed.

Miscellaneous

Gallstone ileus is a disease of the elderly, accounting for 25% of non-strangulated small bowel obstructions in those over the age of 65. The classic radiographic triad of small bowel obstruction, air in the biliary tract and ectopic gallstone is seen in about 20% of the patients on plain abdominal radiographs.

Intraoperatively more than one stone will be found in the intestines in 20% and cholecystoduodenal fistulas are encountered in around 80%. Other fistulas are rare. While mortality has declined over the years, it remains high at around 10–15%. This is largely due to the co-morbidity in elderly patients. Some surgeons feel that relief of the obstruction is all that is required. Others argue that the gallbladder and biliary–enteric fistula must be removed to prevent future recurrence (a one-stage procedure). In one series, the one-stage procedure carried a mortality of 16.9%, compared to 11.7% for simple enterolithotomy. Morbidity after enterolithotomy is low. The recurrence rate of gallstone ileus is less than 5% and only about 10% of patients will require reoperation for continued symptoms related to the biliary tract. Other, rarer causes of SBO include luminal obstruction due to bezoars, which are concretions caused by ingested hair, medication, milk curd or fruit and vegetable matter. Unmasticated food may act as a bolus, as may foreign objects that are usually swallowed by children, alcoholics or the insane. Pica is a condition where a patient will ingest food and non-food substances in an obsessive, compulsive manner. The condition tends to affect children, pregnant women, the intellectually challenged and patients with anaemia or renal failure.

Blunt abdominal injury may cause mural haematomas of the duodenum leading to obstruction and similarly, mural haematomas have been reported after warfarin therapy, usually affecting the jejunum. Subclinical blunt injury to the small bowel may heal with a stricture which can lead to delayed small bowel obstruction. Helminth infection with *Ascaris lumbricoides* or *Strongyloides stercoralis* may also cause small bowel obstruction.

Investigation of suspected small bowel obstruction

Suspected mechanical SBO may account for 20% of acute surgical admissions. Decision making may be difficult as diagnosis is not easy and the differentiation of strangulation from simple obstruction is not clearcut. Mechanical SBO from causes other than adhesions usually requires surgical intervention; however, adhesions may spontaneously resolve and conservative management may be successful. The goal of treatment for SBO is to identify those patients for whom surgery is necessary as soon as possible. Institution of a regime of nasogastric aspiration, intravenous fluids and clinical observation is required to maintain physiological stability while spontaneous resolution occurs and, most importantly, to detect deterioration as strangulation of bowel is associated with poor outcomes.

SBO may be suspected from the history and examination of the patient. Typical features include colicky pain, abdominal distension and reduction in passage of flatus and stool. Vomiting is a common feature and may be described as faeculent, due to fermentation of small bowel content. Abdominal distension is the most common physical sign and raised temperature, tachycardia, abdominal tenderness and a raised white blood cell count may signify strangulation.

A plain, supine radiograph of the abdomen is the first investigation of choice but may be unreliable if the obstruction is proximal, the bowel loops full of fluid or the radiograph taken at an early stage. Erect abdominal radiographs are generally considered to be unnecessary.

Water-soluble contrast studies have been used to predict the need for operative intervention in adhesional SBO. Water-soluble agents are chosen as they are non-toxic and have high osmolarity and can accelerate the resolution of adhesional SBO. In one study, plain X-rays were taken sequentially after oral or nasogastric ingestion of water-soluble contrast. All patients in whom contrast had reached the ascending colon at 24 hours were successfully treated non-operatively.

CT has high sensitivity in accurately diagnosing moderate to high-grade obstruction and is useful to identify small amounts of extraluminal gas or in excluding other pathology thought to be SBO. MR imaging has been used to investigate suspected SBO but requires further evaluation.

Long-term follow-up of patients with SBO reveals poor outcomes. In a series of 309 patients with SBO, 49% underwent laparotomy. In the operated group, postoperative morbidity occurred in 51%. The in-hospital mortality of all the patients was 5.5%. At a mean follow-up of 52 months, 21% of the operated group had recurrence of SBO, significantly less than the non-operated group, with a recurrence rate of 36%.

Adhesional SBO is a serious, common, costly complication of surgery. There is evidence that by using powder-free surgical gloves, avoiding trauma to the bowel serosa with minimal handling and careful use of gauze swabs and not closing the peritoneum, adhesion formation is minimised. Much effort has been expended in developing pharmacological methods of minimising adhesion formation, either by inhibition of adhesion formation or by membrane-like barriers that prevent adhesion between sites of injury. These strategies hold promise for reducing the financial and human impact of postoperative adhesions.

SMALL BOWEL BLEEDING

The small intestine is an uncommon site of GI bleeding, with only 3–5% of patients with GI bleeding having a small bowel source distal to the second part of the duodenum. In addition to its relative rarity, small bowel bleeding may be difficult to diagnose as the bleeding may be intermittent or slow and the small bowel is relatively inaccessible to radiological and endoscopic examination. Only approximately 5% of small bowel follow-through examinations detect a small bowel bleeding site.

Vascular lesions are the most common cause of small intestinal bleeding, accounting for 70–80%. Of these, angiodysplasia is the most common. Angiodysplasias are dilated vessels that develop with ageing and may be found throughout the bowel in the mucosa or submucosa.

Osler–Rendu–Weber syndrome (hereditary haemorrhagic telangiectasia) is the most common cause of intestinal telangiectasia. The patients present with mucocutaneous lesions in their teens and 20s and epistaxis is the most common feature; 15% or so will develop GI bleeding.

Tumours are the second most common cause of small bowel bleeding. Bleeding is the presenting complaint in 25–53% of patients with small bowel tumours.

Bleeding from a Meckel's diverticulum is the cause of bleeding in two-thirds of men less than 30 years who present with bleeding from the small bowel.

Ulcerative diseases of the small bowel also cause bleeding, of which Crohn's disease is the most common. Gross bleeding is uncommon in Crohn's, occurring in 4–10% of patients with ileitis. Transmural inflammation can erode into submucosal vessels and cause massive bleeding. These episodes are usually self-limiting and occur in the context of other symptoms of inflammatory bowel disease.

Although it is estimated that only 5% of people with jejunal diverticula bleed from them, when it does occur bleeding can be massive and may be associated with a mortality of up to 20%.

Bleeding from aorto–enteric fistulas arising from previous abdominal aortic aneurysm surgery can be life threatening. While primary fistulas do occur, they are rare. So-called 'calibre-persistent' arteries that fail to narrow as they penetrate the submucosa may be found throughout the GIT but the most common location is in the gastric fundus where the anomaly is known as a Dieulafoy lesion.

RADIATION ENTERITIS

Radiotherapy for pelvic and abdominal malignancy is powerful and effective, but at the cost of GI side effects. Walsh described the first patient with radiation enteritis in 1897, only two years after Roentgen's description of using radiation. The effect of radiation on the bowel is twofold. First, there is a direct effect on the gut wall itself and second, there is a progressive, obliterative vasculitis, which may produce ischaemic intestinal problems many years later. Preexisting mesenteric vascular compromise appears to predispose to radiation-induced enteritis. Diabetes, hypertension and cardiovascular disease are all significantly more common in patients with radiation enteritis. Previous abdominal operations or sepsis also seem to predispose to radiation enteritis.

Radiation-induced intestinal injury is often subclinical. In a study of 17 patients attending a radiotherapy follow-up clinic, 12 had permanent alteration in bowel habit and 16 had evidence of malabsorption. However, only about 5% of patients will require surgical intervention. Radiation enteritis is progressive and relentless. In a large study the most common presenting feature of small bowel injury was obstruction due to stricture (71%); fistula occurred in 17%, perforation was seen in 10%, haemorrhage in 2% and 22% had associated colorectal injury.

The incidence of anastomotic leakage is increased after resection of affected bowel and therefore, postoperative complications add to morbidity associated with radiation-induced intestinal injury. Anastomotic leak rates of small bowel to small bowel anastomosis can be as high as 25%. Less than two-thirds of patients undergoing surgery for radiation-induced small bowel injury survive over two years; some will succumb to tumour progression but approximately one-third die from progressive radiation injury.

The latent period from radiation to presentation varies greatly. The median latent period for small bowel lesions is two years, but may vary between 0 and 18 years. Extraintestinal radiation-induced lesions are also common. Radiation cystitis and obliterative arterial disease of the iliac vessels may occur and radiation to para-aortic nodes (for example, in testicular malignancy) may lead to radiation myelitis.

PERFORATION OF THE SMALL BOWEL

Perforation of the small intestine may be:

- iatrogenic
- traumatic
- secondary to perforation of intestinal tumours, diverticula, inflammatory or ischaemic segments of bowel
- secondary to infection, such as typhoid
- due to migration of ingested foreign bodies.

Iatrogenic perforation

In several large series, small bowel injury occurred in 0.2% of laparoscopic procedures. The risk of this complication may be reduced by open insertion of the trocars. Laparoscopic surgery has recently been advocated for adhesional small bowel obstruction, but the rate of intestinal injury during trocar insertion at this procedure is much higher, at around 4%.

Endoscopic sphincterotomy during retrograde pancreatography carries a risk of duodenal perforation of approximately 1–2%. The management of duodenal perforation after ERCP is controversial.

Some patients with posterior retroperitoneal perforations will settle with conservative management. However, open anterior perforations with delayed operative intervention result in sepsis and very poor outcomes. Duodenal perforation may be treated successfully without surgery when the symptoms are mild and improve rapidly with medical treatment, but surgery should be undertaken if generalised pain and abdominal signs are prominent, if suppuration is suspected or if symptoms do not improve after a brief period of non-operative management.

Traumatic injury

The proportion of blunt and penetrating injury in abdominal trauma shows a marked geographic variation. In the UK, blunt injury is predominant but this is not the case in South Africa or the United States.

After penetrating injury to the abdomen, the small bowel is the organ most commonly affected, being injured in approximately 60% of cases. Injury to the small bowel is graded according to the America Association for the Surgery of Trauma (AAST) organ injury scales (Box 6.2). Isolated low-grade injuries can be repaired primarily. High-grade or multiple injuries should be treated by resection and primary anastomosis. Outcome depends primarily on extent and severity of associated injuries.

In surgery for trauma, injuries missed at initial operation have the potential to cause disastrous complications and have been called 'the nemesis of the trauma surgeon'.

Damage to the small bowel is the most commonly missed visceral injury. Careful examination of the entire small bowel is mandatory during a laparotomy for penetrating trauma and unpaired holes in bowel are a marker for a missed injury. Although the small bowel is the third most commonly injured organ after blunt abdominal trauma, small bowel injury occurs in only 1–5% of blunt trauma victims. Direct, focused blows to the abdomen increase the risk of blunt small bowel injury (such as falling directly onto the handlebar of a bicycle) and in restrained occupants of motor vehicle accidents of sufficient force to produce visible abdominal wall contusion and vertebral column fracture, the incidence of intestinal injury may exceed 50%.

The increasing trend towards use of CT to screen for abdominal injury and non-operative management of solid-organ injury has heightened concerns about the potential for missing hollow

Box 6.2	Small bowel injury scale
Grade 1	Contusion or haematoma without devascularisation or partial thickness laceration with no perforation
Grade 2	Laceration <50% of circumference
Grade 3	Laceration >50% of circumference without transection
Grade 4	Transection of the small bowel
Grade 5	Transection of the bowel with segmental tissue loss or vascular injury with a devascularised segment

visceral injury. Physical examination, plain X-ray and abdominal CT may be unreliable in the diagnosis of blunt intestinal injury; indeed, only one-third of patients with blunt intestinal perforation display pneumoperitoneum on abdominal X-ray or CT. Delayed diagnosis increases complications and may result in death of the patient. An awareness of the difficulties in diagnosis of blunt small bowel injury, liberal use of radiological screening techniques and repeated, careful clinical examination by an experienced surgeon are the key to successful outcome. Diagnostic peritoneal lavage has a definite place in the investigation of suspected blunt small bowel injury.

Duodenal injuries merit special attention as they are much less common and are frequently associated with other highly lethal injuries. An AAST organ injury scale also classifies duodenal injuries. Most lower grade duodenal injuries can be treated by primary closure after debridement but resection and anastomosis, pyloric exclusion and pancreatoduodenectomy may be required for complex injuries, which often involve the distal common bile duct and pancreatic head.

Typhoid fever

Typhoid fever is caused by *Salmonella typhi*, a Gram-negative bacillus acquired by ingestion of contaminated water or food. The disease has a seasonal variation, peaking at times of heavy rainfall, and is prevalent in developing countries with poor sanitation and contamination of water sources. During the second week of symptomatic illness, bacteria localise in the Peyer's patches in the gut and ulceration occurs. Perforation classically occurs on the antimesenteric border of the terminal ileum. In 20% perforations may be multiple and can be small, with an average diameter of 5 mm. Typhoid perforation is commoner in men and in those under 40. The classic signs of perforation may be absent in the very toxic and if doubt persists after repeated abdominal examination, exploration should be undertaken. Patients have usually been ill and febrile for a week or more and vigorous, preoperative resuscitation with fluids, nasogastric aspiration and antibiotics is advised.

Chloramphenicol is the antibiotic of choice but resistance is recognised, particularly during epidemics, and combination therapy of chloramphenicol with ampicillin, metronidazole and gentamicin is usual. Quinolone antibiotics may give improved results.

The mortality of typhoid perforation may be up to 40% and the surgical procedure of choice is primary repair of the perforation. Segmental resection may be required for multiple perforations or for perforation of the caecum.

Foreign objects

The small bowel may be perforated by ingested material, such as sharp bones, clips or any other foreign object.

SMALL BOWEL DIVERTICULOSIS

Small bowel diverticulosis is rare, usually discovered incidentally during laparotomy, endoscopy or by imaging studies. Small bowel diverticula were first described by Soemmering and Baillie in 1794. The diverticula may be congenital or acquired; 45% occur in the duodenum and approximately 25% are Meckel's diverticula. Jejunal and ileal diverticula are less common. Nearly 80% of jejunoileal diverticula occur in the jejunum, 15% in the ileum and 5% in both. The majority of non-Meckelian diverticula are thought to be acquired, false diverticula in that they lack a true muscular wall. They are pulsion diverticula resulting from intestinal dyskinesis and the site of herniation appears to occur where paired blood vessels penetrate the mesentery into the bowel wall. Jejunoileal diverticular disease may present with malabsorption, bleeding, diverticulitis, perforation and obstruction (Figure 6.6). Rarely, enteroliths form within the diverticula, which may obstruct the lumen in the manner of gallstone ileus.

Symptomatic duodenal diverticula are usually treated with diverticulectomy. Resection and anastomosis is the treatment of choice for symptomatic jejunoileal diverticula.

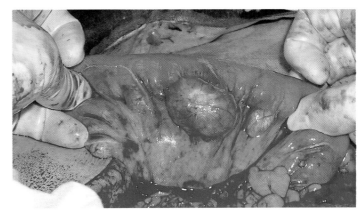

Figure 6.6 Jejunal diverticulum, an incidental finding at laparotomy.

Meckel's diverticulum

Johann Meckel described the diverticulum that bears his name in 1809 (Figure 6.7). Meckel's diverticulum is the most common congenital anomaly of the GI tract. A remnant of the vitellointestinal duct, it is found in 1–4% of individuals at postmortem. Meckel's diverticulum arises from the antimesenteric border of the ileum approximately 40 cm from the ileocaecal valve in adults; 75% will be between 1 and 5 cm long and may contain ileal, gastric, pancreatic or duodenal mucosa. In children, the most common complications are GI bleeding and bowel obstruction. Ectopic gastric secretions act on unprotected ileal mucosa, causing ulceration and bleeding. Radionuclide scanning with technetium-99m pertechnetate can usually be diagnostic by labelling parietal cells within ectopic gastric mucosa. In comparison, 50% of adults will present with acute inflammation of the diverticu-

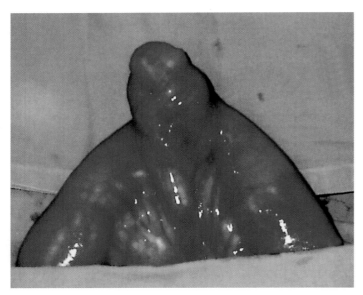

Figure 6.7 Meckel's diverticulum with a focus of ectopic gastric mucosa at the top.

lum, one-third present with bowel obstruction and <20% with rectal bleeding. Obstruction may be due to intussusception, bowel entrapment or kinking due to a mesodiverticular band, adhesions or a fibrous band connecting the tip of the diverticulum to the umbilicus. Rarely, neoplasms may arise in a Meckel's and umbilical suppuration may be the presenting feature. As a rule, asymptomatic Meckel's should not be resected.

SMALL BOWEL PATHOLOGY IN CHILDREN

The following conditions are seen in children.

- Necrotising enterocolitis
- Meconium ileus
- Intussusception
- Congenital abnormalities
- Milk curd obstruction (lactobezoar).

Necrotising enterocolitis

Necrotising enterocolitis (NEC) is the most common surgical emergency in the newborn. Up to half of babies with NEC develop advanced disease requiring surgical intervention. Options include peritoneal drainage under local anaesthetic, enterostomy only, resection and enterostomies, and resection with primary anastomosis. The primary risk factor for NEC is prematurity. Clinical features are abdominal distension, apnoeic attacks, refusal to feed, bloody diarrhoea and fever. Findings on plain abdominal

films include small bowel distension, gas in the portal venous system and pneumoperitoneum. The pathogenesis of NEC is multifactorial but is hypothesised to be due to an immature (inappropriate) enterocyte response to bacterial stimuli.

Meconium ileus

Meconium ileus (MI) affects 15% of neonates with cystic fibrosis. Clinical presentation includes abdominal distension, bilious vomiting and delayed passage of meconium. Uncomplicated MI can be managed non-operatively by Gastrografin™ enema. T-tube irrigation with n-acetylcysteine or pancreatic enzymes can be an effective and safe treatment if Gastrografin™ enema fails. Bowel resection with primary anastomosis may be necessary and occasionally stoma formation is employed.

Intussusception

An inflamed Peyer's patch may become the lead point for an intussusception, where a portion of bowel telescopes into an adjoining portion of bowel. Other causes of intussusception are tumours, worm boluses and Meckel's diverticulum. The mean age is around two years and the male to female ratio is generally around 4:1. The quartet of abdominal pain, bloody mucoid stools, abdominal mass and palpable rectal mass is present in around 70%. Ileo-colic intussusception is most common, occurring in 50% of children. Hydrostatic reduction (sometimes with ultrasound guidance) is the ideal first-line treatment for childhood intussusception. The success rate is around 80%.

Congenital abnormalities

Bilious vomiting in newborns, with or without abdominal distension, is an initial sign of intestinal obstruction. Mid-gut malrotation and volvulus, duodenal atresia, jejunoileal atresia, meconium ileus and NEC are the most common causes of neonatal intestinal obstruction.

Intestinal malrotation is a common cause of upper gastrointestinal obstruction and presents with duodenal obstruction caused by volvulus of the mid-gut loop. Patients are therefore at risk of catastrophic mid-gut infarction. Ladd's procedure is the treatment of choice.

Plain abdominal radiographs may show a double-bubble shadow in the duodenal atresia. The usual treatment for duodenal atresia is end-to-end anastomosis. Jejunoileal atresia can be divided into four groups:

- group I, membranous
- group II, interrupted
- group III, multiple
- group IV, apple peel.

Group I patients can be treated with membranectomy or bowel resection and anastomosis, group II with resection of the dilated bowel, group III with multiple anastomosis to preserve bowel length and group IV with minimal bowel resection and bowel anastomosis.

Annular pancreas is a rare congenital anomaly that usually presents in childhood with symptoms of duodenal obstruction.

Alimentary tract duplication cysts are rare congenital malformations, found primarily in children under the age of 15 years. Heterotopic gastric tissue has been reported in as many as one-third of patients with small intestine duplications and ulceration may lead to perforation.

Milk curd obstruction

Milk curd obstruction typically occurs in preterm infants aged 5–14 days who are being fed concentrated feeds. Improvements in the care of low-birthweight infants have seen a dramatic reduction in this complication.

OPERATIVE SURGERY

Small bowel resection

Historical background

The first recorded operation for small bowel obstruction was performed by Praxagoras in the third century BC when he relieved a strangulated inguinal hernia. Hieronymus Brunschwig undertook the first recorded bowel repair in 1525. However, progress in abdominal surgery was slow, with Baron Dominique Larrey, Surgeon-in-Chief to the French army under Napoleon, reporting only a single successful bowel repair throughout his distinguished career.

Travers was one of the first surgeons to consider intestinal repair in a scientific manner and published his 'Enquiry into the process of nature in repairing injuries to the intestine' in 1812. Lembert advocated careful approximation of the serosal surfaces of the bowel and devised his method of suturing in 1826. It was ten years, however, before Dieffenbach reported the first successful anastomosis of the small intestine using Lembert's method. In 1880, Czerny advocated an inner layer to achieve precise mucosal application and reduce the risk of leakage.

Despite this work, during the Boer War (1899–1902) the dismal results of laparotomy led Sir William MacCormac, the senior British surgeon, to advocate a non-operative strategy for penetrating abdominal wounds. In what became known as MacCormac's aphorism, he wrote: 'A man wounded in the abdomen dies if he is operated on and remains alive if he is left in peace'.

This thinking clouded the minds of military surgeons and at the outbreak of the First World War surgeons practised a non-operative

strategy in penetrating abdominal wounds. The mortality rate of this conservative policy was high (>80%). It was not until 1915 that the value of laparotomy and intestinal repair was established. Owen Richards, working with the British Expeditionary Force, introduced laparotomy for penetrating injuries to the abdomen with resection of damaged small bowel (to reduce the risk of stenosis) and primary repair of duodenal and colonic wounds. The mortality of small bowel injuries fell from 86% to 39%. Since then, progress in surgery has been rapid and intestinal repair, resection and anastomosis are now commonplace.

The word 'anastomosis' is derived from Greek meaning 'mouth to mouth' and there are many described techniques of joining two pieces of bowel together. The sutured techniques have changed little from their original description by Lembert and Czerny, except for evolution in the suture material. Hautefeille first described the single-layer continuous anastomosis in 1976. It has been demonstrated that the single-layer continuous technique is similar in safety to the double layer, but can be constructed in considerably less time and at lower cost. In recent years mechanical stapling devices have become popular but other anastomotic methods have been used, such as biofragmentable rings and even a skin stapler.

Surgical technique

Under general anaesthesia with full muscle relaxation and antimicrobial prophylaxis, the abdomen is opened via a mid-line incision. A careful, sequential examination of the intraabdominal organs is carried out and the small bowel pathology identified. Non-crushing bowel clamps are gently placed to occlude the lumen up- and downstream of the site of proposed bowel section. Care must be taken not to occlude the mesentery. The site of resection should be isolated from the rest of the laparotomy wound by the placement of swabs. The mesentery of the small bowel is then divided between clips, ensuring that the mesentery of the remaining bowel extends up to the wall at right angles to maintain adequate perfusion of the bowel ends. After resection of the specimen, the bowel ends to be joined together are approximated, ensuring they lie next to each other without tension and with no twists. The mesenteric borders should lie together.

Sutured anastomosis

The suture is a continuous, double-needle 3–0 polypropylene beginning at the mesenteric border. All layers of the bowel wall are incorporated, except the mucosa. Each bite should include 4–6 mm of the seromuscular wall, the larger bites being taken at the mesenteric border to ensure an adequate seal. Each stitch is advanced approximately 5 mm. To avoid ischaemia at the anastomosis, the surgeon must ensure that enough pressure is applied to approximate the ends of the bowel and ensure a watertight seal. The suture is tied at the antimesenteric border with care being taken to tie a square knot, so as not to create a pursestring effect.

Stapled anastomosis

Resection of the diseased segment of small bowel can be achieved very simply with a GIA stapler™. The ends of the bowel are then placed side to side, with the mesenteries together, and a small hole made in the suture line at the end of the bowel at the antimesenteric border. A limb of the GIA stapler™ is placed down each length of bowel and the device is closed together. Once the device is fired a side-to-side but functionally end-to-end anastomosis is created.

However the anastomosis is constructed, the mesenteric defect should be closed, avoiding placement of sutures through vessels supplying the anastomosis. The abdomen may be lavaged with water or saline at body temperature and the abdomen is then closed in the usual manner.

Postoperative care

Postoperatively, the patient should be managed on a surgical ward. Traditionally, oral intake would be restricted until the postoperative ileus had resolved and GI motility restored. However, there is increasing evidence that controlled oral intake is not harmful to anastomotic integrity even from very early in the postoperative course. Early mobilisation and chest physiotherapy are important to reduce thromboembolic and respiratory morbidity. Epidural catheters placed by the anaesthetist have made a great contribution to postoperative analgesia.

FURTHER READING

Caplin ME, Buscombe JR, Hilson AJ, Jones AL, Watkinson AF, Burroughs AK. Carcinoid tumour, *Lancet* 1998; **352**:799–805

Coleman MG, Moran BJ. Small bowel obstruction. *Recent Adv Surg* 1999; **22**:87–98

Crump M, Gospodarowicz M, Shepherd F. Lymphoma of the gastrointestinal tract. *Semin Oncol* 1999; **26**(3):324–337

Danzig JB, Brandt LJ, Reinus JF, Klein RS. Gastrointestinal malignancy in patients with AIDS. *Am J Gastroenterol* 1991; **86**(6):715–718

Desai DC, Neale KF, Talbot IC, Hodgson SV, Phillips RKS. Juvenile Polyposis. *Br J Surg* 1995; **82**(1):14–7

Fakhry SM, Brownstein M, Watts DD, Baker CC, Oller D. Relatively short diagnostic delays (<8 hours) produce morbidity and mortality in blunt small bowel injury: an analysis of time to operative intervention in 198 patients from a multicentre experience. *J Trauma* 2000; **48**(3):408–415

Lev D, Kariv Y, Issakov J et al. Gastrointestinal stromal sarcomas. *Br J Surg* 1999; **86**:545–549

Lewis BS. Small intestinal bleeding. *Gastroenterology Clin North Am* 2000; **29**(1):67–95

McGarrity TJ. Peutz–Jeghers syndrome. *Am J Gastroenterol* 2000; **95**(3):596–604

Useful websites

American Association for the Surgery of Trauma: www.aast.org

7

Acute pancreatitis: pathophysiology

Derek A. O'Reilly, Taiichi Otani, Andrew N. Kingsnorth

A clinically based classification system for acute pancreatitis was adopted at the Atlanta symposium of 1992. This defined acute pancreatitis as 'an acute inflammatory process of the pancreas, with variable involvement of other regional tissues or remote organ systems'. The development of complications distinguishes a mild attack from a severe one, irrespective of whether the complications are local (e.g. necrosis, abscess or pseudocyst) or systemic.

Despite extensive research efforts, the pathogenesis of acute pancreatitis remains poorly understood. This is attributable to the inaccessibility of the pancreas to observation. Consequently, much of the understanding of acute pancreatitis is derived from animal models of the disease. Although this has facilitated great progress in the delineation of the events that occur in acute pancreatitis, therapies derived from these models have proved to have low translational potential when applied to the human condition. With this important proviso in mind, the pathophysiological events that occur in acute pancreatitis are described below.

THE PATHOPHYSIOLOGY OF ACUTE PANCREATITIS: OVERVIEW

Acute pancreatitis is a disease of varied aetiology (Box 7.1), yet each produces a similar pattern of disease, indicating that they all converge at a common point, to initiate a cascade of events resulting in pancreatitis. The overwhelming evidence indicates that this common event involves the activation of pancreatic proenzymes (zymogens) and the retention of active enzymes within the acinar cell. These activated enzymes injure the acinar cells, which initiate secretion of cytokines and chemokines, resulting in the recruitment of inflammatory cells, such as neutrophils and macrophages. This further amplifies the inflammatory reaction and the extent of pancreatic injury. The degree to which these mediators escape into the circulation determines the nature of the systemic inflammatory response. Finally, if resolution fails to occur pancreatic infection may supervene (Figure 7.1).

Acinar cell events

In 1896, Chiari postulated that the underlying pathophysiological mechanism of the disease was pancreatic autodigestion, suggesting that the pancreas of patients with acute pancreatitis 'succumbs to its own digestive properties'. Evidence that the protease/inhibitor mechanism is of prime importance in the early stages of pancreatitis includes the identification of mutations in the genes encoding cationic trypsinogen and its inhibitor, serine protease inhibitor, Kazal type 1 (SPINK1), in hereditary and idiopathic pancreatitis. In addition, prophylactic treatment with the synthetic serine protease inhibitor gabexate mesilate (FOY) reduces the incidence of acute pancreatitis related to endoscopic retrograde cholangiopancreatography (ERCP).

Box 7.1 Known aetiology factors for acute pancreatitis. The most frequent aetiologies are gallstones and alcohol. In 10–30%, the aetiology remains unknown (idiopathic acute pancreatitis). CFTR, cystic fibrosis transmembrane conductance regulator.

Mechanical causes (obstruction)	Gallstones
	Gastric/biliary surgery
	Pancreas divisum
	Trauma
	ERCP
	Tumours
	Helminthic infestation
	Duodenal obstruction
Metabolic causes	Alcohol
	Hypertriglyceridaemia
	Hypercalcaemia
	Drugs, e.g.
	azathioprine
	sulphonamides
	tetracycline
	oestrogens
	frusemide
	5-ASA compounds
	corticosteroids
	Scorpion venom
Infective causes	Mumps
	Coxsackie B
	Cytomegalovirus
	Cryptococcus
	HIV
	Yersinia enterocolitica
	Salmonella
Vascular causes (ischaemia)	Cardiopulmonary bypass
	Periarteritis nodosa
	Embolism
Genetic causes	Hereditary pancreatitis
	CFTR mutations

The mechanism whereby pancreatic proteases are prematurely activated remains controversial. The two most prominent theories are the cathepsin B activation of trypsinogen and trypsinogen autoactivation hypotheses.

Using the caerulein-induced model of pancreatitis in rats, Steer and co-workers have demonstrated that co-localisation of lysosomal hydrolase (cathepsin B) and zymogen (trypsinogen) occurs during the early stages of pancreatitis. It is proposed that a sorting error occurs such that cathepsin B is directed away from the normal regulated secretory pathway and that this is linked to a blockade of acinar cell secretion. As cathepsin B can activate trypsinogen and trypsin can activate each of the other proenzymes, a pathway to premature digestive enzyme activation can be established. Cellular injury occurs when the organelles containing activated enzymes become fragile and rupture, releasing their contents into the cytoplasm.

As predicted by this hypothesis, co-localisation and trypsinogen activation precede other early changes of caerulein-induced pancreatitis, such as hyperamylasaemia and pancreatic oedema, and trypsinogen activation occurs within the vacuoles that contain co-localised cathepsin B and trypsinogen. In addition, the cathepsin

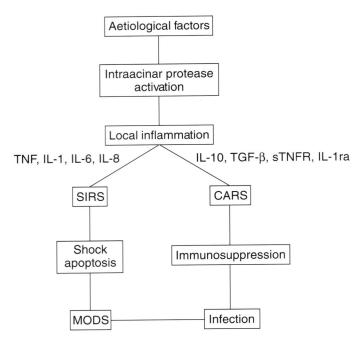

```
           Aetiological factors

        Intraacinar protease
            activation

           Local inflammation

TNF, IL-1, IL-6, IL-8        IL-10, TGF-β, sTNFR, IL-1ra

      SIRS              CARS

    Shock          Immunosuppression
   apoptosis

    MODS               Infection
```

Figure 7.1 Overview of the pathophysiological events that may occur in acute pancreatitis. Homeostasis may be restored if balance between the pro- and anti-inflammatory responses is achieved. SIRS, systemic inflammatory response syndrome; CARS, compensatory antiinflammatory response syndrome; MODS, multiorgan dysfunction syndrome.

B inhibitor E64D prevents *in vitro* caerulein-induced trypsinogen activation.

An alternative explanation for trypsinogen activation suggests that activation occurs at some point along the normal protease secretory pathway. In this model, trypsinogen activation occurs under conditions of low pH and in the presence of calcium, the process becoming pathological with secretory blockade. This hypothesis emphasises the unique features of human trypsinogen, which has the ability to autoactivate. Thus, human trypsinogen may not require lysosome–zymogen co-localisation for pancreatitis to occur. Evidence supporting this hypothesis includes studies that show that zymogen processing takes place in a low pH compartment that overlaps with granule membrane protein 92 (GRAMP-92), a marker of lysosomes and recycling endosomes, suggesting that zymogen processing occurs outside the classic secretory pathway.

Finally, both zymogen activation and retention of activated enzymes may be needed to cause pancreatitis. Disruption of the secretory mechanism and the apical actin cytoskeleton may result in active enzymes being retained in the acinar cell.

Local inflammation

Inflammation is the body's initial non-specific response to tissue injury produced by mechanical, chemical or microbial stimuli. The inflammatory process consists of four major events: vasodilatation, increased microvascular permeability, cellular activation/adhesion and coagulation. Cytokines are the physiological

messengers of the inflammatory response. These are peptides and lipids, released from cells to act by autocrine, paracrine and endocrine means, to mediate inflammation and its resolution. The principal proinflammatory cytokines involved are tumour necrosis factor (TNF), interleukins (IL-1, IL-6), interferons (IFN) and colony-stimulating factors (CSF). Neutrophils, monocytes/macrophages and endothelial cells are the cellular effectors of the inflammatory response. Leucocyte activation leads to increased leucocyte aggregation and tissue infiltration, where further cytokines and other inflammatory mediators are produced. Endothelial cells also become activated and express adhesion molecules and receptors on their surface.

It has become increasingly recognised that the body also launches an antiinflammatory response in an attempt to ensure that the effects of proinflammatory mediators do not become destructive. Antiinflammatory agents include IL-4, IL-10, IL-11, IL-13, soluble TNF receptors, IL-1 receptor antagonist (IL-1ra) and transforming growth factor beta. Antiinflammatory mediators are known to alter monocyte function, impair antigen-presenting activity and inhibit the production of proinflammatory cytokines.

Systemic inflammation

Terminology and new concepts

The American College of Chest Physicians (ACCP)/Society of Critical Care Medicine (SCCM) consensus conference of 1991 standardised the terminology used concerning systemic inflammation, sepsis and its sequelae (Box 7.2). The rationale for the use of

---

Box 7.2 Definitions of SIRS, sepsis and MODS. Modified from: American College of Chest Physicians/Society of Critical Care Medicine Consensus Conference. Definitions for sepsis and organ failure and guidelines for the use of innovative therapies in sepsis. *Crit Care Med* 1992; **20**: 864–874.

Systemic inflammatory response syndrome (SIRS): This response is manifested by two or more of the following conditions:
  Temperature >38°C or <36°C
  Heart rate >90 beats/min
  Respiratory rate >20 breaths/min or $PaCO_2$ <4.3 kPa
  White blood cell count <4000 or >12 000 cells/mm³ or >10% immature (band) forms.

Sepsis: This response is manifested when two or more of the above conditions occur as a result of infection.

Severe sepsis: Sepsis associated with organ dysfunction, hypoperfusion or hypotension. Hypoperfusion abnormalities may include, but are not limited to, lactic acidosis, oliguria or an acute alteration in mental status. Hypotension is a systolic BP of <90 mmHg or a reduction of >40 mmHg from baseline.

Septic shock: Sepsis with hypotension, despite adequate fluid resuscitation, along with the presence of hypoperfusion abnormalities.

Multiple organ dysfunction syndrome (MODS): Presence of altered organ function in an acutely ill patient such that homeostasis cannot be maintained without intervention.

the term SIRS to describe the clinical condition produced by infectious insults and non-infectious causes is based upon their similar pathogenesis and their similar, or even identical, clinical picture.

It has become increasingly recognised that the ACCP/SCCM model contains a fundamental flaw: an overemphasis has been placed on proinflammatory mediators while the opposite and compensatory antiinflammatory response (CARS) has been ignored. If CARS is sufficiently severe, it will manifest itself clinically as an inadequate immune response and increased susceptibility to infection.

New theories have been proposed to integrate both sides of the inflammatory response. Proinflammatory and antiinflammatory mediators can be viewed as opposing forces, which often become unbalanced. If the mediators balance each other at the local inflammatory level, homeostasis is restored. If this does not occur, spillover of mediators into the systemic circulation will result. If balance cannot be established there and homeostasis restored, SIRS or CARS will develop. A range of clinical sequelae may then follow. If SIRS predominates, cardiovascular shock, organ dysfunction and apoptosis may develop, whereas immune suppression is the characteristic feature of a predominant CARS. Restoration of homeostasis results if SIRS and CARS achieve equilibrium.

Pathophysiology

Loss of control of local inflammation results in the systemic response, SIRS. Whilst vasodilatation and increased microvascular permeability occurring in a localised inflammatory process result in a beneficial increased delivery of oxygen and other nutrients, systemic microvascular activation produces hypotension and extravascular fluid loss. Coupled with the circulatory changes, cardiac contractility is depressed. Failure to correct this adverse haemodynamic response, either physiologically or therapeutically, results in end-organ hypoperfusion, oedema, initiation of anaerobic metabolism and end-organ dysfunction, i.e. MODS.

Other microcirculatory changes also contribute to the development of end-organ dysfunction. As the circulation becomes flooded with inflammatory mediators, capillary wall integrity is lost. This allows activated leucocytes and cytokines to escape into end organs, producing additional sites of damage.

Decreased capillary blood flow results from decreased perfusion pressure, a failure to allow the normal passage of blood cells and adherence of leucocytes to the endothelium, creating increased resistance to flow. Coupled with this, a procoagulant environment is produced. These profound microcirculatory changes lead to the development of microthrombi, further obstructing blood flow and producing an exacerbation of MODS.

Inflammatory mediators and acute pancreatitis

The following is a brief and selective account of some inflammatory mediators whose antagonism shows therapeutic promise.

Tumour necrosis factor

Tumour necrosis factor (TNF) is a proximal mediator of the host response to infection and inflammation. TNF is produced predominantly by macrophage/monocytes in response to a variety of inflammatory stimuli. It binds to two receptors, which are expressed on nearly all nucleated cells. TNF receptor signal transduction employs intracytoplasmic proteins, such as the transcription factor nuclear factor-kappa B (NF-κB). Expression of NF-κB increases the transcription rate of a great variety of genes encoding cytokines, adhesion molecules and enzymes.

A number of studies have examined the relationship between TNF and acute pancreatitis in humans. However, assaying serum TNF levels in acute pancreatitis is problematic, due to its short half-life and phasic release, the masking effects of circulating inhibitors and its mainly paracrine level of function. Therefore, in order to avoid the pitfalls associated with measuring this cytokine in serum, leucocyte *in vitro* TNF secretion has been measured. Peak lipopolysaccharide-stimulated TNF secretion has been shown to be significantly higher in patients who develop systemic complications than those with an uncomplicated course. An alternative strategy is to assay the soluble TNF receptors (sTNFR), on the basis that this reflects the degree of TNF-induced inflammation. Recent studies have confirmed the value of sTNFR as a severity marker in acute pancreatitis and strengthened the view that TNF is a central mediator in the development of SIRS and MODS in acute pancreatitis.

A number of experiments have examined the consequences of TNF inhibition in animal models of pancreatitis. Using transgenic knockout mice, deficient in TNF type 1 receptor, IL-1 type 1 receptor or both, a nearly identical beneficial effect on the severity and mortality of acute pancreatitis was observed when TNF or IL-1 activity was prevented. Using another novel approach, the molecule CNI-1493, which is known to inhibit macrophage production of TNF and IL-1 by inhibiting translation of TNF mRNA into protein, was shown to inhibit cytokine gene processing in both mild and severe models of acute pancreatitis. This posttranscription blockade of TNF production resulted in dramatic reductions in tissue damage and disease severity.

Most studies have examined pre-treatment regimens. This does not directly relate to the clinical situation where TNF antagonism must show benefit after the disease has commenced. The future role of TNF antagonism in acute pancreatitis remains unclear but those investigating it must take into account the beneficial antimicrobial action of TNF, evidence of adverse outcome with its antagonism and the failure of this modality in sepsis.

Interleukin-1

The interleukin-1 family consists of three distinct proteins: IL-1α, IL-1β and IL-1 receptor antagonist (IL-1ra), a naturally occurring inhibitor of IL-1. The macrophage is the primary cell of IL-1 production. The effects of IL-1 include increased cytokine production, enhancement of haematopoiesis and activation of neutrophils, monocytes, platelets and the endothelium.

As a prototypic multifunctional cytokine affecting nearly every cell type, IL-1 is believed to be at the forefront of the cascade of mediators that lead to SIRS and MODS in AP. The temporal dynamics of IL-1 in acute pancreatitis have recently been evaluated in 50 consecutive patients, by serial determination of serum concentration within the first week of admission. The median peak value of IL-1 was reached on day 1 and thereafter decreased rapidly. Levels on days 1, 2, 3, 4 and 7 were significantly higher in severe than in mild pancreatitis. Imbalance of the ratio of circulating IL-1β to IL-1ra has also recently been demonstrated in patients with severe acute pancreatitis and pulmonary failure.

IL-1 inhibition has been extensively investigated in many models, by means such as IL-1ra administration, IL-1 receptor gene targeting and IL-1 converting enzyme (ICE) inactivation. These experiments indicate that IL-1 antagonism may be a promising therapeutic strategy. Importantly, delayed administration of an effective dose of IL-1ra has been shown to be almost as protective as prophylactic administration. Studies with knockout mice, genetically deficient in the IL-1 receptor, have elegantly demonstrated the extent to which IL-1 contributes to the propagation of pancreatitis.

Chemokines

Chemokines are chemotactic cytokines that mediate the movement and activation of leucocytes in inflammation. Over 40 chemokines have been identified to date. Chemokines bind to specific G-protein coupled cell-surface receptors on target cells. These receptors activate multiple signalling pathways, which regulate the actin-dependent intracellular machinery that propels the cell in its chosen direction. The capacity to control precisely the movement of leucocytes during an inflammatory process suggests that chemokines and their receptors may provide novel targets for therapeutic intervention.

Interleukin-8 (IL-8) is a chemokine that is chemotactic for neutrophils and stimulates their activation. In clinical studies, IL-8 is detected early in the course of acute pancreatitis. Levels are higher in severe pancreatitis compared with the mild form of the disease and precede, by several hours, the rise in serum polymorphonuclear elastase levels that indicate neutrophil activation. A recent study has shown that the activation of chemokine genes is an important early event in experimental pancreatitis. The cellular source of pancreatic chemokine expression was identified as the acinar cells, rather than infiltrating leucocytes.

Interleukin-10

Interleukin-10 (IL-10) is a global inhibitor of cytokine production. It is elaborated from multiple sources and has diverse cellular effects to regulate immune and inflammatory responses. IL-10 has

therefore attracted much attention because of its therapeutic promise as an immunomodulating and antiinflammatory agent.

Endogenous IL-10 is produced during the course of experimental pancreatitis and plays a protective role during the local and systemic evolution of the disease. The short half-life of IL-10 has prompted some groups to attempt gene therapy delivery systems with viral and human IL-10. This demonstrated a protective effect in caerulein pancreatitis amongst animals with prior IL-10 transfection.

Some reports concerning serum levels of IL-10 during the clinical course of human pancreatitis suggest significant elevation in mild but not in severe disease. This finding supports the view that down regulation of the compensatory antiinflammatory response occurs in those who develop severe acute pancreatitis. In contrast, others have found IL-10 to be an early marker of severity. This may be indicative of a role for T lymphocyte activation in early acute pancreatitis. As IL-10 has the capacity to modulate inflammatory and immune pathways at multiple points in the inflammatory cascade, it deserves further evaluation as a damage-limiting agent in acute pancreatitis.

Infection

Acute necrotising pancreatitis occurs in 15–20% of patients with AP. Infection occurs in 40–70% of this group. Organisms responsible for infection of pancreatic and peripancreatic necrosis consist primarily of Gram-negative bacteria, i.e. *Escherichia coli*, Pseudomonas spp, Klebsiella spp and Proteus spp. Infection with Gram-positive organisms, such as *Staphylococcus aureus* and *Streptococcus faecalis*, is also significant. There is recent evidence that anaerobic and fungal infection is increasing, since the advent of widespread antibiotic use. The recognition that it is colonic bacteria that frequently cause pancreatic infection fits with the theory of bacterial translocation, whereby the gut acts as a reservoir from which bacteria can pass to colonise pancreatic necrosis and acute fluid collections, resulting in infected necrosis and abscess formation.

Pharmacokinetic studies reveal that imipenem alone or combinations of metronidazole with either ciprofloxacin, ofloxacin or mezlocillin have the highest bactericidal activity in pancreatic infection and achieve optimal therapeutic levels in pancreatic tissue and necrosis. Antibiotic prophylaxis to prevent infected pancreatic necrosis is supported by a number of studies and is widely practised but still awaits validation by a large-scale, prospective, randomised, double-blind, placebo-controlled trial.

Individual susceptibility to pancreatitis and pancreatitis severity

Genetic factors substantially influence the production of cytokines. In acute pancreatitis, polymorphisms associated with low production of IL-1ra have been associated with severity of acute pancreatitis. Polymorphisms associated with high TNF and low

IL-10 production have also been associated with a worse outcome. Mutations of the cationic trypsinogen gene have been determined to be disease-causing genes in hereditary pancreatitis, which is characterised by recurrent episodes of acute pancreatitis progressing to chronic pancreatitis. SPINK1 is a disease-modifying gene that may lower the threshold for developing pancreatitis amongst those who possess it. Both genes have also been identified in patients with idiopathic chronic pancreatitis and, to a lesser extent, other sporadic forms of pancreatitis. Mutations of the cystic fibrosis transmembrane conductance regulator gene have also been associated with idiopathic chronic pancreatitis but the clinical significance of this remains unclear. The genetic elucidation of susceptibility to and severity of acute pancreatitis remains in its infancy. Further research should reveal a broad range of susceptibility genes that influence the onset and course of this condition.

POTENTIAL THERAPEUTIC IMPLICATIONS

Damage control

Although inhibiting the deranged intracellular processes that occur within the acinar cell during acute pancreatitis, e.g. with serine protease inhibitors, may seem an attractive therapeutic proposition, clinical trials have not realised this promise. The failure of this approach has been attributed to the fact that patients present some hours to days after the onset of pancreatitis. Such drugs may be effective in damage prevention, e.g. ERCP-induced pancreatitis, but not in damage control. Thus, attention has been redirected at treatments that limit the propagating factors. In this regard the antagonism of selected inflammatory mediators is an approach which shows therapeutic promise.

Genetic factors

The success or failure of anticytokine therapy will depend upon our ability to deliver the right drug, at the right time, to the right patient. This means much more than simply identifying agents that are effective against the inflammatory process in experimental models. The inflammatory profiles of patients with AP require much greater delineation. Account must also be taken of how these profiles may alter during the course of the disease. Ultimately, clinically applicable tests are required that will accurately profile the correct systemic inflammatory state of an individual patient. The propensity for interindividual variation in the nature of the inflammatory response mounted, against injury or infection, also needs to be considered, as this appears to have a significant genetic basis. A knowledge of an individual's genetic programming may allow us to target, with even greater accuracy, those who may benefit from novel therapies directed against the endogenous mediators of inflammatory disease.

The interventional window

An optimal timing for delivering damage-limiting interventions has recently been proposed. This 'interventional window' exists between the time of patient presentation and the onset of the development of organ dysfunction (Figure 7.2). Typically, the former occurs at 12–18 hours after disease onset whilst, for the latter, the incidence rises rapidly on the second and third day, distinguishing those likely to have a complicated attack from those likely to have a mild attack. Cytokine production begins shortly after disease onset but does not peak until 36–48 hours later. This scenario provides a potential therapeutic window of opportunity that begins at hospital presentation and may last for 2–3 days, during which inflammatory mediator antagonism could be employed in an attempt to attenuate the development of MODS. Current clinical trials utilise such a framework to dictate the timing of the intervention.

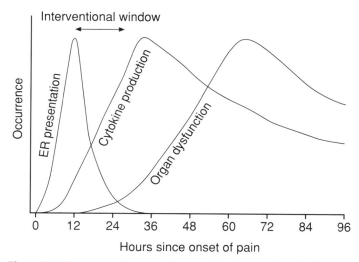

Figure 7.2 Time course of pancreatitis progression demonstrating the therapeutic or interventional window. During this period, inflammatory mediator antagonism could be administered to attenuate or block the development of organ dysfunction. Reprinted from Norman J *Am J Surg* 1998 **175**: 76–83, with permission from Excerpta Medica Inc.

FURTHER READING

Gorelick FS, Otani T. Mechanisms of intracellular zymogen activation. *Baillière's Clin Gastroenterol* 1999; **13**:227–240

Karne S, Gorelick FS. Etiopathogenesis of acute pancreatitis. *Surg Clin North Am* 1999; **79**:699–710

Norman J. The role of cytokines in the pathogenesis of acute pancreatitis. *Am J Surg* 1998; **175**:76–83

O'Reilly DA, Kingsnorth AN. Damage-limitation strategies in acute pancreatitis. In: Wig JD, ed. *The Pancreas*. Chandigarh: Azad Printers, 1999: 117–167

Whitcomb DC. Early trypsinogen activation in acute pancreatitis (selected summaries). *Gastroenterology* 1999; **116**:770–773

8

Surgical complications of acute pancreatitis

Dhia Al-Musawi, Geoffrey Glazer

Despite the apparent improvements in the management of acute pancreatitis, including the availability of dynamic computed tomography (CT), advances in the intensive therapy unit (ITU) care of the critically ill patient and the improvement in operative strategy for septic complications, the overall mortality has remained unaltered at around 10–15% for the last 20 years. The disease is usually mild and self-limiting, but in one-fifth to one-quarter of patients it is severe, with systemic or local complications. Approximately 1 in 4 patients who developed complications will die. The UK guidelines for management of acute pancreatitis recommend that complex or severe pancreatitis should be managed in specialist units.

DEFINITIONS

An international symposium in Atlanta on acute pancreatitis developed clinically based definitions of the disease and its local complications. Many of the previous terms, such as phlegmon, haemorrhagic or oedematous pancreatitis, have now been abandoned.

The Atlanta group defined the severity of the disease as follows.

- *Mild acute pancreatitis* is an attack with minimal organ dysfunction and an uneventful recovery. It constitutes 80% of all attacks and is usually predicted as mild by different scoring systems.

- *Severe acute pancreatitis* is associated with organ failure and/or local complications. It is characterised by three or more Ranson criteria or eight or more APACHE II (Acute Physiology and Chronic Health Evaluation) points. These patients are critically ill, have longer hospital and ITU stay and often require surgery with aggressive organ and ventilatory support. Many patients do, however, die in the first few days of a severe attack from multiple system and organ failure.

SURGICAL COMPLICATIONS OF SEVERE ACUTE PANCREATITIS

The following are important local complications of severe acute pancreatitis.

- Acute fluid collections
- Sterile pancreatic/peripancreatic necrosis
- Infected pancreatic/peripancreatic necrosis
- Pancreatic abscess
- Pseudocyst

Acute fluid collections

Acute fluid collections occur early in the course of acute pancreatitis, are located in or near the pancreas and always lack a wall of

granulation or fibrous tissue. These fluid collections occur in 30–50% of patients with severe acute pancreatitis. The majority are multiple and may communicate with each other and/or the pancreatic duct. They are rarely demonstrable by physical examination and are usually discovered with different imaging techniques including ultrasound (US), computed tomography (CT) or magnetic resonance imaging (MRI).

The precise composition of these collections is variable. The fluid may be clear or thick with inflammatory debris from the pancreatic or peripancreatic necrotic tissues. The amylase content is high. The wall is thin, ill-defined and usually made from the adjacent serosal and omental membranes in the lesser and/or greater sac of the peritoneal cavity. Occasionally these fluid collections occur in the paracolic gutters, mediastinum, pleural cavity or the pericardium. More than half resolve spontaneously. The remainder which persist may develop into a pseudocyst. Infection is not uncommon in these collections and usually presents with fever, abdominal pain and raised inflammatory markers (white cell count and C-reactive protein). Occasionally low-grade infection over a period of a few weeks may lead to a true pancreatic abscess.

Rupture of one or more of these localised collections into the peritoneal cavity may also occur. This can cause sudden abdominal pain, vomiting, tachycardia and a tender abdomen. The serum amylase and CRP may increase. The treatment at this stage remains conservative as the fluid is gradually absorbed from the peritoneal cavity, usually without systemic major side effect. However, if there is a large communication with the pancreatic duct, the fluid leak into the peritoneal cavity or even the pleural cavity may continue and this will lead to pancreatic ascites (Figure 8.1).

In summary, the outcomes of acute fluid collections are:

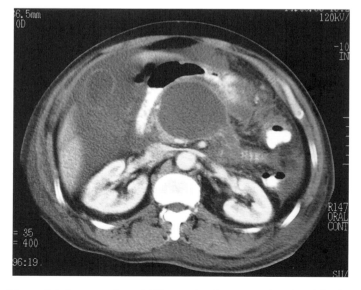

Figure 8.1 Contrast-enhanced CT scan showing pancreatic ascites following rupture of multiple fluid collections. This was treated conservatively.

- resolution

- rupture

- infection

- pseudocyst

- pancreatic ascites.

Management of acute fluid collections

The management of acute fluid collections is basically observation along with routine conservative and supportive therapy. Octreotide (a long-acting somatostatin analogue) reduces pancreatic secretions and may be used occasionally if there is a ductal leak. As the majority of acute fluid collections resolve spontaneously, they do not require specific surgical or interventional therapy in a stable patient. Percutaneous drainage in the absence of sepsis is not required. Such unnecessary intervention merely increases the risk of introducing infection. The possibility of infection in acute fluid collection must be actively pursued by the use of CT (or ultrasound) guided fine needle aspiration. The aspirate should be examined by urgent Gram stain and culture. If sepsis is suspected, the initial treatment may be empirical with antibiotics like cefotaxime and metronidazole to cover Gram-negative coliforms, Gram-positive cocci and anaerobes. Appropriate antibiotics are used once positive culture results are obtained. Imipenem is an alternative critical antibiotic as it has a good pancreatic penetration. Subsequent management is determined by the extent of any underlying necrosis (see below).

Sterile pancreatic/peripancreatic necrosis

Definition

Pancreatic necrosis is a diffuse or focal area(s) of non-viable pancreatic parenchyma, which is typically associated with peripancreatic fat necrosis. It is one of the serious consequences of a severe form of the disease because of the risk of infection. The development of pancreatic and peripancreatic necrosis is a critical factor in the course of acute pancreatitis and is a main determinant of the prognosis.

Diagnosis

Pancreatic and peripancreatic necrosis can be diagnosed by bolus intravenous contrast-enhanced computed tomography (CT) at an early stage in the disease. In contrast to the normal pancreas, the necrotic area(s) does not take up the contrast and looks underperfused on CT scanning. The sensitivity of CT improves after a week of the onset of symptoms, as the demarcation of necrosis in the pancreatic region will take place. The usual policy is to perform contrast-enhanced CT within the first week after admission for patients with predicted severe pancreatitis. Heterogeneous densities in the peripancreatic fat represent a combination of fat necrosis, fluid collections and haemorrhage. As a result, the extent of peripancreatic fat necrosis cannot be reliably determined with CT. Whether MRI will add to the detection of pancreatic or peripancreatic necrosis is uncertain at this time.

Many serum markers have been proposed as indicators for pancreatic necrosis such as CRP, polymorphonuclear neutrophil elastase and trypsinogen activation peptide (TAP), but none has proved to be totally reliable.

Management of sterile pancreatic necrosis

The clinical distinction between sterile and infected pancreatic necrosis is important as the development of infection in the necrotic tissue results in a trebling of mortality risk. Furthermore, whilst many patients with sterile necrosis can be treated without surgical intervention, infected necrosis requires surgical debridement and drainage. The initial management of patients with sterile necrosis is conservative. This includes full organ support and continuous monitoring, preferably in a high-dependency unit. The majority of these patients with documented sterile necrosis recover gradually without surgical intervention. However, in a small number of cases, the clinical condition may continue to deteriorate and these patients may benefit from operation even in the absence of documented infection. The decision to operate is a finely balanced one. The operation involves debridement of the necrotic tissue and drainage of the pancreatic region (pancreatic necrosectomy).

The timing of intervention is variable and it reflects two schools of thought: enthusiasm for early aggressive surgery or a preference for delayed intervention. The literature is confusing, as many series comprise a mixture of patients with either infected or sterile necrosis. The co-morbid state of these patients is also variable. What seems clear is that early operation (i.e. radical surgery within 1–2 weeks) is associated with high morbidity and mortality. It is preferable to nurse the patient through the initial multiple system organ failure and to allow the acute systemic effects of pancreatitis to subside.

The onset of infection may be marked by rapid deterioration and drainage (surgical or radiological) will then be necessary (see below). Patient selection for surgery is critical and difficult prior to a 'septic collapse'.

Possible indications for intervention in pancreatic necrosis without proven infection include the following.

- Deterioration in clinical condition despite full intensive therapy ('failure to thrive').

- Persistent organ failure despite maximum ITU treatment.

Infected pancreatic necrosis

Definition

Infected pancreatic necrosis is an infection of devitalised pancreatic and/or peripancreatic, retroperitoneal tissue which is proven by a positive smear or culture for bacteria or fungi.

Incidence

Overall infection rates in acute pancreatitis do not exceed 10%, but infection occurs in up to 70% of patients with a necrotising pancreatitis and is associated with a high mortality rate up to 60%. Animal and human studies have shown that bacterial contamination can occur in the first few days of acute necrotising pancreatitis, but this may not manifest itself until the second or third week of the illness. The infection rate increases with the extent of parenchymal necrosis, number of acute fluid collections and the duration of the disease. Patients with three or more acute fluid collections or with 50% or more of the gland necrosis have a 70% chance of becoming infected.

Bacteriology

Animal and bacteriological studies have demonstrated that the most likely source of pancreatic infection is bacterial translocation from the small intestine and colon. The most frequently isolated organisms in infected pancreatic necrosis are Gram-negative bacteria, such as *Escherichia coli* and Enterobacter. Other organisms include *Staphylococcus aureus* and Enterococcus and fungi such as *Candida albicans* are also reported. Patients with infected necrosis may have a high fever, tachycardia, tachypnoea, leucocytosis and one or more organ failures.

Diagnosis

In view of the high morbidity and mortality associated with infection, the diagnosis is critical. CT scan or plain abdominal radiography may occasionally show gas bubbles in the necrotic area consistent with anaerobic infection, but this is a sign of advanced infection. The diagnosis should be made earlier with CT or ultrasound-guided fine needle aspiration with Gram staining and culture of the aspirate from the necrotic area. This test for infected pancreatic necrosis has a high sensitivity and specificity.

Prevention

Part of the initial treatment of patients with severe acute pancreatitis will be an attempt to prevent infection in the retroperitoneum. The routine prophylactic use of antibiotics soon after admission is recommended, usually in the form of cefuroxime and metronidazole or imipenem. The evidence is based on a number of small trials which have not all shown significant improvement in survival. However, the ethical and practical problems of now running a further trial mean that antibiotics are currently an accepted therapy in patients with necrotising pancreatitis.

Other methods to prevent bacterial translocation from the gut have included selective gut decontamination or early enteral feeding via a nasogastric or nasojejunal tube. These reports are based on small studies and have shown improvement in inflammatory markers and a reduction in septic complication but no reduction in overall mortality.

Management of patients with infected pancreatic necrosis

These patients should be managed in an ITU with continuous monitoring and full systems support. All patients with documented infected necrosis need surgical intervention as the mortality without surgery is high, approaching 80–90%. The goal of surgical therapy is to remove the necrotic extrapancreatic and pancreatic tissue, preserve intact vital pancreatic tissue and to allow postoperative irrigation and drainage of the pancreatic bed. Percutaneous drainage procedures may temporise but do not usually allow proper debridement.

Three surgical techniques have been described.

Pancreatic necrosectomy and free closed drainage

This involves surgical debridement/resection of the necrotic tissue, simple drainage of the peripancreatic bed and closure of the wound. The overall mortality with this technique is 30–50% and one-third of patients require reoperation for persistent infection or abscess.

Pancreatic necrosectomy and open drainage (laparostomy)

This entails debridement/resection of the necrotic tissue followed by packing of the cavity. The wound is left open and the packing changed every 24–48 hours in the theatre under anaesthetic, but subsequently in the ITU under sedation. The morbidity from repeated dressing and debridement is high and, including intestinal and pancreatic fistula and haemorrhage, the overall mortality is 20–30%.

Pancreatic necrosectomy and closed irrigation/lavage

This is currently the most popular procedure. Operation is via a bilateral subcostal incision, the lesser sac is explored and the extent of necrosis is carefully assessed. Excision of all devitalised tissue is performed either digitally or with forceps, combined with meticulous haemostasis and extensive saline lavage. Two large-bore silicone tubes are inserted into the lesser sac via each flank before abdominal wall closure. Continuous saline or Hartmann's solution irrigation and drainage are applied in the postoperative period. Subsequent debridements are carried out as necessary. The complications are less frequent and overall mortality with this procedure is reported to be 7–15%.

Recently percutaneous endoscopic and also laparoscopic debridement of pancreatic necrotic tissue have been described but the benefit and outcome of these two techniques need to be analysed further with more studies.

Pancreatic abscess

Definition

A pancreatic abscess is a circumscribed intraabdominal collection of pus, usually in proximity to the pancreas, containing little or no pancreatic necrosis, which arises as a consequence of acute pancreatitis.

Pathogenesis

The possible origin of pancreatic necrosis is as follows.

- Limited pancreatic/peripancreatic necrosis followed by infection, liquefaction and subsequent pus formation.

- Low-grade infection in a localised acute fluid collection.

- Infected pancreatic pseudocyst.

The presence of pus and little or no pancreatic necrosis differentiates a pancreatic or peripancreatic abscess from infected pancreatic necrosis. The distinction is important as the treatment and outcome differ. Patients with pancreatic abscess have a low APACHE II score and the mortality is half that of patients with infected necrosis. The clinical picture of pancreatic abscess is one of sepsis. Pancreatic abscess tends to occur later in the course of an acute attack of acute pancreatitis, often after four or more weeks. The diagnosis is confirmed by dynamic CT scanning and the abscess can often be managed by a percutaneous catheter drainage technique. However, surgical drainage and debridement may be required in recurrent abscesses or failed percutaneous drainage, particularly when the pus is thick.

Pseudocyst

Definition

Acute pseudocyst is a collection of pancreatic juice enclosed by a wall of fibrous or granulation tissue, lacks an epithelial lining and arises as a consequence of acute pancreatitis or pancreatic trauma.

The presence of a well-defined wall distinguishes a pseudocyst from an acute fluid collection (Figure 8.2). Formation of a pseudocyst requires four or more weeks from the onset of acute pancreatitis and arises as a result of persistence and maturation of an acute fluid collection. More than 80% of acute pseudocysts are located within or adjacent to the pancreas in the lesser sac. They have also been reported in the mediastinum and pelvis. In contrast, chronic pseudocysts have a well-defined wall within the pancreatic capsule (intrapancreatic) and tend to arise in patients with chronic pancreatitis with whom there may not be an obvious recent episode of acute pancreatitis (Table 8.1).

Pseudocysts develop in about 2% of cases of acute pancreatitis. They are solitary in 85% of cases and multiple in the remainder. The clinical features include continued abdominal pain and a

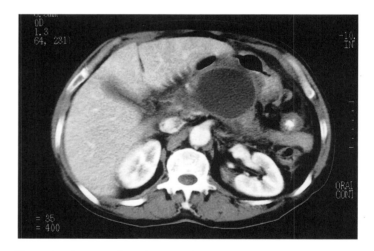

Figure 8.2 Contrast-enhanced CT scan showing an acute pseudocyst in the lesser sac and adherent to the posterior wall of stomach. This was drained into the stomach (cystogastrostomy).

Table 8.1 Differences between acute and chronic pseudocyst		
	Acute pseudocyst	**Chronic pseudocyst**
History	Acute pancreatitis or trauma	Chronic pancreatitis
Shape	Irregular (sometimes)	Circular
Site	Lesser sac or distant sites	Lesser sac only
Relation to pancreatic capsule	Extrapancreatic	Intrapancreatic
Pancreas	Oedematous and inflamed – no calcification	Bulky or atrophic with calcification
Pancreatic duct	Collapsed	Dilated with strictures
		Irregular or absent side branches
Communication with the pancreatic duct	Unknown (but most likely)	50%
Spontaneous resolution	Possible	Rare
Overall mortality	5–10%	3–5%

tender epigastric mass. Vomiting is variable but may arise from duodenal obstruction or gastric irritation. Jaundice may reflect compression of the bile duct. An elevated serum amylase is present in about half of cases.

A CT scan is the best diagnostic tool to assess the size, shape and the relationship of the pseudocyst to other viscera, while US scan is useful for repeated follow-up. An ERCP is indicated in chronic pseudocysts and when there are suspected abnormalities of the bile or pancreatic ducts shown on other imaging or the results of liver function tests. The duct may be dilated and require surgical drainage in conjunction with the drainage of the pseudocyst. An ERCP requires antibiotic cover as there is a risk of infection. An upper gastrointestinal contrast study or endoscopy may be performed to rule out duodenal obstruction in patients with vomiting.

Complications of pseudocysts

Established pseudocysts are at risk of complications.

Infection

Infection of the pseudocyst can occur and results in fever, chills and leucocytosis. Occasionally, this follows endoscopic placement of a pancreatic stent as a treatment for pseudocyst. Immediate removal of the stent and US-guided percutaneous drainage are required if the initial treatment with antibiotics has failed. Internal drainage into stomach or jejunum with gross infection is contra-indicated because of the risk of an anastomotic leak.

Rupture

Less than 5% of pseudocysts rupture spontaneously into either the peritoneal cavity or an adjacent viscus like the stomach, colon or jejunum. Occasionally rupture occurs into the pleural or pericardial cavity. Sudden perforation into the free peritoneal cavity produces a severe chemical peritonitis with board-like rigidity and severe pain. If the diagnosis is confirmed, conservative treatment (octreotide, intravenous fluids, antibiotics) may suffice. If laparotomy is required then irrigation, biopsy of the wall and probably internal rather than external drainage of the pseudocyst is performed.

Haemorrhage

Bleeding may occur into the pseudocyst cavity or an adjacent viscus following erosion of its wall. It usually follows erosion of an adjacent artery and formation of a pseudoaneurysm in the cyst wall. The treatment of choice is arteriographic embolisation of the bleeding vessel which is usually splenic or the gastroduodenal artery. If bleeding continues, then emergency surgery is performed to either suture ligate the bleeding vessel in the cyst wall, followed by internal drainage of the cyst, or, if possible, to excise the cyst to avoid the risk of recurrent bleeding. Pseudoaneurysms in the head of pancreas are best treated by angiographic embolisation.

Treatment of pseudocysts

Operation is recommended for pseudocysts greater than 6 cm in size and of six weeks duration or longer. The procedure of choice is internal drainage into the stomach for the pseudocyst which is adherent to the posterior wall of the stomach (cystogastrostomy). Non-adherent pseudocysts require drainage into a Roux-en-Y loop of jejunum (cystojejunostomy). Some pseudocysts, particularly giant lesions (more than 10 cm), are preferably drained into a jejunal loop as the drainage is more dependent and the complications are less frequent. Pseudocysts in the head of pancreas can be drained directly into the duodenum. Excision is the most definitive treatment, occasionally performed for pseudocysts in the head of pancreas, but more commonly for chronic pseudocyst in the tail of the gland.

Laparoscopic and endoscopic cystogastrostomy are new techniques and require long-term evaluation. Percutaneous catheter drainage is indicated for infected pseudocyst, extraanatomical pseudocyst and also in symptomatic patients who are not fit for surgery. Endoscopic placement of pancreatic stent may have a role in patients with pseudocyst and stricture in pancreatic duct as this improves internal drainage of the pseudocyst. The risk of infection, however, is high.

A proportion of apparently established pseudocysts may resolve spontaneously but prolonged delay of operation increases the chances of complications. About 5% of those treated by surgical cystogastrostomy will recur. The recurrence rate of the other new procedures awaits evaluation.

The diagnosis of cystic tumour of the pancreas should always be borne in mind when dealing with a possible pseudocyst. The preceding history of acute pancreatitis is one of the simplest and most reliable signs for differentiating acute pseudocyst from a cystic tumour. It is often more difficult to differentiate neoplasm from a chronic pseudocyst, especially in the idiopathic group. Cystic tumours are associated with a solid component, are thick walled and usually septate. Calcifications may be present, especially with non-functioning neuroendocrine tumours. Cystic tumours can be hypervascular or hypovascular and are associated with raised tumour serum markers like CA19–9 and CA 125. It is recommended that a biopsy is taken from the wall of the pseudocyst routinely during operation to exclude malignancy. The distinction between a pseudocyst and a cystic tumour can sometimes become difficult in spite of preoperative imaging techniques and operative assessment; complete excision of the cystic lesion may be required to reach the final tissue diagnosis.

OPERATIVE SURGERY

Cystogastrostomy

Indications

A moderate sized to large pseudocyst that is adherent to the posterior wall of the stomach.

Preoperative investigation and preparation

CT scan should be performed to define the anatomy and the relationship of the pseudocyst to the posterior wall of the stomach and also the nature and extent of any other complications. Regular follow-up of the pseudocyst with serial ultrasound scans should be performed during the maturation phase of its wall. Barium or Gastrograffin meal is valuable when gastric outlet obstruction by the pseudocyst is suspected. ERCP is only indicated when there is obstructive jaundice or a question about the pancreatic duct. Antithrombotic prophylaxis with subcutaneous heparin and intravenous antibiotics in the form of cefotaxime and metronidazole are given on induction of anaesthesia.

Anaesthesia

Operation is under general anaesthesia.

Procedure

- *Surgical access.* Abdominal incision may be mid-line, paramedian, upper transverse or gable incision and should be large enough to allow complete inspection and assessment of the whole pancreas and the biliary system (Figure 8.3).

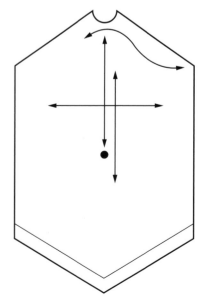

Figure 8.3 Surgical access.

- *Exposure.* On exploration of the abdomen, the pseudocyst is usually encountered protruding behind the stomach. A thorough exploration is performed, in particular to assess the pancreas, bile duct and gallbladder for gallstones. Gallstones must be treated by cholecystectomy and if necessary common bile duct exploration (if not removed by preoperative ERCP).

- *Anterior gastrostomy.* The anterior wall of the stomach is opened longitudinally with a cutting diathermy point or using a stapling device. The gastrostomy should be positioned directly over the palpable pseudocyst (Figure 8.4). Any major vessel in the submucous layer is ligated with catgut or Vicryl.

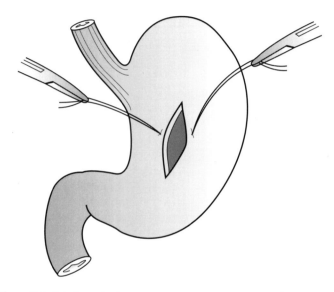

Figure 8.4 Anterior gastrostomy.

- *Exposure of posterior gastric wall.* Upon examination of the posterior wall of the stomach, an 18-gauge needle is inserted into the most dependent bulging area of the cyst and fluid aspirated. Intraoperative ultrasound is useful to define the precise relationship of the pseudocyst.

- *Opening the cyst.* The electrocautery is used to excise a full-thickness disc of posterior gastric wall of approximately 3 cm in length: the cyst is entered and the fluid aspirated with suction. A sample of fluid should be sent for culture and biopsy of the wall taken for histology to exclude malignancy. Necrotic debris is removed by suction, sponge holders or dissecting forceps. Adherent slough in the base of the cyst is best left undisturbed as severe haemorrhage can occur from disruption of the underlying vessel. The edge of the cystogastrostomy is sutured with a continuous chromic catgut or Vicryl haemostatic suture (Figure 8.5).

- *Closure of gastrostomy.* The anterior wall of the stomach is closed in two layers with chromic catgut or Vicryl. Alternatively the gastrostomy is closed with a 55 mm linear stapler. An abdominal drain is not usually necessary.

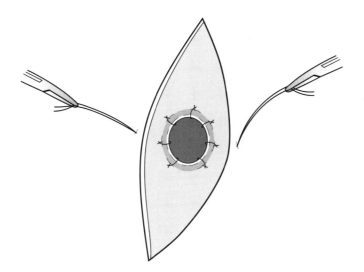

Figure 8.5 Cystogastrostomy following suture.

Postoperative management

Postoperative pain control is with either epidural or patient-controlled analgesia.

The nasogastric tube is usually left for 24 hours to prevent vomiting and aspiration into the lung. Antibiotics may be continued for 48 hours. Free fluids are commenced from the second day and a soft diet followed by normal diet are given when bowel sounds are present.

FURTHER READING

Bradley EL III. A clinically based classification system for acute pancreatitis. *Arch Surg* 1993; **128**:586–590

Glazer G, Mann D. United Kingdom guidelines for the management of acute pancreatitis. *Gut* 1998; **42**:(suppl 2):1–13

Glazer G, Mann D. Acute pancreatitis in: Monson J, Duthie G, O'Malley K (Eds). *Surgical Emergencies*. London: Blackwell Science 1998

Johnson CD, Imrie CW (eds). *Pancreatic Disease Towards the Year 2000*, 2nd edn. London: Springer, 1999

9

Chronic pancreatitis

Chris Russell

Chronic pancreatitis comprises a spectrum of pancreatic disorders that ranges across:

- a subclinical morphological derangement

- intermittent inflammatory exacerbations

- chronic persistent pain

- fibrotic obstruction of structures adjacent to the pancreas (bile duct and duodenum, portal, mesenteric and splenic veins)

- end-stage exocrine and endocrine failure.

It is a disease with various causes, overwhelmingly alcohol abuse, yet in a substantial number of cases no currently identifiable predisposing factor is found. The disease has an unpredictable clinical course and at present treatment remains pragmatic. In many patients, chronic pancreatitis is clinically silent, yet other patients have severe abdominal pain. Because of the variable nature of chronic pancreatitis its prevalence is unclear; the best estimates suggest that it has a prevalence of less than 30 cases per 100 000 population. Recent reports suggest that in males the incidence has increased from 10 to 43 per million population in the last 30 years. A study from Finland reported a fourfold increase in alcohol consumption between 1960 and 1989 associated with a 20% increase in the incidence of chronic pancreatitis – from 10.4 to 13.4 cases per 100 000 population. In developed countries, 60–70% of patients with chronic pancreatitis have a long history (6–12 years), often with a background of heavy alcohol consumption (150–175 g per day). Alcohol-induced pancreatitis is most common among men and has a peak incidence at the age of 35–45 years.

PATHOPHYSIOLOGY

Chronic pancreatitis is characterised by the presence of chronic inflammatory lesions, the destruction of exocrine and endocrine parenchyma and fibrosis. The molecular and pathobiochemical mechanisms resulting in the focal inflammation and fibrosis of the pancreas are largely unknown. A common feature histologically is infiltration by leucocytes, pancreatic main duct and side branch duct alterations, focal necrosis and extensive fibrosis. Leucocytes release cytokines and growth factors (e.g. IL-1, IL-6, TNF-α and EGF), which are thought to induce the proliferation of mesenchymal cells. Overexpression of EGF and TGF-α and -β and acid and basic FGF (fibroblast growth factors) is observed. Activated cytotoxic cells and their mediators are considered to play a key role in the chronic inflammatory process.

Upper abdominal pain, the leading clinical symptom, is related to an increase in duct and tissue pressure of the pancreas. Clinically this increase in pressure has been observed in the tissue at operation, by the dilatation of the main ducts and by the relief of pain after decompression of the duct. These pathomorphological changes possibly produce in the sensory nerves an increase in

nerve diameter, perineural infiltration of inflammatory cells and an increase in the neurotransmitter substance P and calcitonin gene-related peptide such that each is considered to be causally related to the 'pain syndrome' in chronic pancreatitis. A significant correlation has been found between nerve growth factor (NGF), mRNA expression and the amount of pancreatic fibrosis, as well as the degree of acinar cell destruction; the TrkA transmembranous tyrosinkinase receptor, binding NGF, and the intensity of pain are correlated. The increased activity of the NGF/TrkA signal cascade suggests a role in the pathway involved in nerve proliferation and the pain syndrome in chronic pancreatitis. On long-term follow-up, the natural course of chronic pancreatitis reveals persistence of pain in 85% of patients five years after diagnosis. The progression of exocrine and endocrine insufficiency, frequently observed, has a limited influence on the pain syndrome. Local complications such as pseudocyst, common bile duct stenosis, inflammatory mass in the head of the pancreas and compression of anatomic structures surrounding the pancreatic head are observed frequently. Long-term follow-up reveals that patients with chronic pancreatitis have a five-year survival rate of 70% and a 10-year survival rate of 40%. The death rate directly related to chronic pancreatitis is between 12% and 20%.

Epidemiological studies of patients with chronic pancreatitis have demonstrated a coincidence with pancreatic carcinoma in 1.8–4% and with extrapancreatic cancers in 4–13%.

AETIOLOGY

Alcohol accounts for 70–80% of all cases of chronic pancreatitis with the remainder being idiopathic (10–20%) or due to diverse causes (5–10%).

Alcohol

Contrary to popular belief, the type of alcohol and the manner of consumption do not seem to be important factors. The risk of chronic pancreatitis does, however, increase with the duration and amount of alcohol consumed. Ingestion of 150–200 ml of greater than 40% ethanol per volume daily for 10–15 years is needed for clinically significant chronic pancreatitis to develop. Despite such estimates, there is no doubt that some cases of so-called 'idiopathic' pancreatitis may actually be alcoholic pancreatitis in sensitive patients; however, it is a mistake to call all patients with idiopathic pancreatitis 'secret drinkers' or accuse the social drinker of being an alcoholic. The fact that only 5–10% of heavy drinkers develop pancreatitis suggests a role for genetic or nutritional factors.

In alcoholics a diet high in protein and fat may predispose to chronic pancreatitis although others suggest that malnutrition, particularly in those patients with pancreatitis in the Third World, may well be a factor. Dietary deficiency of trace elements such as selenium and zinc may predispose to pancreatic injury by decreased production of antioxidant enzymes.

The mechanism by which ethanol causes chronic pancreatitis remains unclear. Duct obstruction by protein plugs has been suggested as a trigger by which the plugged ducts raise the pressure and cause intracellular activation of pancreatic enzymes which give rise to acinar damage. A further suggestion is the 'flow-reflux' hypothesis in which it is suggested that alcohol reduces the tone in the sphincter of Oddi and allows reflux of duodenal juice, which contains activated pancreatic enzymes, into the pancreatic duct in a manner similar to the experimentally produced pancreatitis model of creating a closed-duodenal (Pfeffer) loop. Such a hypothesis would fit with 'binge' drinking in association with 'binge' eating, but it is unlikely to be the cause of chronic pancreatitis. More likely is the toxic metabolic hypothesis which suggests that excessive stimulation of acinar cells by alcohol could derange intracellular protein transport, leading to an admixture of digestive enzymes and lysosomal hydrolases. Fatty degeneration of the acinar cells, rather than ductal obstruction, could then lead to periacinar fibrosis. Alternatively, the lipophilic substrates metabolised by cytochrome P450 monooxygenators increase the oxidative stress and thus pancreatic cell damage. Free radical activity in acinar cells may have key importance in the pathogenesis. Unfortunately, in many individuals with chronic pancreatitis of alcohol aetiology, the condition may progress even after cessation of alcohol consumption.

Idiopathic

Epidemiological evidence suggests that idiopathic chronic pancreatitis is a distinct entity from alcoholic pancreatitis. There is a bimodal distribution of age at presentation; the juvenile type begins between 10 and 20 years of age and the senile type between 50 and 60 years of age. About equal numbers of men and women are affected and in contrast to alcoholic pancreatitis, delayed progression of endocrine and exocrine insufficiency is a feature of this group. A mutation in the cystic fibrosis transmembrane conductance regulator gene has been identified in some adult patients with idiopathic chronic pancreatitis, none of whom have cystic fibrosis. Due to the prevalence of this gene mutation it is difficult to know the meaning of this finding, but evidence is accruing in carefully controlled comparative studies that this may be an important predictive factor of chronic pancreatitis.

Hereditary

In a small number of families, chronic pancreatitis is inherited as an autosomal dominant condition with penetrance of about 80%. More than 80% of affected individuals develop clinical disease before the age of 20 years. The point mutation in the cationic trypsinogen gene of chromosome 7 is associated with hereditary pancreatitis in most affected families. At least two further muta-

tions have now been described. The mutation interferes with the trypsin inactivation mechanism and allows activated trypsin to autodigest the pancreas. The importance of this finding is that the genetic abnormality reveals a probable pathophysiological mechanism of pancreatic injury.

Tropical

In parts of Africa, south-east Asia and the subcontinent of India, pancreatitis is not alcohol related. The disorder usually presents in childhood leading to endocrine and exocrine insufficiency in adolescence. Pain is not prominent and indeed, deficiency of endocrine and exocrine function may be the presenting feature. The cassava fruit has been implicated, which fits nicely with the oxidant hypothesis as cassava contains certain toxic glycosides that are converted to cyanogens when exposed to stomach acid. As cyanogens inhibit a variety of antioxidant enzymes, it is postulated that cassava ingestion may promote unchecked free radical generation with toxic effects.

Hyperparathyroidism

Ten to fifteen percent of patients with hyperparathyroidism will develop pancreatitis. Routine measurement of serum calcium concentration is a required part of the investigation of all patients with pancreatitis. Treatment of hyperparathyroidism will resolve the pancreatic problem.

Trauma

Blunt and penetrating trauma to the abdomen can result in pancreatic injury. Indeed, complete disruption of the main pancreatic duct can occur, particularly in road traffic accidents or incidents in which a bicycle handlebar compresses the neck of the pancreas against the lumbar spine. Unless carefully considered, this injury can be easily missed.

Pancreas divisum

This anomaly is found in 7–8% of individuals of European origin. The anomaly arises due to the failure of the two buds of the primitive foregut to fuse correctly together to form the pancreas. Because only a small percentage of individuals with pancreas divisum develop pancreatitis there is debate as to whether or not pancreatitis is secondary to damage of the accessory papilla giving rise to papillary hypertension or merely an idiopathic pancreatitis in individuals with this anomaly. The matter remains controversial (Figure 9.1).

Other causes

A variety of other causes of pancreatitis are outlined in Box 9.1.

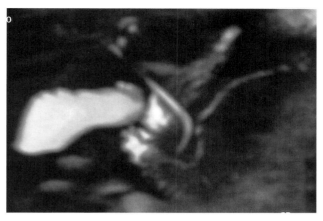

Figure 9.1 An MRI scan showing the main pancreatic duct draining into the accessory papilla with the common bile duct entering the major papilla. The duct of Wirsung was not imaged by ERCP or MRI.

Box 9.1 Aetiology of chronic pancreatitis

Alcohol	Metabolic
Idiopathic	Hyperlipidaemia
Obstructive	Hyperparathyroidism
Pancreas divisum	Hereditary
Ampullary stenosis	Tropical
Hamartoma	Juvenile kwarshiorkor
Parasites	Biliary
Duodenal wall cysts/diverticulae	Choledochal cyst
Ectopic pancreas	Choledochocoele
Pancreatic or ampullary tumour	Miscellaneous
Congenital intrapancreatic cyst	Cystic fibrosis
Duct damage/scarring	In association with PSC/
Past acute pancreatitis	inflammatory bowel disease
Trauma	Abdominal radiotherapy
Annular pancreas	Exposure to certain chemicals

CLINICAL FEATURES

The principal symptom of chronic pancreatitis is pain. It is a deep boring epigastric and left subcostal discomfort that radiates through to the back. It can range from mild to severe and tends to fluctuate in severity during the course of the disease. It will vary from week to week. In the early phases there may be definite acute episodes of pain but as the disease progresses so a more chronic pattern of pain may ensue.

Two typical patterns of pain have been identified.

- Type A pain, a pattern typically observed in acute relapsing pancreatitis, is characterised by short-lived pain episodes usually lasting less than 10 days and separated by long pain-free intervals. Such intermittent episodes are of varying severity but many will require hospital admission.

- Type B pain is characterised by prolonged periods of persistent daily pain and/or clusters of recurrent severe pain exacerbations. Typically the severe pain occurs for two or more days

per week. Type B pain tends to be associated with more advanced morphological change. The potential causes of the pain are outlined in Box 9.2.

Box 9.2 Causes of pain in chronic pancreatitis

Pancreatic	*Extrapancreatic*
Acute inflammation	Bile duct obstruction
Increased intrapancreatic pressure	Duodenal stenosis
Intraductal	Peptic ulcer
Parenchymal	
Pseudocyst	
Neural inflammation	

Some differences in pain patterns among the presentations of chronic pancreatitis (early-onset idiopathic, alcoholic and late-onset idiopathic) are the age at onset (mean age 21, 45 and 55 years respectively) and the incidence and severity of the pain. At the beginning of disease pain is present in approximately 75% of patients with alcoholic chronic pancreatitis, 50% of those with late-onset idiopathic chronic pancreatitis and all patients with early-onset idiopathic chronic pancreatitis. Pain is less severe in the late-onset group. Overall 40% of patients with alcoholic chronic pancreatitis and 60% of patients with idiopathic chronic pancreatitis require surgery to relieve the pain. The remainder can be treated with medical, non-surgical therapy. Pain eventually decreases in 75% of patients with or without surgery.

Food consumption may increase the severity of the pain. Appetite is decreased and hence weight loss occurs. Narcotics taken for pain relief become addictive and are a major feature of the disease. Cigarette smoking appears to be a coexistent factor often associated with intractable disease.

Pancreatic insufficiency is progressive with clinically significant protein and fat deficiency. Stools become loose, foul smelling and difficult to flush away. Bloating, abdominal cramps and flatus are additional disabilities. It is important to remember from the nutritional point of view that many patients with alcohol dependence may be thiamine deficient and Wernicke's encephalopathy in association with pancreatitis is well described.

Diabetes mellitus becomes progressively more frequent and, in the severe pancreatitic, eventually almost universal. Patients who have diabetes secondary to chronic pancreatitis behave in a manner identical to other diabetics and appear to develop the same complications.

Physical examination reveals few signs other than tenderness in the epigastrium. Occasionally a mass is present if a pseudocyst has developed but more usually there is no defining clinical sign. Erythema *ab igne* may give some indication of the severity of the pain.

The differential diagnoses for patients with suspected chronic pancreatitis are outlined in Box 9.3 and the criteria for the evaluation of pain in Box 9.4.

Box 9.3   Differential diagnosis

Neoplasia
Peptic ulcer disease
Biliary tract disease
Irritable bowel syndrome
Mesenteric vascular disease
Endometriosis
Abdominal pain syndrome

Box 9.4   Criteria for the evaluation of pain

Duration of pain dating back to the first episode
Character of pain: intermittent versus daily; frequency if intermittent
Subjective estimation of intensity of pain: mild, moderate or severe (e.g. 1–5; 1–10)
Use of narcotics and other medications to treat pain
Evaluation of addiction to narcotics
Documentation of exclusion of other diseases that could be causing abdominal pain
Measurement of quality of life including work performance, social interaction and family interaction

INVESTIGATION

Blood investigations

- Serum amylase, lipase and elastase are all unhelpful in the diagnosis of chronic pancreatitis. These enzymes may be elevated in the early stages of the disease with acute episodes, but are of little value in the patient with severe chronic pancreatitis.

- C-reactive protein is a good indicator of inflammation and is useful for following the progress of the disease.

- Routine haematology, a coagulation screen and routine biochemistry including a lipid and bone profile and an estimate of the glycated haemoglobin level should be performed as a baseline in all patients.

- Secretin stimulation testing, PABA testing and the pancrealauryl estimation are all performed but are of little help in surgical practice. Appropriate questioning concerning bowel habit is of more value.

Imaging

- Ultrasonography should be performed to exclude gallstones.

- The prime investigation is contrast-enhanced helical computed tomography scanning (CT) of the pancreas (Figure 9.2). A protocol specific for the pancreas recommends imaging thin sections using large volumes (100–150 ml) of pressure-injected intravenous contrast (5 ml/sec) to achieve the best results. Water is taken orally to delineate the gastrointestinal tract. The CT scan should reveal the outline of the gland and any changes in contour; the duct should be clearly defined and its

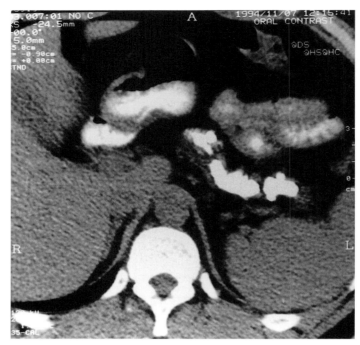

Figure 9.2 A CT scan of the tail of the pancreas and hilum of the spleen with oral contrast alone demonstrating calcification within the atrophic pancreas. Good-quality non-enhanced scans to show calcification are essential in the patient with suspected pancreatitis.

diameter measured with the variation in diameter throughout the pancreas noted (Figures 9.3, 9.4). Finally, attention should be turned to adjacent organs and evidence of inflammation and compression, and splenic hypertrophy with or without abnormal blood vessel formation noted.

- The progressive improvement in images achieved with an appropriate protocol makes magnetic resonance imaging (MRI) now almost equal in value to CT scanning. Further, the MRI images will enable an outline of the biliary tree and

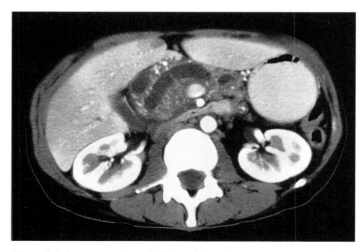

Figure 9.3 A contrast-enhanced CT scan delineating a 15 mm pancreatic duct in the head of the pancreas and a relatively atrophic pancreas.

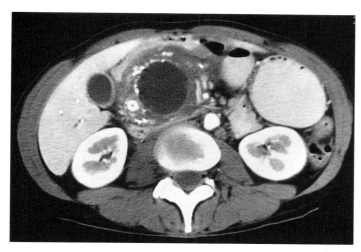

Figure 9.4 CT scan showing a stone in the main pancreatic duct and a cyst within the head of the pancreas. With conservative therapy the cyst resolved and a Frey procedure was performed with removal of the stone.

pancreatic ducts to be obtained without injection of contrast, though agents such as gadolinium, secretin and cholecystokinin are used to improve the images by some radiologists. The accuracy of the images achieved enables pancreas divisum to be confidently diagnosed (Figure 9.1). It is assumed that much of the value of diagnostic endoscopic retrograde cholangiopancreatography (ERCP) will be replaced by imaging by MRI.

- ERCP should be performed only if the CT or MRI scan suggests that there is further information to be gained by outlining the ducts or some interventional procedure such as biopsy, brush cytology or dilatation of a stricture and stent insertion is deemed appropriate.

- Endoscopic ultrasound (EUS) is of value and has largely replaced routine angiography to define involvement of the main vessels by the inflammatory process.

DIFFERENTIAL DIAGNOSIS

Chronic pancreatitis is a common 'label' for the patient with chronic abdominal pain. It is important that the term 'pancreatitis' is not attached to such patients without evidence of pancreatic disease or an attack of acute pancreatitis that has progressed to chronic pancreatitis. The pain can be confused with other causes of chronic abdominal pain such as those outlined in Box 9.2.

Complex peptic ulcer disease can easily be missed in this era of effective therapy for peptic ulcer. The unusual retroperitoneal perforation can be most confusing. A major challenge has been the differential diagnosis between cancer of the pancreas and an inflammatory mass. Both can occur for the first time in the older patient, both can occur in the patient who is a heavy social drinker and both may show an indolence which suggests benign disease. Unless the diagnosis of benign disease is certain for the

mass in the head of the pancreas, a pancreatoduodenectomy is now an accepted therapy provided the operating surgeon has a mortality rate well below 5%.

MANAGEMENT

Chronic pancreatitis is poorly understood and its management is controversial. There is an increasing appreciation that pain patterns differ among the types of chronic pancreatitis and may be due to different mechanisms. Contributing to the treatment controversy is the paucity of information about the basic mechanisms producing pain, lack of information about the character of pain and when to intervene with treatment and what treatment to use. It is increasingly apparent that the nature of the pain (e.g. constant versus intermittent) confounds response to treatment.

The algorithm in Box 9.5 defines a management pathway that will help decide the surgical treatment. There is now a general consensus that endoscopic treatment, such as the use of stents to overcome bile duct stenosis or pancreatic fistulae, rarely effects long-term cure and endotherapy in conjunction with extracorporeal lithotripsy for stones is rarely effective. Interventional radiology for cysts, abscesses and collections can be of value in the treatment of complications but rarely influences the overall course of the disease. Angiographically guided embolisation for haemorrhage due to splenic artery aneurysm rupture or other visceral aneurysm is of value in the acute situation.

Surgical treatment

A proper patient selection is based on the individual presentation. The history, the age, the associated complications and the physical status of the patient influence selection. Because of the multifaceted picture of the disease, this selection should be based on an interdisciplinary consensus for the individual patient (Box 9.6).

- Intractable pain remains the most important indication for surgical intervention.

- Surgery is also indicated to control complications related to adjacent organs such as the distal common bile duct stenosis and segmental duodenal obstruction.

- Occasionally, the inability to exclude pancreatic cancer necessitates surgery.

The goals of surgical treatment for pancreatitis are as follows:

- pain relief

- control of pancreatitis-associated complications of adjacent organs

- preservation of exocrine and endocrine pancreatic function, social and occupational rehabilitation and improvement of quality of life.

Box 9.5 Guidelines for the treatment of pain in chronic pancreatitis

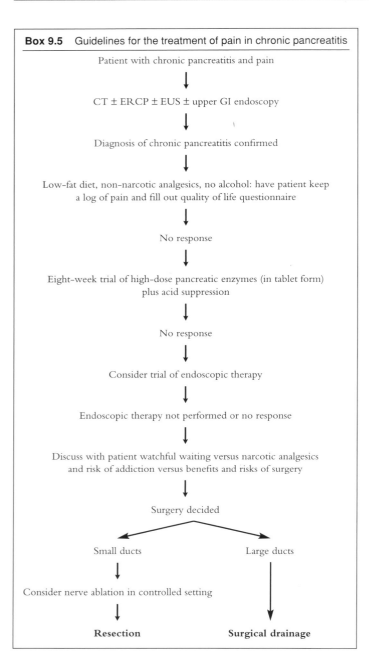

Patient with chronic pancreatitis and pain

↓

CT ± ERCP ± EUS ± upper GI endoscopy

↓

Diagnosis of chronic pancreatitis confirmed

↓

Low-fat diet, non-narcotic analgesics, no alcohol: have patient keep a log of pain and fill out quality of life questionnaire

↓

No response

↓

Eight-week trial of high-dose pancreatic enzymes (in tablet form) plus acid suppression

↓

No response

↓

Consider trial of endoscopic therapy

↓

Endoscopic therapy not performed or no response

↓

Discuss with patient watchful waiting versus narcotic analgesics and risk of addiction versus benefits and risks of surgery

↓

Surgery decided

Small ducts   Large ducts

↓   ↓

Consider nerve ablation in controlled setting

↓

Resection   **Surgical drainage**

Box 9.6 Indications for surgical intervention

Severe intractable pain
Pancreatitis-associated complications of adjacent organs
  Distal common bile duct stenosis
  Duodenal stenosis
Endoscopically unmanageable pancreatic pseudocysts with ductal pathology
Internal pancreatic fistulas and pancreatogenic ascites
Exclusion of malignancy despite extensive work-up

Type of operation

The operative approach must be influenced by the pattern of the disease encountered. The choice of operation is predicated on the two anatomical variants of the disease, which are distinguished by the size of the main pancreatic duct.

- Large duct disease (greater than 6 mm diameter) accounts for approximately 40% of cases and is thought to develop from increased pressure in the pancreatic ductal system. In this circumstance drainage procedures have been the treatment of choice, benefiting close to 80% of patients.

- Patients with small duct disease (less than 6 mm diameter) generally are thought not to be candidates for duct drainage and require pancreatic resection. Because of the historical ineffectiveness of distal resections and the complications associated with total pancreatectomy, resections targeting the head of the pancreas are the primary operations for patients with chronic pancreatitis of the small duct form that is refractory to medical treatment.

Three main types of operation are available to these patients:

- the Whipple-type of pancreatoduodenectomy (with antrectomy)

- the pylorus-preserving pancreatoduodenectomy

- the Beger duodenum-preserving pancreatic head resection (Figures 9.5–9.7).

Regarding pancreatoduodenectomy for chronic pancreatitis, controversy exists with respect to the choice of operation and the expected rate of successful outcomes. The pylorus-preserving pancreatoduodenectomy was first described by Watson in 1944 and reintroduced by Traverso and Longmire in 1978 to improve on the nutritional deficiencies associated with the classic pancreatoduodenectomy. However, large published series report successful maintenance of nutritional parameters in more than

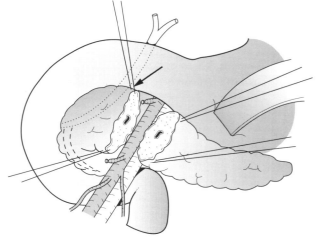

Figure 9.5 Beger operation: the neck of the pancreas is divided and the head of the pancreas removed, preserving a rim of pancreas and the bile duct (arrow).

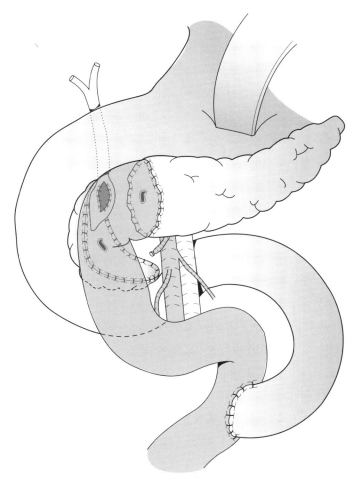

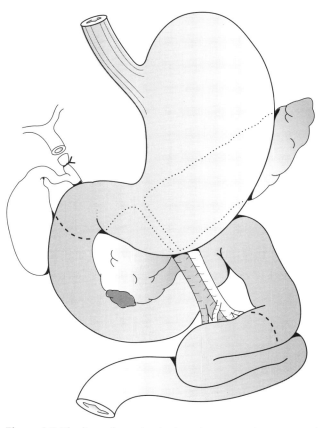

Figure 9.7 The lines of resection in the pylorus-preserving pancreatoduoden-ectomy.

Figure 9.6 Beger operation: the completed procedure with a Roux loop drain-ing the body of the pancreas, the bile duct and the rim of remaining pancreatic tissue within the 'C' loop.

80% of patients after both operations. Comparison of the two operations shows minimal difference in outcome.

Current data suggest that preservation of the gastroduodenal pas-sage and common bile duct described in the Beger (Figures 9.5, 9.6) and Frey (Figure 9.8) procedures is a better alternative for the management of patients with pancreatic disease. The reason why these procedures work is that both remove a section of the head of the pancreas which appears to be critical in the development of the disease. This critical area lies between the pancreatic duct, the portal vein and the common bile duct. This region is removed in both the Frey and the Beger procedure but not in the simple drainage operations without some resection. It appears that limited local pancreatic head excision is crucial in this critical triangle.

In summary, patients who have small duct disease are preferably managed either by a duodenum-preserving resection of head of the gland of the Beger type or, probably less ideally, by a pylorus-preserving pancreatoduodenectomy, while those patients with a duct that is larger than 6 mm in diameter are preferably managed

by a Frey procedure excising the critical triangle of tissue. This is almost certainly preferable to the Puestow procedure in which no resection of tissue is undertaken although the duct is opened from the tail of the pancreas to the head (Figure 9.9).

Other procedures such as sphincterotomy of the major or minor papillae are rarely, if ever, indicated and cyst drainage is now the domain of the endoscopist or the minimally invasive interven-tionalist.

Outcome

The success of an operation for pancreatitis now rests with an assessment of the morbidity of the procedure and its mortality and standard measures of outcome. The morbidity remains high with up to 50% of patients having a named complication following a pancreatoduodenectomy, while for a Frey procedure the morbid-ity is half that. Both procedures will be undertaken with a mortality of 1–3%. The long-term outcome depends on the severity of the pancreatitis and whether or not diabetes and enzyme deficiency develop. There is no evidence that any opera-tion will preserve or prevent the loss of exocrine or endocrine function. Thus, the main criteria of successful outcome must be pain relief, rehabilitation, quality of life and return to active work.

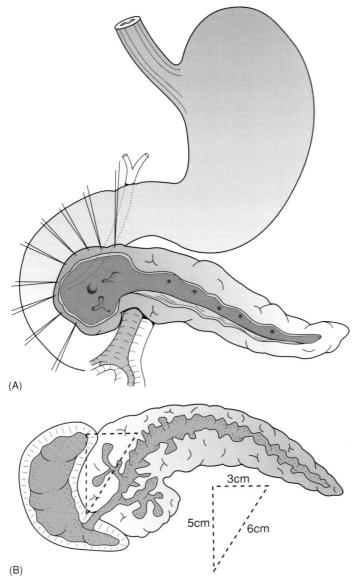

(A)

(B)

Figure 9.8 The Frey procedure. (**A.**) The dilated duct in the body and tail of the pancreas is laid open and the head of the pancreas is 'saucerised' before being anastomosed to a jejunal loop. (**B.**) The tissue between the bile duct, the portal vein and the main pancreatic duct must be excised in order to adequately decompress the head of the pancreas.

The evidence is that if the patient is correctly chosen, 80% will achieve a good quality of life with freedom from symptoms.

Long-term complications relate to the type of procedure. Peptic ulcer disease develops in 9% and 3% after pylorus-preserving pancreatoduodenectomy and Whipple procedures respectively; however, in the latter, this advantage is outweighed by the slight increase in bile gastritis and 'dumping'. Poor surgical results are

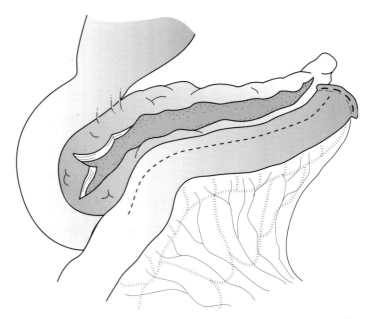

Figure 9.9 The Puestow or, more accurately, the Partington–Rochelle modification, in which the pancreatic duct is laid open longitudinally and anastomosed to a Roux loop of jejunum.

associated with a disease duration of greater than 10 years, an absence of demonstrable pathology in the head of the pancreas, and failed previous surgery. Behavioural characteristics can impair long-term outcome if alcohol consumption, cigarette smoking and poor self-care continue. The late death rate will vary from 12% to 20%.

FURTHER READING

American Gastroenterological Association. AGA technical review: treatment of pain in chronic pancreatitis. *Gastroenterology* 1998; **115**:765–776

American Gastroenterological Association. AGA medical position statement: treatment of pain in chronic pancreatitis. *Gastroenterology* 1998; **115**:763–764

Beger HG, Warshaw AL, Buchler MW et al (eds). *The Pancreas*. Oxford: Blackwell Science, 1998

Buchler MW, Freiss H, Uhl W. Malfertheiner chronic pancreatitis. *Novel Concepts in Biology and Therapy*. Oxford: Blackwell Publishing, 2002

Izbicki JR, Bloechle C, Knoefel WT, Rogiers X, Kuechler T. Surgical treatment of chronic pancreatitis and quality of life after operation. *Surg Clin North Am* 1999; **79**:913–944

Jimenez RE, Fernandez-del Castillo C, Rattner DW, Chang Y, Warshaw AL. Outcome of pancreaticoduodenectomy with pylorus preservation or antrectomy in the treatment of chronic pancreatitis. *Ann Surg* 2000; **231**:293–300

Trede M, Carter DC (eds). *Surgery of the Pancreas*, 2nd edn. Edinburgh: Churchill Livingstone, 1997

Neoplasms of the pancreas

T.R. Worthington, R.C.N. Williamson

Any classification of pancreatic tumours should take into consideration the cell of origin for each individual tumour. Within the pancreas, acinar cells comprise about 80% of the volume, the remainder being made of ducts, stroma, blood vessels and a small amount of endocrine tissue (2%). Despite only occupying a small volume of gland, pancreatic ductal tissue gives rise to approximately 90% of pancreatic tumours in the form of adenocarcinomas. Acinar cells, endocrine tissue and other non-epithelial tissues (fibrous, lymphoid and muscular tissue) give rise to other, much rarer tumours.

This chapter will start by considering the less common and less aggressive types of pancreatic tumour, which should be considered as neoplasms of indeterminate malignancy since they have a variable tendency to invade and metastasise. Frankly malignant tumours will then be discussed, starting with the common type of ductal adenocarcinoma that is so difficult to cure.

NEOPLASMS OF INDETERMINATE MALIGNANCY

Cystic tumours of the pancreas

This heterogeneous group of tumours arises from pancreatic ductal tissue and accounts for barely 1% of all pancreatic neoplasms. Despite their infrequency, they are important because they are eminently curable and they feature in the differential diagnosis of pancreatic cysts or, more commonly, pseudocysts. Most patients with cystic neoplasms present with vague symptoms of mild upper abdominal pain or discomfort. Other symptoms include weight loss, a palpable mass, postprandial fullness, nausea and vomiting.

In general, cystic tumours of the pancreas can reliably be distinguished from the much commoner pseudocysts on clinical and radiological appearances. Both CT and ultrasound can detect the solid components, septa and loculations that are suggestive of a cystic neoplasm (Figure 10.1). Laparotomy is the final arbiter,

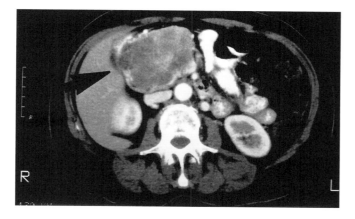

Figure 10.1 CT scan of a 68-year-old woman who presented with epigastric pain and an abdominal mass; she was not jaundiced. The scan illustrates a large cystic tumour of the head of pancreas. She underwent a pylorus-preserving proximal pancreatoduodenectomy and made an uneventful recovery.

however, and if there is any doubt as to the nature of a cystic lesion at operation, it should be excised. It is far better to resect a pseudocyst than leave behind or drain a cystic neoplasm. In brief, there are two main types of cystic neoplasm, mucinous and serous, and a number of much rarer entities such as papillary cystic neoplasm, cystic endocrine tumours and mucinous ductal ectasia.

Mucinous cystic neoplasms

These variants make up about 1% of pancreatic exocrine tumours. The peak age of incidence is 40–60 years with a 6:1 female-to-male ratio. The tumour contains unilocular or multilocular cysts filled with sticky mucin; the surrounding fibrin capsule may be calcified. Characteristically, mucinous cystic neoplasms stain strongly for carcinoembryonic antigen (CEA) and carbohydrate antigen 19–9 (CA 19–9), and each of these molecules can be found in the cyst fluid.

There is a gradation from cystadenoma to cystadenocarcinoma, but in practice all mucinous cystic neoplasms should be considered malignant and treated as such. Biopsy tends to have a high sampling error; thus it is difficult to be certain of a particular tumour's malignant potential until it is excised in its entirety. Resection will involve a pancreatoduodenectomy if the lesion is located in the head of the gland or distal pancreatectomy with splenectomy if located in the tail. The prognosis of mucinous cystic neoplasms is good; depending on histological grade, five-year survival rates following resection are 50–76%. Moreover, patients with high-grade lesions that have metastasised before diagnosis still have a reported five-year survival rate of 18%.

Serous cystadenoma

By contrast with the mucinous type, this is a slow-growing tumour that appears in elderly women. It is also termed microcystic adenoma. Macroscopically, most serous cystadenomas are well-circumscribed, nodular tumours. Numerous cysts give a honeycomb-like appearance to the cut surface. Histologically, there are multiple cysts lined with glycogen-rich epithelium, a vascular stroma, dystrophic calcification and cholesterol clefts. Recent reports have questioned the benign nature of these tumours, but malignant transformation is exceedingly uncommon. In view of their benign nature, less radical surgery has been advocated. Enucleation of such tumours appears to be safe and is associated with a low recurrence rate.

Papillary cystic neoplasm

This rare tumour almost exclusively affects young girls. They usually present with a mass that is either palpable or visible on CT undertaken for investigation of abdominal pain. The tumour contains solid tissue with areas of cystic degeneration. Papillary cystic neoplasms are of low-grade malignancy and are generally cured by wide resection; this may necessitate a pancreatoduodenectomy for lesions in the head of pancreas. The prognosis is excellent following radical surgery, and even patients with liver metastases (a rare event) can survive for many years.

Mucinous ductal ectasia

Mucinous ductal ectasia is characterised by dilatation and filling of the main pancreatic duct or its side branches with thick viscid mucus. The condition is also called intraductal papillary mucinous tumour (IPMT). The mucus is produced by hyperplastic columnar epithelium which lines the duct. In addition to hyperplasia, the epithelium may show a spectrum of changes ranging from mild atypia through carcinoma *in situ* to infiltrating carcinoma. Characteristically, tumours spread along the ducts before invading the pancreatic parenchyma, but in time they may invade the duodenum and bile duct and metastasise to the liver.

Mucinous ductal ectasia tends to occur in males, many of whom are heavy smokers. Although difficult to classify histologically, approximately 50% of tumours are malignant. Treatment should involve pancreatic resection, both to relieve symptoms and avoid development or progression of any malignant process. Total pancreatectomy may be required.

Endocrine tumours of the pancreas

Pancreatic endocrine tumours are uncommon, occurring at a rate of less than 1 per 100 000 population per annum. Insulinomas are the commonest single type, accounting for about 50%. Gastrinomas make up 20% and the rarer tumours only 5%; the remaining 25% do not secrete any active substances and are thus designated 'non-functioning' endocrine tumours; they tend to be much larger than functioning endocrine tumours because their lack of a clinical syndrome delays the diagnosis.

In general these tumours are slow-growing neoplasms of indeterminate malignancy. Often it is difficult to establish malignant potential on histological grounds, and a definitive diagnosis of cancer is made by the radiologist or surgeon who observes infiltration of adjacent structures or metastatic spread (usually to regional lymph nodes or the liver). Similarly, to establish the truly benign nature of a tumour, prolonged follow-up will be required, as metastases may appear some years after removal of the primary.

Insulinoma

Insulinomas comprise half of all pancreatic endocrine tumours and have an equal sex distribution. The incidence is highest between the ages of 30 and 60 years.

Pathology

Most insulinomas are benign, malignancy occurring in only 4–16% of tumours. They virtually all arise within the pancreas; only 1% are ectopic. An insulinoma arises from the beta-cells of the pancreatic islets. At least 90% are solitary, and these measure between 2 and 50 mm in diameter. Multiple insulinomas should prompt a search for multiple endocrine neoplasia type 1 (MEN-1), in which pancreatic (or duodenal) tumours are associated with hyperparathyroidism and sometimes pituitary tumours. Malignant insulinomas tend to be larger, and one-third of them will have metastasised by the time of initial diagnosis.

Insulin can be detected immunohistochemically in almost all tumours, except those with an insulin concentration below 1.0 units/g tissue. Approximately half of insulinomas are plurihormonal on immunohistochemical staining; they may contain glucagon, pancreatic polypeptide and gastrin as well as insulin.

Presentation and diagnosis

Symptoms are intermittent and are caused by hypoglycaemia or neuroglycopenia, which develops during fasting or after severe exercise. Onset of hypoglycaemia can be rapid, but it is more often gradual. Neuroglycopenia presents with a strange constellation of symptoms including confusion, automatism, epileptic seizures or transient paralysis and may lead to patients being labelled as psychiatrically disturbed. As eating often relieves the symptoms, many patients will gain weight.

The diagnosis of insulinoma is established by demonstrating Whipple's triad, namely:

- hypoglycaemic attacks occurring in the fasting state
- blood glucose levels <2 mmol/l during the attack
- relief of symptoms by the administration of glucose.

This triad forms the basis of the fasting test, which is the best provocative test for insulinoma. The diagnosis is confirmed by demonstrating hypoglycaemia with simultaneous elevation in blood insulin levels (>50 pmol/l). The patient is fasted for 24 hours, though rarely it is necessary to prolong the fast for 48 or even 72 hours. During this period simultaneous determinations of blood glucose and immunoreactive insulin are obtained at six-hourly intervals and/or when symptoms occur. Insulinoma patients have an autonomous source of the hormone so that the insulin level is not suppressed during fasting. In the presence of hypoglycaemia (<2.2 mmol/l), therefore, even a 'normal' or slightly elevated insulin level is inappropriately high. Insulin and C-peptide are stored in islet cell granules and are released into the circulation, molecule for molecule. Thus the plasma concentration of C-peptide is an index of endogenous insulin secretion. Measurement of C-peptide can be used to rule out artificial hypoglycaemia produced by exogenous administration of insulin (hypoglycaemia artefacta).

Localisation of the tumour

- The single most sensitive technique is selective pancreatic arteriography, which can detect up to 90% of tumours (Figure 10.2).

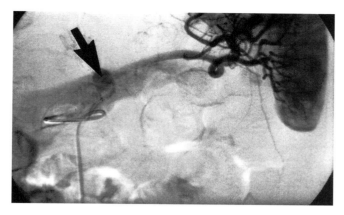

Figure 10.2 A 55-year-old male presented with recurrent attacks of hypoglycaemia. A selective splenic arteriogram was performed which revealed a vascular tumour in the neck of pancreas (arrow).

- CT and ultrasonography are less sensitive but can still be useful. CT should be used with intravenous contrast, and images should be taken in the arterial phase of perfusion as endocrine tumours are highly vascular.

- Percutaneous transhepatic portal venous sampling can be used to measure insulin concentrations in the venous tributaries of the pancreas and can thus identify the part of the pancreas from which the excess insulin is released. It is an invasive test, however, and its use should probably be restricted to those patients in whom other diagnostic tests have failed, i.e. those with MEN-1 syndrome and those requiring reoperation.

- A somewhat less invasive test involves selective intraarterial injection of calcium. A small dose of calcium is given into each artery in turn, i.e. the gastroduodenal and splenic arteries and their tributaries; the insulin concentration of hepatic venous blood is measured synchronously. A rise in hepatic venous insulin is only seen when calcium is injected into an artery supplying tumour tissue; thus a tumour can be localised to the area supplied by the relevant artery. It is less invasive but may also be less precise than portal venous blood sampling with regard to anatomical location of the tumour concerned.

- Endoscopic ultrasonography is another recent technique that is particularly sensitive at detecting small tumours localised to the pancreas. It is quite a difficult method that requires a skilled endoscopist to obtain plenty of experience, but it can then prove invaluable.

- Ultrasound scanning can also be used intraoperatively to detect insulinomas that elude palpation and to determine the relation of the tumour to the pancreatic duct and blood vessels. This information can help a surgeon decide between resection or enucleation of the insulinoma and whether to cover the cavity in the pancreas with a loop of jejunum to reduce the risk of pancreatic fistula, pseudocyst and abscess.

Because of the failings of each individual procedure, some workers have argued that preoperative localisation is not as good as meticulous surgical exploration. Perhaps with the advent of intraoperative ultrasound, preoperative localisation procedures will decrease in importance.

Treatment and outcome

Surgical removal of the tumour represents the only prospect of cure and should therefore be performed unless there are clear-cut contraindications. Insulinomas can be removed either by enucleation or by formal pancreatic resection. Even in the presence of liver metastases, excision of the primary tumour still has a place in reducing hypoglycaemic symptoms, in combination with adjuvant therapy such as embolisation, chemotherapy or perhaps partial resection of the liver. Medical treatment with diazoxide can control symptoms by inhibiting insulin release from tumour cells, but response is variable and side effects are common; its use should therefore be restricted to patients who are unfit for anaesthesia.

Preoperative localisation procedures can give the operating surgeon some idea of the site of tumour, but examination of the pancreas at laparotomy is the final determinant. The pancreas must be fully exposed to allow thorough inspection and palpation of the gland. Exposure of the head entails full mobilisation of the second and third parts of the duodenum (Kocher's manoeuvre), while exposure of the body and tail involves incision of the peritoneum along the superior and inferior borders of the gland. The tumour should be palpable in at least 90% of cases. Multiple tumours are present in about 10% of patients, and this fact should be remembered once the main lesion has been found. Intraoperative ultrasound is invaluable in picking up these additional tumours in patients with MEN-1. If the tumour cannot be found, blind resection is seldom advisable; a further attempt at localisation is recommended after an interval of 6–12 months.

The ideal surgical procedure for solitary insulinoma is enucleation because it preserves the maximum of normal pancreatic parenchyma. After enucleation, the cavity should be inspected for damage to the pancreatic duct which, if unrecognised, will result in a postoperative pancreatic fistula. If there is any suggestion of a duct leak, a Roux-en-Y loop should be brought up and anastomosed to the margins of the cavity. Whatever the procedure carried out, a drain should be placed in close proximity to the relevant area. If a tumour is located in the tail of the gland, distal pancreatectomy is an appropriate alternative to enucleation; the spleen can often be preserved. Pancreatoduodenectomy is generally too radical a therapy for benign insulinoma of the head of pancreas.

The commonest postoperative complication is pancreatic fistula, which occurs in up to 10% of cases. Acute pancreatitis and pseudocyst are much rarer problems. The operative mortality rate for insulinomas is low and cure is usually achieved. Hospital mortality rates of 2% have been described in one recent review, but the rate can rise to nearly 6% for reoperations following a failed laparotomy. Without operative excision, insulinomas can prove fatal; death results from intractable hypoglycaemia.

Gastrinoma

It was in 1955 that Zollinger and Ellison suggested a cause-and-effect association between recurrent ulcer disease, gastric hypersecretion and non-β-cell pancreatic endocrine tumours. Five years later Gregory in Liverpool extracted gastrin from these tumours and identified the reason for this link. Gastrinomas, which represent 20–25% of pancreatic endocrine tumours, occur at a rate of 1 per 1000 among patients with duodenal ulcer disease. They generally present between 30 and 50 years of age but can occur at almost any age. They are commonly malignant, and between 60% and 70% of tumours arise in males.

Pathology

Gastrinomas are small tumours, usually less than 2 cm in diameter. They are typically oval or round in shape with a smooth tan appearance. Most arise within the pancreas, but a previously unrecognised group of patients has recently been described who have microadenomas (1–5 mm in diameter) in the duodenal wall. This subgroup, which was found among a study of Zollinger–Ellison patients with negative laparotomy, may account for as many as 40% of all gastrinomas. Gastrinomas may also occur in the stomach and jejunum and, more surprisingly, in the omentum, liver and ovary. Nearly 90% of gastrinomas are to be found in the 'gastrinoma triangle', which is bounded by the junction of the cystic duct and common bile duct above, the junction of the second and third parts of the duodenum below and the junction of the neck and body of pancreas medially.

At least 60% of gastrinomas are malignant, although this term can be confusing. Histological appearances are of little help. The presence or absence of metastases (usually nodal or hepatic) is the only reliable criterion. Approximately one-third of patients with gastrinomas have MEN-1. This autosomal dominant syndrome usually comprises a combination of pancreatic and parathyroid tumours, and the gastrinoma is likely to be malignant.

Presentation and diagnosis

The usual clinical presentation is of peptic ulceration, which is often multiple and atypical in site, including the oesophagus, distal duodenum and upper jejunum. Complications, which used to occur in a high proportion of patients, include perforation, pyloric stenosis, haemorrhage and fistula. With the introduction of H_2 receptor antagonists, however, many patients have a less dramatic presentation with chronic abdominal pain; indeed, the duration of ulcer symptoms before diagnosis now averages 4–5 years. Diarrhoea occurs in up to 60% of patients and is caused by acid inactivating pancreatic lipase in the proximal jejunum and causing severe mucosal irritation.

The availability of H_2 receptor antagonists and proton-pump inhibitors means that some gastrinoma patients receiving long-term ulcer therapy may be escaping detection. Moreover, it is now accepted that patients with the Zollinger–Ellison syndrome succumb more often to the malignant nature of the disease than to ulcer complications. The early detection of gastrinoma is vital, therefore, to allow localisation and surgical resection of the tumour before it disseminates.

The clinician should be alerted to the diagnosis of Zollinger–Ellison syndrome when one of the following is present.

- Peptic ulcer disease in the young
- Virulent peptic ulcer disease
- Peptic ulcer disease occurring at an unusual site, such as in the third and fourth parts of the duodenum
- Stomal ulceration following a gastric operation for peptic ulcer
- Unexplained diarrhoea
- A family history of peptic ulcer and/or diarrhoea

The combination of an elevated fasting gastrin (usually >100 pg/ml) and an elevated basal output of gastric acid (15 mEq/h) is required for the diagnosis of gastrinoma. An elevated gastrin level is also seen in patients with achlorhydria or renal failure, in patients after vagotomy or those taking H_2 receptor antagonists. Provocative tests for gastrin release have been advocated, and the secretin stimulation test is probably the best method to distinguish between Zollinger–Ellison syndrome and other conditions resulting in increased gastrin levels.

Tumour localisation

- CT will detect up to 80% of tumours, but smaller tumours (less than 1 cm), which typically occur in the duodenum and in patients with MEN-1 syndrome, are liable to be missed.
- A combination of CT and highly selective visceral angiography probably gives the highest detection rate (approximately 90%).
- Selective portal venous sampling for gastrin has been claimed as a reliable though difficult means of localising gastrinomas, but it is unlikely to be more sensitive than conventional imaging techniques.
- Radioactive indium[111]-labelled somatostatin analogues have been used and can visualise up to 80% of gastrinomas.
- Another localising strategy involves provoking gastrin secretion by selective intraarterial injection of secretin. The splenic and gastroduodenal are selectively cannulated and small doses of secretin are given. When the artery supplying the gastrinoma is injected with secretin, there is a rise in gastrin levels in hepatic venous blood (the hepatic veins are selectively cannulated at the same time). Imamura and co-workers have reported some success with this procedure, but it is cumbersome, moderately invasive and not very precise in its localisation of the tumour.

- Intraoperative ultrasound can visualise tumours, though often these lesions are easily palpable at laparotomy. As with insulinomas, its main use lies in pinpointing the relation of the tumour to the pancreatic duct and surrounding vessels.

- Finally, intraoperative endoscopy with transillumination of the duodenal wall has been advocated in the detection of duodenal gastrinomas, where it may be more sensitive than either CT or angiography.

Treatment and outcome

Surgical cure of the tumour can often be achieved if there is either a single resectable gastrinoma or spread that is confined to the duodenopancreatic nodes. Surgical cure in this context means resection of all gastrinoma tissue so that the patient becomes eugastrinaemic, requires no antiulcer medication and has no evidence of recurrent disease on long-term follow-up. Superficial pancreatic tumours in the head of the pancreas can be locally excised, taking care to avoid damage to the pancreatic duct. If they are too deeply placed for safe enucleation, pancreatoduodenectomy should be considered, especially if adjacent involved nodes confirm the malignant nature of the tumour. Tumours of the body or tail should be amenable to distal pancreatectomy with or without splenectomy.

When there are multiple tumours (as in MEN-1 syndrome) or local metastases, cure is very unlikely. Palliative surgery, including radical debulking of liver metastases, will sometimes prolong survival, but such high-risk operations should be confined to those with symptomatic disease. Gastric hypersecretion can usually be controlled by omeprazole, though the requisite dose may be as high as 120 mg/day. Such treatment has reduced the need for total gastrectomy, yet since the long-term effects of this drug are not yet established there may still be a place for lesser acid-reducing operations such as vagotomy and antrectomy if full tumour clearance seems unlikely.

Chemotherapy is usually based on 5-fluorouracil. In patients with metastatic disease, response rates both as high as 60% and as low as 5% have been reported. Octreotide, a long-acting somatostatin analogue, can also relieve symptoms when given by regular subcutaneous injections, but it does nothing to control the liver metastases. Hepatic artery embolisation or even metastasectomy may provide good palliation in selected patients, but embolisation requires a patent portal vein and an expert radiologist.

In patients with Zollinger–Ellison syndrome who have MEN-1, omeprazole treatment has been recommended because the surgical alternative of total pancreatectomy was considered too severe. However, it now appears that MEN-1 gastrinomas often arise outside the pancreas and are of uncertain malignant potential. Patients with MEN-1 gastrinomas should therefore undergo the same localisation procedures as those with solitary sporadic tumours to show whether exploratory laparotomy is indicated.

Lengthy survival can generally be achieved even in the presence of small metastatic deposits in regional lymph nodes. A five-year survival rate of 20% in patients with metastases to the liver or extraabdominal sites compares with one of 80% or more in those with a single resectable lesion. Nevertheless, a reasonable quantity and quality of life can be enjoyed despite a large tumour bulk.

Other rare endocrine tumours

Sophisticated improvements in immunohistochemical techniques and biochemical assays have shown that tumours of neuroendocrine origin can produce several normal or 'ectopic' pancreatic hormones such as glucagon, vasoactive intestinal polypeptide, somatostatin and adrenocorticotrophin. Moreover, plurihormonal tumours, that produce a combination of hormones, are not as rare as previously thought.

Non-functioning neuroendocrine tumours

Approximately one-third of endocrine tumours do not secrete any active substances and are thus designated 'non-functioning'. They are generally much larger (>5 cm in diameter) than functioning tumours at the time of diagnosis, and most of them are malignant with evidence of local invasion or metastasis to adjacent nodes and/or the liver. Localisation is usually a straightforward matter, therefore, and CT is the most versatile modality.

The diagnosis of neuroendocrine tumour should be suspected under the following circumstances.

- The tumour is large, but the patient remains in good health.

- The tumour is situated in the head of the pancreas, but jaundice is absent or minimal.

- There is evidence of marked vascularity or calcification on imaging. Thus angiography can have a valuable diagnostic as well as staging role in such cases; liver metastases may also 'blush' with intravenous contrast.

Treatment and outcome

Since the diagnosis is often delayed, these tumours tend to be large by the time of presentation, yet surgical resection is the best treatment if possible. It can be curative and may provide useful palliation in the presence of metastatic disease. The relatively indolent progress of the malignancy justifies palliative resection, unlike the situation in ordinary pancreatic ductal carcinoma.

Resection of a non-functioning neuroendocrine tumour will entail distal pancreatectomy with or without splenectomy for lesions of the left pancreas and pancreatoduodenectomy with or without antrectomy for lesions of the right pancreas. A curative resection rate of about 50% can be anticipated, but the substantial size and vascularity of these tumours will often make for a technically difficult operation.

MALIGNANT TUMOURS

Carcinoma of the pancreatic duct

Incidence

About 6000 Britons die from pancreatic cancer each year. Among the leading causes of cancer death in the UK and USA, pancreatic cancer occupies between fourth and sixth place. Over the last 50 years the incidence has increased two- or threefold, though it has now reached a plateau.

Apart from small tumours confined to the pancreatic head, ductal cancer is exceedingly difficult to cure and any attempt demands a moderately high-risk operation. Regardless of therapy, median survival is usually a paltry 2–3 months from diagnosis. The overall survival rate at one year (about 10%) and five years (less than 3%) reflects the fact that approximately 90% patients will have metastases at the time of first diagnosis. Only better imaging or screening techniques would seem likely to improve the situation.

Epidemiology

Pancreatic cancer is uncommon under the age of 45 years, and most cases arise between the ages of 60–80 years. Worldwide, men are affected approximately twice as often as women with a ratio of at least 1.5:1. The highest incidence of pancreatic cancer is to be found in affluent countries including Japan, Israel, Canada, Sweden, UK and USA. In areas of low incidence, the rates are roughly similar for each sex, whereas in areas of high incidence men predominate. Unlike other gastrointestinal cancers, socio-economic status has a negligible effect on susceptibility to pancreatic cancer. Neither income nor education has a consistent effect.

Racial groups at a higher risk include New Zealand Maoris, native Hawaiians and black Americans, who have an incidence of 14.4/100 000 compared to 9.5/100 000 in whites. Indeed, throughout the USA, black Americans have incidence rates that are 1.5–2.0 times higher than those of the white population; Connecticut is the one exception. Since this trend is not mirrored in African populations, environmental factors must play a part in the aetiology of the disease.

Aetiology

- Cigarette smoking is the most established risk factor. Smokers are two or three times more likely to develop pancreatic cancer than non-smokers, and they develop the disease about 15 years earlier. There is a linear relationship between the number of cigarettes smoked and the increase in risk.

- The next most important risk factor is probably diet, which could also account in part for the wide variations in incidence found in different geographical regions as well as the altered risk in migrant populations. High-fat diets enhance pancreatic carcinogenesis in rats exposed to azaserine, and there is a positive correlation between per capita consumption of fats and incidence of pancreatic cancer in man. By contrast, foods with high levels of protease inhibitors (fruit and vegetables) have a protective effect.

- Among occupational factors, chemical plant workers exposed to betanaphthylamine and benzidine were reported to have a fivefold increase in mortality rate. Likewise, atomic energy workers and radiologists may be more susceptible, though none of these cases has been proved.

- There are numerous reports of pancreatic cancer among several family members of the same generation, yet any disease that is so frequent in the general population is likely to display chance aggregations. Autosomal dominant disorders that predispose to pancreatic cancer include hereditary pancreatitis, Gardner's syndrome and Lynch syndrome type 2.

- Diabetes mellitus is difficult to evaluate as a risk factor because glucose intolerance may be an early feature of pancreatic cancer. Since resection can improve endocrine function, the intolerance may reflect insulin resistance caused by a soluble factor liberated from the tumour. Nonetheless, those that have been diabetic for more than one year may have twice the normal risk of developing pancreatic cancer.

- Pancreatic cancer generally leads to (obstructive) pancreatitis in the upstream gland. While chronic pancreatitis is probably itself a premalignant condition, concomitant hyperplasia of the pancreatic duct increases this risk. K-ras mutations at codon 12 and 13 have been identified in up to 95% of pancreatic cancers as well as those patients with chronic pancreatitis who also have ductal hyperplasia. There could therefore be a genetic basis for the progression from chronic pancreatitis to pancreatic cancer.

Pathology

As already stated, ductal tissue comprises a relatively small proportion of the pancreatic mass, yet it gives rise to nearly 90% of the tumours. Established cancers often have areas of adjacent ductal carcinoma in situ in the resected specimen. Two-thirds of cases of ductal adenocarcinoma arise within the head of pancreas. The other tumours in the body and tail may be more advanced at presentation because of the absence of jaundice. Pancreatic cancers spread by direct invasion. They have a predilection for perineural invasion both within and beyond the gland and also for rapid lymphatic spread.

Duct cell carcinoma is characterised immunohistochemically by the expression of CEA, CA 19–9 and the keratins 7, 8, 18 and 19 and histologically by a mucinous pattern and marked desmoplasia. Haemorrhage, fat necrosis and acinar atrophy are other common features.

Clinical presentation

As with most cancers, the size and stage of a pancreatic cancer at the time of presentation profoundly influence the clinical outcome. Resectability rates seldom exceed 10–20%. Although very small tumours (2 cm diameter) may be associated with a five-year survival rate of 37%, identification at this stage is exceptional.

The first symptoms of a pancreatic cancer are often vague and non-specific: malaise, anorexia, weight loss, change in bowel habit and epigastric discomfort. Pain is common but seldom severe, although penetrating pain to the back is a sinister symptom that may indicate posterior extracapsular extension of the tumour.

The timing of obstructive jaundice reflects the precise site of the tumour, being early with tumours close to the papilla but slower to develop with those that arise in the neck of pancreas. Generally, the jaundice is remorselessly progressive. A palpable gallbladder in obstructive jaundice is a useful physical sign because it implies a malignant obstruction rather than gallstones (Courvoisier's law). Since patients with concomitant gallstones and cancer can still have a palpable gallbladder, it is probably the intensity of obstruction rather than the inelasticity of the gallbladder wall that explains this phenomenon.

A recent onset of diabetes mellitus should be regarded with suspicion, likewise a sudden increase in the insulin requirement of an established diabetic. Occult bleeding is usually present in pancreatic cancer and accounts for the frequent mild anaemia. The occasional patient with pancreatic cancer presents with acute pancreatitis or migratory thrombophlebitis (Trousseau's syndrome).

Investigation

Increasingly, improvements in imaging are enhancing the ability to diagnose pancreatic cancer and select the appropriate treatment for affected patients.

Ultrasound scanning is usually the first investigation and is particularly effective at demonstrating duct dilatation and the level of obstruction. Tumours appear as hypoechogenic areas, and cancers as small as 2 cm can sometimes be detected; overlying bowel gas often obscures clear views of the pancreas, however. Portal venous blood flow can be assessed by the use of pulsed Doppler scanning.

Contrast-enhanced spiral CT scanning is currently the premier modality for pancreatic imaging. It is excellent at identifying tumours >2 cm in size (sensitivity >90%) and in assessing the major vessels for the presence of local tumour invasion. It will also demonstrate dilatation of the bile duct and/or pancreatic duct. CT is of limited value in assessing smaller primary tumours and in detecting the presence either of liver metastases less than 1 cm in size or peritoneal seedlings. Sometimes it can be difficult to distinguish the tumour itself from the distal obstructive pancreatopathy that it causes.

Gadolinium-enhanced magnetic resonance imaging (MRI) is claimed to be particularly effective at identifying subtle changes in pancreatic contour and overall vascularity of the gland. Magnetic resonance cholangiopancreatography offers the potential of delineating the biliary and pancreatic ducts without requiring endoscopic cannulation and contrast injection. This technology is rapidly improving with time.

In the hands of an experienced operator, endoscopic retrograde cholangiopancreatography (ERCP) has a 95% sensitivity and an 85% specificity in detecting pancreatic cancer. An obstructed pancreatic duct or bile duct may not be caused by cancer, however. Rigid duct encasement (the 'double duct sign') may sometimes be the result of chronic pancreatitis, though benign biliary strictures tend to be longer and smoother on cholangiography. In addition, a normal pancreatogram does not completely exclude the diagnosis of pancreatic cancer, nor does it confer a better prognosis. A variety of tissue sampling methods may be utilised during ERCP. Aspiration of pancreatic duct fluid for cytology, passage of brushes into the duct for cytology, fine needle aspiration or endoscopic biopsy can each provide material for confirmation of malignancy, though the sensitivity rates are still disappointingly low. The use of polymerase chain reaction technology to detect K-ras mutations in cytological brushings and pancreatic juice obtained at ERCP enables DNA to be analysed at minute concentrations and should thereby increase the positive yield and perhaps identify tumours at an earlier stage.

A tissue diagnosis may be gained by biopsy via the endoscopic or percutaneous route. Though specific, these methods are relatively insensitive, negating their potential for excluding malignancy. Concern also arises about seeding along a percutaneous biopsy route, though the use of endoscopic ultrasound may avoid this risk; we do not recommend preoperative biopsy of potentially resectable lesions at present, therefore.

Serological tumour markers have been assessed for their possible roles in the screening, diagnosis and follow-up of pancreatic cancer. CA19–9 and CEA are often elevated in pancreatic cancer, but unfortunately they do not have a high enough degree of diagnostic accuracy to be used as a true screening test. It is larger tumours that tend to give positive values, and these can be picked up by other methods. Tumour markers can help to differentiate between benign and malignant disease and to indicate tumour recurrence before it becomes clinically apparent.

Improvements in CT and ultrasound technology have reduced the need for routine visceral angiography to determine vascular invasion. Circumferential involvement of the portal vein or its tributaries and encasement of the hepatic or superior mesenteric arteries are usually taken to indicate irresectability. Angiography remains a useful test if there is suspicion of major vascular involvement and it can also provide additional helpful information about anatomical anomalies such as a replaced right hepatic artery. As previously mentioned, it may also refine the diagnosis of the exact tumour type if it shows a hypervascular lesion.

Despite the many investigations available, clinicians are still limited in their ability to pick up small and potentially resectable tumours. Novel imaging techniques emerging include laparoscopic ultrasound, which is potentially the most sensitive method for detecting small liver metastases and in addition may indicate vessel encasement. A recent paper has reported improved assessment and preoperative staging when this technique was used in conjunction with diagnostic laparoscopy. It is of concern that laparoscopic biopsy may precipitate peritoneal seeding; it should therefore probably be avoided in potentially resectable tumours.

Endoscopic ultrasound enables visualisation of the pancreas and surrounding structures and can provide access for fine needle aspiration (FNA) of suspicious lesions. A recent study reported better detection of patients for curative resection and better preoperative identification of patients with regional nodal disease, thereby enabling their inclusion in appropriately designed clinical trials. The detection of distant metastases is hampered by the limited depth of penetration of the ultrasound probe, however. The long-term place of endoscopic ultrasound may be in the localisation of smaller, well-localised pancreatic tumours, such as pancreatic endocrine tumours.

Although modern imaging techniques are increasingly reliable in the detection of advanced disease, up to a third of patients are still found to have metastatic disease in the liver, omentum or peritoneum at laparotomy. Laparoscopy can be used to detect such metastatic disease and avoid unnecessary laparotomy, although it usually involves an additional anaesthetic. Since laparotomy provides excellent palliation in selected cases, with appropriate bypass if the expected curative resection is not possible, laparoscopy is not routinely performed in all centres.

Surgical management

Preoperative preparation

Pancreatic cancer patients will often have had obstructive jaundice for three weeks or more by the time they reach a pancreatic surgeon; thorough preoperative preparation is essential, therefore. Clotting abnormalities caused by vitamin K deficiency should be corrected, with normalisation of the prothrombin time. Vigorous fluid rehydration will prevent the development of the hepatorenal syndrome. Undeniably, jaundiced patients with frank cholangitis or impending renal failure need urgent biliary decompression. The use of preoperative biliary drainage to reverse the other ill effects of cholestasis is still a debatable issue, however. Although theoretically attractive, prospective controlled studies have not confirmed this potential benefit because of the complications that can arise from transhepatic or transpapillary drainage. Acute pancreatitis or a bile leak can hamper the subsequent resectional operation, and the obstructed biliary tree is inevitably contaminated with bacteria.

Resectability

Between 80% and 90% of patients with pancreatic cancer have irresectable primary tumours (Figure 10.3) or distant metastases by the time the diagnosis is established, and the five-year survival for this group is a fraction of 1%.

For the minority with resectable tumours, perioperative mortality rates of less than 10% and five-year survival rates of up to 24% have been reported in specialist units. The only cure for pancreatic cancer is successful surgical resection; for practical purposes this is confined to patients with disease arising from the head of pancreas (60% of tumours). Resectability rates have improved recently in major centres either because the diagnosis is established earlier or because of selected referral patterns.

Most cancers of the neck, body and tail of the pancreas are irresectable because of involvement of the splenic vessels and/or distant metastases. A few of these tumours (perhaps 5%) can be resected by means of distal pancreatectomy and splenectomy, but subsequent recurrence is the rule. The five-year survival rate of ductal carcinoma outside the head of pancreas approximates to zero.

- The assessment of resectability starts with a thorough history and physical examination. Back pain is a sinister symptom. There may be evidence of distant metastases in the form of supraclavicular lymphadenopathy, an umbilical nodule or ascites.

- Ultrasound and CT may show liver metastases, and laparoscopy may show peritoneal spread.

- Doppler ultrasound, MR imaging and visceral angiography are useful for demonstrating a patent portal vein without collateral circulation and thus a potentially resectable tumour.

- Any laparotomy for pancreatic cancer should start with the exclusion of distant metastases followed by a trial dissection to confirm that the portal vein is not grossly involved.

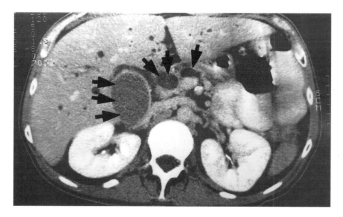

Figure 10.3 A 47-year-old male presented with epigastric pain and jaundice. CT scan demonstrated an irresectable carcinoma of head of pancreas, with a dilated gallbladder (triple arrow), dilated common bile duct (double arrow) and dilated main pancreatic duct (single arrow).

Proximal pancreatoduodenectomy

Since the 1940s the standard resection for carcinoma of the head of pancreas has been a proximal pancreatoduodenectomy with distal gastrectomy (Whipple's operation). In essence, the head of pancreas, including the uncinate process, is excised as far as the neck of pancreas *en bloc* with the duodenum and the lower common bile duct. The rationale for including a gastrectomy is to reduce gastric acidity and prevent the potentially lethal complication of stress ulceration and bleeding in the postoperative period; some surgeons remove half the stomach, others combine a lesser resection (antrectomy) with truncal vagotomy.

A modification that preserves the stomach and duodenal cap is the pylorus-preserving proximal pancreatectomy or PPPP that was described by Watson in 1944 and has gained popularity in several centres since the 1970s. Preservation of an intact pylorus and duodenal cap should prevent enterogastric reflux, erosive gastritis and postoperative bleeding and in theory offers less physiological disturbance of the gastric reservoir. Despite the retention of nodes along the greater and lesser curves of the gastric antrum, the survival rate of pancreatic cancer patients is similar to that of patients undergoing the standard Whipple resection.

Extent of lymphadenectomy

The extent of lymphadenectomy that should accompany a pancreatoduodenectomy for pancreatic cancer remains controversial. Skeletonisation of the hepatic and/or superior mesenteric arteries can be undertaken in every case or be reserved for younger and fitter patients with a more favourable prognosis. Some surgeons routinely include an *en bloc* resection of the regional soft tissues (especially posteriorly) and have a low threshold for resection of any or all of the three major vessels near the neck of pancreas: portal vein, superior mesenteric artery and coeliac axis. Such radical surgery extends the proportion of patients that can undergo resection (up to 40%), who otherwise could only be palliated. Obviously it must carry an increased risk, and there is little evidence to suggest that survival is improved over conventional pancreatectomy. Given that pancreatic cancer affects elderly patients, there seems little justification for such radical surgery in routine practice, but it may be appropriate in selected cases.

Alternatives to proximal pancreatoduodenectomy

Interest in total pancreatectomy as an alternative to the traditional Whipple procedure has centred on its theoretical benefits. It avoids the difficult pancreaticojejunal anastomosis and deals with multicentric tumours that may occur in 25% or more of cases in some but not all series. In practice, recurrence is seldom seen within the residual pancreas. There are three arguments against total pancreatectomy for cancer.

- Higher operative morbidity and mortality rates.

- A lack of improvement in five-year survival.

- The obligate diabetes and total exocrine failure.

The procedure should therefore be reserved for those already on insulin or those with a positive resection margin at the pancreatic neck, as shown by intraoperative histology.

Surgical outcome

Despite marked improvements in postoperative mortality rates, median survival for patients undergoing resection is only of the order of 11–15 months. Long-term survival following resection rarely exceeds 7–10% at five years and is usually much lower. Better results have been seen in the highly selected group of patients with tumours less than 2 cm in size, who had a five-year survival rate of 37% in one series. The patients included in this study accounted for only 5% of the total number treated for pancreatic cancer, however.

The pattern of recurrence following apparently curative resection gives an insight into the natural history of the disease. In one series, all resections that failed to cure the patient were associated with intraabdominal recurrence. Nineteen percent of recurrences were local only, i.e. affected the pancreatic bed, regional nodes, adjacent organs and immediately adjacent peritoneum, while 73% had a component of local failure. Peritoneal deposits (42%) and hepatic metastases (62%) were other common sites of tumour recurrence. Total pancreatectomy neither altered the rate of local failure nor appeared to prolong survival.

Adjuvant therapy

It is clear that local control of disease is an elusive goal, no treatment being very successful in this regard. There have been several studies of the use of postoperative external beam radiotherapy (EBRT) or intraoperative radiotherapy (IORT), with or without concomitant chemotherapy, but the results have been inconclusive. The superiority of IORT to EBRT is questionable, since IORT prolongs the operative procedure to nine hours or more. In all trials conducted local recurrence has been reduced, but without any commensurate improvement in survival.

An alternative adjuvant therapy was investigated by the North American Gastrointestinal Tumor Study Group (GITSG), in which patients who underwent curative resection were randomised to receive either supportive care or adjuvant treatment. Treatment consisted of 40 Gy EBRT, with bolus 5-fluorouracil (5-FU) as a radiosensitising agent, followed by weekly bolus 5-FU for two years or until recurrence. The two-year survival rate among 21 patients randomised to treatment was double that of the 22 given supportive care alone (40% versus 20%). Unfortunately, in a British study that followed the same GITSG regimen in 40 patients, the two-year survival rate of 36% was similar to survival data in other British studies following resection alone.

Despite the plethora of adjuvant therapy trials in pancreatic cancer, the issue of what therapy (if any) should be given remains unanswered. At present, the European Study Group for Pancreatic Cancer (ESPAC) is conducting a trial comparing the benefits of radiotherapy (40 Gy with 5-FU as a sensitising agent), chemotherapy for six months (5-FU and folinic acid) or a combination of these treatments. The results of this trial should help to show whether the additional burden of adjuvant therapy is justified by a real improvement in both survival and quality of life.

Palliative procedures

These are appropriate in the 80–90% of patients with irresectable tumours. Palliation has three objectives.

- To abolish jaundice and the associated bile salt pruritus.
- To treat or prevent vomiting from duodenal obstruction.
- To control pain.

Most patients with pancreatic cancer present with jaundice and many are elderly, so a prosthetic stent is theoretically attractive. Stents may be placed via the transhepatic route (for high strictures) or via the endoscopic route (for low strictures); the primary cancer usually invades the distal bile duct, but sometimes nodal metastases obstruct the hilum. Transhepatic stenting can cause bleeding, cholangitis and biliary peritonitis. Endoscopic stenting can cause bleeding, duodenal perforation and acute pancreatitis. The late complications of either technique include cholangitis, stent blockage or stent migration. A recent study investigating the safety and efficacy of self-expanding metal stents has reported a 30-day mortality rate of 4.3% following stent placement, deaths occurring from both disease progression and iatrogenic arterial injury. These figures can be compared with a recent series of surgical bypass procedures with a 30-day mortality of zero and a similar median survival.

Operative palliation has the advantage that all three of the therapeutic objectives can be achieved at one sitting. The simplest type of operative biliary decompression is a side-to-side chole-cystojejunostomy, but the risk of subsequent cystic duct obstruction makes this procedure inappropriate unless the patient's anticipated survival time is very short (in which case non-operative stenting would be better). In most cases the best procedure is transection of the hepatic duct above the tumour, followed by a hepaticojejunostomy using a Roux loop. Biliary bypass procedures that involve anastomosing either the gall-bladder or bile ducts to the duodenum (cholecystoduodenostomy or choledochoduodenostomy) should be avoided because of the risk of subsequent duodenal invasion.

Duodenal invasion may be uncommon at initial presentation, but a review of reported series demonstrated that the subsequent incidence of gastric outflow obstruction in patients treated with biliary bypass alone varied between 4% and 44% (mean of 17%).

As the addition of a gastroenterostomy does not appreciably increase operative risk, a good case can be made for performing it routinely. A further attraction of a formal operative approach is that a permanent coeliac plexus block (using alcohol or phenol) can be accurately placed to relieve pain. Alternatively, percutaneous coeliac plexus blocks may be effective at pain relief for a period of 4–6 months, followed by repeat injections if necessary. Furthermore, division of efferent nerve fibres in the chest by thoracoscopic splanchnicectomy may have a role in those with intractable pain. Finally, pain relief can be achieved in up to 60% of patients with the use of single-modality treatment such as external beam radiation or intraoperative radiation therapy with electrons or brachytherapy. Unfortunately this symptomatic improvement does not translate to improved long-term survival.

Other pancreatic cancers

Giant cell carcinoma (pleomorphic carcinoma, carcinosarcoma)

This tumour is characterised by the presence of bizarre giant tumour cells with sarcomatous elements. Epithelial elements and mucin are also present. Patients present with advanced disease and median survival is about two months.

Acinar cell carcinoma

This distinct variant is characteristically grey or tan in colour and firm in consistency with areas of necrosis. Histologically, acinar cells are present with a small central lumen. Metastatic fat necrosis is occasionally seen, with elevated blood levels of pancreatic enzymes. Median survival is similar to that for tumours of ductal origin.

Other types of cancer

Anaplastic carcinoma, mixed cell type and connective tissue cancers are all very rare, and experience with such tumours is limited. Occasional pancreatic metastases have been reported in patients with primary tumours in a variety of sites including lung, breast and kidney.

PERIAMPULLARY TUMOURS

The term 'periampullary tumour' is generally used to denote tumours that arise either in the pancreatic head or in one of the nearby organs, either the ampulla, the distal bile duct or the duodenum itself. More precisely, the term relates to neoplasms arising from the ampulla and its immediate vicinity and excludes pancreatic head tumours.

These tumours present in a similar fashion to cancer of the pancreatic head, but with the following distinctions:

- jaundice is seldom as intense

- the resectability rate is higher

- the prognosis is rather less dismal, especially in the case of carcinoma of the ampulla.

One drawback for the surgeon, however, is that the pancreatic duct may not be obstructed (dilated), so that there is an increased risk of leakage from the pancreatojejunostomy after resection.

OPERATIVE SURGERY

Proximal pancreatoduodenectomy

Preoperative preparation

See above.

Procedure

Incision

The authors employ a 'gable' (bilateral subcostal or 'rooftop') incision for all operations on the pancreas. It provides excellent access and may cause less postoperative respiratory embarrassment than a vertical incision.

Proximal pancreatoduodenectomy can be subdivided into two phases, resectional and reconstructive, each lasting 2–3 hours on average.

Resection

The operation starts by examining the liver, peritoneal cavity and adjacent nodal areas for metastatic disease, sending any suspicious material for frozen-section examination by a histopathologist.

The surgeon proceeds to a thorough examination of the pancreas. The head of pancreas is examined after wide mobilisation of the duodenum (Kocher's manoeuvre) and gentle cleaning of the peritoneum that covers its anterior aspect. The neck, body and tail of pancreas are exposed by entering the lesser sac through the greater omentum. Incision of the peritoneum along the upper and lower borders of the pancreatic body will allow examination of its posterior surface, if needed. The uncinate process is relatively inaccessible but can be exposed by identifying the right-hand border of the superior mesenteric vein as it runs towards the tunnel behind the neck of pancreas. Delineation of this tunnel is the key step in nearly every pancreatic resection.

The superior mesenteric vein is identified below the pancreas by following the middle colic vein towards its termination and by dissecting the underlying areolar tissue with great care. The portal vein is identified above the pancreas by mobilising first the bile duct and then the origin of the gastroduodenal artery from the common hepatic artery and then exploring deeply between them. Obvious portal vein invasion (despite favourable preoperative imaging) is usually an indication to abandon resection and perform a bypass procedure (Figure 10.4).

Sometimes the surgeon encounters adherence of tumour to the right border of the superior mesenteric or portal vein late in the procedure. The choice then lies between a palliative resection (marking the remnant tumour with metal clips to facilitate post-operative localisation by the radiotherapist) or proceeding to a localised resection of portal vein with end-to-end reconstruction. Further dissection will often reveal extension of tumour to surround the superior mesenteric artery as well, in which case there is little purpose in undertaking a major vascular reconstruction. Moreover, some apparent involvement of the vein wall turns out merely to be inflammatory rather than true mural invasion when the segment of portal vein is examined post-operatively.

For tumours of the lower head and uncinate process, the authors prefer PPPP, while cancers in the upper head will require a Whipple resection to ensure adequate clearance.

In a standard PPPP:

- the pancreas is divided in front of (or just to the left of) the portal vein

- the duodenum is divided 3–5 cm beyond the pylorus

- the bile duct is divided above the entry of the cystic duct with removal of the gallbladder

- the jejunum is divided 20–30 cm distal to the ligament of Treitz.

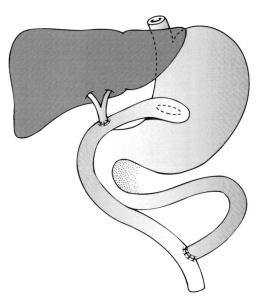

Figure 10.4 Illustration demonstrating the authors' preferred method of single-loop biliary and gastric bypass for irresectable pancreatic carcinoma.

Gastric resection is limited to the distal one-third in Whipple's operation.

It is advisable to send tissue from the pancreatic, bile duct and duodenal resection margins for frozen-section examination to ensure adequate oncological clearance.

Reconstruction

Reconstruction of intestinal continuity involves:

- anastomosis of the proximal jejunum to the pancreatic duct (which can be technically difficult), followed by

- the common bile duct and then

- the gastric outlet, either the stomach or duodenum.

There are many different methods for reconstructing the upper gastrointestinal tract and the authors' standard arrangement is shown in Figure 10.5. The most important anastomosis is the pancreatojejunostomy, for leakage at this point can cause lethal complications (pancreatic fistula, sepsis and haemorrhage). Some surgeons prefer end-to-side pancreatojejunostomy or even pancreatogastrostomy to the reconstruction shown.

The difficult case is one in which the pancreas is completely unobstructed and presents a friable cut surface with a tiny duct. Techniques to reduce leakage in this circumstance include:

- a two-layer invaginating anastomosis using non-absorbable sutures

- a transanastomotic stent that is firmly secured in the duct

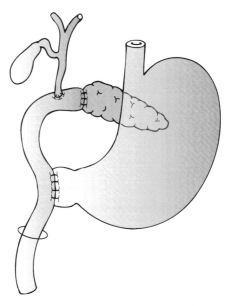

Figure 10.5 Illustrated is the authors' preferred method for reconstruction after pylorus-preserving proximal pancreatoduodenectomy (PPPP). Following resection of the pancreatic head, continuity is restored by anastomosing the pancreas, bile duct and duodenal stump to the upper jejunum.

- the potential use of a separate Roux loop (so that any leak is of pure pancreatic juice only)

- the prophylactic use of octreotide.

The end-to-side biliary–enteric anastomosis is usually straightforward in a patient with malignant biliary obstruction as most patients have a dilated bile duct. Most surgeons remove the gallbladder to ensure a clear bile duct margin. In PPPP it is usually possible to preserve 3 cm of healthy duodenum for anastomosis (end-to-side) to the upper jejunum, but if the pylorus and antrum are resected (for reasons of ischaemia or oncological clearance) then a gastroenterostomy is performed.

Postoperative care

At the end of every pancreatoduodenectomy care must be taken to ensure good haemostasis, and at least two tube drains should be left in the region of the pancreatic anastomosis. If the preoperative serum albumin is low (<30 g/l), then an enteral feeding tube should be carefully considered, whether a direct-access feeding jejunostomy or a nasojejunal tube.

In experienced hands the postoperative mortality rate should not exceed 5–10%, and most patients are fit to leave hospital within two weeks of operation. By contrast, when this operation is done by a surgical team that only occasionally performs the procedure, the operative mortality may be 20% or greater, with a commensurate rate of complications.

The early complications of this operation are septic collections adjacent to the anastomoses, pancreatic and biliary fistulas, hepato-renal failure (especially in deeply jaundiced and inadequately rehydrated patients), postoperative haemorrhage, gastric outflow obstruction, acute pancreatitis and (rarely) diabetes. The most serious problem, a leaking pancreatic anastomosis, should be suspected if the patient develops a tachycardia and fever at 5–8 days and especially if discoloured fluid rich in amylase is observed in a drain. Small leaks may settle with conservative measures including nil by mouth, antibiotics, nutritional support and subcutaneous octreotide. Otherwise, it is necessary to proceed to laparotomy and completion pancreatectomy.

Aside from disease recurrence, the late complications are anastomotic stricture, particularly of the biliary anastomosis, poor nutritional status with loss of exocrine pancreatic function and gastric outflow problems, and postoperative adhesions.

FURTHER READING

Born P. Biliary stenting in pancreatic disease. *Hepatogastroenterology* 1998; **45**:833–839

Fernandez del Castillo C, Warshaw AL. Cystic tumors of the pancreas. *Surg Clin North Am* 1995; **75**:1001–1016

Gregory R, Morley J, Tracy H. Extraction of a gastrin-like substance from a pancreatic tumour in a case of Zollinger–Ellison syndrome. *Lancet* 1960; **1**:1045–1048

Isla A, Worthington TR, Williamson RCN. A continuing role for surgical bypass in the palliative treatment of pancreatic cancer. *Digest Surg* 2000; **17**(2):143–146

Lynch H. Familial pancreatic cancer: A review. *Semin Oncol.* 1996; **23**:251–275

Neoptolemos J, Kerr D. Adjuvant therapy for pancreatic cancer. *Br J Surg* 1995; **82**:1012–1014

Neoptolemos J, Russell RC, Bramhall S, Theis B. Low mortality following resection for pancreatic and periampullary tumours in1026 patients. UK Survey of Specialised Units. UK Pancreatic Cancer Group. *Br J Surg* 1998; **85**:425–428

Stabile B, Morrow D. The gastrinoma triangle: operative implications. *Am J Surg* 1984; **147**:25–31

van Heerden J. Total pancreatectomy for ductal adenocarcinoma of the pancreas: an update. *World J Surg* 1998; **12**:658–662

Watson K. Carcinoma of ampulla: successful radical resection. *Br J Surg* 1944; **31**:368–373

Williamson RCN. Conservative pancreatectomy. *Br J Surg* 1985; **72**:801–803

Williamson RCN. Pancreatic cancer: the greatest oncological challenge. *BMJ* 1988; **296**:445–446

Worthington TR, Williamson RCN. Tumour markers in pancreatic cancer. *World J Surg* 1999; **23**:230–232

Zollinger R, Ellison E. Primary peptic ulcerations of the jejunum associated with islet cell tumours of the pancreas. *Ann Surg* 1955; **142**:709–723

11

The liver

J.N. Baxter

PATHOPHYSIOLOGY AND CLINICAL FEATURES

Surgeons commonly encounter patients with liver disease. The clinical features of the liver disease are influenced by the cause, e.g. biliary obstruction causing jaundice, chronic hepatic failure resulting in a low serum albumin and clotting disorders, a wide variety of pathologies causing portal hypertension, etc. Sometimes a combination of these liver conditions may occur in the same patient. It is important to understand the typical patient scenarios which the surgeon may encounter.

Chronic biliary obstruction

In this situation the surgeon is usually referred a patient who has obvious cholestatic jaundice (high direct bilirubin and alkaline phosphatase) with relatively normal liver enzymes. The crucial diagnostic investigation for the surgeon is to determine whether it is a 'surgical jaundice', i.e. dilated ducts, or a medical cause (undilated ducts), often due to drugs.

- A history of gallstones or symptoms suggestive of a pancreatic neoplasm are uppermost in the surgeon's mind although there are several other causes of obstructive jaundice.

- Previous biliary surgery suggests a retained bile duct stone or a possible bile duct stricture.

- Jaundice which occurs following the resection of a gastro-intestinal tumour is suggestive of liver metastases, the patient often presenting with weight loss and anorexia.

- A history of a fever with rigors is strongly in favour of a cholangitis secondary to bile duct obstruction.

Generally the rate of increase in serum bilirubin is slower in surgical jaundice compared to acute viral hepatitis or cholestatic drug jaundice.

Occasionally the gallbladder is palpable in a distal malignant bile duct obstruction (Courvoisier positive).

Ultrasound of the liver to detect dilated intrahepatic ducts will usually decide the matter although in patients with cirrhosis sometimes the intrahepatic ducts will not dilate when there is an extrahepatic cause for the obstruction. If the ducts are dilated the ultrasonographer can then image the bile duct and head of pancreas to try and determine the cause of the obstruction. A good ultrasonographer will often make the diagnosis without recourse to endoscopic retrograde cholangiopancreatography (ERCP) or percutaneous transhepatic cholangiography (PTC), both investigations being diagnostic in the large majority of patients. Increasingly, magnetic resonance cholangiopancreatography (MRCP) and computed tomography (CT) scanning are also used to image the biliary system, the former because it is less invasive and the latter to obtain further information about the cause.

Although the jaundice is self-evident, it has other effects on the patient that must be borne in mind by the surgeon since if an operation is contemplated, then the patient may experience further complications. For example, the kidneys have an increased susceptibility to hypoxic damage, cardiovascular responses are abnormal, wound healing is abnormal, platelets may be abnormal and peptic ulceration is more common. In addition, endotoxaemia and immunosuppression are more common in jaundiced patients than those with normal bilirubin levels.

Chronic hepatic failure

The surgeon is often called upon to manage patients with some degree of liver failure, often secondary to cirrhosis of the liver. In the UK the most common cause of cirrhosis is alcoholic liver disease. Depending on the degree of liver decompensation, the patient may exhibit a general malaise with weakness and easy fatiguability.

- The typical patient with cirrhosis often has the stigmata of chronic liver disease (spider naevi, liver palms, pale nails, liver tremor, anaemia, hepatosplenomegaly, ascites, hypogonadism, hirsutism, gynaecomastia, scratch marks).

- There is usually a history of the aetiology, e.g. alcohol abuse, hepatitis, primary biliary cirrhosis, etc.

- The patient may have a history of catastrophic haematemesis from gastro-oesophageal varices.

- A history of easy bruising should alert the surgeon to a possible bleeding diathesis which is usually of a complex nature with thrombocytopenia (often $60–90 \times 10^9/l$) secondary to hypersplenism, reduced synthesis of clotting factors and inhibitors of coagulation and enhanced fibrinolytic activity, to name but a few.

- In addition, these patients, if they have decompensated liver disease (Childs' B/C) will often be malnourished with a low serum albumin, have ascites and exhibit a symptomatic anaemia of chronic liver failure.

- Furthermore, they may exhibit a degree of cholestatic jaundice from sinusoidal block which is usually directly related to the severity of the liver failure.

- In severe decompensated liver disease they will also exhibit the neurological features of chronic hepatic encephalopathy such as liver flap, personality change, intellectual deterioration and disturbed consciousness.

- A hyperdynamic circulation may also be evident although renal blood flow, especially to the cortex, is reduced.

- In approximately one-third of patients with decompensated cirrhosis a hepatopulmonary syndrome develops which is characterised by a reduced arterial saturation which occasionally results in cyanosis.

- Also, about one-third of decompensated patients have a low-grade fever, probably secondary to cytokine release from chronic inflammation.

- Septicaemia occurs often as a terminal event in these patients. Endotoxaemia from gut translocation is much more prevalent in decompensated cirrhosis. Because these patients are immunosuppressed they should receive prophylactic antibiotics for all invasive procedures.

MANAGEMENT OF CHRONIC HEPATIC FAILURE

Although surgeons will usually ask for assistance from a gastroenterologist in the management of chronic hepatic failure they should have some knowledge of the principles involved. All treatment is generally symptomatic unless a liver transplant is contemplated. Any factor which aggravates hepatocellular function can cause decompensation so a thorough search must be made, looking for reversible factors such as hypotension following surgery, acute infections, electrolyte dislocations from any cause.

All patients should have bedrest during a decompensating phase since this reduces the metabolic requirements of the liver. Some form of dietary protein restriction may be advisable, usually 80–100 g of protein daily. Sometimes in the alcoholic who has not been taking a good diet, a high-protein diet may be desirable. In the alcoholic cirrhotic further alcohol abuse must be avoided, the patient usually being advised to avoid all alcohol permanently. If the patient has a symptomatic anaemia this may require transfusion if <10 g/100 ml.

If the patient has an exacerbation of hepatic encephalopathy then precipitating causes must be excluded and some form of treatment started which reduces gut production and absorption of toxins. This usually involves reducing the dietary protein further to around 20 g daily until there is improvement. Neomycin or metronidazole is usually given orally to decrease intestinal ammonia production. For reasons which are not entirely clear, lactulose is effective in addition to antibiotics. Purgation with an effective regime is also recommended. Some patients who have had a shunt of some form inserted may, if their encephalopathy is very severe, be considered for reversal of the shunt which may require some other form of treatment to prevent variceal bleeding.

Occasionally the surgeon is asked to assist in the management of ascites or may have to operate on a patient who has ascites. The former is usually due to refractory ascites and the latter because the patient is a surgical emergency. For refractory ascites a peritoneo-venous shunt is very effective but it is not without its complications, e.g. disseminated intravascular coagulation, variceal bleeding, pulmonary oedema. If it is essential to operate on patients with ascites invariably the ascites will become worse after the surgery for a period before it settles down. It is very important to close the abdomen tightly, especially the deep layers, to prevent a chronic ascitic leak. Usually the patient has a poor

prognosis after the emergency surgery since ascites is a marker of the severity of the liver disease.

In general, following surgery you should consult a gastroenterologist about the management of the ascites which would generally involve fluid restriction (1 l/day), sodium restriction (22 mmol/day), and administering spironolactone 200 mg daily. If this does not work after four days then add frusemide 80 mg daily. Patients should have bedrest and be weighed daily which is the best indicator of progress. Monitoring of electrolytes is necessary. If the ascites is very uncomfortable or causing respiratory embarrassment then a paracentesis should be carried out removing 5–10 l whilst giving at the same time salt-poor albumin (6 g/l ascites removed).

The coagulation defect that most of these patients have must be treated if surgery is contemplated. Vitamin K_1 10 mg i.m. for three days is usually prescribed. This will be effective in about three hours for those patients with cholestatic jaundice who have vitamin K malabsorption. If the prothrombin time and partial thromboplastin time are excessively elevated (>1.5 × normal) then fresh frozen plasma can be given which will restore clotting factors for a few hours during the surgery. Platelet transfusions can also be given although the author does not advise this unless the platelet count is <50 × 10^9/l.

The hepatorenal syndrome (functional renal failure) may occur in these patients due to sensitivity of the renal vasculature to the circulating toxins. There is an intense renal vasoconstriction which causes reduced glomerular filtration rate in the face of normal tubular function. It is usually precipitated by some event such as surgery in a poorly hydrated patient or some other cause which results in hypovolaemia. Initially it may be quite mild and not recognised but then rapid uraemia develops with a general deterioration of the patient. The serum urea and creatinine levels increase.

PORTAL HYPERTENSION

The most common cause of portal hypertension in the Western world is cirrhosis secondary to alcoholic liver disease. The intra-hepatic vascular resistance is raised due to the pathology which causes raised portal pressure and the development of collaterals (shunts) where blood is shunted around the liver through the anatomical portal–systemic shunts, of which those at the gastro-oesophageal junction are the most important. These augmented shunts give rise to gastro-oesophageal varices which have a high propensity to bleed, giving rise to life-threatening haemorrhage. The shunts also lead to a hyperdynamic circulation which results in an increase in portal venous inflow which helps to maintain the elevated portal pressure despite the development of collateral shunts. These patients who are already ravaged by chronic severe liver failure have a high mortality from their first bleed. Indeed, when varices are diagnosed before they have bled some thought should be given to primary prevention of variceal bleeding by commencing propranolol therapy.

Over the last 20 years the management of a variceal haemorrhage has gradually shifted from the domain of the upper gastrointestinal surgeon to the gastroenterologist due largely to the high success of endoscopic means of stopping bleeding. However, the surgeon may still be called upon to stop a variceal haemorrhage by endoscopic means or, if this fails, by surgical means if transjugular intrahepatic portal–systemic shunting (TIPS) is not available. When bleeding is brought under control endoscopically it is important to remember that further treatment is necessary to prevent recurrent haemorrhage (secondary prevention) because of the high likelihood of recurrent haemorrhage without further treatment.

Acute variceal haemorrhage

The algorithm for the management of an acute variceal bleed is shown in Figure 11.1. When variceal haemorrhage is first suspected as a possible diagnosis, IV glypressin (1 mg if <50 kg weight; 1.5 mg if patient 50–70 kg weight; 2 mg if >70 kg weight) should be immediately administered, with a transdermal glyceryl trinitrate patch (10 mg over 24 hour) being applied. Alternatively, native somatostatin can also be administered with a 250 μg bolus followed by a 250 μg/h infusion, taking care not to interrupt the infusion between bag changes. Resuscitation must be carried out with two IV lines being established and close monitoring of the urinary output and CVP. Resuscitation can be carried out with IV colloid until whole blood becomes available.

The patient should then be endoscoped immediately by an experienced endoscopist, if available. If there is any delay in obtaining an endoscopy and the patient is haemodynamically unstable, balloon tamponade of the oesophagus should be instituted. At endoscopy when the diagnosis of variceal bleeding from oesophageal varices is confirmed then injection sclerotherapy or banding should be carried out (see below). If bleeding is torrential and endostasis cannot be carried out then a balloon tube should be inserted and the procedure carried out again after 12–24 hours of tamponade. It is important to let the oesophageal balloon down after 12 hours of compression (leaving the gastric balloon inflated) to avoid ischaemia of the oesophageal mucosa. Should bleeding recur then it is only necessary to reinflate the oesophageal balloon.

Following successful endostasis (sclerotherapy or banding) there may be some mild ooze which is usually acceptable without insertion of a balloon tube. The patient should then be monitored very closely and a repeat injection or banding applied in one week. Ideally glypressin should be administered continuously for this week. Management of the acute bleed is only considered finished after the second course of endostasis. The patient should then have their varices obliterated by repeat sclerotherapy/banding every three weeks until the varices disappear.

The acute variceal bleed can usually be controlled in 90% of cases by two courses of sclerotherapy/banding. In around 10% of cases, despite attempts at endostasis bleeding will not stop and other means must be employed. A TIPS procedure should then be carried out

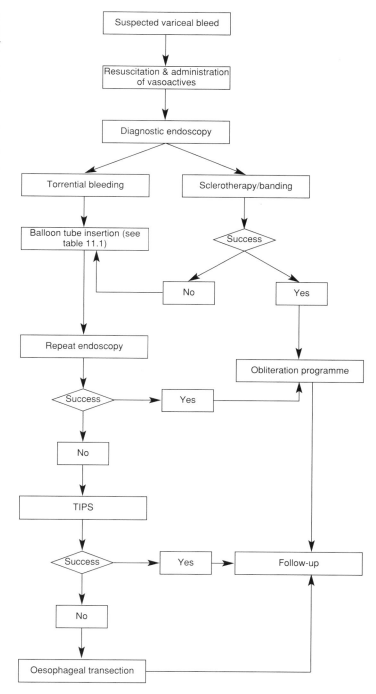

Figure 11.1 Algorithm for acute variceal haemorrhage.

as a semi-urgent procedure whilst a balloon tube controls the bleeding (Table 11.1). In centres where this procedure is not available a decision must be made whether to transfer the patient to a centre where this technology is available or, alternatively, consider an oesophageal transection (see below). Prior to development of the TIPS procedure, oesophageal transection was the preferred method for stopping variceal bleeding although some surgeons preferred an emergency portocaval shunt (often a small-diameter H-graft). The latter is a skill that few surgeons outside specialised

Table 11.1 Balloon tube insertion for bleeding gastro-oesophageal varices

- Use 4 lumen tube of Minnesota or Sengstaken-Blakemore type (if time, stiffen by putting in refrigerator for 30 minutes)
- Test balloons before insertion
- Lubricate tube well with KY jelly
- Insert through mouth with patient in head down position and an endoscopy mouth guard in place – ask patient to swallow
- Listen to air insufflation into stomach with stethoscope before inflating gastric balloon
- Use only air in gastric balloon (around 250–300 ml) – pull back to gastro-oesophageal junction
- Use fluid (mixed with contrast) in oesophageal balloon to pressure of 35 mm Hg – monitor by direct measurement
- Apply artery clamps to all oesophageal and gastric balloons
- Apply low pressure suction to oesophageal aspiration channel
- Put gastric channel on free drainage
- Apply light traction with a spatula taped to tube at the level of the mouth
- Let down oesophageal balloon after 12 hours compression (leave gastric balloon inflated)

centres have nowadays, hence oesophageal transection is the preferred option because it is technically much less demanding.

BLUNT LIVER INJURIES

General surgeons doing an acute on-call rota will occasionally come across a serious liver injury which they will often struggle to deal with due to inadequate experience and/or poor specialised support. In general terms we are currently in an era of doing little as possible in order to stop the bleeding then transfer the patient to an experienced liver centre or, alternatively, get a liver surgeon to come and help with the procedure. Ideally most hospitals should have a surgeon with a working knowledge of how to deal with serious liver injuries available for assistance when needed. It is important to remember that blunt liver injuries are often associated with other injuries (polytrauma) which may delay the diagnosis of the liver injury.

Initially rapid resuscitation is carried out in the usual manner. If after 1–2 l of resuscitation fluid the patient is stable they can then have further assessment of their putative abdominal injury. If resuscitation is not succeeding then the patient should be transferred to theatre immediately for laparotomy.

Non-operative management

For the 'stable' patient a contrast-enhanced CT scan should be urgently requested. CT scanning has reduced the laparotomy rate for liver injury by one half. If contrast is seen outside the liver substance then bleeding is likely to be active and laparotomy is advised although arteriography followed by embolisation may be successful. If a non-operative policy is employed then close monitoring of vital signs is necessary but with a low threshold for surgical intervention if continued bleeding is suspected.

Operative management

A mid-line incision is usually recommended because this allows adequate assessment of all abdominal organs for other injuries. A cell-saver, if available, is very useful to avoid the need for massive exogenous blood transfusions with all the problems of banked blood. Two suckers are useful while the extent of intraabdominal injuries is rapidly assessed. The surgeon should initially concentrate on the site where most bleeding is coming from in order to allow haemodynamic stabilisation. All injuries are dealt with on their merits but we will assume here that only the liver is damaged. If the liver damage is discovered as part of a laparotomy for other injuries then often it will have stopped bleeding and not require any surgical treatment. Do not explore a non-bleeding liver fracture since this will almost inevitably cause further haemorrhage. If a fractured liver is bleeding compress the fracture for 20 minutes and then reassess. If bleeding has stopped do no more.

The real problem is when the surgeon is faced with a shattered lobe which is actively bleeding. In this situation the surgeon needs to decide on a policy of 'pack and pray' or of active management by exploring the injury and even a possible liver resection. Naturally, the policy will depend on the surgeon's skill and experience and also that of colleagues available for assistance. There is no shame in calling a senior, more experienced colleague to help when you are out of your depth.

One important factor in determining the operative strategy is the site and extent of liver injury. If injury is confined to the left lobe to the left of the falciform ligament (segments II/III) then most surgeons would feel comfortable with removing these segments by a left lobectomy. However, more usually the right lobe is involved and in order to obtain better access to assess the right liver, you will need to extend the mid-line incision to the right with a subcostal incision. This is not necessary if you have decided on a 'pack and pray' approach. Packing should be carried out with large laparotomy packs and placed so as to compress liver tissue, not open it. If packing is used the patient should then be very closely monitored in the intensive care unit (ITU) with the objective of removing the packs in 72 hours when the patient is haemodynamically stable. If despite packing the patient continues to bleed in the ITU, do not be afraid to return to theatre for reassessment and repacking if necessary. During this time the management team needs to assess whether to transfer the patient to a liver unit.

If the surgeon/surgeons feel confident to explore the fracture after a failed compression test or the liver lobe is completely shattered then a Pringle manoeuvre should be tried using a soft bowel clamp on the hepatoduodenal ligament. If this controls the bleeding then by intermittently releasing the clamp the bleeders can be identified and suture ligated. If inflow occlusion does not stop the bleeding then hepatic venous bleeding is the only other possibility. In order to deal with this you may be able to identify the venous bleeders with good suction but often it will be necessary to fully mobilise the right lobe by dividing the right triangular ligament right up to the inferior vena cava and then rotating the right lobe of the liver into the wound. This is a very useful manoeuvre which will result in the surgeon being able to compress the right hepatic veins manually from behind and slow down or completely stop hepatic venous bleeding.

The most difficult situation is when the hepatic veins at the back of the liver are damaged – a frequently fatal condition. If expertise is available then a direct attack on the bleeding site by direct suture may stop the bleeding but speed is vital. A decision has then to be made whether the right hepatic vein has been compromised to such a degree that a formal resection will be necessary which may then be undertaken if the surgeon/surgeons are sufficiently confident that they can perform the procedure. If bleeding cannot be stopped then packing should be carried out and the abdomen closed. The team managing the patient should then consult a liver centre for advice about the preferred management, taking into account logistics and distance.

During the surgery it may become apparent that a coagulopathy has developed due to the usual multifactorial reasons of massive transfusion, hypothermia, acidosis, etc. Even following successful control of major bleeding from the liver there is often continual oozing from the liver surface which may require packing for a few days until the coagulopathy has been reversed. An argon plasma coagulator is useful in this situation.

Intensive therapy unit management

Generally severe liver injuries will require positive pressure ventilation in the ITU postoperatively. A broad-spectrum antibiotic should be administered prophylactically and for at least three days postoperatively. During this period rewarming the patient and correcting coagulopathy and acidosis is important. Bile leakage through drains may be apparent but will usually settle without the need for any further treatment. Liver function tests will be deranged for a period and the patient will need total parenteral nutrition.

LIVER CYSTS (INCLUDING HYDATID DISEASE)

The most common true liver cyst is a simple lesion probably similar to the origin of those seen in polycystic disease. The next most common is a hydatid cyst which is more common in areas where this disease is endemic. Finally neoplastic cysts are occasionally seen such as cystadenomas, cystadenocarcinoma or a malignant cyst of a different cell origin. There are many small print causes which are too numerous to mention here. Pseudocysts of the liver lack an epithelial lining and usually are due to neoplastic growth or occur following trauma.

Most hepatic cysts are asymptomatic and are diagnosed incidentally on CT or ultrasound scanning. When they enlarge to a size sufficient to cause symptoms these are usually vague with pain in the right upper quadrant, dyspeptic symptoms and, rarely, obstructive jaundice. Occasionally the cysts are palpable.

Investigations

MRI, CT and ultrasound scanning are the most useful modalities for diagnosis. Expert gastrointestinal radiologists can usually differentiate between the various causes of liver cysts. For example, hydatid cysts often have daughter cysts and partial calcification of the cyst wall. Hydatid cyst diagnosis is usually complemented by performing an antigen test which is usually positive. Laparoscopic ultrasonography allows better discrimination than all externally applied modalities.

MRI is especially useful if haemorrhage into a cyst is suspected because the patient gives a history of increasing pain. If sclerosis of a cyst is contemplated then an ERCP must be carried out to exclude connection with the biliary tree.

Treatment

Most simple cysts which are not causing symptoms can be left. It is common to image them for 2–3 years and if they remain unchanged in size, the patient can be discharged from follow-up. Symptomatic cysts should be aggressively treated since they will often grow further and symptoms may become worse. In general, the principles of treatment involve aspiration with or without sclerosant insertion, external drainage, internal drainage, cyst excision, deroofing with marsupialisation (with or without omentoplasty) and liver resection.

Cyst aspiration is usually non-curative, resulting in recurrence although many workers have recently reported good results with insertion of sclerosants such as ethanol or tetracycline. If this technique is to be used then cyst communication with the biliary tree, neoplastic causes and hydatid disease need to be excluded although the latter is debatable (see below). External drainage, and to a lesser extent, internal drainage may lead to infection. Deroofing of the cyst with marsupialisation of the edges (also called fenestration) is the most traditional treatment which has stood the test of time. Before this procedure is undertaken the surgeon should be reasonably sure that a neoplastic lesion has been excluded – these being better resected by a liver surgeon. Where the diagnosis is not certain then it is better to treat the cyst as neoplastic. All roof linings must be examined histologically to exclude neoplasia. Any bile observed within the cyst must be assumed to come from a biliary connection and the source looked for so that it can be closed with fine sutures. The deroofing should be as wide as possible with removal of as much of the lining as possible. In polycystic disease only the large and symptomatic cysts should be treated.

Importantly, in this modern era simple cysts can be deroofed with a laparoscope in the same manner as carried out by open surgery. This has the important effect of considerably reducing the access trauma and hence the postoperative morbidity. A laparoscopic approach allows for close inspection of the cyst wall and biopsies to exclude malignancy. Use of laparoscopy will depend on the position of the cyst and the confidence of the surgeon to deal with it by a laparoscopic approach. Simple deroofing with or without omentoplasty and cyst excision are all possible. Further experience is needed with this technique before it can be widely recommended. However, the author believes that if infectious and neoplastic cysts have been excluded and the cyst is superficial on the anterior, lateral or inferior surface of the liver then it is reasonable to attempt deroofing laparoscopically, converting readily to an open procedure if indicated.

For some cysts resection of the cyst or part of the liver including the cyst may be indicated, especially if neoplasia is suspected. The precise approach will depend on the position of the cyst.

Benign cystadenomas are most commonly found in young to middle-aged women and must be suspected when septations are found on CT scanning. Biopsy of the wall will confirm the suspicion by finding cuboidal epithelium although this may not be present in all parts of the cyst hence all projections must be biopsied. Treatment is by complete enucleation of the cyst wall, a procedure which is often a little bloody and can be greatly facilitated by using an argon beam for haemostasis.

HYDATID DISEASE

Most hydatid cysts are asymptomatic. However, if they rupture, a fatal anaphylaxis may occur if not aggressively treated. Rupture may also seed viable scolices into the peritoneal cavity resulting in further development of troublesome cysts. Increasing cyst size may cause discomfort and occasionally they may rupture into the biliary system, causing jaundice. Usually the diagnosis is easy with a characteristic appearance on CT scanning of septal loculations and daughter cysts. The patient may have an eosinophilia in addition to positive antigen tests, although the latter is only positive in 80% of cases. If the cyst has a completely calcified wall there is a good chance that it does not contain live scolices, particularly if the antigen tests are negative or low in titre. These cysts should be left alone as the risk of complications is very low.

Medical treatment with mebendazole or albendazole has been shown to be effective in 30–50% of cases but such drugs have toxic side effects. Medical treatment is often preferred for lung hydatids where drug penetration is better. Nevertheless, there is an increasing trend to use the drugs as an neoadjuvant treatment prior to surgery to kill scolices and hence reduce the morbidity if any are spilled during drainage.

Recently there have been many reports of successful treatment with percutaneous aspiration with immediate instillation of alcohol. There are various techniques for this procedure which are described in detail in the radiological literature. Surgery is still the standard treatment with the objectives of removing all cyst contents including the laminar membrane (Figure 11.2) whilst protecting against cyst spillage. Briefly the procedure is carried out as follows.

- Determine exact location of cyst (using intraoperative ultrasound if necessary).

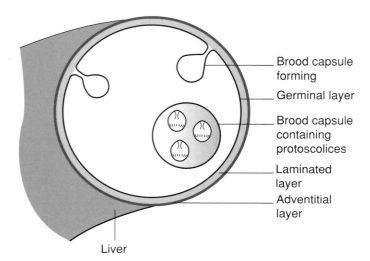

Figure 11.2 Hydatid cyst.

- Carefully pack off the area of the cyst wall to be incised.

- Incise the cyst wall and suck out contents as soon as visible with two high-pressure suckers.

- Open the cyst widely to ensure all contents are removed and extract the laminar membrane.

- Perfuse with cetrimide solution for 10 minutes and then aspirate.

- Close any biliary connections with fine sutures.

- Use a pedicled omental flap to fill the cavity, suturing in place through the edge of the cyst wall.

- Only use a drain if bile has been encountered.

LIVER ABSCESS

Pyogenic liver abscess is a relatively uncommon condition since portal pyaemia is rare nowadays. However, biliary tract lesions responsible for cholangitis may result in the occasional liver abscess. Other miscellaneous causes are arterial blood spread and in continuity spread from an adjacent abscess. A single liver abscess has a 15% mortality, rising to 41% for multiple abscesses. However, in many centres of excellence these figures are considerably lower. Multiple abscesses are often due to biliary drainage problems, malignancy or liver surgery.

Pyogenic liver abscess usually presents as a toxic illness with some local symptoms of abdominal pain. Leucocytosis is common and the alkaline phosphatase is usually elevated. Jaundice is uncommon unless there is a biliary cause. Interestingly, in some series up to 40% of patients are afebrile at the time of diagnosis. Imaging is usually carried out in the first instance using ultrasound which is sensitive if the abscess is large. A CT scan may be necessary, especially if a small abscess is suspected. Needle aspiration should be performed to obtain pus for culture and antibiotic sensitivity analysis. After consultation with the surgeon, the radiologist should consider percutaneous drainage at the same time as diagnostic aspiration since this has become the main form of treatment for liver abscess. A pigtail catheter is usually inserted and instructions left on how to manage it. The catheter should be irrigated with small amounts of sterile saline to prevent blockage. In general percutaneous drainage is 90% effective. In a very small abscess aspiration can be performed without insertion of a pigtail catheter. This latter approach with appropriate antibiotic treatment has a high success rate.

There have been recent reports of using aspiration only plus antibiotics instead of pigtail insertion for abscesses of any size. This may be more acceptable to the patient and is particularly useful in multiple liver abscesses and obviously does not have the problem of catheter blockage or displacement. Multiple aspirations are often necessary with this technique.

Multiple organisms are usually encountered in at least 50% of patients so broad-spectrum antibiotics should be administered first until antibiotic sensitivities based on aspirated pus become available. Prolonged treatment with antibiotics may be necessary according to the patient response. There is no place for antibiotics alone in the management of liver abscess.

In the Western world amoebic liver abscess is uncommon but may be encountered in travellers returning from abroad. Generally if the diagnosis is suspected it can be confirmed by the very specific imaging features coupled with positive serology. Occasionally diagnostic aspiration is necessary to distinguish a pyogenic from an amoebic abscess. There is hardly ever a need to leave a pigtail catheter in an amoebic abscess because of the very good results from antiamoebic chemotherapy.

Surgery is generally only used where there is some other abdominal condition which must be treated in order to allow the abscess to settle (appendicitis, etc.) or where percutaneous drainage has failed. The abscess is localised at laparotomy, then incised and pus evacuated using a sucker. The cavity is then washed out and a drain inserted.

OPERATIVE SURGERY

Variceal sclerotherapy and banding technique

Injection sclerotherapy

Injection sclerotherapy may be carried out as an emergency or electively as part of a variceal obliteration programme. The description here will apply to the emergency situation which is more complicated than elective sclerotherapy.

- Diagnostic endoscopy is usually carried out under light sedation to determine the cause of a haematemesis.

- When bleeding oesophageal varices are encountered they may be bleeding profusely or may have stopped temporarily and

you may see signs of a recent variceal bleed such as a bluish bleb on the varix which has bled. Concurrent administration of vasoactive drugs such as somatostatin or glypressin may make injection easier by reducing or stopping the bleeding.

- The aim of the injection technique is to inject the sclerosant intravariceally to initiate an inflammation which causes a thrombosis although some endoscopists prefer to place the injections paravariceally to cause a tamponade of the bleeding varix rather than attempt direct injection (Figure 11.3). In reality probably a combination of both occurs.

- The use of a twin-channel endoscope is recommended since it allows aspiration whilst at the same time allowing the injection needle to be passed down the other channel. The author recommends using 5% ethanolamine oleate although other substances are equally useful. The aim should be to attack the bleeding varix first (if it is recognised) by injecting 5 ml of sclerosant into the varix. Up to 20 ml of sclerosant can be used if there is more than one varix. Injections must be placed as low as possible in the oesophagus immediately above the gastro-oesophageal junction (GOJ) if success is to be obtained. Sometimes the varix is bleeding too profusely and it is useful to try and inject a smaller volume (2 ml) paravariceally immediately above the varix which often tamponades the varix and allows a clearer view to proceed with intravariceal injection. All columns must be treated. A complete endoscopy must also be performed to exclude any other potential causes of bleeding.

- In <10% of cases bleeding is so profuse that the endoscopist cannot safely inject. They should then pass a balloon tube and repeat the attempt at injection treatment 12–24 hours later. Vasoactive treatment should be continued for at least one week to reduce the incidence of rebleeding.

Using this technique, >70% control of the acute bleed should be achieved with one injection. Around 30% will rebleed in the first

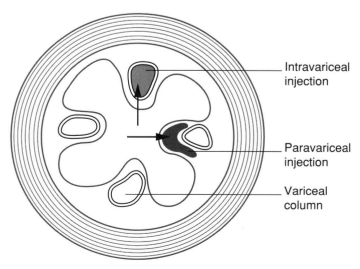

Figure 11.3 Injection sclerotherapy.

Intravariceal injection

Paravariceal injection

Variceal column

week and a second injection will usually lead to further control, giving an overall control rate of >90%. A second injection should always be carried out at one week following the first treatment before the patient is discharged. The patient should then receive injections every three weeks until variceal obliteration is confirmed endoscopically.

Some variations on technique are worth mentioning. Although most endoscopists use sedation it is the author's contention that general anaesthesia is not used enough, especially where the patient is encephalopathic and in danger of aspirating. The injections are much easier to perform, are less rushed and more controlled. An overtube of the Williams or Kitano type can also be used if desired, which is very helpful in dealing with the actively bleeding patient.

Post sclerotherapy, the patient is kept nil by mouth for 24 hours and then allowed free fluids. Some retrosternal discomfort is common, as is a low-grade fever for a few days.

Banding technique

Endoscopic band ligation (EBL) has in many centres taken over from injection sclerotherapy although ideally both techniques should be mastered, as they are complementary in many situations. In general, band ligation is now considered to have fewer complications and produce faster obliteration than injection sclerotherapy. Many workers find that injection sclerotherapy is better in the acute situation with EBL being easier in the elective situation. However, with experience they are mutually interchangeable. Gastric varices are much more safely managed with EBL than with injection sclerotherapy which may make them bleed.

The EBL device has undergone several changes since it was first introduced in 1986, with single banding devices being replaced by multifiring devices which obviate the need for an overtube and multiple insertions of the endoscope. Often the endoscopic view is limited by the endoscopic device on the end of the endoscope but with experience this is not a problem for the endoscopist.

As with injection sclerotherapy, varices should be banded serially as close as possible to the GOJ. There is no evidence that using a combined technique of EBL with injection sclerotherapy improves the results – indeed, there is some evidence that the results are worse with a combination technique.

If EBL is being used in the acute situation the endoscopist should first attempt to directly band the bleeding varix. If this proves difficult it is usual to try and band proximal and distal to the bleeding site. Up to 4–6 bands can be applied at the one sitting. Essentially suction is used to pull the varix into the endoscopic banding device and the band released by pulling a trip wire which allows a band to be released similar to banding second or third-degree haemorrhoids.

Oesophageal transection technique

The aim of this operation is to disconnect the portal and azygous connections in the region of the GOJ by transecting the oesophagus immediately above the GOJ. Since most variceal bleeds occur within 1 cm of the GOJ it is important that the transection is kept as low as possible to avoid recurrent bleeding (Figure 11.4).

- The abdomen should be opened through a mid-line incision. It is helpful to have a sternal retractor of the Omnitract® type. If the left lobe of the liver is very enlarged or stiff then a deep blade is very helpful to elevate the liver.

- The peritoneum is then very carefully divided over the lower oesophagus and all venous channels ligated. It is important to be patient since a hurried mobilisation will cause profuse bleeding and make further progress difficult.

- The oesophagus is then elevated by passing a finger behind from left to right in a similar way used for mobilisation of the oesophagus for a truncal vagotomy procedure. A tape or catheter is useful to sling the oesophagus. It is helpful to also divide the gastrophrenic ligament as far as possible to elevate the fundus of the stomach and hence allow for further mobilisation of the oesophagus. A strong ligature is then passed around the gullet to replace the sling.

- A gastrotomy is performed as high as comfortably possible on the anterior wall of the stomach. A quick check is made to establish that the cause of bleeding is from oesophageal varices and not gastric varices.

- A 25 mm circular stapler is then inserted into the oesophagus and the anvil and head separated by unscrewing the device. The ligature is then tightened around the shaft of the instrument between the anvil and the head, being careful to maintain the position of transection immediately above the GOJ (Figure 11.4).

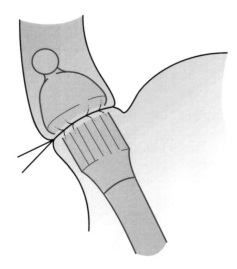

Figure 11.4 Oesophageal transection.

- The instrument is then closed and a careful check made around the oesophagus to ensure that only the oesophagus is included in the stapler.

- The instrument is then fired and removed by unscrewing and removing carefully. Only one doughnut is found in this case and it should be complete.

- Any gastric varices which are seen emerging from the oesophagus and radiating into the stomach should be underrun with an absorbable suture as an insurance policy against rebleeding from this source.

- The gastrotomy is then closed in two layers with a continuous absorbable suture, taking care to make the closure haemostatic.

- The author would also recommend ligating any other obvious large venous tributaries in the region of the GOJ and fundus which serve to divert blood away from the area. In particular, it is worth dividing the left gastric (coronary) vein along the lesser curve of the stomach.

- The abdomen is then closed with a mass closure technique using a continuous non-absorbable suture. If the patient has ascites a leak may occur if the closure is not tight. Ascites may even occur transiently in those patients who did not have ascites preoperatively but usually resolves in 3–4 weeks.

Postoperative care must pay attention to correction of coagulopathy and general supportive care.

FURTHER READING

S Ch Yu, R Hg Lo, PS Kan and C Metreweli. Pyogenic liver abscess: Treatment with needle aspiration. *Clin Radio* 1997; **52**:912–6

Klinger PJ, Gadenstatter M, Schmid T, Bodner E and Schwelberger HG. Treatment of hepatic cysts in the era of laparoscopic surgery. *Br J Surg* 1997; **84**:438–444

Parks RW, Chrysos E and Diamond T. Management of liver trauma. *Br J Surg* 1999; **86**:1121-35

Strong RW. The management of blunt liver injuries. *Aust NZ J Surg* 1999; **69**:609–616

Taylor BR and Langer B. Current surgical management of hepatic cyst disease. *Adv Surg* 1998; **31**:127–148

Neoplasms of the liver

Cornelis H.C. Dejong, O. James Garden

In recent years, surgical management of liver neoplasia has become increasingly important due to three factors.

- The incidence of some benign and malignant tumours is increasing.

- The routine use of sophisticated modern imaging techniques leads to early detection of hepatic tumours either in 'screening' programmes or as incidental findings.

- Our increasing knowledge of hepatic anatomy and physiology, combined with improvements in surgical and anaesthetic technique, has made liver resections possible for a greater number of patients with low morbidity and mortality rates.

The first part of this chapter will address surgical aspects of benign hepatic neoplasms. Subsequently, the management of primary and secondary malignancies of the liver will be reviewed. Finally, the technique of a common hepatic resection, right hepatectomy, will be described.

BENIGN TUMOURS

Benign hepatic tumours are rare and can be separated into solid and cystic lesions with the latter being infectious or non-infectious. Benign liver lesions may require surgical treatment for relief of symptoms, prevention of haemorrhage or to exclude malignancy. The four most common benign lesions are liver cysts, liver cell adenoma, focal nodular hyperplasia and haemangioma. Generally speaking, benign lesions do not need surgical treatment unless they cause symptoms, if there is a risk of malignant transformation or because of diagnostic uncertainty.

Simple cysts

Although liver cysts (Figure 12.1) are equally distributed over both sexes, for some yet unexplained reason, symptomatic cysts are 10 times more common in females, presenting usually between the ages of 50 and 60 years. Asymptomatic cysts do not require treatment but can develop complications. They can become infected or haemorrhage and the cysts can cause mechanical problems. Pain, nausea, vomiting and early satiety are the predominant symptoms. Percutaneous aspiration of cysts generally leads to recurrence and carries the risk of introducing infection into the cyst. Symptomatic simple cysts are best dealt with by either laparoscopic or open radical deroofing. Laparoscopic deroofing is indicated for large superficial cysts that are easily accessible. Open deroofing is the treatment of choice for centrally located cysts and those that are inaccessible to the laparoscope. Three-year symptomatic recurrence rates after laparoscopic or open deroofing are reported at about 10% and 30%, respectively, although there are few reports of long-term follow-up for the laparoscopic approach. The higher recurrence rates after open deroofing are probably attributable to case selectivity.

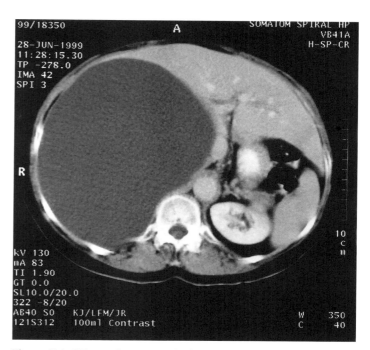

Figure 12.1 CT scan of a patient with a large simple cyst in the right hemiliver.

Polycystic liver disease

This is an autosomal dominant, inherited disease with varying penetrance and expression (Figure 12.2). With advancing age the cysts increase in number and size, generally giving rise to symptoms by the age of 40. About 50% of patients also have cysts in their kidneys. Treatment is indicated for symptoms such as

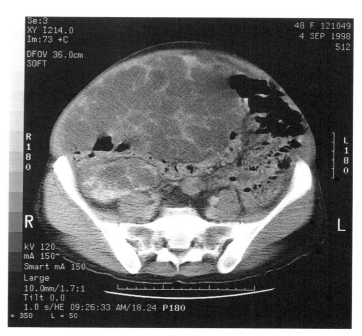

Figure 12.2 CT scan of a patient with polycystic liver disease extending into the pelvis.

epigastric fullness and discomfort, which are generally of a mechanical nature. The liver can increase to an enormous size, sometimes reaching into the pelvis (Figure 12.2). Laparoscopic or open deroofing may not control symptoms and three-year recurrence rates in our experience are around 70% and 20% for laparoscopic and open deroofing, respectively. Formal hepatectomies should be considered in the treatment of these patients. However, the morbidity rate of these procedures is high in this patient group. Experience with liver transplantation is limited and probably one should be reluctant to consider transplant because of the risk of further renal impairment in these already compromised patients.

Focal nodular hyperplasia

Focal nodular hyperplasia (FNH) is an uncommon benign tumour predominantly encountered in females during their fertile years. It is usually an incidental finding in asymptomatic patients undergoing imaging or laparotomy for extrahepatic problems. Like hepatocellular adenoma (see below) its incidence has steadily increased since the 1960s. This might be attributable to improved imaging systems but there is also an apparent association with the increasing long-term use of oral contraceptives. Unlike liver cell adenoma, there is no known risk of malignant transformation. Conservative management is therefore justified, when the diagnosis is certain, since 80–90% of patients are asymptomatic and complications are rare.

Unfortunately, the currently available imaging modalities lack diagnostic specificity. CT scanning and ultrasonography are equally sensitive in the detection of focal nodular hyperplasia. However, FNH and liver cell adenoma (see below) can give a very similar picture using these imaging techniques. In view of the fact that FNH is not a premalignant condition, whereas hepatocellular adenoma has the potential for malignant degeneration, a definitive diagnosis is crucial. Typically, ultrasound shows a hypoechoic tumour with a central scar and CT scans with contrast enhancement show a hypervascular, usually solitary tumour located peripherally in the liver. The value of MRI, angiography and technetium scintigraphy remains to be established, but all of these may assist in differentiating FNH from liver cell adenoma. Percutaneous biopsy of asymptomatic liver masses to differentiate between FNH and liver cell adenoma is not without risk considering the propensity of hepatocellular adenoma to bleed.

Liver cell adenoma (hepatocellular adenoma)

Liver cell adenomas are rare, usually solitary tumours composed of hepatocytes. Multifocality is more common (up to 30%) than for FNH. They do not contain bile ducts and the blood supply is mainly through the hepatic artery. The pathogenesis is unclear, although a clear relation with the use of oral contraceptive medication exists. Prolonged use of oral contraceptives (>10 years) increases the incidence of hepatocellular adenoma 25-fold. From

this it is evident that this tumour is predominantly found in females in the fourth decade.

It can be very difficult to discriminate between liver cell adenoma and focal nodular hyperplasia or hepatocellular carcinoma and in fact, there is no single laboratory test or imaging modality with appropriate accuracy short of biopsy. Biopsy carries a high risk of inducing haemorrhage from adenomas and it should be borne in mind that biopsy of hepatocellular carcinoma carries a 3% risk of puncture site metastases. Hepatocellular adenoma has been reported to regress and even disappear after stopping oral contraceptives. Based on these observations, some authors have proposed conservative management of lesions <5 cm. Others, however, feel that surgery should not unnecessarily be postponed for two reasons. These tumours are known to have a high risk of spontaneous rupture (especially in patients using oral contraceptives) and very often this is the initial mode of presentation. Second, there is a clear risk of malignant degeneration, especially in patients with positive hepatitis B or C serology. The natural history of liver cell adenoma is still incompletely understood, but since over 75% of patients present with symptoms and 30% have acute symptoms from haemorrhage or rupture, we feel surgical therapy is indicated for every liver cell adenoma that does not regress after stopping oral contraceptive steroids.

Surgical treatment for bleeding adenomas should consist of emergency laparotomy and tamponading of the bleeding. Emergency liver resection has a high morbidity (8%) and mortality (5%) even in experienced hands. Definitive treatment should be performed in specialised centres under well-controlled circumstances.

Haemangioma

This is the most common of all benign liver tumours (Figure 12.3). The tumour probably has a prevalence of around 5% and is

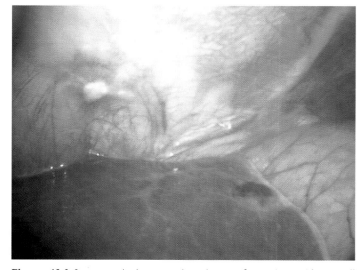

Figure 12.3 Laparoscopic intraoperative picture of a patient with a small haemangioma detected during laparoscopy in the work-up for liver resection for colorectal metastases. Note small peritoneal metastasis on diaphragm.

more common in females than in males. Haemangiomas can be small and multiple, but they can also reach a substantial size. There appears to be an inverse relation between size and age, presumably as a consequence of repeated infarcts in the haemangioma. Haemangiomas rarely cause symptoms and usually are discovered incidentally. The risk of spontaneous rupture of even large haemangiomas is probably less than was formerly thought and only approximately 30 such cases of life-threatening haemorrhage had been described in the literature before 1995. Giant haemangiomas can give rise to coagulopathy as part of the so-called Kasabach–Merritt syndrome, where there is an increased consumption of clotting factors and thrombocytes in the cavernous haemangioma. Haemangiomas do not transform into malignant tumours. Therefore, it seems justified in asymptomatic patients to follow these patients up by repeated ultrasound examinations. Ultrasound has a 60–80% sensitivity in detecting haemangiomas compared to sensitivities of CT, angiography and MRI of 75%, 85% and 92% respectively. Biopsies should not be undertaken in view of the risk of bleeding.

Surgery is rarely indicated for haemangiomas. Persistent growth of lesions, severe symptoms or the development of the Kasabach–Merritt syndrome would represent an indication for intervention. In these cases, the lesion can usually be removed by limited resections with or without selective clamping of the portal and arterial blood supply. Haemangiomas can usually be dissected out of the liver because there is a fibrotic plane between the tumour and the normal liver.

Bile duct adenoma (hamartoma)

These are usually small tumours located beneath the capsule of the liver. Very often they give rise to diagnostic confusion during laparoscopy or laparotomy. They are composed of nests of bile ducts. The natural history is benign and usually without complications. There is no risk of malignant degeneration and consequently they do not need surgical treatment.

Other benign tumours

Apart from the tumours mentioned above, there are various extremely rare benign tumours of the liver. These include lipomas, fibroma, mesothelioma, teratoma, myxoma, leiomyoma, hepatic pseudotumours and mesenchymal hamartomas (see Further Reading).

This chapter concentrates on surgical treatment of neoplasms. A discussion of hepatic abscesses as well as parasitic cysts (hydatid, amoebiasis) is beyond its scope. The interested reader is referred to the Further Reading section at the end of this chapter.

MALIGNANT TUMOURS

In recent years, screening programmes have led to a relative increase in the number of resectable liver malignancies. This is the case for both primary and secondary hepatic malignancies. The feasibility of liver resection in the treatment of malignant liver tumours is limited by anatomic and functional restraints. Thus, a small tumour in an inaccessible location can make resection technically impossible. Similarly, multiple bilobar metastases are often beyond resectability. Finally, extensive resection in a functionally normal liver or even small resections in a cirrhotic liver may not leave sufficient liver to support vital functions. Although the ancient Greeks appreciated that liver can regenerate (Prometheus, chained to the mountains, was assaulted every day by an eagle, which ate his liver daily until Hercules liberated him), this is not the case for cirrhotic liver. This limits the applicability of resectional therapy in patients with liver cirrhosis.

Primary malignant tumours

Hepatocellular carcinoma

By far the most common primary malignancy of the liver is hepatocellular carcinoma (HCC). The tumour, as the name indicates, consists of malignant hepatocytes. Its incidence varies throughout the world, being very high in Asia (30/100 000 per year) and low in Europe (2/100 000 per year). Hepatocellular carcinoma is nearly always (90%) associated with liver cirrhosis and HCC is commonly associated with hepatitis B and C in endemic areas. The annual incidence in patients with cirrhosis is about 5%. The natural course of this tumour is very aggressive, although to some extent it shows a geographic distribution. The tumour is generally considered to have a dismal prognosis without treatment. In Asia the median survival without treatment is seven weeks, whereas in Europe patients may survive for four months following diagnosis. It is well established that smaller tumours (<3 cm) have a better prognosis.

Ultrasound and a raised plasma alpha-fetoprotein level are usually sufficient to confirm the diagnosis, although 30% of patients have a normal alpha-fetoprotein. Spiral CT scans or CT angioportography (CTAP) are helpful in defining the relation of the tumour to surrounding structures and may exclude any additional tumours. Lipiodol-CT is very sensitive in the detection of small nodules since blood supply of the tumour is mainly through the hepatic artery. The tumour has a tendency to invade the portal vein and may metastasise locally in this way in the liver. Hepatic vein involvement is not a common mode of tumour spread, but sometimes the tumour does invade into the vein and inferior caval vein (Figure 12.4).

Although many hepatocellular carcinomas are discovered earlier as a consequence of intensive screening, only a minority of cases (maximally 30%) are amenable to surgical treatment by hepatic resection. This is mainly because 90% of patients with HCC have cirrhosis. Liver function in cirrhotic patients can be classified according to a modification of the Childs' classification, based on the presence or absence of ascites, encephalopathy and on albumin, bilirubin and prothrombin levels. Patients graded Childs B

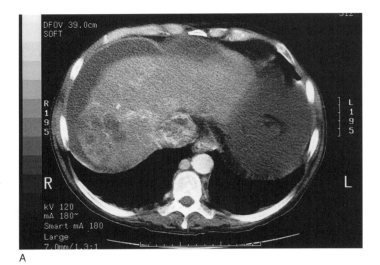

Figure 12.4 A. CT-scan picture of a hepatocellular carcinoma extending into the inferior vena cava (reprinted from: Wigmore SJ, Garden J. *Hepatology* 1999; **31**: 160, with permission). **B**. Intraoperative laparoscopic view of a multifocal hepatocellular carcinoma in the right hemiliver.

rates of around 75% have been reported, resulting in demands for less stringent transplant criteria. The results for larger multifocal tumours are, however, less promising.

Other primary malignancies

These are very rare and their clinical presentation and treatment will not be discussed here. The most common of these tumours in the Western hemisphere is fibrolamellar carcinoma. This tumour is equally common in males and females and is not usually associated with underlying liver disease. Alpha-fetoprotein levels are not raised in 95% of cases and the tumour is assumed to have a better prognosis than HCC. Another not uncommonly encountered primary malignancy is cholangiocarcinoma of the intrahepatic biliary tree (as opposed to hilar cholangiocarcinoma). Other primary malignancies include angiosarcomas, epithelioid haemangio-endothelioma and primary hepatic lymphoma.

Secondary malignant tumours

Hepatic resections for metastatic tumours are mainly performed for three tumour categories. Metastases from colorectal cancers form the majority of cases of hepatic resections. Liver resection for metastatic neuroendocrine tumours may also be considered. Finally, there have been some recent suggestions that there may be an indication for liver resection in the treatment of non-colorectal, non-neuroendocrine metastases.

Colorectal cancer metastases

Colorectal cancer is one of the most common cancers in the Western world. Approximately half of the patients with colorectal cancer will ultimately develop liver metastases and the prognosis of such patients without treatment is poor. Median survival is approximately 10 months after diagnosis. There is growing evidence that, unlike any other currently available therapy, hepatic resection for colorectal metastases can provide long-term survival and even cure. Based on very large series of patients treated by hepatic resection, it has been shown that 10- and 20-year survival rates are 20% and 15% respectively (including operative mortality). Considering the low morbidity and mortality rates of liver surgery in specialist centres, liver resection should be offered to all patients with resectable disease.

Until recently, most hepatobiliary surgeons would use four main criteria to assess resectability. The patient should be fit enough to undergo major surgery and there should be no evidence of extra-hepatic disease. Free resection margins of at least 1 cm should be obtainable and there should be no more than four metastases, preferably located on one side of the liver. Based on these criteria, 25–30% of all patients with colorectal metastatic disease would be candidates for liver surgery.

and C are not normally considered for hepatic resection in view of the high perioperative morbidity and mortality. In Childs A grade patients, only segmental resections may be possible.

Survival rates after partial liver resection for HCC have improved in recent years. Currently, most European and Asian centres publish five-year survival rates, which vary between 20% and 65%. The better survival figures are usually associated with smaller tumours.

In recent years, liver transplantation has been proposed as a treatment for HCC in cirrhotic patients, when tumours are less than 3 cm in size and when there are other indications for transplantation. Currently, 12% of all liver transplantations in Europe are performed for HCC. Initial results for both graft survival and disease-free patient survival are promising and five-year survival

However, debate has recently arisen as to whether one should adhere very stringently to these criteria. Thus, studies have shown that although the presence of five or more metastases adversely affects resectability, this factor does not influence overall or disease-free survival if radical resection has been achieved. Equally, it has been argued that wide resection margins are not strictly necessary, taking into account the fact that satellite metastases are not common in colorectal cancer metastasis. Clearly, positive resection margins affect outcome adversely, but there is no convincing evidence that patients with resection margins of less than 1 cm fare less well than patients with margins of 1 cm or more.

In larger series, five-year survival rates have been reported to range between 40% and 50% after curative resections with disease-free survival rates of around 35%. However, median survival of patients with macroscopic or microscopic residual disease after hepatic resection is approximately 14 months. Tumour recurrence after hepatic surgery occurs in 60–70% of patients, but does not imply that further surgical treatment is impossible. Recent data suggest that repeat hepatectomies and sequential hepatic and pulmonary resections for colorectal metastases are warranted in a highly selected patient group.

Hepatic metastases of colorectal primaries are usually asymptomatic but an increasing number of patients with hepatic metastases are identified earlier due to intensive follow-up screening programmes. Serum carcinoembryonic antigen (CEA) levels are useful in the follow-up of colorectal carcinomas, particularly if they have been elevated prior to resection of the primary tumour. Ultrasound is said to be sensitive in the detection of hepatic metastases, but intravenous contrast-enhanced CT scan, especially the newer generation of spiral CTs is vital for assessing the number of metastases and their anatomic relations to vital structures in order to develop a treatment strategy. The exact role of MRI (Figure 12.5) in the work-up of hepatic colorectal metastases remains to be determined, although it does not seem to be more accurate than spiral CT scan. Laparoscopic assessment including laparoscopic ultrasound provides very useful information concerning the presence or absence of peritoneal metastases and the number and localisation of the hepatic metastases. Intraoperative ultrasound is crucial in modern treatment of hepatic metastases in those patients submitted to laparotomy, because it helps to detect small tumours. In addition, the hepatic anatomy can be more clearly defined to enable safe resection.

Immediate postoperative complications include atelectasis and chest infections. Intraoperative blood loss may be significant, but transfusion is usually required in less than a third of cases. Postoperative bile leaks may occur and, if persistent, can usually be effectively controlled by endoscopic stenting. Long-term outcome is adversely affected by the grade of differentiation and lymph node status of the primary tumour, the presence of synchronous metastases, hepatic metastases greater than 5 cm, positive hepatic resection margins, extrahepatic disease and hepatic resections by non-anatomic procedures.

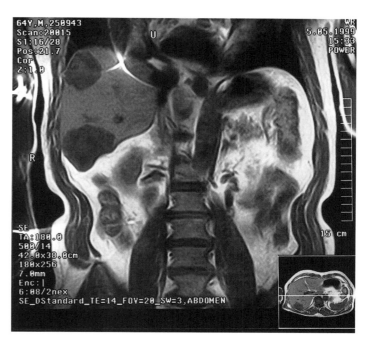

Figure 12.5 Coronal MRI of a patient with two colorectal cancer metastases in the right hemiliver.

Neuroendocrine metastases

Metastatic neuroendocrine tumours to the liver are rare. The primary tumours arise from neural crest cells and are usually intestinal or pulmonary in origin. Neuroendocrine tumours may or may not be hormonally active. The vast majority of these tumours have a carcinoid differentiation and they may produce serotonin, giving rise to the characteristic symptoms of carcinoid syndrome. Less frequently, insulinomas, gastrinomas, glucagonomas and vasoactive intestinal polypeptidomas (VIPomas) are encountered. Pancreatic polypeptidomas and somatostatinomas are exceedingly rare.

Modern ultrasonography and contrast-enhanced spiral CT scanning are usually sufficiently sensitive and specific to confirm the diagnosis of hepatic metastases of neuroendocrine primaries. Mesenteric angiography and selective portal vein sampling using calcium still have a place in cases where it is vital to find the primary tumour. Endoscopic ultrasonography may play a role in the detection of pancreatic islet cell tumours. Intraoperative ultrasound or laparoscopic ultrasound can be extremely valuable in localising small primaries or detecting liver metastases. More recently, indium-labelled octreotide scanning, with or without single photon emission computed tomography (SPECT) scans, has been suggested to be very promising in detecting primary tumours and the presence of extrahepatic disease. Plasma and urine hormone screening and histochemical staining of biopsies can be used to typify the tumour. In addition, if the tumour actively secretes a particular hormone, this can be used as a marker to follow the effect of treatment.

Significant long-term palliation can be achieved by debulking resections for neuroendocrine tumours for both tumours with endocrine activity and those with mechanical symptoms. Hepatic artery (chemo-) embolisation may be considered in providing symptom relief, since these tumours are almost exclusively supplied by the arterial system. Finally, octreotide and especially its long-acting counterpart (Lanreotide, Sandostatin LAR) is very effective in reducing symptoms and some authors have even suggested that there might be an effect on tumour growth. Neuroendocrine tumours and their metastases are slow-growing tumours with a relatively benign behaviour and surgical treatment should therefore be limited to selected patients in whom benefit is likely.

Non-colorectal, non-neuroendocrine metastases

For a long time, most hepatobiliary surgeons have been fairly stringent in their criteria for surgical resection of metastatic liver tumours. Thus, only patients with colorectal cancer metastases were offered treatment. The fact that resectional treatment can nowadays be performed with a very low morbidity and a mortality well below 5% has led to a more liberal policy in treating metastases from other malignancies. There is still a paucity of data, but preliminary results would suggest that resectional therapy might be advantageous in renal cell carcinoma, Wilms' tumour and adrenal tumour metastases. The applicability of resectional surgery for metastases from non-colorectal gastrointestinal as well as gynaecological and breast malignancies does not appear to prolong survival but awaits further assessment.

NON-SURGICAL MANAGEMENT

There are several alternative treatment modalities for liver tumours. Most of these are used for irresectable lesions. It is beyond the scope of this chapter to cover all these forms of treatment in detail. So they will only briefly be discussed.

Radiotherapy

Most primary and secondary liver tumours are not particularly radiosensitive. In addition, the surrounding liver cells are more susceptible to the effects of radiation than the tumour itself. It may well be that more sophisticated techniques of delivering high-dose radiotherapy to selected areas of liver parenchyma may increase the applicability of this treatment in the near future, but this treatment is not frequently used for hepatic tumours.

Alcohol injection

Direct absolute alcohol injection into hepatic malignancies causes dehydration and in this way kills the tumour. The technique is probably only effective in small (<3 cm) tumours. Using this technique repeatedly, five-year survival rates of 30–40% have been obtained for selected patient groups with less than three small tumours. The effectiveness of the therapy is dependent on delivering the alcohol accurately and because of the high tendency to recurrence (63% at three years), this technique has never gained widespread acceptance.

Cryotherapy

In recent years, several reports have appeared on the safety and efficacy of this treatment. The technique involves intraoperative ultrasound-guided placement of a probe in the centre of the tumour. Liquid nitrogen is subsequently passed through the probe until the tumour and a circumferential margin of 1 cm of normal liver tissue is frozen. The development of an ice ball can be checked with ultrasound. The method is safe and can be done at either open or laparoscopic surgery. Current estimates are that approximately 10–15% of patients with irresectable metastases would be candidates for cryotherapy, but the results of long-term follow-up studies are awaited. For irresectable hepatocellular carcinomas of <5 cm, five-year survival rates as high as 50% have been reported. Similarly, one- and two-year survival rates for colorectal cancer metastases treated by cryotherapy were between 50% and 70%, although recurrence rates are greater than 50%. Future improvements in this technique, including the use of multiple array probes, might further increase the effectiveness of this treatment.

Interstitial laser coagulation

Interstitial laser coagulation was introduced in the early 1980s. Through recent advances this technique has now become a minimally invasive procedure. Essentially, the principle is similar to cryotherapy, although interstitial laser coagulation uses heat to induce tumour necrosis. The heat is delivered over no more than 20 minutes by a low-power laser light probe. Unfortunately, the effects are difficult to monitor in real time, but it has become clear that because of the temperature gradient in the tumour, only lesions less than 5 cm can be treated. It has been suggested that portal inflow occlusion during interstitial laser coagulation may increase the efficacy of this treatment. Long-term survival rates are now being reported. Although three-year survival rates of around 40% can be obtained, recurrence rates are high.

Radiofrequency interstitial thermal ablation

This is a relatively new technique that is gaining popularity. A radiofrequency electrode is percutaneously inserted into the tumour under ultrasound guidance or during laparoscopy. The local application of the radiofrequency leads to thermal ablation of the tumour. The technique appears to be safe and effective, but results from long-term follow-up have not yet been presented.

Chemotherapy

Chemotherapy can be given either systemically or regionally via a hepatic artery catheter connected to a subcutaneously implanted port. Systemic chemotherapy has been reported to offer effective palliation to patients with irresectable malignant tumours. Chemotherapy may prolong the duration of survival with response rates of approximately 40% being reported with a mean survival of 12 months. There is no apparent proven benefit of adjuvant chemotherapy after liver resections. However, chemotherapy has been used with a view to reducing tumour volume in large tumours in order to improve resectability.

Chemoembolisation

Chemoembolisation can be undertaken via the hepatic artery by selectively injecting a combination of chemotherapy and occluding agents (gelfoam, coils, microspheres). The rationale behind this treatment is that many hepatic tumours derive their blood supply from the hepatic artery. Arterial chemoembolisation usually gives rise to a postchemoembolisation syndrome, consisting of abdominal pain, nausea, fever and leucocytosis. Its effectiveness in the treatment of colorectal metastases is not greater than chemotherapy alone. Recently, some centres have used portal vein embolisation as part of a multimodality treatment protocol (see below).

Immunotherapy

The use of immunotherapy in the treatment of liver tumours remains to be established.

Multimodality treatment

Various combinations of treatments have been tried. Preoperative chemotherapy can be used to downstage hepatic tumours prior to resection, but chemotherapy in the postoperative period is not of any apparent additional benefit. Percutaneous transhepatic portal vein embolisation has been used prior to surgery. The principle is that embolisation will lead to atrophy of the affected liver lobe and hypertrophy of the future remnant liver. This would facilitate more extensive liver resections with a lower risk of postoperative liver failure. *In situ* isolated liver perfusion is a relatively novel approach combining surgery and chemotherapy. Preliminary data suggest that disease-free survival rates are very good, but this is achieved at the expense of high morbidity and a 10% mortality rate.

FUTURE DEVELOPMENTS

The feasibility of extensive liver surgery ultimately depends on residual liver function after surgery. There is a good correlation between volume and function in the normal liver and it is generally believed that in this situation about 70% of the liver can be removed. However, it is often difficult to predict whether a liver is entirely normal and what the residual function will be after resectional therapy. This has led to a large number of human and animal studies evaluating various methods to assess liver function before surgery, with the aim of predicting liver failure post resection. Unfortunately, none of these, sometimes very sophisticated, liver function tests have been proven specific enough to rely upon and the clearance of indocyanine green is currently considered the gold standard. From these studies, however, it has become clear that there is a very good correlation between liver volume and function for the normal liver.

Recent improvements in CT scanning have enabled the very accurate measurement of liver volume as a guide to decision making in liver resections (Figure 12.6). Marescaux and colleagues have taken this one step further and applied the concept of virtual reality to three-dimensional reconstructions of the liver from volumetric CT scan pictures. This enabled them to three-dimensionally reconstruct the complex anatomy of the liver and use this for surgical planning and real-time interactive training. It remains to be established what the precise implications of this new technology are for surgical training, but at the very least it is a promising concept.

Notwithstanding this, hepatic resection is unlikely to be the sole answer to the problem of hepatic malignancy since the majority of tumour recurrence occurs outwith the liver.

OPERATIVE SURGERY

Hepatic Resection

The final part of this chapter will describe how we carry out the most common of all hepatic resections for malignancies: right hepatectomy.

Preoperative work-up

One of the crucial points in liver resections for colorectal metastases is patient selection with respect to local resectability, general fitness of the patient and evidence of extrahepatic disease. Liver metastases, unless very large, do not in themselves give rise to symptoms. Hence, weight loss and abdominal complaints usually point to more advanced disease. Particular attention is also paid to previous cardiorespiratory problems. Diabetic and obese patients are at increased operative risk.

Renal function and hepatic function are assessed with particular attention being paid to the prothrombin time. Preoperative tumour markers (CEA, alpha-fetoprotein) should be assessed. Abdominal ultrasound, chest radiograph and colonoscopy may have already been performed to confirm the presence of hepatic metastases and exclude recurrent colonic or metastatic pulmonary

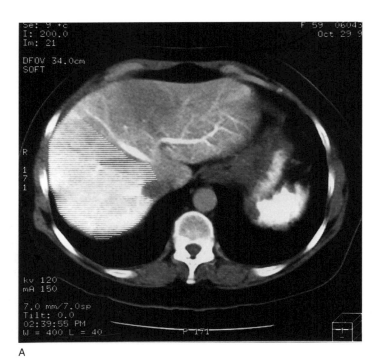

A

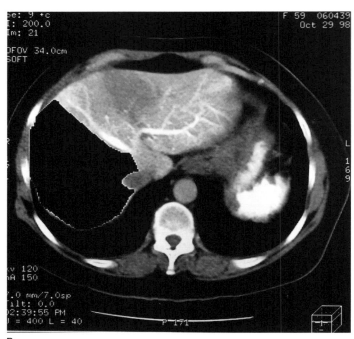

B

Figure 12.6 A. Example of volumetric assessment of the liver using spiral CT scanning in a patient with colorectal metastases in his right hemiliver prior to right hepatectomy **B.** Situation after virtual right hepatectomy.

disease. CT angioportography or spiral CT scan and chest CT scans are undertaken to determine the exact number and localisation of the metastases and exclude pulmonary metastases. In our centre, the patient undergoes laparoscopy and laparoscopic ultrasound to exclude peritoneal dissemination and define the exact anatomic relations of the metastases with respect to hepatic segmental anatomy as defined by Couinaud (Figure 12.7).

Liver resections can be subdivided into anatomic and nonanatomic resections. The latter are usually subsegmental or wedge resections and the outcome of such resections has been shown to

be less favourable than for the classic anatomic resections. Nonanatomic resections are only rarely performed in our institution. The anatomic resections can be classified as right hepatectomy (segments V–VIII), left hepatectomy (segments II–IV), extended right hepatectomy (segments IV–VIII), extended left hepatectomy (segments II–V and VIII) and various (poly-)segmentectomies (Figure 12.8). The principal plane dividing the liver into a right and left hemiliver is the line of Cantlie, which is a virtual line between the gallbladder and the suprahepatic inferior vena cava. The following section gives a description of how a right hepatectomy is undertaken.

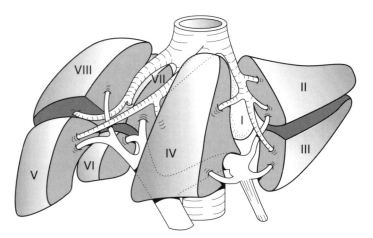

Figure 12.7 Segmental anatomy of the liver according to Couinaud (reprinted with permission from Garden OJ, Bismuth H. Anatomy of the liver. In: Carter DC, Russell RCG, Pitt HA, Bismuth H, eds. *Rob & Smith's Operative Surgery. Hepatobiliary and Pancreatic Surgery.* London: Chapman and Hall Medical, 1996).

Right hepatectomy

- The patient is fully informed about the potential benefits and risks of the operation and written consent is obtained.

- Blood is crossmatched but blood is not routinely available in theatre.

- An epidural catheter is inserted and the patient is anaesthetised and endotracheally intubated, following which a central line, arterial line, nasogastric tube and a urinary catheter are inserted.

- Prophylactic low molecular weight heparin is administered to prevent deep vein thrombosis and compression stockings are applied.

- The patient's abdomen is shaved in theatre and broadspectrum antibiotic prophylaxis (cefotaxime 1.5 g) is administered.

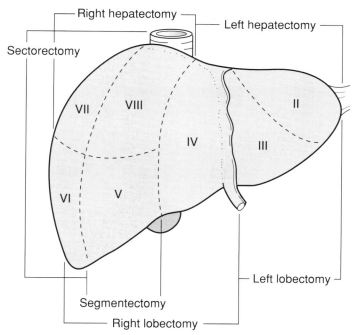

Figure 12.8 Nomenclature of hepatic resections (reprinted with permission from Garden OJ, Bismuth H. Anatomy of the liver. In: Carter DC, Russell RCG, Pitt HA, Bismuth H, eds. *Rob & Smith's Operative Surgery. Hepatobiliary and Pancreatic Surgery*. London: Chapman and Hall Medical, 1996).

- During the procedure, central venous pressure is maintained below 5 mm Hg to minimise venous bleeding.

- The patient is in the supine position, the surgeon on the right side and the assistant and scrub nurse on the left side.

Procedure

- A bilateral subcostal 'roof-top' incision is normally used that extends on the left side to the lateral border of the rectus abdominis muscle.

- The costal margins are retracted upwards using Doyne's blades attached to posts secured beneath the drapes at the cranial end of the table.

- All adhesions are taken down to expose the liver and exclude extrahepatic disease.

- Exposure is further improved by means of an Omni Tract device.

- The falciform ligament is taken down and subsequently an intraoperative ultrasound is performed to delineate the exact anatomy and exclude other small lesions.

- The liver is further mobilised by division of all peritoneal attachments on the right side. The retrohepatic inferior vena cava is exposed after dissecting peritoneal attachments and without ligating the right adrenal vein. The extrahepatic part of the right hepatic vein is exposed and controlled by

encircling it with a vessel loop. The hepatic venous segment I branches to the inferior vena cava (IVC) and other venous tributaries are secured and divided to the sagittal plane (to avoid congestion of segment I).

- The gallbladder is removed to allow the portal vein to be identified and followed to its bifurcation. The right branch of the portal vein is secured between clamps, divided and suture-ligated with 4-0 polypropylene (Prolene) sutures. Following identification of the left hepatic artery, the right hepatic artery is dissected, suture-ligated and divided. At this stage, the right hemiliver becomes avascular and usually shows a clear line of demarcation with the left side (Figure 12.9).

- Transection of the liver parenchyma is performed using the Cavitron Ultrasonic Surgical Aspirator (CUSA) once the liver capsule has been incised with diathermy. During the parenchymal transection, the argon beam coagulation is used to coagulate small vessels, whilst absorbable polydioxanone (PDS) clips and ties are used to control larger branches. Special care is taken to avoid injury to the preserved middle hepatic vein. The right hepatic duct is suture-ligated with 4-0 polydioxanone sutures and divided. The right hepatic vein is clamped, cut and oversewn with 4-0 Prolene. The cut surface of the liver is spray-coagulated with the argon beam coagulator.

- The abdominal cavity is then washed with saline and a large-bore drain is left in the right upper quadrant.

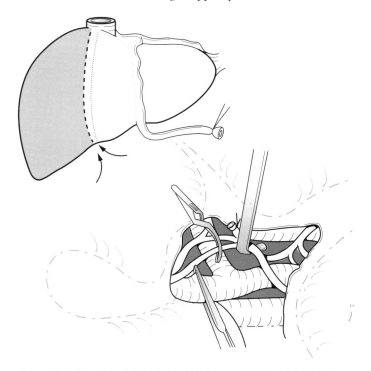

Figure 12.9 Clamping of the right branch of the portal vein and the right hepatic artery leads to a clear line of demarcation (reprinted with permission from Garden OJ, Bismuth H. Hepatic resection. In: Carter DC, Russell RCG, Pitt HA, Bismuth H, eds. *Rob & Smith's Operative Surgery. Hepatobiliary and Pancreatic Surgery*. London: Chapman and Hall Medical, 1996).

Intraoperative problems are usually the consequence of excessive bleeding, which may be related to an elevated central venous pressure. On the other hand, care must be taken to adhere to meticulous control of bleeding vessels during hepatic transection. Air embolism is a rare complication and is usually avoidable if bleeding is limited.

In the immediate postoperative period patients are nursed in the high-dependency unit. No efforts should be made to raise central venous pressure excessively, because this may precipitate haemorrhage. Hepatic insufficiency is rare after right hepatectomy for colorectal cancer in patients without previously impaired liver function. Blood glucose and lactate levels can be monitored if there are concerns about hepatic insufficiency. Prothrombin time should be checked regularly. The nasogastric tube can usually be removed on the first postoperative day and the drain is usually removed a day later.

After the epidural catheter has been removed, patients are put on patient-controlled analgesia and transferred to the regular ward.

Acknowledgements

C.H.C. Dejong is a recipient of a Research Fellowship Grant from the Niels Stensen Foundation (Amsterdam, The Netherlands). The help of Dr D.N. Redhead in providing the CT scans for some of the illustrations is greatly appreciated.

FURTHER READING

Bismuth H, Nakache R, Diamond T. Management strategies in resection for hilar cholangiocarcinoma. *Ann Surg* 1992; **215**:31–38

Elias D, Debaere T, Roche A, Bonvallot S, Lasser P. Preoperative selective portal vein embolizations are an effective means of extending the indications of major hepatectomy in the normal and injured liver. *Hepatogastroenterology* 1998; **45**:170–177

Farges O, Daradkeh S, Bismuth H. Cavernous hemangiomas of the liver: are there any indications for resection? *World J Surg* 1995; **19**:19–24

Finch MD, Crosbie JL, Currie E, Garden OJ. An 8-year experience of hepatic resection: indications and outcome. *Br J Surg* 1998; **85**:315–319

Garden OJ, Bismuth H. Hepatic resection. In: Carter DC, Russel RCG, Pitt HA, Bismuth H, eds. *Rob & Smith's Operative Surgery. Hepatobiliary and Pancreatic Surgery*, 5th edn. London: Chapman and Hall Medical, 1996

Garden OJ. Hepatobiliary and pancreatic surgery. In: Carter DC, Garden OJ, Paterson-Brown S, eds. *A Companion to Specialist Surgical Practice*. London: WB Saunders, 1997

Geoghegan JG, Scheele J. Treatment of colorectal metastases. *Br J Surg* 1999; **86**:158–169

Heisterkamp J, van Hillegersberg R, Ijzermans JNM. Interstitial laser coagulation for hepatic tumours. *Br J Surg* 1999; **86**:293–304

Kubota K, Makuuchi M, Kusaka K et al. Measurement of liver volume and hepatic functional reserve as a guide to decision-making in resectional surgery for hepatic tumors. *Hepatology* 1997; **26**:1176–1181

Lehnert T, Knaebel HP, Duck M, Bulzebruck H, Herfahrt C. Sequential hepatic and pulmonary resections for metastatic colorectal cancer. *Br J Surg* 1999; **86**:241–243

Marescaux J, Clement J-M, Tassetti V et al. Virtual reality applied to hepatic surgery simulation: the next revolution. *Ann Surg* 1998; **228**:627–634

Martin IJ, McKinley AJ, Currie EJ, Holmes P, Garden OJ. Tailoring the management of non-parasitic liver cysts. *Ann Surg* 1998; **228**:167–172

Mazziotti A, Cavallari A. *Techniques in Liver Surgery*. London: Greenwich Medical Media, 1997

Nagorney DM. Benign hepatic tumors: focal nodular hyperplasia and hepatocellular adenoma. *World J Surg* 1995; **19**:13–18

Ohto M, Yoshikawa M, Saisho H, Ebara M, Sugiura N. Nonsurgical treatment of hepatocellular carcinoma in cirrhotic patients. *World J Surg* 1995; **19**:42–46

Paye F, Farges O, Dahmane M, Vilgrain V, Flejou JF, Belghiti J. Cytolysis following chemoembolization for hepatocellular carcinoma. *Br J Surg* 1999; **86**:176–180

Sangro B, Herraiz M, Martinez-Gonzales MA et al. Prognosis of hepatocellular carcinoma in relation to treatment: a multivariate analysis of 178 patients from a single European institution. *Surgery* 1998; **124**:575–583

Schwartz SI. Hepatic resection for noncolorectal nonneuroendocrine metastases. *World J Surg* 1995; **19**:72–75

Seifert JK, Morris DL. Indicators of recurrence following cryotherapy for hepatic metastases from colorectal cancer. *Br J Surg* 1999; **86**:234–240

13

Biliary tract

James Toouli

Disorders of the biliary tract make up some of the most common digestive conditions requiring management. The majority of the disorders are secondary to benign conditions such as gallstones but in addition, a significant percentage of congenital and malignant problems originate in the biliary system.

CHOLELITHIASIS

Prevalence

Gallstones are very common in Western-type communities and account for a large percentage of health-care expenditure. A number of studies in the USA and Europe have documented an overall gallstone prevalence ranging between 10% and 20% in the population. During the reproductive years, there is a female-to-male ratio of 2:1, but the ratio narrows with increasing age as the prevalence increases with age so that at age 70, the prevalence for females is approximately 30% and for males 20%. Hereditary aspects are associated with an increased prevalence, with the Pima Indians of North America having an overall prevalence of approximately 50% rising to greater than 75% in females in the third decade of life. Other factors which influence prevalence include familial risk which doubles the risk, Western-type diet, rapid weight reduction and factors which may influence gallbladder motility, such as parenteral nutrition and truncal vagotomy.

Composition

Gallstones are classified into three types according to the composition and mechanism of formation:

- cholesterol stones
- brown pigment stones
- black pigment stones.

Cholesterol stones

Approximately 80% of gallstones occurring in a Western-type community are of the cholesterol type. These stones have cholesterol as their major component but, in addition, have variable concentrations of calcium which is bonded to bilirubinate phosphate or carbonate. Consequently the common 'cholesterol stone' is a mixed stone which has a multifaceted appearance, whilst the pure cholesterol stone is more rounded and is quite uncommon.

Cholesterol gallstone formation is a multifactorial process which involves metabolic aspects of hepatic cholesterol secretion as well as physical elements associated with biliary tract motility. Hepatic bile cholesterol is derived from three sources: chylomicrons which transport dietary cholesterol to the liver cell, low-density lipoproteins that deliver cholesterol from extrahepatic tissues, and hepatocyte synthesis of cholesterol from acetate. This latter

process is controlled by the enzyme 3-hydroxy-3-methyl-glutasyl coenzyme A (HMG CoA) reductase. Regulatory mechanisms maintain the hepatic cholesterol at a constant concentration so that it is soluble in bile. Changes in these regulatory mechanisms may be influenced by exogenous factors such as diet, obesity and drugs or endogenous influences such as advancing age, hyperlipidaemia or genetic predisposition.

Cholesterol is insoluble in water so transport mechanisms are necessary in order to retain it in a soluble form in bile. Human bile is an isotonic aqueous solution which contains electrolytes and organic solutes. The solutes are made up of 67% bile salts, 4% cholesterol, 22% phospholipids, 4.5% protein and 0.3% bilirubin. Hepatic bile is secreted by hepatocytes, transported into the gallbladder where it is concentrated by an active mechanism which extracts water and expelled by slow gallbladder contraction into the duodenum via the bile duct and sphincter of Oddi.

Cholesterol is maintained soluble in bile as it is transported in the form of vesicles and simple micelles which are aggregates of cholesterol bile salts and phospholipids. Cholesterol interchanges between micelles and vesicles, the latter being the more stable of the two structures. In circumstances which promote super-saturation of cholesterol, vesicle and micelle formation can no longer maintain the cholesterol in a soluble state, resulting in precipitation of cholesterol from solution and the formation of cholesterol crystals which lead to the formation of gallstones. Factors which promote the precipitation of cholesterol are not only confined to cholesterol supersaturation but are also enhanced by gallbladder hypomotility which promotes stasis of bile, mucin hypersecretion which provides a nucleating factor for the precipitation of cholesterol, plus an increase in concentration in bile of arachidonyl lecithin and biliary calcium.

Pigment stones

These stones are formed when free bilirubin binds to calcium to produce calcium bilirubinate. Normally bilirubin is secreted in the form of bilirubin diglucuronide which is water soluble. Deconjugation by the enzyme beta-glucoronidase promotes pigment stone formation as it releases insoluble bilirubin. There are two types of pigment stones, occurring at different sites and having different composition and aetiology.

Black pigment stones

These occur primarily in the gallbladder. They result from an increase in bilirubin levels mainly following haemolytic anaemia. Rarely, they may also be found proximal to a biliary stricture and, in this instance, are a result of stasis.

Brown pigment stones

These calcium bilirubinate stones have a soft, earthy consistency and are primarily found in the bile duct. They are associated with stasis and infection, be it parasitic (e.g. *Ascaris lumbricoides* or *Clonorchis sinensis*) or bacteria (e.g. *Escherichia coli* or *Klebsiella pneumoniae*). The bacteria possess beta-glucuronidase activity which promotes deconjugation of bilirubin diglucuronide.

CLINICAL PRESENTATION AND MANAGEMENT OF GALLSTONES

Cholelithiasis

Approximately 50–80% of patients with gallbladder stones remain asymptomatic and thus do not require treatment. In at least two longitudinal studies it has been demonstrated that 'silent' gallstones do not require treatment and it is safe to await the development of symptoms prior to implementing therapy.

The main symptom associated with gallbladder stones is biliary pain. Characteristically the visceral component of the pain is sited in the epigastric region. The pain is constant with some fluctuation. It usually begins some 2–3 hours following a meal. It may radiate to the right upper quadrant and under the tip of the right scapula posteriorly. It may be associated with nausea which induces vomiting, but these symptoms on their own are not diagnostic of cholecystolithiasis. The pathophysiology of pain production is thought to follow obstruction of the gallbladder outlet by a stone impacting in Hartmann's pouch. Resolution of the symptoms occurs when the stone disimpacts. However, the symptoms usually recur as the stone impacts again on subsequent occasions.

In circumstances where the stone remains impacted in Hartmann's pouch, the initial 'chemical' inflammation progresses. Oedema and total obstruction of the gallbladder may result in a mucocoele of the gallbladder. Bacterial infection also may occur in up to 20% of patients and an empyema of the gallbladder may form.

Clinical signs depend on the severity of the inflammation and the time when the clinician examines a patient following presentation. Typically a patient with recurrent biliary-type pain may present to a clinician in between episodes of pain. Abdominal examination may not detect tenderness but on deep inspiration, the patient may feel a twinge of pain as the clinician palpates the right upper quadrant. This set of events, i.e. no tenderness on abdominal palpation followed by pain in the right upper quadrant on deep inspiration, is known as a positive Murphy's sign.

In patients with continuing abdominal symptoms of pain, abdominal examination will generally reveal tenderness in the epigastrium and right upper quadrant. In addition, if a mucocoele or empyema is present, a gallbladder mass may be palpable.

In most patients with symptomatic gallstones, the temperature is not elevated. However, when it is abnormal, this sign suggests severe inflammation and possible bacterial infection. In patients with gallbladder empyema, a swinging temperature characteristic of pus collection may be evident. Uncommonly the inflammation

surrounding an acutely inflamed gallbladder may impinge on the bile duct to produce cholestatic jaundice. This is known as Mirizzi syndrome.

Diagnosis of cholecystolithiasis is most commonly made by abdominal ultrasonography (Figure 13.1). Real-time ultrasonographic examination of the gallbladder is more than 95% accurate in diagnosing gallstones. In addition, ultrasonography may indicate the presence of associated pericholecystic oedema or the collection of fluid. The specificity of these latter signs in the diagnosis of mild to severe gallbladder inflammation has not been well determined, hence these signs should not be given undue emphasis.

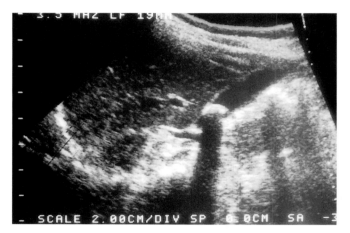

Figure 13.1 Upper abdominal ultrasound illustrating a large gallstone in the gallbladder. Note the 'typical' acoustic shadow of the gallstone.

Other investigations

A variety of other radiological investigations are used in the investigation of patients with biliary-type symptoms, when ultrasonography fails to make the diagnosis or in instances where the clinical diagnosis is not matched by the ultrasonographic findings.

Plain abdominal radiograph

In 10–15% of patients, gallstones will be evident on plain abdominal radiograph as their calcium content produces radio-opacity. Rarely, the presence of air in the gallbladder and/or bile ducts may be evident if a cholecystoduodenal fistula exists.

Oral cholecystogram

This is an excellent and 95% accurate investigation for the diagnosis of gallstones. However, it has been superseded by ultrasonography and is now only rarely used. It requires the ingestion of oral contrast at least 12 hours prior to the radiographic examination.

Scintigraphy

Technetium-labelled iminodracetic acid (^{99m}Tc IDA) administered intravenously is secreted in bile and may be detected by a gamma camera. This quality can be used to demonstrate cystic duct obstruction and may be of occasional use when the clinical diagnosis of acute cholecystitis may be in doubt.

The investigation is now more commonly used in conjunction with intravenous infusion of the hormone cholecystokinin in patients with suspect acalculous gallbladder disease. After initial uptake of the isotope in the gallbladder, an abnormal delay to gallbladder emptying, as calculated by determination of the gallbladder ejection fraction, is strongly indicative of a gallbladder motility abnormality and acalculous gallbladder disease.

CT Scan and MRI

These investigations have little place in the diagnosis of gallbladder disease.

Treatment

The acute treatment of a patient with symptomatic gallstones depends on the severity of clinical presentation. A patient who presents with severe abdominal pain associated with epigastric to right upper quadrant tenderness usually requires hospital inpatient management. Initial treatment includes nil by mouth, intravenous fluids plus intravenous analgesia. Traditionally pethidine (meperidine) has been used as the preferred analgesic over morphine in the belief that this prevented stimulation of the sphincter of Oddi which might aggravate symptoms. Manometric studies have shown that, in analgesic doses, pethidine effects on the sphincter of Oddi are similar to morphine. Hence, there is no contraindication to morphine use as an analgesic.

Definitive treatment in patients with symptomatic gallstones is cholecystectomy. The timing of the operation will largely depend on local circumstances and availability of resources. Numerous studies have shown that, for either open or laparoscopic cholecystectomy, there is no advantage to delaying surgery. Consequently the recommendation is for cholecystectomy at the same admission, but not necessarily as an emergency unless clinical circumstances dictate such an approach.

Choledocholithiasis

Unlike gallbladder stones, once stones have either migrated into the bile duct or developed in the duct, they invariably produce symptoms. Bile duct stones clinically present in a number of ways.

Recurrent biliary-type pain

Similar to gallbladder stones, pain is felt in the epigastric region and radiates into the back. It may be associated with epigastric tenderness and serum biochemistry may reveal a cholestatic picture. It needs to be appreciated that the earliest serum markers that become elevated with a stone in the bile duct are the transaminases (aspartate transaminases (AST) and alanine transaminase (ALT). The alkaline phosphatase (ALP) becomes elevated with more prolonged cholestasis.

Jaundice

A bile duct stone may obstruct the bile duct to produce obstructive jaundice. This usually is associated with biliary pain and serum biochemistry reveals an abnormal serum bilirubin level as well as a cholestatic picture with a rise in transaminases and alkaline phosphatase.

Cholangitis

Infection of the obstructed bile produces cholangitis. The clinical triad of Charcot, i.e. biliary pain, jaundice and fever, is suggestive of cholangitis due to stone obstruction of the bile duct. Severe cholangitis is clinically characterised by Reynold's pentad: pain, fever, jaundice, hypotension plus mental confusion. This finding heralds a surgical emergency requiring urgent intervention to treat the infection and drain the biliary system.

Biliary pancreatitis

A stone which has migrated into the bile duct may migrate further into the channel of the sphincter of Oddi and either pass into the duodenum, impact in the ampulla or return back up into the bile duct. In so doing, the stone invokes a dysmotility of the sphincter of Oddi which in some individuals produces acute pancreatitis. The pathophysiology of acute pancreatitis in these patients is thought to be a combination of obstruction of pancreatic juice outflow and hypersecretion against this obstruction. Clinically the patient presents with severe epigastric pain which may radiate into the back. Dependent on the severity of pancreatitis, there may be associated clinical features of haemodynamic shock. Serum biochemistry will indicate an abnormally elevated serum amylase and, dependent on the severity of the pancreatitis, blood glucose may be elevated, serum calcium decreased and liver enzymes have a cholestatic pattern.

Investigations

Ultrasonography

Ultrasonography may diagnose a stone in the bile duct but in general this investigation is of low sensitivity due to the position of the bile duct adjacent and posterior to the duodenum. An abnormally dilated bile duct is suggestive of biliary obstruction in keeping with a stone. Consequently, a positive diagnosis of a stone by ultrasonography is useful but non-visualisation of a stone does not exclude its presence.

Endoscopic retrograde cholangiopancreatography (ERCP)

The endoscopic approach to the bile duct is best for the diagnosis and subsequent treatment of bile duct stones (Figure 13.2). A side-viewing duodenoscope is positioned in the duodenum to visualise the common opening of the bile and pancreatic ducts. Selective cannulation of the bile duct via a catheter introduced through the working channel allows radiological visualisation of the biliary tract after infusion of radioopaque contrast. The biliary tract is visualised in real time using a high-quality image intensifier. Stones or other biliary pathology may be recorded with high accuracy. Following the detection of stones in the bile duct, the catheter may be exchanged for a papillotome which can then be used to divide the sphincter of Oddi (Figure 13.3), thus providing access into the bile duct for the removal of stones. This approach to bile duct stones has revolutionised the management of stones in the bile duct and has converted to a day case what previously required lengthy hospital stay and at least two weeks of an indwelling tube in the bile duct.

ERCP and endoscopic sphincterotomy have few contraindications when carried out in expert units. This is the optimal approach for the management of patients with severe cholangitis, with dramatic results in the very sick patient with Reynold's pentad, following the removal of stones and drainage of the bile duct. In addition, prospective clinical studies have shown that early ERCP and sphincterotomy are associated with improved

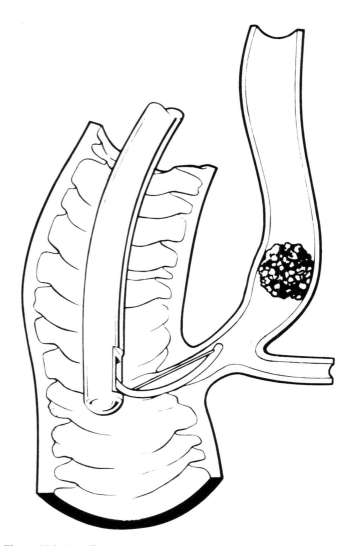

Figure 13.3 A papillotome positioned to perform a sphincterotomy for removal of a stone from the bile duct.

outcome for patients with severe biliary pancreatitis when compared to conservative management of pancreatitis.

Percutaneous cholangiography

In instances where the anatomical arrangement precludes the use of ERCP (e.g. Roux-en-Y gastroenterostomy, some Polya gastrectomies), the biliary tract may be accessed via a percutaneous, transhepatic route using a fine needle. It may also be possible to treat stones in the biliary system via this approach but the potential morbidity is significantly higher than the endoscopic route.

CT cholangiography and MR cholangiography

There are developing diagnostic modalities for bile duct stones. The sensitivity and specificity approach that of ERCP but these

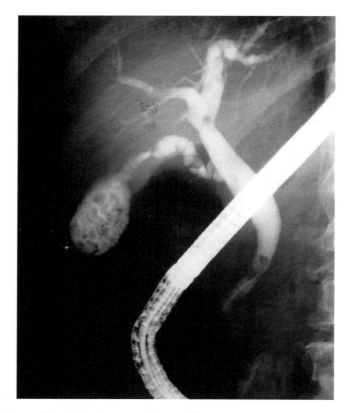

Figure 13.2 ERCP showing radiolucent filling defects in both the gallbladder and bile ducts, representing stones.

techniques do not allow for therapy and the patients would need a separate procedure for therapy. A more likely use for these radiological techniques would be for diagnosis in individuals where the likelihood of stone disease is low.

Treatment of bile duct stones

Patients who present with symptoms and signs of bile duct stones require initial resuscitation and treatment with analgesics for pain. If cholangitis is diagnosed, broad-spectrum intravenous antibiotics with coverage for Gram-negative bacilli and anaerobes should be commenced. The optimal treatment of bile duct stones in patients who have had a previous cholecystectomy is via an endoscopic approach which allows the removal of the stones following endoscopic sphincterotomy. In patients with an intact biliary tract (i.e. no cholecystectomy) and in whom it is intended to undertake cholecystectomy, bile duct stones may be treated during the same procedure as the cholecystectomy. In those patients undergoing laparoscopic cholecystectomy, bile duct stones may be treated by introduction of instruments through the cystic duct (Figure 13.4). Bile duct stones may be either extracted via this route or manipulated into the duodenum. Alternatively, in patients with a bile duct diameter greater than 10 mm, laparoscopic choledochotomy may be done to remove the stones. Another variation is to introduce a duodenoscope at the time of the laparoscopic operation and perform a sphincterotomy to remove stones aided by instruments and fluid introduced via the cystic duct.

Endoscopic sphincterotomy for the management of bile duct stones has revolutionised the treatment of this condition. As in any surgical procedure, it is associated with a significant morbidity and mortality but these are significantly lower when compared to open surgical approaches for patients with comparable co-morbidities.

The major complications of endoscopic sphincterotomy include pancreatitis (3%), cholangitis (1%), haemorrhage (1%) and retro-duodenal perforation (0.5%). The most severe of these complications is that of retroperitoneal perforation. This complication may require treatment via laparotomy.

Overall mortality for endoscopic sphincterotomy for patients with and without co-morbidities is approximately 3% at 30 days with less than 1% being procedure related.

BILIARY INFECTION

The biliary tract, liver and bile are sterile under normal circumstances. However, bacteria may colonise and subsequently proliferate and infect the biliary tract following biliary stasis, obstruction, altered anatomy or presence of a foreign body.

The organisms most commonly found in the biliary tract include *Escherichia coli*, *Klebsiella pneumoniae*, enterococcus and, under certain circumstances, the anaerobe *Bacteroides fragilis*. In acute cholecystitis, two-thirds of the organisms will consist of Gram-negative aerobes, the remainder being made up of enterococcus. Anaerobes are only rarely involved in acute cholecystitis, but may be isolated in patients with empyema of the gallbladder and emphysematous cholecystitis. However, in patients with cholangitis secondary to bile duct stones, anaerobes may be cultured in up to 30%. Furthermore, anaerobic bacteria are outlined in patients with bile duct strictures and those with biliary endoprostheses. Viral and parasitic infections of bile are uncommon but they have been isolated from patients with immune deficiency syndrome.

Treatment

Patients presenting with recurrent biliary colic have no evidence of infection and hence do not warrant treatment with antibiotics. However, at the time of cholecystectomy, a single dose of antibiotic is administered intravenously in order to prevent wound infection due to contamination of the wound by organisms in the gallstone-containing gallbladder. An antibiotic with cover for Gram-negative aerobes and enterococcus is most appropriate.

In patients with acute cholecystitis, the bile is infected in approximately 50%. In these patients, there is an elevated temperature and a leucocytosis. Treatment with antibiotics which act against Gram-negative aerobic bacilli and enterococcus should be used

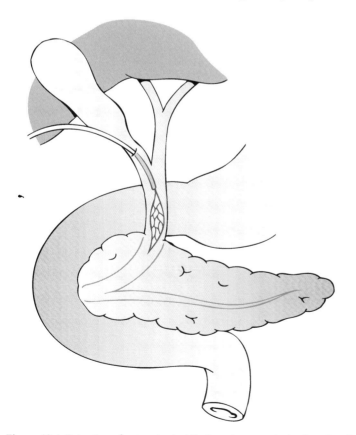

Figure 13.4 Extraction of a stone in the bile duct via a stone basket introduced into the bile duct from the cystic duct.

163

up to and including the perioperative period. If there is evidence of empyema or the rare emphysematous cholecystitis, anaerobic organism treatment should be used.

In patients with cholangitis, either as a result of stones in the bile duct or stasis due to malignant or benign strictures, broad-spectrum antibiotics providing anaerobic cover should be used. In addition, in the absence of cholangitis but in patients undergoing surgery or endoscopic procedures on the bile duct, intravenous prophylaxis with broad-spectrum antibiotics including anaerobic cover should be utilised.

BENIGN BILIARY STRICTURES

A number of conditions are associated with the formation of benign biliary strictures, which may be single or multiple depending on the cause. A summary of causes of benign strictures of the biliary tract is given in Box 13.1.

Box 13.1   Causes of benign biliary tract strictures
Congenital, e.g. biliary atresia
Bile duct injuries
Postoperative
Post cholecystectomy
Post bile duct exploration
Post bilio-enteric anastomosis
Other abdominal surgery
Pancreatic operations
Gastrectomy
Traumatic (blunt or penetrating)
Postinflammatory
Gallstones
Chronic pancreatitis
Duodenal ulcer
Parasitic infestation
Recurrent cholangitis
Primary sclerosing cholangitis
Radiotherapy
Sphincter of Oddi stenosis

The most common causes for the formation of benign biliary tract strictures are secondary to inflammation or as a result of injury to the bile duct. For a single stricture the level along the bile duct determines its complexity, approach to treatment and consequently long-term outcome. The Bismuth classification (Figure 13.5) is accepted as a useful anatomical means of classifying strictures.

Type 1   Low common hepatic duct; stump >2 cm
Type 2   Middle common hepatic duct; stump <2 cm
Type 3   High (hilar), no hepatic duct; confluence of right and left hepatic ducts intact
Type 4   Destruction of hilar confluence; right and left hepatic ducts separated
Type 5   Involvement of sectoral right branch alone or with common hepatic duct

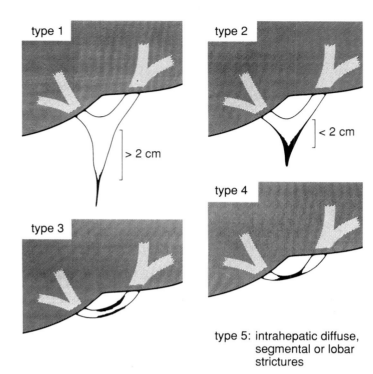

Figure 13.5 Bismuth classification of bile duct strictures.

Bile duct injuries

The prevalence of bile duct injuries has increased with the advent of laparoscopic cholecystectomy. In some series it is at least double the prevalence which was recorded with open cholecystectomy. However, the accuracy of the figures with open cholecystectomy needs to be questioned as minor injuries to the bile duct probably were not recorded but repaired at the time of injury. Despite this, there has undoubtedly been an increase in major duct injuries with laparoscopic surgery. There are many reasons for this and, in the section on operative technique below, strategies which assist in avoiding duct injury will be discussed.

Bile duct injuries recognised at the time of operation should be repaired at the time of recognition, provided the surgeon has had adequate experience in dealing with complex biliary anastomoses. The first repair should be the best repair and certainly the first attempt at repair provides the best opportunity for a satisfactory outcome.

Chronic strictures

Benign bile duct strictures may not present until some time after the event which initiated the stricture. Ischaemia of the bile duct probably contributes to most of these strictures, whether they follow cholecystectomy, exploration of the bile duct or bilio-enteric anastomosis. The blood supply of the bile duct runs in three vascular columns, one posterior and two lateral, out of which small branches feed the duct. The blood supply to the distal bile duct is well supplied by collaterals, whilst the blood supply to the more proximal (i.e. hepatic end) duct is more tenuous. Indeed, the proximal duct depends on blood supplied by the three vascular columns and which originates in the more distal segment (Figure 13.6).

Ischaemia of the bile duct may follow excess devascularisation of the bile duct in preparation for bile duct exploration or it may follow ligation of one or more of the vascular columns. In a bilio-enteric anastomosis, if the common hepatic duct stump is long, stricturing may occur at the anastomosis due to inadequate blood supply from the proximal end of the duct.

Patients with chronic biliary tract strictures present clinically with symptoms and signs of recurrent cholangitis. The most appropriate initial radiological investigation is ultrasonography. This may demonstrate a dilated biliary system. However, if the disease is chronic and the liver has become cirrhotic, intrahepatic ducts may not be dilated. Accurate assessment of the site and nature of the stenosis is mandatory and a cholangiogram is required. This investigation may be done either via an endoscopic approach (ERCP) or, if the anatomical arrangement does not permit, via a percutaneous approach. Other radiological investigations which may be useful in the assessment of a biliary stricture include scintigraphic assessment of flow through the stricture, CT cholangiography and magnetic resonance cholangiography.

Biliary strictures require treatment as, left untreated, the patients continue to have episodes of recurrent cholangitis, ultimately leading to cirrhosis of the liver and its complications. In general, biliary strictures should be treated by open operation and the performance of a bilio-enteric anastomosis between the vascularised proximal common hepatic duct and a Roux-en-Y jejunal loop. In instances where open surgery may be hazardous or in patients with short acute strictures, endoscopic dilatation of the

stricture with a period of intraluminal stenting has been associated with good results on limited follow-up. Consequently, for the latter patients, a policy of initial endoscopic therapy appears appropriate, reserving open operative treatment if this fails.

Inflammatory strictures

These may occur following acute inflammation of the gallbladder (Mirizzi syndrome) or the pancreas and generally involve the lower bile duct. Patients may present either with jaundice or cholangitis. Diagnosis is usually made by ERCP. In general, the most appropriate therapy is endoscopic sphincterotomy and drainage of the biliary system via a replaceable endoprosthesis. Dilatation of the stricture also may be necessary.

Sphincter of Oddi stenosis

Sphincter of Oddi dysfunction is a motility disorder of the sphincter of Oddi which, in some patients, may lead to a fixed fibrotic stenosis of the sphincter. These patients may present clinically with recurrent abdominal pain and cholestatic liver enzymes. ERCP demonstrates a dilated bile duct and manometry of the sphincter of Oddi shows elevated sphincter of Oddi basal pressure. Division of the sphincter by endoscopic sphincterotomy usually is associated with excellent long-term results.

CHOLEDOCHAL CYSTS

This is an uncommon congenital abnormality of the biliary tact with a higher prevalence in East Asia, particularly Japan. The reason for the higher frequency in this region is unknown but in Japan up to 2.5% of benign biliary tract disease is associated with the presence of choledochal cyst. The condition not only involves the bile duct, but also may extend to involve the intrahepatic ducts. Choledochal cysts have been classified according to Alonso-Lej with a more recent addition to include the intrahepatic component as modified by Todani (Box 13.2).

Box 13.2	Choledochal cyst classification
Type 1	Cystic dilatation of the common bile duct
Type 2	Diverticulum of the common bile duct
Type 3	Cystic dilatation of the terminal common bile duct within the duodenal wall (choledochocoele)
Type 4A	Multiple cysts of intra- and extrahepatic ducts
Type 4B	Multiple cysts of extrahepatic bile duct
Type 5	Single or multiple intrahepatic bile duct cysts with normal extrahepatic duct (also known as Caroli's disease)

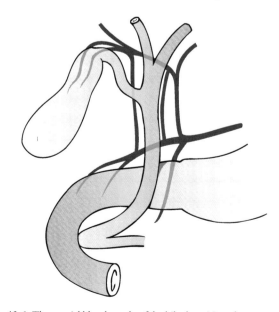

Figure 13.6 The arterial blood supply of the bile duct. Note that most of the flow arises from the distal end of the bile duct.

Choledochal cyst is associated with an abnormality of the pancreatobiliary junction where the bile duct joins the pancreatic duct proximal to a common channel and sphincter of Oddi. This anomalous arrangement promotes reflux of pancreatic juice into the bile duct. It is thought that the enzymatic action of activated pancreatic juice acts on the epithelial lining and wall of the bile duct to produce the cystic change. As a result of stasis, chole-dochal cysts often contain gallstones (30–40% of adults with choledochal cyst). Furthermore, the cyst lining has a 20-fold higher predisposition to malignant transformation, the incidence of this in the Japanese population of patients with choledochal cysts approaching 15%.

The majority (60%) of choledochal cysts present in children before age 10. The classic presentation is that of abdominal pain, jaundice and abdominal mass. The remaining patients present in adulthood usually with symptoms suggestive of choledocho-lithiasis.

Diagnosis is made by ultrasonography and the features of the cyst determined by cholangiography. The latter investigation may be achieved via either ERCP or percutaneous access.

Treatment of choledochal cyst demands its total excision in order to prevent recurrence and tumour formation. However, dependent on the type of cyst, total excision may not be possible. In such an instance, bilio-enteric anastomosis to the proximally dilated hepatic ducts is achieved in order to enhance bile drainage. The cyst is removed to its junction with the pancreatic duct.

Long-term prognosis depends on the type of cyst and the time of intervention. Types 1, 2 and 3 are readily resectable, with excellent long-term results. Types 4 and 5 cannot be totally resected and these patients may redevelop symptoms.

TUMOURS OF THE BILIARY TRACT

Cancers of the gallbladder and bile duct are uncommon malignancies which have an incidence ranging between 0.1% and 0.5%. They are typically adenocarcinomas which have a fibrous consistency and thus are relatively slow growing when compared to other adenocarcinomas of the digestive system. Spread is often by local extension, although as the disease progresses, metastases to the liver and peritoneal cavity are seen. The presentation, diagnosis and treatment of gallbladder and bile duct cancers are different so their description will be discussed under separate headings.

Gallbladder cancer

This is a disease of the elderly and seen in the seventh decade or later. It is an uncommon cancer but most commonly diagnosed as an incidental finding at cholecystectomy.

Aetiology/pathogenesis

Gallbladder cancer is almost always associated with the presence of gallstones, hence gallstones have been implicated in its aetiology.

However, gallstones are very common in elderly patients and it is uncertain to what degree the gallstones contribute to the patho-genesis of gallbladder cancer. With the prevalence of gallbladder cancer being less than 0.5% in the population, prophylactic cholecystectomy cannot be recommended in patients with asymptomatic gallstones in order to prevent cancer as the mortality from cholecystectomy in elderly patients (approximately 0.5%) would outweigh any potential benefits. The exception is in patients with 'porcelain gallbladder' who have been shown to have a higher likelihood of developing cancer when compared to other patients with gallstones. Porcelain gallbladder is demonstrated on a plain abdominal X-ray which shows the gallbladder as a radioopaque organ due to calcium deposition in the gallbladder wall. In addition, a higher incidence of gallbladder cancer has been noted in patients with gallstones from Chile and the Pima Indians of North America. Both of these populations have a high prevalence of gallstones but it is unknown how this contributes to the high prevalence of gallbladder cancer.

Occasionally ultrasonography may demonstrate one or more polyps in the gallbladder, either with or without stones. There is good evidence to suggest that gallbladder polyps are associated with the development of malignant change and ultimately gall-bladder cancer. The likelihood of malignant change increases with polyp size, being more likely with polyps having a diameter greater than 1 cm. Therefore, it is recommended that cholecyst-ectomy be performed in these patients in order to prevent the development of gallbladder cancer.

Surgical pathology and complications

Adenocarcinomas of the gallbladder are staged according to the degree of spread beyond the gallbladder.

Stage I   Cancer confined to the gallbladder mucosa and not invading the muscularis
Stage II   Cancer spread to the muscularis but not beyond the serosa
Stage III Cancer spread beyond the serosa of the gallbladder and into the adjacent liver
Stage IV   Distal spread of cancer with metastases in the liver and porta hepatis

Stages I and II are associated with the best prognosis and potential cure with total removal of the gallbladder and cancer. In most instances, cancer in stage I and II is diagnosed as a coincidental finding after examination of the gallbladder following chole-cystectomy.

The major complication with gallbladder cancer occurs with stages III and IV with involvement of the adjacent bile duct. Obstruction of the bile duct occurs either due to direct encroach-ment of the tumour on the bile duct or secondary to metastatic involvement of the porta hepatis nodes and the patient presents with jaundice.

Clinical presentation

The common symptom of a patient with gallbladder cancer is obstructive jaundice. This occurs in patients with either stage III or IV disease when the cancer has spread to involve the bile duct either by direct extension or due to metastatic involvement of lymph nodes in the porta hepatis.

Uncommonly a patient may present with pain in the epigastrium and right upper quadrant and on examination a mass may be palpated in the region of the gallbladder. The mass may be tender due to associated cholecystitis.

Investigation

There are no specific investigations for gallbladder cancer as the presentation is either with symptoms similar to that of symptomatic gallstones or jaundice. Consequently the investigations are directed at the diagnosis of either jaundice or pain in the epigastrium to right upper quadrant.

Ultrasonography may demonstrate a mass in the region of the gallbladder which may suggest gallbladder cancer. A CT scan of the liver may provide further information by demonstrating whether there has been extension into the liver or development of metastases in the porta hepatis.

In a jaundiced patient, a mass in the gallbladder area associated with obstruction of the bile duct is strongly suggestive of gallbladder cancer. Cholangiography performed either via an endoscopic approach (i.e. ERCP) or via a percutaneous transhepatic route is the most accurate investigation for demonstrating the level of obstruction.

Treatment

In stages I and II, cholecystectomy is curative in the majority of patients and no further treatment is warranted. Unfortunately, it is quite uncommon for stage I or II gallbladder cancer to be diagnosed other than as a coincidental finding in a patient who has had cholecystectomy performed for the treatment of symptomatic gallstones.

Most patients with gallbladder cancer present with complications as the cancer spreads beyond the gallbladder to produce jaundice. In patients with stage III disease, the spread may be confined to the adjacent right lobe of the liver and in this instance it may be possible to surgically remove not only the gallbladder but also the adjacent liver either by a non-anatomic resection of the involved liver parenchyma or via a formal right hepatic lobectomy.

In patients with porta hepatis involvement and jaundice, resection of the tumour mass is not feasible and therapy is directed at palliation.

Chemotherapy and radiotherapy have not been demonstrated to have a role in the treatment of gallbladder cancer.

Operative management

Patients with either polyps of the gallbladder or stage I and II gallbladder cancer are treated by removing the gallbladder, usually via a laparoscopic approach. In order to prevent implantation of cancer cells at the site of gallbladder removal from the abdomen, if gallbladder cancer is suspected, it is important to place the specimen in a plastic bag prior to its removal through the portal incision.

In patients with direct extension into the liver parenchyma, hepatic lobectomy is done.

Prognosis/results

In patients with stage I or II disease where gallbladder cancer is diagnosed as an incidental finding following cholecystectomy, the prognosis is good and the majority of patients (>60%) will be free of cancer at five years. Indeed, up to 100% five-year survival has been reported with stage I cancers.

Even in patients with stage III disease, five-year survival for patients with resectable tumours approaches 30%. However, the majority of patients on presentation have stage IV and in these patients life expectancy beyond one year from diagnosis is uncommon.

Conclusions

Gallbladder cancer is an uncommon disease which in most instances is diagnosed late and often spreads beyond the gallbladder. Best results are obtained firstly by its prevention, i.e. cholecystectomy in patients with 'porcelain gallbladder' and in patients with gallbladder polyps. However, where gallbladder cancer has been diagnosed as an incidental finding in patients undergoing cholecystectomy for gallstones, the majority of patients are cured by the operation.

Bile duct cancer

This is an uncommon adenocarcinoma which occurs in people primarily in the sixth decade and older. It is generally a fibrous tumour which causes stricturing and obstruction of the involved part of the bile duct.

Aetiology/pathogenesis

There are no specific casual agents for bile duct cancer but patients with choledochal cyst or primary sclerosing cholangitis have a significantly higher incidence for the development of bile duct cancer when compared to the normal population. In patients with choledochal cyst, tumours occur early in the third decade and the risk increases with age so that prevalence approaches 30% in adults.

In patients with primary sclerosing cholangitis (a fibrotic stricturing disease of the bile duct) there is an increased propensity for developing bile duct cancer. The diagnosis is often difficult as the malignant stricture is difficult to differentiate from the strictures associated with sclerosing cholangitis. However, in any patient with sclerosing cholangitis who develops rapidly evolving jaundice, development of malignant change should be suspected. An uncommon association which is seen in underdeveloped countries is with chronic infestation of the liver by *Clonorchis sinensis* or liver fluke.

Surgical pathology/complications

Bile duct cancer is subdivided according to its site of growth in the bile duct (Figure 13.7). Bile duct cancers may be intrahepatic or extrahepatic. The latter are subdivided as follows:

- High bile duct cancer occurring in the proximal or upper bile duct at the bifurcation of right and left hepatic ducts and extending into either of these ducts. At this site, it is also known as a Klatskin tumour, after the pathologist who first described it as an entity at this site.

- Mid bile duct cancer involves the bile duct in the region of its junction with the cystic duct and usually involves the cystic duct. The cancer is confined to the supraduodenal part of the bile duct but does not involve the duct adjacent to the hepatic duct bifurcation.

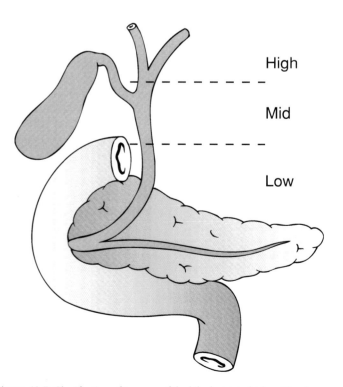

Figure 13.7 Classification of tumours of the bile duct into high, mid or low.

- Low bile duct cancer involves the terminal one-third of the bile duct, which is situated in a groove of the head of the pancreas.

In general, adenocarcinomas of the bile duct exhibit a large fibrous component on histology. They are relatively slow growing and produce stricture obstruction of the duct. Uncommonly, adenocarcinoma of the bile duct may develop in conjunction with a villous, mucus-secreting adenoma of the bile duct. These tumours are more cellular and anaplastic.

Clinical presentation

The most common presentation of bile duct cancer is a patient with painless jaundice. Occasionally, if there is associated infection of the bile, cholangitis may occur and this is characterised by epigastric to right upper quadrant pain, jaundice and fever.

Examination confirms the jaundice. It is uncommon for there to be other signs as usually the tumour is quite small in size.

Investigation

Investigations are those which are directed at the diagnosis of obstructive jaundice. Specific investigations include an ultrasound examination of the liver and bile duct. Dilated intrahepatic ducts will be demonstrated and, if the tumour is in the upper or middle third of the bile duct, the gallbladder may be collapsed. A tumour sited in the distal bile duct will produce a distended gallbladder.

Cholangiography either via ERCP or percutaneous transhepatic cholangiography usually provides a diagnosis by demonstrating the typical appearance of a malignant stricture (Figure 13.8). If the endoscopic approach has been used (i.e. ERCP) a cytology brush may be inserted into the duct and brushings taken to examine for malignant cells. Carcinomas of the bile duct (cholangiocarcinomas) often do not shed sufficient cells to give a cytological diagnosis so a negative result does not necessarily mean that a stricture demonstrated on cholangiography is benign.

CT scan of the liver may be normal in patients with bile duct cancer. However, it should be performed in order to evaluate the liver and the rest of the abdomen for any metastatic extension.

Magnetic resonance cholangiopancreatography (MRCP) and spiral CT provide information on the extent of infiltration into the parenchyma as well as the extent of vascular involvement.

Treatment

Surgical resection of the cancer is associated with the best outcome. However, even if this is not possible, palliation of jaundice is indicated as these tumours are slow growing and survival up to five years even with non-resectable tumours is not uncommon.

These tumours do not respond to treatment with either radiotherapy or chemotherapy.

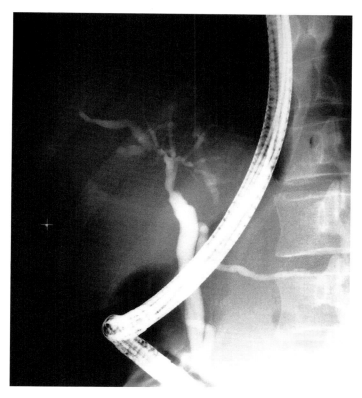

Figure 13.8 ERCP illustrating a large cholangiocarcinoma at the hilum of the liver.

metal stent that may be inserted through the stricture by either an endoscopic (ERCP) or percutaneous (PTC) route.

Prognosis/results

Due to their 'strategic' position, bile duct cancers of the middle or distal duct present relatively early when compared to other hepatobiliary pancreatic tumours and to proximal bile duct cancers. Therefore, resection is often possible with an acceptable prognosis of survival greater than 30% at five years. However, Klatskin tumours tend to have spread into either the left or right lobe of the liver by the time of presentation so even if resection is feasible, survival is not much better than 10% at five years.

Due to the slow growth of Klatskin tumours, even palliative therapy is associated with survival figures not unlike those for resection. However, the only long-term survivors, i.e. beyond five years, are those patients in whom resection has been possible.

Conclusions

Bile duct cancers are uncommon tumours of the digestive tract. They present as one of the differential diagnoses of jaundice. Surgical resection provides the best opportunity for achieving cure so early diagnosis is important.

Operative management

Surgical resection and type of operation are dependent on the site of the cancer. High bile duct cancers may be resected by removing the common hepatic duct, plus part of the left and right hepatic duct. An anastomosis is then performed to a Roux-en-Y jejunal loop of small bowel so that bile flow is reconstituted. More commonly, however, the cancer involves one or other of the left or right hepatic ducts. In this instance that part of the liver, i.e. left or right, is removed also; hence a left or right hepatic lobectomy is done in order to achieve clearance of the tumour.

For cancers of the mid bile duct, it may be possible to remove the tumour along with the common hepatic duct and down to the lower bile duct. Bile flow is reconstituted by anastomosis of the proximal bile duct to a Roux-en-Y jejunal loop of small intestine.

Cancer of the distal bile duct is treated by resection via a pancreaticoduodenectomy (Whipple's operation).

In patients in whom surgical resection for cure is not possible, either a bypass or stent insertion is used for palliation. For patients in whom open surgery is being done to resect the tumour but resection has not been possible, bypass is achieved by anastomosis of a loop of bowel to either the dilated left or right hepatic duct.

If the diagnosis of inoperability has been made prior to attempted resection, drainage of the liver can be achieved via a plastic or

OPERATIVE SURGERY

Open cholecystectomy

Patient preparation

A single dose of intravenous antibiotics is given on induction of anaesthesia. Antibiotics are broad spectrum and in most instances cover Gram-negative rods, enterococcus and anaerobic organisms. A combination of gentamicin, ampicillin and metronidazole fulfils these requirements.

Subcutaneous heparin is commenced on induction and continued whilst the patient is relatively immobile. The dose is 1000 units twice daily.

Anaesthesia and position

Most commonly, muscle relaxant general anaesthetic with endotracheal intubation is used. The patient is positioned supine with a mild reverse Trendelenburg elevation of the head of the operating table. The table is also tilted towards the left.

The surgeon is positioned to the right of the patient, the assistant on the left and, opposite the surgeon, the scrub nurse stands to the left of the assistant.

Incision

The author prefers a right transverse incision situated in the midline at the mid-point of the xiphisternum and umbilicus, extending laterally towards to the tip of the 12th rib. Some surgeons prefer a right subcostal incision which runs approximately 2 cm below the right costal margin.

Once the skin has been incised, the anterior rectus sheath is divided. The rectus abdominis is then divided transversely to expose the posterior sheath which is also divided to enter the peritoneal cavity. The incision is extended laterally by dividing the lateral oblique group of muscles.

Procedure

- Following a brief laparotomy, particularly of the upper abdominal structures, adhesions to the gallbladder are gently divided. A hand is introduced above the liver which usually separates the liver from the diaphragm by introduction of air. Some surgeons insert a tissue pack above the liver in order to encourage its downward retraction.

- What is more important is the placement of two subhepatic packs, one to retract the colon hepatic flexure away from the porta hepatis and the second over the line of the bile duct and duodenum medially. The assistant's left hand is placed over this pack and retraction downwards in the direction of the bile duct is maintained. The gallbladder is grasped just proximal to Hartmann's pouch using a large sponge holder. This instrument is held in the surgeon's left hand positioned over the costal margin. Manipulation of the gallbladder holder opens Calot's triangle and aids in the dissection.

- The liver also requires upward retraction and this is achieved by a broad flat retractor usually held either by the assistant or by mechanical fixation to the operating table.

- The dissection begins by incising the anterior peritoneum over the neck of the gallbladder on the edge of the triangle of Calot (Figure 13.9). A reliable landmark is the cystic artery lymph node which is usually enlarged by inflammation. The incision should be made on the gallbladder side of the node and the node with surrounding adipose tissue gently swept away from the gallbladder in the direction of the bile duct. The peritoneum on the posterior aspect of the gallbladder is also incised at an equivalent position and extended upwards at the junction between the gallbladder and liver. This manoeuvre frees the gallbladder from the liver bed and assists in further opening of Calot's triangle.

- The cystic duct and cystic artery are identified and the duct ligated at its junction with the gallbladder. A transverse incision is made on the anterior aspect of the cystic duct, bile allowed to flow freely and any small calculi 'milked' so as to pass from the duct. A cholangiogram catheter is then introduced and secured (Figure 13.10).

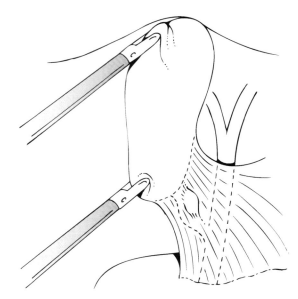

Figure 13.9 Gallbladder cystic duct junction showing the cystic duct node. The dotted line illustrates the site where initial dissection is commenced.

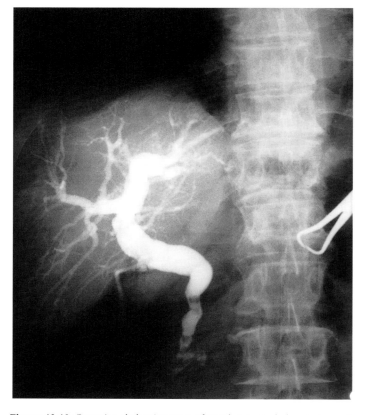

Figure 13.10 Operative cholangiogram performed at open cholecystectomy. A number of radiolucent stones are shown in the bile duct.

- Operative cholangiography is mandatory during cholecyst-ectomy. Angiograffin at 30% dilution is slowly infused under real-time screening of the biliary tract using an image intensifier.

- Cholangiography demonstrates the anatomy of the intrahepatic and extrahepatic biliary tract, ensuring that an inadvertent injury to the bile duct has not occurred. Furthermore, any gall-stones which migrated into the duct may be detected plus any other pathology not expected from the clinical presentation.

- On completion of the cholangiogram, the cholangiogram catheter is removed. An absorbable ligature is passed distal to the cystic duct incision and the duct ligated. It is then divided. Similarly the cystic artery is now ligated and divided.

- The gallbladder may be dissected from the gallbladder bed using diathermy, either in a fundus down direction or from the cystic duct upwards and towards the fundus. The author prefers the former approach as this allows the surgeon to remain close to the gallbladder, thus avoiding any injury to the surrounding structures.

- It used to be taught that the cystic duct–bile duct junction should be identified in gallbladder surgery. There is ample evidence that refutes this teaching. Indeed, in most instances, such dissection may cause injury to the bile duct as a result of ischaemia following division of small arterial tributaries.

- On completion of gallbladder removal, haemostasis is achieved. Normal saline solution may be used to wash out the right subphrenic and subhepatic regions and the abdominal incision closed by mass closure of the muscle and muscle sheaths using non-absorbable synthetic suture. Skin is closed via subcuticular absorbable suture. A peritoneal or sub-cutaneous drain is not normally used.

Postoperative management

Patients have nil by mouth until the postoperative ileus resolves, which is usually 12–24 hours. Fluids are given intravenously. Appropriate analgesia is given.

It is usual for patients to remain in hospital for 3–5 days following open cholecystectomy and to have up to three weeks rehabilita-tion following discharge home.

Laparoscopic cholecystectomy

Patient preparation is similar to that for open cholecystectomy.

Anaesthesia and position

General relaxant anaesthesia with endotracheal intubation is used.

The surgeon stands to the left of the patient and the assistant is on the surgeon's left side, so as to freely hold the laparoscope. The scrub nurse stands to the right of the patient.

The patient is supine with the head of the table elevated and rotated 15° to the left. A single video monitor is positioned to the right of the patient at the head of the table in line with the surgeon's and assistant's direct vision.

Incisions

The size and site of the port incisions are illustrated in (Figure 13.11). The laparoscope is introduced via the umbilical port.

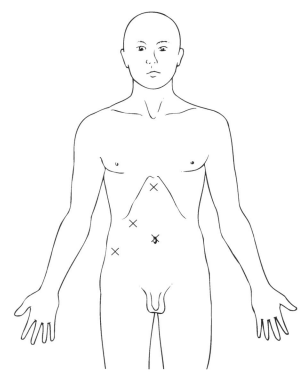

Figure 13.11 Sites (✕) used for the ports to perform a laparoscopic cholecystec-tomy.

Procedure

- Open introduction of the initial port is mandatory for safety. A vertical incision is made below the umbilicus which is elevated by skin tissue forceps. The incision is deepened by a fine scalpel so as to traverse extraperitoneal fat and through the peritoneum. The opening is enlarged using fine forceps and a blunt introducer inserted so that it passes freely into the peritoneal cavity. The 10–12 mm port without sharp trocar is then introduced over the blunt rod. The laparoscope and camera are then introduced as slow CO_2 insufflation begins. Once the position inside the peritoneal cavity is confirmed, the rate of insufflation may be increased to rapidly attain the desired intraabdominal pressure.

- The other ports, i.e. for gallbladder retraction and operating instruments, are introduced under vision.

- The dissection of the gallbladder, cystic duct and artery follows similar principles to those for open cholecystectomy.

- As in the open procedure, the anterior peritoneal incision begins at the junction of the cystic duct node and gallbladder. The tissue is then gently separated along the line of the gallbladder wall both anteriorly and posteriorly so as to lift the gallbladder out of the gallbladder fossa.

- Operative cholangiography is done routinely and the principles are the same as for open cholecystectomy.

- On completion of a normal cholangiogram, the catheter is removed, the cystic duct is secured with metal clips and divided. Similarly the cystic artery is double ligated and divided.

- The gallbladder is dissected from the gallbladder bed using diathermy. It is removed from the peritoneal cavity via the umbilical incision, which may need to be enlarged if the gallbladder contains large stones. A plastic bag may be used to assist gallbladder extraction and may prevent wound contamination by the inflamed gallbladder.

- As for open cholecystectomy, a drain is not routinely used once haemostasis has been achieved.

Postoperative management

Following laparoscopic cholecystectomy recovery is rapid. Within 8–12 hours patients are able to move freely out of bed and are usually happy to ingest oral fluids and a light diet.

Patients are usually discharged home after one night in hospital. The majority require 1–2 weeks' rehabilitation at home before returning to normal activities.

Exploration of the common bile duct

Patient preparation

This is similar to that for open cholecystectomy.

Anaesthesia and position

Similar to open cholecystectomy.

Incision

Exploration of the common bile duct usually occurs in the setting of an open cholecystectomy when a stone is detected in the bile duct by the operative cholangiogram. Consequently the incision is the same as that for open cholecystectomy.

If the bile duct is to be explored *de novo*, then again the optimal incision is the same as that for open cholecystectomy. An upper mid-line incision may be used but this is not the author's preference.

Procedure

- In order to explore the bile duct for the presence of stones, it should be only minimally exposed, hence minimising ischaemia of the duct. The bile duct is identified after the gallbladder is removed and the cystic duct is ligated. However, maintaining a long ligature on the cystic duct stump may assist in the dissection and identification of the bile duct, especially when the surrounding tissues are oedematous as a result of inflammation. If there is any doubt regarding the anatomical orientation of the bile duct and surrounding structures, aspiration of the duct contents via a fine-bore needle can clarify the duct position.

- In most instances it is not necessary to mobilise the duodenum by the Kocher manoeuvre in order to successfully explore the bile duct.

- The bile duct should be incised by scalpel in between two stay sutures. The incision is usually 1–2 cm in length and situated as close to the upper border of the duodenum as can be allowed without extensive dissection.

- On making the initial incision, there is usually an outflow of bile which is often accompanied by the offending gallstones either coming into view in the duct or passing out of the duct through the incision.

- The next manoeuvre in safely extracting stones from the bile duct is the gentle insertion of a Fogarty-style balloon catheter first towards the distal duct and then proximally towards the liver. The tip of the catheter with balloon deflated is negotiated through the sphincter of Oddi into the duodenum. The balloon is then inflated and withdrawn. As the sphincter is passed the balloon needs to be deflated but then again immediately inflated, thus trapping before it any stone in the distal duct. As the catheter is withdrawn, any stone passed in the duct will precede the inflated balloon. The manoeuvre is again repeated proximally.

- Instead of the above procedure, or in addition, choledochoscopy is carried out. A sterile flexible choledochoscope is introduced into the bile duct and the distal end initially inspected. On visualisation of a stone, a stone basket is inserted via the working channel in order to entrap the stone. It is then removed on extracting the endoscope. The procedure is repeated in order to inspect and clean the proximal biliary system.

- A number of other manoeuvres have been described and are used for stone removal, some with advantages but also potential hazards.

- A large-bore catheter may be used to flush normal saline both distally and proximally in order to encourage the passage of stones out of the duct along with the fluid. The danger of this manoeuvre is that a small stone may impact in the ampulla of Vater distally or in the small intrahepatic ducts proximally.

- Rigid stone-grasping forceps have been used to remove stones. These are effective, but may produce mucosal damage inside the biliary system if not used with care.

- Dilators have been used in the past to dilate the sphincter of Oddi and encourage passage of stones into the duodenum. This practice has caused injury to the lower bile duct and the creation of false passages and thus cannot be justified.

- On successfully clearing the bile duct of stones, a small T-tube is placed in the bile duct and the incision closed by interrupted fine absorbable sutures. Any air bubbles in the duct are expelled and a completion T-tube cholangiogram done to demonstrate a clear duct.

- The long arm of the T-tube is exteriorised in as direct a route to the bile duct as possible, thus allowing for subsequent percutaneous access if this becomes necessary postoperatively.

Postoperative management

The T-tube is left open to drain bile and a cholangiogram done 3–4 days after the operation. On demonstrating a normal duct with no stones and normal flow into the duodenum, the external limb of the T-tube may be shortened, occluded and secured under a dressing. This allows the patient free mobility and they may be discharged from hospital. The T-tube is usually removed 3–4 weeks after operation in the consulting suite.

Biliary bypass: bilio-enteric anastomosis

Roux-en-Y choledochojejunostomy is the optimal biliary bypass operation that may be used for a number of indications including non-resectable malignancy of the pancreatic head and lower bile duct, benign strictures or inadvertent division of the bile duct at laparoscopic or open cholecystectomy.

Patient preparation

This is similar to that for open cholecystectomy. In patients who may be jaundiced, coagulation needs to be checked and, if a clotting defect exists, vitamin K should be administered to arrest this.

Anaesthesia and position

Similar to open cholecystectomy.

Incision

- A bilateral subcostal incision with an upper mid-line extension is the most useful incision for all upper abdominal major

surgery. This incision runs approximately 2 cm under the costal margin bilaterally, made longer on the right side as compared to the left (i.e. on the left it does not need to be extended laterally much beyond the lateral edge of the rectus abdominis). A short mid-line upper extension may be added if exposure necessitates.

- Division of the various layers is the same as for open cholecystectomy, but bilaterally. Once the peritoneal cavity is entered the mid-line falx peritonei is divided between haemostatic clamps, the divided ends are ligated but the suture to the hepatic end is left long as it can be used to assist in retraction.

- Fixed frame retraction is used in order to elevate both costal margins. In addition, a fixed frame malleable retractor is useful for elevating the liver in order to expose the upper bile duct in the porta hepatis.

Procedure

- A laparotomy is done to determine the extent of the disease.

- If the gallbladder has not been previously removed, cholecystectomy is done as described previously.

- The common hepatic duct is exposed as high as possible, remembering that its blood supply is best close to the hilum. At least 2 cm of common hepatic duct is exposed anteriorly and two stay sutures are inserted. The duct is incised vertically using a scalpel in between the two stay sutures. Alternatively, the bile duct may be divided, its distal portion resected (if a tumour is present) or oversewn when the operation is done for treating a stricture.

- A Roux-en-Y jejunal limb is next prepared. The duodenal jejunal flexure is identified in the infracolic compartment and to the left of the superior mesenteric vessels. The site of division of the jejunum is defined by visualising the arcuate blood supply and ensuring that both ends of the jejunum are adequately perfused. This point on the jejunum is usually identified 15–20 cm distal to the duodenojejunal flexure.

- A linear stapler and cutter is used to divide the jejunum and the arcuate vessels in the mesentery are divided and ligated between haemostats. It is important to extend the division of the mesentery as close to its base as the arterial supply will allow.

- The distal jejunal limb can now reach to the site of anastomosis with the common hepatic duct either in an antecolic position (favoured if the bypass is done for cancer) or retrocolically by passing through a window in the mesocolon to the right of the middle colic vessels. The jejunal limb should lie in position adjacent to the common hepatic duct without tension.

- The anastomosis is made between the incision in the common hepatic duct and a 2 cm longitudinal incision made on the antimesenteric border of the jejunal limb. The jejunal incision is situated approximately 1–2 cm from the stapled end of the jejunum. The anastomosis is made using interrupted absorbable sutures positioned between the posterior cut of the jejunum and bilaterally in the inferior half of the choledochotomy before tying the knots which are situated inside the lumen (Figure 13.12). Once these ligatures are knotted, the anterior interrupted sutures are inserted and these knots ligated so that the knots are extraluminal.

- A stent is not required.

- A jejunum-to-jejunum anastomosis is next done in order to complete the Roux-en-Y loop. A side-to-side anastomosis may be readily performed using a reloadable linear stapler. However, the anastomosis may also be done using single-layer continuous absorbable sutures.

- In the case of a malignant obstruction of the bile duct by pancreatic cancer, a prophylactic or therapeutic gastroenterostomy may be necessary. This is done as a side-to-side gastroenterostomy between the stomach and the proximal limb of the jejunal loop. A linear stapler will facilitate this anastomosis.

- The bilateral subcostal incision is closed in a similar manner to the open cholecystectomy wound.

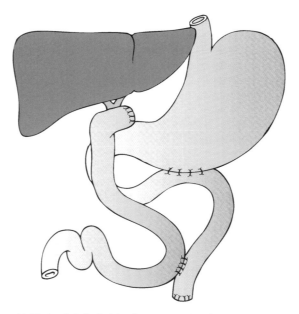

Figure 13.12 A choledochojejunal anastomosis using a Roux-en-Y loop anastomosis.

Postoperative management

This is similar to open cholecystectomy. Paralytic ileus will be prolonged, reflecting the greater extent of surgery. If a nasogastric tube had been inserted to decompress the stomach, consideration for its removal should be given as early as possible.

Enteral nutrition usually commences within 3–5 days from the operation and the patient may leave hospital 7–10 days following the operation.

Repair of biliary injuries

Biliary injuries vary in severity and depend on the mechanism of injury. The operations described already are used to repair any bile duct injuries and the operation used depends on the injury.

Incision into the bile duct or simple ligation by a staple without duct transection may be simply corrected when recognised. It is such instances that illustrate the value of operative cholangiography in that more severe injury to the bile duct can be avoided.

Where a minor injury such as described is recognised, the staple can be readily removed, usually with little to no effect on the bile duct. If the bile duct has been incised, the incision may be closed by interrupted sutures inserted either laparoscopically or via an open approach. A T-tube may be placed in the duct as described previously for open bile duct exploration.

Total transection of the bile duct should not occur if an operative cholangiogram is correctly executed and read correctly by the surgeon. The reason for this view relates to the strong recommendation that no duct should be divided prior to viewing the operative cholangiogram. If such a policy is followed, the worst that can happen in a situation where the common bile duct is mistaken for the cystic duct is a stapled ligation plus incision for inserting the cholangiogram catheter. Such a complication may be repaired as above.

Complete transection of the bile duct is a major complication which may have disastrous effects on the patient. When recognised, it is best treated by a surgeon competent in high bile duct anastomosis as the patient's best chance of successful resolution lies in an ability to make this the first and only operation required. The difficulty of this operation resides in the size of the resected duct or ducts, which often are of small diameter.

The operation is similar to that described previously, i.e. a Roux-en-Y bilio-enteric anastomosis. If the duct transection has occurred above the hilar junction, both left and right hepatic ducts require anastomosis to the Roux-en-Y loop.

The only addition to the operation previously described is to mark a site on the jejunal loop through which a percutaneous approach may be accessed if the anastomosis were to narrow. The mark is created simply by using a fine stainless steel suture placed on the antimesenteric aspect of the jejunal limb which is anastomosed to the bile duct. It is placed at a position on the limb which can comfortably be attached to the inner aspect of the anterolateral abdominal wall so that it may be detected radiologically if it becomes necessary to intervene at a future date.

FURTHER READING

Blumgart LH, Kelley CJ. Hepaticojejunostomy in benign and malignant high bile duct stricture: approaches to the left hepatic ducts. *Br J Surg* 1984; **71**:704–708

Boer HU, Stain SC, Dennison AR, Eggers B, Blumgart LH. Improvements in survival by aggressive resection of hilar cholangiocarcinoma. *Ann Surg* 1993; **217**:20–27

Brook I. Aerobic and anaerobic microbiology of biliary tract disease. *J Clin Microbiol* 1989; **27**:2373–2375

Geenen JE, Hogan WJ, Dodds WJ, Toouli J, Venu RP. The efficacy of endoscopic sphincterotomy in post cholecystectomy patients with sphincter of Oddi dysfunction. *N Eng J Med* 1989; **320**:82–87

Gracie WA, Ransohoff DF. The natural history of silent gallstones: the innocent gallstone is not a myth. *N Eng J Med* 1982; **307**:798–800

GREPCO (Rome Group for the Epidemiology and Prevention of Cholelithiasis). Prevalence of gallstone disease in an Italian adult female population. *Am J Epidemiol* 1984; **119**:796–805

GREPCO. The epidemiology of gallstone disease Rome Italy part I. Prevalence data in men. *Hepatology* 1988; **8**:904–906

Halpern Z, Dudley MA, Lynn MP, Nader JM, Breuer AC, Holzbach RT. Vesicle aggregation in model systems of supersaturated bile: relation to crystal nucleation and lipid composition of the vesicular phase. *J Lipid Res* 1986; **27**:295–306

Kawai K, Akasaka Y, Murakami I, Tada M, Kohle Y, Nakajima M. Endoscopic sphincterotomy of the ampulla of Vater. *Gastrointest Endosc* 1974; **20**:148–151

Klatskin G. Adenocarcinoma of the hepatic duct at its bifurcation within the porta hepatis: an unusual tumour with destructive clinical and pathological features. *Am J Med* 1965; **38**:241–256

Northover JMA, Terblanche J. A new look at the arterial blood supply of the bile duct in man and its surgical complications. *Br J Surg* 1979; **66**:379–384

Todanic T, Watanabe Y, Narusne M. Congenital bile duct cysts: classification operative procedures and review of thirty-seven cases including cancer from choledochal cyst. *Am J Surg* 1977; **134**:263–268

14

Spleen, lymph nodes, soft tissue sarcomas and retroperitoneal tumours

P. O'Dwyer

SPLEEN

Functions of the spleen

Haemopoiesis

The spleen is involved with haemopoietic function only during intrauterine life. After birth no blood formation takes place in the spleen. However, there may be a reversion to the fetal pattern of erythropoiesis in cases where the marrow production of red cells is defective, e.g. in myeloproliferative disorders.

Filtration of blood cells

This function has to do with the destruction of abnormally shaped or rigid red cells, by 'culling' and 'pitting' in the red pulp. 'Culling' is the filtering and phagocytosis of all red blood cells which have either been damaged or contain inclusions such as nuclei, Howell-Jolly bodies (nuclear remnants), Heinz bodies (denatured haemoglobin), Pappenheimer bodies (iron granules), target cells and spherocytes. 'Pitting' is the removal of specific inclusions such as red blood cell nuclei or malarial parasites from red blood cells, without destroying the cells, and the return of those red cells to the circulation. Therefore after splenectomy Howell-Jolly bodies, siderotic granules and cells with changes in shape and size, such as acanthocytes and target forms, may be seen in the peripheral blood.

Phagocytosis of foreign substances by macrophages and histiocytes

These substances include bacteria, fungi, protozoa and also bacteria coated with antibody or opsonic proteins. In the case of bacteria with no existing antibody present in the blood circulation of the host, the spleen acts as a major site for clearance of these bacteria, as well as an initial site of synthesis of immunoglobulin M (IgM).

Platelet storage

The spleen is an important site for platelet sequestration and in a normal situation it contains approximately 30–40% of the total body platelet volume. In conditions of splenomegaly, sequestration can rise to approximately 80% and, in combination with the accelerated platelet destruction, can result in thrombocytopenia. The phagocytosis of platelets is a normal function of the spleen, but can be accelerated in certain conditions such as a idiopathic thrombocytopenic purpura.

In some animals the spleen contains a reverse of red cells, which can be released into the circulation by contraction of the muscular capsule following a hypoxic stimulus, providing therefore a kind of autotransfusion. This function is less marked in humans.

Immunological functions

The spleen accounts for the largest single accumulation of lymphoid tissue in the body. It contains 25% of the total T lymphocyte population and 15% of the B lymphocyte population. There is a proliferation of T lymphocytes and antibody-forming B lymphocytes within the lymphatic sheaths and the lymphatic nodules respectively. As a result there is an increased production of humoral immune factors of both B and T cell origin. Circulating antigens are trapped in the marginal zone of the white pulp, thus triggering IgM production in its germinal centres.

The spleen also accounts for the largest production of tuftsin, opsonin, properdin and interferon. Tuftsin is a tetrapeptide which stimulates phagocytosis by neutrophils. Opsonins are antibodies and other proteins, which make fungi and bacteria more susceptible to phagocytosis. Properdin is an immunoglobulin that fixes complement to bacterial and fungal surface polysaccharides prior to phagocytosis. Finally, interferon is a glycoprotein, which stimulates the activity of killer cell/macrophages by exerting an antiviral effect.

Haematologic disorders

Thrombocytopenic purpura

Immune thrombocytopenic purpura (ITP) is a haemorrhagic disorder characterised by low platelet count, as a result of platelet destruction in the reticuloendothelial system by circulating IgG antiplatelet factors. Normal or increased megakaryocytes, on bone marrow examination, and absence of systemic disease or medications capable of inducing thrombocytopenia also characterise ITP.

Female patients are three times more likely than male patients to develop this disease, with an age range of 15–50 years, and may develop either an acute or a chronic syndrome. The acute syndrome is found mostly in children and occurs usually after the patient's recovery from a viral or an upper respiratory tract illness. The chronic syndrome is more troublesome and is found mostly in young women.

Most patients with ITP present with easy bruising and petechiae or ecchymoses of the skin. Other symptoms include epistaxis, bleeding gums, gastrointestinal bleeding, haematuria or, rarely, intracerebral haemorrhage. The spleen is almost always of normal size and is palpable in only 2–3% of cases. The symptoms of ITP depend on the degree of thrombocytopenia. Bleeding is not likely to occur with a platelet count between $50\,000\,mm^3$ and $100\,000\,mm^3$, while platelet counts between $20\,000\,mm^3$ and $50\,000\,mm^3$ may result in bleeding after minor trauma or surgery. Spontaneous bleeding with purpura, petechiae, mucosal bleeding and menorrhagia may often occur when the platelet count is below $20\,000\,mm^3$ and particularly below $5000\,mm^3$. There are specific laboratory findings that characterise ITP. The platelet count is usually less than 100 000 mm³ and there may even be a complete absence of platelets. Although the bleeding time is prolonged, the clotting time remains normal. Platelets frequently appear larger than normal on the blood film, while increased numbers of megakaryocytes, which are frequently small with few nuclear lobulations, are observed during bone marrow examination. There is usually no significant anaemia or leucopenia. The presence of autoimmune haemolytic anaemia together with ITP constitutes what is known as Evans syndrome, which is found in approximately 5% of cases.

In the treatment of ITP the patient's age, the severity and duration of the thrombocytopenia and its underlying cause are very important factors. Acute ITP has an excellent prognosis in children. Sixty percent of these patients recover in 4–6 weeks and over 90% recover within 3–6 months. Spontaneous remission is, on the other hand, unusual in chronic ITP patients.

The administration of glucocorticoids is the most common method of treatment. Prednisone 60 mg\day is given to the patients for a period of six weeks to two months with a progressive reduction of the dosage when possible. The platelet count tends to increase within a week. Although controversial, some specialists will withhold glucocorticoids until the platelet count drops below 20 000 mm³.

When, despite a high dose of glucocorticoids, an adequate level of platelet count cannot be reached, an elective splenectomy is indicated. Seventy five percent of patients who undergo splenectomy will have a satisfactory response after the operation. During the splenectomy, care must be taken to search for and remove any accessory spleens, which may be the cause of relapse of the disease after the operation. Emergency splenectomy is most commonly performed in patients who are critically ill and do not respond to any other measures for the improvement of haemostasis.

Patients who, despite the administration of glucocorticoids or splenectomy, still have dangerously low platelet levels should receive immunosuppressive drugs. Although they may have serious side effects, drugs like cyclophosphamide, azathioprine, vincristine and vinblastine may be beneficial. The administration of intravenous immunoglobulin has been used with limited success.

Haemolytic anaemias

Hereditary spherocytosis

Hereditary spherocytosis is the most frequently found hereditary haemolytic anaemia in Europe. It is an autosomal dominant disorder and is characterised by a deficiency in spectrin, one of the main structural components of the membrane skeleton that keeps the shape, strength and reversible deformity of the erythrocyte the same. As a result of this deficiency red cells lose their flexible biconcave shape and become small, thick and spherical. These spherocytes are trapped in the red pulp of the spleen and destroyed by reticuloendothelial cells.

The most prominent characteristics of this disorder, which may develop at any age, are anaemia, reticulocytosis, jaundice and splenomegaly. The severity of these features may vary. The disease can be so mild as to go unnoticed during childhood but can also become so severe that repeated blood transfusions may be required and even fatal aplastic crises may occur. Gallstones occur in 30–60% of patients and are rare under the age of 10.

The diagnosis is made by examination of the peripheral blood film where spherocytes and reticulocytes are demonstrated in more than 60%. The Coombs test is negative and osmotic fragility is increased while serum bilirubin levels are usually higher than normal.

Splenectomy is the treatment indicated for almost all the patients and eliminates all clinical symptoms. In order to minimise the risk of postsplenectomy infection, splenectomy should be avoided under the age of six. Although splenectomy does not affect the shape of the red cells it results in a normal red cell survival time. The gallbladder should be examined prior to splenectomy with an ultrasonogram and during the operation by the surgeon. Where gallstones are present a cholecystectomy should be performed at the same time.

Hereditary elliptocytosis

Hereditary elliptocytosis is a disorder of the red cell membrane which results in the abnormal oval shape and deformability of the cells. Most of the patients develop no symptoms through their lifetime and mild haemolysis. Examination of the peripheral blood film reveals the presence of elliptical erythrocytes. Splenectomy should be carried out in symptomatic patients and has good results, although it does not affect the abnormal erythrocyte morphology.

Thalassaemias

Thalassaemias are hereditary haemolytic anaemias, caused by defects in the haemoglobin chain synthesis. The disease is classified as minor, major or intermediate. Minor or heterozygous thalassaemia is a mild disorder, in which the affected child receives an abnormal gene from only one parent. It is usually asymptomatic and is often detected during blood examinations for unrelated problems. Major or homozygous thalassaemia is a severe disorder where the affected child receives an abnormal gene from each parent. Its main symptoms are anaemia with jaundice and splenomegaly. Death occurs early in life as a result of complications. Thalassaemia intermedia characterises heterozygous patients with more moderate anaemia than usual, as well as homozygous patients with a milder than usual anaemia.

The clinical manifestations of major thalassaemia can be observed within the first year of life. These are pallor, retarded growth, enlarged head, leg ulcers, jaundice, bony abnormalities predisposing to fractures, splenomegaly and hepatomegaly. As a result of defective iron utilisation together with increased iron absorption and continual transfusions, iron overload is a typical complication of the disease. In thalassaemia major, examination of the peripheral blood film reveals microcytosis, hypochromia, basophilic stippling and normoblasts. Electrophoresis of haemoglobin reveals almost complete absence of HbA and persistence of HbF. Radiographs may show expansion of bones with a typical 'hair on end' appearance of the skull.

The treatment of thalassaemia major consists of blood transfusion and iron chelation therapy. Even though the basic haematologic disorder will not alter, splenectomy may reduce both the haemolytic process and transfusion requirements and relieve any discomfort or pain caused by excessive splenomegaly. Thalassaemia minor requires genetic counselling, especially in countries where the disease is common.

Sickle cell disease

Sickle cell disease is a hereditary haemolytic anaemia, which occurs predominantly among the black population and is characterised by the replacement of the normal haemoglobin A by haemoglobin S which is less compatible with oxygen. When not enough oxygen is available, red cells with HbS acquire the sickle shape. The extended adhesion of the sickle cells to the vascular endothelium raises blood viscosity, leading to stasis and further reduction in oxygen, resulting in further sickling. The primary consequence of this stagnation is thrombosis which results in ischaemia, necrosis and organ fibrosis.

Even though the sickle cell trait is identified in about 9% of the black population, the majority present with no symptoms and a moderate haemolytic anaemia. The clinical features may be acute or chronic. Infarctive crises may occur in any organ and are very painful. In proportion to the vessels affected by the occlusion, patients may present with severe abdominal pain or peritoneal irritation similar to those caused by surgical illnesses, bone or joint pain, priapism, neurologic symptoms, haematuria and leg ulcers. Diagnosis is established by examination of the peripheral blood film which reveals characteristic sickled red cells. Haemoglobin electrophoresis shows predominately HbS, variable amounts of HbF and no HbA, as well as the presence of the trait in both parents. There is no specific treatment and most patients are treated palliatively. The spleen's role in sickle disease is not well established. Although most patients undergo autoinfarction of the spleen, due to recurrent sickle crises, splenectomy is rarely indicated for patients who present with increased splenic red blood cell sequestration or splenomegaly.

Autoimmune haemolytic anaemia (AIHA)

AIHA is an acquired haemolytic anaemia, characterised by the production of an antibody against red cells. It may be caused by exposure to a variety of drugs, viral infections, collagen vascular or rheumatic diseases or by other unknown factors. Two main types of anti-red blood cell antibodies can be distinguished in this disease: a warm reactive antibody (often IgG, less often IgM or IgA), which facilitates the destruction of red blood cells in the spleen, and a cold reactive antibody (often IgM, less often IgA or IgG), which results in the destruction of red blood cells outside the spleen. AIHA develops mostly after the age of 50 and is found twice as often in females as in males.

The symptoms are non-specific and similar to those seen in congenital haemolytic anaemias. They may include mild jaundice, pallor and abdominal pain. The spleen is enlarged in 50% and gallstones are present in 25% of cases. The diagnosis is made by the demonstration of anaemia, reticulocytosis and spherocytosis in the blood smear, shortened erythrocyte survival time and a positive Coombs test.

AIHA has an acute self-limiting course and requires no specific treatment. If the anaemia is severe, blood transfusions and corticosteroid therapy may be indicated. The removal of the causative agent and the treatment of any responsible disease are also mandatory. Splenectomy should be considered only in the warm type of AIHA when corticosteroids are not effective, the patient develops complications due to long-term steroid treatment or there are contraindications to administrating corticosteroids. Splenectomy results in a complete haematologic remission in approximately 80% of patients.

Hypersplenism in other disorders

Felty's syndrome

Felty's syndrome is characterised by severe rheumatoid arthritis, splenomegaly and granulocytopenia. It occurs only in a few patients with chronic rheumatoid arthritis, who are also prone to developing recurrent infections and leg ulcers. Blood films reveal persistent leucopenia and steroid treatment is used to reverse the neutropenia. Splenectomy is effective in most patients and has excellent haematologic results. It should be considered in patients with serious infections, severe leg ulcers and those who require transfusions.

Myeloid metaplasia

Myeloid metaplasia and myelofibrosis are unusual disorders characterised by connective tissue proliferation within the bone marrow and simultaneous proliferation of haemopoietic elements in the liver, spleen and long bones. Myeloid metaplasia, together with polycythaemia vera, chronic myelogenous leukaemia and idiopathic thrombocytosis, belong to the group of myeloproliferative disorders. Myeloid metaplasia, occurs in middle-aged patients and the presenting symptoms usually are abdominal fullness and discomfort due to splenomegaly, intermittent abdominal pain caused by splenic infarction, spontaneous bleeding, recurrent infections, bone pain, pruritus, complications of hyperuricaemia and hepatomegaly in 75% of the patients. Examination of the peripheral blood film reveals increased red blood cell fragmentation, immature red cells, poikilocytosis and anisocytosis. The white blood cell count is usually elevated and hyperuricaemia is also present. Thrombocytosis with a platelet count over $1\,000\,000\,mm^3$ occurs in 25% of patients. Bone marrow biopsy shows varying degrees of fibrosis. Treatment consists of blood transfusion, corticosteroid therapy, chemotherapy and splenic irradiation and aims to correct the anaemia and splenomegaly. Splenectomy is indicated in patients with increased transfusion requirements, abdominal pain due to splenomegaly, bleeding due to thrombocytopenia and cardiac failure. Mortality is high in patients who undergo splenectomy at the late stages of the disease. There is also a high incidence of thromboembolic complications which makes the preoperative correction of thrombocytosis and postoperative use of antiplatelet drugs especially significant.

Chronic leukaemias

Chronic leukaemias can be classified as chronic lymphocytic leukaemia (CLL) and chronic myeloid leukaemia (CML) and must be taken into consideration in the differential diagnosis of splenomegaly. The clinical manifestations are characteristic for both disorders and the diagnosis is established by examination of the peripheral blood and marrow films. The basic treatment is chemotherapy and/or radiotherapy. Splenectomy is indicated in selected patients and aims at the palliation of severe anaemia and thrombocytopenia and the relief of the symptoms of splenomegaly. Higher mortality and morbidity rates are associated with splenectomy in patients with CLL.

Hairy cell leukaemia is an uncommon form of chronic leukaemia, characterised by pancytopenia and splenomegaly without significant lymphadenopathy. It occurs mostly in males over 50 years of age. Symptomatic patients present with abdominal discomfort due to splenomegaly, weight loss, weakness, easy bruising due to thrombocytopenia or recurrent infections due to neutropenia. The diagnosis is confirmed by the presence of characteristic malignant mononuclear cells in the bone marrow. Splenectomy is indicated in patients with associated thrombocytopenia, increased transfusion requirements and splenomegaly. A complete response occurs in 65–75% of patients.

Trauma

Although the spleen is protected by the lower ribs of the chest wall, it is the most commonly injured intraabdominal organ. The causes of splenic injury may be blunt, penetrating or iatrogenic trauma, whereas in some cases the spleen can rupture spontaneously as a result of excessive splenomegaly caused by various disorders or infections. The possibility of splenic injury should be considered in all patients with a history of blunt abdominal trauma, fractures of the left lower ribs and penetrating injury to the upper abdomen or left lower thorax. Pathologically enlarged spleens tend to rupture more easily after a minor injury, while normal-sized spleens do not. Delayed splenic rupture occurs rarely and usually after an interval of more than 24 hours from the injury and is the result of the tear of the splenic capsule due to an expanding subcapsular haematoma.

Much effort has been made to grade splenic injury, in order to predict which type of injury can be repaired or managed nonoperatively (Table 14.1).

The signs and symptoms of splenic injury depend on the severity of the injury and can be divided in two groups.

Rapid exsanguination and death

In this group there is a complete avulsion of the spleen from its pedicle, where the patient exsanguinates and dies before any attempt at resuscitation or laparotomy can be made. It is very rare and is usually associated with other abdominal injuries.

Table 14.1 Splenic Injury Scale

*Grade	Type of injury†	
	Haematoma	**Laceration**
1	Subcapsular, non-expanding, <10% surface area	Capsular tear Non-bleeding, <1 cm parenchymal depth
2	Subcapsular, non-expanding,10–50% surface area Intraparenchymal, non-expanding, <2 cm diameter	Capsular tear Active bleeding
3	Subcapsular, >50% surface area expanding or Ruptured Intraparenchymal haematoma, >2cm or expanding	>3 cm parenchymal depth or involving trabecular vessels
4	Ruptured intraparenchymal haematoma with active bleeding	Laceration involving segmental or hilar vessels producing major devascularisation (>25% of the spleen)
5	Completely shattered or devascularised spleen	Completely shattered or devascularised spleen

* Advance one grade for multiple injuries to the same organ
† Based on the most accurate assessment at autopsy or through laparotomy or radiographic study
Modified from Shackford SR, Molin M. Management of splenic injuries. *Surg Clin North Am* 1990; **70(3)**: 595

Hypovolaemic shock, initial recovery and signs of intraabdominal bleeding

This type is the most common. The signs and symptoms of hypovolaemic shock correspond to the extension of the injury and include increasing pallor, rising pulse rate, tenderness of the abdomen or of the left upper quadrant and referred left shoulder pain (Kehr's sign). There is often abdominal distension, bruising in the left hypochondrium and signs of localised peritonism, which may later spread if the bleeding continues.

Laboratory evaluation usually reveals decreased haematocrit and increased white blood cell count. These findings, however, are not especially helpful, since they do not exclude other injuries. A plain abdominal film may reveal enlargement of the splenic shadow, obliteration of psoas shadow and a medial displacement of the stomach. A chest radiograph may reveal lower rib fractures, elevation of the left hemidiaphragm, pleural effusion and associated pneumohaemothorax. The stable patients should be further investigated with:

- abdominal ultrasound (US)
- computed tomography (CT)
- splenic scintiscanning
- angiography
- diagnostic peritoneal lavage (DPL).

CT of the abdomen is the technique that best defines the anatomic details of the spleen and its relationship with the surrounding organs, with a high degree of accuracy. It may reveal a subcapsular or perisplenic haematoma, lacerations of the spleen and free intraperitoneal fluid, which could indicate splenic injury.

US reveals information about the size and the consistency of the spleen and is also used in the diagnosis and follow-up of traumatic injuries of the spleen.

Radioisotope scans using ^{99}TC-labelled colloid is similar to US and can reveal information about the position, size and presence of occupying lesions of the spleen. Both isotope scans and US, however, have poorer resolution than contrast-enhanced CT scan but may still be useful if a CT scan is not available.

Arteriography is mostly used for the diagnosis of splenic artery pseudoaneurysms and splenic vein thrombosis and for the embolisation of the splenic artery when indicated.

DPL is a very useful method for detecting a significant haemoperitoneum. It is safe, quick and thus of great use in urgent situations where there is an immediate need to know if a haemoperitoneum is present and an emergency operation for associated injuries is indicated. Although DPL is very sensitive in detecting haemoperitoneum, it is not organ specific.

Having clinically assessed the degree of blood loss and resuscitated the patient properly with blood or colloids, a management plan should be followed.

Operative management

If despite adequate resuscitation continuous blood loss is evident or if associated injuries to other organs are suspected then a laparotomy is indicated. The intraoperative management of the splenic injury depends on its extension and on the experience of the surgeon in splenic conservation techniques. The main aim of surgical treatment is the control of any active bleeding and the second is preservation of the splenic tissue when possible.

During laparotomy the extent of the splenic injury is evaluated, after the spleen has been completely mobilised from its attachments.

- Superficial tears of the splenic capsule can be controlled with the use of haemostatic agents.
- Lacerations of the splenic surface can be controlled with splenorrhaphy, using absorbable sutures tied gently over pledgets.
- Extended lacerations involving only one pole of the spleen should be treated with partial splenectomy.
- Finally, extended hilar injuries and pulverised splenic parenchyma are usually treated with splenectomy.

Estimates of the successful splenic preservation following splenic injury depend on the injury grade (Table 14.2).

Table 14.2 Successful splenic preservation following splenic injury	
Injury grade	**Successful preservation (%)**
I	90–100
II	80–90
III	40–70
IV	10–25
V	Minimal

From Moore EE, Shackford SR, Pachter HL et al. Organ injury scaling: spleen, liver and kidney. *J Trauma* 1989; **29(1)**: 664

Non-operative management

Non-surgical management of splenic injuries is the most common method of splenic conservation and has initially proved useful in children with success rates of over 90%. This method has also been applied successfully in adults, although some controversy exists regarding the selection criteria of patients. The percentage of cases suitable for nonoperative management varies between 13% and 60% according to various series. Patients selected for non-operative management should be victims of blunt abdominal trauma who after adequate resuscitation are haemodynamically stable, should not have a coagulopathy or other associated intraabdominal injuries, should not have any neurological damage and must have radiographic confirmation of the degree of the injury with CT scan. Patients with an altered state of consciousness caused by injury, medication, alcohol or drugs are poor candidates for non-operative management.

The success rate of non-operative management has been found to be 93% in patients aged less than 55 years, haemodynamically stable, with a grade III or less injury and with no associated abdominal injuries. Patients selected for non-operative management should be adults with grade I or II injuries. For non-operative management very careful clinical and laboratory observation is essential and should be carried out in an intensive care unit. Bedrest is crucial for 48–72 hours after the injury. As the patient may deteriorate suddenly and unexpectedly, crossmatched blood should always be available because an urgent laparotomy will then be required. It is essential that these patients are observed for a period of two weeks, during which a repeat CT scan must be performed a week after the injury. An additional CT scan or US should be performed 6–8 weeks after the patient is discharged.

According to various series 0–30% of patients managed non-operatively will finally require surgery. As surgeons have become more at ease with non-operative management of splenic injuries, a tendency to liberate the selection criteria has been observed. As a result, in many recent series the age of the patient and the presence of head injury are not considered to be contraindications, while patients with a single stab wound may be treated non-operatively. Most of the patients who fail non-operative management will require surgery within 48–72 hours after the injury although significant and potentially life-threatening complications may occur after this period. Delayed bleeding can be caused by rupture of a subcapsular haematoma or secondary to the lysis of clotted blood at the site of the primary injury. Other delayed complications include splenic abscess and the formation of a splenic artery pseudoaneurysm.

Overwhelming postsplenectomy infection

The most serious late complication in asplenic patients or in patients with insufficient splenic function is the development of an overwhelming postsplenectomy infection. After splenectomy the patient becomes more susceptible to infections for two reasons. First, the spleen's architecture makes it quite efficient at removing encapsulated bacteria and exogenous organisms through phagocytosis and second, the spleen's white pulp is a site of bacterial opsonisation and antibody production.

Although the precise incidence of severe postsplenectomy infection is unknown, various series have found an overall incidence of 4–5%. The risk of infection is higher in children than in adults and is also higher when splenectomy is performed for haematological diseases (25%) than for trauma (1–2%). It usually occurs within three years after the operation, although it has been described even 30 years later. The most common organisms responsible are *Streptococcus pneumoniae*, *Haemophilus influenzae*, *Neisseria meningitidis*, *Escherichia coli*, Staphylococcus and Streptococcus in decreasing frequency. Other implicated organisms are *Capnocytophaga canimorsus*, Enterococcus, Salmonella, Bacteroides and *Pseudomonas pseudomallei*. The mortality rate is between 50% and 75% and is higher in cases of *Streptococcus pneumoniae* infections.

The syndrome that characterises severe sepsis is called OPSI and progresses so rapidly that a healthy individual may die within 24 hours. Although the first signs are similar to those of a non-specific viral illness, patients may very quickly become quite ill with high fever, nausea, vomiting, headaches and confusion and may even fall into a coma. Blood cultures occasionally reveal the causative organism. Disseminated intravascular coagulation and electrolyte balance are often present, while multiorgan haemorrhage and Waterhouse–Friedrichsen syndrome can be seen at autopsy.

The minimum amount of splenic tissue needed to prevent postsplenectomy sepsis is thought to be between 30% and 50%. All patients undergoing splenectomy should receive vaccination against pneumococci, *Haemophilus influenzae* and meningococcus 2–3 weeks before an elective operation. In emergency cases the vaccination should be performed postoperatively. The response to the vaccination of an asplenic patient is less than 50% that of a patient with an intact spleen. Protection from vaccination is not guaranteed, because many subtypes of microorganisms are not covered. The use of antibiotics in prophylaxis is controversial. Oral penicillin is given postoperatively for periods which may vary from three years until the onset of puberty, in cases where splenectomy is performed in a child. Antibiotics such as amoxicillin/clavulanic acid, trimethoprim/sulphamethoxazole or cefuroxime may also be used. The major problem of long-term prophylaxis is the patient's compliance. As a patient runs a greater risk of developing infection during the first 2–3 postoperative years, antibiotics should be given for that period of time. All patients should be informed of their condition and advised to seek medical attention at the first signs of any illness or the development of fever. If appropriate precautions are taken, overwhelming postsplenectomy infection should be largely preventable.

LYMPH NODES

Inflammation

Acute and chronic infections commonly produce lymphadenopathy. The source of acute infections is usually bacterial but can be viral or parasitic. Such lymph node enlargements are usually self-limiting or respond to antibiotics.

Chronic infection such as tuberculosis can produce considerable lymphadenopathy. This is particularly the case in primary bovine tuberculosis where large cervical lymph nodes are present. Sarcoidosis may also produce cervical adenopathy, as can chronic fungal infection. Cat scratch fever usually presents with a single tender lymph node and is not usually associated with splenomegaly.

Generalised lymphadenopathy due to inflammation is usually of viral origin. The common viral illnesses causing such lymphadenopathy include infectious mononucleosis, influenza, cytomegalovirus infection and rubella. Autoimmune diseases also produce generalised lymphadenopathy, such as collagen and vascular disorders and hypersensitivity reactions.

While some texts suggest that the only place where non-diseased lymph nodes can be palpated is the groin, this is not strictly true as both cervical and axillary lymph nodes may also be palpated in normal subjects. Enlarged occipital lymph nodes usually indicate chronic scalp infection.

Neoplastic disorders

Metastatic carcinoma is the most common neoplastic disorder of lymph nodes. When one suspects that a lymph node is neoplastic, a fine needle aspirate should be performed. This is particularly important in the head and neck region where an incisional biopsy will often make subsequent definitive surgery difficult. It is also important in these areas to exhaust all means to identify a primary site. For example, in the head and neck area every patient should have a chest radiograph, direct and indirect laryngoscopy, oesophagoscopy and bronchoscopy.

Hodgkin's disease

Hodgkin's disease usually presents with enlargement of the anterior cervical lymph nodes. Axillary, inguinal or mediastinal lymphadenopathy may be the presenting site in up to 30% of patients. It occurs predominantly in males and has a peak incidence in the second and third and sixth and seventh decades. The patient may be asymptomatic or have systematic systems such as weight loss, sweating, intermittent fevers or pruritus. The diagnosis of Hodgkin's disease is confirmed by lymph node biopsy. Biopsy should preferably be incisional, ensuring that an intact node is sent fresh to the pathology department for cytogenetic and immunohistochemical staining. Staging is by chest and abdominal CT. Staging laparotomy is rarely used nowadays as chemotherapy has become the treatment of choice for all but stage 1A disease. Stage 1A patients are treated by radiotherapy with salvage chemotherapy for those that relapse. Combination chemotherapy with agents such as cyclophosphamide, vincristine, prednisolone and procarbazine (MOPP) is still used as first-line treatment, reserving agents such as adriamycin, vinblastine and bleomycin for relapse. Ninety percent of patients with Hodgkin's disease will be cured by such treatment modalities.

Non-Hodgkin's lymphoma

The majority of patients with this disease present with painless enlargement of one or more superficial groups of lymph nodes. Less commonly, extranodal regions such as skin, gastrointestinal tract or nervous system are involved. Approximately a quarter of patients will present with retroperitoneal adenopathy. The diagnosis in most of these patients is confirmed by lymph node biopsy for superficial lymph node involvement and by CT-guided biopsy for retroperitoneal tumours. Again, these patients will be staged by CT and bone marrow biopsy. Staging laparotomy has no role in this disease as all patients are treated medically. As with lymph node biopsy for Hodgkin's disease the node should be removed intact and sent fresh to the pathologist so that cytogenetic and immunohistochemical staining can be performed to enable the exact pathologic type to be determined. For practical purposes these are defined as low, intermediate and high-grade tumours and may be of B or T cell origin. While most patients will be treated with chemotherapy, in rare instances low-grade tumours may be observed if asymptomatic. Approximately 40% of patients will be cured by such treatment modalities.

SOFT TISSUE SARCOMAS

Soft tissue sarcomas are a heterogeneous group of malignant neoplasms, which arise from mesenchymal tissues excluding bone and cartilage. The term 'sarcoma' is derived from the Greek word *sarkoma*, which means fleshy tumour. Soft tissue sarcomas are relatively uncommon neoplasms, comprising 0.5–1% of the malignant tumours, and their incidence rate is approximately two per 100 000 of the population. They can arise in any anatomical site of the body and show a great variety in terms of their histology and biological behaviour and their potential for local infiltration and distant metastases. All soft tissue sarcomas take their name from the tissue type that they most closely resemble (Table 14.3). There is a slight preponderance of soft tissue sarcomas in males. They are more common in people greater than 55 years old, whereas rhabdomyosarcomas almost always arise in children.

Table 14.3 Soft Tissue Sarcomas

Resemble mature tissue type	Tumour
Fat	Liposarcoma
Lymphatic tissue	Lymphangiosarcoma
Blood vessel	Angiosarcoma, Kaposi's sarcoma
Fibrous tissue	Malignant fibrous histiocytoma
Neural sheath	Malignant schwannoma
Smooth muscle	Leiomyosarcoma
Fascia	Fibrosarcoma
Synovium	Synovial sarcoma
Skeletal muscle	Rhabdomyosarcoma
Mesothelium	Mesothelioma
Uncertain	Epithelioid sarcoma, alveolar soft part sarcomas

Aetiology

The aetiology of soft tissue sarcomas is largely unknown. However, cytogenetic studies provide new information concerning genetic deletions and translocations that may change the function of oncogenes and tumour suppressor genes. The involvement of genetic factors plays a role in the pathogenesis of certain types of soft tissue sarcomas. There is a 7–10% risk that patients with neurofibromatosis (von Recklinghausen's disease) will develop a neurofibrosarcoma during their lifetime while patients with Gardner's syndrome may develop a desmoid tumour or fibrosarcoma. Patients with Li–Fraumeni cancer family syndrome are susceptible to develop sarcomas, breast cancer, brain tumours, adrenocortical carcinoma and leukaemia. Maffucci's syndrome is also associated with the development of chondrosarcomas.

Radiation therapy may lead to the development of sarcomas in the radiated area 2–25 years after the exposure. The frequency increases with the radiation dose and the most common histopathological type is a malignant fibrous histiocytoma. Lymphangiosarcoma can arise in women with a prolonged lymphoedematous extremity after mastectomy and axillary dissection performed for breast cancer with or without radiation (Stewart–Treves syndrome). Environmental factors such as chemical carcinogens are believed to cause certain types of sarcomas. Industrial exposure to polyvinyl chloride, for example, may cause angiosarcoma of the liver, while asbestos is associated with the development of pleural and peritoneal mesotheliomas.

Diagnosis

Physical examination

The physical examination of the patient is of great importance. The site, size and possible extension and fixation of the lump to the surrounding structures must be defined precisely. Although soft tissue sarcomas can arise in any region of the body, 55% of them occur in the extremities (40% in the lower and 15% in the upper extremities). Approximately 20% occur in the chest and abdominal wall, 15% in the head and neck and 10% in the retroperitoneal area. The deeper and larger the lump and the more firmly it is fixed to the surrounding structures, the greater the possibility that it is malignant.

The majority of patients present with a painless, slowly enlarging lump of variable duration, which is usually situated to fascia deep rather than in subcutaneous tissues. Pain is rarely present, particularly in the advanced stages of a disease, and is the result of nerve infiltration or compression. Infiltration of an artery is uncommon because soft tissue sarcomas tend to displace rather than infiltrate the vascular structures as they expand. Distal oedema of a limb may indicate venous compression. Signs of widespread disease such as weight loss and cachexia are very rarely present. Regional lymph node involvement is rare in soft tissue sarcomas and ranges between 3.9% and 5.9% in various series. However, specific histological types of soft tissue sarcomas like epithelioid sarcoma are associated with a higher incidence of lymph node involvement.

Diagnostic studies

Laboratory investigations

A complete blood count and urinalysis must be obtained from all patients. If the lesion is in the abdominal or pelvic cavity, liver function tests and a liver scan should also be performed.

Tumour imaging

Plain radiographs are not very helpful and their use is limited in detecting soft tissue sarcomas. Sometimes, however, certain characteristics such as periosteal reaction or involvement of adjacent bones may be revealed, helping in the differential diagnosis. CT provides excellent definition of the extent of the lesion and its relation to the surrounding structures (bones, muscle groups and neurovascular structures). It can also provide some evidence about the tumour's grade, since low-grade soft tissue malignancies have homogeneous density, while high-grade tumours have heterogeneous density with areas of central necrosis. CT scan is also important in detecting or excluding pulmonary metastases, if they have not already been revealed in the chest radiograph. Magnetic resonance imaging (MRI) is considered to be the imaging modality of choice for staging soft tissue sarcomas. It gives superior resolution of muscle, fat, fibrous tissue and adjacent vascular structures. It is the best way to discriminate adequately between fibrous scar tissues and other soft tissues and is therefore helpful in evaluating patients for a possible recurrence in the region of a previous operation.

Biopsy

Biopsy plays a significant role in the diagnosis and institution of proper therapy. Fine needle aspiration (FNA) cytology will often result in a diagnosis of malignancy, but classification and grading of the sarcoma cannot be performed on the basis of the cells alone. Its usefulness is therefore limited in establishing the presence of a recurrent tumour and ruling out a metastatic sarcoma.

Because a large sample of tissue is required to diagnose and grade a sarcoma, an adequate core or open biopsy is indicated. The open biopsy may be incisional or excisional depending on the size and location of the soft tissue tumour. Incisional biopsies are almost always advocated for soft tissue sarcomas when there is uncertainty on the core biopsy, unless the lesion is very small (<2 cm) and situated in an accessible site. The drawback of excisional biopsies in soft tissue sarcomas is that these tumours are surrounded by a pseudocapsule which contains tumour cells that are left behind. The excisional biopsy usually contaminates tissue planes and makes the final resection wider than necessary. Lesions that are larger than 3 cm in diameter and deeply located should be considered as possible malignant tumours and should be removed by an incisional biopsy. Incisional biopsy has to be performed by an experienced surgeon, bearing in mind that the placement of the biopsy incision should comply with the principles of a major operation (Figure 14.1), which will eventually follow if the lesion is proven to be a sarcoma.

General anaesthesia is preferable to local anaesthesia because of the deep location of the tumour and the possible discomfort of the patient. The biopsies of extremity tumours should be oriented longitudinally, while at other sites the incision of the biopsy should be placed parallel to the direction of the underlying muscle. To avoid heat artefacts, cautery should not be applied

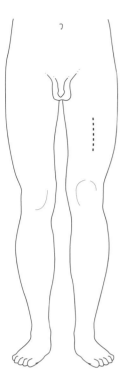

Figure 14.1 Direction of incision for biopsy of soft tissue sarcoma in the left thigh.

Box 14.1	Staging soft tissue sarcomas

Definition for TNM
Primary tumour (T)
    T1 Tumour 5 cm or less in greatest dimension
    T2 Tumour more than 5 cm in greatest dimension
Regional lymph nodes (N)
    N0 No regional lymph node metastasis
    N1 Regional lymph node metastasis
Distant metastasis (M)
    M0 No distant metastasis
    M1 Distant metastasis
Histologic grade (G)
    G1 Well differentiated
    G2 Moderately differentiated
    G3 Poorly differentiated
    G4 Undifferentiated

Staging

Stage IA	G1, T1, N0, M0
Stage IB	G1, T2, N0, M0
Stage IIA	G2, T1, N0, M0
Stage IIB	G2, T2, N0, M0
Stage IIIA	G3, G4, T1, N0, M0
Stage IIIB	G3, G4, T2, N0, M0
Stage IVA	Any G, any T, N1, M0
Stage IVB	Any G, any T, Any N, M1

Modified from American Joint Committee on Cancer: *Manual for staging of cancer*, 4th edn, Philadelphia: JB Lippincott, 1993.

until after the specimen is removed. After haemostasis is secured, the wound is closed in layers without the use of a drain.

Staging

Although in the classification of solid tumours the TNM system is used, in soft tissue sarcomas the most important factor in prognosis is the grade of the tumour. This is based on the number of mitotic figures per 10 high-power fields, the presence of necrosis, the cellularity and the extent of stroma. The American Joint Committee on Cancer uses the tumour grade in combination with the TNM system to stage soft tissue sarcomas (Box 14.1).

Management

The main goal in the management of soft tissue sarcomas is the eradication of disease at the primary site. Various approaches have been used in the management of soft tissue sarcomas: surgery alone, surgery combined with radiotherapy, radiotherapy alone and chemotherapy.

Surgical management

Sarcomas can be managed surgically by marginal resection, radical resection, wide resection, amputation, debulking and surgery combined with brachytherapy.

Marginal excision is an enucleation of the tumour having as a plane the tumour's pseudocapsule. But, as the pseudocapsule of the tumour is in almost all cases a compressed fibrous tissue infiltrated by the tumour, there is a very high incidence of local recurrence, occurring in 80–90% of patients. This option must therefore be followed by radiotherapy.

Radical excision is the removal of the entire musculofascial compartment containing the tumour and is the procedure of choice in the surgery of soft tissue sarcomas. This procedure is impossible in many anatomical sites but has the smallest local recurrence rate, varying between 5% and 20%.

Wide excision is the removal of a margin of normal tissue at least 2 cm in size in all directions around the tumour when possible. The surgeon should incise through healthy tissues during the operation and should remove the tumour encompassed by healthy tissue. The incidence of local recurrence after wide excision is around 40%.

The extent of the margins removed by resection depends on the anatomical relationships of the tumour with the surrounding structures. As a result, in the case of a head or neck tumour it is usually impossible to remove more than 1 cm margin in all directions around the tumour. In order to achieve free microscopic margins, a margin of at least 1 cm around the tumour is necessary. In high-grade tumours a more extensive marginal resection is mandatory. All cases with macroscopic or microscopic disease in the resected margins are associated with unacceptably high recurrence rates.

Although *amputation* was considered to be the treatment of choice in the past, since the introduction of multimodality treatment for soft tissue sarcomas, its rate for extremity sarcomas has fallen over the last two decades to 4–16%. Today amputation is performed in cases of extensive sarcomas involving a bone or a joint and where conservative surgery is inadequate. Specific tumour locations that are better treated by amputation are the foot and ankle regions (high grade). Other tumour cases for which amputation must be considered are large or recurrent tumours lying at the inguinal ligament, in the buttock or high in the medial compartment. Hemipelvectomy may be required for pelvic tumours, for tumours growing through the sciatic or obturator foramina and for those involving the common femoral or iliac artery.

When complete excision of the sarcoma is impossible tumour *debulking* procedures may be performed, to be followed by radiotherapy to the tumour bed and possibly by chemotherapy.

Brachytherapy is the implantation of afterloading catheters to the tumour bed after complete surgical resection. These catheters are placed at approximately 1 cm intervals, encompass the tumour bed with a 2 cm margin and are secured in place with cat-gut sutures. A drain is then placed and the wound is closed. The radioisotope iridium-192 is loaded on the sixth postoperative day. Earlier loading is associated with higher incidence of wound complications.

Radiotherapy

Although in the past soft tissue sarcomas were thought to be radioresistant a significant improvement in their management came through the series of Suit who demonstrated that radiotherapy is effective in sterilising subclinical tumour deposits. Combination of local surgery followed by radiotherapy has achieved similar local control rates to those of cases where complete resection was performed.

Radiotherapy can be administered preoperatively or postoperatively. The advantages of preoperative administration of radiotherapy are that it reduces the tumour size, making the treatment volume smaller, it causes no delay in the start of radiation and by reducing the number of viable tumour cells, it eliminates the possibility of an autotransplantation in the surgical bed. The main disadvantage of preoperative radiotherapy is the increase in wound complications due to delayed healing.

Usually postoperative radiotherapy begins 2–4 weeks after the operation. The advantages of postoperative radiation are that it can be planned once histological grading is available and delivered directly to the tumour bed which has been marked with clips by the surgeon. Small grade I tumours (<5 cm) removed with 1 cm margin will not require radiotherapy. Larger tumours (>5 cm), even if low grade, require radiation, similar to grade II or III tumours. High-dose radiotherapy 6–7000 rads delivered in 6–7 weeks, with or without limited surgical excision, has been proven to be effective in patients with small low-grade soft tissue sarcomas.

Chemotherapy

The value and justification of postoperative adjuvant chemotherapy have long been questioned. Various agents are effective in producing partial or occasionally complete remission in patients with local recurrence and/or metastatic disease. The most effective agent is doxorubicin, which has been used either alone or with ifosfamide, with a response rate of 25%.

Although regional chemotherapy by intraarterial infusion is performed in some centres it is not usually used as a routine procedure for extremity sarcomas. The tumours most responsive to chemotherapy are embryonal rhabdomyosarcomas in children, in which the successful use of combination chemotherapy (actinomycin D, doxorubicin and cyclophosphamide) for metastatic disease has resulted in its routine use as an adjuvant treatment after radiotherapy and/or surgery for these tumours.

Many randomised trials evaluating adjuvant doxorubicin have failed to demonstrate any benefits in terms of overall survival following surgical resection for soft tissue sarcomas. Additionally, trials of combination chemotherapy (cyclophosphamide, vincristine, doxorubicin and dacarbazine) have also failed to demonstrate any significant survival benefit. As a result, chemotherapy remains useful only in the palliative treatment of metastatic sarcoma, with response rates around 50%.

The management of metastatic disease includes surgical resection, when possible, and chemotherapy. Carefully selected patients may remain free of disease for many years following resection of the metastatic lesions. Twenty to 30% of the patients who undergo resection of pulmonary metastases are still alive five years after the operation.

RETROPERITONEAL TUMOURS

The retroperitoneal space is large and is bounded anteriorly by the posterior parietal peritoneum, posteriorly by the spine, psoas and quadratus lumborum muscles, superiorly by the diaphragm, inferiorly by the levator muscles of the pelvis and laterally by the flank muscles. Several organs are contained in the retroperitoneal space: kidneys, ureters, pancreas, adrenal glands, abdominal aorta, inferior vena cava and portions of the duodenum and the ascending and descending colon. In this space are also contained portions of the autonomic and peripheral nervous systems and of the lymphatic, fatty and fibrous connective tissues. From all the above-mentioned structures primary tumours, either benign or malignant, can develop (Table 14.4).

Primary retroperitoneal tumours are uncommon, with a rate of 0.3–3%. Most of these tumours (60–80%) are malignant. Between 35 and 45% of all retroperitoneal masses are found to be soft tissue sarcomas, 25–35% are lymphomas, 5% are of extragonadal germ cell origin and 5% are carcinomas. The retroperitoneal soft tissue sarcomas comprise 10–15% of the soft tissue sarcomas and about 0.1–0.2% of all malignancies. The most common

Table 14.4 Classification of primary retroperitoneal tumours

Tissue of origin	Neoplasm
Neurogenic	
Nerve/nerve sheath	Neurofibroma/ neurofibrosarcoma Neurilemmoma/malignant schwannoma
Sympathetic ganglia	Ganglioneuroma/ganglioneuroblastoma
Ectopic adrenal tissue	Paraganglioma, extraadrenal phaeochromocytoma
Mesenchymal	
Adipose tissue	Lipoma/liposarcoma
Smooth muscle	Leiomyoma/leiomyosarcoma
Striated muscle	Rhabdomyoma/rhabdomyosarcoma
Fibrous tissue	Fibroma/fibrosarcoma/malignant fibrous histiocytoma
Lymphatics	Lymphangioma/lymphangiosarcoma
Vascular tissue	Haemangioma/angiosarcoma/ haemangiopericytoma
Mucoid tissue	Myxoma/myxosarcoma
Gland tissue	Adenoma/carcinoma
Embryonic remnants	
Germ cell	Teratoma/seminoma/choriocarcinoma

histopathological type is liposarcoma (50%) with 60% having a high histological grade.

Clinical presentation

Because the retroperitoneum is a quite big and distensible space, tumours usually reach a considerable size before they produce any signs and symptoms. Almost a quarter of the patients has evident metastases at the presentation. Most patients complain of a pain or discomfort in the abdomen or back, while a non-tender abdominal mass is palpable in 75% of the cases. Other signs and symptoms depend on the structures that are compressed or infiltrated by the tumour. These typically include obstructive symptoms of the gastrointestinal or urinary tracts, symptoms of venous obstruction from occlusion or compression of major venous structures and symptoms from stretching or compression of the lumbar or pelvic plexuses. Occasionally weight loss, fever and weakness may occur. On physical examination a non-tender abdominal mass is usually present. The regional nodal groups must be examined carefully for lymphadenopathy, as well as the scrotum in men to evaluate the possibility of testicular neoplasm spread to the retroperitoneal nodes. Vaginal and rectal examination may also reveal the presence of a pelvic tumour.

Diagnostic studies

Laboratory investigations

Laboratory evaluation includes blood count, urinalysis, liver and kidney function tests and the common serum markers of germ cell tumours like B-human chorionic gonadotrophin (B-hCG) and alpha-fetoprotein (AFP). In addition, cortisol and urinary catecholamines must be measured if a large adrenal tumour cannot be excluded.

Tumour imaging

Computed tomography remains the primary modality in the evaluation of retroperitoneal tumours. CT scan can reveal the extension of the tumour, possible infiltration of the surrounding organs or vascular structures and the presence of metastatic disease in the retroperitoneal space or in the abdominal cavity. It can also reveal heterogeneous areas, which are formed by the presence of necrosis within the tumour. These can narrow the differential diagnosis because the above-mentioned appearance is more likely to appear in a retroperitoneal sarcoma, whereas lymphomas have a homogeneous multinodal involvement (Figure 14.2A).

MRI provides a generally superior definition of fascial planes by enhancing the contrast between tumour and muscle and tumour and adjacent blood vessels.

Arteriography is not routinely used, but is helpful as it reveals the blood supply of the tumour and possible displacement of major vascular structures.

Intravenous urography is also helpful in demonstrating the possible infiltration of the ureters and the functional state of the kidneys, in cases where a nephrectomy may be required for curative resection.

A preoperative chest CT should also be performed in order to detect pulmonary metastatic lesions.

Biopsy

Preoperative biopsy of a retroperitoneal mass is not indicated, because it will not modify the plan of treatment and surgical exploration will follow in the majority of cases. However, if there is a clinical suspicion of lymphoma (lymphadenopathy, fever, night sweats) a CT scan or a US-guided needle biopsy should be performed.

Treatment

Surgery is the treatment of choice for retroperitoneal sarcomas. Complete removal of the tumour is the primary factor for a successful outcome.

All patients should undergo mechanical and antibiotic preparation, because a partial resection of the colon or the rectum may be required in order to achieve complete tumour resection. Although the mid-line incision is the incision of choice, in some patients with tumours in the upper retroperitoneum a thoracoabdominal incision is preferable. After the abdomen is opened a careful exploration follows to determine whether the tumour is resectable or not and to find out if there are metastases to the liver or the peritoneal cavity. If the patient has obvious inoperable disease or a

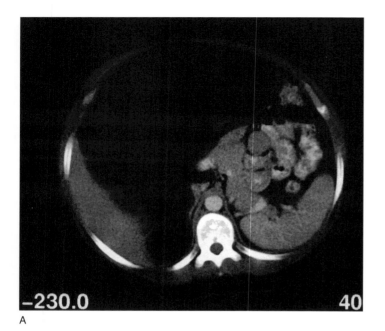

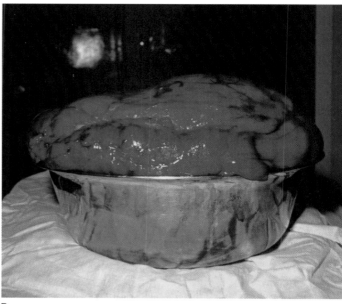

A

B

Figure 14.2 A. CT scan demonstrating a large retroperitoneal soft tissue sarcoma. **B.** Resection specimen from lesion demonstrated on CT scan.

lymphoma is suspected, an incisional biopsy of the tumour should be carried out. If the tumour is resectable, it has to be removed *en bloc* with the surrounding involved organs in order to achieve a complete resection (Figure 14.2B). The most commonly resected organs *en bloc* with the tumour are the kidneys, the adrenal glands, the colon, the pancreas and the spleen, required in 50–80% of the complete resections. The aim for the surgeon is to excise the tumour with adequate margins, taking care not to violate the pseudocapsule. There may be great difficulty in excising these tumours because of the surrounding vital organs and major vascular structures. *En bloc* removal of multiple organs should be avoided when the tumour's margin is the aorta or the vena cava. Debulking surgery is usually not important for the long-term survival of a patient.

The operative mortality is less than 5% and the most common postoperative complications are haemorrhage, bowel ileus and intraabdominal abscess. Resectability rates vary in recent series between 50% and 95% and depend on the relative number of primary versus recurrent sarcomas. The rate of radical resection does not seem to relate to the histological type, grade or tumour size. When the tumour is completely excised the five-year survival rate ranges between 54% and 64%, while in patients with partial resection it ranges between 10% and 35%.

Local recurrences occur in 46–59% of the patients with complete resection either alone or with metastatic disease. The average time for recurrence is 15 months for high-grade tumours and 42 months for low-grade tumours. Local retroperitoneal recurrence is best treated with complete reexcision as this is possible in up to 44% of patients with median survival time of 41 months. The use of radiotherapy together with operative resection may contribute into the reduction of the local tumour recurrence rate after the

operation. Due to the low tolerance of the adjacent vital organs, the patient can receive only a limited dose of external beam irradiation. Radiation is beneficial for local control in doses greater than 6.000 cGy. However, since this dose can cause several complications to the surrounding structures, it is preferably given intraoperatively (IORT). IORT offers several potential advantages over conventional external beam radiation because it delivers a single large radiation dose directly to the tumour and protects the healthy surrounding tissues.

Radiotherapy alone is indicated only in patients with an inoperable disease as a palliative treatment for pain. The use of chemotherapy has not proven to be beneficial for the adjuvant therapy of retroperitoneal sarcomas.

OPERATIVE SURGERY

Splenectomy

Elective splenectomy

Preoperative preparation

In order to give proper preoperative preparation, the nature of the disease for which splenectomy is indicated must be considered carefully. The indications for splenectomy are shown in Box 14.2. The preparation for splenectomy is similar to that of other abdominal operations, with the exception that close consultation with the haematologist is essential, in order to ascertain very thoroughly the patients' haematological findings, clotting parameters and liver enzymes.

Box 14.2 Indications for splenectomy

- Rupture of the spleen   Accidental trauma
       Iatrogenic trauma
       Spontaneous rupture
- Primary hypersplenism   Idiopathic thrombocytopenic purpura
       Hereditary spherocytosis
       Hereditary elliptocytosis
       Autoimmune haemolytic anaemia
       Sickle cell disease
       β-thalassaemia major
- Secondary hypersplenism   Chronic lymphocytic leukaemia
       Chronic granulocytic leukaemia
       Hairy cell leukaemia
       Myelofibrosis
       Felty's syndrome
       Banti's syndrome
- As part of surgical resection   Total gastrectomy
       Distal pancreatectomy
       Conventional splenorenal shunt
- As part of staging laparotomy   Hodgkin's disease
       Other lymphomas
- Diagnostic splenectomy   Splenomegaly of unknown cause
       Pyrexia of unknown origin (PUO)
- Other   Splenic cysts
       Splenic abscess

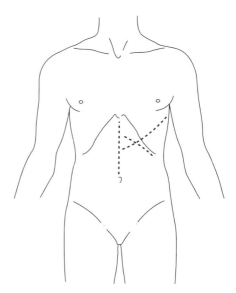

Figure 14.3 Incisions for access for open splenectomy (a mid-line incision must always be used for emergency spenectomy).

Packed red blood cells and platelets, if thrombocytopenia is present, are reserved for the patient in the blood bank. In most cases of idiopathic thrombocytopenic purpura platelet counts are transiently elevated before operation as a result of maximal medical treatment (gamma-globulin, steroid therapy). Two weeks before surgery all patients should receive pneumococcal vaccine.

Anaesthesia and positioning

The patient is positioned supine on the operating table under general endotracheal anaesthesia and muscle relaxation. Care should be taken during intubation to avoid any trauma to the mouth and upper respiratory passages, which may result in haemorrhage in thrombocytopenic patients.

Incision

After administration of prophylactic antibiotics (penicillin or second-generation cephalosporin), access to the peritoneal cavity is gained through a left subcostal incision or upper mid-line in patients with a narrow subcostal angle when the spleen has a normal size or is slightly enlarged. In cases of massive splenomegaly a left thoracoabdominal approach is preferable (Figure 14.3).

Procedure

After the peritoneal cavity is opened, a general exploration of the abdomen follows. This exploration includes a careful search for any adhesions, the presence of lymph node enlargements and tumour infiltration. In patients with haematological disorders the presence of gallstones and accessory spleens should also be excluded. As a general rule it is wise to perform this operation with two assistants. If only one is available then a stationary upper abdominal retractor is helpful.

The spleen is mobilised by dividing its ligamentous attachments. After searching for subdiaphragmatic adhesions, the surgeon uses the left hand to pull up the spleen towards the abdominal incision, so that the lienorenal ligament is well demonstrated. With the right hand the surgeon incises the ligament with scissors or diathermy (Figure 14.4A), allowing the posterior surface of the spleen and the contents of the hilum to be drawn up to the wound. The gastrosplenic ligament is then ligated and divided between artery forceps, taking care not to include the stomach wall in the ligatures. Each individual vessel should be ligated with an absorbable suture (Figure 14.4B). After dividing both ligaments the splenic pedicle can be identified. Individual double ligation of the splenic artery and vein are performed, again with an absorbable suture such as polyglactin, taking care not to damage the tail of the pancreas (Figure 14.4C). Dissection around the splenic artery and vein is best performed by gentle separation of tissues with a right-angled dissector such as a Lahey.

Many surgeons, especially in cases of massive splenomegaly and hypersplenism, ligate the splenic artery at the upper border of the pancreas, before mobilising the spleen. This technique allows the blood to drain from the spleen, thus providing an autotransfusion, which causes the spleen to reduce in size and makes resection easier.

After ligation of the pedicle, the spleen is removed and a careful check for adequate haemostasis is performed.

The abdominal wound is then closed in layers, usually without the use of a drain. If there is oozing or suspected damage to the tail of the pancreas, a closed suction drain can be put in the splenic bed for 24–48 hours.

191

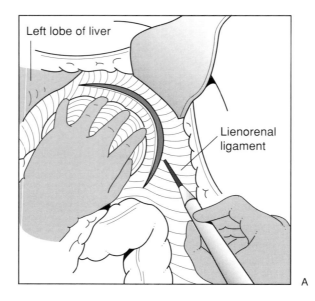

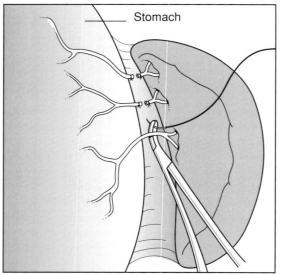

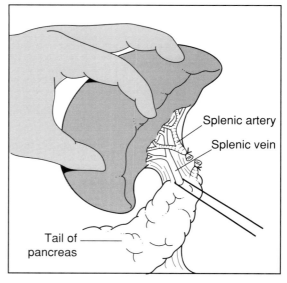

Figure 14.4 Elective splenectomy procedure.

Laparoscopic splenectomy

There are no significant differences regarding the indications for laparoscopic splenectomy and those for open splenectomy. Relative contraindications for laparoscopic splenectomy are a large spleen, prior upper abdominal surgery, splenic injury, a splenic artery aneurysm, splenic abscess, portal hypertension and ascites. An absolute contraindication is an uncorrectable coagulopathy.

The most common indication for laparoscopic splenectomy is idiopathic thrombocytopenic purpura, especially in patients with a normal or slightly enlarged spleen. The preoperative preparation of a patient undergoing laparoscopic splenectomy is similar to that for open splenectomy.

Anaesthesia and positioning

After the introduction of general anaesthesia the patient is positioned supine on the operating table. Many surgeons prefer the patient in anti-Trendelenburg (head up) position and rotated 25–30° to the right, with a bean bag used to elevate the left flank. The omentum and the colon thus fall away from the spleen, with the help of gravity.

Procedure

- A 10 mm port is inserted halfway between the umbilicus and the xiphoid process, using an open method of laparoscopy.

- The abdominal cavity is then insufflated with CO_2 and a 30° laparoscope is inserted, taking care not to damage an enlarged spleen.

- A 12 mm port is then inserted in the left iliac fossa with two further 5 mm ports, one in the anterior axillary line below the costal margin and the other in the mid-line just below the level of the xiphistenum (Figure 14.5).

- After all trocars are inserted under direct vision, the abdomen is inspected for accessory spleens and adhesions. Omental adhesions to the spleen are divided and the splenic flexure of the colon is taken down.

- The short gastric vessels are ligated, usually between clips, and then divided and the splenic hilum is identified. The tail of the pancreas is then identified and the splenic artery and vein ligated and divided using an endoscopic vascular stapler introduced through the 12 mm port in the left iliac fossa.

- The table is then tilted further, placing the patient in the lateral decubitus position and allowing the spleen to fall anteriorly. After the lateral peritoneal attachments are divided, a strong plastic bag is introduced into the peritoneal cavity. The spleen is then placed into the bag and morcellated. If an intact specimen is required for pathology enlargement of the left ilial fossa port site is required. Care must be taken to avoid tearing the bag with subsequent spillage into the peritoneal cavity and the development of splenosis.

- After the removal of the bag and a check for adequate haemostasis, the fascial and skin incisions are closed.

The overall morbidity of laparoscopic splenectomy is minimal in experienced hands, with 10% of patients developing perioperative complications. The major complications of laparoscopic splenectomy are intraoperative or postoperative haemorrhage and pancreatitis. Conversion to open splenectomy due to an excessive haemorrhage occurs in 10–20% of patients. Gastrointestinal and respiratory complications that are common in open splenectomy are infrequent in laparoscopic splenectomy patients. Most authors agree that the operative time, which may be significantly longer in laparoscopic than in open splenectomy, can be reduced by 50% with increased operating experience. Hospitalisation is significantly longer after open than after laparoscopic splenectomy.

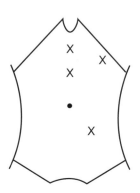

Figure 14.5 Port sites for patients undergoing laparoscopic splenectomy (specimen is usually retrieved through left iliac fossa port site).

Many studies have been published comparing the use of laparoscopic and open splenectomy in the treatment of haematological diseases. In general, laparoscopic splenectomy is superior to open splenectomy in terms of postoperative pain, parenteral analgesic use, length of hospitalisation and recovery time, whereas open splenectomy requires shorter operating times and has lower costs.

Emergency splenectomy

The principles of operation are the same as those in the elective method. Here, however, the additional problems are the initial control of the haemorrhage, splenic conservation when possible and the identification of co-existing abdominal injuries.

The incision of choice is a mid-line incision, which can be extended rapidly if other abdominal injuries are discovered.

The first aim of the surgeon, when the abdomen is opened, is the control of bleeding. After removal of blood and clots from the left hypochondrium by scooping, mopping and suction, the surgeon confirms that the source of the bleeding is the spleen. If the patient is bleeding heavily, the surgeon can compress the vascular pedicle between thumb and finger to control bleeding. At the same time the anaesthetist corrects the hypovolaemia. If compression of the pedicle has to be prolonged, non-crushing intestinal clamps can be used.

When the patient's situation is stabilised and the surgeon estimates that the damage to the spleen is so extensive that no form of conservation is possible, a splenectomy is carried out in a manner as near as possible to that described for elective splenectomy. The surgeon must avoid applying forceps in a blind fashion and mass ligature of structures in the splenic hilum to avoid damaging the tail of the pancreas and the wall of the stomach.

After other abdominal injuries are excluded and haemostasis is secured by diathermy or ligation sutures, the abdominal wall is closed in a usual manner. A low-pressure closed suction drain should be placed in the left hypochondrium if an injury to the tail of the pancreas is suspected.

Splenic conservation

During the past two decades, the role of the spleen in immune function has been studied extensively and having taken into consideration the relatively low incidence but highly fatal syndrome of overwhelming postsplenectomy sepsis, surgeons adopted a more conservative approach to the management of splenic injuries. Various techniques have been described for splenic conservation.

Haemostatic agents

Various topical applications, combined with digital pressure, are usually sufficient for small superficial tears of the splenic capsule without parenchymal damage.

- Fibrin glue is the most suitable haemostatic agent for splenic tears. Fibrin sealing is based on the conversion of fibrinogen to fibrin, creating a reaction similar to that of the last stage of blood clotting. Fibrin glue is sprayed on the injury or injected into or over the fractured area.

- Microfibrillar collagen activates platelets by trapping them. It is known to be hypoallergenic, causes a small amount of tissue reaction and is absorbed between three and six weeks.

- Other haemostatic agents include gelatin foam, cyanoacrylate adhesive, bovine collagen and thrombin. All these agents should be used on a surface temporarily free of blood, otherwise they will not adhere. Following their application pressure should be applied for five minutes.

The major advantage of haemostatic topical applications is that they can be used in combination with all other splenic repair techniques.

Splenic artery ligation

In order to reduce blood loss during massive bleeding, the splenic artery can be ligated at the upper border of the pancreas. Ligation of the splenic artery does not lead to splenic infarction and loss of function, because there is adequate inflow from the short gastric vessels, when these are intact. Haemostatic agents or splenorrhaphy may then be used to stop the residual haemorrhage. After splenic artery ligation careful examination of the spleen should take place, in order to remove any devitalised splenic tissue by sharp dissection, diathermy or blunt finger dissection.

Splenorrhaphy and partial splenectomy

After the abdomen is opened the spleen has to be fully mobilised in order to reveal the extent of the injury. If the tear is in the splenic capsule, as stated previously, it can be easily managed with haemostatic agents and compression for 6–8 minutes.

If there is a deep parenchymal laceration, sutures are required. Because splenic tissue is quite friable, simple suture of the laceration may result in further bleeding. The most effective method therefore is the use of mattress interrupting absorbable sutures, which are inserted gently and tied with caution over Teflon bolsters (pledgets). Alternatively the adjacent omentum can be mobilised on a viable vascular pedicle, in order to fill the cavity created by the laceration. The haemostatic effect can be intensified by topical application of any of the agents already described.

When both extensive hilar and diaphragmatic tears are discovered, haemostasis is gained by splenorrhaphy and use of a compressive mesh. After the spleen is completely mobilised a piece of absorbable mesh is wrapped around it. A window is created in the mesh to accommodate the splenic vessels and its free edges are then approximated with the use of sutures, taking care to produce haemostasis without compromising intraparenchymal

circulation. After compression of the splenic surface for 10 minutes and if no active bleeding is identified, the spleen is returned to the left upper quadrant and the wound is closed in layers.

When the splenic injury is extensive but involves only one pole, a partial resection may be appropriate. The bleeding from an extensive polar injury can be controlled by identifying and isolating the appropriate artery and vein within the hilum, which supplies that region (Figure 14.6). After dividing the gastrosplenic ligament, the surgeon identifies the splenic artery and controls bleeding by applying a bulldog clamp across the artery. The major vessels leading to the injured splenic pole are identified and ligated securely. The damaged section of the pole of the spleen is recognised by a change in its colour and is excised by diathermy or finger dissection. The bulldog clamp on the splenic artery is then released. Any further

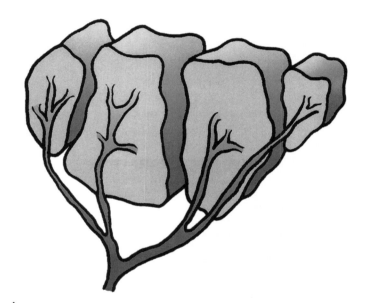

A

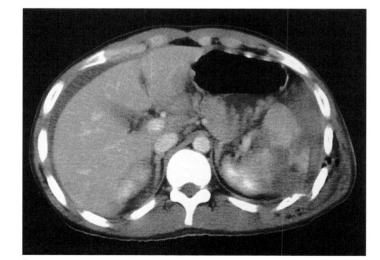

B

Figure 14.6 A. Segmental anatomy of spleen with two polar and two central segments. **B.** CT scan of ruptured spleen with contrast enhancing one segment only.

active bleeding from the cut surface of the spleen is controlled with the use of through-and-through sutures tied over pledgets. Haemostatic agents or viable omentum can also be applied to achieve better haemostatic result to the surface. An alternative solution to partial splenectomy is the use of stapling techniques. The use of a TA 55 stapler during a resection is simple and reduces the operating time and the blood transfusion necessary.

Splenic autotransplantation

When no kind of splenic preservation is possible and splenectomy is inevitable, splenic autotransplantation may be performed, as a potential way to preserve some of the immune functions of the spleen. Four to five fragments of the spleen ($40 \times 40 \times 3$ mm) can be implanted in the abdominal wall or enclosed within a greater omental pouch. These implants will develop a blood supply. However, their immunological function and efficacy in preventing postsplenectomy infections remain to be answered. This technique should be considered especially in children, when splenectomy is inevitable.

Complications of splenectomy

- The most common complication of splenectomy is atelectasis of the left lower lobe, especially in patients with rib fractures. Therefore all the patients should receive physiotherapy soon after the operation.

- Serous effusion in the left hypochondrium usually revolves spontaneously.

- Subphrenic abscess occurs in 3–13% of patients, with a higher incidence in those series where a drain was used. The patient develops pyrexia and complains of left shoulder pain. A CT scan may reveal downward displacement of the stomach from the diaphragm. If the symptoms do not resolve, a CT-guided drainage should be performed.

- Postoperative bleeding may occur after either splenectomy or splenic repair techniques. Reoperation for haemorrhage is rare, occurring in approximately 2% of splenic trauma patients, and is more frequent after splenorrhaphy than splenectomy.

- Damage of the gastric wall and the tail of the pancreas can cause fistula and pancreatitis respectively, which are usually treated conservatively. Although the risk of an acute gastric dilatation is quite small, postoperative nasogastric suction for 24 hours is a sensible precaution.

- Other complications include pneumonia, wound infection and portal or mesenteric venous thrombosis.

- Thrombocytosis is also common after splenectomy. It occurs 2–10 days after the operation, usually peaking between seven and 12 days. The platelet count often increases to between $600\,000$ and $1\,000\,000/cm^3$, particularly in patients with myeloid metaplasia. Although this factor has been implicated in the greater incidence of thromboembolic disease, many series have failed to prove any correlation between these complications and the platelet count. The platelet count usually returns to normal levels within 12 weeks. Although it is controversial, the administration of antiplatelet agents (aspirin, dipyridamole) is recommended in patients with platelet counts exceeding $800\,000$ to $1\,000\,000/cm^3$.

As discussed above, overwhelming postsplenectomy infection is an important late complication of splenectomy.

FURTHER READING

Brady MS, Gaynor JJ, Brennan MF. Radiation associated sarcoma of bone and soft tissue. *Arch Surg* 1992; **127**:1379

Bridgen ML, Pattullo AL. Prevention and management of overwhelming postsplenectomy infection – an update. *Crit Care Med* 1999; **27**:4

Brunt I, Langer G, Quasebarth MA et al. Comparative analysis of laparoscopic versus open splenectomy. *Am J Surg* 1996; **172**:596

Casson AG, Putnam JB, Natarajan G et al. Five year survival after pulmonary metastasectomy for adult soft tissue sarcoma. *Cancer* 1992; **69**:662

Cullingford GL, Watkins DN, Watts ADJ, Mallon DF. Severe postsplenectomy infection. *Br J Surg* 1991; **78**:716–721

Feliciano DV, Spjut-Patrinely V, Buch JM et al. Splenorrhaphy: the alternative. *Ann Surg* 1990; **211**:569–582

Heslin MJ, Lewis JJ, Nadler E et al. Prognostic factors associated with long term survival for retroperitoneal sarcoma: implications for management. *J Clin Oncol* 1997; **15**(8):2832–2839

Li FP, Fraumeni JF Jr. Soft tissue sarcomas, breast cancer and other neoplasms: a familial syndrome? *Ann Intern Med* 1969; **71**:747

Malerba M, Doglieto GB, Pacelli F et al. Primary retroperitoneal soft tissue sarcomas: results of aggressive surgical treatment. *World J Surg* 1999; **23**(7):670–675

Uranus S, Mischinger HT, Pfeifer J et al. Haemostatic methods for the management of spleen and liver injuries. *World J Surg* 1996; **20**:1107–1112

Watson D, Coventry B, Chin T et al. Laparoscopic versus open splenectomy for immune thrombocytopenic purpura. *Surgery* 1997; **121**:18

Weber T, Hamsch E, Baum RP et al. Late results of heterotopic autotransplantation of splenic tissue into the greater omentum. *World J Surg* 1998; **22**:883–889

Section 2

Lower gastrointestinal surgery

Large bowel obstruction

Janos Nagy, Michael H. Lyall

15

LARGE BOWEL OBSTRUCTION

Large bowel obstruction accounts for 15% of all cases of intestinal obstruction. It is most commonly seen in the sigmoid colon and complete obstruction of the colon is most often caused by carcinoma. In adults, carcinoma of the colon accounts for 65% of all cases. The remaining 35% of cases are due to diverticular disease (20%), volvulus (5%) and miscellaneous conditions (10%) which include stricture, acute colonic pseudoobstruction, hernia, adhesions, and faecal impaction (Table 15.1).

Table 15.1 Causes of acute large bowel obstruction

Cause	Percentage
Primary colorectal cancer	65
Diverticular disease	20
Volvulus	5
Other causes:	10
• extrinsic obstruction from metastatic carcinoma	
• hernia	
• faecal impaction	
• pseudoobstruction	
• adhesions	
• stricture	
• undetermined	

Pathophysiology

Intestinal obstruction results in progressive distension of proximal bowel with fluid and gas. Intestinal secretions that are normally absorbed in unobstructed intestines become sequestered in the obstructed intestine so that dehydration occurs. Lesions which obstruct at the ileocaecal valve behave as small bowel obstruction. In 10–20% of patients the ileocaecal valve is incompetent and colonic pressure is relieved by reflux into the small bowel. In these instances the small bowel distends and large volumes of fluid and electrolytes are lost through faeculent vomiting. In 80% of patients, the ileocaecal valve is competent and a closed-loop obstruction occurs. Because the small bowel continues to empty, the colon progressively distends. At high luminal pressures circulation is impaired and gangrene occurs.

The caecum is particularly susceptible to perforation due to its thinner wall, greater luminal capacity and hence greatest wall tension (law of Laplace). When caecal diameter reaches 10–12 cm the possibility of rupture may be imminent. Once the capacity of the right colon is exceeded, the serosa between taeniae split, patches of haemorrhage and infarction are seen and punctate mucosal perforations occur. Colonic perforation may also occur at the site of obstruction, particularly when the carcinoma is present. Patients with large bowel obstruction have increased numbers of both aerobic and anaerobic organisms in the intestine. This may be responsible for the increased incidence of septic complications seen postoperatively in these patients.

Clinical findings

Symptoms

Patients with large bowel obstruction generally present with colicky abdominal pain, constipation and abdominal distension. Visceral cramping pain is usually suprapubic in distribution. Lesions at fixed points of colon are often located by position of the organ, e.g. caecum, hepatic or splenic flexures. Severe or continuous pain suggests ischaemia or peritonitis. Complete or incomplete constipation of stool or flatus is the most frequent complaint. A history of progressive alteration of bowel habit over weeks or months suggests the diagnosis of carcinoma whereas a sudden onset of marked abdominal distension suggests volvulus. Vomiting is a late symptom of large bowel obstruction and may not occur if the ileocaecal valve is competent.

Signs

The presence of grossly tympanitic abdominal distension suggests large bowel obstruction. The bowel sounds are often increased. A mass may be detected, suggesting neoplasm, faeces, inflammatory phlegmon or gross caecal dilatation. An abdomen without bowel sounds with minimal tenderness and pain suggests acute colonic pseudoobstruction. Rectal examination may demonstrate mass or impacted faeces. More commonly, the rectum will feel dilated and empty. The presence of blood should alert the clinician to the presence of tumour or ischaemic bowel. Detection of perforation or bowel ischaemia is largely based on clinical findings. Pyrexia, persistent tachycardia despite rehydration or peritoneal tenderness strongly suggest perforation or strangulation and require urgent laparotomy. Other causes of obstruction such as abdominal wall hernias should be excluded.

General management

Treatment of patients with large bowel obstruction involves resuscitation, investigation and definitive management.

Resuscitation

Patients with large bowel obstruction are volume depleted and require rehydration with intravenous crystalloid. Hourly urine volumes should be measured once the patient is catheterised. A central venous line may be necessary where fluid overload is a concern or when hourly urine volumes are inadequate despite adequate initial resuscitation. A complete obstruction may be partially relieved by several enemas whilst the patient is being rehydrated.

Investigations

History and full clinical examination complemented by serum electrolytes and blood count are performed. A marked leucocytosis suggests ischaemia or perforation. Abdominal radiology confirms the clinical diagnosis of large bowel obstruction but may not be accurate in detecting the site or cause. The supine plain abdominal film will demonstrate colonic distension which is identified by its peripheral position and haustral markings that do not cross the colon completely (Figure 15.1). Colonic gas 'cut-off' is often seen at the site of obstruction. Sigmoid and caecal volvulus have characteristic radiological appearances. Massive pneumoperitoneum is

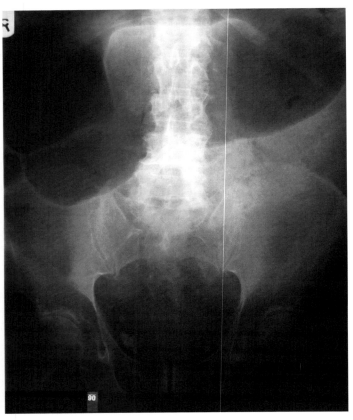

Figure 15.1 Abdominal radiograph showing typical appearance of colonic obstruction.

often due to colonic perforation. There is sufficient evidence to support the routine use of water-soluble contrast enemas in all patients with clinical and radiological signs of large bowel obstruction. A high proportion of these patients have other diagnoses following contrast enema, including acute colonic pseudoobstruction.

Definitive treatment

The principal aim of management is relief of obstruction before perforation occurs (Table 15.2). Secondary objectives include treatment of underlying condition with restoration of bowel continuity. Wherever possible, the minimum number of operations should be performed. Patients with perforation or clinically suspected perforation or ischaemia require urgent laparotomy. For patients without such indications, laparotomy may still be required if they do not improve or if caecal distension increases through the following 12–24 hours of resuscitation. Perioperative antibiotics with good anaerobic and Gram-negative cover, deep venous thrombosis prophylaxis and preoperative stoma marking are required. Specific surgical strategies depend on the site of obstruction, condition of the patient, presence of peritonitis and expertise of the surgeon. The presence of peritonitis, impaired circulation or tension will necessitate a staged approach. Anastomosis between distended ileum and normal colon is usually safe. However, anastomoses between distended colon and normal colon should only be considered in optimal circumstances.

MALIGNANT LARGE BOWEL OBSTRUCTION

This is the most common cause of large bowel obstruction in Europe and North America. It is a disease of the elderly and is most frequently seen in the left colon, particularly the sigmoid colon and splenic flexure. The ascending colon is the next most common site. Obstruction of the rectum is rare. In advanced cases the colon may perforate either through the tumour or secondarily at

Table 15.2 Summary of surgical strategies for acute large bowel obstruction

Causes	Treatments
Colorectal cancer	
Right-sided obstruction	Right hemicolectomy with primary anastomosis★
Transverse colon obstruction	Extended right hemicolectomy with primary anastomosis★
Left-sided obstruction	Hartmann's procedure†‡
Diverticular disease	
Abscess/free perforation	Hartmann's procedure
Fibrous stricture	Intraoperative lavage, resection and primary anastomosis
Colonic volvulus	
Sigmoid	Preoperative decompression followed by resection and primary anastomosis★
Caecal	Right hemicolectomy with primary anastomosis★
Pseudoobstruction	Sigmoidoscopic or colonoscopic decompression. Caecostomy if non-operative treatment fails★

★ Resection with exteriorisation of bowel ends if perforation or gangrene is present
† Intraoperative lavage following resection with primary anastomosis if patient condition is optimal and experienced surgeon present
‡ Proximal stoma if the patient is severely ill or surgical team inexperienced

the caecum. Patients presenting with obstructed carcinomas often have a poorer prognosis compared to non-obstructed disease at a similar stage.

Investigations

History, examination and plain supine abdominal radiology should indicate the presence of large bowel obstruction. When possible, a single contrast enema should be performed to confirm the diagnosis (Figure 15.2).

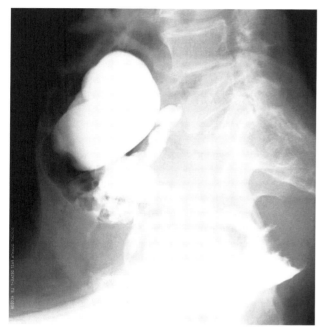

Figure 15.2 Single-contrast enema demonstrating colonic stricture.

Preoperative management

Patients with large bowel obstruction exhibit dehydration and concomitant electrolyte disturbances. These should be corrected with intravenous fluid therapy and monitored by hourly urine output. Central venous pressure assessment is necessary if urine output does not respond quickly. Co-existent medical problems should be optimised. Nasogastric tube and suction may be used to decompress the stomach and small bowel and prevent further air becoming swallowed and trapped. Decompression of the bowel may occur following contrast enema or sigmoidoscopy, allowing more detailed preoperative staging investigations.

General treatment

Several general points can be made that facilitate the operative management of patients with malignant large bowel obstruction. Patients with right-sided lesions should be positioned supine whereas lithotomy or the Lloyd-Davies position is often more

convenient for left-sided lesions. A generous mid-line incision should be made. This is especially important when mobilisation of the splenic flexure is necessary. Decompression of the colon is often essential to facilitate progress in these operations. If the ileo-caecal valve is incompetent, milking bowel content into the stomach via small bowel and out through a large-bore nasogastric tube is possible. When the bowel is very tense, decompression may be achieved through a 16 gauge needle inserted obliquely into antimesenteric taenia of the colon. Having done this, a thorough laparotomy is performed to identify primary tumour, exclude synchronous lesions, stage disease and assess operability. If operable, standard techniques of radical cancer surgery should be employed. In the presence of metastases, resection of primary carcinoma should be considered and gastrointestinal continuity restored whenever possible. Staged procedures should be avoided if possible in patients with limited life expectancy.

Right-sided obstruction

The treatment of choice for right-sided obstructed colon cancers is right hemicolectomy with primary anastomosis. In the Large Bowel Cancer Project, the anastomotic leak rate was 10% in patients with obstruction compared to 6% of patients without obstruction. In patients who are severely ill or with general peritonitis resection with ileostomy and exteriorisation of proximal colon should be considered because an anastomosis may increase the risk of death. In the patient with unresectable locally advanced disease, ileotransverse bypass may be performed.

Anastomotic technique in these cases depends on the surgeon's own preferences and experience. Where there is disparity in diameter of bowel ends, the anastomosis may be facilitated by:

- antimesenteric small bowel cut-back

- end-to-side anastomosis

- functional end-end anastomosis using a linear cutting stapler. However, the use of staplers in oedematous, thickened bowel should be avoided as staples may cut out, with consequent anastomotic failure.

Transverse colon obstruction

Extended right hemicolectomy with ileocolic anastomosis is most frequently performed in this condition. Mobilisation of the splenic flexure will facilitate formation of the anastomosis. Omentectomy should be considered for total disease clearance. However, locally advanced tumours often invade the mesocolon, limiting disease clearance.

Left-sided obstruction

Opinion is still divided on whether initial decompression followed by staged resection or immediate resection with or without anastomosis should be performed in patients with obstructing carcinoma of left colon. Concern over the safety of primary resection and anastomosis has led to three approaches for this condition.

Three-stage procedure

This consists of colostomy (usually loop transverse), resection of tumour at second operation and closure of colostomy at around six weeks. Formation of colostomy, thereby relieving obstruction, is a lesser procedure in often unwell patients. The patient's overall condition may be improved by second operation and the anastomosis is protected by colostomy. Although this method of treatment may be reserved for the frail patient there are several problems with this approach. The loop transverse colostomy may be difficult to manage and 25% of these patients are too unfit for further surgery for their neoplasm. Furthermore, the hospital stay for this treatment ranges between 30 and 55 days which is greater than two- and single-stage procedures.

Two-stage procedure (Hartmann's procedure)

This consists of primary tumour resection and formation of end colostomy followed by reversal of colostomy some months later. Removal of the neoplasm at the first operation may improve overall prognosis. The overall hospital stay ranges from 17 to 30 days which is shorter than the three-stage procedure. The overall mortality of around 10% is similar to around 11% for the three-stage procedure. Anastomosis at time of emergency surgery with its attendant risks is also avoided. However, only 60% of patients proceed to closure of colostomy. Reversal of colostomy may also be technically difficult. Dense adhesions may be present and the rectal stump may be difficult to identify or mobilise. Reversal of colostomy following surgery for obstruction should be deferred until six months after primary operation as anastomotic leak rates decrease after this time period has relapsed.

Single-stage procedure

This consists of resection of tumour with primary bowel anastomosis. Two procedures may be performed: segmental resection and subtotal colectomy with ileosigmoid or ileorectal anastomosis. Operative mortality and hospital stay associated with these procedures are similar, at around 10%. The SCOTIA Study Group conducted a prospective randomised clinical trial comparing subtotal colectomy with segmental resection in patients with malignant large bowel obstruction. The mortality and complication rates did not differ between these two groups but patients with subtotal colectomy experienced significantly higher number of bowel movements at four months. Therefore subtotal colectomy should be reserved for cases where the tumour is at the splenic flexure, synchronous lesions are detected or when the caecum has perforated secondary to left-sided obstruction.

When performing segmental resection, the colon should be washed out with on-table irrigation. This process may be facilitated if both flexures are mobilised. The resection should be performed first and the whole colon emptied into a suitable sterile bag. The colon is then attached to suitable effluent-collecting equipment and 2–3 litres warm saline irrigated through a Foley catheter inserted in the caecum. The anastomosis is then completed after the lavage.

In summary, patients with left-sided obstruction should be considered for single-stage procedure whenever possible. This is dependent on the presence of a surgeon experienced in emergency colorectal surgery. Anastomoses should be avoided whenever factors are present that impair wound healing. Patients at risk of anastomotic leakage or who are too unwell for lengthy procedures should undergo Hartmann's procedure or loop colostomy.

Preoperative colonic decompression

The operative mortality for patients with malignant large bowel obstruction remains higher than in elective cancer resections despite advances of intraoperative lavage followed by resection with primary anastomosis. In view of this, attention has been focused on decompressing the colon before surgery. This allows the conversion of a patient with obstruction to a more elective situation with all pathophysiological changes of obstruction to reverse. Several techniques have been described, including laser ablation of tumour centre, endoscopic stent insertion, balloon dilatation and transluminal tube decompression. Long-term survival data on patients initially decompressed by these techniques are not available. Furthermore, these techniques may cause tumour fracture or tumour embolisation which theoretically may adversely influence long-term survival.

Palliative treatment

Patients with obstruction secondary to disseminated primary or recurrent colorectal cancer require palliative surgery where possible. Resection is the best treatment for patients with dissemination. Each patient requires individualised evaluation because the best option for high-risk patients with peritoneal carcinomatosis or liver metastases could be enterocolic bypass or proximal diversion ileostomy or colostomy. Patients with abdominal or pelvic recurrence are often not suitable for resection thus internal bypass, so proximal diversion or endoscopic stenting techniques should be considered.

DIVERTICULITIS

This condition usually presents as localised left iliac fossa pain and peritonism. However, degrees of incomplete large bowel obstruction may also be present. Acute diverticulitis with pericolic abscess can cause obstruction by compression and spasm.

Less frequently, complete obstruction may occur due to stricturing of an oedematous segment or at an adherent loop of adjacent small bowel. This condition is often difficult to differentiate from an obstructing colon cancer. Most cases are treated conservatively with bowel rest and intravenous antibiotic therapy. Both aerobic and anaerobic organisms should be targeted and antibiotic combinations such as cefuroxime and metronidazole are effective. It is important to exclude the diagnosis of carcinoma by performing double-contrast barium enema and flexible sigmoidoscopy once the patient has recovered. When conservative measures fail, laparotomy with resection and end colostomy (Hartmann's procedure) is the safest course of management. Pericolic abscess, in patients too unwell for operation, may be drained percutaneously with resection later if the obstruction resolves.

VOLVULUS OF THE COLON

Acute volvulus, an axial twist of the colon around its mesentery, is a surgical emergency accounting for 5% of cases of large bowel obstruction in Europe and North America. It is a more common cause of obstruction in the rest of the world. Sigmoid volvulus accounts for 65% of all cases and caecal volvulus 33%. The presence of an elongated mesentery about which the bowel can rotate is fundamental to the pathogenesis of volvulus. Colonic gangrene, which increases mortality three- to fourfold, should not be allowed to evolve.

Sigmoid volvulus

In this condition the sigmoid colon rotates either clockwise or anticlockwise through 180–720° to produce a volvulus. This condition is often associated with mental illness, Hirschsprung's disease and non-specific motility disorders of the colon. The patient presents with abdominal pain, bloating and constipation. Peritonism, tachycardia and hypotension when present suggest colonic ischaemia. A history of previous attacks may be evident in around 50% of patients. Plain supine abdominal radiology often demonstrates the characteristic massive sigmoid loop distension with an inverted U appearance from pelvis to right upper quadrant (Figure 15.3).

Many patients with sigmoid volvulus can be managed by non-operative decompression followed by elective surgery. A nasogastric tube should be inserted to decompress the stomach and small bowel. These patients are often dehydrated with electrolyte disturbance, requiring careful intravenous fluid therapy.

Non-operative management

In the absence of signs suggesting colonic ischaemia, sigmoidoscopic decompression is the treatment of choice for sigmoid volvulus. A soft, well-lubricated catheter is pushed through the

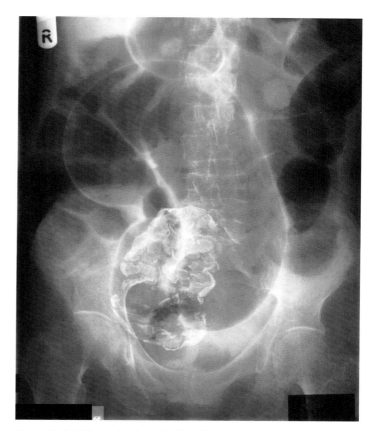

Figure 15.3 Abdominal radiograph of large bowel obstruction caused by sigmoid volvulus.

twist via a rigid sigmoidoscope. The colon will usually derotate at this point. The catheter should be left *in situ* for 24–72 hours to prevent early recurrence. Decompression can also be performed using a colonoscope. The dangers of this procedure are decompressing gangrenous colon and perforation. Presence of blood-stained bowel content or development of abdominal signs should alert the clinician. Recurrence of sigmoid volvulus after decompression is reported in up to 90% of cases and carries a significant mortality. Definitive treatment should be considered during the same hospital admission in patients sufficiently fit for surgery.

Operative management

Emergency

Failure of non-operative treatment or the development of abdominal signs requires urgent laparotomy once the patient is adequately resuscitated. If the colon is gangrenous, then Hartmann's procedure with end colostomy and closure of rectal stump is recommended. Resection of the sigmoid with primary anastomosis has been described. However, this should only be considered in systemically well patients without peritoneal contamination in the presence of an experienced surgeon.

Elective resection

Many patients may experience recurrent volvulus following non-operative management. If the patient is sufficiently fit, elective surgery to prevent further volvulus should be recommended. The most widely accepted procedure is sigmoid colectomy with primary anastomosis following full bowel preparation. This operation is associated with an operative mortality of 2–3%.

Volvulus of the transverse colon

Volvulus of the transverse colon is uncommon and often mistaken for sigmoid volvulus. It is associated with pregnancy, chronic constipation, distal colonic obstruction and previous gastric surgery. The diagnosis is usually made at the time of laparotomy where the transverse colon is untwisted. Evidence of distal colonic obstruction should be excluded. Transverse or extended right hemicolectomy should be performed. Primary anastomosis is not recommended if the bowel is gangrenous or where there is peritoneal contamination.

Caecal volvulus

Caecal volvulus usually takes place in a clockwise direction around the ileocolic vessels. It will involve the ascending colon and ileum so that the caecum will lie above and to the left of its original position. Incomplete mid-gut rotation with excessive length of mesentery may be responsible for this condition. It is often associated with pregnancy, adhesions and distal colonic obstruction. The patient presents with colicky abdominal pain and vomiting. Some patients may describe recurring symptoms. The abdomen is distended. Plain supine abdominal radiology may demonstrate a comma-shaped distended caecum in mid abdomen or left upper quadrant with concavity to the right iliac fossa. Otherwise radiological features of proximal large bowel obstruction are seen, requiring single-contrast enema to make the diagnosis.

Most patients require laparotomy after resuscitation. If the right colon is gangrenous then right hemicolectomy should be performed. There is increased mortality in patients with caecal volvulus associated with gangrene. Unless conditions are optimal, exteriorisation of bowel ends should be performed instead of primary anastomosis. A number of surgical options are available in patients where the caecum is viable after derotation. However, recurrence is frequent when no further action is taken. Right hemicolectomy with primary anastomosis should be considered in patients that are fit for this procedure. In less well patients, a combination of caecopexy and caecostomy may be considered.

ACUTE COLONIC PSEUDOOBSTRUCTION

This term describes a severe form of ileus with massive colonic distension in the absence of an obstructing lesion. Plain abdominal radiography demonstrates a 'cut-off' in gas pattern in 80% of cases. However, no mechanical cause for obstruction is demonstrated on contrast radiology. It is associated with patients having pelvic surgery, trauma, cardiorespiratory disease and puerperium. The risk of perforation is high and the colon should be decompressed. Furthermore, a high mortality is attached to this condition as many of these patients are often elderly or medically unwell. The aetiology of this disease is unclear but may involve an imbalance between sympathetic and parasympathetic activity. Pelvic trauma may interfere with the stimulatory parasympathetic nerve supply of colon. Any condition which results in increased inhibitory sympathetic drive may also influence this condition. Serum electrolyte concentrations are often abnormal.

Clinically the patient presents as large bowel obstruction. The plain supine abdominal radiograph often demonstrates a 'cut-off' at the splenic, rectosigmoid or, less frequently, at the hepatic flexure. The caecal diameter should be noted; distension exceeding 12 cm is associated with perforation. Wherever possible, water-soluble contrast enema should be performed to exclude mechanical obstruction.

Non-operative treatment

These patients are often dehydrated with electrolyte disturbances. Intravenous fluids and hourly urine measurements should be commenced. A nasogastric tube should be passed to prevent further air entering the intestines. Stimulant enemas may be helpful in early cases and the diagnosis should be confirmed by single-contrast enema. Medications such as opiates that reduce peristaltic activity should be limited or withdrawn. The condition resolves in many patients but may take a week to fully recover. Serial clinical and plain abdominal radiographs are necessary to monitor progress. Caecal diameter of 12 cm or more necessitates active intervention. Acute colonic pseudoobstruction has been treated pharmacologically using the combination of guanethidine (adrenergic blocker) and neostigmine (parasympathomimetic). However, further evaluation of this treatment is necessary.

Operative management

Colonoscopy

Colonic decompression using a colonoscope is successful in up to 90% of patients with pseudoobstruction. The perforation rate is around 2%. Necrotic patches on colonic mucosa that herald impending perforation may be seen, preempting laparotomy. However, colonoscopic decompression is a difficult procedure requiring a skilled colonoscopist. Furthermore, up to 29% of patients will proceed to recurrence of pseudoobstruction. These patients may be managed by repeated colonoscopic decompression.

Surgical management

In the absence of peritonitis, patients with a distended caecum who fail to be decompressed with colonoscopy should proceed to tube caecostomy. This can be performed through a standard right iliac fossa grid-iron incision. When clinical signs suggest the possibility of caecal perforation, laparotomy and right hemicolectomy should be performed. If the situation is favourable primary anastomosis should be considered, otherwise bowel ends should be exteriorised.

In summary, these patients can be managed conservatively unless caecal diameter reaches 12 cm or peritonism is detected. In these cases colonoscopic decompression should be attempted. If this should fail a caecostomy can be performed. However, should abdominal signs develop or progress, a laparotomy will be necessary.

COLOSTOMY CARE AND COMPLICATIONS

A colostomy is a surgically created opening of the colon onto the body surface. End colostomies are formed by bringing out divided colon through the abdominal wall and anastomosing to skin. Loop colostomies are created from mobile parts of colon (transverse or sigmoid) and are often used to protect anastomoses or to relieve obstruction. They are often temporary and, due to their bulk, difficult to manage.

Colostomy care

Several issues require attention when a patient is subjected to stoma formation. Preoperative siting and psychological preparation are highly desirable but may not be possible in the acute setting. The quantity and type of stomal output change with time after surgery and an appreciation of these is helpful in patient management. An understanding of stomal appliances is also important. A multidisciplinary approach should be applied to stoma planning and care, involving a stoma therapist, surgeon and nursing staff.

Stoma site

The optimum site for any permanent stoma must be defined preoperatively for easy application of appliances. This should apply equally to temporary stomas as well as permanent whenever possible. Patients should be assessed in their daily clothes, lying, sitting and standing positions. The patient must be able to see and reach the stoma. To prevent leakage from the appliance, bony prominences, deep skinfolds, scars and the umbilicus should be avoided.

Psychological preparation

The prospect of a stoma may be difficult for many patients to accept so it is important to offer these patients an opportunity for further discussion and counselling. The acceptance of a stoma is often dependent on the patient's previous experiences: those who feel relatively well with few symptoms experience more problems than those with prolonged debilitating disease. Patients need to be given a clear outline of the proposed surgery and the plan of care. Early referral to a stoma therapist who can provide physical, psychological and social support to both patient and family is desirable.

Postoperative period

Patients with colostomies tend to experience fewer metabolic complications compared to patients with an ileostomy. Approximately 1500 ml of fluid are delivered to the colon daily. The colon will absorb most of this fluid so that stool contains only 200 ml of water. A transverse colostomy begins to function around the third or fourth postoperative day. Descending colon stomas begin to function around the fifth postoperative day. In patients with active bowel sounds failure to function beyond these time periods should alert the clinician to mechanical obstruction or excessive opiate analgesia. When a colostomy first begins to function, the output is liquid and steadily increases in volume. After 10–14 days the consistency of the effluent becomes more solid. Postoperative appliances should be transparent to allow frequent inspection of the stoma. Diet should be unrestricted, the patient being able to recognise specific foods that increase stomal output or flatulence. A programme of self-care can be introduced after a few days under the guidance of a stoma therapist.

Stoma appliances

These must be secure and comfortable. They need to incorporate adhesives that protect the skin, be made of odour-proof plastic films and be available in a range of sizes and capacities. Two types of appliance, either one piece or two piece, are available. The two-piece appliance comprises a base plate that may be left in place for several days onto which a stoma bag is clipped. Some patients are able to dispense with stoma bags by using a colostomy plug, a small foam plug which clips to a flange attached to skin. Once inserted, the plug expands, filling the lumen of the bowel and blocking the passage of faeces for 8–12 hours. This helps to restore a degree of control over bowel function and reduces the sound of passing flatus.

Complications

Early colostomy complications (Table 15.3) include ischaemia and parastomal abscess.

Ischaemia is caused by a compromised mesentery as a result of the abdominal wall defect being too tight and causing compression of the mesenteric vessels. The initial management is conservative. If the stoma functions without retraction or immediate breakdown, observation is all that is necessary. However, if the stoma fails then

Table 15.3 Complications of colostomy

	Complication
Early	Ischaemia
	Parastomal abscess
Late	Prolapse
	Stenosis
	Parastomal hernia
	Obstruction

resiting must be performed. Separation of the colostomy is caused by tension at the mucocutaneous junction. Spontaneous healing may be expected provided the separation is less than half the circumference of the colostomy.

Parastomal abscess is the result of an infected haematoma. This should be drained and loosely packed.

Late colostomy complications include:

● prolapse

● stenosis

● parastomal herniation.

Properly constructed end stomas have a lower incidence of prolapse than do loop stomas. Stomal prolapse is often associated with parastomal hernia. The prolapse may interfere with fixation of the appliance, resulting in leakage. The development of stomal prolapse is insidious rather than sudden, while the prolapsed stoma is prone to injury and ulceration may develop. Patient-related factors include obesity, increased intraabdominal pressure, COAD and abdominal wall weakness.

During the construction of a stoma it is important to bring bowel through the rectus abdominis muscle. Stomas sited outside this muscle have been associated with development of both prolapse and parastomal hernia. An oversized body wall aperture may predispose to prolapse so the aperture should be about 2–2.5 cm in diameter or two finger breadths for most situations. Failure of fixation of bowel mesentery at the level of the internal opening has been suggested as a possible cause for prolapse. Fixation of the colon to the posterior rectus sheath does not prevent prolapse and the sutures used may in fact encourage fistula formation. Patients with minimal or asymptomatic prolapse should be managed expectantly. Surgical options include local parastomal procedures and intraabdominal procedures. If the stoma is temporary, consideration should be given to restoring intestinal continuity. Patients with permanent stomas with significantly symptomatic prolapse require laparotomy and resiting of the stoma. Incarceration of prolapse is often difficult to reduce because of oedema and patient anxiety. In the presence of tissue necrosis, an urgent laparotomy with resection of compromised bowel and resiting of stoma should be performed if there are abdominal signs. Otherwise a parastomal approach can be considered.

Stenosis of a stoma usually occurs at the mucocutaneous junction and is associated with local ischaemia or sepsis. This complication may be corrected by excising a ring of skin and any other scar tissue that may be present.

Parastomal hernias are incisional hernias at the site of an intestinal stoma and develop in 5–10% of colostomies. The majority of instances can be managed conservatively. Surgery, when required, is complex and local procedures often give poor results. A number of factors appear to participate in parastomal hernia formation. Stomas fashioned through rectus abdominis demonstrate a lower incidence of herniation than stomas placed laterally or through an abdominal incision. Extraperitoneal stomas are not associated with a lower incidence of hernia than transperitoneal stomas. A higher rate of hernia in stomas has been observed in patients undergoing emergency surgery. Other factors such as obesity, postoperative wound infection, abdominal distension and radiotherapy are also implicated. The majority of parastomal hernias are true hernias, having a peritoneal sac that protrudes through the enlarged fascial opening. Small bowel and omentum commonly occupy the hernia, although almost any intraperitoneal organ can enter it. Pseudohernias, including subcutaneous prolapse of bowel or weakness of abdominal wall with intact fascial ring, can also occur. Parastomal hernias present as a bulge on straining or standing. Pain at the stoma site is common. There may be symptoms and signs of intestinal obstruction or ischaemia. The diagnosis is usually clinical but CT scan may be diagnostic if clinical signs are equivocal.

The majority of patients with asymptomatic or mildly symptomatic hernias can be managed conservatively. Non-operative management centres on the use of a well-designed colostomy belt that maintains the hernia in a reduced state. Up to 20% of patients with parastomal hernia come to surgery.

● Absolute indications include incarceration, strangulation and intestinal obstruction.

● A history suggesting incarceration or obstruction, pain, difficulty in maintaining stoma seal, concomitant prolapse, stricture or other indication for revision is a relative indication for surgery.

Patients with advanced malignancy or severe co-morbid factors should not be considered for surgery. Operative repair of parastomal hernia includes simple repair with suture or mesh and relocation of the stoma. Local repair of parastomal hernia involves exposing and reducing the hernial sac and repairing the fascial defect with interrupted non-absorbable sutures. The results of this type of surgery are often poor and up to 65% of repairs will fail. Mesh (Marlex or other non-absorbable mesh) repair of parastomal hernias has been described. Mesh can be placed in the extrafascial, preperitoneal or intraperitoneal plane and bowel brought through the centre or beside the mesh. Preoperative antibiotics should be used and the stoma excluded from the operative field. The mesh must be secured to strong fascial tissues. The results of this type of repair are similar to those of relocation. Infection of mesh appears not to be problematic and may be controlled without removal.

Relocation of the stoma is the preferred surgical option of many surgeons. This involves laparotomy, division of adhesions and fashioning of a new stoma. The long-term success rate of this approach appears to be around 70%.

OPERATIVE SURGERY

Reversal of Hartmann's Procedure

Reversal of Hartmann's procedure can be a difficult operation and should only be considered when the patient's general condition is satisfactory. This operation should be deferred for at least three months to allow any sepsis or inflammatory reaction to subside if present at the time of the original procedure. Deferring reversal for a period of six months or greater has been associated with significant reduction in anastomotic leak rates for patients with previously obstructed bowel.

Patient preparation

Fully informed consent regarding this procedure must be obtained. Bowel preparation facilitates the operation and is associated with reduced wound and anastomotic complications. A low-residue diet is commenced 48 hours prior to surgery and the bowel emptied the day before surgery using an osmotic purgative such as Klean-Prep, bearing in mind that the patient will have to evacuate into a colostomy bag. Preoperative washouts of the rectal stump with warm saline should be performed. Preoperative work-up including urea and electrolyte, FBC, grouped and save, chest radiograph and ECG should be obtained. Antibiotic prophylaxis has reduced wound infection rates from 70% to 10% and serious intraabdominal sepsis from 20% to less than 5% in patients undergoing colonic surgery. Antibiotics should be given at the time of induction and repeated if the operation lasts longer than 3–4 hours. There is no advantage to giving more than three postoperative doses. The antibiotic regime should cover both anaerobes and aerobes. All patients should be considered for DVT prophylaxis in the form of compression stockings and subcutaneous heparin (or equivalent).

Anaesthesia and positioning

The patient is placed in the Lloyd-Davies position. Full general anaesthesia is required. An indwelling urinary catheter is passed, abdomen, groin, perineum and thighs are prepped according to the surgeon's preference and the stoma is covered with a Tegaderm/Opsite dressing. Drapes are then applied, allowing access to the anus.

Procedure

Incision

The previous mid-line incision is opened. Great care should be taken not to perforate bowel as adhesions are often present.

Adhesiolysis

A full adhesiolysis may then be performed to allow identification of the rectal stump and colon. The small bowel is then packed away.

Mobilisation of the stoma

Three to four strong stay sutures are spaced evenly around the mucocutaneous junction of the stoma. This is then dissected from the abdominal wall with sharp dissection, taking care not to perforate the bowel. The stoma is then placed in a sterile glove to protect the abdominal wall from faecal contamination during its replacement into the peritoneal cavity.

Mobilisation of the rectal stump

This may be difficult as inflammatory and fibrous reaction may result in fibrous contraction of the rectum. This dissection may be facilitated by passing an obturator from a small sigmoidoscope through the anus. Care should be taken not to injure bladder, ureters and vagina. The rectal stump is then mobilised and two long stay sutures placed at right and left corners.

Mobilisation of the colon

The distal colon is then inspected. Further mobilisation is often necessary in order to bring the colon down into the pelvis without tension. The descending colon is mobilised by division of lateral peritoneal attachment in the left paracolic gutter. This may be performed by scissor or diathermy dissection followed by blunt dissection with swab. The gonadal vessels followed by the left ureter are identified and preserved. A sling may be placed around the ureters for easy identification and added safety. The splenic flexure will almost certainly require mobilisation to provide a suitable length of colon for a tension-free anastomosis. Care should be taken during this mobilisation to prevent tearing of the splenic capsule. Should this occur, haemorrhage should be controlled by packing and inspected at the end of the operation. In most instances, bleeding will have stopped. Otherwise suture repair or even splenectomy will be necessary. Occasionally extra mobilisation may be gained by division of the inferior mesenteric pedicle. In these situations, the distal colon survives through its marginal artery and viability must be confirmed before considering any anastomosis.

The anastomosis

This may be performed by either suture or using a circular stapler.

Sutured anastomosis. One-layer suture technique

The bowel ends to be anastomosed require preparation. The distal colon and rectal stump are divided transversely between crushing bowel clamps using a scalpel. The bowel ends should bleed vigorously, confirming adequate blood supply. This is controlled by careful diathermy and ligation. A single layer of interrupted 3/0 controlled release non-absorbable sutures is positioned on the posterior wall of the bowel ends. A vertical mattress technique produces good suture security and inversion of bowel (Figure 15.4). However, a sero-submucosal suture is equally effective. The suture is placed 6 mm from the cut edge of the bowel, starting from the mucosal aspect of the colon and traverses all layers to the outer surface. The suture is then inserted in a corresponding position through all layers of the rectal wall from outside to in. The suture is then returned from rectum to colon through mucosa only. The needle is removed and the suture ends clipped with artery forceps. Firstly, two vertical

mattress stay sutures are placed at the lateral margins of the bowel ends and separately clipped. This is followed by the posterior layer of interrupted sutures placed 5 mm apart, the artery clips being held by the assistant in order of placement on a 'nappy pin'. The colon is then 'parachuted' down onto the rectal stump. The sutures are then tied in turn (Figure 15.5). The correct tension is achieved by forming a slip-knot with the first two throws and locking this with three conventional throws of the knot. All but stay sutures are cut, the knots being on the mucosal surface. The anterior layer can then be closed using interrupted vertical mattress sutures but this time starting from outside to in with knots on the serosal surface (Figure 15.6). Alternatively, an interrupted sero-submucosal suture can be used to close the anterior layer.

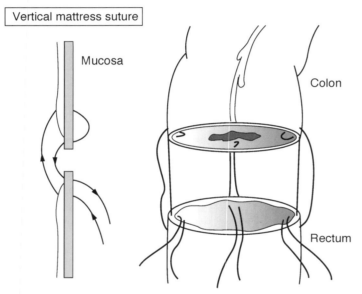

Figure 15.4 Placement of vertical mattress sutures along posterior circumference of bowel wall.

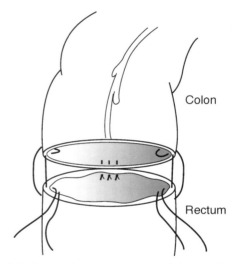

Figure 15.5 Colonic stump 'parachuted' on to rectal stump and sutures tied with knots on mucosa.

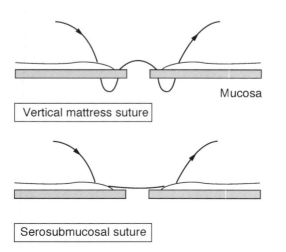

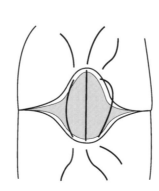

Figure 15.6 Placement of vertical mattress sutures along anterior circumference of bowel wall. A sero-submucosal suture can also be used. Sutures are tied with knots on serosa.

Circular stapling technique

The correct size of circular stapler is assessed by using sounds of various diameters passed into the colonic stump. The widest diameter stapler that comfortably fits the distal colon should be chosen. The anvil of the stapler is obtained by opening the device. An end-end anastomosis is fashioned. First a pursestring suture of 3/0 synthetic monofilament is passed starting from outside to in, spaced at 5 mm intervals close to the seromuscular margin, taking all layers. The pursestring suture is finished with a loop on the mucosa to bring the distal end of the suture on the outside. The anvil of the stapler is then placed in the colon and the pursestring suture tied. The central shaft of the stapler is then closed, the stapler well lubricated and passed per anum by an experienced assistant. The central shaft is then propelled forward through the rectal stump at its centre. The anvil is then connected to the central shaft with care so that the colon is not twisted. The stapler is then closed until the correct gap is indicated. The surgeon should check that no other tissue has been included by the gun. The stapler is then fired and the gap opened according to the manufacturer's instructions. The stapler can then be removed and the anastomosis checked. Two complete 'donuts' must be retrieved from the anvil, otherwise the integrity of the anastomosis is suspect. To check, the pelvis can be filled with warm saline, a soft bowel clamp placed just proximal to the anastomosis and air introduced per rectum. Bubbles may be seen at the site of defect allowing completion of the anastomosis using interrupted sero-submucosal sutures. If the defect is extensive the anastomosis should be repeated by suture technique.

Closure

A sound, tension-free anastomosis with viable bowel ends should be confirmed. The pelvis is washed out with warm saline. Some surgeons will place a silicone drain at the anastomosis. Haemostasis should be confirmed before closure. The stoma site should be repaired first. The fascial defect is repaired using strong interrupted sutures. Skin may be closed if not heavily contaminated; otherwise delayed primary closure should be considered. The abdomen is closed using mass closure technique. The skin is closed.

Postoperative care

The patient is recovered and sent to the ward. Oxygen and intravenous fluids are given as anastomotic healing is dependent on a good supply of oxygenated blood. Two further doses of antibiotics are given and DVT prophylaxis continued. The patient should be allowed to drink clear fluids as desired. Diet may be commenced once the patient's bowel has functioned.

Anastomotic breakdown can happen at any time following surgery. Any unexplained pyrexia, tachycardia, hypotension or abdominal signs should alert the clinician to this. In these instances an emergency single-contrast water-soluble enema should be performed. Where the leak is small and signs localised, conservative management with bowel rest and antibiotics can be instituted. However, any deterioration in clinical condition requires emergency laparotomy. Patients with large leaks, generalised abdominal signs and sepsis should undergo immediate laparotomy and takedown of anastomosis and formation of stoma.

FURTHER READING

Campbell KL, Munro A. Acute conditions of the large intestine. In: *Emergency Surgery and Critical Care*. London: WB Saunders, 1997

Chapman AH, McNamara M, Porter G. The acute contrast enema in suspected large bowel obstruction: value and technique. *Clin Radiol* 1992; **46**:273–278

Keighley MRB, Williams NS. *Surgery of Anus, Rectum and Colon*. London: WB Saunders, 1993

Koruth NM, Koruth A, Matheson NA. Place of contrast enema in the management of large bowel obstruction. *J Roy Coll Surg Edinb* 1985; **30**(4):258–260

Lopez-Kostner F, Hool GR, Lavery IC. Management and causes of acute large-bowel obstruction. *Surg Clin North Am* 1997; **77**(6):1265–1290

MacKeegan JM, Cataldo PA. *Intestinal Stomas. Principles, Techniques and Management*. Missouri: Quality Medical Publishing, 1993

Pearce NW, Scott SD, Karran, SJ. Timing and method of reversal of Hartmann's procedure. *Br J Surg* 1992; **79**:839–841

Phillips RKS, Hittinger R, Fry JS. Malignant large bowel obstruction. *Br J Surg* 1985; **72**:296–302

Stewart J, Finan P, Courtney DF, Brennan TG. Does a water soluble contrast enema assist in the management of acute large bowel obstruction: a prospective study of 117 cases. *Br J Surg* 1984; **71**:799–801

The SCOTIA Study Group. Single-stage treatment for malignant left sided colonic obstruction: a prospective randomised clinical trial comparing subtotal colectomy with segmental resection following intraoperative irrigation. *Br J Surg* 1995; **82**:1622–1627

Crohn's disease

N.J. Mortensen, N.R. Borley

Crohn's disease was originally described by Crohn, Ginzberg and Oppenheimer in 1932 although it had probably been recognised as an entity separate from other chronic inflammatory conditions of the gastrointestinal tract before this.

There is an increasing recognition of the diagnosis of Crohn's disease, probably due to a genuinely increasingly incidence coupled with a greater public awareness and education regarding the disease.

EPIDEMIOLOGY AND AETIOLOGY

The main peak of diagnosis occurs in the period from the late teens to early 30s although symptoms can often be traced for years prior to diagnosis and the time of disease onset is often difficult to ascertain. A diagnosis of Crohn's is rare in childhood, especially under the age of 10, although cases have been reported as young as under one year old.

The annual incidence in the UK is up to 10 per 100 000 although the prevalence is fairly constant at 50–100 per 100 000 of population.

The highest incidence is recorded in Caucasian populations worldwide (although particular ethnic groups such as some Jewish populations may demonstrate regionally exceptional figures).

Mycobacterial infection

Despite original data suggesting an association with the presence of *Mycobacterium paratuberculosis* in the affected bowel, no clear serological, immunocytochemical or polymerase chain reaction evidence exists for the mycobacterial theory of causation.

Viral origins

Following the observation that many cases of Crohn's disease exhibit the presence of granulomatosis vasculitis in the diseased bowel, the possibility of an association with viral infection has been suggested since granulomatous vasculitis is a common finding in measles virus and similar infections. Some evidence exists for the presence of viral inclusion bodies and immuno-histochemically identified viral antigens and RNA in the endothelium of submucosal vessels in Crohn's diseased ileum. This has not, however, been reliably reproduced and the findings may be due to unidentified host proteins mimicking viral antigens.

The role of measles immunisation as a risk factor for subsequently developing Crohn's disease is highly controversial and there is currently no consistent evidence to support this as a cause.

The role of the gut luminal contents

Interest has waxed and waned regarding the role of the contents of the gut lumen. Luminal contents are complex with a wide mix of bacterial products and derived particles as well as whole organisms. There appears to be a definite role for chyme in the exacerbations if not causation of disease. Diversion of the faecal stream from areas of severely affected bowel leads to improvement in both the symptoms and the histological appearance of the disease in a high proportion of patients. Reintroduction is also frequently associated with relapse. The source of this effect appears to be from particles greater than $0.22\,\mu$m in size since their removal from the chyme renders it innocuous again, although what these particles represent is still unclear. It may be that this effect is a secondary phenomenon exacerbating inflammation in already damaged mucosa rather than having a primary role in causation.

Genetic susceptibility

Family history does play a role in determining the susceptibility of individuals to Crohn's disease, with 8–10% of index cases having one family member affected. In monozygotic twins there appears to be up to a 50% risk. Overall, this is equivalent to a 1% risk for a first-degree relative of a sufferer compared to around a 0.01% risk in the general population.

Despite much work which has focused on the human leucocyte antigens (HLA), precisely which HLA genotypes may have associations with susceptibility is unclear although there seems to be a protective role for the DRB1*03 genotype.

Despite initial suspicions, interleukin receptor genes have not been clearly implicated.

Genomic studies from several centres have suggested a susceptibility linkage to the pericentromeric region of chromosome 16 (termed IBD1). What this site may represent is unknown although weaker links have also been demonstrated to a site on chromosome 12 which includes genes for interferon gamma and the vitamin D_3 receptor.

Pathology

Macroscopic features (Figure 16.1)

Generally, Crohn's disease tends to be patchy, demonstrating the classic skip lesions of affected segments interspersed with normal bowel. The disease has a characteristic macroscopic appearance including advancement of the mesenteric fat onto the bowel serosa (fat wrapping), a thickened mesentery and fleshy mesenteric lymph nodes. The bowel itself is often a bluish colour, with fine spiral serosal blood vessels and a grossly thickened wall.

Internally, changes may range from simple aphthous ulceration to longitudinal 'rake' ulceration which is classically found in the line of mesenteric vascular entry on the mesenteric border of the lumen. Confluent ulceration, cobblestoning of the mucosa with a thickened mucosa and submucosa are also common features.

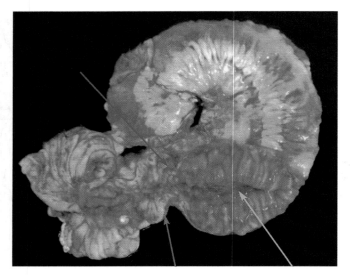

Figure 16.1 Internal macroscopic features of Crohn's disease. Note the longitudinal ulceration in the line of mesenteric vascular entry (green arrow), the wall thickening (red arrow) and patchy ulceration (blue arrow).

Inflammatory masses in the region of the terminal ileum are highly suggestive of Crohn's disease and often contain occult interenteric fistulae.

Microscopic features (Figure 16.2)

Non-caseating granulomata are neither a consistent nor an independently diagnostic finding but are highly characteristic of the disease. Inflammatory changes are usually transmural, particularly in the form of lymphoid aggregates which frequently occur

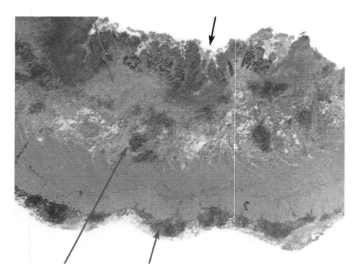

Figure 16.2 Microscopic features of Crohn's disease. Note the mucosal ulceration (black arrow), submucosal fibrosis (red arrow) and transmural inflammation in the form of lymphoid aggregates (blue arrows), including subserosal 'Crohn's rosary' of aggregates.

in the subserosa, giving the classic 'Crohn's rosary' pattern. Perineural chronic inflammation, submucosal fibrosis and neo-muscularisation with the formation of disordered smooth muscle cell bundles are other common findings.

CLINICOPATHOLOGICAL MANIFESTATIONS

Several terms are used in describing the presentation of Crohn's disease although these are broad terms and do not necessarily imply distinct disease forms since different features are often present in the same patient on the same occasion or at different times in the course of their disease.

Perforating/fistulating presentations

Free perforation in Crohn's, fortunately, is rare. It is sometimes the first presentation of the patient with acute abdominal peritonitis (Figure 16.3). Occasionally perforated Crohn's disease may be mistaken for acute appendicitis, with the diagnosis becoming apparent at laparotomy. Often the subtle preceding history is masked by the acute presentation.

Contained perforations are more common. Formation of intra-mesenteric, interenteric, retroperitoneal or paracolic abscesses may occur. These often present with symptoms of occult sepsis, namely weight loss, swinging fever, anaemia, anorexia and abdominal tenderness with or without a palpable mass.

Fistulation may occur either to other segments of gastrointestinal tract or to other organs. Enteroenteric fistulas may present with symptoms of 'blind loop syndrome' due to bacterial overgrowth causing diarrhoea, malabsorption, weight loss and malaise but are often incidental findings during investigation for Crohn's disease and are associated with minimal or no symptoms. The presence of enterovaginal fistulation is usually clear due to passage of faeces or ileal content per vaginam (PV) although flatus PV may be

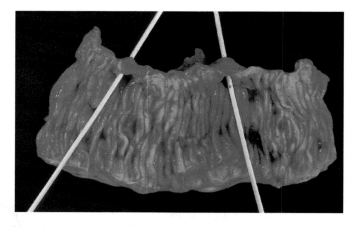

Figure 16.3 Appearances of a perforated specimen of disease. The probes mark sites of free perforation of fistula formation.

the only symptom of a small fistula. Enteroureteric fistulation is rare although enterovesical fistula should be considered in Crohn's patients with recurrent urinary tract infections, ascending urinary sepsis or atypical causative organisms in otherwise 'simple' cystitis.

Enterocutaneous fistulas are often the most distressing for the patient although gross multiple fistulation is fortunately rare.

Fistulation in the context of inflammatory bowel disease is effectively diagnostic of Crohn's disease provided that iatrogenic and malignant causes have been excluded.

Fibrostenosing presentations

Connective tissue changes and thickening in the mucosa and submucosa of affected bowel can lead to areas of stenosis (Figure 16.4). The presence of fixed stenoses in Crohn's disease is characterised by predominantly obstructive symptoms. These are classically: colicky abdominal pain after meals accompanied by abdominal distension, nausea, bloating and borborygmi. Patients may lose weight due to 'food fear' and frequently chronically adapt their diet to counter the symptoms of progressive luminal narrowing. This usually involves the reduction of the daily fibre intake and in exceptional circumstances, patients may become dependent on a 'sloppy' or liquidised diet.

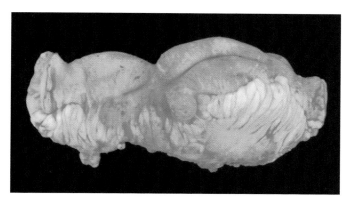

Figure 16.4 Appearances of a stenosed specimen of disease. The stenosed segment is obvious with pronounced associated fat wrapping.

Inflammatory presentations

'Simple' inflammatory presentations can occur. These may take the form of increasing stool frequency associated with anaemia, low-grade fever, anorexia and abdominal tenderness. A mass may be felt although where this is the case, there is a high risk of occult perforating complications and small intramesenteric or interenteric abscesses are often found between the matted loops of bowel at surgery. Occasionally the inflammatory changes present with bleeding per rectum or through an end ileostomy although major haemorrhage is rare. This more often leads to chronic anaemia due to iron deficiency.

In Crohn's colitis, acute toxic dilatation may complicate the disease, as in ulcerative colitis, usually early in the course of the disease but may occur during any acute exacerbation.

Extraintestinal manifestations

Patients with Crohn's disease may suffer from a wide range of non-gastrointestinal manifestations of disease (Figure 16.5). Broadly they can be divided into those in which the severity or activity of, correlates with periods of intestinal disease activity and those which tend to occur independently of the progress of enteric disease.

Eye and skin manifestations can be most symptomatically troublesome for patients. Pyoderma gangrenosum is not common but can be widespread, involving large areas of skin ulceration with secondary bacterial sepsis, extensive destruction and subsequent scarring in severe cases. Treatment is by a combination of the eradication of secondary infection together with topical and systemic steroid administration.

The arthritis of inflammatory bowel disease is characteristically a seronegative, non-deforming arthropathy although ankylosing spondylitis can be particularly troublesome in young men. A destructive small joint polyarthropathy is a rare association.

Sclerosing cholangitis is a highly significant extraintestinal manifestations and may be associated with both a more aggressive disease course and a shortened life expectancy. The presence of portal hypertension resulting from the hepatic cirrhosis may also add to the technical difficulties involved in subsequent surgery.

Aphthous stomatitis is often taken to indicate a diagnosis of Crohn's disease in the context of gastrointestinal disease. However, it is such a common finding in any debilitating condition, of whatever cause, that it is of little use diagnostically and is a relatively poor indicator of disease activity where the diagnosis is established.

DISTRIBUTION

Crohn's disease may affect anywhere in the gastrointestinal tract from mouth to anus (Figure 16.6) but several patterns of distribution are well recognised.

Ileocaecal

Ileocaecal disease is by far the most common with 80% of patients having disease present within two feet of the ileocaecal valve at presentation. In addition to symptoms due to the disease complications, the loss of functioning terminal ileum either due to disease or subsequent surgery may cause steatorrhoea, vitamin B_{12} deficiency and an increased risk of gallstone formation. The macrocytic anaemia of B_{12} deficiency may take two or more years

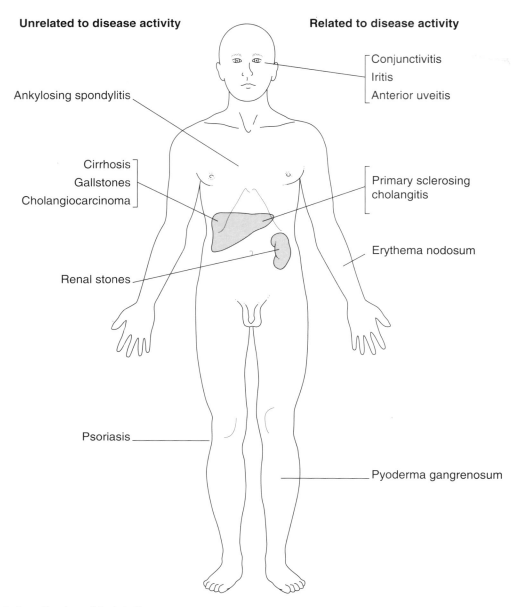

Unrelated to disease activity

Ankylosing spondylitis

Cirrhosis ⎤
Gallstones ⎬
Cholangiocarcinoma ⎦

Renal stones

Psoriasis

Related to disease activity

Conjunctivitis ⎤
Iritis ⎬
Anterior uveitis ⎦

Primary sclerosing
cholangitis

Erythema nodosum

Pyoderma gangrenosum

Figure 16.5 Extraintestinal manifestations of Crohn's disease.

to manifest due to high hepatic stores of the vitamin but can easily be treated by regular supplement injections.

Ileal

Ileal disease is the next most common pattern of involvement. The small bowel may be affected in an isolated segment or there may be many skip lesions involving a large proportion of the small intestine. Depending on the clinicopathological manifestations of the disease, this may pose significant problems for the surgeon. Repeated or extensive resections may render the patient susceptible to short bowel syndrome and in this pattern of disease conservative surgery is even more important than ever. Where

the small bowel is multiply stenosed, preservation of length may be possible using multiple strictureplasties (see below). Exclusion of large lengths of ileum due to ileo-ileal fistulas may give rise to severe symptoms of 'blind loop syndrome' (see above).

Colonic

Crohn's colitis may involve the colon alone or in conjunction with ileal or other sites of disease. The large bowel may be affected by either a segmental disease distribution or a pancolitis. Symptomatic strictures are somewhat less common in the colon than the small bowel although this may simply reflect the larger initial luminal diameter of the colon rather than intrinsic

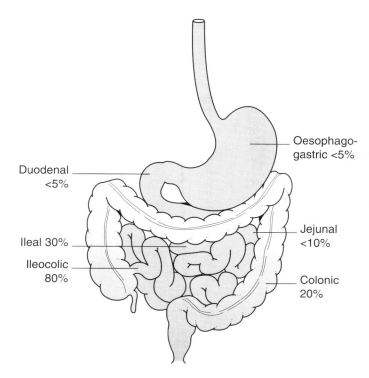

Figure 16.6 Distribution of disease. The figures relate to the percentage of sufferers who manifest with disease at that site.

differences in patterns of disease between the two sites. In cases of extensive colitis, the differential diagnosis with ulcerative colitis may become difficult although the presence of rectal sparing with anal involvement is particularly suggestive of Crohn's disease.

Other sites

Anal

The anus in Crohn's disease is worthy of particular consideration (see below). It may be a primary site of disease or affected by changes secondary to more proximal colonic disease. Occasionally the anus is the site of first diagnosis of the disease.

Jejunal

Diffuse jejunoileal disease is not common but may manifest as panenteric involvement causing problems of malabsorption and severe systemic upset. It is particularly difficult to treat surgically due to its extensive nature.

Duodenal

The duodenum is a primary site in less than 5% of cases. Crohn's duodenitis may occasionally present with fistulas, e.g. duodeno-colic. Duodenal stricturing which may result is somewhat more difficult to treat than ileal strictures. Strictureplasty has been used

although with somewhat variable results and gastrointestinal bypass may worsen the symptoms of gastrointestinal hurry or malabsorption due to small bowel disease.

Oesophagogastric

Interestingly, most patients with an established diagnosis of Crohn's disease have microscopic evidence of chronic features of disease on gastric biopsy although this is an uncommon site for isolated disease. Oesophageal Crohn's may be particularly troublesome due to dysphagia during acute exacerbations, necessitating gastrostomy or jejunostomy feeding.

DIAGNOSIS AND ASSESSMENT

The diagnosis of Crohn's disease is usually made on the basis of a combination of clinical, radiological and histopathological findings. Differentiation from other chronic intestinal inflammations is usually straightforward in the small bowel but it is occasionally difficult, particularly in the situation of widespread colonic disease where the differentiation from ulcerative colitis may only be ascertained with the evolution of the disease over time (see below).

Clinical features

Despite the manifold presentations of Crohn's disease, several clinical entities strongly suggest it.

- Multiple sites of intestinal involvement with apparently uninvolved segments between

- Anal involvement with rectal sparing in the absence of prior topical steroid treatment

- Skip lesions in colonic disease

- Multiple enteric fistulas in the absence of infective causes

Scoring systems

Many systems have been developed to 'score' or evaluate Crohn's disease. The fact that there are such a number indicates that none is ideal. It is important to remember that most systems have been derived as tools to observe the progress of individual patients at serial clinical visits. They are not primarily designed to allow direct comparisons between patients since many of the numerical values are obtained subjectively. Neither should the scores be interpreted as absolute measures of 'disease activity' since different patterns of disease manifest with different symptoms and most tend to underestimate the severity of symptoms due to obstructive complications (Table 16.1). One major role for these 'indices' of disease is in clinical trials and research to allow common, reproducible definitions of 'relapse' and 'disease activity' to be used in the delineation and analysis of groups of patients.

219

Table 16.1 Elements of the Crohn's Disease Activity Index

Category	Symptom or sign scoring	Basic score multiplying factor
1. No of liquid or very soft stools per day	1 point per stool	×2
2. Abdominal pain each day	0 = none, 1 = mild 2 = moderate, 3 = severe	×5
3. General well-being each day	0 = generally well, 1 = slightly under par 2 = poor, 3 = very poor 4 = terrible	×7

4. Number of associated categories	1 for each of:
	   Arthritis/arthralgia
	   Iritis/uveitis
	   E. nodosum/P gangrenosum/aphthous stomatitis
	   Anal fissue/abscess/fistula
	   Other fistula
	   Fever over 37.8°C during past week
		×20

5. Taking lomotil/opiates for diarrhoea	No = 0 Yes = 1	×30
6. Abdominal mass	0 = none, 2 = questionable, 3 = definite	×10
7. Haematocrit	Males (47-result), females (42-result)	×6
8. Body weight	percentage below standard predicted weight in kg	×1

Histopathology

Although the histopathological features of Crohn's disease may be characteristic, it is uncommon for histopathology alone to be used to diagnose the disease. Care should always be exercised where granulomata are found on biopsy since they may occur in other conditions, including ulcerative colitis. Transmural inflammation does occur in association with other conditions but is a strong pointer to the diagnosis of Crohn's.

There is little evidence that histopathology can be used to subdivide Crohn's disease patients into groups. The presence of both granulomata and perineural chronic inflammation has been suggested as a marker of disease which is more likely to recur although this is not generally accepted.

Radiology

Radiological investigation can be very useful in Crohn's disease both during diagnosis and for assessment of the disease (at both diagnosis and follow-up). Several different studies may be utilised in Crohn's disease.

Small bowel studies

The small bowel may be investigated using a simple barium meal and follow-through or by small bowel enema (enteroclysis). Generally the small bowel enema is preferred since it is performed by intubation of the duodenum/proximal jejunum, allowing the small bowel to be filled with contrast under some pressure. This helps to delineate the extent of disease, may offer characteristic mucosal features highly suggestive of Crohn's disease and

delineates high-grade/fixed stenoses which *may* correlate with clinical symptoms. It is usual to perform a small bowel enema prior to surgery for obstructive symptoms to obtain a picture of disease location and severity. Ulceration, fissuring, cobblestoning and the presence of stenosis are all identifiable radiologically. Fistulas and inflammatory masses may also be demonstrated.

Barium enema

Both single- and double-contrast barium enemas of the colon may be used to demonstrate the extent of disease (Figure 16.7), particularly where a distal stenosis precludes the passage of a flexible endoscope (see below). Suspected colovaginal or colovesical fistulas may not be demonstrated using a barium enema and cystoscopy or MRI may be required.

Fistulography

Direct fistulography is occasionally used in the context of entero-cutaneous or anal fistulas to demonstrate the course and involvement of the tract. It has the disadvantage that it may be uncomfortable for the patient.

Compute tomography (CT) scanning

With advances in hardware and software technology and in particular the advent of high-resolution spiral scanners, CT scanning provides an important tool in the assessment of disease. The presence of inflammatory masses, abscesses and the extent of bowel involvement can all be evaluated using CT. Most patients being considered for surgery for inflammatory masses or

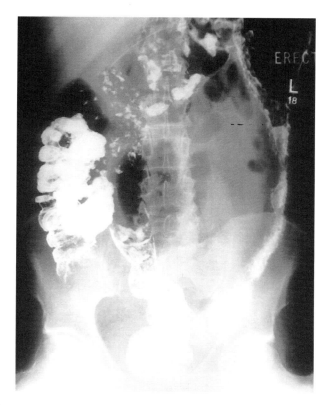

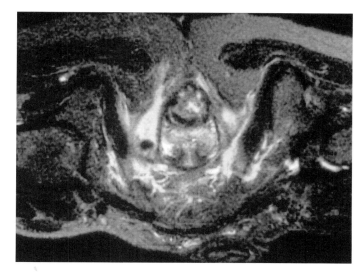

Figure 16.8 Magnetic resonance imaging scan of pelvic sepsis in Crohn's disease. There is extensive high-signal intensity indicating perirectal inflammation with extensive tracking of the sepsis anteriorly.

Figure 16.7 The appearance of Crohn's disease on barium enema. The descending colon is ulcerated, cobblestoned and narrowed.

contained perforating complications should have a CT scan to provide the maximum information about disease location and extent prior to the operation. CT-guided drainage of smaller abscesses is also possible, thus avoiding surgery, at least temporarily, in some patients, particularly the acutely unwell where surgery may be especially hazardous.

Magnetic resonance imaging (MRI) scanning

MRI (Figure 16.8) is most useful in the evaluation of complex perianal disease (see below) but may also be helpful for delineating the tracts in complex abdominal wall fistulas or the extent of pelvic sepsis.

Endoscopy

Flexible endoscopy is mainly used in the context of colonic disease. However, it is also of value where there has been a previous ileocolic resection, since the 'neo' terminal ileum can be visualised. It is an ideal tool for assessment of disease extent and severity as well as for monitoring the progress of the disease and the response to treatment since it can be repeated as often as necessary and allows biopsies to be taken. It is, however, associated with a greater risk of perforation than barium enema although the absolute risk of perforation in Crohn's disease is low

due to the presence of mural thickening. Endoscopy may be better able to identify subtle early changes of disease recurrence than radiological methods.

There is some evidence that the speed of appearance and the nature of the endoscopic features of recurrence present in the early period following resectional surgery can be used to identify groups of patients at higher risk of early symptomatic recurrence. Indeed, several clinical trials have used endoscopic findings as endpoints.

Endoscopy is also the tool of choice in the surveillance of the colon in patients at risk of longer term malignant change in Crohn's colitis.

It is also now recognised that gastric biopsies taken at upper gastrointestinal endoscopy may be abnormal in large numbers of patients with more distal disease although the significance of this is unclear.

MANAGEMENT

Principles

Since Crohn's disease is a life-long, incurable condition, management should be directed towards restoring the patient to acceptable levels of health with the minimum of intervention. This involves physicians, surgeons, stoma therapists, dietitians, nurses, radiologists and many other personnel. The team approach is vital to allow good communication and planning of management strategies. Surgery should generally be reserved for life-threatening complications or situations where reasonable medical therapy has failed.

Medical treatment

The goal of medical therapy is to control episodes of inflammatory complications and the prevention of complications or recurrence of disease where possible.

Corticosteroid therapy

Corticosteroid therapy offers some of the most potent anti-inflammatories available and forms the backbone of acute medical therapy. Steroids reduce many aspects of the cytokine inflammatory network involved in the disease.

In general the principles of steroid use are:

- to employ high doses over the short term to gain control over acute exacerbations of disease

- to rapidly reduce the dose of steroid to avoid the complications of prolonged high-dose regimens (such as immunosuppression with ensuing atypical infections, poor protein biosynthesis and poor wound healing)

- to gradually 'tail off' steroid therapy over a minimum of several weeks to avoid 'rebound' disease activity.

Parenteral hydrocortisone is the most widely used first-line therapy in acute situations although oral prednisolone can be used where the enteral route is available thereafter.

Where the main site of disease is colonic, topical therapy is possible with steroid suppositories and enemas, including newer high-retention foam enemas which penetrate as far as the splenic flexure. Systemic effects may still be significant despite the topical application since high serum levels may result from absorption of the active steroid across the inflamed mucosa.

Generally, the well-known side effects of systemic corticosteroids limit their longer term use and until the development of newer steroids (see below) they have not been extensively used in the longer term control of disease or the prevention of recurrence.

Salicylic acid derivatives

Salicylic acid derivatives possess quite powerful antiinflammatory properties and have been used in the treatment of inflammatory bowel disease for many years. Sulphasalazine was among the first and most used although it has several side effects attributable to the sulphapyridine ring (such as nausea and rash) which led to the development of other compounds possessing the 5-amino salicylic acid (5-ASA) active moiety. These derivatives have very similar antiinflammatory properties but fewer side effects although there is some evidence that sulphasalazine may be more efficacious in colonic disease. Although less toxic than corticosteroids, 5-ASA preparations still possess potentially life-threatening side effects such as bone marrow suppression and patients on long-term treatment need regular monitoring of their full blood count.

One of the main uses of 5-ASA compounds in the semiacute setting is to reduce the dose of steroids required to control the disease (steroid-sparing effect). The addition of 5-ASA preparations may also help in the induction of remission.

Several preparations have been developed which contain pH-sensitive formulations to allow targeted release of the active 5-ASA in the terminal ileum or ascending colon (where the pH is highest), so preventing inactivation of the 5-ASA in the upper gastrointestinal tract.

5-ASA derivatives are also available in enema form for use in colonic disease.

Immunosuppressives

Methotrexate and azathioprine are potent immunosuppressives which are effective in Crohn's disease although their use is limited by both immunosuppressive and bone marrow toxicity side effects. They are most commonly employed as third-line therapy in the treatment of resistant disease exacerbations. Introduction of these drugs may allow patients who are steroid sensitive but steroid dependent to be weaned from steroid treatment. Occasionally they may be used for longer term courses in attempts to reduce the risk of recurrence or relapse but the effect is uncertain and limited due to toxicity.

Immunotherapy

A central role for tumour necrosis factor alpha (TNF-α) in the inflammatory process of Crohn's disease has become well recognised in recent years. The development of commercially available anti-TNF-α antibodies suitable for therapeutic use has made targeted immunotherapy possible. The evidence for the efficacy of the drug is limited but some data suggest that there may be a role in the treatment of active fistulas and severe inflammatory exacerbations although its place in simple disease exacerbations is uncertain.

Antibiotics

Despite the uncertain role of microorganisms in the causation of the disease, some patients do benefit from both antituberculous regimens or treatment with metronidazole. This may be due to an effect on disease activity either through antimicrobial activity or the immunosuppressive activity possessed by both classes of drug. In many cases the reduction in patients' symptoms may also be due to the treatment effect on bacterial overgrowth in diseased segments, especially where symptoms exist in the absence of objective evidence of ongoing inflammation such as raised inflammatory markers.

Nutritional measures

Maintenance of the patient's nutritional status can be a profound problem in any form of Crohn's disease.

There is no evidence that augmenting nutrition in any particular way results in a reduced severity or duration of disease exacerbations but nutrition may be critical to the management of the patient, particularly one coming to surgery. A systematic approach to the nutrition of the Crohn's patient results in the optimal use of expensive and potentially hazardous resources such as parenteral nutrition.

- Enteral nutrition is generally preferable wherever possible since this acts to maintain the normal bile and pancreatic juice flow. It may also promote the normal enteric flora.

- Oral intake may be supplemented using fine-bore nasogastric or nasojejunal feeding overnight. This is useful where the patient's appetite results in inadequate calorific intake or if there is oro-oesophageal disease.

- Percutaneous gastrostomy or jejunostomy feeding may be considered for oro-oesophageal disease.

- Where the patient is grossly malnourished or severe jejunoileal disease (including fistulas) prevents use of the enteric route, peripheral or total parenteral nutrition (TPN) may be necessary. TPN itself may be associated with life-threatening complications (Table 16.2) and its use should be restricted to situations where it is strictly indicated.

Dietary modifications may be necessary due to the effects of the disease, e.g. low-residue diets in the presence of intestinal stenosis. Some patients may exhibit particular intolerance to dairy products but there is no evidence that these are involved in disease activity *per se*. In severe active disease, there is some role for the use of elemental diets but this is generally of limited value.

Table 16.2 Complications related to total parenteral nutrition

	Catheter related	Nutrition related
Early	Pneumothorax★ Arterial injury★ Misplaced catheter★ Major vein thrombosis Catheter-related sepsis	Hyper/hypoglycaemia
Late	Major vein thrombosis Pulmonary emboli Catheter-related sepsis	Hepatic dysfunction Biliary stasis Pancreatic stasis

★ Associated with catheter insertion

Surgery

Principles

Surgical intervention in Crohn's disease has been aptly described as a brief episode in a lifetime of disease. Despite the likelihood that patients will require one or more operations during their lifetime, surgical intervention should be closely directed toward well-defined problems with clear objectives. Eradication of the disease is, of course, not possible and asymptomatic affected segments do not usually require attention.

With respect to technical principles, several guides should be borne in mind.

- Mid-line incisions are usually best. The iliac fossae are best reserved for the formation of stomas which may be needed in future.

- The minimum amount of tissue required to manage the current problem should be dealt with and incidentally noted lesions avoided.

- Localised intraabdominal sepsis should be drained and anastomosis avoided in these circumstances if possible.

- Scrupulous care and gentle handling of tissues are required due to increased friability and risk of bleeding.

- Anastomosis is safe in grossly unaffected bowel.

- There is no clear evidence for the superiority of any particular method or configuration of anastomosis.

- Combined resectional and non-resectional surgery should be utilised where possible.

Indications for surgery

Indications for surgery can be divided broadly according to the time course of presentation and include the following.

Acute/emergency

Truly acute indications for surgery are uncommon.

- Acute haemorrhage

- Free perforation

- Acute colonic dilatation in Crohn's colitis

Subacute

- Inflammatory mass failing to respond to medical therapy

- Symptomatic or complicated fistulas or intraabdominal abscesses

Elective

- Obstructive symptoms with radiological evidence of one or more stenoses

- Chronic disease activity resulting in chronic ill health/malnutrition

- Growth retardation in children

The role of surgery in the chronically symptomatic but stable patient is debatable. There is some evidence that the majority of these patients will ultimately require definitive surgery and that a 'delay' using medical therapy does not offer any advantage in terms of either a reduction in the extent of resection required or an extension in the time period before any subsequent recurrence appears. Since the aim of surgery is to remove or correct the disease causing current symptoms, it can be argued that the patient can be returned to a 'higher level' of health by planned surgery in these circumstances.

Although there is some evidence for an increased risk of colonic carcinoma in chronic Crohn's colitis the role of prophylactic colectomy is less well defined than in ulcerative colitis, although the presence of a neoplasm is obviously an indication for surgery.

Resectional surgery

Regional resection

Most resectional surgery will be in the region of the ileocaecal valve. Ileocaecectomy (or ileocolonic resection) is the most common single resection in Crohn's disease. Short segment ileal resections are also common but care must be taken to preserve ileal length to prevent short bowel syndrome (see below). Segmental colonic resections may be undertaken where the disease is genuinely localised. Upper gastrointestinal Crohn's disease is rarely amenable to resectional surgery due to the difficulty in safely anastomosing macroscopically unaffected bowel.

Total colectomy

Crohn's colitis involving the entire colon may require colectomy. Proctocolectomy with permanent ileostomy is often indicated where there is significant anal involvement. Subtotal colectomy with ileorectal anastomosis may be used in adults where there is clear rectal sparing although there is a risk of both diarrhoea and subsequent Crohn's proctitis requiring further surgery and it should not be undertaken where there is gross perianal involvement. In adolescents, ileorectal anastomosis may be used as a temporising measure to allow the completion of their studies and continued growth, avoiding both a pelvic dissection and an ileostomy. This may provide satisfactory control of symptoms for years although there is a high lifetime risk of requiring some further surgery.

Total colectomy and ileostomy with preservation of the rectal stump may be necessary in the acute setting where a rectal dissection is deemed too hazardous in an ill patient. Proctectomy is often required subsequently for continued proctitis even with the use of topical steroid therapy.

Proctectomy

Proctectomy after total colectomy and ileostomy is undertaken either for continued symptoms (for the convenience of the patient due to persistent rectal discharge), for persistent anal sepsis or due to the long-term risk of malignancy. Proctectomy alone with formation of an end left iliac fossa colostomy is occasionally undertaken for severe perianal disease where the rectum is heavily involved but the colon is relatively spared (see below).

Conservative surgery

It goes without saying that wherever possible, conservative surgery should be used.

Strictureplasty

Where the bowel is involved by chronic fibrosis and stricturing rather than acute inflammatory narrowing, effective widening of the lumen may be achieved by performing a 'strictureplasty'. There is no evidence that the leak rate from strictureplasty is any greater than following anastomosis after resection and there is no greater recurrence rate at these sites. In fact, recurrence has been noted to occur in previously unaffected bowel proximal to the site of strictureplasty. Several principles are important in the undertaking of this procedure.

All clinically significant strictures should be identified and treated. This usually requires preoperative contrast imaging and intraoperative assessment of the degree of luminal narrowing throughout the *whole* small bowel. Palpation by the surgeon may identify areas of major stricturing but it is usual to pass a Foley or similar balloon catheter via an enterotomy to formally assess the minimum luminal diameter of each segment. Strictures failing to pass a balloon of diameter 20 mm or less are likely to be significant and should be marked for treatment after the entire bowel has been assessed. Occasionally intraoperative enteroscopy is used to assess the severity of disease in segments where resection is considered since the external features of disease do not necessarily correspond with the internal findings.

Short strictures (up to around 35 mm) are suitable for a 'Heineke–Mikulicz' type of procedure (Figure 16.9). Longer strictures may be suitable for an extended or 'Finney' type of closure although truly long strictures may best be treated by resection since the majority of the involved segment is likely to be non-functional in absorptive terms and the relative loss of healthy tissue at the margins is less. Groups of strictures closely adjacent may also be resected to avoid serial suture lines in close proximity.

Care should be taken during balloon measurement of the luminal diameter since this can cause significant bleeding from areas of ulceration or inflamed bowel.

Defunctioning stomas

As suggested previously, there is some evidence to indicate that the enteric contents contain factors which are involved in the disease process during exacerbation. Defunctioning affected

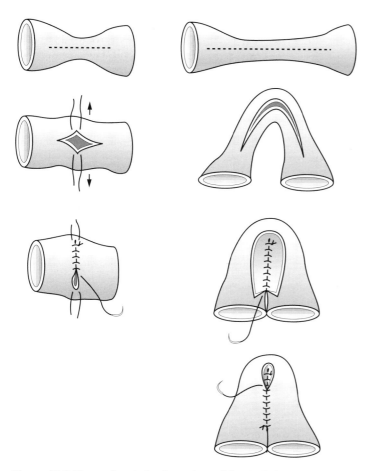

Figure 16.9 Types of surgical strictureplasty. (*left* – 'Mikulicz' type for short strictures; *right* – 'Finney' type for long lesions).

bowel has been shown to reduce the inflammation and may be used particularly in colonic Crohn's disease resistant to medical therapy to avoid the need for colectomy. Unfortunately, the disease activity often recurs promptly once the stoma is closed and the ultimate rate of colectomy may be little altered. It may, however, offer an opportunity to improve the general health of a patient with severe colitis prior to colectomy. 'Split' stomas rather than 'loops' have been used in the past to ensure that the distal bowel is totally defunctioned although the benefit of the separation of the bowel ends is uncertain.

Other interventional procedures

Balloon dilatation

Dilatation of strictures using a fixed pressure balloon has been undertaken with some success. This may be performed per-operatively or occasionally under radiological control. Although the short-term results appear as good as for surgery, it may be that the early 'restenosis' rate is higher for this procedure.

Stenting

Some low colonic or rectal strictures may be suitable for the placement of an expanding wall stent inserted under radiological guidance. This is particularly appropriate for patients unsuitable for general anaesthesia or unwilling to contemplate resection. The rate of stent failure and slippage in the context of Crohn's disease is unknown.

OTHER ISSUES

Cancer complicating Crohn's disease

The evidence for patients with Crohn's disease being at an increased risk of ileal or colonic neoplasia is less clear than for ulcerative colitis. In part, this is due to the difficulty in studying any sizeable population of Crohn's colitis for the necessary length of time as many come to surgery for other complications. As with carcinoma in ulcerative colitis, tumours show a predominance of right-sided lesions and are often diagnosed late due to the symptoms being attributed to disease exacerbations. The role of colonoscopic surveillance in Crohn's colitis is even less clear than in ulcerative colitis. Ileal carcinoma is also a rare complication of ileal disease and is usually associated with proximal chronic active disease. It has a very poor prognosis, partially because of the inherent problems of recognising the diagnosis before the disease is far advanced.

Crohn's disease and the appendix

Crohn's disease may occur in relation to the appendix in several ways.

Terminal ileal Crohn's disease may be diagnosed during appendicectomy for acute right iliac fossa pain. In these circumstances, the disease should be treated as for Crohn's discovered any other way. Resection is not necessarily indicated unless there are local complications which would otherwise require excision of the affected segment.

The diagnosis of Crohn's disease in the appendix may be made by the pathologist after an apparently conventional appendicectomy. This may be due to other granulomatous diseases and not Crohn's. If there is evidence of Crohn's disease in the appendix without involvement of the resection margins (i.e. truly confined to the appendix), the risk of recurrence is much lower than for any other presentation of disease and it tends to run a very benign course.

Acute obstructive appendicitis may occur due to caecal disease. In these circumstances the decision to proceed to a resection rather than simple appendicectomy depends on the severity of the ileo-colic disease although there is some evidence that a high proportion of patients with this presentation will come to surgery in the following year if no resection is performed.

Intestinal failure in Crohn's

Intestinal failure in Crohn's disease is characterised by a combination of problems. In part this is due to:

- failure of salt and water retention leading to diarrhoea

- failure of nutrient absorption with effective calorie and/or protein malnutrition

- micronutrient deficiencies, including selenium, zinc, manganese, copper and hypovitaminoses.

This failure may be due to disease involvement of the small bowel causing hypofunction of the affected segments, surgical resection reducing the overall available absorptive area or a combination of the two. The risk of 'short bowel syndrome' increases with reducing small bowel length but is very uncommon above lengths of 200 cm. Lengths below 100 cm are at high risk of significant symptoms. Strategies for prevention include:

- minimising the use of resectional surgery

- measurement and documentation of the remaining ileum during all laparotomies

- dealing with symptomatic enteroenteric fistulas which are resulting in the functional exclusion of lengths of ileum

- preservation of the ileocaecal valve where possible in proximal disease to preserve the ileal 'brake' on chyme flow.

Ileo-anal pouch formation in patients with Crohn's disease

A diagnosis of Crohn's disease is usually considered a contra-indication to ileo-anal pouch formation. This is true where there is any small bowel involvement. Some success with ileo-anal pouch formation has been reported by some groups for patients with exclusively colonic disease without anal involvement although a proportion of these patients may have had a diagnosis of 'indeterminate colitis – with features of Crohn's disease'. Results are worse than for pouches in which the diagnosis of ulcerative colitis is certain but there may a subset of Crohn's colitis patients in whom the risk of pouch failure is low enough to warrant consideration of restorative surgery in younger, motivated and compliant patients.

Recurrence in Crohn's disease – risk and prevention

Crohn's disease is recognised as a potentially life-long illness but the risk of recurrence quoted to patients depends on the definitions of recurrence used. Definitions exist based on radiological findings, clinical findings or the need for further surgical intervention. Data on recurrence risk are up to 20 years old but most indicate that 75% of patients undergoing surgery for Crohn's disease will suffer a clinical relapse over the following 20–25 years.

Most of these will require some form of surgery. Attempts to define subpopulations at higher risk have been problematic. The evidence that there may be an 'aggressive' and 'indolent' form of the disease is divided. More recently, the suggestion that those presenting with a 'perforating' rather than a 'fibrostenosing' complication have a higher risk of recurrence is also debatable. At present there is no consensus that differing 'phenotypes' of the disease exist or can be recognised clinically.

In recent years oral steroids which have a very high first-pass metabolism in the liver have been developed. Since these compounds remain topically active in the terminal ileum and colon but produce minimal adrenocortical suppression, they offer the potential for long-term therapy which may reduce the long-term recurrence risk without the inherent risks of steroid treatment.

Indeterminate colitis

In situations where inflammation is confined to the colon with no evidence of other intestinal disease, the problem of the differential diagnosis with ulcerative colitis arises. Although there may be clear features of one or other disease present on colonic biopsies, a small proportion of patients may be labelled as having 'indeterminate colitis'. This may be further qualified by the addition of 'suggestive of Crohn's disease' or ' suggestive of ulcerative colitis'. Even after colectomy, the diagnosis may not be certain. This influences the surgical management options, in particular what advice the patient should be given regarding the possibility and risks of reconstructive (pouch) surgery. In difficult cases, the fate of the isolated rectal stump may help to differentiate the two conditions and in other patients close observation over a period of time may reveal other intestinal lesions pointing to a diagnosis of Crohn's disease.

Life expectancy in Crohn's disease

Despite the chronic and often debilitating nature of the disease, there is good data to suggest that the life expectancy of Crohn's patients is little different from the normal population.

PERIANAL CROHN'S DISEASE

Patterns of involvement

Perianal disease in Crohn's disease is usually due to active disease in the anus although occasionally simple perianal sepsis or excoriation occurs in relation to increased stool frequency caused by Crohn's colitis (Figure 16.10).

The initial primary lesion may be ulceration, fissuring and inflammation of the anal canal and perianal skin. Deeper cavitating ulceration may result in destructive involvement of the sphincter complex.

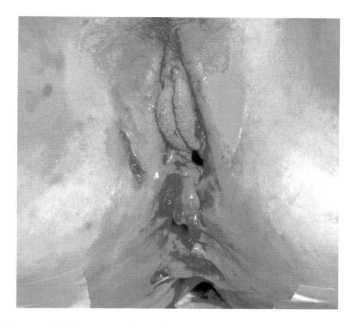

Figure 16.10 Appearance of perianal Crohn's disease. The anus is discoloured with multiple atypical fistulous openings visible.

Secondary phenomena such as abscess formation, fistulation to the rectum, vagina, urethra or bladder may result from uncontrolled sepsis. Large, multiple bluish discoloured skin tags are also secondary lesions caused by the repeated episodes of inflammation and attempts at healing. Severe fistulation is, fortunately, relatively rare in perianal disease but where it is present it can be both life-threatening, due to extensive pelvic sepsis, and disabling for the patient with continued leakage and discharge.

Perianal inflammation may be related to active proximal colonic disease and anal exacerbations may be worsened during episodes of colitis, particularly if the rectum is heavily involved with disease.

Diagnosis and assessment

The overall aim of diagnosis and assessment of the perianal disease is to obtain a clinical and anatomical understanding of the extent of involvement of the anus and surrounding/proximal tissues.

Clinical assessment

This involves a careful documentation of the state of disease as well as a careful evaluation of the severity of the patient's symptoms since treatment is only directed at asymptomatic disease which poses a threat to life or the integrity of the continence mechanism.

Scoring systems

A scoring system similar to those developed for enteric disease exists although it is most useful for serial comparison of the state of the anal disease and for clinical trials.

Histopathology

Biopsies of anal ulceration may confirm the presence of granulomata or other features highly suggestive of active Crohn's disease, particularly when the characteristic skin tags of perianal Crohn's are sampled. However, biopsies may reveal only non-diagnostic inflammatory slough. The absence of features of Crohn's disease in the biopsy should not alter the plan of management. Examination of the biopsies for the presence of atypical infective pathogens such as herpes virus, parasites or other bacterial causes of a deterioration in symptoms is probably as important as the presence of features of disease since these are contraindications to systemic steroid therapy and indicate that the super-added infection should be treated initially.

Endoscopy

Flexible endoscopy is used to evaluate the extent and severity of proximal colonic disease. Severe rectal involvement should be documented as this is a frequent indication for consideration of surgical intervention. Occasionally the proximal openings of complex fistulas can be identified at endoscopy.

Contrast studies

Barium enema

The main role of a barium enema is to evaluate the extent of colonic disease in patients where colonoscopy is either contra-indicated or impossible due to the presence of a rectal stricture. The study may also demonstrate the presence of colorectal fistulation although it is not the investigation of choice for the investigation of perianal fistula.

Fistulogram / sinogram

Fistulas which may be high or complex can be identified and assessed using contrast exams injecting media down the fistula tract although this has effectively been superseded by ultrasound and MR scanning.

Endoanal ultrasound

Endoanal ultrasound (Figure 16.11) has several advantages over fistulography in the assessment of the perineum.

- Fistulas can be identified and tracked with a high degree of accuracy.

- The sensitivity of the technique can be improved with the use of hydrogen peroxide injected into the tract, forming 'echopoor' gas bubbles which can be seen on the scan.

- It offers the ability to visualise the sphincter complex directly.

- It is more comfortable than more invasive techniques.

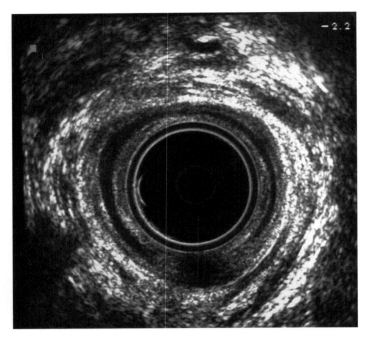

Figure 16.11 Endoanal ultrasound of Crohn's disease.

Magnetic resonance imaging

MR scanning has a high sensitivity for the detection of fistulas and is probably the best investigation for the delineation of the complex or supralevator fistula. It also offers the advantage of being non-invasive. Its main role is in situations where there is complex pelvic sepsis or for suspected fistulas where fistulography or ultrasound has failed to define a track.

Aims of treatment

The basic aims of treatment have remained unchanged for many years.

- Where there is acute sepsis, adequate drainage must be established.
- Chronic sepsis should be controlled and allowed to drain freely.
- Asymptomatic fistulas other than to the urinary tract do not require treatment.
- Tissue should be preserved unless no alternative.

Medical treatment

Control of colonic disease may do much to ameliorate anal symptoms. Topical or systemic therapy should be used where appropriate. Antibiotics such as ciprofloxacin and metronidazole have a role in the treatment of chronic perianal sepsis and metronidazole may act to reduce the disease process itself by its immunosuppressive effect.

More recently, severe perianal disease in combination with rectal involvement has been treated using anti-TNF-α antibody immunotherapy with some success.

Surgical treatment

Setons

Seton sutures remain the mainstays of surgical therapy. They are almost always used for drainage of sepsis and are tied loosely. Their placement may allow an acutely infected and inflamed anus to be controlled sufficiently for medical therapy to be effective. Cutting setons are special setons which are tied tightly and should only be used in very experienced hands since the risk of damage to the continence mechanism is a constant worry in severe perianal disease. In general setons should be used with the following principles in mind.

- Identify and treat all significant tracks.
- Use setons wherever there is doubt about the involvement of the anal sphincter complex.
- Setons may be left for months or even years if symptoms are adequately controlled.

Defunctioning stomas

In the face of severe sepsis, perianal disease with acute active Crohn's proctitis or where seton treatment is failing to control symptoms, formation of a defunctioning colostomy or ileostomy may provide the opportunity to control the perianal disease without recourse to major excisional surgery. Unfortunately, closure of the stoma is often associated with disease relapse.

Fistulotomy

Other than the most superficial of fistulas, generally fistulotomy should only be used by experienced surgeons after thorough investigation of the perianal region. It is useful to have a detailed evaluation of the sphincters by ultrasound or MR scanning prior to surgery.

Advancement flaps

Where there is marked anal disease but the rectal mucosa is uninvolved, a flap or even a sleeve of mucosa can be mobilised on the submucosa or as a full-thickness flap of rectal wall and brought down into the anal canal. This may be used to close off the internal opening of a fistula resistant to seton treatment during fistulectomy (particularly for anterior or anovaginal fistulas). Anorectal advancement flaps may also be used to help recreate the anal mucosa where recurrent sepsis has led to anal stenosis although they should not be used in the presence of acute sepsis due to the high risk of flap breakdown.

Proctectomy

The ultimate control of perianal symptoms is by proctectomy. If there is widespread colonic Crohn's disease then this may form part of a total proctocolectomy. However, proctectomy does have associated problems. Where there is colonic involvement which is not resected, the end colostomy may have a much more fluid output than a standard colostomy, which may pose difficulties.

Failed healing of the perineal wound may also be a problem, particularly where the rectum is severely involved. Sometimes it may be necessary to perform a wide excision of all areas of sepsis and fistulas, leaving the wound open rather than attempting a primary closure. Continued problems from the perineal sinus can usually be controlled conservatively but occasionally a rotational myocutaneous flap from the buttock may be necessary to achieve healing.

Summary

Crohn's disease can be a complex problem diagnostically, requires careful medical management and offers demanding technical challenges to the surgeon. A multidisciplinary team approach is necessary to optimise the management of these patients and the judicious use of surgery is required to offer patients the best chance of a long and 'normal' life.

FURTHER READING

Borley NR, Mortensen NJ, Jewell DP. Preventing postoperative recurrence of Crohn's disease. *Br J Surg* 1997; **84**(11):1493–1502

Crohn BB, Ginzberg L, Oppenheimer GD. Regional ileitis: a pathologic and clinical entity. *JAMA* 1932; **99**:1323–1329

de Dombal FT, Burton I, Goligher JC. Recurrence of Crohn's disease after primary excisional surgery. *Gut* 1971; **12**(7):519–527

Goebell H, Wienbeck M, Schomerus H, Malchow H. Evaluation of the Crohn's Disease Activity Index (CDAI) and the Dutch Index for severity and activity of Crohn's disease. An analysis of the data from the European Cooperative Crohn's Disease Study. *Med Klin* 1990; **85**(10):573–576

Greenstein AJ, Lachman P, Sachar DB et al. Perforating and non-perforating indications for repeated operations in Crohn's disease: evidence for two clinical forms. *Gut* 1988; **29**(5):588–592

Harms HK, Blomer R, Bertele HR, Shmerling DH, Konig M, Spaeth A. A paediatric Crohn's disease activity index (PCDAI). Is it useful? Study Group on Crohn's Disease in Children and Adolescents. *Acta Paediatr* 1994 (Suppl); **83**(395):22–26

Harper PH, Lee EC, Kettlewell MG, Bennett MK, Jewell DP. Role of the faecal stream in the maintenance of Crohn's colitis. *Gut* 1985; **26**(3):279–284

Hughes LE. Clinical classification of perianal Crohn's disease. *Dis Colon Rectum* 1992; **35**(10):928–932

McLeod RS, Wolff BG, Steinhart AH et al. Prophylactic mesalazmine treatment decreases postoperative recurrence of Crohn's disease [see comments]. *Gastroenterology* 1995; **109**(2):404–413

Post S, Herfarth C, Bohm E et al. The impact of disease pattern, surgical management, and individual surgeons on the risk for relaparotomy for recurrent Crohn's disease. *Ann Surg* 1996; **223**(3):253–260

Present DH, Rutgeerts P, Targan S et al. Infliximab for the treatment of fistulas in patients with Crohn's disease. *N Engl J Med* 1999; **340**(18):1398–1405

Stebbing JF, Jewell DP, Kettlewell MG, Mortensen NJ. Long-term results of recurrence and reoperation after strictureplasty for obstructive Crohn's disease. *Br J Surg* 1995; **82**(11):1471–1474

17

Ulcerative colitis

Ian G. Faragher, Robert J.S. Thomas

INTRODUCTION

Ulcerative colitis and Crohn's disease are both classified under the general heading of inflammatory bowel disease (IBD). Both are diseases of unknown aetiology but in the majority of cases they can be separated on the basis of their clinical features and distinctive pathological changes in the gastrointestinal tract. Occasionally, however, no definite diagnosis can be made, in which case the disease is classified as indeterminate colitis.

Ulcerative colitis is more common than Crohn's disease and both these conditions are most prevalent in Caucasian populations, being uncommon in Asia and Africa. The prevalence of the disease does not seem to be increasing.

The disease usually occurs in the young to middle age groups although it can occur at all ages.

Ulcerative colitis is essentially a disease confined to the large intestine with variable systemic manifestations. However, Crohn's disease may involve the entire gastrointestinal tract although commonly it involves the small intestine, colon and perineum.

Where possible, a clear diagnosis is important as the therapy differs for each disease, in particular the surgical options are quite distinct. Crohn's disease almost universally recurs after surgical excision whilst ulcerative colitis is cured by total colectomy. Thus the importance of pursuing the correct definitive diagnosis cannot be overemphasised.

The remainder of this chapter will be concerned with the condition of ulcerative colitis.

AETIOLOGY

The aetiological factors involved in the development of ulcerative colitis are not known. There is a slight familial incidence but no studies have defined any genetic abnormality to account for the family link.

Ulcerative colitis is an inflammatory process and is associated with lymphoid infiltration in the colon. It has extracolonic manifestations which are similar to other immunologically related diseases. However, extensive investigation of possible immunological and inflammatory disorders has not defined specific defects. Changes in cell-mediated immunity have been demonstrated. A complex of inflammatory changes in the colonic mucosa with expression of cytokines and other inflammatory mediators, for example prostaglandin, has been described. However, despite a vast body of literature there is still not a precise definition of the key aetiological factors inducing this disease. A variety of immunological mechanisms have been postulated as causing tissue injury in this situation.

PATHOLOGY

Ulcerative colitis is characterised by an inflammatory process involving the mucosa of the colon. This process is variable in extent and descriptive terms used to describe this disease based on its extent and severity include the following.

- *Proctitis*: if the inflammatory change is confined to the rectum, the diagnosis is of proctitis. Proctitis alone is usually excluded from the classification of ulcerative colitis.

- *Ulcerative colitis*: if the inflammation extends to the colon, then the diagnosis is of ulcerative colitis. Almost invariably the inflammation in ulcerative colitis starts distally and extends in a continuous fashion proximally.

- *Pancolitis*: this inflammation might involve part of the colon or the entire colon, in which case the condition is defined as pancolitis.

- *Localised ileitis*: there may be some backwash into the terminal ileum, producing a localised ileitis.

Ulcerative colitis occurs in a continuous fashion, in comparison to Crohn's disease which often consists of discrete areas of the disease with normal mucosa in between these abnormal areas. These areas of abnormality are known as 'skip' lesions. Crohn's disease commonly involves the small intestine but may involve any part of the gastrointestinal tract.

In ulcerative colitis the macroscopic appearance of the mucosa, seen at either colonoscopy or sigmoidoscopy, is of redness, loss of the normal vascular pattern, the presence of mucus and slime on the mucosa and variable degrees of ulceration (Figure 17.1). In the chronic stages of the disease, the macroscopic appearance may be close to normal.

The histological examination in the acute phase of the illness shows diffuse infiltration with inflammatory cells usually limited to the mucosa. The chronic changes of ulcerative colitis include a flattened, potentially dysplastic mucosa with goblet cell depletion and atrophy of the mucosa.

As ulcerative colitis primarily involves the mucosa of the colon, regenerating islands in mucosa separated by linear ulcers can look like colonic polyposis. However, these are not true polyps and the condition is known as pseudopolyposis. This is an inflammatory and not a neoplastic process (Figure 17.2).

Where the condition is severe and widespread, so-called fulminant ulcerative colitis, the inflammatory process extends through the entire wall into the serosa. When this sequence of events occurs inflammation results in dilatation of the bowel and this life-threatening process is known as toxic megacolon.

Where the inflammation is severe and extensive, the patient may be dehydrated and show signs of sepsis.

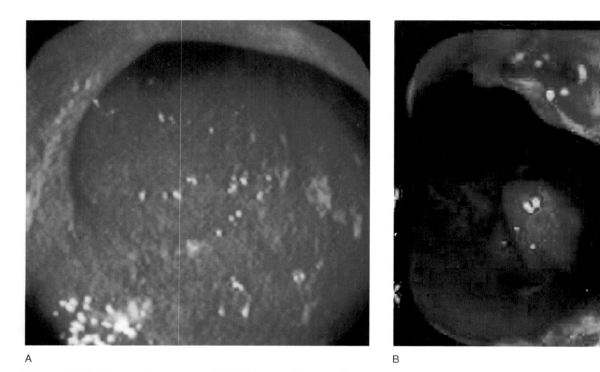

A   B

Figure 17.1 A. Colonoscopic appearance of mild ulcerative colitis. **B.** Colonoscopic appearance of severe ulcerative colitis

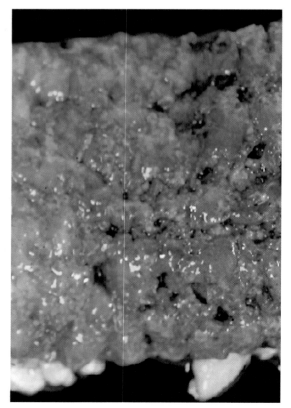

Figure 17.2 Macroscopic appearance of severe ulcerative colitis following emergency colectomy

Potential for malignant change

An important feature of chronic ulcerative colitis is the potential for malignant change. The risk of cancer in total or pancolitis is about 3% after the condition has been present for 10 years and increases slightly in the years that follow. This is usually associated with the development of dysplasia of the mucosa but occasionally it occurs without dysplasia being recognised. The detection of dysplasia by histopathologists is always prone to interpretation error although the absence of dysplasia and high-grade dysplasia are much more definitely identified. In about 10% of cases of severe long-standing total colitis, dysplasia can be identified.

Malignancy is more commonly associated with the presence of a mass lesion or stricture in the colon. If a stenosis or mass lesion is detected at colonoscopy, there is very likely to be an associated cancer, even if superficial biopsies show only normal tissue or low-grade dysplasia. This type of abnormality is known as dysplasia-associated mass lesion (DALM). Benign stricturing is not a feature of ulcerative colitis and is a major point of comparison with Crohn's disease where stricturing is common.

To add to the diagnostic difficulty, carcinoma in ulcerative colitis can occur without any evidence being seen on macroscopic examination and it can only be detected by histological examination.

The fact that cancer can occur where dysplasia has not been recognised introduces problems in relation to surveillance for the development of cancer. Although surveillance is commonly practised, there is no definite evidence that there is a survival benefit from surveillance in chronic ulcerative colitic patients.

Although patients with total colitis show the greatest risk of the development of cancer, there is also a risk in patients with left-sided colitis and this is particularly significant after 20–30 years of the disease being present. A particular group to be checked by surveillance are those where there is a rectal stump present after subtotal colectomy for extensive ulcerative colitis.

The recommendations of the American Society of Gastrointestinal Endoscopy are as follows.

- Surveillance is commenced after seven years in a patient with pancolitis and after 10 years with left-sided colitis.

- Colonoscopy and biopsy should be performed every 1–2 years to identify dysplasia.

- Where dysplasia is identified in these patients, surgical removal of the colon and rectum should be undertaken.

CLINICAL FEATURES

The clinical features of ulcerative colitis relate to both the local colonic disease and the extracolonic manifestations. The seriousness of the symptoms depends upon the severity and extent of the disease. The symptoms of the bowel disturbance are given in Box 17.1.

Box 17.1 Symptoms and signs of ulcerative colitis

Bright bleeding per rectum
Diarrhoea
Mucus and slime per rectum
Tenesmus
Cramping abdominal pains
Fever
Anorexia
Weight loss

There are four typical modes of presentation of ulcerative colitis related to the severity of the disease process.

- Presentation with rectal bleeding and some diarrhoea and without any systemic effects. A patient with inflammation limited to the rectum may present in this way.

- Presentation with tenesmus, cramping abdominal pain and more severe diarrhoea when the inflammation extends into the more proximal colon.

- Presentation with very severe diarrhoea, with 10–12 bowel actions per day, cramping abdominal pain and tenesmus, rectal bleeding with general symptoms of fever, vomiting and weight loss. This occurs in the patient with a pancolitis and severe-onset ulcerative colitis.

- Presentation with acute megacolon or toxic colitis. This is a severe illness with a patient presenting with usually an acute

onset of diarrhoea, anaemia, dehydration and evidence of infection. Electrolyte disturbances include hyponatraemia, hypokalaemia and alkalosis. Examination reveals abdominal distension and tenderness and evidence of circulatory insufficiency. An abdominal radiograph will reveal a dilated colon usually exceeding 6 cm on plain abdominal radiography. This type of patient requires urgent resuscitation and medical management and may also require urgent surgery.

The extraintestinal manifestations of ulcerative colitis are shown in Box 17.2. These manifestations may occur singly or in combination.

Box 17.2 Extraintestinal manifestations of ulcerative colitis

Skin: erythemanodosum and pyoderma gangrenosum
Eyes: iritis
Mucous membranes: aphthous ulcers
Joints: flitting arthralgia or more severe sacroileitis and ankylosing spondylitis
Hepatobiliary system: sclerosing cholangitis, cirrhosis and chronic active hepatitis
Haematopoietic system: anaemia and leucocytosis

INVESTIGATION AND DIAGNOSIS

The patient with ulcerative colitis presents with a fairly typical history. Sigmoidoscopy in the office can usually demonstrate abnormal rectal mucosa and a biopsy can be taken at that time to confirm the diagnosis of inflammation. This biopsy also helps to exclude other causes of proctitis listed below.

The demonstration of the extent of the process through the colon can be made by colonoscopy or barium enema (Figure 17.3).

In the chronic stage of the disease the colon is shortened and loses its haustral pattern and shows a classic picture on a barium examination. Colonoscopy is the investigation of choice because of the ability to take biopsies around the whole length of the colon and visualise the mucosa.

The differential diagnosis for a person presenting with the typical acute symptoms includes the following.

- Infective causes: this requires stool examination for Salmonella, Shigella, Campylobacter and Yersinia as well as ova, cysts and parasites.

- Pseudomembranous colitis: there is usually a history of recent antibiotic use. This can be diagnosed by detection of *Clostridium difficile* toxin in the stool and by biopsy of the rectal mucosa.

- Ischaemic colitis, radiation colitis and rectal and colon cancer should be considered and excluded on the basis of the history and examination findings, as well as the colonoscopic findings.

- Irritable bowel syndrome may present with diarrhoea and abdominal discomfort but the patient is rarely ill and characteristically blood is not present in the faeces.

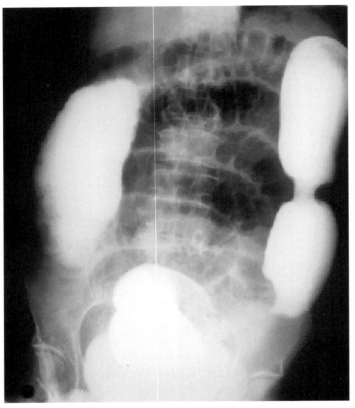

Figure 17.3 This patient with longstanding ulcerative colitis presented with a bowel obstruction. Gastrograffin enema shows stenoses in the descending colon and in the proximal sigmoid colon. Both lesions proved to be carcinomas.

The patient requires full investigation which includes assessment of the general state of the patient, a full blood examination, erythrocyte sedimentation rate, serum electrolytes and liver function tests.

As noted earlier, distinguishing between ulcerative colitis and Crohn's disease is occasionally not easy. Histological findings may not allow differentiation between the two diagnoses. The presence of severe perianal disease is commonly associated with Crohn's disease.

MANAGEMENT

Ulcerative colitis is a disease of remission and relapses. It is of variable severity and variable chronicity.

Medical management

Medical management is the mainstay of treatment for most patients except those presenting with the most severe fulminant form of the disease. The medical therapy has to be 'tailored' to the particular needs of each individual patient.

The aims of the therapy are to reduce symptoms, induce remission and then maintain the patient in remission. The following agents are used to control the disease.

Sulphasalazine and 5-aminosalicylic acid (5-ASA)

Sulphasalazine consists of sulphapiridine and 5-ASA linked by an azobond. 5-ASA is the active moiety and is liberated in the colon where the azobond is cleaved by colonic bacteria. Sulphasalazine is given in a dose of 4 g per day and helps induce remissions in moderate colitis and maintain these remissions in the long term. 5-ASA and related compounds may be given by enema, an effective treatment for distal disease.

The main drawback to its use are the side effects which occur in 20% of patients and include nausea, anorexia, headache and dyspepsia. More serious allergic reactions can occur including rash, fever and haematological side effects. Monitoring for these side effects is essential. Abnormalities in spermatogenesis are also associated with the intake of this drug. For those patients who do have side effects, use of the newer 5-ASA compounds is indicated although these agents still have side effects, including abdominal pain and diarrhoea.

Corticosteroids

Corticosteroids are valuable in inducing a remission in ulcerative colitis but are not effective in maintaining remission. Doses of up to 30–40 mg of prednisolone per day may be necessary. Steroid enemas are also effective in distal disease.

Immunosuppressants

Azathioprine is effective in inducing remission where control of the disease has been difficult with the other drugs. Combined drug regimes may result in disease control with fewer side effects, e.g. lower doses of steroids. However, significant complications occur, including nausea, vomiting and bone marrow toxicity.

Cyclosporin A has a role in deferring surgery in patients with acute exacerbations of ulcerative colitis that have not responded to steroids. Approximately two-thirds of patients will recover from the acute illness but half of this group will come to colectomy within six months. This may be particularly useful in a severe first presentation of ulcerative colitis where the patient has had little time to come to terms with colectomy. Serious complications such as renal impairment, seizures, lymphopenia and reduced T cell function may occur and require continuous clinical and laboratory monitoring.

These patients are also advised about management of stress and the use of diet. Occasionally the exclusion of dairy products improves symptomatology in ulcerative colitis. The use of an elemental diet has been shown to improve outcomes in ulcerative colitis.

This group of patients require considerable psychological support and may show evidence of psychiatric disturbances, possibly related to the presence of the disease. The management of the whole patient, including the use of diet, exercise and replacement therapy, is essential for a successful outcome in severe chronic ulcerative colitis.

Surgical management

Indications for surgery

Indications for surgery are summarised in Box 17.3.

Box 17.3 Indications for surgery

Absolute
Perforation associated with toxic megacolon
Cancer
High-grade dysplasia

Relative
Failure of acute disease to respond to medical therapy
Side effects of medication or recurrent refractory chronic disease
Haemorrhage
Growth retardation or incipient puberty
Cancer risk
Inability to perform normal activities (work, schooling)

Development of colorectal cancer is an absolute indication for surgery. The diagnosis of high-grade dysplasia on random colonic biopsies is also an indication for surgery. This diagnosis should be made by an experienced gastrointestinal pathologist and if there is any doubt a second pathologist's opinion should be sought. Colectomy for dysplasia is associated with a significant rate of unexpected colorectal carcinoma in the colectomy specimen.

Emergency operations are indicated for acute disease; that is, toxic megacolon with or without perforation. Occasionally haemorrhage is an indication for surgery. The operation performed is usually total colectomy and end ileostomy.

Elective operations for chronic disease include construction of a neorectum – the ileoanal pouch procedure (also called restorative proctectomy) – as well as mucosectomy, loop ileostomy and perineal proctectomy.

Total colectomy and ileoanal pouch (restorative proctectomy) has replaced both proctocolectomy with end ileostomy or the Koch pouch, and colectomy and ileoanal anastomosis as the most frequent operation in patients with ulcerative colitis. The relative merits of the three surgical options are summarised in Table 17.1.

OPERATIVE SURGERY

Preoperative care

Time should be spent discussing the surgical options for patients with ulcerative colitis who may come to surgery. For patients considering a pouch, the expected functional outcome and medium to long-term complications, specifically pouchitis and small bowel obstruction, should be discussed, in addition to perioperative complications. Further education by a stoma therapist and a meeting with another patient with an established pouch are helpful. Regardless of the surgeon's preferences for the use or otherwise of a covering loop ileostomy, the patient should be carefully reviewed. There is a small chance that the pouch will not adequately reach into the pelvis and in such an eventuality the procedure cannot then be completed.

Box 17.4 Guidelines for siting a stoma

- Away from the incision, other scars, bony landmarks, the umbilicus and future incisions.
- Within the rectus abdominis muscle.
- Fit an appliance and recheck with the patient sitting and lying down that the site doesn't include a skin crease or significant concavity.

Perisurgical care includes steroid cover, prophylactic antibiotics, subcutaneous heparin and antithromboembolic stockings. Operations should be performed under general anaesthesia, with an endotracheal tube. Placement of an epidural catheter which can be used postoperatively for analgesia should be considered. The patient should be positioned supine on the operating table,

Table 17.1 A comparison of surgical options for the treatment of ulcerative colitis			
	Proctocolectomy and ileostomy	**Colectomy and ileorectal anastomosis**	**Total colectomy and ileal pouch–anal anastomosis**
Advantages	Curative One operation No anastomosis	Continent, average 2–4 motions/day No stoma, no pelvic dissection	Curative and continent Average 4–6 motions/day, 0–1/night May use pad at night Function may improve over first year
Disadvantages	Permanent stoma Intubation required for Koch ileostomy	Residual disease Proctectomy may be required	Variations in pouch function Requires good sphincter function
Complications	Stoma revision 25% Delayed perineal wound healing	SBO in 20%	Pouch complications: fistulas, sepsis, stenosis, pouchitis, SBO in 20%, late diagnosis of Crohn's disease
Contraindications		Incontinence, severe rectal inflammation, rectal malignancy	Crohn's, rectal cancer, poor sphincter function in elderly

SBO, small bowel obstruction

with their legs in Lloyd Davies stirrups. A urinary catheter should be inserted.

Useful equipment includes a headlight and specific retractors. A St Mark's retractor is essential for deep pelvic dissection; an Eisenhammer retractor is of great assistance with mucosectomy; additional exposure for the perineal operation may be gained from a Lone Star™ retractor or a Norfolk-Norwich retractor. Longer instruments, particularly scissors and a diathermy extension, are needed for pelvic surgery.

Total colectomy and end ileostomy

A total colectomy with end ileostomy is recommended in the setting of an acute flare of ulcerative colitis in an unwell patient on significant doses of steroids or immunosuppressive agents.

Colectomy

- Careful handling of the inflamed colon is important to avoid perforation during resection.

- The terminal ileum and its blood supply should be preserved by division of the terminal branches of the ileocolic artery adjacent to the caecum and the division of the ileum adjacent to the ileocaecal valve. This maximises the length of ileum with an intact blood supply for later construction of a J-pouch that reaches to the anal canal. The rectum should be left *in situ*; the mesorectal plane should not be opened as this only increases the difficulty of subsequent proctectomy.

- The rectal stump may be divided at the rectosigmoid junction with a linear staple and left intraperitoneal. For patients with significant rectal inflammation, it is safer to divide the colon in the distal sigmoid. This permits the rectal stump to be exteriorised via the lower end of the wound as a mucus fistula. Intraperitoneal leakage of the rectal stump due to increased pressure from continuing inflammatory secretions and bleeding is thus avoided. The anal canal may be decompressed with a proctoscope at the end of the case, thus draining any intraluminal contents. It may be necessary to repeat this during the early postoperative course.

End ileostomy

- The ileum is appropriately divided, either abutting the ileocaecal valve, if an ileoanal pouch is considered, or 5–10 cm from the valve in the absence of ileal disease. Use of a linear cutter stapler reduces the chance of contamination. Allis tissue forceps are placed just below the dermis and on the rectus fascia at the level of the stoma site in the primary incision. This prevents lateral tunnelling during dissection.

- A 2 cm diameter circular incision is made through the skin at the marker site. The incision may be continued with diathermy to the rectus sheath, removing a core of subcutaneous fat. The anterior rectus sheath is incised vertically. The rectus fibres are split longitudinally and retracted transversely with the aid of Langenbeck retractors. Take care to avoid the inferior epigastric vessels at this time. The posterior rectus sheath and peritoneum are incised vertically with diathermy whilst the abdominal contents are protected underneath.

- Small lateral incisions in the rectus sheath may be required to accommodate the ileum. In general, it should be possible to pass the tips of the surgeon's index and middle fingers from inside the abdomen to above the skin. A Babcock tissue forceps is used to gently draw the end of the ileum through the stoma site – check the ileal mesentery is not twisted. About 4.5 cm of ileum should project above the skin level, curving slightly cephalad. One or two 3/0 chromic sutures may be placed between either the anterior or posterior sheath and the ileum.

- After the mid-line incision is closed, the staple line is trimmed from the ileum. Four 3/0 chromic sutures are placed equidistant around the stoma. Each suture starts with picking up the dermis from inside to outside, next the end of the ileum, again from inside to outside, before lastly picking up a bite through the serosa of the ileum, just above the level of the skin. As these sutures are tied, with some gentle encouragement, the ileum everts to form a 2 cm spout pointing slightly cephalad. Further simple sutures between the subcuticular layer of the skin and edge of the ileum complete the stoma. A temporary appliance is fitted and the end of the bag is clipped shut.

Postoperative care

Immunosuppressive agents are ceased and steroids are gradually reduced.

Time should be taken to verify the histological diagnosis on the complete specimen with the pathologist.

Ileostomy care

Stoma education lessons should include skin care and preparation, sizing of the stoma, cutting the appliance base to size and securing the reservoir to the base plate (for two-part appliances).

The patient is followed by the enterostomal nurse for several months as the stoma may change slightly in size. The patient should also be encouraged to drink plentifully to reduce dehydration, particularly in hot weather. A simple self-check is for the patient to monitor their urine colour and aim to keep it dilute. Some patients may require loperamide, lomotil or codeine if high output from the stoma remains a problem. Another common concern is skin irritation by the ileal contents. Simple problems may be addressed by scrupulous skin care, a well-fitting appliance and wiping the skin with an antacid solution.

Late complications may include ileal prolapse, parastomal hernia, ileostomy retraction and fistula. These problems may be managed by the enterostomal nurse but may require local revision or even relocation of the stoma.

Total colectomy and ileoanal pouch (restorative proctectomy)

Colectomy

See above.

Ileoanal pouch

The principle of the operation is to create a 'neorectum' or reservoir from ileum that is anastomosed to the dentate line. In practice, the stapled J-pouch has superseded the more complex 'S' and 'W'-shaped pouches due to its relative simplicity. The pouch anal anastomosis is most commonly a double stapled anastomosis as it is technically easier and quicker for most surgeons than the alternative – routine mucosectomy and a handsewn pouch anal anastomosis from below.

Preoperatively issues of functional outcome and medium to long-term complications, specifically pouchitis and small bowel obstruction, should be discussed with the patient in addition to discussion of perioperative complications. Further education by a stoma therapist and a meeting with another patient with an established pouch are helpful. Regardless of surgeon preferences for the use or not of a covering loop ileostomy, the patient should be sited in advance. There is a small chance that the pouch will not adequately reach into the pelvis and the procedure could not then be completed.

Following either colectomy, or mobilisation of the end ileostomy and division of adhesions, the operation proceeds as follows.

Mobilisation of the rectum

Rectal mobilisation is easiest in the mesorectal plane. Care is taken to identify the presacral nerves in order to preserve sexual function. The risk of nerve damage may be reduced by dissection close to the rectum. The majority of surgeons would mobilise in the mesorectal plane.

Mucosectomy (see below for details of surgical technique)

Mucosectomy is indicated if cancer has developed in the colon and may be considered in patients with high-grade dysplasia. Advocates of routine mucosectomy point out that a small number

of cancers in the world literature have arisen in rectal mucosa between the stapled anastomosis and the dentate line. There is little evidence of any functional differences between patients with double stapled pouch anal anastomosis and those with mucos-ectomy and a handsewn anastomosis.

Construction of the pouch and (tension-free) pouch anal anastomosis

The J-pouch is constructed by selecting the apex of an ileal loop that reaches furthest to the symphysis pubis. The limbs should be approximately 15–20 cm in length and may require three or four firings of a linear cutter stapler. The efferent limb is stapled shut and the anvil belonging to the circular staple is inserted via the apex of the loop and held in place with a pursestring (Figure 17.4A–E).

Additional techniques may be required to allow the pouch anal anastomosis to sit without tension. These include:

- full mobilisation of the ileal mesentery back to above the duodenum

- scoring the visceral peritoneum overlying the ileal mesentery perpendicular to the line of tension

- selective division of vascular arcades/vasa recta whilst preserving a good blood supply – this may gain an additional centimetre

- rarely, the S-pouch may be used as the efferent limb reaches relatively further. However, a long efferent limb is associated with difficulties in emptying the S-pouch which may even require revision of the pouch.

Loop ileostomy

Use of a covering loop ileostomy varies. It is indicated if there are any technical concerns about the pouch anal anastomosis and in patients on 20 mg prednisolone or more. The majority of surgeons favour loop ileostomy to avoid the poorer functional outcome which is associated with pelvic sepsis due to a leaking anastomosis. Timing of closure of the loop ileostomy varies from two weeks to six months.

Loop ileostomy

- The intestine exteriorised as a loop is often proximal ileum as the distal ileum is used to form the pouch in the pelvis. The loop of intestine that reaches the site of the stoma with the least tension and is closest to the pouch should be selected.

- A vessel loop or tape is passed around the mesenteric border of the ileum and brought out through the stoma site.

- The ileum is gently pulled into position so the mesentery can just be seen above the skin and sits without undue tension.

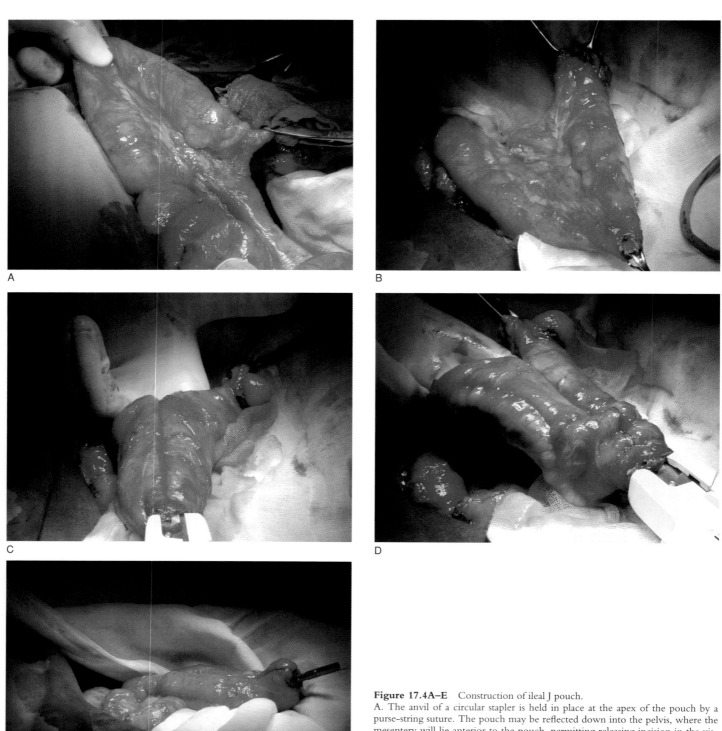

Figure 17.4A–E Construction of ileal J pouch.

A. The anvil of a circular stapler is held in place at the apex of the pouch by a purse-string suture. The pouch may be reflected down into the pelvis, where the mesentery will lie anterior to the pouch, permitting releasing incision in the visceral peritoneum as required.

B–C. The ileal pouch is created with three or four firings of a linear cutter stapler. Take care to staple along the antimesenteric border of the ileum. The surgeons index and middle finger assist in maintaining the orientation of the ileum.

D. The ileum is reflected towards the patient's head. An enterotomy is made at the apex of the ileal loop.

E. The midpoint of the distal loop reaches the symphysis pubis. The limbs should be 15–20 cm long.

- The serosal surface of the ileum is marked differently with diathermy, on either side of the vessel loop, to identify the afferent and efferent limbs of the stoma.

- After the mid-line incision is closed, the ileal loop is opened on the efferent limb side of the vessel loop, close to the skin.

- A 3/0 chromic suture placed between the proximal ileal cut edge and the furthest skin edge everts the proximal ileum into a small spout (Figure 17.5). This suture may also pick up the serosa of the proximal ileum adjacent to the skin to secure the everted limb to the skin. Simple sutures approximate the rest of the spout to the margin of the ileostomy site, leaving only a small space for the distal limb to be sutured to the skin.

- The vessel loop is removed and a temporary appliance is fitted.

As there is often less intestine above a loop ileostomy, the stoma output is often higher. Care must be taken to monitor fluids and electrolytes after discharge from hospital. Timing of closure of the loop ileostomy varies from two weeks to six months.

Mucosectomy

- The patient is positioned to allow good access to the anus, which is irrigated with an antiseptic solution.

- A solution of 0.5% marcaine with 1/200 000 adrenaline is then infiltrated in the submucosal plane.

- Beginning at the dentate line, the mucosa is dissected with scissors from the internal sphincter muscle. This is most easily done quadrant by quadrant with the aid of an Eisenhammer retractor. The appearance of fat in this plane indicates the upper level of dissection at the pelvic floor.

- The abdominal surgeon can remove the remainder of the bowel and subsequently deliver several sutures attached to the apex of the ileal pouch.

- The pouch may be positioned in the pelvis and a handsewn pouch anal anastomosis completed at the dentate line.

Perineal proctectomy

Proctectomy may be part of total proctocolectomy or may be performed some time after colectomy. It is less frequent due to the increasing use of ileal pouches. Some patients will end up with a permanent ileostomy and the remaining rectal mucosa needs to be removed to prevent cancer.

- The patient is positioned in Lloyd Davies stirrups.

- The rectum is irrigated with an antiseptic solution and the anus closed with a 0 monofilament pursestring suture.

- A circumferential incision is made at the anal verge and deepened in the intersphincteric plane (between the internal and external anal sphincters). Dissection may be helped by infiltrating a solution of 0.5% marcaine with 1/200 000 adrenaline; this helps to define the plane, reduce bleeding and relax the sphincter muscles. Initial dissection usually proceeds from lateral to posterior on each side.

- Anteriorly in the female, the rectum is dissected from the vagina until the pouch of Douglas is opened. Anteriorly in the male, the upper fibres of the external sphincter are divided where they decussate and the rectum is dissected from the posterior surface of the prostate. Any remaining part of the lateral ligaments can be divided and the rectum removed.

- The wound is copiously irrigated, haemostasis secured and a low-pressure suction drain brought out laterally.

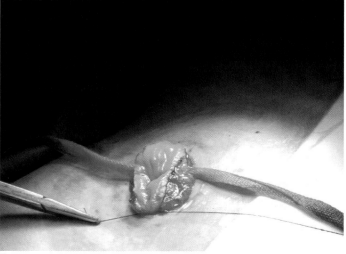

A

B

Figure 17.5 Construction of loop ileostomy. **A.** The ileum is opened close to the skin on the efferent side of the loop. **B.** The mucosal edge is sewn to the skin edge. This suture is being placed on the efferent limb of the stoma.

- The levator ani muscles are approximated and the subcutaneous space closed. Mattress sutures may assist skin edge eversion.

FURTHER READING

Ardizzone S, Molteni P, Bollani S, Porro GB. Guidelines for the treatment of ulcerative colitis in remission. *Eur J Gastroenterol Hepatol* 1997; **9**(9): 836–841

Ardizzone S, Porro GB. A practical guide to the management of distal ulcerative colitis. *Drugs* 1998; **55**(4): 520–538

Frizelle FA, Burt MJ. The surgical management of ulcerative colitis. *J Gastroenterol Hepatol* 1997; **12**: 670–677

Kornbluth A, Present D, Lichtiger S, Hanauer S. Cyclosporin for severe ulcerative colitis: a user's guide. *Am J Gastroenterol* 1997; **92**(9): 1424–1428

Marion J, Present D. The modern medical management of acute, severe ulcerative colitis. *Eur J Gastroenterol Hepatol* 1997; **9**(9): 831–835

Podolsky DK (ed). Inflammatory bowel disease. *Curr Opin Gastroenterol* 1999(4): 283–370

Thompson-Fawcett MW, Jewell DP, Mortensen N. Ileoanal reservoir dysfunction: a problem-solving approach. *Br J Surg* 1997; **84**: 1351–1359

18

Diverticular Disease and Colonic Bleeding

Ronald A. Keenan, Zygmunt H. Krukowski

DIVERTICULAR DISEASE

Sigmoid diverticular disease is a common condition with an increasing prevalence with advancing age: 5% in the 5th decade rising to 60% in the 9th decade and symptomatic complications occur in 10–30% of patients. It is remarkable, therefore, how infrequently patients are admitted for either elective resection or with inflammatory complications of this common disorder. For a population aged under 64 years it accounts for 0.5 deaths/100 000 rising to 6.2 deaths/100 000 in the age group 65–74 years. Continuing high morbidity and mortality rates may be obscured by infrequency in the absence of sustained and determined effort prospectively to document outcomes.

Morbidity and death in diverticulitis relate to the degree of sepsis at presentation aggravated by coincidental degenerative disease in aged patients which may be reduced but cannot be eliminated by optimal operative and supportive treatment. Only 17% of patients with diverticular disease develop diverticulitis and less than 1% require surgery. Consequently management is focussed on identifying patients who will benefit from operation whilst avoiding unnecessary and inappropriate interventions. In contrast to the emergency situation in which there may be a tendency to precipitate surgery there may be a contrasting reluctance to offer elective surgery to patients with continuing symptoms, or at risk of recurrent sepsis.

There is, in addition, a new factor exerting an important influence on rates of surgery for both complicated and uncomplicated diverticular disease. The introduction of laparoscopic colonic resection may have had an impact on the indications for surgery. Whatever the chosen approach the challenges in managing diverticular disease remain those of timing of surgery and selection of the appropriate operation.

The published literature is substantial but the quality of the evidence base for therapy in diverticular disease is striking in its paucity. There are only two published randomised controlled trials, and one major consensus document from the American Society of Colon and Rectal Surgeons. The vast majority of papers published between 1965–99 are retrospective.

Aetiology

Acquired sigmoid diverticular disease is generally held to be a consequence of a chronic dietary deficiency in vegetable fibre, but structural changes in the ageing colon with hyperelastosis and altered collagen structure also contribute. High intraluminal pressure secondary to segmentation of the narrow calibre sigmoid colon results in the characteristic protrusion of the colonic mucosa through the weak points in the bowel wall where the terminal arterial branches penetrate the circular muscle. Diverticula comprise mucosa and serosa except within the mesocolon when they may also be surrounded by fat (Figure 18.1). The major complications of sigmoid diverticular disease are sepsis, haemorrhage, obstruction and fistula formation.

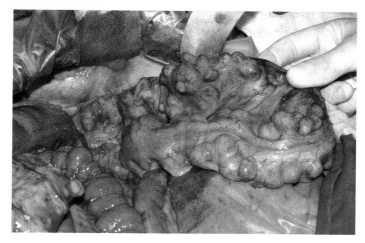

Figure 18.1 Operative photograph of extensive sigmoid diverticular disease.

Obstruction of a diverticulum encourages bacterial proliferation with development of a local abscess. Minor episodes may be self-limiting but progression occurs in a minority. NSAIDs increase this risk of sepsis. A phlegmonous mass results if diffuse cellulitis without suppuration involves a length of colon. The evolution of the disease depends on the rate of progression of sepsis and the initial site. For example faecal peritonitis may follow the 'blow-out' of a previously uninflamed diverticulum or result from the slow progression through abscess formation with late intraperitoneal rupture. A complex suppurative mass incorporating colon, small bowel, bladder, uterus, ovaries, tubes and occasionally ureter may develop with fistulation to any of these structures. The extent of peritonitis associated with diverticular masses varies and although there may be extensive fibrinous exudate and inflammatory peritoneal fluid, this may contain few bacteria.

Comparison between series requires consistent description of the pathology (Box 18.1) and some form of risk stratification. The most widely quoted staging of the severity of the intraabdominal sepsis is that of Hinchey, although this has never been rigorously

---

Box 18.1 Classification of pathology of 'acute diverticulitis'

- Abscess
  peridiverticular
  mesenteric
  pericolic (pelvic)
- Perforation
  free
  concealed (indirect)
- Gangrenous sigmoiditis
- Peritonitis
  (a) serous
    purulent
    faecal
  (b) local
    pelvic
    generalised (diffuse)

Adapted from Killingback (1983).

validated, and recent work includes more sophisticated physiological parameters. The importance of stratifying the inflammatory process is well illustrated in Haglund et al. In 392 patients admitted with acute diverticulitis, 97 (25%) underwent emergency operation. Within the operative group, 31 patients had phlegmonous inflammation with no evidence of suppuration or perforation and the mortality was 3%. By contrast, in 66 patients with evidence of perforation the mortality was 33%. The relevance of this observation is that if the threshold for operation is inappropriately low more patients with mild disease and a good prognosis are subjected to surgery and a low mortality for surgery is reported. High-quality reports of surgery for diverticulitis should be prospective and describe the population under study, the operation rate and the extent of sepsis, if the analysis of outcome is to be valid.

CLINICAL PRESENTATION

There are a number of different patterns of presentation of sigmoid diverticular disease. Many patients present with symptoms of lower abdominal pain, distension and altered bowel habit and prove to have diverticular disease whilst excluding colorectal cancer. However, in a study of 'normal' individuals 31% complained of symptoms which could be related to colonic disease and 14% had symptoms relieved by defaecation. In a small number of patients, failure of medical management while symptoms continue in the absence of complications over a number of years prompts surgery. Resection of the colon does not guarantee relief of pain in all these patients and by inference an underlying bowel motility problem coexists.

Acute diverticulitis

The patient with this typically presents with a history of a few days of increasing lower abdominal pain which localises in the left iliac fossa with variable nausea, altered bowel habit and irritation of pelvic viscera. Pain and tenderness can be maximal to the right of the midline and may mimic appendicitis.

In the majority of patients, signs in the left iliac fossa support a working diagnosis of acute diverticulitis although a number of other disease processes affecting the large or small bowel, the genitourinary system, major arteries and abdominal wall can produce left iliac fossa pain. The differential diagnosis should also include gangrenous sigmoiditis, Crohn's disease and diverticular colitis. Gangrenous sigmoiditis has been considered a complication of diverticular disease with prolonged severe muscle spasm. A more plausible explanation is a vascular occlusive problem. Crohn's disease may be diagnosed in conjunction with diverticular disease. This may be suggested by the recognition of multiple complex fistulas on contrast studies or by the histological findings of granuloma in resected specimens of colon for diverticular disease. While the two diseases may co-exist, granulomatous changes can be identified in association with diverticular disease limited to

the sigmoid colon and not associated with any other current or subsequent manifestations of Crohn's. Diverticular colitis is a recently described entity in which there is chronic focal mucosal sigmoid colitis occurring in the presence of diverticula. It presents with rectal bleeding and may be difficult to differentiate from other colitides.

Fistula

A fistula may develop between an inflamed diverticulum and any abutting viscus. Although fistulae occur between colon and appendix, ovarian tube, uterus, ureter, skin and both large and small bowel, the most common are colovesical (65%) and colovaginal (25%) and incidence can vary from 5% in district general hospitals to over 30% in referral centres. Colovaginal fistulas are characterised by discharge of flatus, faeces and pus often in association with lower abdominal pain. It is more likely after hysterectomy, which allows the diseased colon to adhere to the vault of the vagina. When a diverticular abscess adheres to and subsequently ruptures into the vault of the bladder, a colovesical fistula results, with typical symptoms of pneumaturia (60%) and urinary infection (75%). Lower abdominal pain may be absent in over one-third of patients. Sigmoid diverticular disease is the most likely cause of a colovesical fistula but Crohn's disease, and colon or bladder cancer must be excluded.

Abscess

Patients with pericolic, pelvic or mesocolic abscesses secondary to diverticular disease usually present with signs often localised to the left iliac fossa. The degree of systemic upset, pain and tenderness depends on the extent of inflammation. Although a classical pelvic abscess palpable through the anterior rectal wall may be clinically obvious, most diverticular abscesses are detected on urgent contrast enema, ultrasound or CT scanning (Figure 18.2A & B). In some patients the development of an abscess may be obscure, identified only in retrospect when an elective barium enema reveals an abscess communicating with the bowel lumen.

Haemorrhage

Bleeding from colonic diverticular disease is typically painless, profuse and bright red, although the colour depends on the site of bleeding in the colon. Bleeding from the left side of the colon presents as bright red blood with clots, whereas that from the right side of the colon is darker and plum coloured. The incidence varies widely occurring in between 3–27% of patients in reported series. Fortunately colonic bleeding is rarely exsanguinating and stops spontaneously in approximately 70% of cases. Continuous or recurrent bleeding requires transfusion and ultimately operation. Not uncommonly there may be no prodromal symptoms before the onset of profuse rectal bleeding.

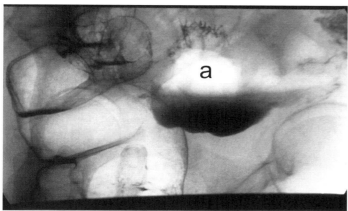

A

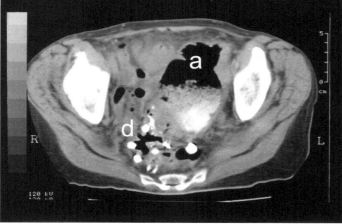

B

Figure 18.2 A Contrast enema showing a large abscess with a gas/fluid level secondary to diverticular disease (a – abscess cavity), **B** CT scan showing large abscess in the same patient (a – abscess cavity, d – diverticular disease).

Obstruction

Obstruction due to diverticular disease is uncommon. Patients presenting with left-sided colonic obstruction due to fibrous stricturing in the sigmoid colon present in a similar manner to a carcinoma with progressive distension and constipation. Investigation and management are essentially identical and depend on the demonstration of typical features on plain abdominal radiographs with confirmation of the site of the obstruction on an urgent water-soluble contrast enema. The benign nature of the stricture may be suspected but in the presence of complete obstruction requiring urgent intervention the diagnosis may only be confirmed after resection, examination of the opened bowel and subsequent histology. Indeed the converse is rather more likely that a presumed malignant large bowel obstruction is only shown to be fibrotic in nature after resection.

Intestinal obstruction may also result from adhesion of loops of small bowel to an inflammatory pericolic mass and the features of small bowel obstruction may obscure the diagnosis of the underlying colonic pathology.

INVESTIGATION

The value of a careful history and physical examination should never be underestimated. If a few minutes are spent determining the nature and site of onset of lower abdominal pain the embarrassment of making an inappropriate incision in a patient with sigmoid diverticulitis can be avoided. Furthermore, clinical features in patients with mild disease may be sufficient to define management with minimal investigation. Plain radiography of the abdomen and chest often provide indirect evidence of major inflammation: the most obvious being a pneumoperitoneum or subdiaphragmatic gas. The demonstration of a small amount of intraperitoneal gas, a traditional sign of generalised peritonitis, is not an absolute indication for operation and management depends on the clinical assessment of the extent of peritoneal contamination. It is important to realise that a high fever and leucocytosis may not be indicative of an abscess. Occasionally soft tissue changes, including evidence of obstruction, thickening of bowel wall and extraluminal masses suggest acute diverticulitis.

Although digital rectal examination is an important preliminary to contrast radiology and may detect a low rectal tumour, it is an opportunity to assess the quality of the anal sphincter. This may influence the proposed operation, especially in the elderly female. The authors do not advocate routine sigmoidoscopy prior to an emergency contrast study, although this should be performed before a laparotomy. Patient discomfort is minimised if sigmoidoscopy is performed under general anaesthesia prior to opening the abdomen. Sigmoidoscopy is necessary to exclude anorectal conditions which may also influence the proposed operation.

When clinical features do not warrant immediate laparotomy the clinical diagnosis of acute diverticulitis must be confirmed as soon as is clinically appropriate. There has been a major shift in choice of imaging modality in the investigation of possible acute diverticulitis during the last five years, with a trend towards spiral CT (Figure 18.3). The arguments in favour of this change to CT in preference to ultrasound or a single contrast enema are persuasive and should be performed shortly after admission in patients

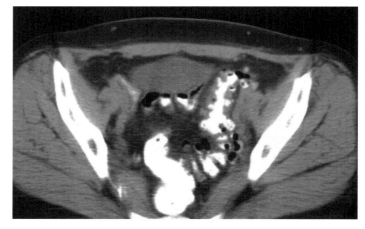

Figure 18.3 CT scan of pelvis showing contrast in the colonic lumen and sigmoid diverticulae.

suspected of having acute diverticulitis. A recent prospective study involving 420 patients compared CT and contrast enema in patients who did not require urgent surgery. CT had superior sensitivity (98% vs 92%) and permitted better grading of the severity of inflammation (26% vs 9%). However the authors considered that the examinations should be complementary and not exclusive. The amount of ionising radiation in CT, especially if usage is 'early and frequent', should remain a concern and be weighed against the impact on management.

When access to spiral CT is limited a water-soluble contrast enema remains a practical alternative. Although dilute barium gives superior mucosal definition it is undesirable if perforation may be present and is more difficult to eliminate from the bowel lumen in the event of operation. Contrast enema may show thickening, mucosal oedema, irregularity and occasional extravasation of contrast. Extravasation, if present, is usually localised but free perforation into the peritoneal cavity may be seen. The examination should be limited to confirming the diagnosis, although if the imaging is restricted to the left side of the colon, the possibility of synchronous pathology must be subsequently excluded by formal colonoscopy or barium enema in the convalescent period. The information derived from an urgent enema, although valuable in determining management, cannot be considered definitive and the possibility of carcinoma being co-existent with the inflammatory mass or elsewhere in the colon must be excluded after resolution of the acute episode. When the left colon is excised as an emergency for presumed diverticular disease, a colon cancer may be found within the mass in 20–25% of cases.

Whilst CT has advantages over a single contrast enema in demonstrating the extraluminal changes secondary to acute diverticular disease and alternative diagnoses it is clear that the threshold for requesting CT varies. In one series of 150 patients with suspected diverticulitis this proved to be the final diagnosis in only 64 (43%) compared to possibly more discriminating use when 66–77% of patients had the disease. However because of the diagnostic accuracy of CT and its ability to detect alternative pathology when the clinical diagnosis of diverticulitis is unclear, the authors have moved towards requesting a spiral CT as the first investigation when imaging is indicated.

Whilst the improved imaging and diagnostic yield of routine CT is an advantage in terms of diagnosis the impact on early management may not be so striking. Demonstration of extravasation of contrast on either enema or CT increases the likelihood that operation will be required during the acute admission but is not an absolute indication for operation. Only five (11.4%) of the most recent 44 patients admitted under the care of one of the authors required an operation during the emergency admission. The routine first investigation during this period was a water-soluble contrast enema. CT was reserved for patients in whom management decisions were not clear on the basis of the single contrast enema. This is somewhat less than the operative rate of 24% reported when CT is routine although there must be uncertainty about the comparability of the patient populations. CT also

detects more abscesses than would otherwise be diagnosed although only a minority of these require intervention.

Ultrasound scanning has been employed effectively in some centres but the variability of interpretation and dependence on operator skill reduces its general applicability as the first investigation. When surgical staff have received training in this modality it significantly enhances diagnostic accuracy. Sonography is of value in following the progression of abscesses or masses.

The contribution of contrast enema, CT and ultrasound scanning to the diagnosis of acute diverticulitis, depends on different physical features. Contrast enema depends on intraluminal changes and leakage of contrast and may underestimate extramural disease; nevertheless sensitivity is high (approximately 90%). Ultrasound and CT are more sensitive in demonstrating bowel wall thickening, non-communicating abscesses and extraluminal disease than a contrast enema but the impact on patient management should be similar. The choice of imaging modality will reflect local expertise and facilities. The results of imaging investigations must be interpreted in light of the patient's clinical condition to avoid unnecessary intervention. Any of these urgent investigations may suggest malignancy but scanning of whatever modality, or a single-contrast water-soluble enema, cannot be relied on to differentiate malignancy from inflammation. Follow-up colonoscopy or barium enema should be performed to exclude cancer.

Obstruction

If a plain abdominal radiograph raises the possibility of left-sided colonic obstruction, a single-contrast enema is mandatory because of the unreliability of determining the level of obstruction and the problem of pseudo-obstruction.

Fistula

Diagnosis of a colovesical fistula is often straightforward and made on the history. A barium enema will diagnose the underlying pathology in many patients but demonstration of the fistulous tract is less reliable, varying between 5–80% in colovesical fistula. Similarly cystoscopy tends to show inflammation, only detecting the opening in 46% of patients. Increasingly, a CT scan is used as the first investigation and may reveal some of the rarer fistulas to uterine tube or ureter for example. Colovaginal fistula is much commoner if a patient has had a prior hysterectomy and a vaginal fistulogram may be more sensitive.

Haemorrhage

Continuing or repeated episodes of bleeding require either urgent mesenteric angiography, radionucleotide scintigraphy or colonoscopy. Angiography should include visualisation of both the superior and inferior mesenteric circulation. Demonstration of a bleeding point (Figure 18.4) permits targeted resection limited to

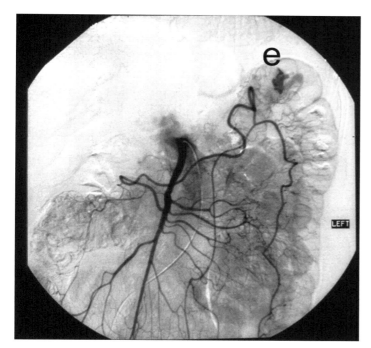

Figure 18.4 Inferior mesenteric angiogram with extravasation (e) of contrast into the colonic lumen secondary to bleeding from a diverticulum at the splenic flexure.

one-half of the colon rather than blind subtotal colectomy. The development of superselective arterial catheterisation allows embolisation with reduced risk of intestinal infarction. Local facilities and expertise dictate which diagnostic modality can be used. Radionucleotide scintigraphy although useful in the stable patient is contraindicated in active bleeding. Skilled colonoscopy can now make a diagnosis even in patients who are actively bleeding. In the debilitated patient unfit for resectional therapy, there may be a role for endoscopic haemostasis if the bleeding diverticulum can be identified. When these preoperative manoeuvres fail to identify the source or massive bleeding precludes investigation, on-table colonic irrigation with colonoscopy may identify the source and avoid subtotal colectomy. Furthermore, transillumination of the colon may show the characteristic features of angiodysplasia.

MANAGEMENT

The management of acute diverticulitis continues to evolve and more discriminating attitudes to operation, improved supportive therapy and increasing confidence in single-stage definitive surgery in the emergency situation continue to modify contemporary practice. Yesterday's heresy evolves into current convention. There are many influences on interventional and operative patterns in both the elective and emergency situation in diverticular disease. Individual and institutional interest and, possibly, income can positively influence the rate of treatment. Conversely, lack of resource may be a subtle negative pressure on activity in a technically benign condition. Furthermore, the

variable interpretation of the available evidence on optimal patient selection and timing of surgery allied to reluctant acceptance or lack of awareness of these evolving concepts implies that the optimal balance between emergency and elective procedures has yet to be achieved. Unlike colonic cancer, in which diagnosis almost always demands surgery, only a minority of patients with sigmoid diverticular disease require operation. The imprecise boundary between the two groups makes decision making difficult and demands experience and judgement. Although perceived to be a common problem, a recent prospective audit encompassing some of the surgical units of 30 hospitals in the UK revealed that an average of only 10 patients were admitted to each unit with complicated diverticular disease over a four-year period. An individual consultant general surgeon, therefore, is unlikely to admit more than two or three patients with the most severe forms of acute diverticulitis in a year (Figure 18.5). Accumulating and maintaining experience is difficult particularly when decision making is delegated, as is still sometimes the case, to trainees.

Elective

In elective surgery, the indications for operation, in the absence of prior emergency admissions with complications, are prolonged failure of medical treatment with continuing symptoms. Careful follow-up after elective resection for uncomplicated sigmoid diverticular disease, however, reveals continuing symptoms in one-quarter of patients. This presumably reflects an underlying problem in gut motility in which sigmoid diverticula are the most obvious abnormality. The risk of postoperative symptoms should be explained to patients before elective surgery is considered. The

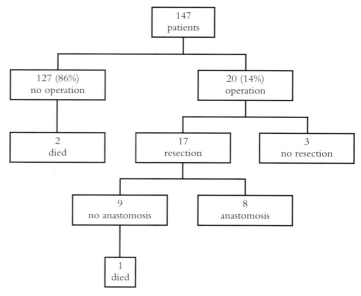

Figure 18.5 Prospective audit of outcome in 147 emergency admissions (1991–2000) with diverticulitis under the care of one consultant (ZHK). (The two deaths in the 'no operation' category were in moribund aged patients for whom active treatment was considered inappropriate: diagnosis made at autopsy).

extent of resection depends on the distribution of the diverticular disease, but should never be less than a formal sigmoid colectomy with colorectal anastomosis at the level of the peritoneal reflection. The distal resection must include all the affected bowel, failing which, the incidence of recurrent disease is unacceptably high. Resection of the entire left colon is required when this is extensively involved but the occasional diverticulum placed more proximally can be ignored. When there is pan-colonic involvement by diverticular disease the aetiology is different from acquired sigmoid diverticular disease and the reasons for operation need to be clear. Subtotal colectomy with ileorectal anastomosis for diverticular disease is rarely indicated unless there is more than one pathology present in the colon.

Operation for colovesical fistula depends on the persistence of the fistula in a patient fit for major surgery and conservative management may prove successful in the aged and infirm by avoiding surgery altogether. The majority of patients will require a definitive procedure. Sigmoid colectomy with end-to-end colorectal anastomosis and interposition of pedicled greater omentum between the anastomosis and the defect in the bladder is essential. The fistulous opening in the bladder wall is usually small and easily repaired with a catheter draining the bladder postoperatively. Recurrence of a fistula after a definitive procedure is uncommon and reflects anastomotic failure which should only occur after around 1% of high colorectal anastomoses. In contrast, simple detachment and repair of the fistulous opening carries an unacceptably high recurrence rate of the order of 30–50%.

Emergency

The management of acute diverticulitis is directed to the control of peritoneal sepsis and a simplified scheme of the surgical options is shown in Box 18.2. Surgery has a role in patients who present with overwhelming sepsis or fail to settle on conservative therapy. The major management decisions in managing acute diverticulitis may be addressed by answering the three questions:

- when to operate?
- when to resect?
- when to anastomose?

Box 18.2 Surgical options in perforated diverticulitis

- Conservative
  suture of perforation
  drainage
  transverse colostomy
- Exteriorisation
- Radical
  resection – anastomosis
  resection + anastomosis
  resection + anastomosis + colostomy

From Krukowski and Matheson (1984).

When to operate?

This is the most difficult of the three questions. When systemic upset is limited and abdominal signs confined to the left lower quadrant, few would advocate urgent surgery. Equally, when there is evidence of widespread peritoneal contamination with generalised peritonitis and free gas, urgent operation based on a diagnosis of generalised peritonitis of unknown origin is indicated. For the remainder, a policy of vigorous resuscitation and antibiotic therapy is the better option. It is remarkable how rapidly patients with extensive signs of peritoneal contamination can improve on such a regimen. During the last 15 years several patients with radiological evidence of free perforation have settled with conservative non-operative measures.

Optimal management requires serial assessment with a degree of observer continuity or very detailed handover. A trial of conservative management with early confirmation of the diagnosis by appropriate imaging also requires regular review in the light of the evolving clinical response. As a general rule the authors persist with conservative management for a maximum of three days before opting for surgery. In contrast to North American practice the authors rarely drain abscesses percutaneously and the majority of those less than 5 cm in diameter resolve with conservative measures. Evidence of extravasation on contrast studies increases the likelihood of surgery during the emergency admission but is not an absolute indication for urgent operation.

Laparoscopy has been described in the evaluation and treatment of acute diverticulitis but, although the authors have on occasion observed phlegmonous inflammation during diagnostic laparoscopy for suspected appendicitis, this seems unnecessarily invasive in diverticulitis when management can be determined by alternative methods. This conservative policy resulted in a substantial reduction in the frequency of urgent operation for sigmoid diverticular disease over the last 20 years with low overall mortality and morbidity (Figure 18.6).

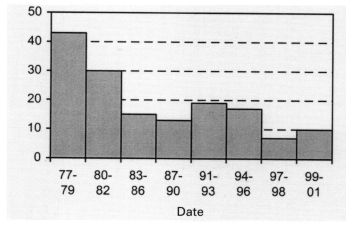

Figure 18.6 Percentage of patients undergoing urgent surgery during the emergency admission with acute diverticulitis.

When to resect?

When the indications for operation are generalised or there is faecal peritonitis or, more commonly, there is failure to resolve with conservative management, then the question of resection of the sigmoid colon is easily answered. Control of bacteraemia and sepsis in the peritoneal cavity requires eradication of the source of infection by resection. Review of published data suggested poorer survival with conservative procedures in which therapy depends on drainage and proximal colostomy without resection compared with emergency resection for patients with the most severe sepsis. A recent randomised clinical trial showed that primary resection is superior to secondary resection in the management of generalised peritonitis. There was less incidence of postoperative peritonitis, fewer reoperations and shorter hospital stays. In 55 patients undergoing primary resection, this took the form of Hartmann's procedure in 52 and only three had a primary anastomosis. The clear recommendation under these circumstances is to resect the sigmoid colon with or without anastomosis.

It is more difficult to decide if the operation has been performed prematurely or when the diagnosis is unexpected. Usually the latter situation arises from a misdiagnosis of gynaecological or appendicular sepsis. Increasingly, however, with the wider use of laparoscopy in the assessment of the acute abdomen, an inflamed left colon may be seen with a variable degree of peritoneal inflammatory response. Under these circumstances it is probably better not to proceed to laparotomy and resection, which may result in a stoma. The more appropriate action is antibiotic therapy in the expectation that the phlegmonous inflammation will resolve. Although this is an infrequent event in the authors' practice this approach has invariably resulted in rapid resolution without re-operation. The redundant manoeuvres of proximal stoma, drainage or, even worse, inappropriate resection with or without anastomosis are unwarranted. Adherence to dogma might dictate resection to eliminate the source of peritoneal contamination but the patient, often elderly and compromised, is subjected to a prolonged procedure with a major bowel resection and possibly a stoma which may prove permanent. Although presented as a life-saving operation, the mortality, morbidity, inconvenience and potential for a second major laparotomy in the authors' opinion outweigh the risks of non-resection under these circumstances.

When the policy is conservative management with urgent investigation whenever required the problem of operating on an inflamed but non-perforated colon rarely arises. Every surgeon with an emergency commitment should be aware that such a conservative option is not only available but usually preferable.

When to anastomose?

If the decision to resect is relatively straightforward when the indications for operation are patients with the most severe or progressive peritoneal sepsis, then the question of timing of anastomosis is more problematic. Considerations of safety have,

for the last 25 years, led to primacy of the Hartmann's procedure as the safest option in the management of left-sided colonic emergencies. Immediate resection without anastomosis eradicates the source of sepsis and the risk of anastomotic leakage albeit with the problems attendant on a stoma and either closure or exteriorisation of the rectal stump. These manoeuvres require the same care and attention to technical detail in fashioning an anastomosis in unfavourable circumstances. A left iliac fossa colostomy brought out under tension, particularly in an obese patient, creates problems as bad as a leaking anastomosis. Impacted faecal loading in the bowel proximal to the stoma or in the rectal stump may cause stercoral perforation or leakage of the rectal stump, particularly if there has been an inadequate resection with a long intraperitoneal rectal stump. Scyballous masses should be cleared both proximally and distally.

Increasing experience with immediate anastomosis after resection and on-table irrigation in the management of the obstructed colon has led to the selective implementation of this manoeuvre in patients considered to be at low risk of anastomotic failure after immediate resection for perforated diverticulitis. The results of two recent studies suggest that this procedure is safe in selected patients with septic complications. In the first study, 124 patients underwent emergency surgery, 49 of whom had a primary anastomosis, 33 had localised peritonitis and 16 generalised purulent peritonitis. There was a 7.2% mortality rate with one anastomotic leak and a morbidity rate of 45%. In the second study 45 patients underwent a similar emergency procedure without on-table colonic lavage. Eight patients were obstructed and 37 had septic complications. In the latter group, seven had phlegmonous disease, 21 localised pelvic peritonitis or pericolic abscess and nine had diffuse faecal or purulent peritonitis. There were three anastomotic leaks in the obstructed group, but only 1 in the septic group and a total of three deaths.

Anastomosis requires a fully resuscitated patient, competent anaesthesia and a surgeon trained in colorectal anastomoses. Access to a high level of postoperative care and supervision encourages early intervention to prevent the cardiovascular instability and hypoxaemia which promote anastomotic failure. A recent study has confirmed the benefits of high-dependency care in patients judged to be at high risk by POSSUM scoring. Circumstances may preclude these prerequisites, in which case considerations of safety should override surgical enthusiasm and anastomosis should be deferred.

Haemorrhage

The site and cause of major colonic bleeding should be identified preoperatively whenever possible either by angiography if actively bleeding or by labelled red cell scan if less acute. When this fails, peroperative colonoscopy should be attempted. Accurate localisation can lead to segmental resection, which may result in lower morbidity. If a bleeding point cannot be found then 'blind' subtotal colectomy must be performed. When this is necessary the patient's condition is usually unstable and it may be unwise to perform an ileorectal anastomosis. Completion of the operation by ileostomy and closure of the rectal stump is the prudent option. The possibility of subsequent restoration of bowel continuity can be considered later.

Practical aspects of management

Conservative management

Rapid resolution of peritoneal signs due to acute diverticulitis is to be expected in the great majority of patients. The author, routine practice for the majority of patients is vigorous conservative management with fluid resuscitation, appropriate monitoring and systemic antibiotics. Although single antibiotic agents may be as effective as combination therapy, none has been shown to be superior and most are more expensive. A tailored response reflecting the degree of contamination has proved successful over the years. A combination of metronidazole and trimethoprim, either orally or initially intravenously is effective against both aerobic and anaerobic organisms and is used for less severe episodes. For major sepsis combination therapy is favoured: gentamicin (7 mg/kg i.v. once daily) for rapid bactericidal activity against Gram-negative coliform organisms and metronidazole (500 mg i.v. t.i.d.) for anaerobic organisms. The authors are no longer convinced of the requirement for activity against enterococci and a penicillin derivative is not used in first-line therapy. Suitable alternative combinations include metronidazole and cefuroxime/ cefotaxime or single agents like coamoxiclav, imipenem or cefoxitin.

Although antibiotics serve as the mainstay of conservative therapy they must always be instituted before operation; the dramatic impact of systemic antibiotics on reducing the viable bacterial population in peritonitis is well documented. Repeated reassessment of the patient preferably by the same surgical team is essential to recognise a deteriorating condition.

Operative strategy

Optimal preoperative preparation of the patient undergoing laparotomy for advanced intraperitoneal sepsis with clinical assessment supplemented by appropriate monitoring must continue through to the postoperative period.

The patient is placed in the modified Lloyd-Davis position with suitable leg padding to prevent injury, especially to the lateral peroneal nerves, and intermittent pneumatic compression cuffs are fitted to the legs. This position also allows optimal access both to the rectum and the splenic flexure if the operating surgeon stands between the patient's legs while his assistants retract. It is usually necessary to mobilise both the hepatic and splenic flexures during on-table colonic lavage and mobilisation of the splenic flexure is often necessary to allow a tension-free colostomy.

Incision

A midline incision for its simplicity, reliable closure and low wound infection rate is used. It also allows easier access to the subdiaphragmatic recesses which are contaminated in generalised peritonitis and a more thorough peritoneal lavage and toilet can be performed. In laparotomy for diverticular disease the skin incision should be to the right of the umbilicus to avoid a subsequent left-sided stoma. Mechanical precautions to minimise contamination of the abdominal parietes from infected intraperitoneal material comprise wound towels, a plastic ring wound protector and institution of a 'red danger towel' technique. Before the peritoneum is opened widely the abdominal wall is elevated to allow aspiration of pus and contaminated peritoneal fluid before it percolates over and inocculates the wound. Whilst these manoeuvres lack individual scientific validation they appear effective as components of a strategy to reduce wound sepsis.

There are only disadvantages to a short incision in this emergency situation not least of which is failure to appreciate and document accurately the extent of peritoneal contamination and colonic disease. Restricted exposure and access inevitably results in inadequate surgery with poor peritoneal toilet and colonic mobilisation. Full access to all quadrants of the abdomen permits thorough assessment and classification of contamination. Inaccurate recording of the severity of peritoneal sepsis may arise because of inexperience, a desire to justify the decision to operate or in anticipation of an unfavourable outcome.

Although the operation is for presumed benign disease, there is little place for wedge excision of a few centimetres of sigmoid colon. If the affected area can be eliminated so readily the need for operation should be re-examined. Mobilisation of the left colon is equivalent to a radical cancer operation. This requires routine (although not invariable) mobilisation of the splenic flexure for tension-free formation of a stoma or anastomosis. The extent of resection of the colon is dictated by the extent of inflammation and adequacy of arterial pulsation at the point of division of the colon. If there is gross faecal loading of the colon and rectum, this should be evacuated, even in a Hartmann's procedure, to avoid stercoral perforation and obstruction proximal to a stoma.

Hartmann's procedure

If conditions preclude safe anastomosis the divided left colon is brought out through a trephined wound in the left lower quadrant, selecting a flat area of the abdomen and preferably emerging through the rectus abdominis muscle. Parastomal herniation may thereby be reduced. Closure of the lateral space is not required and if omitted facilitates subsequent reconstitution of bowel continuity. Closure of the rectal stump can be accomplished by cross-stapling or suturing, although the authors' experience (including closure of the rectal stump after total colectomy for inflammatory bowel disease) suggests fewer leaks in sutured cases. A single layer of continuous 2/0 or 3/0 serosubmucosal monofilament absorbable suture is supplemented with two long non-absorbable sutures at the lateral ends to aid future identification of the rectal stump.

Immediate anastomosis

Although there is debate about the need for mechanical preparation of the colon for left-sided anastomoses, on-table colonic irrigation achieves near perfect cleansing and has aesthetic if unproven clinical appeal (Figure 18.7). The appendix, or if absent the terminal ileum, is intubated with a Foley catheter. In the absence of a custom collection device corrugated anaesthetic tubing is inserted into the colon proximal to the diseased area and tied in place with nylon tape. The rigid corrugated tube, which should be as short as possible, usually results in siphoning with suction of the bowel wall into the tube as irrigation proceeds. This is prevented by inserting a 16 FG needle into the tubing to abolish the low pressure inducing the siphon.

The advantages of radical resection are that unexpected malignancy has been appropriately treated and healthy bowel is obtained for potential anastomosis. However it may be beneficial to keep the superior rectal artery intact when the diagnosis is unequivocally benign because this will improve perfusion of the upper rectum (Figure 18.8). The rectum is irrigated with aqueous chlorhexidine through a catheter passed into the rectum via a proctoscope. A site is chosen for division of the rectum which is usually at a point between the sacral promontory and peritoneal reflection. The proximal colon is divided and an open single layer serosubmucosal end-to-end colorectal anastomosis made with interrupted 3/0 sutures. There is no need for proximal 'defunctioning' stomata in anastomoses at this level.

Topical antibiotic lavage

For many years the authors used tetracycline solution (1 mg/ml 0.9% saline) to lavage the peritoneal cavity and abdominal parietes and this was associated with low wound and intraperitoneal infection rates. The withdrawal of a parenteral preparation of tetracycline from the UK market forced a change to cefotaxime as the topical agent of choice. This has been used for many years in the local paediatric hospital with comparable results and continuing audit suggests equivalence to tetracycline. Several litres may be required for peritoneal toilet and lavage and is repeated at the end of the procedure. The midline incision is closed with a continuous mass suture with 1 polydioxanone and the subcutaneous space is lavaged again before primary skin closure. This strategy, even in such 'dirty' surgery, is associated with a low wound infection rate and the authors have not found delayed primary closure to be necessary at a first laparotomy. Postoperative antibiotics are continued for only three days provided peritoneal contamination has been eliminated. Gentamicin levels are checked daily and if systemic sepsis persists beyond three days, bacteriology

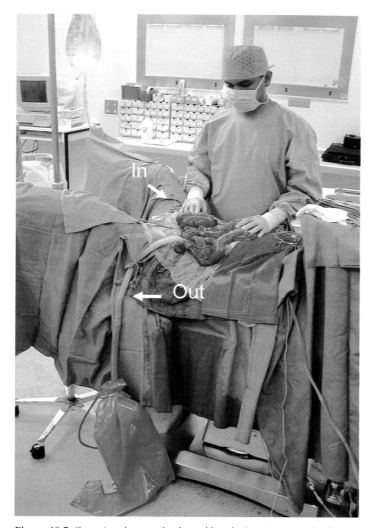

Figure 18.7 Operative photograph of on-table colonic irrigation with 3 l warm saline through a Foley catheter inserted via the appendix (In) with effluent collected in a plastic bag connected to anaesthetic tubing inserted into the distal descending colon (Out).

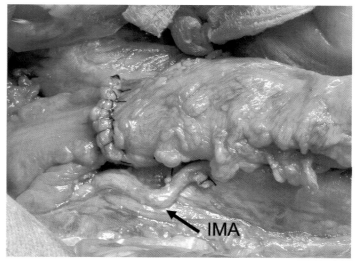

Figure 18.8 Operative photograph showing preserved inferior mesenteric artery (IMA) after emergency sigmoid colectomy with colorectal anastomosis.

and sensitivities from cultures taken at operation will be available to indicate a change of antibiotics.

Controversies in management

Timing of emergency surgery

If every patient with sigmoid diverticular disease was destined to proceed to colonic resection like those with colon cancer, an argument case could be made for early scheduled intervention with, preferably, a single-stage procedure during the acute admission. However, operation is necessary in a minority of patients and such an approach would subject often elderly patients to major surgery with the risk of avoidable mortality, stoma formation and anastomotic leakage. An excessively aggressive approach, whether born of enthusiasm or inexperience, can result in accumulating a large series of patients treated surgically. Such an unselected series should be associated with low mortality and morbidity and a high rate of single-stage procedures. It is possible that some patients with moderate diverticular inflammation are subjected to surgery in the belief, albeit misplaced, that it is a life-saving procedure. Under these circumstances data may be produced which appear to support conservative surgery in the management of complicated diverticulitis. Selection bias in such accounts can only be assessed if the total number of patients managed non-operatively during the study period is reported.

Resection of the source of sepsis

Indirect evidence supports the concept that elimination of the source of sepsis in the most severe forms of peritonitis is historically associated with lower mortality, but one of the two randomised comparative trials which compared primary resection with proximal stoma formation and drainage showed a lower mortality in the conservative group. The study, however, extended over many years and the conclusions are not widely accepted.

Single stage procedures with primary anastomosis

The role of primary resection and anastomosis during an emergency admission is liable to similar biases. If an emergency procedure can be accomplished with a minimal resection and completed with primary anastomosis this might reflect an incorrect decision to operate and an unnecessary resection rather than optimal management. Whilst a single-stage procedure in the presence of diffuse or faecal peritonitis remains controversial it can be used selectively when circumstances are wholly favourable.

Timing of elective surgery

Opinion is polarised on the need for surgery following conservative management of an acute episode of diverticulitis. Ambrosetti

has refined the argument by demonstrating a relationship between the severity of the episode as judged on CT scan with the risk of delayed complications. Patients categorised as 'mild' have a risk of recurrent episodes of 14% and 'severe' forms a risk of 39%. The corollary of this useful observation, however, is that the majority of patients do not suffer a further attack. The unanswered question is whether this level of risk merits subsequent colectomy. The variability of the acute disease and the wide spectrum of patients affected precludes categorical statements and exercise of clinical judgement remains appropriate. For example, the aged and infirm patient with a mild attack settling rapidly on antibiotics should simply be observed in anticipation that recurrence is unlikely.

There is considerable debate regarding the need for surgery in younger patients (variably defined as less than 40 or 50 years of age). The disease is said to run a more virulent course in this group, but this is based on retrospective data. Such reports have described the need for surgery in approximately 61–77% of patients under 40 years old following their first episode of diverticulitis. This contrasts to a rate of 30% for all ages. Others have argued against this aggressive approach based on their experience of these patients. They found that these young patients had few serious complications with subsequent attacks. In one series of 63 patients under 45 years old, only six presented with abscess or peritonitis and two-thirds responded completely to conservative management. This suggests that the disease may not be as virulent as suspected. Furthermore in a study of 40 young patients followed up for 9 years after medical treatment for acute diverticulitis, only 30% required further surgery, all of which were elective one-stage resections. Such conflicting data is variably interpreted as confirming the need for elective surgery or indicating that the majority of patients will not require operation and all should be managed conservatively. Ambrosetti has reported a recurrence rate of 60% for young patients with an initial severe episode of sepsis and even the mild form carried a 23% risk of further complications in their series. If these risks are reproducible elsewhere there would be a more potent argument for advocating routine resection in younger patients with a severe initial episode.

Any patient admitted twice with acute sepsis, albeit of limited extent, should be considered for operation whilst considering coincidental risk factors. Elective surgery in the younger patient is also a matter of judgement but majority opinion favours operation after a single attack. There is some evidence that long-term administration of a poorly absorbed antibiotic may reduce the frequency and severity of episodes of diverticular inflammation and is an option to be considered in the poor-risk patient. Similarly, increased admission rates in patients on non-steroidal antiinflammatory agents (NSAIDs) should encourage critical assessment of the need for these in the elderly.

Laparoscopic surgery in colonic diverticular disease

Laparoscopy has been advocated in the diagnosis and management of acute diverticulitis but the arguments for and against remain anecdotal for the present. Reservations about accurate description of case selection in open surgery apply equally to series of laparoscopic operations. There is an accumulating body of published evidence attesting to the applicability of laparoscopically assisted techniques for elective colectomy (Table 18.1). Although some papers have addressed the comparative costs of laparoscopic surgery for diverticular disease there has been no sophisticated health economic analysis to support or refute a wholesale change to this approach. Furthermore publication bias may present a more favourable picture of laparoscopic surgery in terms of morbidity and conversion rates than actually pertains. Nevertheless when successful a laparoscopic resection for sigmoid diverticular disease appears to be associated with short-term benefits in terms of duration of hospitalisation and convalescence.

The management of complicated diverticular disease requires careful clinical assessment, judicious use of appropriate imaging and a considered surgical strategy which combines a selective approach to surgery with a radical approach once committed if low mortality and morbidity are to be achieved.

COLONIC BLEEDING

Colonic bleeding can present major diagnostic and management dilemmas. Acute massive lower gastrointestinal bleeding, defined as bleeding from a source distal to the ligament of Treitz, accounts for 20% of acute gastrointestinal haemorrhage and 1.5% of all surgical emergencies. The problems of lower GI tract and colonic bleeding are in accurately locating the source of bleeding and deciding on the subsequent management. The difficulty in making the diagnosis is compounded by the fact that in many cases the bleeding is often self-limiting. Access to diagnostic and management options varies between individual institutions and the development of radionucleotide scanning, diagnostic and therapeutic angiography and colonoscopy has led to a moderate improvement in 'targeted' therapeutic modalities.

Table 18.1 Laparoscopic surgery for sigmoid diverticular disease. Review of published series comprising more than 20 procedures.

1st author	Year	No.	Conversion		Died	% mortality*
Burgel	2000	56	8	14.3%	–	
Tuech	2000	22	2	9.1%	–	
Kockerling	1999	304	22	7.2%	3	1.0%
Schlacta	1999	92	6	6.5%	–	
Siriser	1999	65	3	4.6%	–	
Smadja	1999	54	5	9.2%	–	
Berthou	1999	110	9	8.2%	–	
Petropoulos	1998	171	18	10.5%	1	0.6%
Schiedeck	1998	57	8	14.0%	1	1.8%
Carbajo	1988	22	2	9.1%	–	
Eijsbouts	1997	41	5	12.2%	–	
Bruce	1996	25	3	12.0%	–	
Overall		1019	91	8.9%	5	0.5%

*Percentage mortality as a percentage of the number of deaths/number of patients.

Aetiology

Not all patients presenting with profuse rectal bleeding are bleeding from the large bowel (Table 18.2). In a 2-year prospective study performed in an open-access bleeding unit there were 278 admissions (17%) with suspected lower GI haemorrhage: 252 were confirmed and 48% were felt to be significant. A total of 102 (83%) of significant bleeds occurred in patients over 60 years of age. The commonest causes of lower gastrointestinal bleeding are angiodysplasia and diverticular disease.

Table 18.2 Final source of haemorrhage in patients presenting with massive fresh rectal bleeding

Site of bleeding	
Colon/rectum	85%
Upper gastrointestinal tract	10%
Small intestine	5%

Angiodysplasia

Angiodysplastic lesions consist of a small collection of dilated venules and thin-walled capillaries, usually less than 5 mm in diameter, which are only separated from the colonic lumen by a single layer of epithelium. They are considered to be degenerative phenomenon and consequently more common in the elderly. They are produced by obstruction of submucosal veins secondary to colonic distension and peristalsis of the muscularis propria. They are normally found in the proximal colon but have been described in both the transverse colon and distal ileum. This predominance in the right side of the colon may relate to its diameter and wall tension (Laplace's law). The reported incidence varies from 25% in asymptomatic patients over 60 years of age to 0.83% in 964 patients older than 50 years. The incidence depends on how carefully the colon is examined and in one series of 1938 total colonoscopies, only 59 (3.0%) patients were found to have angiodysplasia. These variations may reflect differences in the study populations and reasons for colonoscopy.

Bleeding from angiodysplasia tends to be intermittent with 15% presenting with massive bleeding. Ninety percent stop bleeding spontaneously but bleeding recurs in 25% of patients. These patients may have up to five episodes of haemorrhage before the diagnosis is made.

Other vascular malformations including venous ectasias and various hamartomas also cause major haemorrhage. Cavernous haemangioma can affect the gastrointestinal tract and 50% involve the rectum. The Osler-Weber-Rendu syndrome (hereditary haemorrhagic telangiectasia) is an autosomal-dominant disorder associated with skin, oropharyngeal and gastrointestinal telangiectasia which bleed intermittently.

Inflammatory bowel disease

It is surprising that more patients with inflammatory bowel disease do not present with major colorectal haemorrhage. Massive bleeding tends to be slightly more common in Crohn's disease than ulcerative colitis but is the presenting feature in less than 1% of all patients. The colon is the major source of such haemorrhage and may precipitate urgent colectomy or proctectomy (Figure 18.9).

Colonic neoplasia

Major bleeding from benign colonic neoplasms is unusual unless the patient is anticoagulated *(vide infra)*. Bleeding occurs after less than 1% of colonoscopic polypectomies and can be either reactionary or secondary in character presenting over one week after the initial procedure. The majority can be managed non-operatively.

Colonic carcinoma remains a very rare cause of such major bleeding (Figure 18.10A & B) accounting for 10–15% of bleeding in elderly patients and massive bleeding was reported in 6% of 114 colonic neoplasms in one series. This study is probably an overestimate and may reflect variations in referral patterns.

Ischaemic and other colitis

Ischaemic colitis presents with bloody diarrhoea, typically dark in colour, and major haemorrhage is a rare event. Although it can involve any part of the colon, it predominantly affects the area of the splenic flexure or mid-sigmoid colon in elderly women.

Infective colitis, especially *Escherichia coli 0157*, has been implicated in lower GI bleeding which can vary from blood mixed with stool to frank haemorrhage.

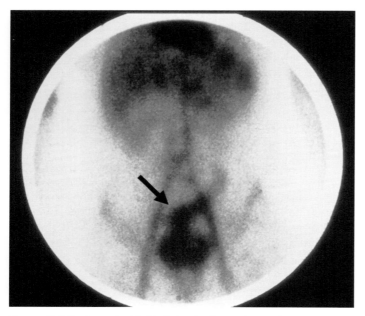

Figure 18.9 Radio-nucleotide-labelled red cell scan showing haemorrhage into rectum in a patient with an ileorectal anastomosis after total colectomy for Crohn's disease several years previously.

Bleeding secondary to radiation enteritis for pelvic malignancies usually presents several months following the completion of treatment. Bleeding tends to be chronic and recurrent with the rectum most commonly affected. Sustained active haemorrhage is fortunately rare because surgical intervention to gain control is a dangerous undertaking.

Miscellaneous causes

Other rare causes of active bleeding are endometriosis, solitary rectal ulcer syndrome and anorectal varices. Dieulafoy lesions, more often described in the upper gastrointestinal tract have been described in the colon and rectum. The lesion presents as small superficial mucosal ulcerations with a protruding submucosal artery and bleeding can be massive.

Anal disease rarely produces substantial acute blood loss. Haemorrhoids and fissures may bleed but this usually of small volume unless associated with coagulopathy or due to secondary haemorrhage. Nevertheless proctoscopy should be performed routinely to rule out an anal source of bleeding.

Pharmacological

Bleeding can be induced or aggravated by medication. Anticoagulation which may be in the therapeutic range can unmask a previously undiagnosed colonic condition including cancer, polyp or angiodysplasia. Coagulation studies should be performed and a cause sought without attributing the bleeding simply to the anticoagulation.

NSAIDs have been incriminated in an increased risk of lower gastro-intestinal bleeding and again may precipitate bleeding from a co-existent mucosal condition. Enteric-coated potassium chloride occasionally produces significant haemorrhage secondary to jejunal ulceration.

MANAGEMENT AND EVALUATION OF MAJOR LOWER GASTROINTESTINAL BLEEDING

Management can be divided into assessment, resuscitation, diagnosis and therapy. These stages are not exclusive and resuscitation may be required during the assessment of a patient bleeding heavily. Furthermore a lucid history may be difficult to obtain from an elderly patient confused due to hypotension and hypoxia secondary to a major bleed. A sense of urgency in resuscitating a shocked patient should not preclude an attempt to obtain an accurate history from either the patient or the patient's relatives.

Assessment

The age of the patient has a major impact on the likelihood of the underlying cause of major haemorrhage (Figure 18.11). It would,

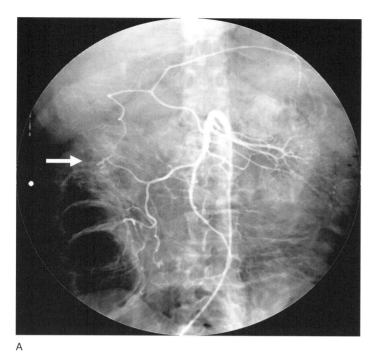

A

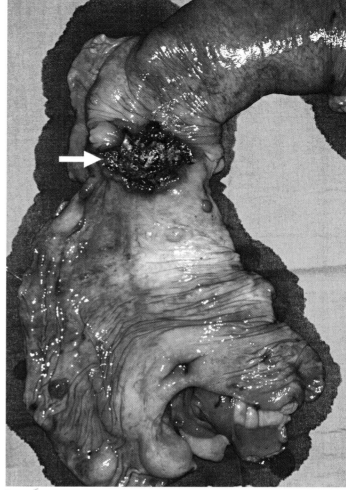

B

Figure 18.10 A Superior mesenteric angiogram in a patient presenting with major colonic haemorrhage showing abnormal pattern in ascending colon (arrow). **B** Resected specimen in same patient with cancer ulcerating into an artery in the colonic wall (arrow).

for example, be rare for a 40-year-old patient to have angiodysplasia, whereas an ulcerated Meckel's diverticulum is more likely in a child. The type of bleeding including colour, intensity, timing and persistence may suggest a possible source, e.g. maroon stools from a proximal colonic source. However both the colour of the stool and patients' descriptions can be an inaccurate guide. Melaena is usually associated with bleeding from the stomach and duodenum but has been found in blood loss from the caecum. Stool colour is influenced by both the volume of blood and transit time in addition to the source of blood loss. In one study of patients with massive rectal bleeding 14% of patients had an upper GI source. Bloody diarrhoea associated with mucus and pus may indicate a colitic process.

Abdominal pain can be a feature of ischaemic colitis, inflammatory bowel disease, radiation enteritis and infective colitis, and anal pain may point to a fissure. Many causes of lower GI blood loss are recurrent and a history of previous bleeds in a middle-aged or elderly patient may indicate diverticular disease or angiodysplasia. Previous investigations and procedures including endoscopy,

contrast studies, colonoscopic polypectomy or haemorrhoidectomy may be significant. Even banding of piles can cause significant blood loss in 0.6% of patients.

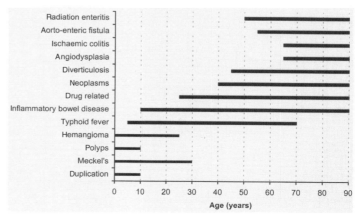

Figure 18.11 Diagrammatic representation of distribution of sources of massive rectal bleeding with age (Adapted from: Jones PF *Emergency Abdominal Surgery* 2nd Edn London Blackwell 1987).

Beta-blockers may affect the vital signs of patients by suppressing the tachycardia associated with major blood loss. In contrast anti-hypertensives may exaggerate the associated hypotension. A history of excess alcohol ingestion raises the possibility of a variceal bleed.

Clinical examination is directed at detecting both the cause and effect of major blood loss. Features of blood loss should be assessed and stigmata of chronic liver disease, splenomegaly and telangiectasia may be identified. Abdominal pain and tenderness are often absent in patients with major rectal bleeding. Anal examination is mandatory. It allows the colour of stool to be assessed and the perianal signs of Crohn's may be identified. Procto-sigmoidoscopy should be performed unless there is immediate access to flexible endoscopy and even this limited examination may detect the cause of bleeding in 10% of cases. Occasionally normal stool can be visualised above an area of bright red blood loss and this can direct investigations appropriately.

Baseline assays of haemoglobin and haematocrit levels are measured, although early in the bleed these may not have equilibrated. Blood is also taken for cross-matching. A clotting screen is necessary and may need to be repeated, especially if large volume resuscitation and transfusion are required. Liver disease and clotting abnormalities which may be aggravated by massive transfusion may require fresh frozen plasma or other clotting factors.

Resuscitation

In patients who are bleeding heavily it is more important to achieve early and good i.v. access to permit rapid infusion of fluids than to secure central venous access for monitoring purposes. Central catheters have a lower infusion rate and early use is not indicated. Crystalloid or synthetic colloid solutions are used according to local protocol until laboratory results are available. These results and the clinical condition will direct blood transfusion. In the unusual event of near exsanguination then group O Rhesus-negative blood can be transfused. Monitoring urine flow is useful in these patients, who are best cared for in a high-dependency or specialised bleeding unit. In such an environment arterial and venous monitoring can be performed as indicated. Fortunately most lower gastrointestinal bleeds stop and invasive monitoring is often unnecessary unless there is significant co-existing morbidity.

Diagnosis

It is not always possible to make either a quick or indeed accurate diagnosis in patients presenting with massive rectal bleeding. The majority of bleeds stop spontaneously and even if recurrent, it can be difficult to pinpoint the cause and site of bleeding. In patients who stop bleeding and remain stable, standard investigations including colonoscopy and barium enema can be used. The dilemma arises in the group of patients who continue to bleed heavily or in whom bleeding recurs.

It is important to consider angiography early in the course of a bleed because this is most sensitive when bleeding is ongoing. The accuracy of angiography depends on the rate of blood loss which should be in excess of 0.5–1.0 ml/min. Selective mesenteric angiography has been successful in identifying a source in up to 80% of investigations. However, rapid access to angiography by skilled interventional radiologists is not universally available particularly out of hours. Routine angiography may not be available and detection rates can fall to 50% even in experienced hands. Pharmacological manoeuvres, e.g. heparin and thrombolytic agents have been used to provoke or exacerbate bleeding, with improvement in detection and a reduction in false-negative investigations, albeit at a small risk of dangerous increase in the rate of blood loss.

Intraoperative angiography has been used especially in small bowel haemorrhage and the angiogram catheter which had been placed preoperatively can be left *in situ* to facilitate operative angiography. The bowel should be marked with metal clips to allow easier identification of a vascular abnormality. Methylene blue, injected via the catheter, has been used to stain the area of an identified vascular anomaly and may be more precise than operative enteroscopy.

Angiography catheters may have a therapeutic as well as diagnostic role. Infusion of vasopressin has been used to control both small and large bowel haemorrhage but there are serious potential side effects, particularly intestinal and peripheral vascular ischaemia. Intraarterial embolisation with, for example, coils and polyvinyl sponge can be selectively used to control haemorrhage and may be superior to vasopressin. Whatever the technique, there is a danger of infarction and perforation which may be an acceptable risk in very high-risk patients or allow surgery to be performed in an elective setting.

Radionucleotide scintigraphy has been used in patients with lower GI blood loss. Sulphur colloid, technetium (99Tc) and technetium-labelled red blood cell scintigraphy have both advantages and disadvantages. They are more useful in recurrent bleeding because the isotope remains in the circulation for over 48 hours but may not be so useful in profuse blood loss. The sensitivity of radioisotope scanning for demonstrating blood loss is high in comparison to angiography, but it lacks precision in accurately localising the site of haemorrhage. Its accuracy can be less than 50%.

Colonoscopy has been advocated as the initial diagnostic manoeuvre with detection rates of 90% being reported. In addition therapeutic colonoscopy can be successful in 50% of cases. In intermittent bleeding its use in a semi-elective setting is indisputable but colonoscopy in massive bleeding is more problematic. Visibility is impaired although novel irrigation techniques and improved suction channels in modern colonoscopes may overcome some of these problems. Enemata or even formal bowel preparation 'if time allows' all improve visibility with high detection rates of up to 90%. Colonoscopy may detect the bleeding site but even when unsuccessful in demonstrating the source may identify an area of concern.

Preoperative detection of angiodysplasia is entirely dependent on good quality colonoscopy which may also permit immediate management with laser, sclerotherapy or diathermy. It is important to note that 20% of patients with an identified vascular lesion can bleed from an alternative site.

Intraoperative colonoscopy with on-table lavage is a useful technique and it may make a diagnosis when preoperative attempts failed. Upper GI endoscopy may also be required and it is useful to have facilities available for both upper and lower GI endoscopy in theatre when a patient with massive bleeding has to proceed undiagnosed to operation.

Therapy

Not all patients require surgery. The majority stop bleeding and the underlying condition once identified may not warrant an operation. Several conditions can be managed locally, e.g. injection of polypectomy site, sclerotherapy for angiodysplasia or by interventional radiological techniques. However some patients do require surgery and in a large series reported from an open access bleeding unit 12.6% of patients over 60 years of age required emergency surgery with diverticular disease being the commonest condition.

If surgery is indicated for continuing or recurrent bleeding the outcome depends on the ability to find the cause and site of bleeding. Mortality rates are markedly reduced when targeted segmental resection of the colon is performed compared to 'blind' subtotal colectomy despite the fact that re-bleeding rates are similar. Transfusion requirements and timing of the surgery influence both the need for surgery and mortality rates. In a series of 96 patients, 88% of patients who required over 1.5 L of blood required surgery whereas none of the patients who received less than this volume of blood required an operation. Whilst the volume of blood transfused may assist in the decision to operate a predetermined level of haemoglobin of 6 gdL has also been used.

Increased transfusion requirement is associated with an increase in mortality and morbidity. There was a 45% mortality rate for those receiving 10 units or more of blood compared to 7.7% for those receiving less. Surgery should be considered, therefore, when there is life-threatening haemorrhage, ongoing hypotension, a transfusion requirement over 4–6 units in a 24-hour period and certainly before 10 units are given and if re-bleeding occurs.

OPERATIVE SURGERY

When operation is indicated the patient should be positioned in a modified Lloyd-Davies position to allow access to the whole abdomen and perineum. Facilities for gastroscopy, colonoscopy and on-table colonic irrigation should be available. Segmental resections should be performed when the diagnosis is made preoperatively and may reduce morbidity. Difficulty arises in

10–50% of patients when there is no diagnosis. In this situation, on-table colonic lavage via a catheter in the appendix with a rigid scope in the rectum is performed. The colonoscope can then be passed *per rectum* and manipulated readily to the caecum or even small bowel if necessary by the abdominal surgeon. Gentle handling is important to avoid trauma to the bowel because petechiae mimic angiodysplasia. The operating lights can be dimmed and the bowel transilluminated to identify small lesions.

The distribution of blood seen during colonoscopy can be helpful in localising an affected segment, if not a precise source of bleeding and define the extent of resection. If fresh blood is seen only in the right colon a right hemicolectomy may be preferred to a total colectomy. Mortality rates can be as low as 5% with re-bleeding, less than 20% if a limited resection can be performed. Patients are thereby spared the disadvantages of diarrhoea and possible incontinence which may follow an ileorectal anastomosis. If re-bleeding does occur completion colectomy may be required although in a number of cases the bleeding is found to arise from the small intestine. For this reason urgent repeat investigation including angiography should be considered.

With all the panoply of modern imaging it is important to remember that a total colectomy may still be necessary when all diagnostic modalities have failed to define the source. Under these circumstances ileorectal anastomosis should only be considered if the patient is in a stable well-resuscitated state.

FURTHER READING

Ambrosetti P. Diverticulitis of the left colon. In Recent Advances in Surgery Vol 20. Eds Taylor I, Johnson CD: 1997: 145–160

Ambrosetti P, Morel P. Acute left sided colonic diverticulitis: diagnosis and surgical indications after successful conservative therapy of first time acute diverticulitis. *Zentralbl Chir* 1998; **123**:1382–1385

Berthou JC, Charbonneau P. Elective laparoscopic management of sigmoid diverticulitis. Results in a series of 110 patients. *Surg Endoscopy* 1999; **13**:457–460

Biondo S, Perea MT, Rague D et al. One stage procedure in non-elective surgery for diverticular disease complications. *Colorectal Dis* 2001; **3**:42–45

Bramley PJ, Masson JW, McKnight G et al. The role of an open-access bleeding unit in the management of colonic haemorrhage. A 2-year prospective study. *Scand J Gastroenterol* 1996; **31**:764–769

Bruce CJ, Coller A, Murray JJ et al. Laparoscopic resection for diverticular disease. *Dis Colon Rectum* 1996; **39**:S1–S6.

Burgel JS, Navarro F, Lemoine MC et al. Elective laparoscopic-assisted sigmoidectomy for diverticulitis. Prospective study of 56 cases. *Ann Chir* 2000; **125**:231–237

Carbajo Caballero MA, Martin del Olmo JC, Blanco JI, de la Cuesta C, Atienza R. The laparoscopic approach in the treatment of diverticular colon disease. *J Soc Laparoendoscopic Surg* 1998; **2**:159–161

Driver CP, Anderson DA, Keenan RA. Massive intestinal bleeding in association with Crohn's disease. *J R Coll Surg Edinb* 1996; **41**:152–153

Eggesbo HB. Jacobsen T, Kolmannskog F et al. Diagnosis of acute left sided colonic diverticulitis by three radiological modalities. *Acta Radiol* 1998; **39**:315–321

Eijsbouts QA, Cuesta MA, de Brauw LM, Sietses C. Elective laparoscopic assisted sigmoid resection for diverticular disease. *Surg Endosc* 1997; **11**:750–753

Foutch PG, Rex DK, Lieberman DA. Prevalence and natural history of colonic angiodysplasia among healthy asymptomatic people. *Am J Gastroenterol* 1995; **90**:564–567

Gledhill A, Dixon MF. Crohn's-like reaction in diverticular disease. *Gut* 1998; **42**:392–395

Gomes AS, Lois JF, McCoy RD. Angiographic treatment of gastrointestinal hemorrhage: comparison of vasopressin infusions and embolization. *AJR* 1986; **146**:1031–1037

Gooszen AW, Tollenaar RAEM, Geelkerken RH. Prospective study of primary anastomosis following sigmoid resection for suspected acute complicated diverticular disease. *Br J Surg* 2001; **88**:693–697

Hinchey EJ, Schall PGH, Richards GK. Treatment of perforated disease of the colon. *Adv Surg* 1978; **12**:86–109

Jensen DM Management of severe lower gastrointestinal bleeding. *Gastrointestinal Endoscopy* 1995; **41**:171–173

Killingback M. Management of perforated diverticulitis. *Surg Clin North Am* 1983; **63**:97–115

Knutsen OH, Wahlby L. Colonic haemorrhage in diverticular disease – diagnosis and treatment. *Acta Chir Scand* 1984; **150**:259–264

Kockerling F, Schneider C, Reymond MA et al. Laparoscopic resection of sigmoid diverticulitis. Results of a multicenter study. *Surg Endosc* 1999; **13**:567–571

Kronborg O. Treatment of perforated sigmoid diverticulitis: a prospective randomised trial. *Br J Surg* 1993; **80**:505–507

Krukowski ZH, Matheson NA. Emergency surgery for diverticular disease complicated by generalized and faecal peritonitis: a review. *Br J Surg* 1984; **71**:921–927

Krukowski ZH, Matheson NA. A ten-year computerised audit of infection after abdominal surgery. *Br J Surg* 1988; **75**:857–861

MacRae HM, McLeod RS: Comparison of haemorrhoidal treatment modalities. A meta-analysis. *Dis Colon Rectum* 1995; **38**:687–694

McGuire HH. Bleeding colonic diverticula. A reappraisal of natural history and management. *Ann Surg* 1994; **220**:653–656

Petropoulos P, Nassiopoulos K, Chanson C. Laparoscopic therapy of diverticulitis. *Zentralbl Chir* 1998; **123**:1390–1393

Pohlman T. Diverticulitis. *Gastrointest Clin North Am* 1988; **17**:357–385

Ogunbiyi OA, Fleshman JW. The limitations and disadvantages of radionuclide scintigraphy. *Semin Colon Rectal Surg* 1997; **8**:161–163

O'Kelly TJ, Krukowski ZH. Acute diverticulitis. Non-operative management. In Crucial Controversies in Surgery Vol 3. Eds Schein M Wise L: 1999: 109–116

Rampton DS. Diverticular colitis: diagnosis and management. *Colorectal Dis* 2001; **3**:149–153

Rao PM, Rhea JT, Novelline RA et al. Helical CT with only colonic contrast material for diagnosing diverticulitis: prospective evaluation of 150 patients. *Am J Roentgenol* 1998; **170**:1445–1449

Rao PM. CT of diverticulitis and alternative conditions. *Semin Ultrasound CT MR* 1999; **20**:86–93

Schiedeck TH, Schwander O, Bruch HP. Laparoscopic sigmoid resection in diverticulitis. *Chirurg* 1998; **69**:846–853

Schlachta CM, Mamazza J, Poulin EC. Laparoscopic sigmoid resection for acute and chronic diverticulitis. An outcomes comparison with laparoscopic resection for nondiverticular disease. *Surg Endoscopy* 1999; **13**:649–653

Siriser F. Laparoscopic assisted colectomy for diverticular sigmoiditis. A single-surgeon prospective study of 65 patients. *Surg Endosc* 1999; **13**:811–813

Smadja C, Sbai Idrissi M, Tahrat M et al. Elective laparoscopic sigmoid colectomy for diverticulitis. Results of a prospective study. *Surg Endosc* 1999; **13**:645–648

The Standards Task Force American Society of Colon and Rectal Surgeons. Practice parameters for sigmoid diverticulitis. *Dis Colon Rectum* 1995; **38**:125–132

Tudor RG, Farmakis N, Keighley MRB. National audit of complicated diverticular disease: analysis of index cases. *Br J Surg* 1994; **81**:730–732

Tuech JJ, Pessaux P, Rouge C et al. Laparoscopic v open colectomy for sigmoid diverticulitis: a prospective comparative study in the elderly. *Surg Endosc* 2000; **14**:1031–1033

Wess L, Eastwood MA, Wess TJ, Busuttil A, Miller A. Cross linkage of collagen is increased in colonic diverticulosis. *Gut* 1995; **37**:91–94

Whiteway J, Morson BC. Elastosis in diverticular disease of the sigmoid colon. *Gut* 1985; **26**:258–266

Wright HK, Pelliccia O, Higgins EF et al. Controlled, semi-elective, segmental resection for massive colonic hemorrhage. *Am J Surg* 1980; **139**:535–538

Zeitoun G, Laurent A, Rouffet F et al. Multicentre randomized clinical trial of primary versus secondary sigmoid resection in generalized peritonitis complicating sigmoid diverticulitis. *Br J Surg* 2000; **87**:1366–1374

Neoplasms of the colon and rectum

R. Al-Mufti, P.B. Boulos, I. Taylor

BENIGN TUMOURS OF THE COLON AND RECTUM

Benign tumours can arise from each component of the colon and rectum. With the exception of mucosal polyps (such as adenomas), other benign tumours are rare.

Colonic polyps

Clinical features

Polyps that are of clinical relevance are the adenomas, because of their malignant potential which depends on the morphology, size and histological cell differentiation. Adenomas are frequently asymptomatic and are detected by chance at sigmoidoscopy, on a barium enema or colonoscopy performed for an unrelated indication. However, when sizeable, excessive mucus secretion and bleeding from mucosal ulceration causing anaemia, become clinically evident, particularly when polyps are in the distal colon or the rectum. The presence of a large adenoma in the recto-sigmoid region can give the sensation of incomplete evacuation with tenesmus and when pedunculated, may prolapse into the anal canal. In the proximal colon large adenomas may intussuscept and cause intestinal obstruction.

Colorectal polyps can be classified as neoplastic (such as adenomas) or non-neoplastic (such as hamartomatous and inflammatory) polyps.

Neoplastic polyps

Neoplastic polyps may be adenomas, carcinomas, carcinoid or mesenchymal tumours. Adenomas are usually polypoid neoplasms. All adenomas start as a neoplastic change in a single crypt (microadenomas) which gradually increases in size. Adenomas should be regarded as foci of intraepithelial neoplasia with the potential to evolve into invasive carcinoma. Adenomas can be tubular, villous or tubulovillous. The genetic predisposition for adenomatous polyps involves mutations or deletions of the APC gene, COX1 and COX2 and DNA methylation, which are discussed later, as they are similar to those that predispose to malignancy.

- *Tubular adenomas* are the commonest type and form up to 65% of adenomas. They have a smooth lobulated surface, more often pedunculated, and are well differentiated, consisting of mostly glandular tissue resembling colonic mucosa, with a stalk which can be 3–4 cm long.

- *Villous adenomas* are less differentiated, less common (only 10% of adenomas) and invariably sessile and consist of long papillary processes covered by epithelium, which secretes mucin, and often carpet many centimetres of the colon. They generally exhibit a frond-like hard surface. Size for size, villous adenomas carry a 10-fold higher risk than purely tubular types for malignant potential.

- *Tubulovillous adenomas (mixed)* form 25% of the adenomas and show mixed features of both tubular and villous types in frequency and morphology.

Malignant changes in a polyp

The malignant potential of an adenomatous polyp depends on the:

- size

- type of the adenoma

- pattern of growth

- number

- degree of epithelial atypia (dysplasia).

Severely dysplastic adenomas have pronounced architectural disturbance of gland formation and cytological abnormality referred to as carcinoma *in situ*. The presence of multiple adenomas will enhance the risk of malignancy. Most adenomas under 1 cm in diameter are benign and the hazard is low, 10% of adenomas with 1–2 cm in diameter show malignant changes and 45–50% of adenomas larger than 2 cm in diameter will show malignant changes. Over 50% of the larger adenomas are found in the rectum. Familial adenomatous polyposis (FAP) syndromes are important examples of neoplastic adenomas. Hyperplastic polyps are unique to the colon, the cause of which is unknown, but are believed to arise from failure of the normal sloughing mechanism of cells at the epithelial surface.

Polyposis syndromes

These present with diarrhoea and rectal bleeding and the diagnosis is based on the appearances at colonoscopy and on tissue biopsy, although in adolescence and young adulthood specific syndromes may show some characteristic features. Classification of familial and non-familial syndromes is determined by histology, which is an essential requirement for management.

FAMILIAL ADENOMATOUS POLYPOSIS SYNDROMES (FAP)

These syndromes occur in 1:8000 to 1:10 000 births in the UK and 1:5000 inhabitants in the USA. They are among the commonest autosomal dominant syndromes predisposing to cancer. Polyps begin to appear in the second decade of life. At the time of maturity, hundreds and thousands of polyps result, which carpet the entire surface of the colon. Polyps usually arise in the rectum, sigmoid and left colon. Left untreated, one or more of the polyps will progress to cancer, which appears before the age of 40 (i.e. at least 20 years earlier than the appearance of cancers among unaffected individuals). FAP can be part of many syndromes. The first described was that by Gardner in 1951.

GARDNER'S SYNDROME

A variant of FAP, which is also autosomal dominant, with polyps appearing in the colon, stomach and duodenum. In addition to the adenomas, the patients develop osteomas of the mandible and skull, multiple epidermoid cysts, supernumerary and impacted teeth, skin fibromas, desmoid tumours and congenital hypertrophy of the retinal pigment epithelium (CHRPE) which presents in early teenage life. Other rare extracolonic manifestations of these syndromes include carcinomas (of the duodenum, pancreas, adrenal gland and thyroid papillary carcinoma) and benign tumours (of the duodenum, pancreas, adrenals and thyroid).

TURCOT'S SYNDROME

A variant of FAP, in which there are also malignant tumours in the central nervous system (including astrocytomas, glioblastoma multiforme and medulloblastomas).

JUVENILE POLYPOSIS

These are hamartomatous polyps, which are usually solitary and can occur in any part of the alimentary tract, but more commonly in the colon and rectum. They most commonly appear in the first five years of life, as rounded smooth-surfaced polyps, 1–2 cm in diameter with a short stalk, and can undergo torsion and present with rectal bleeding and anaemia. There have been rare instances when solitary juvenile polyps have undergone neoplastic changes, with dysplasia and then later invasive carcinoma. Familial juvenile polyposis is inherited and occurs when more than 10 polyps are present.

CRONKHITE–CANADA SYNDROME

This is a rare but fatal condition, with diffuse gastrointestinal polyposis (stomach and colon), skin pigmentation, alopecia and atrophy of nails. The polyps resemble juvenile polyposis, but a notable feature is the microscopic mucus retention cysts in the mucosa and common presenting symptoms include diarrhoea and gastrointestinal bleeding. Adenomas and colorectal carcinoma have been reported in Cronkhite–Canada syndrome.

RUVAKABA–MYHRE–SMITH SYNDROME

This is associated with hamartomatous polyps of the colon and ileum with ectodermal changes which include pigmentation of the penis and macrocephaly. The commonest symptoms are diarrhoea, gastrointestinal bleeding and obstruction. It is regarded as a variant of juvenile polyposis and similarly managed.

PEUTZ–JEGHERS SYNDROME

This is typically more common in the small bowel and stomach, but may be found in the colon and rectum. There are sessile arborising lesions with a core of smooth muscle covered by normal mucosa. In those rare instances where the syndrome is complicated by the development of an adenocarcinoma, the malignancies occur most frequently in the stomach and duodenum, but not in the colon or rectum. Patients with Peutz–Jeghers syndrome present with abdominal colic, intestinal obstruction and anaemia from multiple polyps predominant in the small intestine that develop after puberty. An associated sign is pigmentation in the perioral and buccal mucosa which fade with age. Diagnosis includes gastroscopy and colonoscopy and if the presence of polyps with representative histology is confirmed, a routine barium meal, with 20mg of hyoscine hydrobromide intravenously to stop peristalsis, and compression of the bowel for detail will delineate polyps in the small intestine.

Non-neoplastic polyps

These include metaplastic, hamartomatous, inflammatory and lymphoid polyps.

Metaplastic polyps are synonymous with hyperplastic polyps and occur in the elderly as small pale grey sessile nodules, a few millimetres across. These lack dysplastic features and apparently do not have malignant potential. Metaplastic polyposis can be confused with FAP due to the large numbers of polyps which may be present in both conditions.

Hamartomatous polyps in the colon are of two types: juvenile polyps and Peutz–Jeghers polyps, which may be single or multiple. There is a strong family history, particularly with multiple ones. The presentation is at a young age and hamartomas are frequently associated with adenomatous change and therefore there is a small risk of malignant transformation. Treatment is usually polypectomy via colonoscopy or colectomy. Hamartomatous polyposis includes disorders with polyps of normal epithelium present in abnormal amount and configuration.

Lymphoid polyposis consists of lymphoid aggregates in the rectum which undergo reactive hyperplasia and present a polypoid appearance. This harmless condition is found mainly in young women, probably as a result of viral infection, and in patients with immunodeficiency states.

Inflammatory polyps. This refers to lymphoid hyperplasia and the mucosal appearance in inflammatory bowel disease. The mucosa in the acute inflammatory disease becomes congested and densely infiltrated with leucocytes and plasma cells, with lymphoid aggregates and neutrophils marginating in congested blood vessels. This condition is occasionally referred to as pseudo-polyps. Inflammatory polyposis is more commonly associated with ulcerative colitis than with Crohn's disease and treatment is of the primary disease.

Management of colonic polyps

Treatment is by complete excision and histological examination of the polyp. Polyps are best removed by endoscopic snare polypectomy and a thorough examination of the colon performed at the same time to ensure that it is clear of synchronous polyps.

When a polyp is seen on a routine sigmoidoscopy, a tissue biopsy should be avoided since this will not provide full information on the true nature of the polyp and may result in unnecessary bleeding. Only if the polyp is of such a small size as to allow its complete removal within the cups of the biopsy forceps should this type of biopsy be attempted. Since hyperplastic polyps have low malignant potential, they do not need to be kept under close surveillance and histological confirmation is essential in order to avoid unnecessary colonoscopy in these patients.

However, in about 5% of polyps safe polypectomy may not be feasible because of its size or because the base is too broad. Invariably these are sessile villous adenomas with a high potential for malignancy, which increases from about 1% when an adenoma is 10 mm in diameter to nearly 50% when it is 25 mm or more but this is not ascertainable until the whole specimen is examined histologically. A preoperative biopsy is unreliable as it is more likely to miss the area of invasion. Sessile villous adenomas are common in the rectum and digital examination may not be sensitive enough to detect subtle malignant change. Endoanal ultrasonography identifies evidence of infiltration into the muscularis propria associated with malignancy. It is also a useful preoperative diagnostic aid, as this information will help determine the extent of excision. Endoscopic ultrasonography allows examination of lesions beyond the reach of the endorectal probe.

Growths within 10 cm (lower and mid rectum) which are too large for snare polypectomy are suitable for surgical excision by the technique of endoanal submucosal excision. With an endoanal retractor, the lesion is exposed and stay sutures are placed in the mucosa about a few millimetres away from the edge of the tumour for traction during dissection. The submucosa is infiltrated with saline containing adrenaline in a dilution of 1:300 000 until the mucosa is elevated, to allow dissection along the submucosal plane and the adenoma is excised with a clear margin. Obliteration of the submucosal plane is suggestive of focal malignant infiltration when excision of the full thickness of the rectal wall is required and the defect closed.

When high in the upper rectum and inaccessible for endoanal excision, transanal endoscopic microsurgery (TEM) avoids an abdominal approach. This technique requires special equipment and expertise not widely available. Large circumferential villous adenomas extending proximally require abdominal excision usually by anterior resection. When these are in the colon a standard resection with lymphovascular clearance is the recommended procedure because of the high probability of malignancy.

Management of Peutz–Jegher and Juvenile polyposis syndromes

This Peutz–Jegher syndrome involves clearing the gastroduodenal and colonic polyps larger than 0.5 mm by endoscopy and intra-

operative enteroscopy for polyps larger than 15 mm. There is an estimated 18-fold increased risk of gastrointestinal and extra-intestinal cancers of the breast, ovary and pancreas. Therefore, the advocated follow-up policy is biennial colonoscopy, gastroduodenoscopy and small bowel barium study. For affected females, annual cervical biopsy with biennial pelvic ultrasound and mammography and for prepubertal males testicular ultrasound have been suggested. Unaffected parents and siblings of patients are recommended to have one-time colonoscopy and gastroscopy, as the syndrome is an autosomal dominant disorder that occurs in patients with and without a family history.

Juvenile polyposis, unlike solitary juvenile polyps or mucus retention polyps which are common in children, particularly in the rectum, is often diagnosed in adolescence or early adulthood, based on the presence of at least five gastrointestinal polyps, mostly in the colon and stomach. When in large numbers, it can be confused with FAP. Associated congenital anomalies include heart defects, hydrocephalus, malrotation of the gut, cleft palate and polydactyly. There is a risk of epithelial dysplasia in 47% and a cumulative cancer risk in 68% by age 60 in these patients. However, the data do not justify prophylactic colectomy, unless the polyps' number and rate of growth are beyond endoscopic treatment. Follow-up intervals by colonoscopy and upper gastrointestinal tract screening are determined by polyp number, grade and size. In the absence of a family history, one-time colonoscopy is recommended for at-risk parents and siblings of affected patients.

Management of Familial polyposis syndromes

Clinical screening

It is essential to establish a family register in order to identify members at risk. Flexible sigmoidoscopy commencing at puberty is used in preference to rigid sigmoidoscopy. Colonoscopy is reserved for positive diagnosis of FAP. Detection of APC gene mutation and ophthalmoscopy for congenital hypertrophy of the retinal pigment epithelium (CHRPE) (which is invariably present in FAP and in individuals in the same family of affected patients) have been used to differentiate high-risk patients from low-risk patients. High-risk patients will require biennial flexible sigmoidoscopy followed by colonoscopy until adenoma progression requires colectomy. Low-risk patients are followed up annually until age 35 years and every 3–5 years up to the age of 60 years.

Timing and type of treatment

The average age at which symptoms develop is about 20 years and the average age at which carcinoma is detected is 35 years, although malignancy has been recorded at 15–20 years. It is logical that treatment is not delayed beyond 20 years. The treatment options are pan-proctocolectomy, colectomy and ileorectal anastomosis or restorative proctocolectomy.

Proctocolectomy eliminates all colorectal polyps and therefore the risk of cancer but has the disadvantage of an ileostomy. Pelvic dissection to excise the rectum also carries the risk of pelvic nerve damage which may result in urinary and sexual dysfunction. It is not a procedure that would appeal to many of these young patients. It is for this reason that sphincter-saving procedures are favoured.

A *colectomy and ileorectal anastomosis* maintains gastrointestinal continuity with reasonable bowel function and has been the standard treatment. However, the patient requires biannual examination of the rectal stump and repeated fulguration of residual or newly formed polyps. In addition there is a 2–3-fold risk for rectal cancer which can develop in rectal mucosa not occupied by polyps.

Restorative proctocolectomy, with mucosectomy of the short segment of rectal mucosa above the retained anal canal and an ileal pouch anal anastomosis, eradicates the disease. The gastrointestinal continuity is restored while bowel function and continence are maintained. It is of particular relevance in patients who are unlikely to comply with the strict surveillance required after an ileorectal anastomosis. Although the morbidity and mortality are low, the procedure involves pelvic dissection to excise the rectum with the risk of sexual and bladder dysfunction.

Postoperative management

All patients with ileorectal anastomosis require biannual sigmoidoscopy and fulguration of the polyps in the rectum. A 3–4 monthly follow-up is necessary when the polyp density is high and in patients over 50 years because of the increased risk of cancer. In these patients a restorative proctocolectomy may have to be considered as it obviates anxiety in these patients.

Patients should also undergo gastroduodenoscopy, because of the coexistence of stomach and duodenal polyps. The first examination is performed at the time of admission for colonic surgery and screening commenced at 25 years. If normal or if only fundic gland polyps are identified on biopsy, five-year follow-up is recommended. Patients with significant duodenal polyposis are endoscoped at yearly intervals or more frequently if there is concern. Prophylactic removal of the common non-adenomatous fundic gland polyps is not indicated. Larger polyps should be removed by diathermy excision as the incidence of periampullary carcinoma is 12% and these develop from preexistent adenoma. Early detection of a malignant periampullary lesion by screening offers the only prospect of long-term survival.

Management of extra-gastrointestinal manifestations

Cutaneous skin lesions, osteomata classically in the mandible and maxilla, and fibromata in addition to polyposis, originally described as Gardner's syndrome, is no longer regarded as a separate entity but part of the spectrum of familial adenomatous polyposis. Clinicians should be alert to the possibility of FAP in patients with these lesions. Similarly, hepatoblastoma, thyroid carcinoma and medulloblastoma may alert the clinician to screen at-risk children or siblings with these lesions for FAP.

Management of desmoid tumours

The incidence of desmoid tumours in FAP is between 4% and 12%, and can occur prior to, at the time of or after colectomy. The treatment can be difficult. Desmoids in the abdominal wall should be removed if they are progressively enlarging, if symptomatic or cosmetically unacceptable. Excision may leave large defects that may require prosthetic cover. Intraabdominal desmoids cause intestinal obstruction or hydronephrosis and generally are inoperable or excision is associated with high morbidity. Alternative treatment has included radiotherapy, indomethacin and ascorbic acid, sulindac and tamoxifen since approximately 40% of desmoids are oestrogen receptor positive, but the results have been disappointing. Chemotherapy using adriamycin and vincristine has met with variable success.

COLORECTAL CANCER

Introduction

Carcinoma of the colon and rectum has been a disease of great medical interest ever since the early 20th century when the pioneering studies of the English pathologists Dukes and Cole were initiated. Major improvements in the treatment of this disease have arisen as a result of a better understanding of its natural history and with the introduction of better surgical techniques. Over the past decade, three important advances in the study and treatment of colorectal cancer have occurred. The first was a series of important discoveries on the molecular genetics of this disease. The second was the discovery of effective surgical adjuvant therapy. Finally, detailed biochemical studies of the mechanisms by which fluoropyrimidines interact with tumour cells have resulted in the design of newer chemotherapeutic strategies for advanced colorectal cancer.

Much has been written on the treatment and prognosis of patients with colorectal cancer and its metastases (especially hepatic), but there is little information on the epidemiology of these lesions. Most cancer registries collect information on incidence rather than survival. Approximately 20–25% of patients undergoing resection of primary large bowel cancer will have liver metastases at the time of primary tumour resection and only 10–20% of these may be suitable for liver resection. Up to 50% of all patients who present with colorectal carcinoma will eventually develop liver deposits, in many cases the only site of recurrent disease following a successful resection of the primary tumour. Approximately 75–90% of all patients with recurrent colorectal cancer, who eventually die from their recurrent cancer, have multiple liver metastases.

Epidemiology

Colorectal carcinoma is the fourth most common cause of cancer deaths worldwide and the second most common cancer in Europe, superseded only by breast cancer in women and by prostatic cancer in men. Colorectal carcinoma accounts for 8.5% of all new cases of cancer and 7.5% of all cancer deaths. As a common malignancy, it is predominantly a disease of older people, though it may occur at any age. Less than 5% of patients are under the age of 40 (<4 per 100 000 population) and more than half are over 60, with a peak incidence between 70 and 80 (300 per 100 000 population). There are almost 31 000 new cases each year in the United Kingdom. It is second only to carcinoma of the bronchus as a cause of cancer death, with an annual UK mortality of about 19 000–22 000. There are no noticeable sex differences for colonic cancers, but there is a slight male predominance for rectal cancers. There has been no significant change in mortality from large bowel cancer over the past 40 years and half the cases present beyond surgical cure.

The overall cancer incidence in the United Kingdom is 394 per 100 000 population per year (for all cancers). In England and Wales, there were 22 291 newly diagnosed cases of colorectal cancers in 1974 (10 485 males and 11 806 females), 24 417 new cases in 1984 (11 917 males and 12 500 females), and 27 159 new cases in 1990 (13 492 males and 13 667 females). The rate for colorectal cancer in England and Wales was 22 per 100 000 for males and 23.4 per 100 000 for females in 1974, rising to 27.4 per 100 000 for males and 26.4 per 100 000 for females in 1994. A similar trend has been observed in Scotland (29.8 per 100 000 population in 1993). In Northern Ireland there were 621 new cases of colorectal carcinoma in 1991, with an incidence of 38.8 per 100 000 population (colon: 197 males and 228 females; rectum: 112 males and 84 females). Two-thirds of colorectal cancers occur in the rectum, rectosigmoid junction and sigmoid colon (Figure 19.1).

Aetiology

The exact cause as to why colorectal mucosal cells become malignant remains obscure. Over 90% of colorectal cancers appear sporadically in patients with no previous family history of cancer and are not due to hereditary factors. At least two thirds of patients with colorectal carcinomas will also have benign adenomas of the colon, with a similar distribution to the cancer, and hence the adenoma–carcinoma sequence has been considered an important factor in the aetiology of colorectal cancer.

Risk factors for colorectal neoplasms

Colorectal cancer is causally related to both genetic and environmental factors. The risk factors include a positive family history, meat consumption, smoking and alcohol consumption. Important inverse associations exist with vegetables, NSAIDs, hormone replacement therapy (HRT) and physical activity.

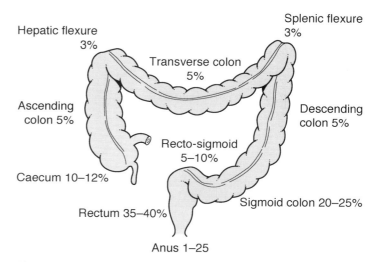

Figure 19.1 Distribution of colorectal cancers.

There are several molecular pathways to colorectal cancer which are important, in both inherited syndromes (familial adenomatous polyposis and hereditary non-polyposis colorectal cancer) and include:

- the APC (adenomatous polyposis coli)–beta-catenin–Tcf (T-cell factor; a transcriptional activator) pathway (Figure 19.2)

- pathway involving abnormalities of DNA mismatch repair

- inhibition of cyclooxygenase-2 by NSAIDs

- specific bloodborne carcinogens from environmental sources such as tobacco smoking and meat.

Some metabolic pathways, e.g. those involving folate and heterocyclic amines, may be modified by polymorphisms in relevant genes. Examples of this are the MTHFR (methylenetetrahydrofolate reductase), NAT1 and NAT2 (N-acetyltransferase 1 and 2). Vegetables, as a source of folate, antioxidants and inducers of detoxifying enzymes, thus offer a protective effect.

Other factors, such as physical activity, remain obscure even when the epidemiology is quite consistent.

Genetic factors

The risk of colorectal cancer increases 2–3 times in a first-degree relative of an affected person. Inherited risk for the development of colorectal cancer falls into three main categories.

FAMILIAL ADENOMATOUS POLYPOSIS SYNDROMES (FAP)

These syndromes are rare and account for less than 1% of colorectal cancers. They are among the commonest autosomal dominant syndromes predisposing to cancer. Polyps usually arise in the rectum, sigmoid and left colon and if left untreated will progress to cancer, which appears before the age of 40 (i.e. at least 20 years earlier than the appearance of cancers among unaffected individuals). Eighty percent of the polyposis-associated cancers occur in the rectosigmoid and left colon region. Synchronous tumours are found in 50% of patients with FAP. Patients usually become symptomatic in the third or fourth decade of life, with a cancer risk of approximately 100%.

HEREDITARY NON-POLYPOSIS COLON CANCER (HNPCC) SYNDROMES

These syndromes may account for approximately 4–8% of all colorectal carcinomas. They include a syndrome characterised by site-specific prediction for colon cancer in the absence of familial polyposis (Lynch type I syndrome), and the cancer family syndrome (Lynch type II syndrome). There is an increased incidence of metachronous (24%) and synchronous (18%) cancers.

- Lynch I syndrome is associated with an increased incidence of colorectal cancer, with up to 75% of these lesions appearing in the proximal (right) colon, at an early age of onset (mean age of onset 45 years).

- Lynch II syndrome shares all the characteristics of Lynch I, but in addition to tumours of the colon, patients are also prone to develop carcinoma of the pancreas, endometrium, ovary, breast and stomach as well as other malignancies. When associated with skin tumours, it is referred to as Muir–Torre syndrome. However, all these syndromes are now collectively known as hereditary non-polyposis colorectal cancer syndromes (HNPCC).

SPORADIC COLORECTAL CANCERS

These account for over 90% of all colorectal carcinomas. Although still associated with family risk factors, they are not associated with the same extensive cancer family genealogies as HNPCC. Studies have supported the dominant inheritance of a susceptibility to colorectal adenomas and cancers with a gene frequency of 19%.

GENES AND GENETIC PREDISPOSITION IN COLORECTAL CANCERS

APC gene

Familial adenomatous polyposis (FAP) is caused by an inherited mutation in the APC gene, which was independently localised in 1987 by Leppert et al and Bodmer et al. It was mapped to chromosome 5q and subsequently cloned and sequenced. The population frequency of truncated forms of APC has been estimated at 1 in 10 000 and lifetime penetrance approaches 100%.

The APC gene is a tumour suppresser gene which requires independent mutation of both alleles for loss of function and such mutations result in loss of proliferative control – 'the gatekeeper' mechanism. The mutations described so far in FAP families are at different sites within the APC gene, but almost all lead to stop codons and thus a truncated APC protein. Mutations at the APC locus are a common and early somatic event in polyps and cancer, i.e. for some patients the first hit is the germline mutation, whereas for others it is a somatic event.

There are several variants of FAP, with correlations between APC mutation sites and the variant phenotypes, e.g. attenuated FAP where the mutations are at the 5' end of the gene, the profuse polyposis syndrome where the inherited mutation normally occurs between codons 1285 and 1465, the appearance of CHRPE with mutations at codons 542-1309, and the multiplicity of extracolonic manifestations with mutations at codons 1465, 1546 and 2621. However, the same mutation may be associated with different phenotypes within members of a single family, which suggests the combination of environmental modifiers and genetic influences on the phenotype. Although inheriting a mutated copy of APC is associated with a highly penetrant phenotype, there are both genetic and environmental influences that modify that penetrance. Even if surgery remains the only treatment for FAP patients for the foreseeable future, such combination of genetic and environmental influences have implications for the management of FAP patients and for the prevention of sporadic cancer.

Genetic mutations in HNPCC

In 1913, Warthin described several different family cancer syndromes. In one of the families, family G, the initial history was of gastric and endometrial cancers. In subsequent generations of this family, there was a high incidence of colorectal cancers which was typical of HNPCC. HNPCC is an inherited autosomal dominant syndrome with no tendency to extensive polyposis, but with a much less well-defined phenotype than FAP. The most distinguishing features of the family history are a tendency to early onset and a pattern of other cancers, particularly those involving the stomach, endometrium, urinary tract and biliary system. Several attempts have been made to provide a specific definition of the syndrome, such as the Amsterdam criteria in 1991 (Box 19.1) using the basic molecular diagnosis which were rather restrictive. The National Cancer Institute workshop expanded these clinical criteria into the Bethesda criteria (Box

---

Box 19.1 Criteria for clinical diagnosis of HNPCC

Amsterdam criteria (1991)
1. Three cases of familial colorectal cancer in which two of the affected individuals are first-degree relatives of the third.
2. Colorectal cancers occurring across two generations.
3. One colorectal cancer diagnosed under age of 50.

Bethesda criteria (1997)
1. Amsterdam criteria individuals.
2. Individuals with two HNPCC-related cancers: synchronous/metachronous colorectal cancers; endometrial, ovarian, gastric, hepatobiliary, small intestine or renal tract transitional cell cancers.
3. Individuals with colorectal cancer and a first-degree relative with one or more of the following:
(a) colorectal cancer diagnosed under the age of 45 years
(b) HNPCC-related cancer diagnosed under the age of 45 years
(c) adenoma diagnosed under the age of 40 years.
4. Individuals under 45 years of age with colorectal or endometrial cancer.
5. Individuals with proximal cancer of undifferentiated type.
6. Individuals under 45 years of age with signet ring cancer.
7. Individuals under 40 years of age with adenomas.

19.1). The clinically defined history can be confirmed by examining the tumour for microsatellite instability or by testing for germline mutations in a family of genes that are involved in DNA mismatch repair (MMR). Microsatellite instability, while common in HNPCC tumours, is nonetheless neither sensitive nor specific. It is unclear whether survival of HNPCC patients is better than or similar to that of patients with sporadic colorectal cancers.

To date, four mismatch repair genes have been identified, hMSH2, hMLH1, hPMS1 and hPMS2. The DNA MMR system identifies and repairs errors that result from the activity of DNA polymerase during replication, in a strand-specific manner. The MMR system recognises the mismatch, binds to it, excises the mismatched region and facilitates the resynthesis of the correct sequence (involving a complex set of proteins). Microsatellite instability is a characteristic feature of genomes that show defects in the MMR system in humans, and was recently recognised in colorectal cancers. The first gene mutation shown in the germline of an HNPCC family (hMSH2) was the human homologue (human MutS) of one of the known bacterial MMR genes (MutS); it was identified on chromosome 2p. Another homologue of the bacterial MutL gene (hMLH1) was identified on chromosome 3q. Mutations in these two genes account for the large majority of HNPCC families identified to date. Two homologues of MutL, namely hPMS1 and hPMS2, account for a small proportion of HNPCC families. One other MutS homologue, GTBP/hMSH6, has been reported to be mutated in HNPCC.

The loss of MMR has several consequences, most crucially loss of 'proof reading' and correction of small deletions and insertions. In addition, colorectal cell lines deficient in MMR show generally higher accumulation of other mutations and deletions. As with the APC gene, somatic mutation or hypermethylation of MMR genes is also a pathway to colorectal cancer.

Other important genes in colorectal carcinogenesis

- *The cyclooxygenase (COX1 and COX2) pathway:* the over-expression of cyclooxygenases (COX1 and COX2) remains an integral early event in the development of colorectal cancer. It appears to occur after the mutation of the second APC gene allele. The cyclooxygenases catalyse the conversion of arachidonic acid to prostaglandin H_2 and malondialdehyde (which is mutagenic) in early polyp formation, promoting further polyp proliferation. COX2 overexpression is extremely common in the progression of colorectal adenomatous polyps and carcinomas. COX1 is overexpressed in 20% of colorectal carcinomas. The NSAIDs, such as aspirin, inhibit cyclooxygenases and so have a potential therapeutic role in the prophylaxis of colorectal carcinoma.

- *DCC gene (deleted on colorectal carcinoma):* the DCC gene is localised on chromosome 18q21 and mutations involving this gene have been recognised in approximately 80% of colorectal cancers and in 50% of dysplastic adenomas. It has structural similarity to the cell adhesion molecule ICAM-1 and plays a role in cell adhesion. Mutation of this gene results in the disruption of cell-to-cell adhesion inhibition, in combination with reduced expression of E-cadherin. This gene has dual functions, since it also acts as a tumour suppresser gene. Inactivation of the gene requires independent mutations of both alleles (like APC and p53), which is consistent with its tumour suppressor activity.

- *DNA methylation – methylenetetrahydrofolate reductase (MTHFR):* DNA hypomethylation has been demonstrated in benign adenomas and in carcinomas of the colon and rectum and the loss of the methyl groups inhibits chromosomal condensation which would facilitate malignant transformation. A diet rich in vegetables is associated with a decreased risk of colorectal cancer and this is thought to be the result of increased levels of folate which is important in the metabolism of the methyl group. This may influence both methylation of DNA and the available nucleotide pool needed for DNA replication and repair. Both folate and vitamin B_{12} are co-factors in the MTHFR pathway and are associated with a reduced risk of colorectal cancer.

- *Ki-ras oncogene:* this protooncogene is a member of the ras family, which forms an integral part of intracellular signal transduction, and is located on the inner surface of the cell membrane. Mutation of the Ki-ras gene occurs in 50–80% of colorectal cancers and results in decreased GTPase activity, leading to a permanent state of ras activation and increased cell division. Mutation of the Ki-ras gene is not expressed in benign polyps, but its expression is increased in dysplastic polyps and in carcinomas.

- *The role of p53:* the p53 tumour suppressor gene has been localised to chromosome 17p and functions as the 'guardian of the genome'. It recognises DNA damage and induces G1 cell cycle arrest until the damage is repaired (through the transcription of p21 protein) or if the damage is irreparable then apoptosis (programmed cell death) will be initiated. Mutation of this gene is rare in adenomas, but is found in approximately 75% of colorectal carcinomas. Mutant p53 in colorectal cancer cells downregulates thrombospondin-1 which leads to tumour vascular endothelial growth factor (VEGF) upregulation. This is an angiogenic stimulatory factor. Therefore, p53 has a role in stimulating tumour angiogenesis, which could enhance bloodborne tumour metastases.

- *SMAD4 gene:* this tumour suppressor gene is similar to the DCC gene and is localised to 18q21. It has a role in the 'landscaper mechanism'. Mutations of SMAD4 are seen in approximately 15% of colorectal cancers (as well as pancreatic and brain cancers). It was initially identified in juvenile polyposis syndromes (JPS), which is an autosomal dominant condition with increased predisposition to the formation of hamartomatous polyps and gastrointestinal malignancies in 9–68% of patients. Mutation of SMAD4 deregulates the normal inhibitory transforming growth factor beta (TGF-β), resulting in stromal proliferation.

- *High prevalence polymorphisms:* meat consumption is associated with increased risk of cancer, particularly for heavily cooked meats. The heterocyclic amines in the meat act as colorectal carcinogens. This raises the question of whether the metabolism of heterocyclic amines, which may be altered by the genetic variability of three main enzymes (NAT1, NAT2 and CYP_{1A2}), might influence the development of colorectal neoplasia. However, recent studies do not support any independent carcinogenic role for NAT1 with cancers or polyps. The combinations of rapid NAT1, NAT2 and CYP_{1A2} genotypes can be associated with increased risk of developing colorectal cancer in the presence of tobacco smoking or high intake of meat.

Inflammatory bowel disease

There is an increased risk of colorectal cancer in patients with inflammatory bowel disease (both ulcerative colitis and to a lesser extent Crohn's disease), and surveillance colonoscopy with mucosal biopsies for dysplasia has been advocated to prevent malignancy or permit its early diagnosis. Cancer occurs at a younger age in patients with long-standing inflammatory bowel disease. The tumours are often mucinous, multiple and located in the left colon. Despite increasing acceptance of surveillance colonoscopy as a recommended strategy in cancer prevention, almost half the patients have their cancers diagnosed because of increased symptoms which led to colonoscopic examination. Eighteen percent of patients develop cancer with less than an eight-year history of inflammatory bowel disease. Patients with mild distal colitis have no greater risk of developing colorectal cancer than the normal population, while patients with severe long-standing disease have a 1 in 2 chance of developing colonic cancer after 30 years.

Environmental factors in colorectal cancer

There is considerable worldwide variation in the incidence of colorectal cancer. It seems to be particularly prevalent in highly developed countries. There is a high rate in the United Kingdom, United States, Australasia and Western Europe, but a low incidence in central Africa and Asia. This geographical variation has been ascribed to environmental factors. It has been suggested that components of our diet play an essential role in carcinogenesis, with the strongest evidence for a dietary role in the induction and growth of tumours or their inhibition. The significant association between diet and the prevalence of colorectal cancer and heart disease suggest that a diet rich in fat and meat is a common factor in both diseases. Initially a low-fibre diet was suggested as the causative factor and subsequently an excess of animal fat or protein. Part of the problem is that there are usually multiple differences in diet between different ethnic groups and it becomes more difficult to know which component is responsible. The paradox is illustrated by the Eskimos, who have a low-fibre, high-fat diet and a very low incidence of colorectal cancer. However, dietary factors do seem to play some part, as when black Africans adopt a Western diet their incidence of colorectal cancer progressively increases.

Fat, cholesterol and bile acids

Strong evidence has been provided to show that a diet rich in fat, and particularly in animal fat, is associated with a high incidence of colorectal cancer. While a fatty diet is the major environmental factor so far identified, fat itself is not a carcinogen. Animal experiments suggest that all fats are mutagenic in very high concentrations, but unsaturated fats are more likely to induce progression from adenomas to carcinoma. The luminal fat and its oxidation products promote colonic epithelial cell proliferation and an increase in crypt cell production rate. Diets high in animal fats are also rich in cholesterol, which is a major substrate for bacterial degradation. There is a correlation between the incidence of colorectal cancer and the volume of the faecal cholesterol. However, it is unlikely that cholesterol *per se* is itself a carcinogen, but its metabolites probably are. Cholesterol and its metabolites have an important endocrine function in the production of sex hormones. Lynch II HNPCC is associated with oestrogen-dependent breast and endometrial cancers, and the polyps in FAP appear at or after puberty when the sex hormones are high. Increased excretion of bile acids (e.g. following cholecystectomy) has been shown to result in a slightly increased risk of right-sided colonic cancer in women.

Fibre

The Western diet is notoriously low in fibre and resistant starch, which results in an increased intestinal transit time. Fibre has been propounded as a protective agent because it decreases bowel transit time, increases stool bulk, alters the bacterial flora in the gut and binds intraluminal carcinogens, which reduces the contact time of any potential carcinogen with the mucosa. Certain bacteria are known to degrade bile salts to form carcinogens. Dietary fibre consists of many substances with different properties, from soluble compounds such as pectins and hemicellulose, to insoluble celluloses and lignins. Indigestible fibre increases the bulk of stool by retaining water and decreases the intestinal transit time in most people (except in patients with colonic irritability and pathologically rapid transit). Fibre alters the quality and quantity of the colonic bacteria and also dilutes and absorbs luminal toxins.

Meat and heterocyclic amines

Proteins (like fats) in the diet are broken down into potential carcinogens such as heterocyclic amines and nitrosamines. Sugimura and Sato originally proposed that specific heterocyclic amines are important in the aetiology of colorectal cancer, as they have been shown to be carcinogenic, including a direct effect on the APC gene. Nitrosamines are also a plausible factor in human colorectal carcinoma, the levels of which are directly related to dietary intake of red meat. These dietary risks might be exacerbated by genetically determined variations in relevant metabolic pathways.

SMOKING

Tobacco smoke is a major source of a variety of carcinogens, including nitrosamines, polycyclic hydrocarbons and heterocyclic amines. These act as bloodborne carcinogens, with possible interactions between smoking and genotypes.

ALCOHOL CONSUMPTION

There is an association between smoking and excessive consumption of alcohol and colorectal neoplasia. Alcohol and its metabolite acetaldehyde both inhibit DNA repair. Alcohol may also exert its effects through associated deficiencies in folate and other nutrients.

COFFEE

Drinking coffee was previously suspected to be involved in colorectal carcinogenesis, but there has been no evidence to support this and it now does not seem to be implicated.

DIETARY CALCIUM

The association between higher intake of calcium and colorectal neoplasia has been explored in experimental studies, which suggest either a reduced risk or no association. Higher intake of calcium is associated with reduced intestinal hyperplasia and reduced crypt cell production rate in animal studies. Calcium reduces the likelihood of metachronous adenomas (by 15–20%) and potentially has a protective effect against colorectal tumours.

NSAIDs

NSAIDs suppress COX_2 and are capable of inhibiting polyp growth even in individuals with FAP. Inhibition of COX_2 produces apoptosis and reduced epithelial proliferation and angiogenesis. NSAIDs (such as aspirin) have been shown recently to suppress the HNPCC-associated mutator phenotype by genetic selection for a subset of cells that do not express microsatellite instability.

HRT

Hormone replacement therapy reduces the oestrogen receptor hypermethylation. HRT has an inverse relationship with polyps and colorectal cancer by replacing the declining endogenous oestrogen levels associated with ageing.

SURGICAL PROCEDURES

Certain gastrointestinal surgical procedures are associated with increased risk of colorectal cancer. A bowel anastomosis increases the risk of a cancer developing at the site of surgery, both in experimental models and at the site of implantation after resection.

Cholecystectomy is also associated with an increased risk of colonic cancer, in particular right-sided lesions in women. The risk is similar after gastric surgery in men. Both operations may exert their effect by increasing the delivery of bile acids within the colon.

Uretero-sigmoidostomy, performed for urinary diversion, is particularly associated with the development of colorectal cancer at or near the ureterocolic anastomosis. The mechanism is uncertain, but it may be caused by the effects of phenols, cresols and other compounds from cigarette smoke, excreted in the urine.

IRRADIATION

Ionising radiations are important mutagens and radiotherapy used for treating cervical carcinoma is associated with a slight increase in the risk of colorectal cancer. Most of the cancers occur in the rectum, within the radiation field, and appear 5–15 years later.

BACTERIA

Bacteria are a major constituent of stool and may have an important role in colorectal carcinogenesis. The two important bacterial enzymes are beta-dehydrogenase and 4,5-nuclear dehydrogenase. The first breaks down harmless primary bile acids into mutagenic secondary bile acids such as lithocholic acid and chenodeoxycholic acid and the second desaturates bile acids into metabolites which are tumour inhibitors and growth promoters. There is a close correlation between the incidence of colorectal carcinoma and faecal secondary bile acids concentration. There is also a close correlation between the carriage of nuclear dehydrogenase-producing *Clostridia* in the colon and the incidence of colorectal cancer.

IMMUNOSUPPRESSION

Long-term immunosuppression is associated with an increased risk of colorectal cancer. Examples of immunosuppression include HIV infection, following transplantation or following chemotherapy for other malignancies such as lymphomas.

OTHER DIETARY FACTORS

A number of dietary constituents have been found to inhibit colorectal carcinogenesis, including vitamins C and E, selenium, retinoids, beta-carotene and plant sterols. Fish consumption has been shown to have a protective effect against digestive tract cancers.

Pathogenesis

There are at least four suggested pathways from normal cell to colorectal cancer. Some of the molecular pathways appear to be common.

Table 19.1 Summary of colorectal cancer promoters and inhibitors

Promoting factors	Effects
Genetic (family history)	FAP → APC pathway
	HNPCC → Microsatellite instability pathway
	Sporadic → Other pathways
	Peutz–Jeghers
	Juvenile polyposis
Diet	
Meat:	Nitrosamines and heterocyclic amines → ?APC & K-ras mutation
Bile acids:	Secondary mutagenic bile acids (powerful tumour promoters)
Fat:	Oxidised luminal fat promotes epithelial proliferation
Smoking	Nitrosamines and heterocyclic amines → ?APC mutation & K-ras mutation
Excess alcohol	Acetaldehyde → DNA damage
	Reduction of folate → defects in DNA repair and replication
Operations	Cholecystectomy: increased bile acids in the colon
	Gastric surgery: increased bile acids in the colon
	Ureterosigmoidostomy: urinary irritants affecting colonic mucosa
Irradiation	Important tumour promoter
Colonic diseases	Ulcerative colitis and Crohn's disease: chronic inflammation

Inhibitory factors	Effects
Diet:	
Vegetables and fibre	Antioxidants → reduced DNA damage
	Folate → DNA integrity
	Fibre → short chain fatty acids → apoptosis
	Reduced colonic transit time → less exposure to carcinogens
Vitamins C and E	Inhibit carcinogenesis
Selenium	Inhibits carcinogenesis
β-Carotene	Inhibits carcinogenesis
Physical activity and low body mass	Reduced growth stimulus and reduced colonic transit time
NSAIDs	Cyclooxygenase-2 inhibition
HRT	? Prevention of oestrogen receptors hypermethylation

Table 19.2 Genes involved in hereditary colorectal cancer

Genes	Chromosome	Function	Abnormality
Genes involved in predisposition to carcinogenesis			
APC gene	5q21	Cell adhesion	Deletion/mutation
DCC	18q21	Cell adhesion	Deletion/mutation
HMSH2	2p16	DNA mismatch repair	Mutation
HMLH1	3p21	DNA mismatch repair	Mutation
HPMS1	2q31-q33	DNA mismatch repair	Mutation
HPMS2	7p22	DNA mismatch repair	Mutation
Genes involved in progression of neoplasia			
T p53	17p13	Transcription	Deletion/mutation
RAS family	12p,1p,11p	Transcription	Mutation
CMYC	8q24	DNA synthesis	Overexpression
SMAD4	18q21	Transcription	Deletion/mutation
Genes with putative role in carcinogenesis			
Examples: MCC, DRA, RB1, NM23 mutations: unproven functions			

ing series of specific chromosomal and genetic changes that accompany the transition from normal colonic mucosa to metastatic carcinoma, which are summarised in Figure 19.2. These include the mutation of K-ras (a protooncogene), changes in methylation patterns and mutation or loss of p53 (a tumour suppressor gene controlling entry into the cell cycle). Other important deletions include possibly DCC and DPC4/SMAD4 on chromosome 18 and the Peutz–Jeghers gene on chromosome 19.

With the identification of the HNPCC genes as being DNA MMR genes, it was expected that mutations of APC, K-ras and p53 would be more likely. However, it became clear that mutations or deletions in other genes take place in HNPCC, such as the MMR genes and TGF-β-R II (transforming growth factor β receptor II gene), and that mutations of APC, K-ras and p53 are less common in HNPCC and in sporadic cancers with microsatellite instability.

In the absence of an inherited APC mutation, the likelihood of developing an adenoma in an individual with a DNA MMR defect may not be greatly different from that in the general population. However, once an adenoma develops, its progression to carcinoma is more rapid with a DNA MMR defect because of the colonic field defect with an irreparable damage. It is possible to lose DNA MMR function not by somatic mutation but by hypermethylation, for example of hMLH1, which now appears to be a very early event in many sporadic colorectal cancers, an event that will in turn lead to a mutator phenotype. The initial hit could be an inherited or an acquired mutation in an MMR gene or hypermethylation specifically of hMLH1, and this pathway will lead to a vicious cycle of increasing microsatellite instability involving the MMR genes themselves and additional deletions of important controllers of DNA and cell integrity.

- The archetypal pathogenic pathway (the adenoma-carcinoma sequence) (Figure 19.2) was first described by Morson et al in the 1970s. It is the accepted early step in the majority of cancers and the key in the mutation of APC (germline or somatic), e.g. in FAP. Mutation or deletion of the APC gene induces polyp formation as a result of loss of orderly cell replication, adhesion and migration. The pathway involves beta-catenin, which binds E-cadherin and activates transcription, and Tcf (T-cell factor) as a downstream transcriptional activator gene. A mutant APC or beta-catenin results in failure of proliferative signal and mutations in beta-catenin can substitute functionally for loss of APC (Tables 19.1 and 19.2).

- It has been shown that the molecular steps after the activation of the APC–beta-catenin–Tcf pathway involve an accumulat-

- The third pathway for colorectal pathogenesis is via ulcerative colitis and, to a lesser extent, Crohn's disease. Although this disease is a minor contributor to the overall population burden of colorectal cancer, patients with ulcerative colitis have a

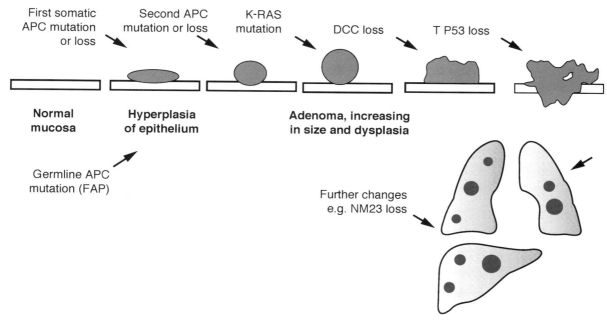

Figure 19.2 Possible pathways of colorectal carcinogenesis.

20-fold excess risk for cancer. This pathway involves the 'dysplasia-carcinoma sequence'. The somatic molecular changes are much less defined, the p53 deletion can occur early and the APC mutations are uncommon. Microsatellite instability may occur in the absence of DNA MMR defects, suggesting perhaps an overwhelming source of mutagenic activity. The chronic inflammation and loss of the epithelial integrity in combination with colonic luminal agents will cause mutation in p53, which can result in aneuploidy and subsequently in the development of dysplasia and carcinoma.

● The fourth pathway has been suggested by the evidence that almost all colorectal cancers arise from cells in which the oestrogen receptor gene (ER) has been silenced. The hypermethylation of the oestrogen receptor gene is an age-related phenomenon. It is not known whether this is an early crucial step or why the deletion of this gene is so critical for colonic epithelial cells. However, the loss of a mitotic checkpoint may be important, as many colorectal tumours have a marked degree of chromosomal instability.

Clinical features of colorectal cancer

The clinical presentation is varied and is dependent on the site of the tumour, although few can be asymptomatic. Bowel symptoms are prominent in cancers of the left colon and rectum which feature as constipation or, alternatively, increased frequency and looseness of the stool. Diarrhoea is more often observed in patients with cancer of the right and transverse colon, although may also present with rectosigmoid cancer associated with a villous adenoma or an enteric fistula. This should be distinguished from 'spurious' diarrhoea due to urgency, sensation of incomplete evacuation, the desire to strain with unsatisfactory result and the passage of blood mixed with stool or mucus, described as tenesmus, usually suggestive of a lesion in the distal sigmoid or rectum. Bleeding is intermittent, rarely profuse, and the blood is passed mixed with the stool or in clots. This is a common presentation of left-sided colonic and rectal cancers while blood loss from caecal and right-sided cancers presents with anaemia or is recognisable as melaena stool or when testing for occult blood. Abdominal pain is more often experienced with right-sided cancers and in stenosing lesions is accompanied by flatulent distension and audible borborygmi, especially after meals. Rectal pain is unusual unless the tumour is advanced and has invaded the sacrum or the major pelvic nerves. Involvement of the bladder or prostate manifests as cystitis or urethritis and fistulation into the bladder or vagina by infiltrating tumour causing recurrent urinary tract infection, pneumaturia and discharge of faeces and flatus per vaginum.

Differential diagnosis

Colon cancer affects both sexes equally, but rectal cancer appears to be more common in males. The disease should always be considered in the elderly patient with bowel symptoms. A history of ulcerative colitis, adenomatous polyps or familial polyposis, or a family background of cancer, should raise the level of suspicion, particularly in the younger patient. The clinical picture of altered bowel habit, abdominal distension, pain and flatulence are recognised features of diverticular disease, that is equally common in the elderly population, and of the irritable bowel syndrome in the younger patient. Blood mixed with the stool, passed in clots or when dark in colour is more consistent with colonic bleeding associated with inflammatory bowel disease, irradiation or ischaemic colitis and diverticular disease. Tenesmus with the passage of blood and mucus is also caused by proctitis either idiopathic or secondary to enteric infections and radiotherapy to the pelvis.

However, patients often do not describe their symptoms clearly and, despite careful questioning and examination, a suspicion of a colonic tumour may not be confidently eliminated. A carcinoma of the colon should be considered as a possible cause of dyspepsia, vague abdominal symptoms, unexplained anaemia and metastatic liver disease. The correct course is to proceed with the appropriate investigations, especially in patients over 40 years of age or with a strong family history.

In general, the diagnosis is based on digital palpation of the rectum, sigmoidoscopy and radiological or endoscopic examination of the large bowel.

Examination

General physical examination involves assessment of the patient's nutritional condition and the cardiovascular and respiratory status. The patient's dependency and mobility, mental state and disability should be noted, as these bear relevance to the management.

Clinical staging starts with inspection for jaundice, palpation for lymphadenopathy in the neck region and examination of the chest, for pleural effusion or signs of consolidation, and the abdomen, for gaseous distension or active bowel sounds, for a palpable mass, an enlarged liver and for the presence of ascites. A caecal cancer is more often palpable than tumours elsewhere in the colon and palpability is usually, but not necessarily, a sign of locally advanced disease, particularly when the tumour is freely mobile.

Digital examination of the rectum detects a lesion within the reach of the finger and, combined with vaginal examination in females, allows assessment of its local extent. Sigmoidoscopy within the length of the 25cm instrument identifies lesions as far as the distal sigmoid colon and allows tissue biopsy. Caution in interpretation of normal findings should be observed with sigmoidoscopy limited to the rectum because of difficulty in negotiating the rectosigmoid junction at 12–15 cm. Streaks of blood on the finger or on sigmoidoscopy with no obvious lesion strengthen the probability that one lies beyond reach.

Diagnostic investigations

Biopsy

It is conventional practice to obtain a tissue diagnosis of lesions within the reach of the sigmoidoscope. This is, however, not mandatory for a more proximal lesion detected on a barium enema, as this requires colonoscopy, unless the radiological appearances are equivocal. Histological sampling in preoperative staging is unreliable, as the degree of tumour differentiation on

biopsy does not correlate with that of the resected specimen. This is of particular relevance in the treatment strategy of rectal cancer.

Imaging of the colon

It is essential that the full length of the colon is visualised, even when a cancer has been recognised by digital examination or sigmoidoscopy, in order to rule out a synchronous cancer, which occurs in nearly 5% of patients, and synchronous polyps which are present in up to 75% of patients with colorectal cancer. The sensitivity of double-contrast barium enema (DCBA) in cancer detection was 65–99% compared with 70–95% in colonoscopy and for detecting polyps less than 1 cm, the best results radiologically were 85–90% compared with 90% for colonoscopy.

A barium enema may not display the rectosigmoid region clearly because of overlapping coils of intestine and in the presence of extensive diverticular disease a neoplastic lesion may be missed. It is advisable, therefore, that patients with diverticular disease should routinely have the sigmoid colon endoscopically inspected, although this may not be successful because of stenosis in the diseased segment. Colonoscopy is probably more suitable than a barium enema for the very old and the seriously ill or disabled patient who is unable to retain the contrast material and who is recognised at attempted sigmoidoscopy which fails for the same reason. In patients with luminal narrowing by tumour, the passage of a colonoscope is impeded and if barium is forced through the stenotic segment, subsequent dehydration of the barium may precipitate colonic obstruction. In these instances, CT colonography, which involves dynamic intravenous contrast-enhanced thin-section helical or multislice CT of the air-insufflated colon with the aid of smooth muscle relaxants, accurately localises cancer and detects all polyps larger than 1 cm and 70% of polyps between 0.5 and 0.9 cm. It allows complete examination of the colon and the abdominal viscera. Thus in a single examination clinical staging is also achieved.

Other investigations

A chest radiograph is performed to rule out pulmonary metastases. An ultrasound examination is a reliable investigation for secondaries in the liver. Helical CT is more sensitive in detecting lesions <1 cm and contrast-enhanced MRI better defines indeterminate lesions. This information is particularly essential when treatment of the metastatic disease is being considered. An intravenous urogram is not routinely required but is of value when the tumour is large and is clinically palpable, in order to eliminate involvement of the urinary tract, particularly if the tumour occupies the pelvic cavity. A preoperative carcinoembryonic antigen (CEA) level is a useful baseline measurement for future reference during follow-up. Routine haematological and biochemical tests are performed as part of the patient's general assessment.

Staging of colorectal cancer

Two staging systems are commonly used – the TNM staging system and Dukes' staging system.

TNM staging

The TNM staging system is as follows.

Primary tumour
Tis: *In situ* carcinoma
T1: Invasion of submucosa
T2: Invasion of muscularis propria
T3: Invasion into subserosa or non-peritonised pericolic or perirectal tissues
T4: Invasion into other structures or perforation of visceral peritoneum

Regional lymph nodes
N0: No involvement of regional lymph nodes
N1: 1–3 pericolic or perirectal lymph nodes involved
N2: Four or more pericolic or perirectal nodes involved
N3: Involvement of apical node (marked by the surgeon)

Metastases
M0: No metastases
M1: Distant metastases

Stage grouping
Stage I: T1/2, N0, M0   = Dukes' A
Stage II: T3/4, N0, M0   = Dukes' B
Stage III: Any T, N1/2/3, M0   = Dukes' C
Stage IV: Any T, any N, M1   = Dukes' D

Dukes' staging system and its modifications

Dukes' staging was originally described for rectal cancer in 1932, but was subsequently extended to include colon cancer.

Dukes' stage A: Tumour into the submucosa or muscularis propria, but not through it
Dukes' stage B: Tumour through muscularis propria, but not involving lymph nodes
Dukes' stage C: Metastatic deposits in the lymph nodes

The first modification was in 1935 by Gabriel et al:

Dukes' stage C1:   Involvement of lymph nodes, but not highest lymph node in the chain at the high surgical tie
Dukes' stage C2:   Involvement of the highest lymph node in the chain closest to the surgical tie

The second modification was in 1954 by Astler and Coller:

Dukes' stage B1:   Into the submucosa or the muscularis propria, but not through the muscularis propria, with no lymph node involvement

Dukes' stage B2:   Through the muscularis propria, with no lymph node involvement

The third modification was in 1967, by Turnbull et al:

Dukes' stage D: Presence of hepatic metastases. Now referred to any distant metastases

The most recent modification was in 1974 by Gunderson and Sosin (used mainly in the USA):

Dukes' stage B3:   Involvement of adjacent structures, with no lymph node involvement
Dukes' stage C3:   Involvement of adjacent structures, with lymph node involvement

Surgical management

Elective surgery

Surgical management is aimed at cure and symptomatic palliation, with restoration of bowel continuity whenever conceivable, at minimal operative risk. Hence, careful selection is crucial and, aided by precise assessment of the extent of the disease, treatment can be tailored accordingly.

Patient selection

Surgical treatment can be curative and offers palliation in advanced disease but this should be balanced against the operative morbidity and the patient's life expectancy, especially in the elderly with associated medical disease. Surgical intervention is unjustified in the asymptomatic patient with limited longevity, because of widespread disease, particularly in rectal cancer as less invasive palliative measures can be offered. The presence of liver secondaries does not preclude treatment, since in a select group resection of the primary lesion and the segment of diseased liver improves survival.

Assessment of resectability

A colonic cancer is rarely palpable and when it is, and even if fixed, this is not essentially a sign of irresectability. The distinction on CT between inflammatory and malignant infiltration is not always clear. Resectability is better assessed at laparotomy which also allows palliative decompression when a tumour is deemed inoperable.

Rectal cancers, being more accessible, allow better clinical and radiological evaluation and this makes it easier to assess the resectability or otherwise of the tumour. Digital palpation measures the circumferential size of the tumour, its depth of invasion into the pararectal fat, the lymph nodes, the adjacent viscera and the pelvic wall. In females, the vagina is digitally examined for tumour infiltration. The extent of local disease, especially fixity, in the conscious patient may not be as accurate as when examination is carried out under anaesthesia. When bladder invasion is suspected, cystoscopy is essential. The distance of the lower margin from the dentate line or anal verge is measured by sigmoidoscopy. However, with an intussuscepting rectosigmoid cancer, or in elderly patients with weak pelvic floor musculature, the level of the tumour may appear erroneously low.

The extent of local invasion of rectal cancer to adjacent organs, when clinically equivocal, is determined by CT. MRI is of no added advantage. However, neither is reliable in determining the extent of rectal wall invasion of an early cancer. Endorectal ultrasonography discriminates cancers within the submucosa (T1), those extending into the muscularis propria but confined to the rectal wall (T2 T3) and those invading the pararectal fat (T4).

Choice of operation

The patient's attitude and ability to manage a stoma are of relevance. While patients with poor sight, arthritis, paralysis or mental handicap are believed to cope poorly with a stoma, it is more convenient for those nursing them. A restorative resection should not compromise the adequacy of cancer clearance. The functional outcome is another consideration which is dependent on bowel function and anal sphincters. Therefore, the patient should be questioned about operations such as vagotomy, gastrectomy or small bowel resection, history of previous anorectal surgery, obstetric injuries and anal trauma, stool frequency and consistency and incontinence, its frequency and severity. The sphincter mechanism is examined digitally for the resting tone of the anus, the contraction strength on squeezing and the integrity of the anorectal angle. In most instances, the skilled clinician's assessment is fairly reliable but, in selected cases, manometric measurements may be necessary.

Further details are provided in the section on Operative Surgery below.

Emergency surgery

Colonic obstruction

Cancer of the sigmoid colon, splenic flexure, transverse colon and, less frequently, rectum can present with partial or complete obstruction and is not often preceded by bowel symptoms or rectal bleeding. Constipation and abdominal distension are the main features but distension may not be pronounced if the colon is decompressed by an incompetent ileocaecal valve and this also reduces the tension in the caecum. The resultant backflow into the small intestine may cause vomiting. Therefore, tenderness over the caecal region in the right iliac fossa, when present, is an ominous sign. The gaseous distension of the colon may, therefore, be seen to involve the small intestine and is obvious on a plain abdominal radiograph film. The distal extent of the colonic gaseous shadow will localise the site of obstruction with a fair degree of accuracy.

Cancer of the caecum, ascending colon and hepatic flexure exhibits insidious symptoms of small bowel obstruction because of the liquid nature of the stool in this segment of the large bowel and acute obstruction is a late event. On a plain abdominal radiograph small bowel distension is a feature.

A palpable abdominal mass or a lesion within reach of the examining digit and the sigmoidoscope is a useful sign. A water-soluble contrast enema is essential to confirm the diagnosis and determine the level of obstruction. It is essential to exclude pseudoobstruction, commonly due to underlying medical illness, particularly in the elderly, and thus avoid an unnecessary laparotomy in these high-risk patients. While an instant barium enema defines the mucosal outline and the nature of the obstructing lesion more clearly, this added information does not influence management and a major disadvantage is that retained barium in the colon makes mobilisation and primary colonic anastomosis hazardous.

Patients with colonic obstruction require resuscitation and immediate surgery. For carcinomas of the lower descending or sigmoid colon, or the rectum, a proximal colostomy should be avoided unless the patient is unfit or the tumour is irresectable, as it entails two further procedures: resection of the primary tumour and subsequent closure of the colostomy. A Hartmann's resection avoids a primary anastomosis in the unprepared colon and the risk of leakage. However, it involves another procedure, which carries a high morbidity. A one-stage procedure shortens the hospital stay and avoids a stoma; however, it is considered with trepidation because of the risk of anastomotic failure in the unprepared obstructed colon. Intraoperative on-table lavage overcomes this problem, but is inadvisable if the patient is a high anaesthetic risk as it prolongs the operation time. A subtotal colectomy with ileosigmoid or ileorectal anastomosis is an alternative option, particularly when the colon is grossly oedematous and distended. It is, however, not suitable for patients with rectal cancer, with poor sphincters.

For carcinoma of the right colon, an emergency right hemicolectomy with primary anastomosis is a safe procedure as the bacterial content of the faecal fluid is low and the resection removes the loaded colon, leaving relatively empty small bowel and distal colon. Extended right hemicolectomy or subtotal colectomy with ileosigmoid anastomosis is the appropriate approach for obstructed carcinoma of the transverse colon, splenic flexure or proximal descending colon.

A short circuiting ileo-colic or colo-colic anastomosis, or a diverting stoma, depending on the level of obstruction, is a reasonable option for the locally advanced and fixed tumour or when there is widespread intraperitoneal disease.

Carcinoma of the colon with perforation and peritonitis

This usually complicates an obstructed left colonic carcinoma, causing a perforation in the caecum. Perforation at or close to the tumour is less frequent. The clinical picture is of abdominal distension, tenderness and guarding in the abdomen, either diffuse or localised to the region of the perforation. The patient exhibits signs of sepsis and may be moribund. A plain abdominal radiograph (or an erect chest radiograph) will, in most instances, demonstrate free gas under the diaphragm. Intensive resuscitation and antibiotic treatment are essential. The surgical management options follow the same line as in obstruction. The resection should include the perforated area, except for a caecal perforation from a distal obstruction which, unless it can be repaired by suturing, is exteriorised as a formal diverting caecostomy with or without resection of the tumour.

The clinical picture in patients with localised peritonitis complicating a perforated carcinoma can mimic acute diverticulitis or acute appendicitis and is more confusing if there is a palpable tender mass. When the acute episode resolves, the large bowel is investigated by either colonoscopy or barium enema. As residual inflammation may distort the morphological appearances, the examination is best carried out after a reasonable lapse of time from the event, for more reliable information. Management follows conventional surgical principles, with a conservative or an interventional approach dictated by clinical criteria. The true nature of the primary pathology may still not be obvious at exploration, as it may not be possible to distinguish a malignant from an inflammatory mass or exclude a co-existent carcinoma with certainty. In these instances, a radical resection is a reasonable and safe option.

Treatment of advanced colorectal cancer

Widespread disseminated disease is usually evident clinically with, for example, gross hepatomegaly, jaundice, ascites or pulmonary effusion, when any operative intervention is unreasonable. Inoperability, however, may only emerge at laparotomy because of extensive liver metastases, intraperitoneal spread, local fixation and involvement of adjacent viscera or a pelvis 'frozen' with carcinoma. Resection of the primary lesion, even if local tumour clearance is not complete, is the better palliative option for the relief of bowel symptoms. When the tumour is unresectable or extensive peritoneal and gross omental deposits preclude a palliative resection, an alternative, particularly when the patient has or is exhibiting symptoms of obstruction, is a short-circuiting anastomosis between the ileum and the transverse colon for a tumour of the right colon or between the transverse and the descending or sigmoid colon for a tumour of the splenic flexure.

Palliation for tumours in the region of the rectum and distal sigmoid is aimed at relieving obstruction, bleeding, discharge, incontinence and pain. Abdominoperineal resection or anterior resection, provided the tumour is deemed resectable, offers the best long-term palliation. However, in the unfit or elderly patient, the benefit must be weighted against the morbidity of the operation, the inconvenience of a colostomy and the life expectancy of the patient. A proximal colostomy close to the tumour is simple and safe but, unless the patient is acutely obstructed, it is reserved should local treatment methods fail.

The methods in vogue until recently have been laser therapy and transanal resection. Nd:YAG laser is administered via a flexible scope, which allows delivery of the laser beam with precision. The procedure is carried out under intravenous sedation and does not require hospitalisation. Several sessions may be required when the tumour is bulky. Transanal resection does not demand special equipment or expertise, is carried out with a resectoscope but requires a general anaesthetic. Although the bulk of the tumour can be resected in a single session, the risk of perforation is higher and, for this reason, treatment is restricted to lesions below the peritoneal reflection. Placement of expandable metallic stents endoscopically under sedation guided by radiological imaging is particularly suited for stenotic lesions in the rectosigmoid region. This modality has proven simple, safe and effective in providing instant symptomatic palliation.

Choice of treatment, therefore, depends on availability, patient's fitness, the level of the tumour and its size. Although effective in relieving symptoms due to obstruction, bleeding, discharge and incontinence, local treatment does not control pain and, in the long term, obstruction may ensue because of extraluminal tumour growth. External beam radiation therapy provides, in a majority of patients, symptomatic relief, particularly from pain due to bone or nerve invasion, although for a limited period, and is used as a treatment alternative or a supplementary to other modalities already discussed.

Local recurrence

Local recurrence is believed to be due to implantation of exfoliated cells in the operative field or to an inadequate clearance of the primary tumour. A local recurrence may be asymptomatic and is detected on routine follow-up examination. However, recurrences are not detected until the patient is symptomatic and do not cause general ill health, unless they are associated with widespread metastases.

Local recurrence after resection for colon cancer is less frequent than after resection for rectal cancer. The patient presents with non-specific abdominal pain, progressing to more pronounced symptoms, owing to visceral involvement. An abdominal recurrence when clinically not evident is identified at CT scanning. Colonoscopy is likely to be normal, as anastomotic recurrence is rare and any visible tumour is more likely to be due to extracolonic infiltration or a metachronous carcinoma. When the recurrence is localised and the patient is in a satisfactory state of general health, re-resection is worth considering, although many cases are found at laparotomy to be unsuitable.

After rectal excision, local recurrence presents with pelvic or sciatic pain, bladder dysfunction due to bone and nerve involvement or oedema of the lower limbs from lymphatic blockage. Following abdominoperineal excision, tumour recurrence may be localised to the perineal wound scar, although this could be an infiltration from a deeper recurrence. Assessment is restricted to CT scanning, which does not always distinguish postoperative tissue changes from a recurrent tumour, and an MRI does not add more information. Positron emission tomography (PET) is more specific in identifying sites of recurrence. In the female, the vagina allows access for digital examination and for a needle biopsy of any lesion palpable in the pelvis. A CT-guided needle biopsy may be resorted to for tissue diagnosis.

After an anterior resection, the patient may also complain of tenesmus, mucus discharge and rectal bleeding. An essential part of the examination is to establish recurrence, as postirradiation proctitis causes similar symptoms, and also to determine whether the recurrence is localised to the suture line or is pararectal. The presence of a palpable extrarectal mass with normal overlying mucosa on digital examination and sigmoidoscopy is consistent with pelvic disease, although the mucosa may sometimes look hyperaemic or superficially ulcerated. Mucosal biopsies are unhelpful and the diagnosis is established by transrectal needle biopsy under general anaesthesia, when the extent of the disease can also be assessed. Subtle changes in the mucosa in the region of the anastomosis, easily recognised by digital examination and sigmoidoscopy with positive biopsies, are features of an anastomotic recurrence. Whether or not it is true suture line recurrence or is secondary to an infiltrating pelvic disease is irrelevant. It is the bulk of the extrarectal tumour and its fixity that will determine operability, as a primary suture line recurrence may grow extrarectally to involve adjacent structures and form a large pelvic recurrence. Hence, an endorectal ultrasound will determine the depth of local disease and a CT scan will outline the extent of extrarectal invasion.

Treatment for an anastomotic recurrence confined to the bowel wall is controversial. An abdominoperineal resection is favoured for its radicality and because it guarantees palliation in case of further pelvic recurrence. However, providing there is no evidence of extrarectal disease at exploration, a restorative resection is acceptable provided it is technically feasible and clearance is not compromised. A primary anastomosis can be deferred until an adequate recurrence-free period is ascertained. Postoperative pelvic irradiation is added for patients who have not been maximally irradiated. This approach provides palliation, with a five-year survival reaching 50%.

Pelvic recurrences are usually extensive and are rarely operable. Resection involves pelvic exenteration, formation of a colostomy and an ileal conduit, and some patients may require excision of the coccyx and a portion of the sacrum. The survival benefit does not justify the high morbidity associated with this approach. Instead, radiotherapy is worth considering, especially for the relief of pain. Palliation is otherwise along the same lines as for advanced rectal cancer, as previously discussed.

Treatment of metastatic disease

Metastases are detected at presentation or after curative treatment of the primary tumour. The liver is the most common site of distant metastases, followed by the lungs, bones and other sites. At the time of diagnosis of the primary disease, 25% of patients have liver metastases and a similar proportion will manifest with recurrence isolated to the liver after curative resection. There is an increasing tendency to actively treat metastatic disease limited to the liver in the younger and the fit patient. With fewer than four metastatic deposits within one lobe, resection is curative and can achieve a 30% five-year survival. When both lobes are involved and provided not more than half the liver substance is replaced, regional hepatic arterial perfusion with a cytotoxic agent, usually 5-FU or FUDR, is the only palliative therapy. In half the patients, tumour bulk is reduced, with alleviation of symptoms, although the mean survival is only 18 months.

Nearly 10% of patients with colorectal cancer will have pulmonary metastases detected during life and 10% of these metastases are isolated. Thus, 1% of patients are suitable for resection, which offers a 20–30% overall survival.

Bone and brain metastases are associated with disseminated disease and isolated brain deposits are rarely resectable. Chemotherapy and radiotherapy are offered for symptomatic relief.

The management of metastatic disease demands careful evaluation by clinical examination and imaging studies to determine the site, extent and distribution of the disease.

Adjuvant therapy for colorectal cancer

Surgical resection for cure fails because of metastatic spread and local recurrence, particularly with rectal cancer. Adjuvant measures in the form of chemotherapy or radiation therapy are aimed at destroying foci of microscopic disease. Clinical trials have compared different treatment protocols and some regimens of adjuvant treatment have been shown to offer survival benefits or reduction in local recurrence.

Radiotherapy for colorectal cancer

Radiotherapy is well established for rectal and anal cancers, as either curative or palliative treatment. Radiotherapy can be preparative, perioperative or postoperative. Preoperative radiotherapy has been combined with surgery for rectal cancer, which markedly reduces local recurrence. The main objective of preoperative radiotherapy is to shrink the tumour and downstage the disease to enable surgical resection. Intraoperative (perioperative) radiotherapy should be considered for selected patients with advanced local lesions and for certain local recurrences. Postoperative radiotherapy can be adjuvant therapy or palliative therapy to achieve relief of symptoms (such as pain). However, heavy irradiation in the lower abdomen can be associated with considerable morbidity such as nausea and vomiting, radiation enteritis, adhesions and cystitis.

Preoperative therapy is associated with an increased incidence of perineal wound breakdown, in abdominoperineal resection. Another disadvantage is that patients with favourable cancers are overtreated unnecessarily and surgery is delayed. However, a short course of preoperative radiotherapy with 25 Gy over 5–7 days, followed immediately by surgery, seems as effective as therapy with 60 Gy over eight weeks with delayed surgery in reducing the local recurrence rate. Postoperative radiotherapy is more favoured, as the therapy is administered after the clinico-pathological staging is confirmed and treatment is limited to patients with lesions who are most likely to benefit. The local recurrence rate is surgeon dependent and is diminished by total mesorectal excision. Thus, individual surgeons must be aware of their failure rates in order to decide whether radiotherapy offers any added advantage to their results.

Adjuvant chemotherapy

Adjuvant chemotherapy is given alone or in combination with radiotherapy and includes preoperative therapy. Most of the chemotherapy regimens use 5-FU (5-fluorouracil) alone or in combination with leucovorin, methotrexate or PALA (N-phos-phonacetyl-L-aspartate). Toxicity and side effects of these chemotherapeutic agents are major problems. Large prospective studies are currently under way to determine whether the efficacy and side effects of the combination chemotherapy can be improved.

Numerous trials over the last 25 years have been designed to assess the efficacy of adjuvant systemic chemotherapy in improving overall survival in patients with resected colorectal cancer. Many of these studies have been underpowered and utilised chemother-apy regimes that have now been shown to be ineffective. In recent years more potent and therefore possibly more effective chemotherapeutic agents have been introduced. Trials which have been larger and more effectively conducted have reported data which in many cases have demonstrated some benefits.

The important prospective randomised trials which have demon-strated unequivocal benefit are usually confined to patients with lymph node-positive colorectal cancer (Dukes' C) The regimes used involve a combination of 5-fluorouracil (5-FU) with either high-dose or low-dose folinic acid. The two major studies demonstrating efficacy are the Impact Trial and the NSABP study.

The Inter Group Study demonstrated a benefit for 5-FU and lev-amisole in patients with Dukes' B2 and C disease. This resulted in widespread utilisation of this regime but subsequent studies have failed to demonstrate unequivocal survival benefit for Dukes' B2. The Impact Trial studied 5-FU combined with folinic acid in patients with both Dukes' B2 and C disease. Data from three dif-ferent but similar studies were amalgamated. Patients with lymph node-positive disease (Dukes' C) had a statistically significant improvement in overall survival with reduced recurrence rates. However, no benefit was obtained for patients with B2 disease. A subsequent metaanalysis of all studies utilising 5-FU and folinic acid in patients with Dukes' B2 disease has been reported. Even though the number of patients in this metaanalysis was significant,

no overall improvements in either recurrence-free survival or overall survival were recognised for Dukes' B2 disease.

For rectal cancer, chemotherapy alone has not demonstrated major improvement but the combination of radiotherapy with chemotherapy, especially for Dukes' C disease, is being increas-ingly recommended. Preoperative radiotherapy for low rectal cancers can downstage the local disease and can make the lesion resectable.

Patients with Dukes' B disease might benefit from adjuvant chemotherapy. The difficulties in demonstrating efficacy in Dukes' B disease may relate to the fewer events. A larger number of patients will therefore be required in a large randomised study to confirm survival improvements. A number of major studies are at present ongoing.

In addition to 5-FU and folinic acid there has been recent interest in other adjuvant drugs such as irinotecan and capecitabine. Further trials are required to demonstrate improvement with these drugs compared to 5-FU and folinic acid. Following resec-tion of Dukes' C colon cancer the evidence supporting adjuvant chemotherapy is now very strong and such patients should be offered 5-FU and folinic acid.

The results of a major UK study (the QUASAR study) are awaited with interest. In this study patients with Dukes' B disease were randomised to surgery only and surgery plus high or low-dose folinic acid with or without levamisole.

There is some evidence of benefit in Dukes' B2 disease from a collaborative USA study in which four trials were amalgamated. In this study the benefits for Dukes' B disease were similar to those obtained in patients with Dukes' C disease.

Screening for colorectal cancer

Colorectal cancer is ideally suited for a screening approach because it is common and lethal, has a very long preclinical phase, accurate diagnostic methods are available and early detection greatly improves prognosis and survival. However, screening is complicated, requiring complex guidelines. This takes into account the effectiveness, cost, risks of intervention, age of patient and co-morbidity, compliance and availability of resources. All screening programmes and guidelines offer good detection rates, but none is 100% effective.

Faecal occult blood (FOB)

Screening for colorectal cancer with FOB has been assessed in several controlled trials. Many have reported a significant reduc-tion in colorectal cancer mortality as a result of screening with FOB, ranging from 15% to 43%. Such studies have also found that screen-detected cancer has a more favourable stage. Despite the reduced mortality from colorectal cancer through faecal occult blood testing, this method is insufficiently sensitive for detecting early colorectal cancer, with 3% false-positive and 22–58% false-negative results. The sensitivity depends on the Haemoccult testing kit used, whether it is non-hydrated (positivity rate of 5%), Haemoccult SENSA (positivity rate of 7%) or rehydrated (positivity rate of 15%). Faecal occult blood screening has a lower sensitivity for detecting colorectal cancers in the distal colon compared to other sites. Studies from the USA and Germany indicate that faecal occult blood screening could reduce mortality by 31–57%. However, poor patient compliance is a major restricting factor.

Flexible sigmoidoscopy screening

Flexible sigmoidoscopy in expert hands should examine to the splenic flexure, which includes up to 75% of colorectal neoplasms. It has been suggested that a baseline flexible sigmoidoscopy at 60 years of age with follow-up restricted to the 5–7% of the population who are likely to develop clinically significant metachronous neoplasia might prevent 50% of colorectal cancers occurring after age 60. Compared to breast cancer screening, costs are similar but effectiveness is much greater. However, only 30% of the eligible population would comply with flexible sigmoidoscopic screening. The presence of hyperplastic polyps at screening sigmoidoscopy is a risk factor for subsequent colorectal neoplasms, which raises questions about whether such patients should have follow-up surveillance colonoscopy.

Surveillance colonoscopy

Colonoscopy offers the convenience of a full examination of the colon with biopsy or polyp removal. However, it is considerably more expensive and time consuming and is associated with morbidity and reported mortality. Colonoscopy requires sedation and full bowel preparation. There is procedure-related discomfort and accidental perforation of the colon occurs in 1 in 1000 examinations. Poor patient compliance is also a problem. Only 38% of patients prefer colonoscopy as a screening method.

Barium enema

A double-contrast enema was considered, in the past, as the gold standard for imaging the entire colon. However, it is expensive and time consuming and associated with considerable discomfort and exposure to radiation. If the barium enema shows any abnormality, e.g. a polyp or a cancer, then colonoscopy will be required for polypectomy or biopsy, which adds to the cost and the morbidity. When asked, only 14% of patients preferred barium enemas to other screening methods.

Air-contrast CT enema/CT pneumocolon

This is a new method for colonic imaging, using the modern spiral/helical or multislice CT scanners, which gives good and rapid colonic imaging, following air insufflation of the colon. In advanced CT scanners, a three-dimensional imaging of the colon can be reconstructed (virtual colonoscopy) and even small lesions (<1 cm) in the colon can be detected. However, this method is still experimental and its long-term efficacy has yet to be calculated. Patients are also exposed to ionising radiation and it is as expensive as a barium enema. Patient compliance and tolerance appear to be much better than with other screening methods.

Magnetic resonance imaging of the colon

Gadolinium-enhanced MRI scanning can achieve good and rapid imaging of the colon, obtained in less than 30 seconds. Small colonic lesions can be detected, with an average sensitivity of 87% and specificity of 96% for detecting polyps. This innovative development is still experimental, but provides assessment of the colon with minimal invasiveness, no radiation exposure and a high level of diagnostic accuracy.

Blood tumour markers

Measurements of circulating antigens released by colorectal cancers, such as carcinoembryonic antigen (CEA) and CA19-9, or less commonly, alpha-fetoprotein have frequently been advocated but have proved of little diagnostic value in the early stages of cancer. However, CEA has a useful role in detecting early recurrences after previous curative surgical resections.

Genetic screening

Genetic counselling and screening are now available in certain centres, for high-risk family members, such as FAP or HNPCC. This includes screening for the APC gene mutations and DNA mismatch repairs seen in HNPCC. However, most of these methods are still experimental.

Criteria and guidelines for screening in colorectal cancer

The crucial decisions for colorectal cancer screening are whom to screen, how often and with what? Many guidelines have been recommended worldwide, such as the guidelines from the American Cancer Society. However, even with such guidelines, cancers are missed despite strict screening programmes. Three groups of patients need to be screened for colorectal cancer.

- High-risk patients (5–10% of the patient population): this includes those with a family history of FAP or HNPCC or inflammatory bowel disease. For patients with FAP, screening begins at puberty and includes surveillance colonoscopy, counselling and genetic testing. If polyps or FAP mutation are found, then total colectomy and ileoanal pouch surgery is recommended. In patients with history of HNPCC, screening begins at age 21 and includes surveillance colonoscopy (every 1–2 years), counselling and genetic testing. For inflammatory bowel disease, surveillance colonoscopy (and biopsies for dysplasia) is advised every 1–2 years, beginning eight years after the onset of pancolitis. If the caecum is not reached on colonoscopy, then a double-contrast barium enema is recommended. In dominant pedigree family members (with three or more first-degree relatives affected), surveillance colonoscopy should be offered early and prophylactic total colectomy is considered.

- Moderate-risk patients (estimated 15–20% of patient population): those patients with a history of adenomatous polyps, curative resection of colorectal cancer or colorectal cancer in first-degree relatives. After polypectomy, surveillance colonoscopy is recommended at one then three years. After curative resection of colorectal cancer, total colonic examination with colonoscopy is repeated at one, three and five years.

- Average-risk patients (70–80% of the patient population): screening should begin at the age of 50 and consist of faecal occult blood testing every year with flexible sigmoidoscopy every five years and total colonoscopy every 10 years.

Lifetime risk of colorectal cancer

The lifetime population risk of developing colorectal cancer in the UK is 1 in 50. However, the risk increases dramatically in relatives of patients with colorectal cancer, with a risk of 1 in 2 in a family of dominant pedigree (where three first-degree relatives are affected). The lifetime risks are summarised in Table 19.3.

Table 19.3 Lifetime risks of colorectal cancer (in relatives of patients with colorectal cancer)

Relatives	Risk
One first-degree relative, aged >45 years	1 in 17
One first-degree and one second-degree relative	1 in 12
One first-degree relative affected, aged <45 years	1 in 10
Two first-degree relatives affected	1 in 6
Dominant pedigree, three first-degree relatives affected	1 in 2
Population risk	1 in 50

Synchronous and metachronous colorectal cancers

Multiple synchronous colorectal cancers are found in approximately 5–7% of patients. Metachronous colorectal cancers have an incidence of 3–9%. There is little consensus regarding the distinction between truly metachronous and missed synchronous large bowel cancers. It is essential that synchronous cancers and polyps are identified before surgery and complete colonoscopy is the optimal method for examining the colon. A lifelong risk of developing metachronous colorectal cancer exists in all patients who have undergone rectal or colonic resection for malignancy. The annual incidence following index surgery is estimated at 0.35% per annum. The cumulative incidence rises to 30% after 41 years of follow-up.

Synchronous and metachronous colorectal cancers are features of HNPCC syndrome, characterised by a genetic predisposition to cancer at an early age, as discussed earlier. Metachronous colorectal cancers arising from mutations in HNPCC genes may develop within 2–5 years of a negative colonoscopy. The time taken for the adenoma-to-carcinoma sequence is probably determined by the precise genetic mutations involved. Microsatellite instability may be useful in recognising patients at high risk of developing synchronous and metachronous colorectal cancer. Multiple colorectal cancers are usually suitable for further curative surgery, with a curability rate of 81%. In a series from St Mark's hospital, London, only 6% were deemed inoperable. While total colectomy eliminates the need for colonoscopic surveillance, vigilance in examining the rectum is still required.

Conclusions

The overall five-year survival after curative resection for colorectal cancer averages about 50%. Prognosis is independent of age or sex and is based on the stage of the disease. Other factors have also been incriminated. Tumours that are histologically poorly differentiated, mucinous and with signet cells or evidence of vascular and neural invasion show poorer prognosis. Patients who present with obstruction or peritonitis have a worse prognosis than those who do not. The surgeon's competence is a recognised independent variable influencing recurrence and survival.

The detection of the disease at an early stage is thus a prime objective. Although early lesions are diagnosed on mass screening by testing for occult blood in the stool, the yield rate does not justify the workload and expense involved. Increased awareness by the public and alertness by clinicians are to be encouraged. Strict surveillance, including colonoscopy, is essential for individuals at high risk of colorectal cancer (as in those with a strong family history).

High ligation of the named vessels remains the standard component of resectional treatment of colorectal cancer. Prophylactic oophorectomy and radical lymphadenectomy do not seem to be of significant advantage. Stapling techniques have promoted sphincter-saving resection for lower rectal cancers, with an outcome comparable to that of abdominoperineal resection. Complete mesorectal excision reduces local recurrence rate and could avoid the need for postoperative radiotherapy.

It is now generally recommended that patients with Dukes' C (lymph node positive) should be offered systemic chemotherapy. At present the optimum regime is 5-fluorouracil with low-dose folinic acid. Patients with Dukes' B disease cannot be unequivocally recommended to undertake six months of chemotherapy. If possible these patients should be randomised into a trial of surgery only versus a surgery and chemotherapy regime. A number of such trials are at present active throughout Europe and the USA.

It should be noted that despite numerous trials over the past 25 years there is still huge controversy with regard to the role of chemotherapy in Dukes' B disease.

An alternative approach is to define adjuvant chemotherapy by portal venous infusion in order to reduce the possible development of liver metastases with survival benefit. A metaanalysis of several trials utilising portal vein infusion has suggested benefits for 'curatively' resected Dukes' B and C disease.

OTHER MALIGNANT COLORECTAL TUMOURS

Squamous cell carcinoma of the colon

Squamous cell carcinoma of the colon is extremely rare and its presentation is the same as adenocarcinoma. When diagnosed, the possibility of the colonic lesion being secondary should be considered and the site of a primary should be excluded. The surgical treatment is the same as adenocarcinoma. However, preoperative radiotherapy should be considered for squamous cell carcinoma of the rectum, as this may allow the tumour to regress sufficiently to allow a sphincter-saving resection. The majority are anal cancers with proximal extension into the rectum. Primary squamous cell carcinoma of the sigmoid colon with metastatic disease to the liver at diagnosis has been described and responded to systemic chemotherapy. Primary squamous cell carcinoma of the colon is a rare malignancy of unknown cause and pathogenesis. Metastatic tumours to the colon should be ruled out in all cases before therapy. Early detection and surgery remain the main therapeutic option and response to chemotherapy in advanced disease is encouraging.

Colorectal lymphoma

Lymphomas of the colon and rectum are rare. Non-Hodgkin's lymphoma (NHL) of the gastrointestinal (GI) tract accounts for 4–20% of all NHLs and is the most common extranodal site of presentation. Immunosuppression after solid-organ transplantation, coeliac disease, inflammatory bowel disease and HIV infection may be risk factors for GI lymphoma. Lymphomas of the colon and rectum are less common than gastric lymphoma. Surgery, radiotherapy and chemotherapy have been used in the treatment of GI lymphomas but the optimal management of these lymphomas has never been determined by prospective randomised clinical trials.

Carcinoid tumours of the colon and rectum

Carcinoid tumours are rare neuroendocrine neoplasms belonging to a more general category of tumours called the APUDomas. Ninety percent of carcinoid tumours are located in the gastrointestinal tract. Abdominal carcinoid tumours are categorised according to the division of the primitive gut from which they arise. Carcinoid tumours originating from the mid-gut develop from the small bowel, appendix and right colon and those originating from the hindgut develop from the distal transverse, left colon or rectum. Among the different organs that may be affected by metastases from carcinoid tumour, special emphasis is placed on the liver. The treatment consists of surgical excision followed by radiochemotherapy.

Small cell carcinoma of the colorectum

Small cell carcinoma of the rectum and colon is an infrequent pathologic finding and its precise incidence is unknown, but is less than 0.2% of all colorectal cancers. This tumour manifests highly aggressive behaviour. The treatment of choice is combination chemotherapy similar to that for small cell carcinoma of the lung, but in small localised tumours, surgery plus chemotherapy is an alternative.

ANAL CANAL TUMOURS

Benign tumours of the anal canal are rare and include anal polyps, skin lesions (such as lipomas, sebaceous cysts and pilonidal sinus) and condylomata acuminata. Fibroepithelial anal polyps are harmless, but occasionally cause irritation and pruritus ani and then require surgical excision.

Condylomata acuminata (venereal warts) are caused by the papilloma virus, as a result of sexual transmission (in homosexual and heterosexual patients). They can occur on the perianal skin, anal canal and lower rectum and are often difficult to eradicate. Typically, they present with cauliflower-type lesions, which can reach enormous sizes (Figure 19.3A), and are associated with penile and perineal lesions which grow slowly. In Figure 19.3, the patient had this lesion for over 10 years. Symptoms include irritation, odour, bleeding, discomfort and difficulty of defaecation.

Before treatment is started, serological testing and culture may be indicated. All treatments are painful and recurrences are frequent. Sexual contact should be stopped during the treatment and examination of sexual partners is advised. Most patients with small lesions require the use of podophyllum resin 25% in compound tincture of benzoin, which causes local discomfort and should be washed off after few hours. For huge lesions (as in Figure 19.3) and for recurrences, a wide local excision and a split skin grafting is recommended. Cryosurgical destruction, electrocoagulation and immunotherapy have been tried in the past, but all have high recurrence rates. Carcinoma has been reported with these perianal condylomata. An unusual variant, giant condyloma (Buschke–Löwenstein tumour), is locally invasive and malignant, although it may look benign on biopsy. Postoperative radiotherapy can be helpful in reducing the rate of local recurrence.

Anal carcinoma

Epidermoid carcinoma

Epidermoid carcinoma comprises 80% of anal carcinomas and histologically squamous cell, cloacogenic and mucoepidermoid

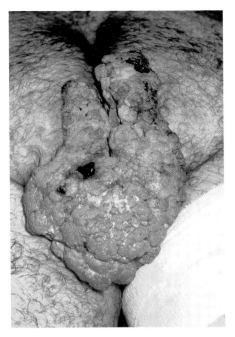
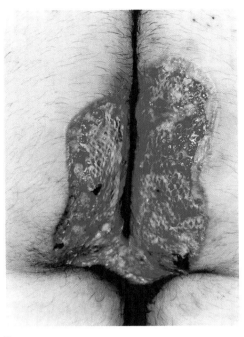
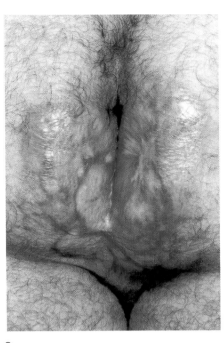

A   B   C

Figure 19.3 A. Giant condylomata (papilloma virus) in the perianal and perineal region (size 24 × 16 × 15 cm). The anal canal was 15 cm deep from the surface. **B.** The wound following excision and early stage of skin grafting. **C.** Subsequently the wound healed well: three months later.

carcinomas can be distinguished although they do not appear to have a different prognosis. Anal carcinoma accounts for less than 4% of anorectal malignancies and is easily misdiagnosed as an anal fissure as the most common symptoms are pain and bleeding. The difference in the age prevalence of these conditions should make the differentiation easier; anal carcinoma is seen in older patients. Faecal incontinence suggests sphincter involvement and infiltration of the posterior vaginal wall and fistulation causes vaginal discharge. The diagnosis is obvious when the lesion is advanced as the appearance of a malignant ulcer and tumour infiltration are evident. Some of these squamous carcinomas exhibit a basilloid pattern resembling rodent ulcers (also called cloacogenic carcinoma).

Digital examination and sigmoidoscopy is often painful. Thus caution should be exercised in making the diagnosis of a fissure in the elderly and when in doubt, biopsy is warranted. Digital palpation for the extent of the lesion and its depth, especially in relation to the anal sphincters, is relevant to the plan of treatment. Examination under anaesthesia provides optimum assessment. Endoanal ultrasonography will aid in determining sphincter involvement in early lesions. In nearly a third of patients, the inguinal lymph nodes are enlarged, especially when the primary tumour is large. Biopsy or fine needle aspiration is mandatory to confirm the presence of tumour. CT scan of the pelvis and abdomen is essential to demonstrate spread beyond the anal canal and exclude lymphatic spread and a chest radiograph to rule out lung metastases.

Radiotherapy (45–60 Gy), with or without the addition of chemotherapy (5-FU and mitomycin C) as a combined modality

therapy (CMT), is the standard primary treatment. Although the actuarial five-year survival is the same (60–70%) for both treatments, there is a significant improvement in local control by the addition of chemotherapy.

Surgery by local excision is reserved for small lesions at the anal margin, provided there is no infiltration into the sphincters. Abdominoperineal excision is the reserved option, when there is tumour residue or recurrence after CMT histologically confirmed by biopsy, and incontinence as a consequence of sphincter disruption or a rectovaginal fistula following regression of a locally extensive tumour.

Inguinal lymphadenopathy, histologically confirmed by tissue biopsy, is treated by radiotherapy or surgery and when present after primary therapy, is most likely to be due to recurrent tumour, when radical dissection will achieve up to 50% five-year survival.

Anogenital intraepithelial neoplasia

This is the better term for Bowen's disease of the anus and leucoplakia, which conveys no specific information. There should be a high level of suspicion, especially in homosexuals or HIV-positive patients with perianal hyperkeratotic lesions, flat, raised or ulcerated. Anogenital HPV-associated lesions are identified by examination with an operating microscope (colposcope) after the application of acetic acid on the skin surface, allowing targeted biopsy, but if unavailable, random incision biopsy or, provided the lesion is not extensive, excision biopsy is necessary to establish the diagnosis. Intraepithelial neoplasia is graded I to III, depending on

283

the proportion of the epithelial thickness involved. In grade III, the full thickness is dysplastic and is referred to as carcinoma *in situ*, for which complete excision should be ensured at the circumferential edges and the deeper layers.

Malignant tumours of the anal canal are rare and can be either a primary cancer or local invasion of a low rectal carcinoma.

Predisposing factors to anal carcinoma

There is an increased incidence of anal carcinoma among homosexuals, those with history of genital warts and infection with papillomavirus (types 16 and 18 DNA incorporated in the genome of their tumour cells). It is expected that with the increase in the incidence of genital human papillomavirus infection, an increased incidence of anal cancer will ultimately result.

Other types of anal cancers

Paget's disease

Paget's disease should be suspected when a demarcated raised erythematous area is associated with pruritus. The diagnosis is made by biopsy. In nearly 50–80% of cases there is an underlying adenocarcinoma, usually of the rectum although rarely of a distant organ; therefore, careful search is required. Treatment is by wide local excision with or without a skin graft, depending on the area excised. Local spread into the anal canal or an associated rectal carcinoma will require an abdominoperineal excision. In patients with widespread or recurrent disease chemotherapy and radiotherapy can be effective. Follow-up is required as local recurrence or metastatic spread may occur years later. In stage I disease, long-term disease-free survival is usual. When associated with adenocarcinoma elsewhere, the five-year survival rate is 50%.

Lymphoma of the anal canal

The diagnosis is made on biopsy and the management is similar to other types of lymphoma, which involves staging and then treatment with radiotherapy and chemotherapy.

Malignant melanoma

Melanoma also occurs rarely in the anal canal and should be borne in mind as it may be confused with a thrombosed external pile. The prospect of cure is minimal because of rapid metastatic spread, such that primary treatment by radical surgery should be considered carefully. The presentation is usually late, with lymphatic metastases (to inguinal lymph nodes). Despite treatment, the prognosis is usually very poor and the average five-year survival is <5%. The treatment involves abdominoperineal excision with block dissection of the inguinal lymph nodes. Adjuvant chemotherapy and radiotherapy offer little benefit.

Anal gland adenocarcinoma

This may result from local extension of a low rectal carcinoma. Such tumours are rare. Treatment involves abdominoperineal excision and radiotherapy, but the prognosis is poor.

Basal cell carcinoma

A rare anal tumour, which requires wide local excision or abdominoperineal excision.

OPERATIVE SURGERY
LARGE BOWEL RESECTION
Preoperative preparation
General health

The patient's general condition is optimised in the usual manner and prophylactic measures are used to reduce the risk of deep vein thrombosis, pulmonary embolism and infection.

Synchronous colorectal neoplasm

It is recommended that patients with colorectal cancer diagnosed by barium enema should have a routine preoperative colonoscopy. Should it fail for technical reasons, enthusiasts have recommended intraoperative colonoscopy. However, the chance of a missed synchronous carcinoma or a polyp larger than 1 cm on a good-quality double-contrast barium enema is exaggerated and double-contrast enema is sufficient to detect the majority of clinically important lesions. The risk of missing an adenoma that may take up to 10 years to develop into carcinoma should be measured against the patient's expected survival. It is logical that colonoscopy, if not employed as the primary diagnostic procedure, be performed during the postoperative surveillance in the younger patients.

Stoma marking

Whenever a temporary or permanent stoma is planned, this should be discussed with the patient. The patient should be visited by a stoma nurse or another patient with a stoma and provided with literature on the subject. With the patient sitting, standing and supine, the stoma site is selected, away from the umbilicus, the belt line, scars, skinfolds and bony prominences, namely the costal margins and the iliac crests. An appliance is fitted to allow siting at a position comfortable for the patient. The stoma site is then marked preoperatively with an indelible marker.

Bowel preparation

A clean bowel facilitates bowel mobilisation and reduces the incidence of septic complications. Methods for mechanical preparation include cathartics such as magnesium sulphate, castor oil, mannitol and whole-gut irrigation. Oral lavage with polyethylene glycol (PEG) or sodium picosulphate (Picolax) is currently the preferred method, as it allows rapid preparation without food restriction until the day prior to the operation. It also avoids the need for enemas. The patient is encouraged to drink plenty of fluids until the faecal effluent is clear. In elderly patients and those with cardiovascular disease, intravenous fluids and electrolytes replacement are monitored to avoid circulatory disturbances. In patients with stenosing lesions, oral purgation should be prescribed with caution as it may precipitate acute obstruction. Intestinal antiseptics administered parenterally further reduce the bacterial flora. A broad-spectrum cephalosporin combined with metronidazole to cover anaerobic organisms is maintained for no longer than 24 hours perioperatively, starting immediately before surgery.

Principles of surgical treatment

The principles of radical resection for cancer involve minimal handling of the primary tumour until its vasculature is interrupted by ligation of the main arterial supply at its origin, to allow removal of the lymphovascular tissues and *en bloc* resection of any involved tissues with clear proximal and distal resection margins.

The primary regional lymph nodes are in the vicinity of the named arteries and veins, which are anatomically related to the site of the primary tumour. Thus, curative resection should encompass all regional avenues of lymphatic spread and the length of the bowel to be resected should correspond to the extent of the vascular and mesenteric lymphadenectomy.

Several techniques have been employed to reduce the risk of colon cancer dissemination during surgical excision, for example:

- the 'no-touch isolation' technique
- using a direct approach to the origin of the artery and vein before mobilising the bowel to limit the potential for venous dissemination
- surgical tapes placed and tied around the bowel a few inches from the line of resection to avoid spillage of intestinal contents upon opening the bowel for anastomosis
- irrigation of the lumen of the bowel stumps with cytocidal agents, such as 1% cetrimide or aqueous povidone iodine, to destroy exfoliated malignant cells before they can be implanted in the suture line.

Cancer of the caecum and ascending colon

The appropriate operation is a radical right hemicolectomy. The right colic, ileocolic and right branches of the middle colic arteries and veins are divided at their origins (Figure 19.4A).

Cancer of the hepatic flexure

While the main route of spread is along the middle colic vessels, the lymph nodes along the right colic vessels may be involved and these vessels are taken at their origin. The resection sacrifices all of the right colon and most of the transverse colon. The ileum is anastomosed to the transverse colon. The operation is referred to as an extended radical right hemicolectomy (Figure 19.4B).

Cancer of the transverse colon

The resection is based on the middle colic arteries, involving both flexures. The right colon is sacrificed for the safety of an ileocolic anastomosis in the descending colon, as an extended right hemicolectomy (Figure 19.4C). A limited transverse colectomy can be used for the very elderly and unfit patient, to reduce the rate of operative morbidity and mortality.

Cancer of the splenic flexure

The middle and the left colic arteries are divided, sparing the inferior mesenteric artery and its sigmoidal branches. The right colon may be sutured to the distal descending or sigmoid colon (Figure 19.4D), although to avoid tension on the anastomosis, the right colon is sacrificed to allow an ileodescending or ileosigmoid anastomosis which is a safer tension-free anastomosis (Figure 19.4E).

Cancer of the descending colon and sigmoid

The resection is based on the origin of the inferior mesenteric artery. The inferior mesenteric vein is divided above the duodenum at the inferior border of the pancreas. Anastomosis of the transverse colon to the upper rectum is facilitated by full mobilisation of the splenic flexure (Figure 19.4F, G).

Cancer of the rectum

Careful evaluation by clinical examination and imaging defines those patients suitable for local excision (T1), those with advanced but resectable cancers (T2 and T3) who will benefit from preoperative adjuvant radiotherapy and those with locally advanced cancers with extrarectal fixity and adjacent organ invasion (T4) where preoperative chemo/radiotherapy may enhance resection. It is particularly helpful in identifying carcinomatous invasion in large villous adenomas, in order to decide on the extent of excision. A T1 or T2 lesion within the mid and lower rectum, not larger than 5 cm and histologically well differentiated, can be locally excised with full wall thickness.

Surgery for T3 and T4 rectal cancer aims at achieving adequate clearance at the several sites of tumour spread. High ligation of the inferior mesenteric artery at its origin or just below the left colic

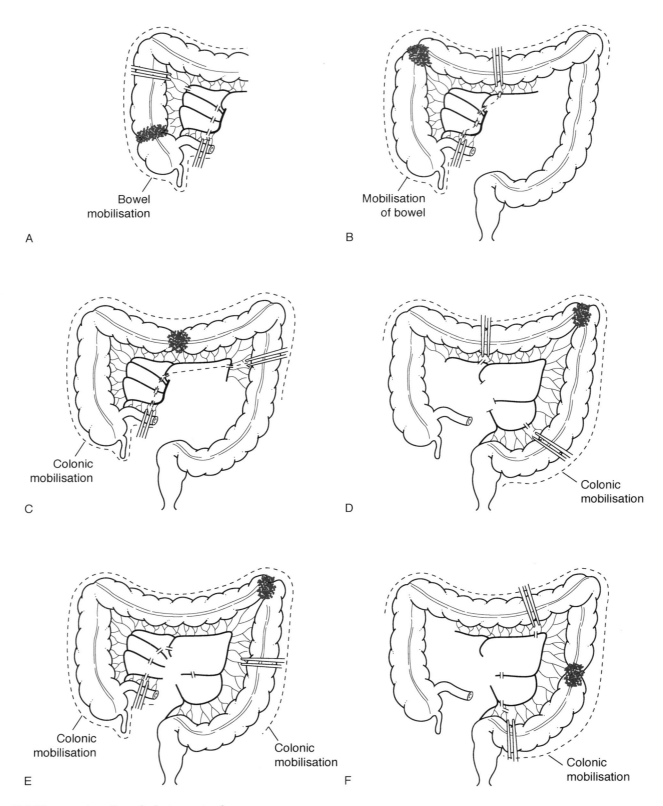

Figure 19.4 Diagrammatic outlines of colonic resection for cancer.

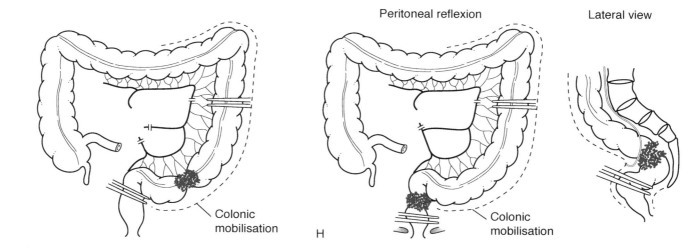

Peritoneal reflexion   Lateral view

Colonic mobilisation

G   H   Colonic mobilisation

branch allows a generous margin of proximal bowel, with its mesentery and maximum cephalad lymph nodes, to be removed (Figure 19.4H). Lateral lymph node excision is part of the dissection of the rectum at its pararectal attachment. Unless the tumour is poorly differentiated, a 2 cm clearance margin below the tumour edge is adequate since distal intramural spread does not exceed a few millimetres and distal lymphatic spread is rare; otherwise a 5 cm distal clearance is required. However, distal deposits can occur in the absence of distal intramural spread in the mesorectum, which should be included in the excised tissue (Figure 19.4H, lateral view).

The anal canal is 3–4 cm long; hence, a restorative resection is feasible for a well- or a moderately differentiated tumour allowing a 2 cm clearance margin down to a minimum distance of 7 cm from the anal verge. Stapling has made it technically possible to perform an anastomosis at even lower levels, as far down as the anal canal. An abdominoperineal resection is rarely necessary unless the tumour is infiltrating the levator muscles or the anal sphincters, or within the anorectal ring, although it is preferable when, for any reason, the functional outcome of a restorative resection is uncertain.

In 10% of patients, local excision or endocavity irradiation can be curative and is most appropriate in elderly patients who are unfit for a major procedure and in those who refuse a colostomy. A T1 or T2 lesion within the mid and lower rectum, not larger than 5 cm in diameter, mobile on digital examination, of favourable differentiation is suitable for local excision. Transanal endoscopic microsurgery (TEM) facilitates excision, particularly when lesions are in the upper rectum.

Diverting stoma

A diverting stoma is a safeguard in patients whose anastomoses are at risk of dehiscence. This includes patients who have received pelvic irradiation, immunocompromised patients and those with a low anastomosis. Complete mesorectal excision appears to increase the likelihood of anastomotic breakdown. A diverting

stoma is not a substitute for a dextrously performed anastomosis and does not prevent anastomotic breakdown, although it reduces the consequences of a leak. For this reason, it should also be considered in elderly patients whose compromised general fitness is judged not to withstand pelvic sepsis, should it occur.

A loop ileostomy is more favoured than a loop colostomy because it is more acceptable to the patient, easier to manage and provides better diversion. It is reasonable to close a diverting stoma after two weeks, once the integrity of the anastomosis is assessed by digital examination and a water-soluble contrast proctogram. However, this may have to be deferred if the tissues are still oedematous, as mobilisation of the stoma and its closure may be technically difficult, with the risk of suture line leak.

Complications

Perioperative complications

Morbidity is due to cardiovascular and respiratory complications, thromboembolism, prolonged ileus and wound and intraabdominal sepsis. Specific complications related to colorectal surgery are discussed further.

Intraoperative bleeding

Severe bleeding from the middle sacral vessels may result from a tear of the presacral fascia during mobilisation of the rectum. Ligation and cautery may stop the bleeding but can often make it worse. Direct pressure and packing the pelvis may control the bleeding but, if it continues, it may be necessary to leave the pack *in situ* for a few days.

Urinary tract complications

Intraoperative injury of the ureter recognised at the time of the operation is immediately repaired. If punctured or clamped but still viable, it should be stented for a few days. When cut, the ends are mobilised and spatulated and an anastomosis is carried out with fine catgut over a stent. An injured lower ureter is reimplanted into the bladder as a neo-ureterocystostomy, by the psoas hitch or the Boari flap technique.

It is important, therefore, to identify the ureters and, when difficulty is anticipated because of a large tumour or previous pelvic surgery, they should be outlined on an intravenous urogram and stents placed cystoscopically at the start of the procedure. If the ureters cannot be identified intraoperatively, stents are placed through a cystostomy.

Injury to the urinary tract is suspected in the postoperative period if the abdomen becomes distended and the urine output is diminished, if there is excessive clear fluid in the drainage bag or leaking through the abdominal wall or perineal wound. The urea and creatinine levels in the drainage fluid, serum and urine will distinguish a peritoneal exudate from urine. An ultrasound examination may show hydronephrosis and an intravenous urogram will localise the injury.

When the bladder wall is breached when involved by tumour, the bladder is closed with absorbable sutures and a urinary catheter drainage is maintained for 7–10 days.

Urinary tract infection associated with catheterisation is common. The catheter should therefore be removed once the patient is mobile and is not demanding nursing. Urinary retention is common in males with previous prostate symptoms and, more frequently, following rectal excision. After several days or weeks of intermittent or continuous catheterisation, a proportion of patients are able to empty their bladder spontaneously, although a few may require transurethral resection of the prostate.

Sexual dysfunction

Impotence and failure of ejaculation are not uncommon after anterior resection and abdominoperineal resection, as a result of injury to the hypogastric plexus, which can be avoided by identifying it at the level of the sacral premonitory where it divides into the right and left bundles lying below the presacral fascia. The pelvic plexus may also be injured during the lateral dissection where the branches run with the middle haemorrhoidal vessels, and their cavernous branches within Denonvillier's fascia anteriorly are also vulnerable.

Females may suffer loss of desire and orgasm and dyspareunia due to neurogenic injury and anatomical changes.

Perineal wound

Primary closure of the perineal wound following rectal excision is the current practice, unless the pelvic cavity is packed because of uncontrolled bleeding. When the pack is removed, the wound is sutured around a corrugated drain. The skin sutures are removed

if infected material or a haematoma accumulates in the pelvic cavity, to allow drainage and regular irrigation. A persistent discharge requires examination under anaesthesia and curettage of the cavity which should be carried out with caution in order not to damage small bowel that may be lying in the cavity. An enteroperineal fistula is excluded with a fistulogram and, particularly in patients who have received radiation therapy, the possibility of bone necrosis is best investigated by CT scanning.

Intestinal obstruction

Early adhesive obstruction is known to occur. The risk of internal herniation is minimised by closing mesenteric defects and the lateral paracolostomy gutter when fashioning an end colostomy. The pelvic peritoneal floor cavity should be closed after total rectal excision. When the peritoneal edges cannot be approximated to close the pelvic cavity without tension, the defect can be filled with omentum or with the caecum, by freeing it from its peritoneal attachment and placing it at the pelvic brim. Small bowel may also get entrapped in a paracolostomy hernia, causing intestinal obstruction, but this usually occurs late.

Colostomy complications

The ostomy aperture for either a temporary or a permanent stoma is best constructed before the abdominal wall incision is made. This allows a vertical core of tissue to be excised within the boundary of the rectus muscle and its sheaths, while the parietes are intact, in order to minimise the risk of a stomal hernia. A transparent stoma bag allows inspection of the stoma in the postoperative period for evidence of ischaemia, bleeding and mucocutaneous dehiscence. Ischaemia confined to the stoma is treated expectantly, but if it extends more proximally, urgent exploration through the stoma wound or main wound is necessary in order to resect the ischaemic segment and construct a new stoma. The extent of the ischaemia is determined by examining the bowel with a rigid or flexible sigmoidoscope passed through the stoma. Ischaemic necrosis of the stoma, mucocutaneous separation and parastomal infection will, in the long term, result in stoma stenosis, requiring refashioning. This should be deferred until a fibrous plane is established, to allow easier dissection between the tissue planes. In the interval, dilatation with the finger or St Mark's dilators may be necessary to avoid blockage.

Anastomotic leakage

Clinically apparent anastomotic leak is far less frequent than a radiological leak for both sutured and stapled anastomosis and is more common in low anastomoses. Anastomotic failure is usually related to technical factors, the adequacy of blood supply and tension on the suture line. A defective stapled anastomosis is suspected when the 'doughnut' rings are incomplete. The anastomosis is examined intraoperatively for a leak by filling the pelvis with saline and distending the anastomosis with air insufflated with a sigmoidoscope. Repairing localised leaks reduces the risk of a subsequent leak.

The management of an anastomotic leak is dependent on the clinical condition of the patient. A routine water-soluble contrast enema, unless for audit purposes, does not influence the management of an asymptomatic patient with a subclinical leak and does not justify the risk of converting a partial to a complete leak or precipitating sepsis by the procedure. A faecal leak through the abdominal wound or the drain site with no systemic disturbance is treated conservatively. Oral intake is restricted to fluids and a low residue diet and is supplemented, if necessary, by enteral feeding or, in the presence of ileus, by parenteral feeding in order to maintain the nutritional state. Should the patient show signs of localised peritonitis, with pain or tenderness, fever and leucocytosis, antibiotics are commenced parenterally. Fluid collection in the pelvis or elsewhere in the peritoneal cavity is identified and percutaneously drained under ultrasound or CT guidance.

Should these measures fail or if a leak is associated with peritonitis and significant sepsis, exploration is necessary. With a minor anastomotic defect, peritoneal irrigation with drainage and a diverting stoma is quite adequate. With a larger anastomotic disruption, the proximal bowel is brought out as an end colostomy and, depending on the level of the anastomosis, the distal end is closed or converted to a mucus fistula. Bowel continuity is restored 3–6 months later.

FURTHER READING

Astler VB, Coller FA. The prognostic significance of direct extension of carcinoma of the colon and rectum. *Ann Surg* 1954; **139**:846–852

Boland CR. The biology of colorectal cancer. *Cancer* 1993; **71**:4180–4186

Bond JH. Colorectal cancer screening. *Curr Opin Oncol* 1998; **10**:461–466

Boulos PB. Colorectal cancer. In: Taylor I, Cooke TG, Guillou P, eds. *Essential General Surgical Oncology*. London: Churchill Livingstone, 1996

Byers T, Levin B, Rothenberger D, Dodd GD, Smith RA. The American Cancer Society guidelines for colorectal cancer screening: have we gone too far (or not far enough)? *Gastroenterology* 1998; **114**:1341–1343

Deans GT, Parks TG, Rowlands BJ, Spence RAJ. Prognostic factors in colorectal cancer. *Br J Surg* 1992; **79**:608–613

Donegan WL. New screening guidelines for colorectal cancer. *J Surg Oncol* 1998; **68**:2–4

Dukes CE. The classification of cancer of the rectum. *J Pathol Bacteriol* 1932; **35**:323–332

Fracasso P, Assisi D, Stigliano V, Casale V. Colorectal cancer complicating ulcerative colitis: an institutional series. *J Exp Clin Cancer Res* 1999; **18**:29–32

Howe JR, Guillem JG. The genetics of colorectal cancer. *Surg Clin North Am* 1997; **77**:175–195

IMPACT (B2) Investigators. Efficacy of adjuvant fluorouracil and folinic acid in B2 colon cancer. *J Clin Oncol* 1999; **17**:1356–1363

Liver Infusion Meta Analysis Group. Portal vein chemotherapy for colorectal cancer: a meta analysis of 4000 patients in 10 studies. *J Natl Cancer Inst* 1997; **89**:497–505

Navaratnam RM, Chowaniec J, Winslet MC. The molecular biology of colorectal cancer development and the associated genetic events. *Ann Roy Coll Surg Engl* 1999; **81**:312–319

Potter JD. Colorectal cancer: molecules and populations. *J Natl Cancer Inst* 1999; **91**:916–932

Sengupta SB, Yiu C-Y, Boulos PB, de Silva M, Sams VR, Delhanty JDA. Genetic instability in patients with metachronous colorectal cancers. *Br J Surg* 1997; **84**:996–1000

Taylor I, Machin D, Mullee M et al. A randomised controlled trial of adjuvant portal vein cytotoxic perfusion in colorectal cancer. *Br J Surg* 1985; **72**:359–363

The anorectum

I.G. Finlay, W.S. Hendry

ANATOMY AND PHYSIOLOGY

Anatomy of the anorectum

An understanding of the anatomy and physiology of the anorectum and pelvic floor is necessary for the successful treatment of patients with anorectal disorders.

The rectum begins as a continuation of the large bowel at the level of the third sacral segment where the taenia coli become diffuse, forming a complete outer layer of longitudinal muscle. The rectum is 15 to 18 cm in length, widening to form an ampulla capable of distension immediately above the levator ani muscles. Although the name is derived from the Latin word 'rectus' meaning straight, the rectum follows two curves in the sagittal plane as it passes through the concavity of the sacrum and the pelvic floor. The inner circular muscles form the Valves of Houston and in the distal three to four cm give rise to the internal sphincter.

The anal canal, which is four cm in length, extends from the anal verge to the anorectal ring (level where the rectum passes through the pelvic floor). This is a practical description of the anal canal which corresponds with clinical and ultrasound examination. On histological examination, however, the anal canal would be much shorter, extending from the anal verge to the dentate line, which is the point where squamous and columnar mucosa meet. At this point there is a transitional zone (ATZ) extending for two cm which comprises modified columnar epithelium. This may have an important role in the sensory component of continence.

Surrounding the anal canal and supporting the ampulla of the rectum lie the muscles of the external anal sphincter (EAS) and pelvic floor. The latter provide a 'sling support' for the rectum and pelvic organs and comprise a sheet of striated muscle (levator ani) which in turn is subdivided into four component parts (puborectalis and pubococcygeus, ileococcygeus and ischiococcygeus). These muscles attach to the pelvic bones, fascial condensations and the coccyx. The puborectalis is particularly important since it forms a loop around the anal canal rectal junction with an origin and insertion in the pubic bones. This loop forms an anorectal angle of approximately 90°. The external anal sphincter is a continuation of the puborectalis and cannot be distinguished from this muscle at surgery. Although the external sphincter is described as having three component parts, the muscle works as a single unit in conjunction with the pelvic floor. There is a distinct avascular space between the internal and external anal sphincters known as the intersphincteric plane. This is anatomically important to surgeons since it allows access to the supralevator space. This space is also important because it contains anal glands which communicate with the anal canal at the level of the dentate line. These glands are particularly prone to infection, which manifests as perianal and ischiorectal abscesses.

Innervation of the rectum, anus and pelvic floor

The anal canal is sensitive to touch, pin prick, heat and cold extending from the anal verge to approximately 15 mm above the anal valves. Although this area has been considered responsible for discrimination between flatus and stool, this ability remains despite local anaesthetic infiltration suggesting an additional mechanism. The anal transitional zone, however, is rich in organised nerve endings such as Krausen bulbs, Meissener's corpuscles and Golgi-mezzoni bodies. Sensory impulses from the anal canal are transmitted via the inferior haemorrhoidal branches of the pudendal nerves to sacral segments 2 to 4.

The rectum is only sensitive to distension which is probably detected by stretch receptors in the pelvic fascia and the muscles of the pelvic floor. It is important to note that distension sensitivity remains after rectal excision as in the ileoanal pouch operation. It is known that the pathway for the recognition of rectal distension is the parasympathetic system via the pelvic plexus to S2, S3 and S4 since rectal sensation is abolished by parasympathetic blockade.

The pelvic floor muscles are innervated by motor neurones which lie in the ventral grey matter of the second to fourth sacral cord segments. The fourth sacral nerve, running above the levator, probably supplies the levator ani muscle. This nerve may be particularly vulnerable in childbirth, either due to traction or ischaemic injury. There remains controversy as to the innervation of the puborectalis, which may have a crossover between the sacral nerves from above and the pudendal nerves from below. The latter carries motor nerves to the EAS by the inferior haemorrhoidal branches of the pudendal nerve. The EAS therefore is under voluntary control as a consequence of the connection between the ventral horn of S2 (Onuf's nucleus) and the corticospinal pathways. The motor neurones of Onuf's nucleus are unusual since they are tonically active during sleep. The integrity of the pudendal nerves and sacral plexus can be easily tested clinically by observing the anocutaneous reflex. This is achieved by stroking the perianal skin; a transient contraction of the external anal sphincter is then observed if the reflex is intact. A similar reflex is observed on coughing when the external anal sphincter spontaneously contracts.

In contrast to the EAS, the internal anal sphincter (IAS) is an involuntary smooth muscle which is under both inhibitory and excitatory control. The sympathetic innervation is excitatory arising from the hypogastric and pelvic plexus. The parasympathetic nerves are inhibitory, arising from S1, S2 and S3. *In vitro* studies have suggested that alpha-adrenergic receptors are excitatory while beta-adrenergic, cholinergic and non-cholinergic/ non-adrenergic receptors are all inhibitory.

There is a clinically important reflex between the rectum and the IAS known as the rectoanoinhibitory reflex. Rectal distension induces reflex relaxation of the internal anal sphincter with a reduction in resting anal canal pressure. This reflex is absent in Hirschsprung's disease, Chagas' disease and after rectal mucosal excision. The reflex is known to be intramural, involving neurones of the myenteric plexus.

Anorectal physiology

Physiologically the principal function of the anorectum is to provide storage of faecal material with a voluntary and controlled mechanism for evacuation of faeces and gas. The mechanism for both continence and defaecation are not yet fully understood. It is, however, a complicated system which can allow the retention of both solid and liquid while gas is expelled in a downward direction.

Continence is dependent upon the complex interaction of the following components:

- IAS
- EAS
- Puborectalis/pelvic floor muscles
- Anal canal cushions
- Sensory innervation of anal canal/pelvic floor
- Consistency of faeces.

The IAS is an involuntary muscle responsible for the majority of the resting anal canal pressure. This muscle in turn keeps the anal canal closed and in conjunction with the anal canal cushions prevents minor leakage. Consequently, loss of IAS produces symptoms of minor leakage of faeces, staining of clothing and irritation of the perianal skin. Loss of the IAS may occur after anal canal surgery. In particular, anal stretch operations have been shown to irretrievably damage the muscle. Other causes include autonomic nerve injury from diabetes or excessive alcohol intake. Similar symptoms may be experienced by patients who have large prolapsed haemorrhoids (anal canal cushions).

The EAS is under voluntary control and on contraction transiently raises the anal canal pressure (30 to 60 seconds). This muscle is considered to be predominantly responsible for averting the call to stool.

The muscles of the pelvic floor, and particularly the puborectalis, are responsible for creating an acute angle between the anal canal and rectum (anorectal angle). Under voluntary control patients can temporarily make the anorectal angle more acute by contracting the puborectalis in conjunction with the EAS. This component of continence is considered to be the most important single factor in the control of formed faeces. Evidence to support this is drawn from the fact that patients who have had a pull-through operation for anal agenesis can be remarkably continent using only the pelvic floor musculature.

Other important factors in the mechanism of continence include the sensory innervation of the anal canal and stool consistency. It is widely accepted that the ATZ of the anal canal has an important role in discriminating flatus and stool by a process known as the sampling reflex, whereby a small quantity of material is periodically allowed to enter the anal canal where discrimination takes place. The mechanism whereby this is achieved, however, remains poorly understood.

Continence for liquid stool is precarious, even for the normal anal sphincter. This is probably because liquids easily flow around 'bends' and in order to achieve control of liquid, a squeeze pressure equal to or greater than rectal pressure must be achieved. Consequently, even minor deficiencies in sphincter integrity will therefore lead to incontinence of liquid stool. It seems probable that since diarrhoea is an abnormal state, no mechanism has evolved for the control of liquid other than voluntary squeeze of the EAS and puborectalis.

Defaecation

It is somewhat surprising that the exact physiological mechanism for the process of defaecation remains poorly understood. It is, however, considered that the urge to defaecate occurs in the superior frontal gyrus. Rectal distension, or more probably levator ani stretch, stimulates IAS relaxation and sampling. Defaecation is deferred by contraction of the IAS and pelvic floor muscles. At an appropriate time evacuation occurs by relaxation of the puborectalis and EAS in association perhaps with contraction of the posterior pelvic floor muscles. In this way the anorectal angle is opened. Simultaneously, the intra-abdominal pressure is increased and the colon and rectum contract. Maintenance of a funnel-shaped outlet is necessary but may be lost in conditions such as rectocele, leading to difficulty in evacuation.

Physiological measurement in the anorectum

Anorectal manometry

An objective assessment of the anal canal tone is obtained by performing manometry. Various techniques are available for this purpose including balloon recording and water perfusion systems. The most up-to-date technique, however, involves the use of a microtransducer system. In this technique the transducer, which is only a few millimetres in diameter, is drawn through the anal canal. In this way the resting anal canal pressure is recorded. Approximately 80% of this value is due to the effect of the tonic contraction of the IAS; the remainder being produced by contraction of the EAS. In addition to providing a numerical value for resting anal canal pressure this technique gives a figure for anal canal length (usually three to five cm).

Voluntary or squeeze pressure is predominantly produced by the EAS. It is higher in men than women and reduces in both sexes with age. There is some concern, however, that results obtained in the laboratory using this technique may not represent the true physiological state. An attempt to overcome this using ambulatory anorectal manometry has been used in the research setting but is rarely available in routine clinical practice.

Electromyography

In patients where the anal sphincter has been shown to be weak by manometric or other testing, it is necessary to identify the cause of this abnormality. There are really two important investigations which are useful in this respect. These are endoanal ultrasound and measurement of pudendal nerve motor latency (PNML). A novel technique to measure PNML was described by Kiff and Swash in 1984. This utilises the fact that the anatomical course of the pudendal nerve allows access to the nerve at the level of the ischial spine immediately prior to the nerve entering the sciatic foramen. In this position the nerve is accessible to stimulation on rectal examination. In order to achieve this, a stimulating anode/cathode electrode is positioned at the tip of the index finger on an examination glove. The ischial spine is palpated but usually the nerve is located by identifying the classical waveform on an EMG machine. A recording electrode at the base of the index finger identifies EAS contraction and the EMG indicates the time interval between stimulation and the contraction, which should be two m or less. Abnormally long PNML times occur classically in neurogenic faecal incontinence, rectal prolapse, chronic constipation, uterovaginal prolapse and in the solitary rectal ulcer syndrome.

Electromyography in the assessment of the anorectum has predominantly been used as a research tool. The technique, however, did find a clinical role in identifying sphincter defects during the process of sphincter mapping. This involved implanting a series of needles in the anal sphincter circumferentially, identifying areas where the normal EMG trace was absent. The technique, however, has become largely redundant with the availability of ultrasound.

Anal and rectal sensation

Measurement of anal canal sensation is a relatively simple and reproducible technique which can be useful in assessment of patients whose major complaint is that of minor faecal leakage. Loss of sensation has been identified in patients with diabetes and after surgical procedures which involve dissection in the anal canal. Measurement of rectal balloon distension and rectal compliance are also relatively easily achieved by inflating a balloon in the rectum and determining the patient's awareness of distension. Patients with megarectum will tolerate a large degree of rectal distension. In contrast, those patients with underlying inflammatory bowel disease or irritable bowel syndrome may be intolerant of the technique with evidence of an irritable rectum.

Endorectal/anal ultrasound

Endorectal endosonography (ERS) was initially developed to stage rectal cancer but now has a number of clinical indications. The technique, however, involves a degree of operator expertise. 'Blind' insertion of the ultrasound probe allows examination of approximately 10 cm of anal canal and lower rectum but higher lesions can be identified using an introducing proctoscope. Although good contact with the rectal wall is required for adequate definition, overdistension of the rectum should be avoided since it limits visualisation of the second mucosal layer.

On endorectal ultrasonography, a five-layer pattern of the rectal wall corresponds with the acoustic reflections from individual layers. These five layers are as follows:

- Mucosa
- Deep mucosa
- Submucosa
- Muscularis propria
- Adventitia.

The technique has predominantly been used to stage early carcinoma with a view to successful local excision of the primary tumour. In this respect the tumours are staged as T_1 to T_4. T_1 are those lesions confined to the mucosa and submucosa, T_2 lesions are limited to the muscularis mucosa while T_3 lesions have breached the muscle and T_4 have invaded adjacent structures. When compared with both CT and MRI, endoluminal ultrasound has been shown to be superior in the identification of T_1 and T_2 lesions. Local excision is predominantly restricted to those lesions which are T_1 since it has been shown that the risk of having associated lymph node involvement is less than 5%. Other uses have included examination of villous adenomas for the presence of tumour.

Anal ultrasound examination has become particularly important in the assessment of the internal and external sphincters. In the anal canal a four-layer pattern is recognised comprising:

- A subepithelial layer
- Internal sphincter
- Longitudinal muscle
- External sphincter.

Using the technique it has become apparent that defects in both the IAS and EAS are much more common than were formerly appreciated. In particular, it is now recognised that as many as 50% of women undergoing childbirth will develop a defect in either the internal or external sphincter after the delivery. This is clinically important since surgery for the correction of a sphincter defect, in the absence of a pudendal nerve neuropathy, has an excellent prospect for a successful outcome. Endoanal ultrasound examination can also be useful in identifying sepsis and fistulas within the sphincter complex. Endoanal ultrasound is an indispensable investigation for patients with faecal incontinence.

FAECAL INCONTINENCE

Loss of voluntary control of faeces is a distressing and disabling symptom affecting all age groups. The incidence is much higher in women and prevalence is highest in patients over the age of 65. The true incidence is difficult to define as many patients are unwilling to admit to symptoms because of embarrassment and minor degrees of soiling may not be regarded as sufficiently troublesome to report. It is estimated that as many as one in three patients in long-term care may suffer from faecal and/or urinary incontinence.

Aetiology

Continence depends on a number of closely related factors including stool consistency, peristaltic activity, rectal compliance, anorectal sensation, an intact rectoanal inhibitory reflex and normal function of the internal and external sphincters. Box 20.1 shows the factors associated with faecal incontinence.

Box 20.1 Faecal Incontinence

Congenital anomalies
Faecal impaction with spurious diarrhoea
Anorectal carcinoma
Proctocolitis
Fistula-in-ano
Rectal prolapse
Sphincter neuropathy
  Demyelination
  Cerebrovascular accident
  Diabetes
  Pudendal nerve neuropathy
Sphincter injury
  Obstetric trauma
  Anorectal surgery
  Trauma

Obstetric causes account for a large number of patients presenting to surgical practice and the underlying problem is related to sphincter damage during delivery or neuropathic damage to the pelvic floor muscles. In many cases there is a history of protracted labour and risk factors include multiparity, prolonged second stage of labour, large babies, and the use of forceps. The incidence of third-degree tears with disruption of the sphincter complex is low and these injuries are immediately recognised and repaired. There are however a number of women who sustain sphincter damage during vaginal delivery with no immediate signs or symptoms that this has occurred. A number of studies using endoanal ultrasound have demonstrated structural damage to one or both sphincter muscles in one-third of women after their first vaginal delivery.

Evidence that nerve damage to the pelvic floor muscles is an important factor relates to the demonstration of an increase in fibrous connective tissue in the external sphincter, puborectalis and levator ani. In addition, a frequent finding in these patients is

a prolonged pudendal nerve terminal motor latency. Damage to the pudendal nerves leads to reduced squeeze pressures in the anal canal and diminished sensation. Perineal descent is a common feature in these patients and this in turn may cause further damage to the pudendal nerves.

Sphincter damage after anorectal surgery is the most common aetiology after obstetric causes. The management of fistula-in-ano can be very challenging, with a high incidence of problems of continence associated with complex fistulae. It is not unusual for patients undergoing surgery for more simple procedures such as haemorrhoidectomy to notice a minor degree of soiling. This is probably due to a degree of sensory impairment although endoanal ultrasound, may on occasion, demonstrate significant structural sphincter damage. Anal dilatation as treatment for chronic anal fissure has been reported to be associated with an unacceptable incidence of incontinence which is seen much less frequently with the alternative procedure of lateral sphincterotomy.

Faecal incontinence is a feature in many neurological disorders such as multiple sclerosis, spinal injury, and diabetic neuropathy. It may also be a manifestation of other colorectal pathology including rectal carcinoma, inflammatory bowel disease and rectal prolapse.

History and examination

Duration and severity of symptoms should be defined and in women, particular care should be taken to establish a careful obstetric history and the time interval between delivery and onset of symptoms. It is important to try to distinguish between incontinence to flatus, liquids or solids. Faecal soiling is typically associated with damage to or dysfunction of the internal sphincter or an abnormality of anal sensation. Urge incontinence is generally associated with external sphincter dysfunction. The history must also include a careful search for any previous anorectal surgery.

General abdominal examination is carried out along with digital examination of the rectum. With the patient in the left lateral position, perineal descent is assessed on straining and the perianal and perineal areas are inspected for evidence of fistulas or previous scars. Rigid or flexible sigmoidoscopy is performed. Digital examination can also provide a reasonable assessment of sphincter tone and the puborectalis sling can be easily palpated by asking the patient to voluntarily contract. Major deficiencies of the sphincter anteriorly are generally easily demonstrated by inspection and palpation.

Endoanal ultrasound and anorectal physiological tests are helpful in defining the cause of incontinence and also in predicting likely outcome of surgical management. Ultrasound can clearly define the anatomical defects in the sphincter apparatus and may also be used to assess the results of surgical repair. MRI may also be indicated particularly when incontinence is associated with fistula-in-ano. The measurement of resting and squeeze pressures is helpful in further defining the site of injury or dysfunction.

Management

Treatment depends on aetiology and severity of symptoms. Patients who have a minor degree of occasional soiling, and in whom no major structural sphincter damage is demonstrated, can be reassured and advised simply on good dietary habits and personal hygiene.

Conservative management is appropriate for many patients, at least in the initial stages. Patients with faecal frequency and urgency may only have difficulty with control if the stool is fluid. A combination of bulking agents and either codeine or loperamide may be sufficient to control their symptoms. Pelvic floor exercises may be helpful, particularly in women who report minor problems with continence following delivery. Biofeedback may be appropriate when the aetiology is sensory loss. The aim is to improve sensory awareness and increase voluntary sphincter response using a combination of visual or auditory feedback signals.

Surgical treatment is aimed towards direct repair of divided sphincters, pelvic floor repair for neuropathic damage or the creation of a neosphincter using transplanted muscle or a synthetic sphincter device.

Surgical treatment

Anterior sphincter repair

This procedure is indicated where a sphincter defect is apparent on clinical examination or where the defect has been defined on endoanal ultrasound. The injury is almost always associated with obstetric trauma and these patients may also have a degree of neuropathic damage to the pelvic floor muscles. Standard bowel preparation and prophylactic antibiotic therapy are used. The prone jack-knife position gives best access. In severe cases the perineal body is completely deficient leaving the posterior vaginal and anterior rectal mucosa confluent. The intersphincteric plane is developed and the external sphincter mobilised from the surrounding scar tissue until the divided ends are defined. The vagina is dissected free from the anterior rectal wall. An overlapping repair of the external sphincter is then carried out in two layers and an anterior levatorplasty may be carried out in addition. The results of this procedure can be very good with continence restored in up to 80% of cases. Those who have a poor functional result can often be shown to have pudendal neuropathy in addition.

Postanal repair

Postanal repair was introduced by Parks. The procedure evolved to address the problems which had been identified in many

patients with idiopathic faecal incontinence. The puborectalis sling is weak, there is evidence of denervation of the pelvic muscles and proctography identifies loss of the anorectal angle. The operation was designed to recreate the anorectal angle by plicating the levator muscles posteriorly. The procedure currently has a decreasing role in the management of incontinence because of poor long-term results.

Preoperative mechanical bowel preparation is again used along with prophylactic antibiotics. The prone jack-knife position gives good exposure. A curved postanal incision is made and the intersphincteric plane identified. Waldeyer's fascia is divided exposing the mesorectum and the two edges of the levator muscle exposed. These are plicated using a series of interrupted sutures and finally the external sphincter is also plicated posteriorly.

Results of this procedure are much less predictable than with anterior sphincter repair. Short-term benefit is seen in up to 80% of cases but this rapidly diminishes with time, with only around 20% fully continent after five years. A large number of studies have failed to show a consistent correlation between preoperative physiological measurements and functional outcome. Prolongation of pudendal nerve terminal motor latency before surgery has been shown to be a bad prognostic sign suggesting that progressive denervation is responsible for the deteriorating results.

Neosphincter

If sphincter repair is not possible or has failed, the use of other muscles or a prosthetic sphincter may be considered. The gluteal muscles have been used but the operation is complex. The gracilis muscle is easier to mobilise and the technique has no major effect on leg function. The mobilised muscle is wrapped around the anal canal and the tendon sutured to the contralateral ischial tuberosity. The main problem with this muscle is that it is composed largely of type 2 fatiguable fibres. An implanted electrical stimulator allows a change in composition to infatiguable type 1 fibres making this a practical, though technically demanding treatment option.

Artificial anal sphincter development is still at an early stage. The artificial urinary sphincter was developed in 1972 with good functional results. Modifications of this model to adapt to anal canal anatomy have been developed comprising a fluid reservoir, valve and cuff placed around the anal canal. The artificial sphincter remains largely a research procedure and is not sufficiently refined to be used outwith that setting.

Colostomy

The formation of a colostomy is still indicated in the management of faecal incontinence if other surgical options have failed or are deemed inappropriate. It may transform the patient's quality of life and allow them to pursue various social activities rendered impossible because of incontinence.

CHRONIC CONSTIPATION

Constipation is a common condition affecting all age groups but the precise definition is often difficult to establish. 'Normal' bowel function varies considerably between individuals and may be influenced by a wide range of emotional, physiological and pathological factors as well as a large number of therapeutic agents. Some patients complain that the stools are too hard or too small. Others complain of difficulty evacuating the stool, often associated with prolonged periods of straining and the need for manual evacuation. A reduction in stool frequency is the most consistent symptom although the variation between individuals is again considerable.

Most people defaecate between once every three days and three times per day. If constipation is defined as the passage of less than three stools per week, around 3% of men and 9% of women will be affected by this condition.

History and examination

A careful history should include the onset and duration of symptoms, associated gastrointestinal symptoms, previous pelvic or abdominal surgery, the use of laxatives, dietary habits and a careful drug history. Patients whose history dates back to childhood may have short-segment Hirschsprung's disease, while those with a history of bleeding, mucus or tenesmus must be considered to have significant colorectal pathology.

Abdominal examination is usually normal although faecal masses are often palpable. Digital examination of the rectum is mandatory to assess intraluminal pathology, check for occult blood and also assess the sphincters.

Investigation

Routine haematology and biochemistry will be normal in the majority of cases but anaemia may be the only manifestation of a colorectal neoplasm and serum calcium, blood sugar and thyroid and renal function tests should be checked as possible endocrine or metabolic causes of constipation.

A plain abdominal radiograph may be helpful to define the extent of faecal loading and a barium enema is usually indicated after either rigid or flexible sigmoidoscopy has been performed. Contrast studies may show a redundant colon, megarectum or other structural abnormality. Colonic transit time may be assessed using radio-opaque markers: 20 small markers are given orally and a plain radiograph taken on days one and five. If markers are still present on day five, a further film may be taken on day 10. The persistence of markers at day five is suggestive of delayed transit and persistence to day 10 diagnostic of significant delay. It is important that patients take normal diet during the study and avoid the use of laxatives. Videoproctography is a further radiological investigation which may be used and patients unable to evacuate liquid barium from the rectum can be considered to have pelvic floor dysfunction.

Anorectal physiological studies have been performed but their use in isolation is often unhelpful. Results often do not correlate with symptoms but they may be useful in conjunction with other investigative techniques in selected cases.

Management

In general terms the management rarely requires any form of surgical intervention. It is helpful to subdivide cases of chronic constipation into those primarily due to disorders of transit (idiopathic slow transit constipation) and those due to functional disorders of the pelvic floor (a number of terms have been used to describe this condition including anismus, outlet obstruction constipation and puborectalis paradox).

The usual cause of constipation is inappropriate diet and faulty habits. Patients must be taught not to ignore the call to stool and to avoid prolonged periods of straining. The importance of dietary fibre must be emphasised and the importance of a high fluid intake to complement this should be explained. Increasing the bulk and volume of the stool stimulates natural peristalsis and has been shown to reduce transit time and lower intraluminal pressure.

Laxative preparations are often of value in addition to addressing dietary factors. A large number of preparations are now available and Box 20.2 lists a few examples of agents which act by different mechanisms.

Box 20.2 Laxatives

Bulking agents
  Bran
  Methylcellulose
  Ispaghula

Stimulant laxatives
  Senna
  Bisacodyl
  Danthron
  Sodium picosulphate
  Castor oil

Faecal softeners
  Paraffin
  Docusate

Osmotic laxatives
  Magnesium sulphate
  Polyethylene glycol
  Lactulose

Faecal softeners lubricate the passage of faeces and are especially helpful if there are associated painful anorectal conditions such as anal fissure. Stimulant laxatives increase colonic motility and may cause unpleasant colic. It is important not to use these agents if there is any suspicion of a mechanical obstruction. Osmotic laxatives act by drawing fluid into the bowel lumen and again must be used in conjunction with a high fluid intake.

Suppositories and enemata are useful in clearing the lower bowel. They act by a combination of mucosal irritation and osmotic effects.

The majority of patients with chronic constipation can be managed conservatively and it is very important to select those who may require surgical intervention with great care.

Idiopathic slow-transit constipation

A number of patients, usually women, have severe constipation which is resistant to treatment with bulking agents and laxatives. They tend to have a bowel motion once every month or less and often become dependent on suppositories, enemata or digital evacuation. The history often dates back to childhood or adolescence. The cause is unknown but recent research suggests that it may be a reflection of a more generalised disorder of gastrointestinal dysmotility.

Radiological marker studies confirm a delay in transit and these patients will have normal videoproctography studies. The first report of surgical treatment for chronic constipation was in 1912, when Arbuthnot Lane carried out a colectomy and ileorectal anastomosis. This remains a treatment option for patients with this condition. However, a number of patients continue to have symptoms of constipation after the procedure and this may be due to concomitant disorders of pelvic floor function or more diffuse disorders of proximal gut motility. It is important therefore to ensure that there is no objective evidence of outlet obstruction before advising subtotal colectomy.

Outlet obstruction constipation

The condition was first described in the mid-1980s and although it is a well-recognised entity, the precise aetiology remains unclear. Again most patients are women and there is no demonstrable delay in colonic transit time. The history is often related to a specific event such as childbirth or pelvic surgery (particularly hysterectomy). Defaecation normally involves relaxation of the puborectalis muscle, which allows the anorectal angle to straighten. Paradoxical contraction of the puborectalis may be demonstrated by videoproctography with a failure of the anorectal angle to open, or by an increase in puborectalis activity on electromyography. The other feature which defines outlet obstruction is the inability to evacuate the rectum of barium paste. It is often possible to demonstrate other abnormalities in these patients such as intussusception or rectocele, although these may result from rather than cause the condition.

Surgical treatment was directed towards partial division of the puborectalis but was abandoned because of poor functional results and an unacceptable incidence of incontinence. Another approach was to reduce anal canal pressure by anorectal myectomy but results were similarly unsatisfactory.

Biofeedback is an alternative approach to manage this condition, and is based on the theory that outlet obstruction in a number of patients is a learned response. It involves a careful explanation of the anatomy and physiology of the pelvic floor. Patients are then taught to learn or relearn various aspects of pelvic floor contraction with visual and auditory feedback using anorectal physiological measurements. The aim is to allow patients to be able to discriminate between rest, squeeze and push. The results of this technique are very variable and there is evidence that it is probably best indicated in those patients who have normal pelvic floor physiological tests.

ANAL TUMOURS

Anal tumours are rare, accounting for around 5% of anorectal cancers. Classification of tumours has generally been divided into those below the dentate line (anal margin or verge) and those at or above the dentate line (anal canal). The median age at presentation is 60 years with a marked female predominance in canal tumours and a male predominance in patients with tumours at the anal margin.

Aetiology

Most tumours arise in patients with no clear predisposing factors. Risk factors which have been associated include previous irradiation, fistulae, leukoplakia and anal condylomata. Epidemiological evidence reports a higher incidence in patients with a history of anal intercourse, suggesting a sexually transmissible agent as an aetiological factor. There is an association in women between anal and cervical carcinoma and human papillomavirus may be an important factor. The disease is also commoner in patients with immunodeficiency.

Clinical features

Most cases present with signs and symptoms indistinguishable from benign conditions. The commonest features are fresh rectal bleeding, anal pain, pruritis and discharge. More advanced cases may present with faecal incontinence, pelvic pain or recto-vaginal discharge. Presentation is often late and the mean size of tumours at time of diagnosis is three to four cm.

Pathology

The WHO histological classification divides anal cancer into epithelial tumours, non-epithelial tumours and malignant melanoma. Non-epthelial tumours include sarcomas and lymphomas. Epithelial tumours are further divided into squamous cell carcinoma (epidermoid tumour) and adenocarcinoma.

Squamous cell carcinoma accounts for 80% of anal tumours. Tumours arising at the anal margin tend to be well differentiated and keratinising and those in the anal canal tend to be poorly differentiated.

Adenocarcinoma may arise from the anal glands or fistulae but most result from down growth from a low rectal adenocarcinoma.

Staging and spread

Dukes' classification of colorectal carcinoma is not applicable to tumours of the anal canal. Classification depends on a combination of clinical, radiological and endoscopic assessment. Examination under anaesthetic is the most important investigation to assess size, fixation to adjacent structures and to obtain histology. The inguinal nodes can be palpated and fine-needle aspiration performed. Transanal ultrasound and imaging either by CT or MRI may be helpful.

Treatment

Adenocarcinoma of the anus can be considered to be the same condition as rectal adenocarcinoma in terms of management.

There are a number of treatment options for squamous cell tumours with a move towards radiotherapy and/or chemotherapy rather than surgery as the primary treatment. The main reason for this is that the results of surgery alone have been disappointing in achieving satisfactory control of local disease in addition to the cost of a permanent stoma. There remains a place for local surgical excision of small tumours at the anal margin but the indication for abdomino-perineal excision of rectum as a primary treatment has now been replaced by other modalities.

Radiotherapy was used alone initially and achieved results which were comparable to surgery in terms of local control and five-year survival.

Combined modality therapy using chemoirradiation was subsequently shown to produce improved results and is currently the treatment of choice. The results from the United Kingdom Coordinating Committee on Cancer Research showed that combined modality therapy resulted in better local control, although there was no significant overall survival advantage. Current evidence suggests that anal squamous carcinoma should be treated with a combination of radiotherapy and i.v. fluouracil and mitomycin. Surgery is reserved for failed or relapsed disease or for specific complications such as incontinence or malignant fistula.

RECTAL PROLAPSE

Rectal prolapse is a protrusion of the bowel through the anal canal. It may be complete when the full thickness of the bowel wall is extruded circumferentially or incomplete if only part of the anterior wall of the rectum passes through the sphincter. The condition can occur in any age group but the highest incidence occurs over the age of 70. This condition is much more common in women. Usually the prolapse is clearly identified by the patient but occasionally it is occult.

Prolapse in childhood is relatively rare and usually associated with constipation. In this age group the incidence is higher in males and the condition tends to be self-limiting, with improvement generally seen with appropriate toilet training. The condition may be associated with cystic fibrosis.

Aetiology

The aetiology is unknown but there are a number of features which are present in most cases. The pelvic floor is usually lax and the sigmoid colon is commonly redundant. There is usually a deep pouch of Douglas and the rectum is loosely attached to the sacrum. Physiological studies tend to suggest that there is dysfunction of the internal sphincter but this may be the result rather than the cause of the prolapse.

Diagnosis

Most patients are aware of a mass prolapsing at the time of defaecation. Initially the prolapse will reduce spontaneously but later will have to be manually replaced. Rectal bleeding and the passage of mucus are common. Impairment of continence is frequently seen and most patients will admit to a long history of constipation prior to the onset of the prolapse.

On examination the diagnosis is usually clear on inspection with the patient in the left lateral position. The sphincters are seen to be lax and, on straining, the full circumference of the bowel wall is extruded. Some patients may be unable to demonstrate the prolapse in this position but may do so when asked to squat. Prolapsed circumferential haemorrhoids can give a similar appearance but there are usually associated external skin tags and the palpable muscle layer between the two mucosal surfaces is diagnostic of full-thickness prolapse.

The main complication is strangulation which can occur if the prolapse cannot be reduced. Most prolapses will reduce with a combination of manual pressure and ice packs to reduce the associated oedema. Strangulation is an indication for urgent surgical resection.

Solitary rectal ulcer

This condition is closely associated with rectal prolapse although in most patients it is occult. Symptoms include prolonged periods of straining and difficulty evacuating the anal canal. Bleeding and the passage of mucus are common and many patients have to digitally extract stool. On sigmoidoscopy the mucosa of the lower rectum is diffusely reddened, usually anteriorly, although the changes may be circumferential. Despite the name given to this condition there need not be true ulceration. The diagnosis is based on a specific histological appearance of replacement of the lamina propria by smooth muscle and fibroblasts radiating at right angles to the muscularis mucosae. Defaecating proctography will often demonstrate an internal intussusception.

Treatment

Most patients with complete rectal prolapse will require surgical treatment to relieve their symptoms. Conservative management is appropriate for those with solitary rectal ulcer and those with anterior wall or mucosal prolapse, at least in the early stages. General advice on a high fibre diet and the avoidance of straining should be given.

The very large number of procedures which have been used to treat rectal prolapse reflects the rather unpredictable outcome after surgical intervention. Perineal procedures were originally described and abdominal procedures subsequently evolved. More recently laparoscopic techniques have been utilised and Table 20.1 lists some of the operations which have been advocated.

The choice of procedure is influenced by a number of factors including the general condition of the patient, the morbidity associated with the procedure and the recurrence rate. The attraction of the perineal procedures is that morbidity tends to be lower, constipation is not so common after the procedure and it is usually not difficult to repeat the procedure in the event of recurrence of the prolapse. Against that, the perineal procedures fail to address the underlying problem of loose fixation of the rectum and the recurrence rate is higher than that seen with abdominal procedures. Perineal rectosigmoidectomy combines many of the advantages of both approaches and will be described in more detail after the following summary of the more commonly used procedures.

Table 20.1 Treatment of rectal prolapse

Perineal procedures	Abdominal procedures
Thiersch wire	Ivalon sponge rectopexy
Delorme's procedure	Ripstein rectopexy
Perineal rectosigmoidectomy	Suture rectopexy
	Resection rectopexy
	Anterior resection

Perineal procedures

Thiersch procedure

Circumferential anal encirclement was first described in the late 19th century. The original material used was silver wire and the advantage of the procedure was that it was simple, could be repeated and did not require a general anaesthetic. Subsequent reports have described the use of monofilament sutures, silicone

impregnated with Dacron and other materials. This operation however only supports the prolapse and does not address the underlying aetiology. Complications include breakage, stretching or infection of the material used and faecal impaction is common. There is little place for this procedure except in a very small number of selected patients who are deemed unsuitable for other treatment options.

Delorme's procedure

The principle of this procedure is to resect the prolapsed mucosa and plicate the underlying muscle. The prolapse is pulled out to its full extent and a circumferential incision made one cm above the dentate line. Dissection is easier if the submucosa is infiltrated with local anaesthetic containing adrenaline. A complete sleeve of mucosa is stripped off the underlying muscle until the apex of the prolapse is reached. By applying traction, more mucosa can be removed from the internal aspect of the prolapse. The mucosal tube is then resected and the exposed muscle is plicated with a number of sutures which are then drawn together. The mucosal edges are then sutured to complete the anastomosis. The morbidity rate is very low but recurrence rates up to 20% have been reported. Many of the recurrences are associated with little or no symptoms and it is not difficult to repeat the procedure if necessary.

Perineal rectosigmoidectomy

This procedure is similar to the Delorme technique except that the full thickness of the prolapse is resected. Following anastomosis, the bowel is fixed to the sacrum by fibrosis. The other advantage is that levatorplasty may be easily performed at the same time, which may help to improve continence. Morbidity is low and recurrence rates are lower than those reported with the Delorme procedure.

Abdominal procedures

Rectopexy

Most abdominal procedures involve posterior rectopexy by mobilisation of the rectum from the sacrum and fixation either by suture or to artificial prosthetic material. Ivalon sponge (Well's operation) or Marlex mesh have been described and Ripstein reported a variation of the procedure with anterior fixation. The recurrence rate is low and the procedure is indicated particularly in younger age groups.

The main problem after surgery is constipation which may be intractable. The aetiology is unclear and may be related to the prosthetic material. These patients often have a redundant sigmoid colon and displacement into the pouch of Douglas may lead to a mechanical obstruction. Another factor which may be important is rectal denervation. There is evidence that preservation of the lateral ligaments leads to a reduced incidence of constipation although this may be at the expense of a higher rate of recurrence.

The other complication of mesh rectopexy is infection, and although the incidence is low, the potential consequences are serious.

Resection rectopexy

A number of studies have shown that the results of suture rectopexy are similar to those of mesh rectopexy in terms of recurrence and that suture rectopexy may have an advantage with improved continence. The addition of sigmoid resection prior to suture rectopexy aims to reduce the incidence of problematic constipation. This procedure is associated with a recurrence rate of two to eight % and may be the treatment of choice in patients who have a background history of constipation.

Laparoscopic procedures

Abdominal operations are generally associated with reduced recurrence rates but higher morbidity in a population often with significant comorbidity. The attraction of laparoscopic surgery is that it might achieve the benefits of rectal fixation and also the advantages of minimal access techniques. Long-term follow-up is not yet available but early results suggest that comparable results can be attained relative to open surgery.

OPERATIVE SURGERY

Surgery for rectal prolapse

Introduction

Although over 100 operations have been described for the treatment of rectal prolapse, these can be broadly described as either abdominal or perineal procedures. Each approach has advantages and disadvantages. The abdominal approach is highly effective in eradicating the prolapse but involves a major operation and may leave patients with troublesome constipation. In contrast, perineal operations are less invasive but have the disadvantage that they are associated with a high prolapse recurrence rate. Both approaches have been described with modifications which involve plication of the sphincter and pelvic floor muscles.

Putative causes of postoperative constipation after abdominal rectopexy include narrowing of the rectum by the fixation procedure, creation of a redundant sigmoid loop and denervation of the colon secondary to division of the lateral ligaments. In an attempt to overcome these complications the operation of resection rectopexy has been advocated and is described later. This operation can be performed either using an open or laparoscopic technique.

Patient selection

The operation of resection rectopexy is appropriate for any patient with a full-thickness overt rectal prolapse who is considered to be fit for an abdominal operation. It is particularly suitable for patients who have other manifestations of pelvic floor neuropathy including uterine prolapse. The resection component of the operation, however, should be used with caution in those patients who are profoundly incontinent or who have a severe sphincter neuropathy.

Preoperative preparation

Patients should be assessed for cardiovascular fitness in the usual way. Where appropriate this may include ECG, chest radiograph and pulmonary function tests, although these would not necessarily be routine. A full blood count and urea and electrolytes should be obtained. It is not usually necessary to cross-match blood for the operation but the patient's blood group should be obtained and serum retained for rapid cross-matching if necessary.

Incision and positioning of patients

The operation is performed in the modified Lloyd-Davies position. A urinary catheter should be inserted. The routine use of central venous and other invasive monitoring is not usually required. DVT prophylaxis should be used; subcutaneous low-dose heparin or compression boots would be appropriate.

Incision

Lower midline or lower transverse.

Procedure

A formal laparotomy is performed. Having confirmed that there is no other intra-abdominal pathology the presence of the classical features of rectal prolapse should then be identified. These include a redundant sigmoid and a very deep pouch of Douglas.

The patient is positioned slightly head down and the small bowel packed away from the pelvis. The sigmoid is then drawn towards the midline and the peritoneal reflection divided. At this stage careful identification and preservation of the ureter is required. This dissection should continue to the pelvic brim, where immediately anterior to the common iliac vein the sacral plexus is often identified. It is the author's preference to perform this dissection using the diathermy, which ensures a bloodless field. Anterior to the nerve plexus is the bloodless mesorectal plane. This can then be followed circumferentially around the rectum. The rectal mobilisation is continued to the level of the pelvic floor. This is a relatively easy dissection due to the attenuation of the tissue planes. Anteriorly the vagina is dissected from the rectum.

Posteriorly the presacral veins should be identified and avoided and the dissection continued to the level of the levator ani. It is the author's preference to preserve the lateral ligament in order that the parasympathetic supply to the hindgut is not disturbed. Some surgeons, however, advocate division of the lateral ligaments, which should be undertaken at this point.

Fixation

Having fully mobilised the rectum it is necessary to achieve fixation to the sacral promontory. It is important not to 'bowstring' the rectum. Rather, it should be allowed to fall into the concavity of the sacrum. Fixation can be achieved by applying two or three sutures to one side of the mesorectum. Care must be taken not to narrow the rectum in this process. Although the use of fixation materials has been advocated, these have been shown in clinical studies to be unnecessary. It is the author's practice, if the uterus remains *in situ*, to also perform a uterosuspension at this point.

Having fixed the rectum in its anatomical position, the redundant sigmoid can then be excised. In performing this procedure the inferior mesenteric vessels are retained since they carry the sympathetic supply to the upper rectum. An end-to-end colonic anastomosis is fashioned using 3/0 vicryl sutures in an interrupted serosubmucosal technique (Figure 20.1). The splenic flexure is not routinely mobilised in this technique.

Closure

The abdominal wall is closed using continuous PDS. A suction drain is applied to the pelvis to prevent haematoma formation.

Postoperative management

The catheter is maintained until the patient is fully mobile and hourly urine volumes are measured for the first 24 hours. IV fluids are maintained until oral intake is established, usually three days

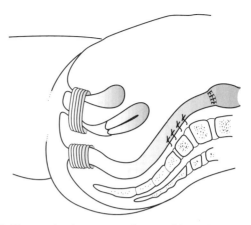

Figure 20.1 The completed rectopexy – fixation of the mobilised rectum to the sacral promontory, resection of redundant sigmoid colon and colonic anastomosis.

after the operation. Diet is introduced as tolerated on approximately the fourth day. DVT prophylaxis is continued until the patient is fully mobile. According to social circumstances, patients are usually well enough for discharge between six to eight days after the operation.

FURTHER READING

Everhart JE, Go VL, Johannes RS et al. A longitudinal survey of self-reported bowel habits in the United States. *Dig Dis Sci* 1989; **34**:1153–1162

Kamm MA. Obstetric damage and faecal incontinence. *Lancet* 1994; **344**:730–733

Kiff ES, Swash M. Slowed conduction in the pudendal nerves in idiopathic (neurogenic) faecal incontinence. *Br J Surg* 1984; **7**:614–616.

Morson BC, Sobin LH. Histological typing of intestinal tumours. In: International Histological Classification of Tumours. No 15. Geneva: World Health Organisation 1976; 67–69

Parks AG. Anorectal incontinence. *Proc R Soc Med* 1975; **68**:681–690

UKCCCR Anal Cancer Trial Working Party. Epidermoid Anal Cancer: results from the UKCCCR randomised trial of radiotherapy alone versus radiotherapy, 5 fluouracil, and mitomycin. *Lancet* 1996; **348**:1049–1054

Therapeutic colonoscopy

Marc Winslet

Colonoscopy is the investigation of choice for most lower gas-trointestinal symptoms. The great advantage of colonoscopy over radiological imaging modalities is that it allows the performance of biopsies and therapeutic manoeuvres. The major disadvantage is the higher complication rate in comparison to other colonic investigations.

INDICATIONS FOR THERAPEUTIC COLONOSCOPY

Colonoscopy is predominantly an elective procedure although urgent or emergency colonoscopy is sometimes required. The indications for therapeutic colonoscopy will be discussed below. Contraindications to therapeutic colonoscopy are few, but include any condition where complications such as perforation or bleeding are highly likely to occur; for example, in the presence of signs of peritoneal irritation or in patients with an uncorrected coagulopathy.

Colonic polypectomy

Colonic polyps may be identified on rigid sigmoidoscopy, barium enema or air contrast CT enema. These require removal to treat symptoms and to allow histological diagnosis. Any polyps identified on surveillance colonoscopy in patients who have previously undergone cancer resections or adenomatous polypectomy should be removed.

Colonic polyps may be removed by hot biopsy or snare polypectomy. Hot biopsy is suitable for polyps of 5 mm or less and snaring for larger polyps up to a maximum of about 5 cm. Large polyps may be removed intact with a single transection if pedunculated, but larger sessile polyps require piecemeal snaring. Sessile polyps of greater than 5 cm diameter, overlying more than two haustra or greater than one-third of the colonic circumference, are best removed surgically to avoid the risk of colonic perforation. This is particularly important in the thin-walled right colon where polyps of greater than 2 cm should be surgically excised.

The ease of access to the rectum allows direct treatment of sessile polyps by per anal local scissor excision and suture of the defect. Large polyps in the sigmoid colon may be snared with a nylon loop and prolapsed through the anus from where they can be easily removed. Colonic polyps rarely present with acute bleeding, but emergency polypectomy may be indicated when this occurs.

Treatment of colonic bleeding

Endoscopic therapy may be employed in the treatment of minor haemorrhage or in massive lower gastrointestinal bleeding (defined as the requirement of 3–5 units blood over 24 hours to maintain cardiovascular stability). Treatment of minor bleeding may require polypectomy or coagulation of areas of angiodysplasia. Laser may be used in the palliation of bleeding malignant tumours.

Identification of the bleeding point is often difficult in massive colonic bleeding, although bleeding stops spontaneously in 85–90% of cases, to allow bowel preparation prior to colonoscopy. After gastroscopy has excluded an upper gastrointestinal source of bleeding, colonoscopy is the best initial investigation in those patients where bleeding stops spontaneously. Angiodysplasia or diverticular disease will be the cause of bleeding in 90% of cases. These are both amenable to endoscopic therapy by diathermy coagulation, laser or adrenaline injection.

In the unstable patient who requires emergency surgery, on-table colonoscopy following lavage may be helpful in identifying the source of bleeding. At this stage therapeutic colonoscopy is best avoided and colonic resection performed, because this abolishes the risk of rebleeding from the same lesion.

Treatment of strictures and tumours

The treatment of colonic strictures and tumours includes both emergency and elective procedures to relieve luminal obstruction and to arrest haemorrhage. The available modalities include

- laser recanalisation
- balloon dilatation
- stent insertion.

Laser recanalisation

Laser recanalisation of the partially obstructed colonic lumen is used in locally advanced, inoperable tumours or in patients with a poor prognosis due to extensive metastatic disease.

Control of haemorrhage may be achieved with laser ablation of irresectable or disseminated colonic malignancies. Curative ablation of extensive villous adenomata has also been performed.

Laser recanalisation has also been used to relieve acute large bowel obstruction to allow staging and a planned elective resection.

Balloon dilatation

Balloon dilatation in the colon is confined to benign stricture, predominantly post anastomotic. More recently it has been used for diverticular strictures and Crohn's disease.

Stents

Endoscopically placed, self-expanding metallic stents have been used in the emergency decompression of left-sided colonic obstruction. This allows full resuscitation and preparation of the patient, including disease staging prior to colonic resection with primary anastomosis as an elective procedure. This reduces the use of the temporary stoma. Also, if the tumour proves irresectable locally or has extensive metastases, surgery can be avoided altogether.

Stents may be placed electively for palliation of obstruction in locally advanced irresectable tumour or disseminated carcinomatosis. It is preferable to avoid surgery and the deleterious effects on quality of life of stoma construction in a patient with limited life-span. For locally advanced disease, radiotherapy may be delivered after stenting the obstruction.

In very elderly or debilitated patients who would not withstand resectional surgery due to co-morbid conditions, stenting avoids the risks associated with general anaesthesia. Stenting is suitable for left-sided colonic tumours but stents in the rectum cause severe tenesmus, making them unsuitable for palliation.

There are reports of the use of stents in benign strictures of the colon, including anastomotic, diverticular and Crohn's strictures, but experience is very limited.

Decompression of colonic dilatation

Decompression of sigmoid volvulus traditionally involved rigid sigmoidoscopy and insertion of a flatus tube into the proximal sigmoid colon. Colonoscopy allows visualisation of the colon, decompression through suction and precise placement of a flatus tube.

Colonoscopic decompression of pseudoobstruction of the colon may be required if the condition does not respond to conservative measures of nasogastric aspiration, intravenous fluids and correction of electrolyte imbalance. Colonoscopic decompression is contraindicated if the caecum is grossly dilated and tender.

EQUIPMENT FOR THERAPEUTIC COLONOSCOPY

Colonoscope

A standard video colonoscope is most useful as this allows simultaneous visualisation of any lesion by the colonoscopist and assistant. A paediatric colonoscope is helpful for the examination of the colon in the presence of tight strictures. Large channel size allows simultaneous aspiration during insertion of instruments through the biopsy channel.

Electrosurgical devices

Electrosurgical units with cut, coagulation and blend circuits with registered power output ratings are useful but only coagulation is essential. The electrosurgical units utilise high-frequency electric currents which are applied to tissue via a monopolar or bipolar electrode.

Snare loops are produced in different sizes and although the standard snare is suitable for most polyps, a mini snare is easier to handle for small polyps. This is connected to the monopolar diathermy circuit.

Hot biopsy forceps are useful for destroying small polyps up to 5 mm in diameter or for electrocoagulation. To achieve electrocoagulation the current flows around the tissue between the forceps and heats the surrounding mucosa, cauterising the area immediately adjacent to the tip of the instrument. A low power setting of 10–15 W for up to three seconds is usually sufficient. Histological analysis of larger polyps removed with hot biopsy can be difficult due to extensive diathermy artefact.

Bipolar electrode probes (BICAP) are used to produce electrocoagulation for bleeding. BICAP reduces the size of the electric field compared with monopolar instruments and hence the depth of tissue being heated. This reduces the risk of perforation.

A heater probe is a Teflon-coated non-stick thermal device which will pass down the instrument channel of the colonoscope. The probe tip delivers a computer-controlled amount of heat as a pulse, effectively sealing blood vessels. A silicon chip in the probe tip produces the heat, generating a temperature of 250°C in 0.2 seconds and cools in 0.5 seconds.

Lasers

The lasers most commonly used in endoscopy are the Nd:YAG (1.06 Nd:YAG) and argon lasers. These emit in the near infrared and blue-green spectrum respectively. Some Nd:YAG lasers (0.532 Nd:YAG) also emit green light.

Lasers produce tumour necrosis by coagulation and volatilisation. Coagulative necrosis raises the temperature of the tissue to 49–99°C in one second, resulting in desiccation and protein denaturation which can be seen as blanching of the tissue. During volatilisation, the tissue temperature is raised to 100–300°C in 0.1 seconds, the tissue water boils, proteins are denatured and smoke is produced with immediate ablation of tumour. The green light is absorbed by the tissues more than the near infrared and therefore produces more superficial effects, predominantly by volatilisation. The predominant effect of the argon beam is coagulative necrosis.

The laser fibre has to be polished and clean to produce a well-demarcated light spot on tissue and most are deployed through the biopsy channel covered by a protective sheath. Argon and 0.532 Nd:YAG lasers emit in the visible spectrum which precludes their use with video endoscopes. Argon plasma coagulators apply non-contact cautery which can be used tangentially. The electrical conductivity of the argon gas passed down a catheter combines with a high-power electrosurgical current to produce a local plasma arc. It generates little smoke and has limited depth penetration, making it safer than conventional laser.

Polypectomy equipment

Excision of the polyp requires a snare and hot biopsy forceps as described above, but several additional devices are needed to retrieve polyps or to aid in identification and removal.

- A polyp retrieval basket or grasping forceps is useful for removing larger polyps although they can often be removed in the snare which avoids changing instruments and the risk of losing the polyp.

- A suction trap for polyp retrieval with an incorporated filter allows capture of the polyp as it emerges from the suction channel.

- A long sclerotherapy needle is needed to inject adrenalin to arrest bleeding or to raise a bleb below a sessile polyp to allow snaring. Injection of India ink may be useful to mark a site of polypectomy for subsequent examination.

- A dye spray cannula allows marking of very small sessile polyps or the margins of diffuse villous adenomata.

Balloon dilators

Balloon dilators are made of polyethylene and either relatively wide 'over the wire' or narrow 'through the scope' in design. Both have a lumen to instil contrast into the balloon to allow fluoroscopic visualisation during dilatation. The balloon is connected to a commercially available manometer to inflate to the desired pressure and maintain it. The balloons are about 8 cm in length and dilate up to about 20 mm.

Stents

The use of stents in the colon is still in its infancy and currently self-expanding stents designed for the oesophagus are being used for colonic strictures. The latest stents consist of a mesh made of nitinol, an alloy of nickel and titanium. This has shape memory so that it can be compressed into a delivery system and returns to a predetermined configuration after deployment. These flexible stents comply with peristalsis in the colon. Most currently available delivery systems are 15 FG in diameter and are inserted after endoscopic placement of a guidewire. Smaller diameter systems to pass down the biopsy channel of the endoscope are being developed.

COMPLICATIONS OF THERAPEUTIC COLONOSCOPY

The complications of therapeutic colonoscopy are early and late and depend on the therapeutic procedure being undertaken. The major complication of diagnostic colonoscopy is colonic perforation which occurs in about 1:1000 colonoscopies, but the rate is increased with therapeutic procedures.

Complications of colonoscopic polypectomy

Bleeding

Primary haemorrhage occurs in 1.5% of polypectomies and is due to inadequate coagulation at the time of snaring or hot biopsy.

Resnaring the polyp and application of pressure for five minutes is usually successful for pedunculated polyps. For sessile polyps cauterisation with the hot biopsy forceps or heater probe should be performed. If this fails, injection of 5–10 ml 1:10 000 adrenaline around the base of the excised polyp provides vasoconstriction.

Secondary haemorrhage complicates 2% of polypectomies and usually occurs between 7–10 days after the procedure. Risk factors for secondary haemorrhage include large polyps removed piecemeal, hot biopsy removal of large polyps, elderly patients and aspirin ingestion. About 99% stop spontaneously and only 2% require blood transfusion. If active bleeding continues, colonoscopy should be performed and local applications to arrest bleeding as described above.

Perforation

Colonic perforation occurs in 0.04–2.1% of polypectomies. This may be subclinical, where air has seeped through a diverticulum, or occur with clinical signs of generalised peritonitis. It should be suspected in patients with increasing abdominal pain following colonoscopy. An erect chest radiograph may show pneumoperitoneum.

Conservative treatment may be successful in carefully selected cases where there is localised peritonitis but generalised peritonitis mandates laparotomy. Conservative treatment involves intravenous fluids, intravenous antibiotics, nil orally and frequent clinical reassessment. Any deterioration in the patient's condition should be treated by laparotomy.

Laparotomy is mandatory if the peritoneal cavity was visualised on endoscopy. Localised peritonitis with pneumoperitoneum is best treated by laparotomy. If the perforation is identified early and there is minimal abdominal soiling at laparotomy, it may be possible to close the perforation primarily, but stoma formation is usually required. Perforation at the site of incomplete polyp resection, tumour or diverticular disease should be treated with resection.

Postpolypectomy syndrome is characterised by localised pain, tenderness, guarding, fever, tachycardia and is associated with a neutrophilia. It complicates about 1% of polypectomies. Symptoms develop six hours to five days following polypectomy. It is caused by transmural burn leading to localised peritoneal inflammation around a self-sealed perforation. It normally responds to conservative treatment.

Complications of treatment of colonic bleeding

The major complications associated with colonoscopic treatment of acute rectal bleeding include rebleeding following therapeutic intervention and colonic perforation. Similar complication rates apply to the different forms of coagulation used to control the bleeding.

The diagnostic yield of colonoscopy in acute colonic bleeding is dependent on the bowel preparation and can be improved by nasogastric whole-bowel irrigation. Figures of 62% to over 70% are quoted.

Rebleeding after endoscopic treatment is common and was documented to occur in 34% of cases following Nd:YAG laser and 50% following diathermy coagulation.

Perforation during coagulation of colonic bleeding sites is the most serious complication and is more common in right colonic lesions. Laser causes perforation in about 6% and diathermy about 7% although most series have small numbers of cases.

Complications of treatment of colonic tumours

Complications associated with treatment of colonic tumours include early perforation, late bleeding and tumour regrowth. Rates of complications for stenting, balloon dilatation and laser for obstructing colonic tumours are difficult to ascertain because all published series contain very small numbers of patients.

Perforation rates for balloon dilation of zero to one out of eight for balloon dilatation are obtained from the literature.

Laser ablation of colonic tumours has been reported to cause one perforation in 26 patients but this is likely to be higher with repeated laser sessions.

The complications of stent insertion to palliate or relieve acute obstruction in colonic tumours include early perforation and late bleeding, stent migration and tumour regrowth causing obstruction.

Complications of the use of colonoscopic decompression of colonic tumours

The major complication of colonoscopic decompression of pseudoobstruction and sigmoid volvulus is perforation. This is a particular problem as the bowel is unprepared, dilated and contains liquid faeces which obscures the view.

The second complication is recurrence which is common in both sigmoid volvulus and pseudoobstruction. Repeat colonoscopy may be required and pseudoobstruction will usually resolve when the patient's general condition improves. Recurrent sigmoid volvulus is best treated by resection, provided the patient is fit enough for surgery.

Continuing caecal distension following repeat attempts at colonoscopic decompression requires surgical decompression with a caecostomy. If there is a question of the viability of the caecum then a laparotomy and colonic resection will be required.

OPERATIVE SURGERY

Techniques in therapeutic colonoscopy

Polypectomy

Colonoscopic polypectomy was a major advancement in the treatment of colonic polyps and the prevention of colonic cancer. It has allowed removal of polyps in an outpatient setting, avoiding the major surgery with its attendant morbidity which had previously been required.

Patient preparation

Patient preparation includes ensuring that the patient is fit for the proposed intervention, an explanation of the procedure and discussion of possible alternatives and risks and cleansing of the colon. These will be discussed below.

PATIENT FITNESS

An adequate history must be taken to ensure that the patient is fit enough to undergo the procedure. This includes the following.

- Personal or family history of bleeding tendency.
- Cardiovascular history with particular reference to heart valve lesions, prosthetic valves, rheumatic fever. These require prophylactic antibiotics, to cover anaerobic and Gram-negative bacteraemia.
- Current medication, with particular reference to anticoagulation. Warfarin should be stopped and the prothrombin ratio checked prior to endoscopic polypectomy. If anticoagulation cannot be safely stopped, for example in patients with mechanical heart valves, warfarin should be replaced by heparin prior to the procedure. Warfarin can be restarted immediately after polypectomy, provided that adequate haemostasis was visualised at endoscopy. Aspirin should be stopped 1–2 weeks prior to the procedure to allow the generation of new functioning platelets. Immunosuppressant medication may mask the signs of postpolypectomy perforation.
- Allergies or adverse reactions to previous sedation.
- A history of obstructive airways disease makes reduced doses of sedation advisable to avoid respiratory depression.
- Details of previous colonoscopies including bowel resection and other abdominal surgery may indicate the degree of difficulty of the procedure. Hysterectomy and other pelvic surgery can cause adhesions in the pelvis which can render the rectosigmoid immobile, preventing the passage of the scope. Barium enema films should be available if the investigation has been performed. If colonoscopy has been performed previously, knowledge of the location of polyp excision or any which remained is useful.

INFORMED CONSENT

A well-informed patient is more tolerant of any intervention. Explanation of the procedure should be instigated in the outpatient clinic by the recommending doctor. This is the best time for discussion of alternatives to endoscopic polypectomy and of the potential risks. Further explanation by a nurse specialist may also be beneficial. This should be reinforced with a written information sheet which the patient can read at leisure. The major risks associated with polypectomy include bleeding and perforation with an incidence of approximately 1% and 0.05% respectively. These will be discussed in detail below.

BOWEL PREPARATION

Good bowel preparation is essential for adequate examination of the colon and hence to allow identification and removal of all polyps. All bowel preparations are unpleasant for the patient to take but especially those which require very large volumes of fluid. A soft diet avoiding fruit and vegetables for 48 hours prior to the procedure allows formation of faeces without large pieces of plant material which can block the sucker channel if aspirated. Polyethylene glycol when taken properly provides good preparation, but the fluid volume and salty aftertaste are unpalatable, causing nausea and poor compliance. Sodium picosulphate may be better tolerated but can cause colicky abdominal pain. All preparations cause profuse diarrhoea and may cause dehydration if oral rehydration is not maintained. Hypokalaemia may also occur. The fluid and electrolyte imbalances may be particularly troublesome in the elderly who often require hospital admission and intravenous rehydration during preparation. Adequate preparation is necessary to reduce to a minimum the volumes of explosive gases generated by the colonic bacteria.

Analgesia and sedation

Most patients require some form of sedation for colonoscopy. However, patient cooperation with position changes is enhanced by keeping this to a minimum. It also allows appreciation of any discomfort which the patient may experience and encourages the endoscopist to modify actions accordingly. Midazolam provides sedation and retrograde amnesia. An initial dose of 5 mg of midazolam is usually adequate. Many endoscopists use opiate analgesics in addition to benzodiazepines but this is not usually necessary. Supplementary oxygen is required and the dose required is indicated by the oxygen saturation monitored by the pulse oximeter. Nitrous oxide and oxygen inhalation are useful additional analgesics.

Procedure

THEORY

Removal of a polyp requires a combination of cauterisation and excision by snaring or biopsy. Cauterisation may be achieved by a blend of coagulation and cutting diathermy or pure coagulation. It has been suggested that blend causes more immediate bleeding and pure coagulation results in a higher incidence of delayed bleeding. Monopolar diathermy is generally used with current flowing from the snare loop and the patient plate. Bipolar circuits are available but not widely used.

The principal requirement for polypectomy is to ensure coagulation of all stalk vessels prior to transection. Heat generation is increased in a cubic manner by snare closure, is directly proportional to the time over which the current is applied and the power setting of the diathermy machine. The aim is to coagulate the stalk fully before section, using low power (15–25 W). However, after approximately 40 seconds of current delivery, there is increased risk of damage to surrounding bowel wall and so it may be necessary to increase the power (30–50 W).

TECHNIQUE FOR POLYP SNARING

- Ensure that the diathermy plate is correctly applied.
- Set the power parameter on the diathermy low to start.
- Mark the snare in the fully closed position to use as a reference point.
- Ensure that the polyp is clearly visualised, that the bowel is sufficiently distended and that the polyp is in an accessible position, usually at about 5 o'clock. This may require torque from an assistant.
- Multiple small polyps may be accentuated with dye spray using 10% washable blue ink introduced via a syringe or a purpose-made spray catheter.

SINGLE TRANSECTION POLYP SNARING

This is suitable for pedunculated polyps greater than 5 mm or sessile polyps less than 1.5 cm. Larger sessile polyps require piece-meal removal.

- Pass the snare over the polyp and use it to assess its mobility and stalk thickness.
- Push the sheath of the snare against the base of the polyp (Figure 21.1) prior to closing to the predetermined mark.
- Electrocoagulate initially at low power for 10–15 seconds and look for burning (whitening) at the base of the stalk. The snare is gently closed as burning progresses. Keep watching the polyp to see where it drops.

With thick-walled large polyps a small area of contact of the polyp head with the opposite colonic wall may lead to preferential current leak, causing contra coup perforation (Figure 21.2). This can be avoided by keeping the whole polyp in view and watching the area of necrosis as it develops.

It may not be possible to coagulate the entire thickness of thick stalked-polyps. Success may be improved by adrenaline injection

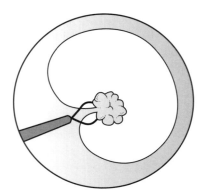

Figure 21.1 Snare applied to base of polyp and gradually closed at base of stalk.

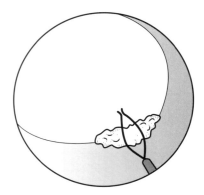

Figure 21.3 Snare applied to distal end of the polyp after submucosal injection of saline to raise a sessile polyp.

as above, nylon loop snare application, metal clip or rubber band application.

PIECEMEAL POLYP SNARING

It is safer to remove large sessile polyps by piecemeal excision because snaring of the entire polyp may result in tenting of the colonic wall and perforation. However, assessment of invasion or completeness of excision may not be possible after piecemeal excision.

Piecemeal excision is recommended for sessile polyps of greater than 1.5 cm diameter in the left colon. The thin wall of the right colon makes this procedure inadvisable because of the high risk of perforation.

- The snare is placed over the polyp with the tip of the catheter at the junction of normal colon and polyp.

- The snare is moved to ensure differential movement between the colonic wall and mucosa.

- Injection of normal saline and adrenaline (1:10 000) generates a submucosal cushion which increases the safety of piecemeal polypectomy, particularly useful in the thin-walled right colon (Figure 21.3).

POTENTIAL DIFFICULTIES

If the snare gets stuck in the wrong position, manipulation or the passage of a gastroscope beside the colonoscope and removal with biopsy forceps should be successful.

If no coagulation occurs, the connections and position of the snare should be checked. Adrenalin injection to the base of the polyp may be helpful.

Pain during polypectomy which persists despite deflation suggests that full-thickness heating is occurring and the procedure should be stopped.

The presence of malignancy in a polyp is suggested by a hard texture during snare manipulation. Complete excision may be achieved colonoscopically. Provided more than 2 mm of normal stalk clearance is achieved, the likelihood of lymph node metastases is very low. Sessile polyps with invasion should be surgically excised. Marking the area with India ink helps identification at laparotomy.

TECHNIQUE FOR HOT BIOPSY

- Small pedunculated polyps of less than 5 mm are suitable for hot biopsy removal. Sessile polyps are unsuitable.

- The power is set at 15–25 W.

- The polyp head is grasped and pulled away from the colonic wall (Figure 21.4).

- The black insulating part of the forceps must be visible outside the endoscope.

- Current is applied and coagulation occurs with necrosis of the polyp stalk (not head) and traction is applied to the forceps.

- If the head coagulates, this suggests that the polyp is too big for hot biopsy and requires snaring. Continued diathermy with biopsy forceps will result in excessive diathermy artefact and may preclude histological diagnosis without removal of the polyp.

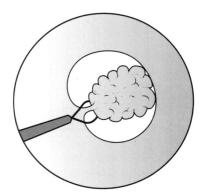

Figure 21.2 Snare closed on to base of polyp. The polyp is lifted clear but care must be taken to ensure that the apex of the polyp is not in contact with the opposite wall as current may preferentially travel in that direction, causing perforation.

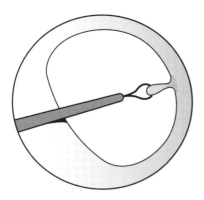

Figure 21.4 Hot biopsy causes coagulation of the base of the polyp provided the polyp is less than 5 mm.

POLYP RETRIEVAL

Retrieval of the polyp depends on its size and position.

- Small polyps, less than 5 mm, can be aspirated into the suction channel and retrieved in a polyp trap (Figure 21.5) or, if they are too large to pass into the suction channel, can be removed with the scope as continuous suction is applied.

- Large and medium-sized polyps can be removed in the snare or with a Dormia basket type device. This unfortunately requires removal of the scope and reintroduction if further polyps are to be retrieved.

- Multiple polyp retrieval may be facilitated with a colonoscope overtube which allows easy reintroduction of the scope after removal with the polyp. The washout technique can be used if all polyps can be delivered to the descending colon; the colonoscope is then passed beyond the splenic flexure and

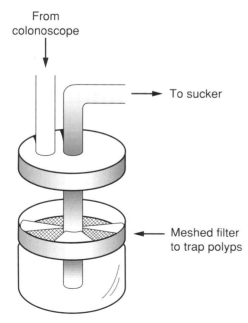

From colonoscope

To sucker

Meshed filter to trap polyps

Figure 21.5 A suction trap for polyp retrieval.

500 ml warm water injected to wash the polyps distally. Evacuation can be aided by a phosphate enema administered via the scope just prior to removal.

Treatment of colonic bleeding

Acute lower gastrointestinal bleeding is common but stops spontaneously in 90% of cases. The commonest cause is diverticular disease followed by angiodysplasia. There is a high mortality because the majority of affected patients are elderly. Diagnostic yield of colonoscopy for acute bleeding is quoted at about 70%. The modalities for the treatment of acute lower gastrointestinal bleeding include polypectomy as described above, diathermy, laser and adrenaline injection.

Patient preparation

Acutely bleeding patients should be resuscitated in the first instance and time should not be wasted attempting to colonoscope an unstable patient.

Clotting disorders should be corrected.

Upper gastrointestinal endoscopy is mandatory to exclude a gastroduodenal source of bleeding; 10% of patients with apparent colonic bleeding will have an upper gastrointestinal source. Nasogastric aspiration is insufficient.

Bowel preparation is not always required as endoluminal blood has a cathartic action, removing any remaining stool. However, coating of the bowel wall with blood may prevent visualisation of arteriovenous malformations. Oral polyethylene glycol solution in a large volume (about 4 litres) is effective to clear blood. Alternatively nasogastric whole-gut irrigation clears blood effectively.

If the patient stops bleeding and is stable, better views can be obtained after full bowel preparation, although this can sometimes restart haemorrhage.

Informed consent must be obtained. The patient needs to be counselled regarding the risks of colonoscopy, including perforation which increases with therapeutic procedures to arrest haemorrhage. The risk of rebleeding must be explained.

SEDATION AND POSITIONING

Most patients will require sedation and antibiotic prophylaxis is required for patients with prosthetic heart valves.

The patient is positioned in the left lateral position with pulse oximetry and cardiovascular monitoring. Inhaled oxygen is administered.

PROCEDURE

The colonoscope is passed and irrigation used as required. It is important to examine the rectum carefully as lesions here are easily missed.

- Bleeding from the left colon is usually from a diverticulum with a single vessel at its apex. Injection of 2–4ml 1:10 000 adrenaline around the neck of the diverticulum (Figure 21.6) produces vasoconstriction and bleeding should be seen to stop. The needle is inserted as far as possible and injection performed on withdrawal.

- Bleeding from the right colon is more often due to angiodysplasia. Injection with adrenaline as above can be performed. Heater probe or electrocoagulation may be more successful.

- Nd:YAG or argon laser has been used with carbon dioxide insufflation to arrest bleeding from arteriovenous malformations although it may have a higher perforation rate than other techniques.

- Bleeding from diffuse areas of the bowel as in inflammatory bowel disease is not amenable to endoscopic treatment.

- Bleeding from a colonic polyp is controlled by polypectomy as described above and postpolypectomy bleeding has been discussed.

The bleeding source may not be identified at colonoscopy. This may be due to coating of the bowel with blood or bleeding may be arising from a lesion in the small bowel. Further investigation will depend on the rate of haemorrhage. Bleeding at 0.1 ml/min may be identified on radioisotope-labelled red cell scan but faster rates of blood loss (1–2 ml/min) are usually needed to identify an abnormality on angiography. If the bleeding stops, small bowel contrast studies can be performed. If not, laparotomy and small bowel enteroscopy should identify the bleeding point.

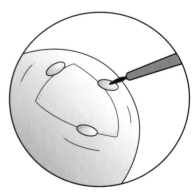

Figure 21.6 Injection of adrenaline into the neck of the bleeding diverticulum to arrest bleeding from vessel in the dome.

Treatment of strictures and tumours

The endoscopic modalities used in the treatment of strictures and tumours include self-expanding metallic stents, balloon dilatation of benign strictures and laser recanalisation of the colonic lumen occluded by tumour. These methods may be required for the relief of acute large bowel obstruction or for palliation of the partially obstructing inoperable carcinoma. Endoscopic treatment of acute large bowel obstruction predominantly involves stents but balloon dilatation and laser have also been used. Palliation in advanced malignant disease is more commonly achieved with laser while benign strictures are usually treated with balloon dilatation.

Self-expanding stents

PATIENT PREPARATION

Acute large bowel obstruction

Patients with acute large bowel obstruction require resuscitation with intravenous fluids, correction of electrolyte imbalance, nasogastric decompression and insertion of a urinary catheter.

Caecal tenderness and evidence of closed loop obstruction on plain film mandates emergency decompression. This can be done by stent insertion but patients with signs of peritonitis require laparotomy.

A water-soluble contrast enema is performed to exclude pseudoobstruction and to identify the position of the obstructing lesion.

Informed consent is obtained. The risks of stent insertion for emergency decompression include perforation and bleeding.

Intravenous antibiotics, comprising a cephalosporin and metronidazole, are administered prior to the procedure. Sedation with midazolam is accompanied by oxygen administration and standard monitoring.

No bowel preparation is required

PALLIATION OF ADVANCED COLONIC CANCER

These patients may not be acutely obstructed but have symptoms of alternating diarrhoea and constipation.

Informed consent is obtained. The early complications of stent insertion for palliation include perforation and bleeding and late complications include stent migration and tumour ingrowth.

Bowel preparation with phosphate enema prior to the procedure is helpful if the patient is not obstructed.

Prophylactic intravenous antibiotics, including a cephalosporin and metronidazole, are administered.

Sedation with midazolam is accompanied by oxygen administration and standard monitoring.

PROCEDURE

The procedure requires a combination of endoscopy and fluoroscopy.

The patient is placed in the left lateral position and the colonoscope inserted to the level of the obstruction with minimal air insufflation.

- A guidewire is passed through the lumen beyond the stricture and its position is confirmed radiologically.

- Contrast is instilled to ascertain the length of the lesion.

- The delivery system for the stent requires a minimum lumen diameter of 15 FG. Balloon dilatation as described below may be required prior to insertion of the stent. Oesophageal balloons have been used.

- Injection of contrast into the balloon allows visualisation of the diameter of the lumen and the result of dilatation. The level of the stricture can be marked.

- Under fluoroscopic guidance, the introducing tube and compressed expandable metallic stent tube are passed over the guidewire (Figure 21.7).

- The stent is passed to 2 cm beyond the stricture and deployed. Gradual expansion occurs over the next 24 hours. Balloon dilatation of the stent may be required if it does not fully expand.

- Water-soluble contrast is instilled following the procedure to verify stent position and to exclude perforation.

- Lesions up to 10 cm are generally considered suitable for stenting but longer strictures can be treated with 2–3 stents flower-potted together.

Following the procedure the patient should be maintained on stool softeners and avoid a high-residue diet.

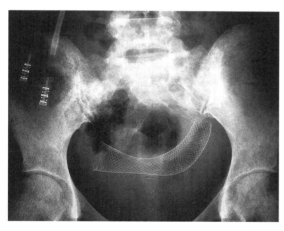

Figure 21.7 Plain radiograph of self-expanding metallic stent.

Laser recanalisation of colonic lumen

PATIENT PREPARATION

Previous endoscopy and biopsy are required as laser resection precludes histological assessment.

A phosphate enema prior to procedure is adequate bowel preparation for most patients.

Prophylactic antibiotics should be given to patients with prosthetic heart valves or valvular disease.

Informed consent is obtained. The major risks of laser treatment are early haemorrhage and perforation and late stenosis of the lumen.

Laser treatment is not painful and there is no special need for sedation for lesions in the rectum and left colon.

PROCEDURE

The patient is positioned in the left lateral position and the endoscope passed to the tumour. For very large tumours snare debulking reduces the laser treatment time.

Overdistension must be avoided because it reduces the thickness of the bowel wall and therefore increases the risk of perforation. A cannula is inserted into the rectum alongside the endoscope to remove gas.

- The laser fibre in its protective sheath is inserted into the biopsy channel of the endoscope.

- Larger tumours are treated with 1.06 Nd:YAG which produces coagulation necrosis which can be seen macroscopically as blanching.

- Smaller tumours are treated with green lasers, argon beam or 0.532 Nd:YAG which induce volatilisation of tumour. Treatment is continued until a flat surface is obtained.

- The distance between the fibre tip and tumour is adjusted frequently to allow for bowel movement and alterations in light absorption by the tumour as treatment proceeds.

- Ablation may take several sessions and can be performed 1–2 times a week, allowing time for coagulated tumour to necrose and separate.

Very large tumours may be debulked with snare electrocoagulation prior to laser treatment.

Colonoscopic Balloon Dilatation

Balloon dilatation is used predominantly for the dilatation of postoperative anastomotic stricture. It is important to obtain a tissue diagnosis prior to dilatation to exclude disease recurrence.

PATIENT PREPARATION

Dilatation produces bacteraemia so patients with valvular heart disease require prophylactic antibiotics.

Informed consent is obtained. The major risk of the procedure is perforation which occurs in about 8% of cases. The patient must understand that should a perforation occur, a laparotomy and colostomy are likely to be necessary. Good success rates have been reported in terms of symptomatic relief and although recurrence of the stricture is a risk, this does not appear to be a major problem in published series.

Bowel preparation consisting of a phosphate enema is sufficient for distal strictures but oral preparation as discussed previously is required for more proximal lesions. Care should be taken in the administration of bowel preparation if obstructive symptoms are present.

Sedation is recommended for all stricture dilatation as this can cause discomfort.

Fluoroscopic facilities must be available.

PROCEDURE

The patient is placed in the left lateral position and the endoscope passed to view the stricture.

Two balloon dilators are available: 'through the scope' and 'over the wire'. 'Through-the-scope' dilators are superior to 'over-the-wire' dilators for the treatment of rectosigmoid strictures because the angulation may be difficult to negotiate with the wire.

Incision of the stricture with the point of the diathermy snare prior to balloon dilatation has been described, with encouraging results.

Through-the-scope

A 'through-the-scope' balloon dilator is lubricated and passed through the biopsy channel and across the length of the stricture. The balloon is advanced past the stricture under direct vision to ensure that the tip is within the bowel lumen. The balloon is dilated up to about 25 mm or to a preset pressure (about 35 psi). Contrast injected into the balloon allows fluoroscopic visualisation of the stricture as it dilates.

Over-the-wire dilator

Under direct endoscopic vision, a guidewire is passed beside the endoscope and across the stricture. The balloon is then passed over the guidewire into the stricture which is dilated as above.

The position of the balloon and the dilatation can be viewed fluoroscopically if contrast is injected into the balloon.

Decompression of colonic pseudoobstruction and sigmoid volvulus

Colonic pseudoobstruction

Pseudoobstruction of the colon is characterised by gross colonic dilatation and usually develops as a complication of concurrent illness, such as following orthopaedic procedures, gynaecological surgery or cerebrovascular accidents. It is more common in elderly patients and has a high mortality, usually due to co-morbid conditions. The differential diagnosis is a mechanical obstruction which must be excluded as the results of surgery for pseudo-obstruction are very poor.

Patient preparation

The diagnosis of pseudoobstruction is usually suggested by the history, clinical signs and plain abdominal film, but mechanical obstruction should be excluded with Gastrograffin enema.

Initial treatment involves stopping oral intake, insertion of a naso-gastric tube and intravenous fluids to correct anaemia and electrolyte imbalances.

If there is no improvement on the above regime and caecal dilatation is apparent, colonoscopic decompression can be attempted.

Recurrence of colonic dilatation is common after simple deflation and better results from decompression are achieved if a flatus tube is left in the colon following the procedure.

Bowel preparation using gentle saline enema may be helpful but stimulants should be avoided.

When obtaining informed consent, it is necessary to explain the risks, including perforation and recurrence of colonic dilatation which may require further colonoscopic decompression. It should be explained that colonic perforation would require laparotomy.

Sedation is usually required and antibiotic prophylaxis is required for patients with cardiac lesions.

If there is clinical evidence of generalised or localised peritonitis then colonoscopic decompression should not be attempted and laparotomy or 'blowhole' caecostomy should be performed.

PROCEDURE

The patient is placed in the left lateral position. The colonoscope is inserted with as little air insufflation as possible. Suction is required to remove large volumes of liquid faeces. Simple suction decompression is associated with recurrence of dilatation in about 30% of cases. This can be improved by the placement of a flatus tube. If a flatus tube is to be inserted, this can be done during the initial colonoscopy.

- A strong nylon thread (e.g. fishing line) at least twice the length of the colonoscope is placed through the proximal end of the flatus tube and tied in a loop. Biopsy forceps are inserted into the biopsy channel and the suture is gripped with the forceps and withdrawn until it emerges from the biopsy channel. The colonoscope and flatus tube are then inserted through the anus and advanced gently along the colon, aspirating as much as possible (Figure 21.8).

- Once the caecum is reached, the nylon loop is snipped and removed, the colonoscope withdrawn and the flatus tube remains in position.

- Alternatively, grasping the end of the flatus tube with the biopsy forceps and leaving them in the biopsy channel during colonoscopy prevents faecal matter from the biopsy channel spraying the colonoscopist, but often results in blockage and inadequate suction.

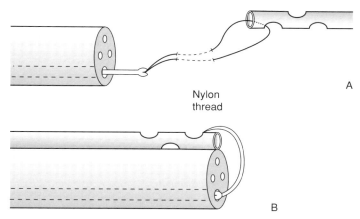

Nylon
thread

A

B

Figure 21.8 A Three-metre nylon thread attached through flatus tube and pulled through biopsy channel. **B** Colonoscope passed through flatus tube alongside and kept in position with nylon thread.

The flatus tube is left in position until the patient is passing flatus spontaneously.

Derotation of sigmoid volvulus

Sigmoid volvulus is a common condition worldwide but is rare in Western populations. In Europe and America it is a condition of the elderly in whom surgery may be hazardous. The diagnosis is usually made from the characteristic appearance on the plain abdominal film. In the acute situation rigid sigmoidoscopic decompression and flatus tube insertion is the standard treatment provided there is no suggestion of colonic ischaemia. Blind insertion of a flatus tube should not be performed as this does not allow visualisation of the colonic mucosa, which may be compromised, and risks perforation of the apex of the sigmoid. Rigid sigmoidoscopy or colonoscopy allows derotation of the volvulus under direct vision.

PATIENT PREPARATION

Resuscitation may be required depending on the length of the history. After 3–4 days the patient may be dehydrated.

Rigid sigmoidoscopy and flatus tube insertion is often easier to arrange than flexible endoscopy in the acute situation and is effective in over 90% of cases.

The rigid sigmoidoscope is inserted gently and usually reaches the site of volvulus at 15–20 cm. At this point, the colonic mucosa is carefully examined; any blue discoloration suggesting gangrenous change will indicate that laparotomy is required. A well-lubricated flatus tube is then passed along the sigmoidoscope under direct vision. As it enters the sigmoid beyond the twist, there will be an 'explosion' of liquid faeces. If the liquid is bloodstained, this suggests ischaemia and laparotomy should be performed.

If the flatus tube cannot be passed at rigid sigmoidoscopy because the volvulus lies beyond the reach of the rigid sigmoidoscope then flexible sigmoidoscopy or colonoscopy is required.

Sedation is not always required and antibiotics only for patients with valvular heart disease.

Informed consent involves a discussion of the possibility of perforation and subsequent laparotomy if necessary.

PROCEDURE

- The patient is placed in the left lateral position.

- The colonoscope is passed to the level of the obstruction with minimal air insufflation and steered around. If bloodstained fluid is aspirated, surgery will be required.

- As deflation occurs the colon will detort spontaneously.

- Large biopsy channel colonoscopes allow a deflation tube with an introducing stiffening wire to be passed down the scope. This can be placed in the colon after the volvulus has been negotiated and left in position when the scope is removed.

- Alternatively, a larger flatus tube can be placed through the colon, as described for decompression of pseudoobstruction. This larger diameter tube is less likely to be occluded with faecal matter.

The flatus tube should be left in position for 24–48 hours and definitive treatment planned as the condition is likely to recur.

FURTHER READING

Akle CA. Endoprostheses for colonic strictures. *Br J Surg* 1998; **85**:310–314

Baron TH, Dean PA. Yates MR 3rd, Canon C, Koehler RE. Expandable metal stents for the treatment of colonic obstruction: techniques and outcomes. *Gastrointest Endosc* 1998; **47**:277–286

Church JM. Analysis of the colonoscopic findings in patients with rectal bleeding according to the pattern of their presenting symptoms. *Dis Colon Rect* 1991; **34**:391–395

Dineen DM, Motson RW. Treatment of colonic anastomotic strictures with 'through the scope' balloon dilators. *J Roy Soc Med* 1991; **84**:264–266

Geller A, Peterson BT, Gostout CJ. Endoscopic decompression for acute colonic pseudo-obstruction. *Gastrointest Endosc* 1996; **44**:144–150

Malthus Vliegan EMH. Laser treatment of intestinal vascular abnormalities. *Int J Colorectal Dis* 1989; **4**:20–25

Rex DK. Colonoscopy and acute colonic pseudo-obstruction. *Gastrointest Endosc Clinics North Am* 1997; **7**:499–508

Schrock TR. Colonoscopic diagnosis and treatment of .lower gastrointestinal bleeding. *Surg Clin North Am* 1989; **69**:1309–1325

Tan CC, Iftikhar SY, Allan A, Freeman JG. Local effects of colorectal cancer are well palliated by endoscopic laser therapy. *Eur J Surg Oncol* 1995; **21**:648–652

Trudel JL, Fazio VW, Sivak MV. Colonoscopic diagnosis and treatment of arteriovenous malformations in chronic lower gastrointestinal bleeding–clinical accuracy and efficacy. *Dis Colon Rect* 1988; **31**:107–110

Truong S, Willis S, Schumpelick V. Endoscopic therapy of benign anastomotic strictures of the colorectum by electroincision and balloon dilatation. *Endoscopy* 1997; **29**:845–849

Waye JD, Lewis BS, Yessayan S. Colonoscopy: a prospective report of complications. *J Clin Gastro* 1992; **15**:347–351

Section 3

Endoscopic surgery

General principles of endoscopic surgery

J.D. Greig

INTRODUCTION

The advent of laparoscopic techniques has created a surgical renaissance which has improved many aspects of patient care where it is used wisely and applied appropriately. This has been made possible by the introduction of advanced video imaging with the associated technological development in instruments and bioprosthetic materials. Many of the common conditions such as gallstones, appendicitis and hernias can be dealt with by modern surgical techniques with little discomfort. Judicious use of new techniques which involve laparoscopic surgery mean less pain and earlier return to normal activities and work for most patients.

INDUCTION OF THE PNEUMOPERITONEUM

Open cut down technique

This is the safest method of establishing a pneumoperitoneum and is mandatory where there has been previous abdominal surgery. A small vertical incision (the size of which will vary with the patient's body habitus) is made below the umbilicus. The subcutaneous fat is incised down to the linea alba. The linea is incised exposing the preperitoneal fat. Using a 1/0 absorbable suture such as polydioxone suture (PDS), the linea either side is grasped by one suture and held up. Using a pair of fine artery forceps the preperitoneal fat is cleared and a small entry point is made bluntly into the peritoneal cavity. The opening is enlarged with the index finger to allow an 11 mm blunt Hassan trocar and port to be inserted into the peritoneal cavity. The Hassan port has a conical outer sheath which sits around the external port and acts as a plug which is held in place in the incision by the two PDS sutures. The CO_2 tubing is connected to the insufflation side hub on the Hassan port and the abdomen is insufflated.

An alternative cut down method involves a transverse or vertical incision around the inferior aspect of the umbilicus. The umbilical tube is followed down and grasped lower and lower as it approaches the linea alba. An incision is made at the base of the tube into the linea alba and entry to the peritoneal cavity is gained in the same manner as described above. The principal advantage of this latter method is that it is easier to hold up the peritoneum to gain access and provides a fixed anatomical landmark to follow.

Veress needle

Veress needles may be disposable or non-disposable (Figure 22.1). They come in lengths of 70 or 120 mm. Disposable needles have the advantage that there is no risk of cross infection. Secondly, disposable needles are always sharp and the spring loading mechanism is intact to allow full retractability of the sharp point when it traverses the peritoneal cavity, whereas there is inevitable wear and tear with reusable needles.

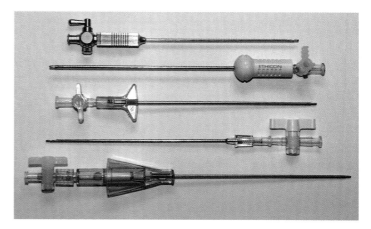

Figure 22.1 Veress needles.

Urinary catheterisation is mandatory for pelvic laparoscopy but optional in patients undergoing other abdominal procedures. If no catheter is used, then percussion of the bladder is required to ensure that a chronic urinary retention has not gone undetected. Following prepping and sterile draping of the abdomen, an incision is made either above or below the umbilicus as the peritoneum is closely adherent to the under surface of the umbilicus at this point. Therefore, this provides a natural anatomical weakness through which the Veress needle can be passed. For this reason the supraumbilical site is probably associated with less risk of rectus sheath insufflation than the subumbilical route. Many surgeons prefer the patient to be in the Trendelenberg position to allow the viscera to fall out of the pelvis and insert the needle in a 45° angle towards the pelvis. The author prefers the patient level and supine. The abdominal wall below the umbilicus is held up by either the operator's left hand or both the operator and the assistant's hand, which ever is easier. The Veress needle is inserted vertically into the peritoneal cavity. The spring-loaded central trocar is pushed back as the needle enters the peritoneal cavity and springs back to cover the sharp point once the peritoneal cavity has been breached. Two clicks can be heard from the Veress needle as it enters the peritoneal cavity. The first as it traverses the rectus sheath and the second as it traverses the peritoneum.

The position of the Veress needle is confirmed by placing a drop of saline over the open hub of the needle. If the needle is in the correct position and the hub is opened, the negative pressure within the abdomen will draw the saline into the shaft of the needle. Alternatively, a small amount of saline can be injected into the needle. If it is easily aspirated, the needle is in the preperitoneal space and needs to be advanced. If the insufflation flow pressure is low then the needle is probably in the peritoneal cavity.

Once it has been established that the Veress needle is in the peritoneal cavity; insufflation begins at 1 l/min. If the pressure remains constant and low, the flow rate can be increased to 2 l/min until the target pressure of 12–15 mmHg has been reached. Because of the fixed diameter of the Veress needle, flow rates of higher than 2 l/min cannot be achieved. When the target pressure has been reached, the needle is withdrawn and a 5 or 11 mm port is inserted into the peritoneal cavity. The sterile CO_2 tubing is connected to the insufflation hub on the port and higher flow rates can now be achieved if required.

One other site which can be used for Veress needle insertion, is 1 cm inferior to the left mid-clavicular point below the costal margin. The skin is drawn inferiorly with the index finger. A small nick is made in the skin to allow access for the Veress needle which is then passed into the peritoneal cavity.

Use of the Veress needle to achieve a pneumoperitoneum is less safe than the cut down technique because of the risks associated with intraabdominal visceral injury. While the cut down technique appears to be more time consuming, laparoscopy can be started immediately as insufflation is much more rapid with the Hassan port.

Remember that a non-operated abdomen can still have intra-abdominal adhesions from the following origins: congenital, primary peritonitis and blunt abdominal trauma.

Insufflator

The insufflator (Figure 22.2) consists of a sophisticated valve mechanism that gates the flow of pressurised gas from the tank into the patient's abdomen. All insufflators have standard functions that can be adjusted and monitored. The gauges indicate rate of flow (l/min); intraabdominal pressure (mmHg); and total litres of gas insufflated. Most modern insufflators can be set so that the flow of gas ceases when a predetermined intraabdominal pressure is achieved. Without this feature, the laparoscopist must be acutely aware because of the higher risks of increased gas absorption, decreased venous return from the IVC, impaired ventilation

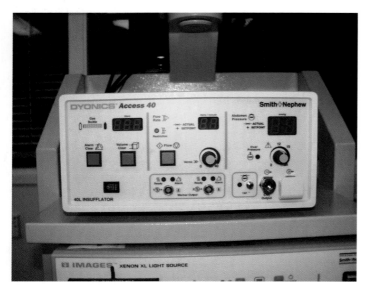

Figure 22.2 Insufflator.

as a result of diaphragmatic splinting, and the development of systemic acidosis where pressures exceed 15 mmHg.

When the insufflator is turned on, the CO_2 pressure should register in the green, indicating sufficient tank pressure. The CO_2 cylinder should be checked to be certain that it contains sufficient gas for the completion of the procedure. If there is any doubt, the CO_2 cylinder should be changed or be easily accessible in theatre.

Following connection of the insufflator tubing to the Veress needle or directly to the Hassan port if an open technique has been used, the flow rate on the insufflator should be adjusted to 1 l/min initially. Next, the volume of gas insufflated is reset to zero, the target pressure of 12–15 mmHg should be set, the pressure in the insufflator tubing should read zero and the gas flow turned on. The abdominal pressure should read between 0 and 5 mmHg while the volume of gas insufflated should be noted at the set rate. If the flow rate is not 1 l/min or the pressure is high, consider that there may be kinking of the insufflator tubing or more likely, the Veress needle is incorrectly placed or lying against bowel or omentum. If the pressure and flow rate are satisfactory, the rate can be increased to 2 l/min. When the pneumoperitoneum has been established and the tubing connected to the side hub of the port, flow rates may be increased to 8–10 l/min.

Choice of insufflatant

A variety of gases have been used as insufflatants but safety versus cost have reduced the list of viable options to two: carbon dioxide (CO_2) and nitrous oxide (N_2O). Air is not used because it is largely insoluble in blood and very little is required to be absorbed to result in a significant air embolus. Oxygen has been avoided because of the risk of explosion when electrocautery is used. Carbon dioxide is preferred for all but short diagnostic procedures. When absorbed, CO_2 rapidly dissolves in blood, thereby decreasing the risk of gas embolism. Furthermore, CO_2 does not support combustion, so electrosurgical instruments can be used safely in its presence.

The main drawbacks of CO_2 are that it is a peritoneal irritant and when it is absorbed significant acidosis can occur. Carbon dioxide is converted to carbonic acid both on the peritoneal surface and in the blood stream. The former situation may cause diaphragmatic irritation and post operative pain; the latter situation results in metabolic acidosis.

Because of these limitations some laparoscopists prefer to use N_2O as the insufflatant, especially for short procedures. Nitrous oxide is not a peritoneal irritant and when absorbed does not result in metabolic abnormalities. However, it is less soluble in blood than CO_2, and theoretically presents a higher risk of gas embolism. Moreover, there is a small but real risk to the patient if N_2O is used in the presence of electrocautery, since it can support combustion.

Dangers of the pneumoperitoneum

Veress needle insertion

Following insertion of the Veress needle, it may lie in the preperitoneal space and cause extensive surgical emphysema. Alternatively, the needle can cause injury to the underlying organs and viscera, together with injuries to the mesenteric and the major abdominal blood vessels including the aorta, iliac vessels and IVC. Inadvertent insufflation of CO_2 into a major vein will cause a CO_2 gas embolus with a potentially fatal outcome from a cardiac dysrhythmia. Use of the open cut down method for establishing a pneumoperitoneum avoids many of these potential risks, as may insertion of the Veress needle into the left upper quadrant.

Trocar insertion

The insertion of the first trocar is essentially blind despite having obtained a satisfactory pneumoperitoneum. Most disposable and many non-disposable trocars have retractable sharp tips. However, control of insertion is still needed with the right hand holding the port and trocar and the left hand placed on its shaft as the insertion proceeds to prevent over-penetration of the peritoneal cavity. Other trocar insertions should be performed under direct laparoscopic vision. A selection of trocars is shown in Figure 22.3a and b.

Abdominal wall bleeding

This may occur from the first port site placement but it is often with secondary port placements where a medium sized vessel has been injured as the trocar passes through the abdominal wall. Most bleeding ceases spontaneously and only infrequently is an external skin suture or formal exploration of a port site needed. Avoidance of this complication can be minimised by identification of the inferior epigastric vessels and transilluminating the abdominal wall with the laparoscope.

Sickle cell anaemia

For patients with this condition, the aims during surgery are to maintain a warm, well-hydrated and well perfused patient with high oxygen saturations. The expected mild hypothermia, reduced cardiac output, high oxygen extraction ratio and venous pooling will mitigate against these aims and thus compromise the patient.

Metabolic

The stress response is reduced in laparoscopic by comparison to open surgery. However, prolonged insufflation may cause a rise in serum potassium levels.

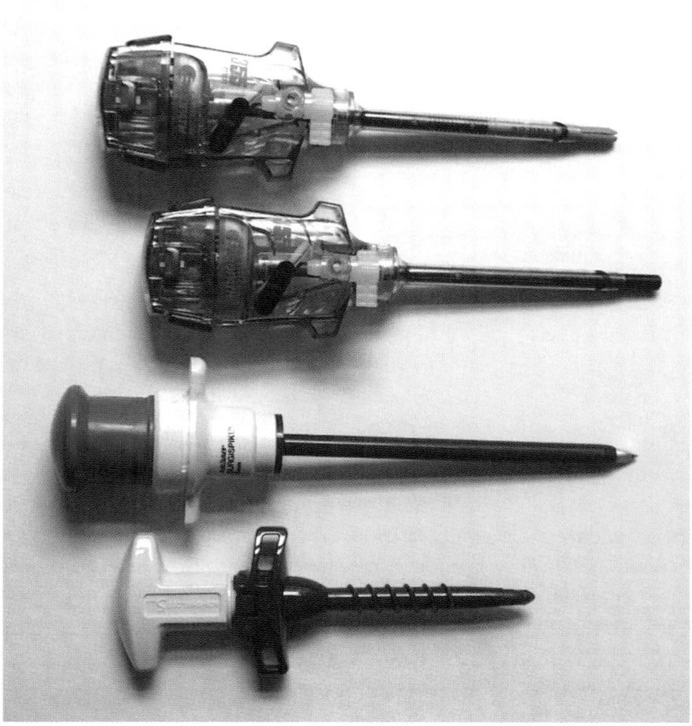

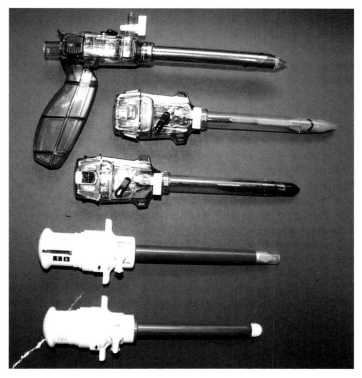

Figure 22.3a 10 mm trocars.

Figure 22.3b 5 mm trocars.

Pneumothorax

A rare complication of pneumoperitoneum is that of pneumothorax and the anaesthetist must be aware to recognise and treat this.

Deep venous thrombosis and pulmonary embolism

The raised intraabdominal pressure reduces venous return to the heart, increases the venous pooling in the lower extremities, and decreases the flow velocities in the larger veins in the legs. Reduced flow velocities in turn may predispose to deep venous thrombosis (DVT). The five principal methods of prevention are:

- preoperative subcutaneous injection of low molecular weight heparin (two hours prior to the procedure)
- below knee graduated compression stockings
- peroperative pneumatic calf and leg compression
- an intraabdominal insufflation pressure of <15 mmHg
- early mobilisation after surgery.

Gasless laparoscopy, using an external lift device inserted through the abdominal wall, may avoid some of the complications associated with the pneumoperitoneum, but this method has not proved popular, particularly as local trauma and haematoma formation at the site of the insertion are recognised problems.

Post-operative shoulder tip pain

This occurs in up to 40% of patients after CO_2 laparoscopy and usually affects the right shoulder. It is believed to be caused by the irritating effects of CO_2 producing carbonic acid locally and affecting the peritoneal lining of the right hemidiaphragm which is in turn is referred to the shoulder. Shoulder tip pain can be significantly reduced by using insufflation pressures of ≤ 9 mmHg.

Port site incisional hernias

Unless the midline 10–12 mm port sites are closed to re-approximate the linea alba, the risk in the short, medium or long term of incisional herniation, remains substantive. Direct visualisation and accurate approximation of tissues minimises this potential complication. Five mm port sites do not require closure. If the newer dilating disposable trocars which separate tissues rather than causing a substantive defect have been used in the midline, they still require formal closure.

PHYSIOLOGY OF THE PNEUMOPERITONEUM

Respiratory physiology

The upward displacement and splinting of the diaphragm leads to an increase in the work of breathing and potential basal collapse of the lungs. Carbon dioxide is absorbed at 70 ml/min for the first 30 minutes and 90 ml/min thereafter. In order to offload the excess CO_2 and to prevent basal collapse, the lungs are overventilated using positive pressure ventilation (PPV) with a raised minute volume.

Patients with pre-existing respiratory disease will retain more CO_2 during surgery. Pulmonary function tests showing a reduced forced expiratory volume, forced vital capacity and impaired diffusion are predictors for intraoperative acidosis. Normally with PPV this is manageable, although with extraperitoneal dissection, where more gas is absorbed (for example, laparoscopic preperitoneal hernia repair), the minute ventilation rates may have to be further increased to compensate.

Where CO_2 retention is perceived to be a potential problem, alternatives include gasless laparoscopy, use of helium as the insufflatant, lower insufflation pressures or a planned open procedure from the start.

It is mandatory to measure end-tidal CO_2 levels during surgery as these correlate accurately with arterial levels of CO_2 tension.

Cardiovascular physiology

Simple clinical measurements of blood pressure and heart rate may give a misleading impression of cardiovascular stability as the effects of the pneumoperitoneum on the cardiovascular system are variable.

Hypertension can occur but may also be the result of hypercarbia following CO_2 absorption from the peritoneal cavity leading to sympathetic nervous stimulation or it may simply be the result of inadequate analgesia or anaesthesia.

Hypotension is not uncommon during laparoscopy and usually indicates a significant decrease in cardiac output due to a decreased venous return to the heart. It must be born in mind that hypotension may also result from gas embolism, pneumothorax or serious dysrhythmia.

Bradycardia is a common rhythm disturbance and is caused either by the vagal effects of distension or manipulation of the pelvic viscera. If it is persistent, it will respond to vagolytic drugs such as atropine.

Raised intraabdominal pressure compresses the abdominal blood vessels causing pooling of blood in the lower extremities, and a decrease in the amount of blood in the abdominal venous system. Both central venous pressure (CVP) and pulmonary capillary wedge pressure are accompanied by a reduction in cardiac output. The 25% fall in cardiac index is because the external pressure of the pneumoperitoneum on the abdominal arterial circulation causes an increase in after-load (increased systemic vascular resistance) which the left ventricle has to overcome. The magnitude of the intraabdominal pressure induced by the pneumoperitoneum affects this.

The degree of Trendelenberg also affects the cardiac filling pressures. A horizontal position and pneumoperitoneum leads to increase of 58% in CVP, 32% in PAOP and 39% in mean arterial pressure (MAP). A 20° head-down tilt is associated with a further 40% increase in filling pressures. A 20° head-up tilt will reduce the filling pressures to the pre-pneumoperitoneum levels. The increased after-load is maintained in both head-up and head-down tilts.

Because of the profound haemodynamic changes, pre-existing cardiovascular disease in some patients may preclude the laparoscopic approach, similarly for the hypovolaemic or shocked patient.

Central nervous system physiology

Laparoscopy is unwise in the presence of intracranial injuries because the pneumoperitoneum will decrease cerebral perfusion pressure (i.e. the difference between MAP and CVP minus the intracranial pressure (ICP). The ICP rises with the pneumoperitoneum due to an increased CVP which in turn affects the ICP. Trendelenberg positioning and intracranial space occupying lesions will exacerbate these effects.

Renal physiology

The pneumoperitoneum decreases renal blood flow and glomerular filtration rate to 25% of baseline. This is as a result of a generalised decrease in splanchnic blood flow and renal vein compression rather than a reduction in cardiac output *per se*. This in turn reduces urine output during surgery, especially in patients with pre-existing cardiac disease.

Peritoneal hypothermia

Carbon dioxide gas is bottled in liquid form at a pressure of around 49 bar (temperature dependent). Sudden vaporisation of the gas produces carbon dioxide snow (−96°C). The insufflator and the connecting tube compensate for this, to a certain extent, and warm the gas to just below room temperature (±20°C). Measurements show that temperature in the abdominal cavity can fall below 32°C during laparoscopy. Furthermore, the rectal temperature may be reduced by as much as 1 to 3°C, depending on the length of surgery and the volume of gas used. If a long laparoscopic procedure is anticipated or where temperature variations may be important to the patient's well-being such as in the elderly, pre-warming of the gas may be considered so that insufflated gas enters the peritoneal cavity at 37°C instead of at 20°C.

INTRAOPERATIVE MONITORING

Routine intraoperative monitoring for patients undergoing laparoscopic procedures consists of an electrocardiogram, non-invasive blood pressure monitor and temperature monitor. Cardiopulmonary derangements (as outlined above) are among the common group of complications encountered during laparoscopy. This fact alone mandates the use of pulse oximetry and monitoring end-tidal CO_2.

For unhealthy patients undergoing a laparoscopic procedure, invasive haemodynamic monitoring is required. Deciding which patients should receive invasive monitoring during laparoscopic procedures involves balancing the risks of placing and maintaining an intravascular catheter against the benefits provided by that particular monitor. Patients with severe pre-existing cardiorespiratory disease who are undergoing laparoscopic procedures should be considered candidates for systemic and pulmonary arterial blood pressure monitoring. However, because of the pressurised pneumoperitoneum and the use of a Trendelenberg position, it should be remembered that central venous and pulmonary artery pressures may not accurately reflect venous return and cardiovascular performance during laparoscopy.

TECHNOLOGY OF VIDEO IMAGING

Laparoscopes

Laparoscopes are designed in two basic configurations: end viewing (0°) and oblique viewing (30° or 45°). The latter are more difficult to orientate but with a little practice this can be rapidly overcome. The oblique viewing laparoscopes are useful when trying to look over obstructing structures down onto the area of attention, such as the anatomy of Calot's triangle, which is often much better demonstrated using an oblique laparoscope.

The diameters of the laparoscopes vary from 1.9–10 mm. The smaller the telescope the greater the limitation of field of view and the greater is the distortion of the images. Use of smaller laparoscopes reduces the size of port site needed and hence the surgical trauma. Most modern telescopes use optics based on the Hopkins rod lens system which provides excellent light transmission, better resolution and contrast, and a large angle of view that leads to a full format video image. They may be sterilised by steam autoclave at 134°C but others (depending on the manufacturer) may not be autoclavable and require glutaraldehyde solution sterilisation. Misting of telescopes is a common problem and easily overcome by warming the laparoscope in warm sterile saline, shifting the CO_2 insufflation port to another which does not bear the laparoscope, and use of a demisting solution on the lens of the laparoscope. Persistent fogging suggests either fluid between eyepiece and camera head, or damage to the rod system of lenses in the telescope.

Light cables

Light transmission can be achieved through fibre or fluid cables. The fibre cables transmit light by glass fibres which are reinforced with a metal spiral making them more rigid and resistant to deformation than fluid cables. They are also autoclavable at 134°C. The diameter of the bundle varies from 1.6–4.5 mm and the length from 1.8–3.6 m. The diameter of the bundle should always be chosen to be slightly larger than the lens system.

Fluid light cables transmit light through liquid permitting a more even transmission of light across the spectrum. They may be used for videotaping or laparoscopic photography. The principal disadvantage is a loss of brightness of 20–30% compared to fibre cables. The diameters available are 3–5 mm and they are 1.8 m in length.

Cold light source

Cold light refers to the spectrum of light delivered. It should be remembered that the light produced from the ends of the fibre-optic cable and the telescope have sufficient heat to burn either the drapes or the patient. Light sources are of the high intensity variety using xenon, tungsten or a halogen vapour bulbs to produce an output of between 100–400 watts. The light intensity can be regulated manually or automatically. Before any procedure is started, a white balance is completed to adjust for colour correction. The light output intensity is controlled at the source. Proper light intensity affords better depth perception and image detail. Light sources are also fitted with an emergency lamp which will automatically cut in case of failure of the primary lamp.

Cameras

Initially, single chip CCDs (charge-couple devices) were developed. These rapidly gave way to three chip CCDs which provided colour resolution for each of the three primary colours, vastly improving the resultant image. Aperture control, a built in zoom facility and manual focussing ring allow the laparoscopist further control of the image. Most centres use cameras which lock onto the eyepiece of the laparoscope and are covered in sterile polythene elephant tubing (Figure 22.4). Cameras are now available which have the laparoscope as an integral part of the imaging system (the so called 'chip on the stick'). Its principal disadvantage is that it does not allow flexibility of switching between different laparoscopes.

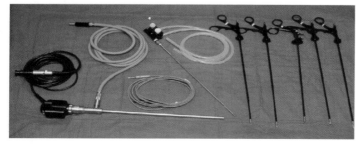

Figure 22.4 Laparoscope with 3 chip CCD camera, light source and a selection of instruments.

Production of image and transmission to a high resolution monitor gives a clear 2D image but laparoscopic surgery involves working in a 3D environment without depth perception. Endoscopic 3D with two optical channels has been available for almost a decade, but all the systems still involve the wearing of red/green glasses or other bulky head sets to produce a stereoscopic image. Most surgeons are able to compensate adequately for the lack of depth perception with practice and using other visual cues, but it is with laparoscopic suturing where the greatest benefit may be observed.

Monitors

Video monitors come from a variety of manufacturers and are available in several standard sizes from 13–19 inches with resolutions of 525–1125 lines. Newer laparoscopic systems have abandoned the concept of having a monitor and rely instead on direct video projection onto a sterile screen mounted just in front of the surgeon which can be touched directly without comprising aseptic technique. It also affords the surgeon with a closer view of the operative field which can be adjusted to provide a more friendly ergonomic environment in which to work.

Voice activated laparoscopy

Systems are now available which allow the operator to control movements of the camera connected to a robotic arm by single voice commands (Figure 22.5). Similarly, control of the image quality can also be adjusted peroperatively by a voice activated menu so that contrast, brightness, aperture control and focussing can also be performed. Control of the insufflator pressures and flow rates can also be made via the same integrated system. Inappropriate activation of the voice command centre is avoided by having the computer recognise the operator's voice during a test session which is then logged onto a hard disk which is personalised to one operator. The computer then responds to the

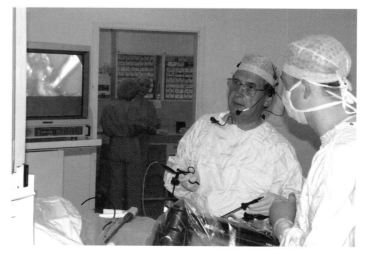

Figure 22.5 Voice activated laparoscopic system.

personalised hard disk which has the operator's voice data on it. This still necessitates the wearing of a light headset during surgery.

Remote console controlled robotic control of laparoscopy

It is now possible that when all the ports are sited and the appropriate laparoscope and working instruments are inserted, that the operator sits down at a remote control ergonomically designed console to perform the surgery and it also lends itself in the future to telemedicine. Instruments still have to be changed manually but it means that difficult procedures could be performed at distance by an 'experienced operator' at a remote site. The technology to allow us to do this is now currently available but because it is available does not necessarily imply it will always be in the best interests of the patient.

LAPAROSCOPIC ANATOMY OF THE ABDOMEN

A port inserted at the umbilicus is the essential central point of the abdomen for conducting a full laparoscopic examination of the peritoneal cavity. Once the laparoscope has been passed through the port and confirmation that a satisfactory pneumoperitoneum has been established, the patient is tilted into the Trendelenberg position to allow inspection of the pelvis and the pelvic viscera. A cursory examination is made of the entire peritoneal cavity to determine the presence or absence of adhesions, obvious intraabdominal pathology or disease of the parietal peritoneum.

The peritoneal folds and inferior epigastric vessels

The first key landmark to orientate the laparoscopist is the midline median umbilical fold (broad based urachus) running down from the umbilicus to the apex of the dome of the bladder on the posterior aspect of the anterior abdominal wall. In some patients this peritoneal fold is not marked and can be difficult to identify but the two medial umbilical folds (obliterated umbilical arteries) are always invariably present lying lateral to the midline. Swinging the laparoscope further laterally, the inferior epigastric vessels are identified lying just superficial to the peritoneum. Location of this vessel bundle is essential as lateral port placement avoids inadvertent damage to them and secondly they are key to identifying potential inguinal hernias.

Following the epigastric vessels caudally towards the pelvis, the external iliac vein can be seen billowing gently with changes in the respiratory cycle along the inner pelvic rim and the associated pulsation of the external iliac artery may be superior or directly behind it.

Potential hernial defects and the bladder
(Figure 22.6)

Having successfully identified the epigastric vessels origin, the deep inguinal ring is readily identified just lateral to this vessel bundle. Indirect inguinal hernias can be diagnosed by bulges in the peritoneum at this point. Confirmation of this landmark is made by identification of the testicular vessels coursing laterally from the posterior peritoneum through the ring and the white vas deferens lying just deep to the peritoneum dropping vertically over the pelvic rim towards the bladder. In the female, once the tubes and ovaries have been identified the round ligament can be

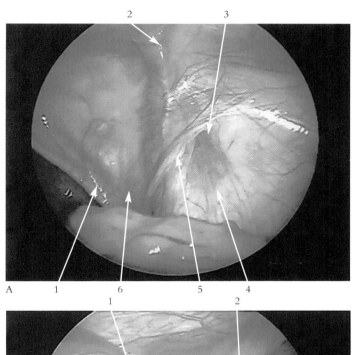

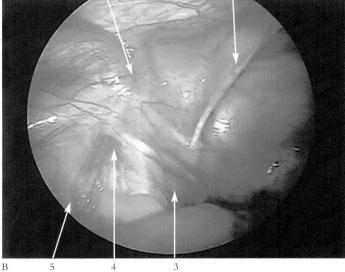

Figure 22.6 Potential hernial defects and the bladder. **a** 1 = (R) medium umbilical fold; 2 = IEP (interior epigastric pedicle); 3 = indirect inguinal hernia; 4 = testicular vessels; 5 = vas deferens; 6 = iliac vessels. **b** 1 = IEP; 2 = (L) medium umbilical fold; 3 = vas deferens; 4 = peritoneal fold at deep inguinal ring; 5 = testicular vessels.

329

followed to its exit from the peritoneal cavity through the deep inguinal ring. If the operator swings the laparoscope to the medial side of the inferior epigastric vessels, the back of the inguinal canal is inspected for the presence of a direct inguinal hernia where the peritoneum does not lie flat along the abdominal wall musculature. On the left, the sigmoid colon may occasionally obscure the deep inguinal ring. No attempt should be made to mobilise the sigmoid colon unless a hernia is suspected. A femoral hernia may be suspected where there are omental or other adhesions to the peritoneum close to the line of the iliac vessels as they exit the peritoneal cavity through the femoral ring. This is marked by the inguinal ligament anteriorly, the lacunar ligament medially and pelvic rim posteriorly. The bladder is identified in the midline by the presence of the catheter balloon in the collapsed bladder and in the female, lying behind the uterus.

Insertion of additional ports

To perform a full laparoscopy, two additional 5 mm ports are used. These are best sited in the right upper and left lower quadrants. This allows satisfactory triangulation of instruments for handling all tissues in the peritoneal cavity. Trocars are passed through the abdominal wall under direct vision lateral to the line of epigastric vessels which the laparoscopist has already identified. Injury to the larger superficial subcutaneous vessels can be avoided by transillumination of the skin with the lighted laparoscope.

The pelvic viscera

Atraumatic graspers are passed into the peritoneal cavity. Any small bowel remaining in the pelvis is gently grasped and removed by traction. In the male, the only contents in the pelvis should be the bladder lying anteriorly and the rectum/sigmoid colon lying posteriorly. In the female, the bladder lies superficial to the uterus in the midline with the rectum lying posterior. Any fluid in the pelvis can be aspirated through the left lower quadrant port prior to any further handling. This may be sent for bacteriological, cytological and biochemical examination. If there is no cervical forceps inserted per vaginally to tip the uterus up, the uterus can be lifted up at the insertion of the fallopian tubes into the uterus by using the atraumatic forceps as elevators rather than graspers of the tubes. Once the uterus is inspected follow the tubes along the pelvic brim. Lightly grasp the distal end of the left and then right tube in turn to allow visualisation of the ovary inferiorly. Using the other grasper, better visualisation of the ovary can be achieved by using this as an elevator to bring the ovary out of the pelvis.

Rectum and sigmoid colon

If rectosigmoid pathology is suspected, the colon can be straightened by grasping the colon and emptying the pelvis. If necessary, partially mobilise the sigmoid off the lateral peritoneum.

However, there are few sigmoid pathologies with the exception of endometriosis which cannot be diagnosed by colonoscopy.

Appendix and right colon

The laparoscope is now directed to the right iliac fossa (RIF). If the appendix is not readily obvious, identify the ascending colon and follow the taenia to their conclusion in the RIF. The caecum can be grasped and elevated to allow inspection of its pole. The appendix base is now identified and followed to the appendiceal tip which is very variable in its position. Unless appendiceal pathology is suspected, no attempt should be made to mobilise a retrocaecal or paracaecal appendix. If there is any difficulty in locating the appendix or the right colon, the patient can be rotated towards the operator with the right side up.

Small bowel

Following location of the appendix, a note will have been made of the medial insertion of the ileo-caecal junction. The ileum is now grasped and elevated for inspection. In many patients the terminal ileum may be attached by short mesentery to the posterior abdominal wall. Again, unless terminal ileal pathology is suspected, no attempt should be made to mobilise this structure as it becomes relatively free within a short distance from the ileo-caecal junction. The whole of the small bowel can now be walked through with the two graspers passing it from hand-to-hand until the duodenal-jejunal flexure is reached. Enlargement of the glands in the mesentery are readily identified by pulling out the left hand towards the pelvis at the ileo-caecal angle to inspect the mesentery or at any other place in the small bowel mesentery where pathology is suspected.

Greater omentum and transverse colon

With the patient in the Trendelenberg position, the greater omentum naturally slides out of the way into the upper abdomen unless it is tethered by adhesions. If it does become problematic, the adhesions can be divided or the omentum simply grasped and placed in the upper abdomen which will, in any case allow external inspection of the underlying transverse colon. However, as with the rest of the colon, the best method of visualisation of the transverse colon, is colonoscopy.

Upper abdominal organs: liver, gallbladder, and their ducts (Figure 22.7)

A reverse Trendelenberg position is now adopted allowing the omentum and small bowel to slide inferiorly towards the pelvis. The two lobes of the liver are identified and split between the falciform ligament hanging off the anterior abdominal wall and running superiorly from the umbilicus in the midline. The falciform enters the liver parenchyma as the ligamentum teres and

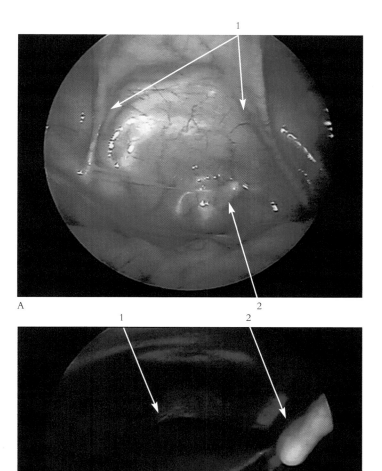

Figure 22.7 Upper abdominal organs: liver, gallbladder and their ducts. **a** 1 = medium umbilical folds; 2 = catheter in bladder. **b** 1 = Liver; 2 = falciform ligament; 3 = stomach; 4 = gallbladder.

posterior aspect of the peritoneal cavity at this point is right kidney and adrenal. Unsuspected enlargement of either of these organs may be detected at this stage.

Oesophageal hiatus

A nasogastric tube is useful to allow deflation of the stomach and act as a palpable marker for the oesophagus as it enters the abdomen. Elevating the under surface of the left lobe of the liver, and gentle downwards traction of the stomach with the other grasper will clearly identify the oesophageal hiatus between the left and right crus of the diaphragm. If a hiatus hernia is present, the peritoneum at this point bulges toward the thorax between the lax crus. The oesophagus must not be handled directly because of the risk of inadvertent perforation.

Stomach, duodenum and spleen

The anterior walls of stomach and duodenum can now be visualised by direct inspection and traction. Pulling the stomach laterally will allow visualisation of the lesser curvature, the overlying lesser omentum and in thinner individuals the body of pancreas can be seen through the lesser omentum. Laparoscopic ultrasound is needed to inspect the liver parenchyma, its ducts and vasculature, the head, body and tail of pancreas. Endoluminal ultrasound may also help fully examine the rest of the upper gastrointestinal tract and its associated lymph node drainage. The spleen is not routinely examined unless there is a specific indication to do so. It can be examined with the patient rotated to the right with the left side up.

Following completion of the laparoscopy, the ports are withdrawn under direct vision, and pneumoperitoneum is released. The umbilical port site is closed with absorbable sutures and the skin with a subcuticular suture. The 5 mm port sites are closed with steristrips only.

SUMMARY

Laparoscopy has made an enormous beneficial impact on the practice of surgery. However, with these benefits comes a specific package of potential complications to catch the unwary. Remember some simple rules:

- If a patient is not fit for open surgery do not attempt to perform the minimalist access surgery in the hope you may get away with a lesser procedure

- Be wary of using the Veress needle

- Use laparoscopic equipment you are familiar with

- Do not use patients to practice and evaluate new laparoscopic equipment on without first test driving it in the abdominal laparoscopic simulator

continues across the superior aspect of the liver as the falciform ligament. The upper surface of the liver is inspected by passing the laparoscope over this. Better visualisation of the posterior aspects of the liver are obtained with the 30° scope. The right lobe of liver is elevated with one grasper and the gallbladder becomes apparent. Gentle traction on the gallbladder assists the inspection of the underside of the liver and the biliary anatomy. Insertion of the cystic duct into the more medially placed common bile duct is often not obvious because of the peritoneal coverings. Obvious hilar lymphadenopathy can often be detected at this stage, if present. In individuals who have very little body fat, the common bile duct, the posterior lying portal vein and further medially placed hepatic artery can all be clearly identified. Lying on the

- If the anaesthetist says the patient has a respiratory or cardio-vascular problem, listen to him and instigate an immediate deflation of the abdomen

- Think about potential complications and try to prevent them

- Maintain and practice your laparoscopic skills to maintain a level of competence especially for laparoscopic suturing

- Think about your ergonomics for standing and operating for long periods to prevent operator musculoskeletal problems now or in the future.

FURTHER READING

Jones, Stephanie B. Anesthesia in ambulatory minimally invasive surgery. *Current Opinion in Anaesthesiology* 2000; **13**(6):637–641

Paterson-Brown S, Garden OJ, editors. *Principles and practice of surgical laparoscopy.* 1994 London: WB Saunders

Targarona EM, Balague C, Knook MM, Trias M. Laparoscopic surgery and surgical infection. *British Journal of Surgery* 2000; **87**(5):536–544

Instrumentation and perioperative management in laparoscopic surgery

K.K. Madhavan, S. Paterson-Brown

For safe laparoscopic surgery to be undertaken it is essential that surgeons understand the various instruments at their disposal, their potential advantages and disadvantages and the underlying operative principles with which they should be used. This chapter will deal with these in turn, in addition to explaining some of the physiological changes which take place during laparoscopic surgery.

LAPAROSCOPIC INSTRUMENTATION

The instruments required for laparoscopic surgery can be divided into the following categories:

- visualisation
- grasping
- retraction
- dissection
- ligation/suturing
- retrieval.

Instruments for establishing and maintaining a pneumoperitoneum are discussed in Chapter 22.

Visualisation

Laparoscopes are based on the Hopkins optical system which uses a series of glass rods with lenses placed at appropriate intervals along the shaft of the instrument. Initial laparoscopic surgery was performed by direct-viewing laparoscopes, often with an operating channel through which instruments could be passed. One of the major drawbacks of this technique was the inability of the assistant to see what was going on but with the advent of video laparoscopy, whereby a small video camera is attached to the end of the laparoscope and images are projected onto a television monitor, this has all changed. Everyone in the operating theatre can now observe the operation, teaching is enhanced and, with advances in telecommunications, these images can now be simultaneously transmitted and viewed by audiences across the world.

Laparoscopes

The initial laparoscopes were 10 mm in diameter but now ones of 2–3 mm are being used in some centres (Figure 23.1). They not only provide visualisation of the surgical field but also various degrees of magnification. The most commonly used laparoscope views directly forward (0°), but increasingly surgeons are using more oblique-viewing instruments (30°) which are particularly helpful for more advanced laparoscopic procedures. These oblique-viewing laparoscopes provide a larger field of vision than the end-viewing instruments and permit the surgeon to view around the side of structures.

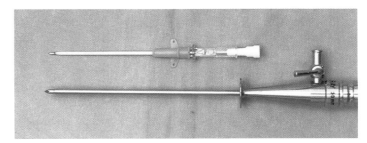

Figure 23.1 Mini-laparoscope (2.8 mm) and port lying beside a 14 gauge venous cannula.

Light source

A fibreoptic cable carries light from a 'cold' source, 100–300 watts, to the laparoscope in order to illuminate the peritoneal cavity. Xenon, halogen or tungsten lamps can be used and although it is called cold light, if it is not attached to the laparoscope, direct contact can cause burns on the drapes and to the patient's skin.

The modern light sources can be set up in manual or automatic mode, the latter adjusting the light intensity according to the picture received. This can also be controlled by opening and closing the iris on the camera attachment adjacent to the laparoscope. When the iris is closed the picture viewed on the monitor becomes less bright and often allows for better viewing. Many cameras now also come with an automatic gain control (AGC) which helps control light intensity.

Video camera system

The video camera is attached by means of a cable to a camera unit, from where the image is projected onto a monitor. The camera is coupled to the end of the eyepiece of the telescope using either 'glass to glass' attachment or attached to the laparoscopic eyepiece. The former is preferred as this prevents water or mist accumulating at this interface. Although the camera can be sterilised by immersion in antiseptic solution, most surgeons now favour using a sterile plastic sleeve through which the camera and cable can be passed as this removes the possibility of moisture entering the camera parts. At the onset of any procedure the camera needs to be 'white balanced', particularly if the three-chip variety (red, blue and green) is being used. Monitors for three-chip cameras have a total of over 1 million pixels, giving a horizontal resolution of more than 600 lines.

Although most laparoscopic surgery can be carried out with a single monitor, two are preferable, sited one on each side of the patient, either 19″ or 21″, mounted at the surgeon's eye level (Figure 23.2). Video recorders can usefully be included within this system to record procedures for later analysis and teaching. Furthermore, the addition of a digital printer will allow a hard copy of any intraoperative view to be made and kept within the patient records. This is particularly useful during diagnostic laparoscopy when the findings need to be conveyed to a third party.

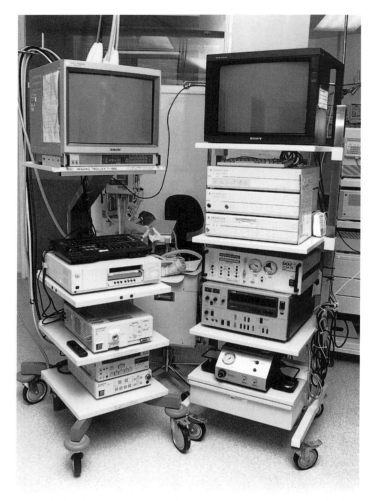

Figure 23.2 Advanced operating stack showing two monitors at eye level. Below the monitor on the right-hand side from above downwards can be seen: laparoscopic ultrasound equipment, the insufflator, a U-matic video recorder and a pressurised suction-irrigation system. Below the monitor on the left-hand side can be seen: a video mixer, a photograph printer, the light source, a super VHS video recorder and the camera unit.

If additional visual sources are being used, such as endoscopes and laparoscopic ultrasound probes (Figure 23.3), these images can be observed on the monitor simultaneously using a mixer device (Figure 23.4). A typical set-up for advanced laparoscopic surgery is shown in Figure 23.2.

Grasping

These instruments function like the assistant's hands and the surgeon's non-dominant hand in open surgery. They provide the

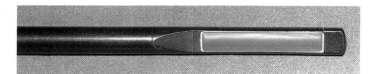

Figure 23.3 A 10 mm diameter linear array ultrasound transducer (Aloka, KeyMed, Southend-on-Sea, UK).

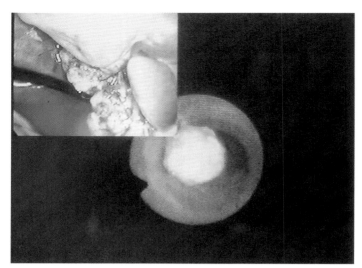

Figure 23.4 A composite image of the laparoscopic view (top left) and the endoscopic view (centre) produced by mixing laparoscopic and choledochoscopic views during a laparoscopic bile duct exploration.

traction and exposure which are so important in laparoscopic surgery. They can broadly be divided into two types – traumatic and atraumatic (Figure 23.5). The former are designed for firmness of grasp and are usually provided with sharp or serrated grasping surfaces. Even without serrated surfaces these grasping forceps can damage delicate structures, such as the bowel, and should only be used to grasp those structures which are either being removed, such as the gallbladder and appendix, or which will not be damaged, such as the crura of the diaphragm. Many of these traumatic graspers are provided with ratchets that can be locked so that the grasp is secure while the assistant uses the long axis of the instrument as a retractor. Spring-loaded graspers are also available which remain closed in their resting state so that they can be engaged on the tissue or organ to be grasped. To release these a coaxial mechanism can be operated from the handle end.

Atraumatic forceps, on the other hand, can be used to pick up and retract bowel, although even then care should be taken not to

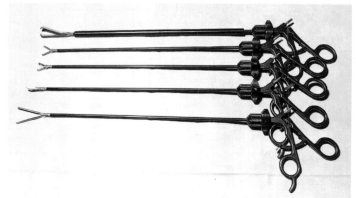

Figure 23.5 Some laparoscopic retractors from above down: 10 mm diameter toothed graspers for removing viscera (such as the gallbladder); non-toothed relatively 'atraumatic' graspers; toothed 'traumatic' graspers; curved (Petelin) grasping forceps also used for dissection; atraumatic bowel-holding forceps.

tear. These forceps may or may not be provided with ratchets; the latter has the advantage that the pressure applied to grasp a tissue or organ is to a large extent dependent on the operator. Some graspers, and indeed other instruments, can be mounted on flexible tips for passage around various structures, such as the oesophagus. However, most surgeons do not find this is a necessity. Other types of grasping forceps, such as those for taking biopsies, are also useful.

Retraction

Most retraction in laparoscopic surgery is done by application of grasping forceps but in special circumstances additional retractors are required. These can take the form of instruments mounted with expandable or inflatable endpieces which can be used through the ports to retract and those which pass through the abdominal wall and are mounted onto a rigid frame attached to the operating table (Figure 23.6). There are also some very ingenious semi-rigid instruments which can be passed down 5 mm laparoscopic ports and then screwed into a different shape, allowing them to be used to retract. Furthermore, sutures passed down laparoscopic ports, around or through intraabdominal structures and then back out are also a useful method of providing retraction. The port can be withdrawn, the suture grasped and then the port reinserted so that it can still be used for instrumentation.

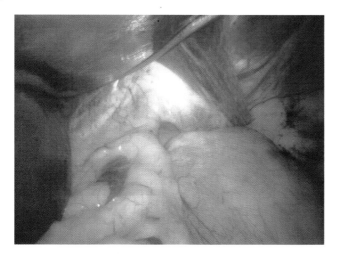

Figure 22.6 An externally fixed 'Nathanson' liver retractor (Cook, UK), shown here retracting the left lobe of the liver during a laparoscopic Nissen fundoplication. Note the hiatus hernia in the centre of the picture.

Dissection

These are instruments usually handled by the surgeon's dominant hand to effect tissue dissection. As in open surgery, tissue dissection can be sharp or blunt and can be achieved by mechanical or other means. The most common instruments for blunt dissection include the curved or 'Petelin' grasping forceps (Figure 23.5) and the 5 mm diameter suction-irrigation device. Rigid probes mounted with small gauze swabs are also available and can be

especially effective in delicate situations. Although most sharp dissection is still carried out using a combination of scissors and electrocautery (either attached directly to the scissors or by using a special diathermy hook) (Figure 23.7), there is now increasing interest in other methods of power supply which coagulate and cut in combination. These include various sources of power which can be used to perform procedures within the body cavity, not just to cut but also to coagulate and even destroy (radiofrequency and cryotherapy).

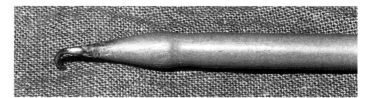

Figure 23.7 A diathermy hook for dissection with electrocautery. For safest use, the insulation should extend as far down the 'heel' as possible.

Electrocautery

Electrosurgical generators (diathermy units) which produce an electrical current of between 500 and 750 kHz remain the workhorses of laparoscopic and open surgery. The power of the electrical current delivered is a product of the interaction of resistance, current, voltage and time. Although 'cutting' and 'coagulating' modes are available, most laparoscopic surgery is carried out using only the coagulating mode with the addition of a lower voltage setting (marked L on the machine). This reduces the tendency for 'sparking' between the tip of the diathermy instrument and the adjacent tissues. Monopolar use tends to be more common but some instruments are available for bipolar use. If the monopolar system is being used care must be taken to ensure that all the instruments are insulated and that short-circuiting between the diathermy instrument and the port through which it passes, causing burns to the patient's skin, does not occur.

Laser

The initial description of laparoscopic cholecystectomy as 'laser cholecystectomy' followed the use of a Nd:YAG laser to remove the gallbladder from the liver. However, it swiftly became apparent that electrocautery was equally efficacious at a fraction of the cost and lasers are now rarely if ever used.

Argon beam coagulation

The argon beam coagulation system (Beacon Laboratory Inc, Colorado, USA) is a modification of diathermy in which a stream of argon gas conducts the coagulating current to the target tissue, providing a more uniform flow of energy with less tissue damage. When applied 2–3 mm away from the tissue surface the argon provides an eschar over the raw surface and is a useful haemostatic tool when there are large raw surfaces, such as following liver resection.

Vibration

The ability to vibrate a dissecting surface at speeds of up to 50 000 oscillations per second means that laparoscopic instruments can be used to coagulate and cut at the same time without resorting to electrocautery (Ultracision, Ethicon Endosurgery, Bracknell, UK: Figure 23.8). This vibration results in denaturing of the tissue with subsequent coagulation and then destruction/division. The advantage over diathermy comes from the smaller area of tissue destruction at the margins of the wound. It is now possible to use 5 mm instruments with this mechanism and vessels such as the short gastric arteries can be safely coagulated and divided without the need for repeated application of titanium clips.

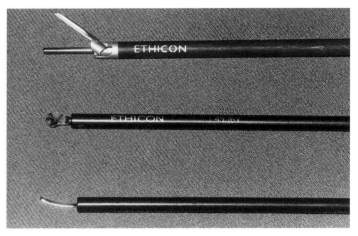

Figure 23.8 Ultracision dissectors (Ethicon Endosurgery, Bracknell, UK). From above down: blades, hook and spatula.

Ligation and suturing

Ligation

Application of titanium or absorbable clips to seal or secure intra-abdominal viscera is common practice in all aspects of laparoscopic surgery. These can be applied using either 5 or 10 mm diameter instruments. Linear staplers which can be passed down laparoscopic ports are also available and can be used across segments of bowel or vascular pedicles, as in open surgery (Figure 23.9).

The recent introduction of a bipolar diathermy ligation device (Ligasure, Tyco Inc, USA) coagulates vessels which can then be cut with scissors. Early reports from experimental studies have been promising and it is now available for both laparoscopic and open surgery.

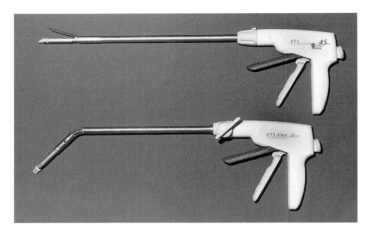

Figure 23.9 Laparoscopic linear stapling devices (Ethicon Endosurgery, Bracknell, UK) with rigid and flexible heads.

Loop ligatures are available with pre-tied Roeder knots and can be used to close off structures too large for the standard clips such as a large cystic duct stump and the base of the appendix.

Sutures

The ability to use sutures for securing haemostasis and closing hollow structures, such as the cystic duct, is as important during laparoscopic procedures as it has always been in open surgery. Time spent mastering the various techniques used to apply sutures will never be wasted.

Extracorporeal suturing

The simplest form of laparoscopic suture ligation involves extracorporeal knotting. This is most commonly used in the form of a pre-tied Roeder knot (Figure 23.10) which is passed over the structure to be ligated and tightened. Alternatively a suture can be passed around a structure and back out of the abdomen where a Roeder or other form of slip knot is tied and pushed down by means of a specially designed pusher (Figure 23.11). Tying a loop externally around a structure allows the structure to be ligated 'in continuity' before division. Alternatively a normal surgeon's knot can be tied and each throw pushed down into the peritoneal

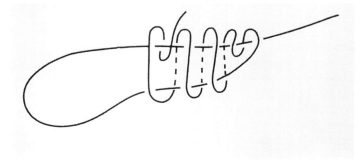

Figure 23.10 A Roeder 'slip' knot which is secured by tightening.

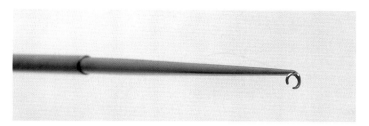

Figure 23.11 A 'pusher' which is used to 'push' the extracorporeal knot down into the peritoneal cavity.

cavity using the pusher. These techniques are particularly useful when a large cystic duct needs to be securely closed.

Intracorporeal suturing

As laparoscopic techniques have advanced and surgeons have become more dextrous and experienced, the majority of sutures are now being tied within the abdominal cavity using laparoscopic needle holders. This method permits both simple and suture ligation to be carried out in addition to procedures which require suture approximation of viscera (fundoplication, bowel anastomosis and common bile duct exploration).

For the novice there are several ingenious instruments designed to help the surgeon carry out intracorporeal suturing and knot tying; however, as experience is gained these usually become unnecessary and needle-holder tying takes over (Figure 23.12). As mounting the needle using two-dimensional imaging can also be a problem during the learning phase, some needle holders have been designed to automatically mount the needle in the correct orientation.

Curved, half-circumference 30 mm needles and smaller, using 0, 2/0, 3/0 and 4/0 sutures, can be passed down most 10 mm ports. The suture is grasped just behind its insertion into the needle using a needle holder and passed into the peritoneal cavity. If only one 10 mm port is being used, the laparoscope will need to be removed and the needle inserted blind. This remains a safe technique if care is taken and the suture grasped rather than the needle. Following

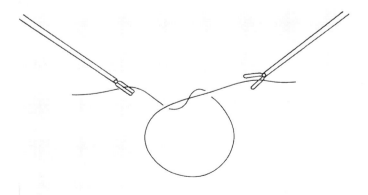

Figure 23.12 An intracorporeal knot tied with needle holders.

tying of the suture, the needle can be removed through a 5 mm port site. The suture is drawn up into the tip of the port under direct vision and then the port and needle removed together as the needle will obviously not pass through the 5 mm port. The 5 mm port is then reinserted under direct vision.

In the earlier days of laparoscopic surgery some surgeons used a 'ski' needle, which was essentially straight but with a small curve at the tip (Figure 23.13). This could be passed and withdrawn down both 5 and 10 mm ports, but is now less commonly used.

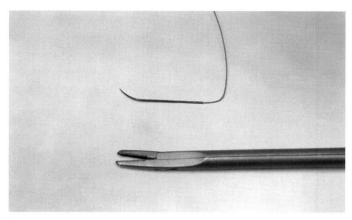

Figure 23.13 A 'ski' needle and standard needle holder.

Retrieval

Instruments for retrieval include the various suction-irrigation devices (Figure 23.14), retrieval bags (Figure 23.15) and large traumatic grasping forceps and 'spoons'.

Suction-irrigation devices

A single 5 mm cannula attached to the aspiration-lavage unit serves both these functions. The irrigation can be set up either with plain saline, a heparinised solution to prevent coagulation or with antibiotics. The desired function can be achieved using controls situated on the handle end of the instrument. Although

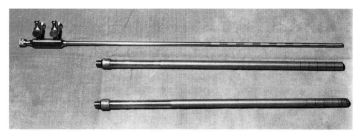

Figure 23.14 Suction-irrigation devices. In addition to the commonly used 5 mm instrument (top) there are 10 mm instruments available with open and 'guarded' tips (bottom). Some head pieces are interchangeable for use with either 5 mm and 10 mm instruments (not shown here).

simple attachment to the suction system and an intravenous administration set suffices, there are several combined pressure or pump action systems which permit rapid suction and irrigation. There are also systems available which permit diathermy to be added. The tips of the suction cannula can be covered by small holes to prevent structures like the omentum from continually occluding the system and, alternatively, larger 10 mm suction cannulas are available to remove large clots and any small stones spilled from the gallbladder (Figure 23.14).

Retrieval bags

These are inserted into the peritoneal cavity and structures to be removed are placed within them before removal. Those which are strong and spring open following insertion are the most user friendly (Figure 23.15). Similarly, they can be applied across the pedicle of a spleen for splenectomy.

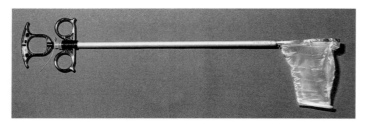

Figure 23.15 A disposable retrieval bag (Ethicon Endosurgery, Bracknell, UK) which is spring loaded so that the bag opens within the peritoneal cavity. There is an attached drawstring which closes the bag before withdrawal.

Miscellaneous advanced instruments

There are a multitude of additional instruments which have been designed for use in specific circumstances. These include expandable balloons to dissect anatomical spaces, such as the extraperitoneal plane for extraperitoneal herniorrhaphy, cholangiography clamps and catheters, Malecot trocars and cannulas for endogastric work, and closed systems whereby the surgeon's hand can be introduced into the peritoneal cavity through relatively small incisions to assist with retraction and remove the specimen. Although this was initially described to aid operations like hemicolectomy and splenectomy, this method is having a significant impact on laparoscopic live donor nephrectomy for renal transplants. The hand port can provide the traction on the organ and can keep adjacent organs retracted and, in the case of kidney retrieval, prevent the dreaded complication of twisting of the kidney with subsequent graft damage.

PERIOPERATIVE CARE

The perioperative care of a patient undergoing laparoscopic surgery is not much different from that of another patient undergoing open surgery under general anaesthesia. More and more of these operations are being done as day cases and patients are discharged early from hospital. Although some simple laparoscopic procedures can be performed under local anaesthesia and sedation, most therapeutic laparoscopy requires general anaesthesia and neuromuscular paralysis. This means that the patient must be fit for a general anaesthetic and patients with severe cardiorespiratory disease often do better with open surgery than laparoscopic surgery due to the physiological changes described below, although the postoperative respiratory complications are less.

Preoperative management

Preparation of patients for laparoscopic surgery includes full informed consent with discussion of the pros and cons of laparoscopic versus open surgery and the risks of the procedure, including the possibility of conversion. There are certain complications specifically related to laparoscopic surgery and these should be fully explained.

There may be a few patients who are clearly not suitable for the laparoscopic approach and the two absolute contraindications are multiple previous laparotomies when the presence of severe adhesions has already been established and severe cardiopulmonary disease. Uncorrected clotting abnormalities should not be an absolute contraindication to laparoscopy but every effort should be made to correct any deficiencies before surgery. The risk of bleeding from open surgery is probably much larger in this group of patients.

In this day and age each unit should be able to discuss with their patients conversion and complication rates. Indeed, many units now provide written information sheets to patients which cover these points. Routine preoperative assessment should be carried out as for all surgical patients and the overall risk for anaesthesia can be estimated using the American Society of Anesthesiology (ASA) score. Patients should be advised of minor postoperative morbidity such as nausea, pain and vomiting. Contraindications to the Trendelenburg position, e.g. increased intracranial pressure, recent head injury and acute glaucoma, should be enquired into and highlighted. A tranquilliser is usually given orally the night before surgery and the morning of the operation.

Peroperative management

Anaesthesia

Therapeutic laparoscopy is best carried out under general anaesthesia with muscle relaxation. However, for diagnostic laparoscopy, which often involves smaller laparoscopes (2–5 mm), it may not be necessary to use muscle relaxation and local anaesthesia might also be possible. If local anaesthesia is used intravenous sedation should also be given. Although carbon dioxide is the most common gas for insufflation as it is inert and rapidly absorbed, nitrous oxide (provides additional analgesia if local anaesthetic is being employed) and air can also be used.

At the onset of anaesthesia a non-steroidal antiinflammatory agent should be given, either sublingually or by rectal suppository. At the end of the procedure all port site incisions should be thoroughly infiltrated with 0.25–0.5% bupivacaine to reduce postoperative analgesic requirement.

During anaesthesia the risks of hypercarbia, due to absorbed carbon dioxide, can be avoided by moderate hyperventilation. An increase in rate of breathing and tidal volume in order not to increase intrathoracic pressure beyond 30 cm H_2O will avoid movement of viscera into the laparoscopic field. If regional anaesthesia is used, it should extend from T4 to L5 because irritation of the peritoneal surface of the diaphragm will cause cervical and scapular pain which can be fairly intense. This type of anaesthesia is reserved specifically for patients with allergies and severe asthma.

Pneumoperitoneum

Raised intraabdominal pressure results in decreased venous return to the heart, a rise in intrathoracic pressure, reduced diaphragmatic movement and hypercarbia. This can lead to significant bradycardia, hypotension and raised ventilatory pressures. Any of these signs should be treated by reducing intraabdominal pressure and hyperventilation with increased inspired oxygen and atropine. Intraoperative monitoring in laparoscopy should therefore include carbon dioxide measurement and pulse oximetry in addition to cardiac monitoring.

The optimal intraabdominal pressure is as low as possible and usually is set between 8 and 12 mmHg. A pressure above 15 mmHg should be avoided. If there is a sudden increase in intraabdominal pressure, gas can be let out by opening the valve at the top end of each cannula. The most common cause of this is inadequate muscle relaxation and immediate remedial action by the anaesthetist will resolve the situation.

Positioning

Although most laparoscopic procedures can be performed with the patient lying supine, tilting the table head up or head down can provide better visualisation for certain procedures. When the patient is put in the Trendelenburg position the cardiac index increases slightly due to an increase in venous return from the lower extremities. However, the position itself does not completely correct the deleterious haemodynamic effects of the pneumoperitoneum. Sudden 'head-up' tilt requested by the surgeon, for example in laparoscopic cholecystectomy, may also be associated with sudden venous pooling in the lower extremities and hypotension. A tilt either way of more than 30° should be avoided.

In the early days of laparoscopic surgery it was customary to decompress the stomach and bladder by means of a nasogastric

tube and urinary catheter. With care taken to produce a pneumoperitoneum safely, and particularly if the open technique is used (see Ch. 24), these manoeuvres are no longer necessary unless specific procedures are being carried out on the bladder and stomach. It would, however, be reasonable to ask the patient to empty their bladder before coming to theatre, especially if a pelvic procedure is to be undertaken.

Thromboembolic prophylaxis

It is now well established that laparoscopic procedures predispose to deep vein thromboses and pulmonary emboli as much as open surgery. The increase in intraabdominal pressure and subsequent venous stasis in the pelvis and lower limbs suggested that there might in fact be a higher incidence in laparoscopic patients although this has yet to be confirmed. It is therefore essential that all patients undergoing laparoscopic surgery receive perioperative prophylaxis against thromboembolism and this should be continued until discharge from hospital.

Port placement and removal

Establishment of pneumoperitoneum and placement of laparoscopic ports have been described in Chapter 24. However, it is a very important aspect of laparoscopic surgery and one on which the success of the operation depends. Standard port placements are described for the common operations but there should be no hesitation to replace badly placed ports or put in additional ports if this is deemed necessary for the adequate exposure and execution of the operation. Additional ports may also be necessary for the placement of additional retractors and to change over from a 5 mm to a 10–12 mm instrument.

All ports other than the camera port should be removed under vision and the port site should be inspected from the peritoneal side to exclude any bleeding. The final port is removed after deflating the peritoneal cavity completely. Gas left behind in the peritoneal cavity can give rise to postoperative shoulder and neck pain and abdominal discomfort. The risk to the surgeon and other staff from the expelled pneumoperitoneum has not been well defined and it is advisable to direct the desufflation away from all theatre personnel. Desufflation has been likened to removal of a tourniquet. In addition to sudden flow of blood rich in metabolites towards the heart, gas embolism may also occur. Hence desufflation should be achieved gently and gradually. Attempts should be made to close all port sites of 10 mm or greater in size to prevent the development of postoperative incisional hernias.

Intraoperative contamination

Spillage of bile and intestinal contents at operation should be avoided as much as possible. However, as in open surgery, if this occurs it should be washed out with a solution of normal saline.

Some surgeons used a mixture of heparinised saline to help prevent blood clots forming around the operative site, which can then be difficult to remove through the 5 mm suction tube. Similarly, if stones are spilled from a torn or ruptured gallbladder every effort should be made to retrieve as much of these as possible. Stones left behind in the abdominal cavity have been found to result in intraabdominal and abdominal wall abscesses. The principle of prophylactic antibiotics is similar to that in open surgery and any operation when contamination is anticipated should receive one intraoperative dose. Recent data have suggested that the incidence of wound infection in clean contaminated cases may actually be lower than for open surgery and routine antibiotics might not be required for operations such as an uncomplicated laparoscopic cholecystectomy.

Postoperative management

The immediate postoperative care of a patient after laparoscopic surgery is no different from that after open surgery. Attention to airway, breathing and circulation should be given in the recovery room and the patient should be transferred to the ward only after full recovery from anaesthesia. Both haemodynamic and respiratory physiology revert back to normal soon after the patient is awake. There is a real risk of hypercapnia and even if $PaCO_2$ is normal an increased 'base deficit' may cause metabolic acidosis as a result of lactic acid released from intraabdominal tissues which have had their venous return interrupted by high intraabdominal pressure. Hypoxia is also common due to depression of ventilation from anaesthetic agents. Routine administration of oxygen is therefore advisable for the first few hours after surgery.

If all carbon dioxide has been removed, a non-steroidal anti-inflammatory agent given and all the wounds infiltrated with bupivacaine, significant postoperative pain is unlikely. Subsequent analgesia will depend on the procedure and the time to resumption of oral intake. However, if there is significant residual pain immediately after surgery additional infiltration of the wounds can be attempted; failing this, an opiate can be given. The presence of persisting pain after surgery, particularly on the first and second postoperative days, should alert the surgeon that a possible intraabdominal complication has occurred and steps should be taken to exclude or confirm this suspicion.

Depending on the procedure, most patients can be discharged on the first postoperative day and some units are successfully performing some laparoscopic operations as day cases. Shared care with the patient's general practitioner is very valuable and can bring to light any undue complication that may present after the patient's discharge from hospital.

Note

As rapid progress continues unabated with ever more sophisticated and ingenious developments, this chapter will quickly become outdated and the reader should make all efforts to remain up to date.

FURTHER READING

Al Fallouji M. Making loops in laparoscopic surgery. *Surg Laparosc Endosc* 1993; **3**:477–481

Bradbury AW, Chan Y-C, Darzi A, Stansby G. Venous thromboembolic prophylaxis for laparoscopic cholecystectomy. *Br J Surg* 1997; **84**:962–964

Higgins A, London J, Charland S et al. Prophylactic antibiotics for elective laparoscopic cholecystectomy. *Arch Surg* 1999; **134**:611–614

Lee A. General anaesthesia for laparoscopic surgery. In: Paterson-Brown S, Garden OJ, eds. *Principles and Practice of Surgical Laparoscopy*. London: WB Saunders, 1994: 23–38

Nyarwaya JB, Samii K. Anaesthesia for laparoscopic digestive surgery. In: Testas P, Delaitre B, eds. *Laparoscopic Digestive Surgery*. Edinburgh: Churchill Livingstone, 1994: 9–17

Basic laparoscopic procedures

Michael Bailey, Guy Slater

INTRODUCTION

The first reported laparoscopic cholecystectomy was in 1987 by a French gynaecologist, Phillipe Mouret. Laparoscopic surgery entered the domain of general surgery and since then has revolutionised surgical practice. The potential advantages of a reduced hospital stay with a shorter period of convalescence and an early return to work caught the imagination of patients, surgeons and government. The subsequent rapid expansion of the field has resulted in many operations now being performed laparoscopically rather than by open surgery.

ANAESTHESIA FOR MINIMAL ACCESS SURGERY

The disruption to the body's normal homeostatic mechanisms, caused by surgery, is minimised by the laparoscopic approach. The anaesthetic technique should complement the surgery to allow an early resumption of diet, discharge the same day, if indicated, and an earlier return to work.

Physiological effects of the pneumoperitoneum

The raised intraabdominal pressure needed for safe laparoscopic surgery affects the cardiovascular and respiratory systems.

Cardiovascular effects

Vagal stimulation secondary to the stretching of the peritoneum during insufflation may cause a bradycardia with a decrease in cardiac output.

Normal venous pressure in the great veins is 4–6 mmHg, the raised intraabdominal pressure of 10–14 mmHg from the pneumoperitoneum can impede venous return decreasing the cardiac output in accordance with Starling's law.

Respiratory effects

The raised abdominal pressure splints the diaphragm, reducing the pulmonary functional residual capacity. In addition, higher ventilation pressures are needed to prevent airway closure with hypoxia secondary to a ventilation: perfusion mismatch. Hypercarbia may result from absorption of the carbon dioxide gas used for insufflation.

These physiological effects need to be considered when planning and maintaining the anaesthesia, as the elderly or patients with preexisting disease may be adversely compromised.

Anaesthetic management

Preoperative assessment should identify patients with significant cardiac or respiratory disease. Although the intraoperative anaesthetic risks for these patients may be slightly higher than for conventional surgery this is outweighed by the reduced postoperative morbidity of minimal access surgery.

Premedications

A long-acting non-steroidal analgesic such as diclofenac sodium should be prescribed for the morning of the operation. A short-acting benzodiazepine may also be prescribed as an anxiolytic, if requested.

Intravenous cannulation

Although blood loss is normally minimal in laparoscopic procedures, it is wise to insert a large-bore 16 G cannula.

Anaesthetic monitoring

In addition to ECG, BP and pulse oximetry, monitoring should also include tidal CO_2. The measurement of end-tidal CO_2 is necessary to assess whether hyperventilation is needed to control hypercarbia. Pulse oximetry ensures that the patient is ventilated sufficiently to counteract the reduced functional residual capacity and any ventilation:perfusion mismatch.

Anaesthetic technique

An anaesthetic technique as used for a routine laparotomy is appropriate.

Endotracheal intubation is necessary for intraperitoneal procedures because the raised intraabdominal pressure increases the risk of regurgitation and aspiration. A pneumoperitoneum is not necessary for totally extraperitoneal hernia repairs and many anaesthetists consider endotracheal intubation unnecessary and use a laryngeal mask airway.

Muscle relaxation is needed to maximise the working space, by increasing the compliance of the abdominal wall.

Postoperative management

Analgesia

Narcotic analgesia should be avoided as it is unnecessary and may contribute to postoperative nausea. Wounds should be infiltrated with a long-acting local anaesthetic such as bupivacaine. Patients rarely have severe pain and most will be pain free within 48 hours. Simple analgesia such as co-dydramol or a regular non-steroidal antiinflammatory drug (NSAID) should be adequate.

Nausea

Nausea postoperatively, although shortlived, may be quite severe and results from a combination of peritoneal stretching and anaesthetic side effects. When planning an individual's anaesthetic, avoidance of nausea should be a priority and can be prevented by routine use of an antiemetic.

OPERATIVE SURGERY

Laparoscopic cholecystectomy

The indications for laparoscopic cholecystectomy are the same as for open cholecystectomy. Contraindications to the laparoscopic approach are relative to the experience of the surgeon. These include previous upper abdominal surgery, cirrhosis of the liver, Mirrizi's syndrome and advanced pregnancy.

Patient preparation

The patient should be fit for a laparoscopic procedure under a general anaesthetic.

Informed consent is obtained for the procedure, with cholangiography if indicated, and for a laparotomy if necessary. It is left to the individual surgeon to decide if cholangiography should be routine or selective. However, most surgeons would perform cholangiography if there is a history of jaundice, abnormal liver biochemistry or dilatation of the common bile duct on ultrasound scan. If bile duct stones are confirmed these may be removed laparoscopically or at a later date by endoscopic retrograde cholangiography (ERCP).

Antibiotic prophylaxis should be given. A single intravenous dose of a second-generation cephalosporin, such as cephalexin, given with induction of anaesthesia is sufficient.

Deep vein thrombosis prophylaxis should also be given. Theoretically the raised intraabdominal pressure and the reverse Trendelenburg position may contribute to deep vein thrombosis.

Simple measures such as thromboembolic deterrent stockings (TEDS) and avoiding prolonged intraoperative compression of the deep veins may be sufficient prophylaxis. However, in a high-risk patient, a subcutaneous low molecular weight heparin regimen is advised.

Patient Positioning

A radiolucent X-ray table is used with the patient in the dorsal decubitus position. For the induction of the pneumoperitoneum and port insertion the patient may be either horizontal or in a Trendelenburg (head-down) position. The cholecystectomy is carried out with the patient in a reverse Trendelenburg (head-up) position, tilted towards the surgeon so that the abdominal contents fall away from the operative field.

The skin is cleaned with an antiseptic solution. Surgical drapes are positioned to widely expose the right upper quadrant. The surgeon and the camera operator stand on the left-hand side of the patient with the scrub nurse and a second assistant on the patient's right. A monitor is positioned on either side of the table at the head end (Figure 24.1).

Procedure

The operation technique may be considered in six steps, with each step needing to be completed before proceeding. 'Alternative manoeuvres' may be needed to complete each step.

Step 1: access and the pneumoperitoneum

INDUCTION OF THE PNEUMOPERITONEUM

This is potentially dangerous. Because the first or primary port is not inserted under direct vision there is always a risk of iatrogenic bowel or vascular injury.

A closed technique or the open (Hassan) technique may be used to create the pneumoperitoneum.

The closed technique has been used for many years by gynaecologists and is still the preferred method for many experienced laparoscopists. A vertical incision is made just above the umbilicus. The abdominal wall is elevated and a Veress needle is inserted into the peritoneal cavity, holding the shaft between forefinger and thumb, aiming inferiorly towards the bifurcation of the aorta. As the needle is passed through the abdominal wall, two 'clicks' will be felt, corresponding to the rectus sheath and the peritoneum.

The open (Hassan) technique is theoretically safer. A vertical skin incision is made above the umbilicus, the subcutaneous fat is retracted and a second mid-line vertical incision is made in the rectus sheath. Blunt dissection is used to separate the rectus muscles, through the linea alba, exposing the peritoneum. The peritoneum is lifted away from the bowel, using two clips, and opened to allow a blunt Hassan trocar to be inserted.

INSUFFLATION

Carbon dioxide is normally used to insufflate the abdomen. When insufflation commences intraperitoneal pressure should be less than 4 mmHg with a gas flow of 1.5–2 litres per minute. A normal-sized adult will need 2.5–3 litres of gas to achieve a satisfactory pneumoperitoneum to insert the primary port in a closed technique; as with the Veress needle, the anterior abdominal wall should be elevated during insertion of the primary port. Carbon dioxide is infused to achieve a working intraabdominal pressure of 12 mmHg.

ALTERNATIVE MANOEUVRES

Previous skin incisions may make the creation of the pneumoperitoneum more difficult. The open technique may be used

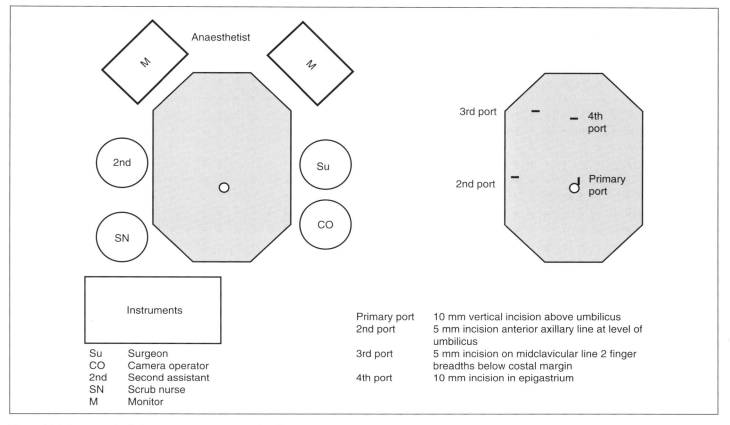

Figure 24.1 Laparoscopic cholecystectomy. Positioning of staff and incisions.

or an alternative site for insertion of the Veress needle can be considered. Inferior to the right costal angle in the mid-clavicular line is a favoured site because the abdominal wall is fixed by the lower ribs above the abdominal contents.

COMPLICATIONS OF PRIMARY PORT INSERTION

Vascular or visceral injuries may occur. Rarely the aorta, inferior vena cava or the iliac vessels may be injured. Such an injury is potentially life-threatening and should be treated with appropriate resuscitation and immediate laparotomy. Injury to mesenteric or omental vessels may require a laparotomy.

Bowel injuries may be obvious or may not be recognised initially.

Step 2: port placement

A full laparoscopy is performed when the primary port has been inserted, to look for adhesions, occult malignancy or coexisting disease. Secondary ports are inserted under direct vision.

- The second port is a 5 mm port. It is normally placed in the right anterior axillary line, at the level of the umbilicus.
- The third port is a 5 mm port placed in the mid-clavicular line, approximately two finger breadths below the costal margin.

- The fourth 12 mm port is placed in the mid-line approximately mid-way between the umbilicus and the xiphisternum, entering the peritoneal cavity just to the right of the falciform ligament.

The optimal position for each port will vary with the body habitus and the position of the intraabdominal structures. If correctly positioned, the working instruments will triangulate at an angle of 60–90°. Experience will guide the surgeon in positioning the ports to always achieve a comfortable working position.

ALTERNATIVE MANOEUVRES

Adhesions to the anterior abdominal wall and old scars may make port placement more difficult. Adhesions should be divided around the planned port sites, if necessary by placing a port away from the adhesions. If, despite adhesiolysis, port placement in the normal positions is not possible, different sites may be used to achieve adequate access.

Step 3: Gallbladder retraction and visualisation

With the patient in the reverse Trendelenburg position, a grasper in the second port is used to retract the gallbladder, superiorly and laterally, towards the right axilla. The surgeon opens up Calot's triangle by retracting Hartmann's pouch inferiorly with a grasping forcep held in the left hand.

ALTERNATIVE MANOEUVRES

If the view of the gallbladder is obscured consider:

- increasing the angle of the head-up position
- tilting the patient further towards the left
- decompressing the stomach with a naso-gastric tube
- using a fifth port placed on the patient's right-hand side to insert a fanned retractor to depress the small bowel.

If the gallbladder is distended, as in a mucocoele, it is decompressed percutaneously.

Step 4: dissection of Calot's triangle

DISSECTING CALOT'S TRIANGLE

The aim is to clearly identify the cystic duct and artery within Calot's triangle and avoid injury to other structures. Starting at the level of Hartmann's pouch, a dissector held in the right hand is used to strip the peritoneum and fat away from the structures in the triangle (Figure 24.2).

The junction between the cystic duct and the gallbladder neck is defined and the cystic artery should be seen in Calot's triangle. If these structures are clearly seen, with bare liver forming the roof of the triangle, then even in the presence of abnormal anatomy an iatrogenic injury should be avoided (Figure 24.3).

The gallbladder neck can be turned over to allow dissection from the posterior aspect of Calot's triangle. Care must be taken with the gallbladder in this position, as the triangle will now be directly over the common hepatic duct.

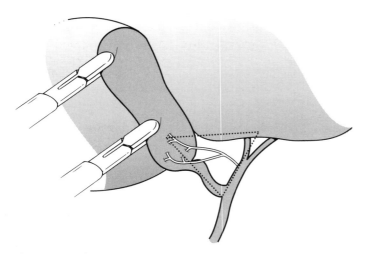

Figure 24.2 Calot's triangle.

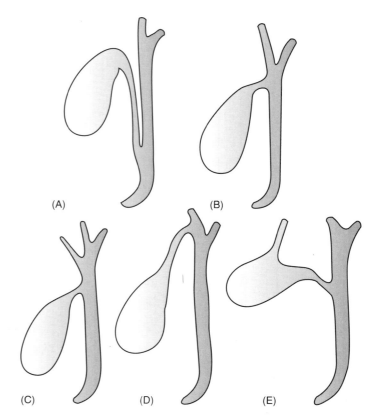

(A) Long cystic duct with low insertion into the common bile duct
(B) Short common hepatic duct with insertion of cystic duct at the bifurcation
(C) Aberrant posterior right hepatic duct
(D) Cystic duct inserted into the right hepatic duct
(E) Duct of Luschka

Figure 24.3 Junctions between the cystic duct and other structures.

DIVIDING THE CYSTIC DUCT AND ARTERY

When the anatomy has been correctly identified the cystic duct and artery can be clipped ready for division. When clipping the cystic duct, the clips must be placed well above its junction with the common bile duct. Two clips are placed at this point and one clip close to the gallbladder neck. The cystic artery is clipped similarly and then both are divided with scissors. It is not essential to demonstrate the junction of the cystic duct with the common bile duct.

ALTERNATIVE MANOEUVRES

These may be necessary if the dissection is difficult. The space in Calot's triangle can be increased by extending the dissection of the peritoneum towards the body of the gallbladder. This dissection will allow Hartmann's pouch to be retracted further away from the liver bed, increasing the working space in Calot's triangle.

A 30° laparoscope may be used to see the posterior aspect of Calot's triangle.

If there is any doubt about the biliary anatomy, this may be helped by an intraoperative cholangiogram.

INJURIES

Injuries within Calot's triangle may be vascular or biliary in nature. If the vascular anatomy is abnormal, the right hepatic artery may lie in Calot's triangle and be mistaken for the cystic artery. More rarely, if the cystic artery is not clearly seen the right hepatic artery may be divided.

Misused diathermy in Calot's triangle may cause a delayed vascular injury. The common bile duct is supplied radially by small arterioles; transmitted diathermy current may cause thrombosis in these vessels and the resultant ischaemia will cause a bile duct stricture.

Biliary injuries are clinically of more concern than vascular injuries. The common bile duct, the common hepatic duct and the right hepatic duct have all been mistaken for the cystic duct and divided.

A stricture of the common bile duct can result from poor placement of the cystic duct clips. If the cystic duct is under tension the common bile duct may be tented up and trapped in the clips as they are applied.

Step 5: gallbladder dissection

DISSECTION OF THE GALLBLADDER

The neck of the gallbladder is retracted superiorly to open up the plane between the gallbladder and the liver bed. Using a combination of diathermy and sharp dissection, the gallbladder mesentery is divided to separate the gallbladder from the liver. The separated gallbladder is then placed above the liver for later removal.

Ducts of Luschka may be seen entering the gallbladder from the liver bed. These ducts should be clipped prior to division.

HAEMOSTASIS AND WASHOUT

At this point the liver bed should be carefully inspected and bleeding vessels should be diathermied if necessary. Spilled blood or bile is removed using a combination of suction and saline wash.

OPERATIVE COMPLICATIONS

- Intraabdominal abscesses, although uncommon, can occur as a result of spillage of gallstones or infected bile during the procedure.

- Subhepatic haematomas present with right upper quadrant pain and normally as a result of incomplete haemostasis of the liver bed.

- Biliary peritonitis or a localised bile collection can result from inadequately placed clips, a biliary tract injury or a leaking duct of Luschka.

Step 6: gallbladder removal and wound closure

The laparoscope is reinserted through the fourth (epigastric) port and guides the surgeon to the gallbladder lying above the liver.

A clean non-infected gallbladder can be removed directly through the camera port. If infected or friable, the gallbladder should be removed using a retrieval bag to prevent wound contamination and spillage of gallstones. The neck of the gallbladder or the retrieval bag is grasped using heavy forceps inserted through the primary (umbilical) port.

The gallbladder neck is firmly introduced into the primary port and the port is removed over the grasping forceps to expose the neck of the gallbladder outside the abdomen. A grasping forceps is used to grip the gallbladder neck, preventing it from slipping back into the abdominal cavity.

It may be possible to tease the gallbladder through the existing incision. Alternatively, to deliver a large gallbladder, the incision can be extended or the gallbladder contents may be removed using a sucker and the Desjardin forceps.

Under direct vision, the remaining ports are removed. The rectus sheath beneath the 10 mm ports should be closed with an '0' soluble stitch, before closing the skin incisions with staples or a subcuticular suture.

When to convert?

Broadly speaking there are two indications for conversion: failure to progress to the next step of the operation despite trying the alternative manoeuvres, and encountering specific complications or unexpected findings such as the following.

- *Bowel injuries* which may be blunt, sharp or secondary to diathermy. The jejunum and ileum are most often injured, followed by the duodenum and colon. A full laparotomy is necessary to look for associated injuries, which can be missed by a laparoscopic examination. Unrecognised injuries are associated with a high morbidity and mortality.

- *Vascular injuries* range from a small bleeding subcutaneous vessel to mesenteric vessel injury and, of most concern, great vessel injury. The decision to convert will depend on the laparoscopic expertise of the surgeon. Unless very experienced, the surgeon should convert for all vascular injuries other than the most trivial abdominal wall vessels.

- *Liver injuries*, if they are slight and the liver is normal, may be easily managed with tamponade and diathermy. If the liver is diseased with cirrhosis or portal hypertension then conversion should be considered, particularly if the bleeding is brisk and it is not possible to gain control of the bleeding or maintain good visibility.

- *Biliary injuries* should be repaired immediately by an experienced biliary surgeon. If adequate expertise in bile duct repair and reconstruction is not available locally, the patient should be transferred to a specialist centre.

- *Unexpected findings* such as gallbladder carcinoma, cholecysto-enteric fistula, biliary and vascular anomalies or a diseased liver may all justify conversion.

Postoperative care and advice

Most patients recover very quickly after a laparoscopic cholecystectomy but some will complain of nausea and drowsiness related to the anaesthetic. The procedure is performed as a day case in many centres.

Postoperatively, patients should drink, eat and mobilise as tolerated. They should be advised not to drive for 24 hours and to return to their normal activities as they feel able.

Abdominal wall discomfort and shoulder tip pain should resolve within 24 hours.

The possibility of a bile leak should always be considered if a patient has unexplained severe abdominal pain associated with peritonism in the early postoperative period.

Operative cholangiography and choledochoscopy

Selective versus routine cholangiography

Intraoperative cholangiography is the most sensitive investigation for the detection of choledocholithiasis. In addition, cholangiography also delineates the extrahepatic biliary tree which can be advantageous when aberrant anatomy is encountered.

A consensus on whether cholangiography should be used selectively or routinely has never been reached. Individual surgeons should choose the most appropriate policy depending on the resources and expertise available locally.

It has been shown that 96% of patients with undetected bile tract stones will require surgery within five years of cholecystectomy. This statistic favours routine cholangiography. However, it has also been shown that only 9% of patients with no clinical features of choledocholithiasis will have stones demonstrated by cholangiography. Even with abnormal liver biochemistry cholangiography will only detect stones in 25% of cases, making routine cholangiography unnecessary for most patients.

A selective policy is probably acceptable if a reliable ERCP service is available to treat stones which subsequently become symptomatic. If a good ERCP service is not easily available then routine cholangiography should be used with removal of detected stones on the same admission.

Cholangiography techniques

Laparoscopic instrument manufacturers have designed many instruments to facilitate cholangiography; the Reddick-Olsen cholangio-catheter introducing forceps, manufactured by Karl Storz, is the instrument used in the authors' unit and is suitable for the method described. The forceps allows a soft flexible cholangiogram catheter to be passed through the instrument's shaft to cannulate the cystic duct and the atraumatic jaws are designed to close around the cystic duct, holding the catheter in position.

- *Calot's triangle* is dissected as previously described until the junction between the cystic duct and the gallbladder is clearly seen. The cystic duct is 'milked' proximally, using the grasping forceps, to ensure that the cystic duct is free of stones. A clip is then applied at the origin of the cystic duct to occlude it.

- *The cystic duct* is partially transected until bile drains from it. The cholangio-catheter forceps is then passed through the mid-clavicular port to enter the abdomen. The catheter is advanced and inserted into the cystic duct. When the cystic duct has been cannulated the catheter is fixed in position by the jaws of the forceps. If the catheter is correctly inserted, normal saline can easily be injected into the biliary tract with no leakage from the cystic duct.

- *A mobile screening unit* is centred over Calot's triangle using the clips as a guide and all remaining instruments are removed.

- *Iodine-based contrast* is injected into the biliary tract while screening. When the biliary tract has been adequately visualised hard copies should be made for the patient's records.

- *A normal cholangiogram* will have no filling defects. The left and right hepatic ducts will be clearly seen and contrast will be seen entering the duodenum through the distal common bile duct.

Filling defects, a dilated common bile duct or absence of flow into the duodenum or any part of the biliary tract is suggestive of a retained stone.

If part of the cholangiogram is obscured a better view can normally be found by moving the cholangio-catheter forceps from side to side. If the cholangiogram is normal, the cannula is removed and the cholecystectomy is completed as previously described.

Laparoscopic choledochoscopy and bile duct exploration

On-table choledochoscopy and bile duct exploration was the treatment of choice for choledocholithiasis before laparoscopic cholecystectomy. The expertise needed for laparoscopic choledochoscopy means that its use is now largely confined to specialist centres.

Choledochoscopes with diameters of 3 mm and 4 mm can be introduced into the biliary tract through the cystic duct rather than needing a separate choledochotomy. With continuous saline irrigation the biliary tract is distended to allow a thorough inspection.

Stones can be pushed into the duodenum using pressure irrigation or may be removed through the cystic duct using a Dormia basket.

A final cholangiogram may be performed to ensure that the biliary tract has been completely cleared of stones.

Laparoscopic appendicectomy

The clinical diagnosis of appendicitis is not always straightforward. Approximately 20% of patients will have a normal appendix following open appendicectomy. Diagnostic laparoscopy can reduce the negative appendicectomy rate, sparing the patient a prolonged period of convalescence and considerable discomfort.

Patient preparation

The clinical suspicion of appendicitis should be high. The patient should be fit for a laparoscopic procedure under a general anaesthetic. Informed consent is obtained, with permission for a laparotomy if necessary.

A urinary catheter is not needed but patients should have voided before leaving the ward for the operating theatre.

Antibiotic prophylaxis decreases the incidence of wound infection and intraabdominal abscesses after appendicectomy. Cover should be aimed at both anaerobic and aerobic organisms. Metronidazole is the antibiotic of choice for anaerobic bacteria while aerobes can be treated with a second-generation cephalosporin or a penicillin. The final choice will be determined by the surgeon and the local antibiotic policy.

With regard to deep vein thrombosis prophylaxis, simple measures including TED stockings and early mobilisation should be used. If the patient is at high risk of a DVT a low molecular weight heparin regimen should also be prescribed.

Patient positioning

The patient is placed on the operating table in the dorsal decubitus position with a Trendelenburg (head-down) tilt. After the skin has been cleaned, the drapes are placed to expose the whole of the lower abdomen.

The surgeon and the camera operator stand on the left-hand side of the patient with the scrub nurse opposite. A single monitor is positioned at the foot of the table (Figure 24.4).

Procedure

There are five steps to complete the operation.

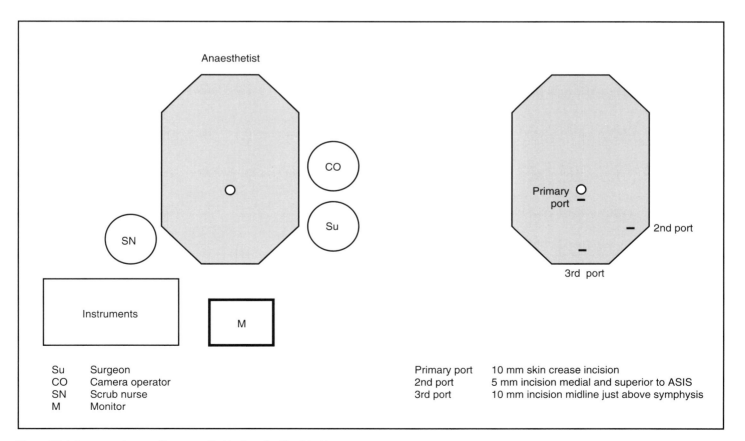

Su	Surgeon	
CO	Camera operator	
SN	Scrub nurse	
M	Monitor	

Primary port	10 mm skin crease incision
2nd port	5 mm incision medial and superior to ASIS
3rd port	10 mm incision midline just above symphysis

Figure 24.4 Laparoscopic appendicectomy. Positioning of staff and incisions.

Step 1: induction of the pneumoperitoneum

The creation of the pneumoperitoneum and insertion of the primary port is carried out by the closed or open method as described for a laparoscopic cholecystectomy.

Step 2: laparoscopy

A full diagnostic laparoscopy is performed. If an adequate examination is not possible with the laparoscope alone, a second port should be inserted in the left iliac fossa. A grasping forceps can be used to move the bowel away from the lower pole of the caecum and to lift the ovaries from behind the uterus for inspection.

In a female patient, gynaecological pathology such as ovarian cysts, endometriosis or pelvic inflammatory disease needs to be excluded.

The normal appendix, in the absence of other pathology, should be removed; publications have shown that an appendix that appears normal laparoscopically may be inflamed histologically.

Step 3: port placement

Two operating ports are needed, a 5 mm port in the left iliac fossa and a 10 mm port suprapubically.

The left iliac fossa port is positioned approximately 2 cm medial to the anterior superior iliac spine, taking care to avoid injuring the inferior epigastric vessels.

The suprapubic port is inserted 2 cm above the symphysis pubis in the mid-line, taking care to avoid the bladder. This port may be difficult to insert as the peritoneum is only loosely attached to the lower abdominal wall at this point.

Step 4: mobilising and excising the appendix

Division of adhesions is necessary if the appendix has been walled off by inflammatory tissue. The appendix tip is held in the left hand with a grasping forceps or a Babcock forceps. A dissecting forceps is used in the right hand to break down all the adhesions until the appendix is fully mobilised and the junction between its base and the caecum is seen. Failure to identify this junction may result in only part of the appendix being removed.

The mesoappendix can usually be divided using diathermy, although some surgeons would recommend clipping it before division. Diathermy should be used judiciously on the appendicular vessels, as transmitted current may cause coagulation in the proximal vessels with subsequent bowel ischaemia. The base of the appendix should be completely cleared of mesoappendix.

The appendix is now ready to be excised. Three endoloops are needed: two are placed proximally on the appendix base and one is placed slightly higher (Figure 24.5). The easiest way to place

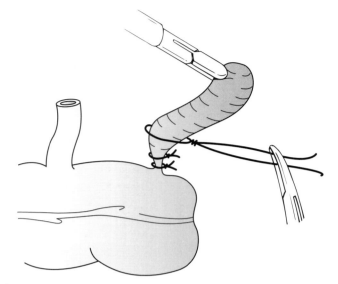

Figure 24.5 Placement of endoloops.

an endoloop is by introducing it through the port and then reducing the size of the snare. A forceps is then passed through the loop and used to grip the tip of the appendix and retract it superiorly. An assistant should maintain this retraction to allow the surgeon to use both hands to accurately position and tighten the endoloop.

When the endoloops have been secured in position the appendix is divided between the ties and the mucosa of the appendix stump is ablated with diathermy. The appendix is removed through the suprapubic port, using a retrieval bag if there is gross inflammation or perforation.

If the appendix base is necrotic it may be buried with a figure-of-eight stitch.

PERITONEAL TOILET

Pus or blood should be washed away with normal saline and suctioned until dry. No drain is required.

Step 5: wound closure

The ports are removed under direct vision. The fascial defect of the 10 mm ports is closed with a soluble stitch before closing the skin wounds.

Complications

Complications may result from the laparoscopic approach but there are no additional complications specific to laparoscopic appendicectomy. As with an open appendicectomy, there is a risk of wound infection and intraabdominal abscess formation.

Postoperative care and advice

The postoperative care for appendicectomy differs from elective minimal access procedures. The patients may be systemically unwell and may have a prolonged ileus secondary to localised intraabdominal sepsis or peritonitis.

Oral fluids can be introduced as tolerated but food should be delayed until any intestinal ileus has resolved.

Anaerobic antibiotics should be continued for five days if the appendix is severely inflamed or there is peritonitis.

When the systemic illness has resolved, patients can be advised to return to normal activities as soon as they feel physically able.

Laparoscopic inguinal hernia repair

Postoperative pain, analgesia requirement and time to return to normal activities are all reduced by the laparoscopic approach for inguinal hernia repair. Recurrence rates of 0–3% also compare favourably. However, the hospital costs are greater for the laparoscopic approach but the total cost to society is probably reduced.

Four techniques of laparoscopic hernia repair have been described.

● Totally extraperitoneal (TEP) repair

● Transabdominal preperitoneal (TAPP) repair

● Intraperitoneal on-lay mesh (IPOM) repair

● Simple closure of the internal ring

IPOM and simple closure of the internal ring have not proven successful and are no longer performed.

Principles of the laparoscopic technique

Stoppa's preperitoneal inguinal hernia repair (Figure 24.6) is the open technique on which both laparoscopic approaches are based. In Stoppa's repair a large mesh is inserted, through a transverse lower abdominal incision, into the preperitoneal space and covers the posterior aspect of all potential hernia sites.

Anatomy of the preperitoneal space

Preperitoneal hernia repairs rely on gaining access to the preperitoneal space. The surgeon is aided by the differing anatomy of the anterior abdominal wall below the umbilicus. Above the umbilicus, the rectus sheath splits into anterior and posterior layers, with the peritoneum closely applied to the posterior layer. Below the umbilicus, at the arcuate line, the posterior layer of the rectus sheath is absent. Here, the peritoneum is in direct contact with the rectus abdominis muscle but only loosely held by areolar tissue. Between the peritoneum and the muscle is the preperitoneal space; a filling bladder expands into this potential space. The

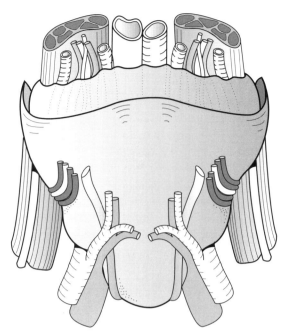

Figure 24.6 Stoppa's preperitoneal inguinal hernia repair.

laparoscopic approaches differ in their method of gaining access to this space.

The TEP repair is much closer to Stoppa's original description. The preperitoneal space is entered, between the rectus muscles and the peritoneum, through an incision just below the umbilicus.

The TAPP repair uses a transabdominal approach and enters the space by incising the peritoneum horizontally adjacent to the internal ring.

Patient selection and preparation

A laparoscopic approach can be used for all non-acute inguinal hernias. Both laparoscopic techniques need a general anaesthetic with full muscle relaxation. If patients are not fit for general anaesthesia they should be managed with a local anaesthetic open repair.

Strangulated or incarcerated hernias should not be attempted laparoscopically because of the difficulty in reducing the hernia and adequately inspecting the hernia contents.

Bilateral hernias are particularly suitable. These patients will benefit most from the decreased pain of the laparoscopic approach.

Recurrent hernias are also particularly suitable. Because the preperitoneal plane has not been entered previously, the repair is no more difficult than for a primary hernia.

Femoral hernias can be repaired laparoscopically, but there are no advantages over the conventional low approach through a small incision.

Previous lower mid-line scars may prevent the development of the preperitoneal space needed for the TEP approach. However, a TAPP repair may still be possible. Appendicectomy or previous open inguinal hernia repair scars are not usually a problem for either method.

Antibiotic prophylaxis should be used, as for any operation where prosthetic material is left in the patient. A single intravenous dose of a second-generation cephalosporin, such as cephazolin, should be given with induction of the anaesthetic. This will provide good cover against both wound infections and prosthetic mesh infection.

Pulmonary embolism and deep vein thrombosis are rare after a TEP hernia repair. This is probably because of early mobilisation and avoidance of a pneumoperitoneum. DVT prophylaxis should be considered for the TAPP repair where a conventional pneumoperitoneum is used.

Patient positioning

For both approaches to laparoscopic inguinal hernia repair the patient is in the dorsal decubitus position with the table horizontal. From this point onwards the operations are totally different so the techniques and specific complications will be described separately.

The totally extraperitoneal hernia repair

The surgeon stands opposite to the hernia with the scrub nurse on the patient's left side at the foot of the table. The camera operator should choose the side of the table on which he or she is most comfortable (Figure 24.7).

The technique is carried out in six separate steps.

Step 1: creating the preperitoneal space

ENTERING THE PRE-PERITONEAL SPACE

A transverse skin crease incision, 15–20 mm long, is made below the umbilicus offset towards the side of the hernia. The underlying rectus sheath is exposed and a further 15 mm transverse incision is made in the anterior rectus sheath on the ipsilateral side to the hernia, exposing the underlying rectus muscle. This muscle is retracted laterally to reveal the posterior rectus sheath.

A dissection balloon is gently introduced and advanced anterior to the posterior rectus sheath until the tip lies just behind the symphysis pubis. The balloon obturator is removed and a 0° laparoscope is introduced. This allows visualisation of the balloon during inflation.

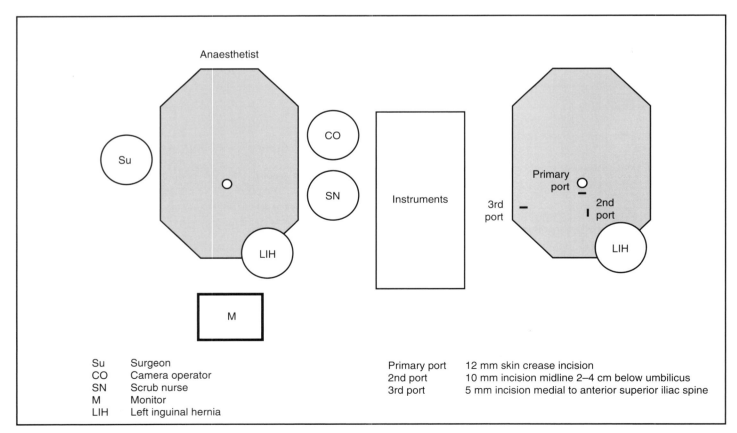

Su	Surgeon
CO	Camera operator
SN	Scrub nurse
M	Monitor
LIH	Left inguinal hernia

Primary port	12 mm skin crease incision
2nd port	10 mm incision midline 2–4 cm below umbilicus
3rd port	5 mm incision medial to anterior superior iliac spine

Figure 24.7 Totally extraperitoneal hernia repair. Positioning of staff and incisions.

Alternatively the space can be created using the laparoscope to break down the soft adhesions between the peritoneum and the anterior abdominal wall.

COMPLICATIONS OF THE CREATION OF THE PREPERITONEAL SPACE

The inferior epigastric vessels may be injured or separated from the anterior abdominal wall by the balloon. If this does occur, they can be stapled and divided or returned to their normal position using a suture passed through the anterior abdominal wall.

Step 2: port placement

A blunt balloon trocar is inserted into the rectus sheath and an air-tight seal is effected at the umbilical incision. Carbon dioxide is insufflated via this trocar into the preperitoneal space to a pressure of 12 mmHg.

The second port (10 mm) is inserted under direct vision in the mid-line, just distal to the tip of the primary port. Blunt dissection is used to separate the peritoneum from the transversus abdominis muscle, lateral to the internal ring, on the contralateral side to the hernia.

The third (5 mm) port is then inserted, under direct vision, just above and medial to the contralateral anterior superior iliac spine.

Complications of port placement should be uncommon but if care is not taken it is possible to puncture the peritoneum or injure blood vessels.

Step 3: reducing the hernia sac and dissection

The aim in this step is to reduce the hernia sac and create sufficient room to position a 13×15 cm mesh over the defect.

Direct and medial recurrent hernias will often reduce spontaneously after the balloon dissection. If not, blunt dissection is used to separate the hernia sac from the transversalis fascia.

Indirect hernias need to be separated from the cord structures. The dissection should start lateral to the internal ring; blunt dissection is used to sweep the peritoneum away from the anterior abdominal wall until the psoas fascia is exposed. When this lateral dissection is completed the hernia sac will be seen entering the internal ring, on the superior aspect of the cord structures. A bimanual technique is used to dissect the sac from the underlying structures and return it to the abdominal cavity.

The lateral and inferior dissection of the peritoneum from the abdominal wall creates space for the mesh. The lateral dissection will expose the lateral cutaneous nerve of the thigh and posterior dissection, below the internal ring, will expose the ilio-inguinal and genitofemoral nerves lying on the psoas fascia. Inferiorly, the peritoneum must be dissected well back to allow adequate space for insertion of the mesh.

COMPLICATIONS OF REDUCING THE HERNIA SAC AND THE DISSECTION

The iliac vessels lie just below the internal ring in the so-called 'triangle of doom'. Care should be taken to prevent injury to these structures, the cord structures and the cutaneous nerves lateral to the internal ring.

Peritoneal tears can cause a pneumoperitoneum with loss of the working space. If this interferes with the operation, the tears can be closed with sutures or staples. Gas trapped in the abdominal cavity is released through an intravenous cannula placed just below the right costal margin as a vent.

Postoperative scrotal haematomas may result from inadequate haemostasis after the indirect sac dissection. In direct hernia the transversalis fascia defect is inverted and stapled onto the pubic ramus to prevent seromas.

Step 4: mesh insertion and placement

PREPARING THE MESH

A 15×13 cm polypropylene mesh is used. To help with orientation and placement, a line is drawn along the middle of the long axis and the lateral corners are rounded.

Insertion of the mesh is done through the second port. Using bimanual manipulation, the mesh is manoeuvred into position.

POSITIONING THE MESH

Medially the mesh should reach the mid-line. Inferiorly the mesh should cover a contour line drawn 2 cm inferior to the internal ring. Laterally, the mesh should extend well beyond the internal ring and the lateral part of the inguinal ligament. Superiorly the mesh will extend above Cooper's ligament onto the posterior aspect of the rectus muscle. For bilateral hernias, two identical meshes or a single large mesh is used to cover the defects. Using two meshes is often easier as a large mesh is difficult to manoeuvre in a confined space.

COMPLICATIONS OF MESH PLACEMENT

Hernias may recur if the peritoneal edge is not sufficiently retracted from the inferior border of the mesh to prevent it being lifted as the peritoneum returns to its normal position.

Step 5: fixing the mesh

The mesh is fixed medially to Cooper's ligament. Superiorly, it may be fixed to the anterior abdominal wall medial to the inferior epigastric artery. The mesh should not be stapled lateral to the inferior epigastric vessels because of the risk of injury or entrapment of the cutaneous nerves. No staples should be placed inferior to the ileopubic tract.

Alternatives for fixation include the following.

- Staples or tacks are most commonly used; the screwing action of the helical tacker is designed to prevent nerve entrapment.

- Suturing is a cost-effective alternative to staples. The mesh is sutured to Cooper's ligament and the rectus abdominis muscle.

- Glue – acyanoacrylate glues may be safer than staples although currently none are licensed for internal use.

No fixation has been advocated.

COMPLICATIONS OF FIXING THE MESH

Failure to adequately fix the mesh may result in folding or migration of the mesh and has been implicated in hernia recurrence. It is important to use a large mesh as there is mesh shrinkage with time.

Chronic pain may result from nerve entrapment or injury and scrotal haematomas may result from inadequate haemostasis.

Step 6: deflation of the preperitoneal space and wound closure

The preperitoneal space should be slowly deflated under vision, using an instrument to keep the lower edge of the mesh in place while the peritoneum expands to cover it.

WOUND CLOSURE

After removal of the ports, the anterior sheath at the 10 mm sites is repaired with an absorbable suture and the skin is closed with a subcuticular stitch or staples.

The transabdominal preperitoneal hernia repair

The final position of the mesh in the TAPP repair is similar to the TEP repair but the approach to the preperitoneal space is different.

The surgeon stands on the left hand side of the table with the camera operator opposite and the scrub nurse on the right at the foot of the bed (Figure 24.8).

This operation is also performed as a sequence of steps.

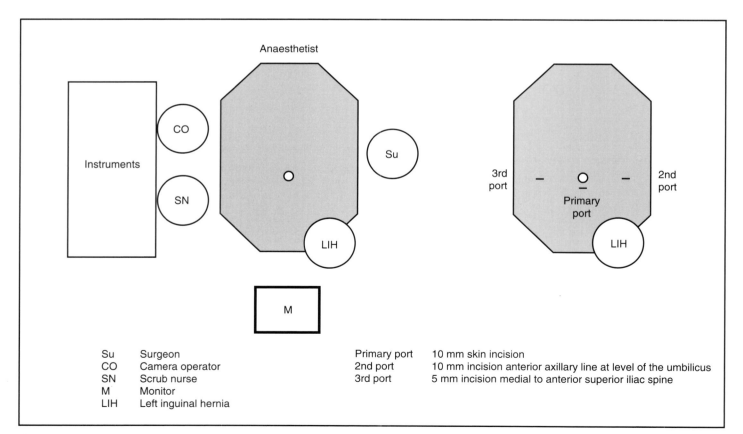

Su	Surgeon	Primary port	10 mm skin incision
CO	Camera operator	2nd port	10 mm incision anterior axillary line at level of the umbilicus
SN	Scrub nurse	3rd port	5 mm incision medial to anterior superior iliac spine
M	Monitor		
LIH	Left inguinal hernia		

Figure 24.8 Transabdominal preperitoneal hernia repair. Positioning of staff and incisions.

Step 1: access and the pneumoperitoneum

Creation of the pneumoperitoneum and primary port insertion is performed as for a laparoscopic cholecystectomy.

Step 2: port placement

Two working ports are used; the exact positioning of each port will be determined by the patient's body habitus and previous abdominal incisions.

The second port (10 mm) is placed on the left of the patient's abdomen on the anterior axillary line at the level of the umbilicus.

The third port (5 mm) is positioned on the right-hand side of the patient, just medial and superior to the anterior superior iliac spine.

Step 3: dissecting the preperitoneal space

A transverse peritoneal incision is made above the deep internal ring, extending from the medial umbilical ligament to a point 4–5 cm lateral to the internal ring. The incision is started medially for left-sided hernias and laterally for right-sided hernias. This incision divides the peritoneum into an inferior and a superior flap.

The inferior peritoneal flap is created by retracting the edge of the flap and by using sharp and blunt dissection to separate it from the abdominal wall, the vas deferens and the testicular and iliac vessels. The flap is extended medially and inferiorly until Cooper's ligament, the ileopubic tract and the myopectineal orifice are widely exposed, creating room for a large mesh to be inserted.

The superior flap is created similarly. The peritoneal sac of an indirect hernia sac is normally circumcised and left *in situ* or can be dissected completely. Medially, this flap should extend almost to the mid-line, exposing the inferior part of the rectus abdominis muscle. Superiorly, the flap should be retracted to a level 4–5 cm above the internal ring.

Step 4: mesh placement and fixation

PREPARATION OF THE MESH

A 10×13 cm mesh is used. As for the TEP repair, the corners are rounded and a line for orientation is drawn down the middle.

Insertion of the mesh is through the left-sided 10 mm port. Bimanual manipulation is used to manoeuvre the mesh into position. The medial edge of the mesh is placed behind the medial umbilical ligament close to the mid-line. The mesh should cover the whole myopectineal orifice and should extend laterally well beyond the internal ring.

SECURING THE MESH

The mesh is stapled to Cooper's ligament. Superiorly, it may also be fixed to the rectus abdominis muscle. It is not stapled laterally because of the risk of nerve damage.

Step 5: closing the peritoneum

The peritoneum is closed over the mesh, taking care not to fold or lift up the edges of the mesh. Sutures or staples can be used for this, taking care to fully cover the mesh.

The ports are removed under direct vision. All the port sites are closed in two layers, using an absorbable suture to close the fascia and a subcuticular stitch to the skin.

COMPLICATIONS OF CLOSING THE PERITONEUM

If the peritoneum is not fully closed bowel may become trapped behind the staples or adhere to the mesh, causing a bowel obstruction.

Port site hernias are a recognised complication of the TAPP repair and occur if the port sites are not adequately closed.

Postoperative care and advice for inguinal hernia repairs

A pneumoscrotum or a gas-filled swelling at the hernia site may be present immediately after the operation and will resolve spontaneously.

Patients should be given the following advice.

- Exercise and lifting are not contraindicated; there is no need to refrain from activity 'to allow the repair to heal'.
- Sexual activity as desired.
- Return to work as soon as the patient feels able.
- Driving should not be allowed for a week.

Complications

The intraoperative complications have been described above. The complications specific to laparoscopic hernia repair are as follows.

- *Wound infections*: these can occur but probably less often than in open surgery. Mesh infection is extremely rare with only a few reported cases.
- *Seromas and haematomas*: seromas can occur at the site of a direct hernia but are usually prevented by stapling the inverted transversalis fascia 'hernia sac' to Cooper's ligament. Seromas are normally asymptomatic and will resolve spontaneously. Scrotal haematomas or haematomas at the hernia site can occur if the surgeon is not meticulous in achieving complete haemostasis.

- *Chronic neuralgia* is less common than with the open operation but may occur due to nerve entrapment.

Recurrences, which occur within the first year of the operation, should be regarded as technical failures. The recurrence rate is less than 2% in trained centres. The reasons for technical failure are:

- incomplete lateral preperitoneal dissection resulting in a furled mesh

- lateral (indirect) hernias that have been missed

- using too small a mesh

- not fixing the mesh.

FURTHER READING

Khoo, DE, Walsh CJ, Cox MR, Murphy CA, Motson RW. Laparoscopic common bile duct exploration: evolution of a new technique. *Br J Surg* 1996; **83**(3):341–346

Liem MSL, van Vroonhoven TJMV. Laparoscopic inguinal hernia repair. *Br J Surg* 1996; **83**(9):1197–1204

McCall JL, Sharples K, Jadallah F. Systematic review of randomised controlled trials comparing laparoscopic with open appendicectomy. *Br J Surg* 1997; **84**(8):1045–1050

25

Intermediate laparoscopic procedures

M.M. Mullins, R.D. Rosin

INTRODUCTION

Having mastered a safe technique for the introduction of a pneumoperitoneum and the insertion of the first port for the telescope and camera, the next skill that will have been learnt is the performance of a thorough peritoneoscopy. Once this has been completed, little can be achieved without secondary ports for the use of the instruments, retractors or changing the camera to another site.

Placement of secondary ports

Port location and size are extremely important, as the surgeon's ability to manipulate the intraabdominal organs is limited, in part, to the location of these ports on the abdominal wall. If the surgeon wishes to approach the operation from a different direction, he or she must reposition the instrument through a separate port. This is often time consuming and usually necessitates reorganising some or all of the retractors and other instruments. Furthermore, unlike open surgery, laparoscopic instruments are severally affected by the fulcrum effect of the cannula across the abdominal wall. This is especially true when operating upon obese patients; often the desired angulation of the instruments cannot be achieved without undue force on the cannula and instruments themselves. The position of the patient (e.g. Lloyd-Davis position) may lead to the inability to manipulate instruments placed through secondary ports because of the elevation of the legs. If the camera needs to be moved or stapling devices introduced, the size of the secondary ports will need to be adequate. With the improved 5 mm telescope and clip applicators this is not as important as it used to be. Of course, smaller ports may always be changed to larger ones for the introduction of large instruments such as a stapling device.

Once pneumoperitoneum has been introduced and the camera inserted through the first cannula, all secondary ports must be introduced under direct vision. Prior to the placement of further ports the surgeon should ensure that no damage to viscera or vessels has occurred while performing a thorough peritoneoscopy. The position and number of secondary ports will depend on the planned procedure. Although for many operations the position of other ports is standardised and may look rigidly adhered to, the anatomy often dictates a slight variation which ensures the procedure is easier. If suturing is necessary one must remember the need for triangulation so that the two working ports and the point at which suturing will take place form a triangle.

There are several guidelines that will facilitate proper port placement. The ports should be spread apart as far as possible across the abdominal wall to minimise the clashing or 'sword fighting' that occurs when instruments are inserted through ports that are too close together. In addition, a good rule of thumb is to place the ports in a semicircle opposite the site of the intended operative dissection. In obese patients the ports should be moved closer to the operative field to lessen the force necessary to manipulate the instruments into proper position, thereby avoiding the potential for instrument breakage and gas leakage around the cannula site.

In general, port placement should be tailored to the patient's external and internal body anatomy. Most surgeons' initial experience with laparoscopic cholecystectomy is a good example of this practice. In the early days of laparoscopic cholecystectomy port placement was often determined by reference to textbook pictures. Surgeons learnt very quickly that such fixed placement of the secondary ports often resulted in difficult angles for the manipulation of the gallbladder and dissection of the triangle of Calot. With experience, surgeons have learned, perhaps unconsciously, to modify their port placement according to the patient's external dimensions. This, together with information from the initial peritoneoscopy, may change the usual port site by even a few centimetres. When starting a new laparoscopic procedure standard port placements are useful starting points. Once the surgeon becomes more experienced port placement will become more individualised, just as incisions are modified with open cases.

The anatomy of the epigastric vessels must be considered when placing ports. One should attempt to identify these vessels and transilluminating the abdominal wall may be helpful in pinpointing their location. The direction of the trocar insertion is also important to avoid injury to these vessels.

Finally, secondary port placement should also be made with the possible need to convert to open operation in mind (Box 25.1). Thus, subcostal port sites should be placed in a line so that they may be joined if conversion is necessary.

The positions of secondary ports for the most commonly carried out procedures are shown in Figure 25.1.

Box 25.1 Secondary port sites
- Ideal position for individual patient
- Preferred port sites
- Clear view on insertion
- Tailor site to anatomy
- Avoid 'sword fighting'

CONTROL OF BLEEDING

Bleeding during laparoscopic surgery is a special problem. Anticipation, recognition and control of haemorrhage are all more difficult under videoscopic views than during an open procedure.

At open surgery palpation of tissues to identify a pulse or the movement of an organ may help identify major vascular structures, thereby preventing bleeding. During laparoscopic surgery this is not possible and also the surgeon's view will be much more limited.

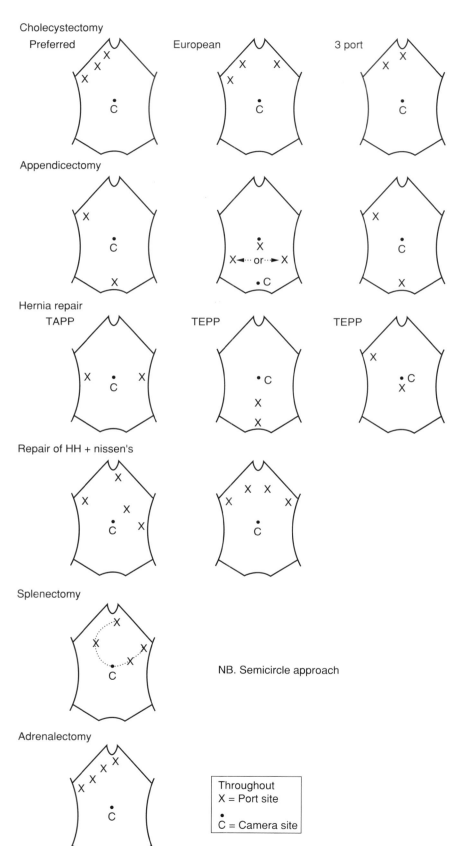

Cholecystectomy
Preferred   European   3 port

Appendicectomy

Hernia repair
TAPP   TEPP   TEPP

Repair of HH + nissen's

Splenectomy

NB. Semicircle approach

Adrenalectomy

Throughout
X = Port site

•
C = Camera site

Figure 25.1 Position of parts for laparoscopic procedures.

Laparoscopy makes identification of the vessels difficult. Very small vessels may be identified and controlled before they are divided but once bleeding starts it takes only a small amount of blood to completely obscure the operative field. The use of suction will decrease the amount of pneumoperitoneum, making the field smaller. The insertion of the suction probe usually requires removal of one of the instruments, which might be helping to control the bleeding vessel. This need to exchange instruments may prevent prompt identification of the bleeding point. Often the bleeding site, once identified with suction and irrigation, is again obscured by the time the suction probe is removed and a clip applicator inserted. In difficult situations a dedicated 'suction port' may be necessary and at times even a new port to insert a second sucker. Large 10 mm suckers can help but tend to remove the pneumoperitoneum rather quickly.

Unlike open surgery, the introduction of large packs is not feasible. However, small sponges can be inserted through larger ports and used to tamponade vessels. Arterial bleeding may cause a 'red-out' by bleeding directly onto the lens of the telescope. This must be removed quickly, cleaned and reinserted in a slightly different direction so that blood will not once again obscure the view. It takes time to reestablish a view of the operative field and identify the bleeding site. This is often very frustrating to the surgeon who must avoid the placement of clips blindly or the use of diathermy without good vision as untold damage could ensue.

Once the bleeding site has been identified, control of the offending vessel or vessels is necessary and often more difficult than at open surgery (Box 25.2).

Although laparoscopic control of bleeding is much more difficult to achieve than at open surgery, it can be safely and efficiently accomplished. A flow-chart of how to deal with minor, moderate and major bleeding is given in Figure 25.2.

Bleeding from the abdominal wall

Vascular injury to the abdominal wall is a relatively infrequent occurrence although its true incidence is probably underreported. It may manifest as oozing externally around an operating port or dripping along the shaft of the cannula into the peritoneal cavity. Much less commonly, delayed presentation as a haematoma of the abdominal wall or rectus sheath may occur. The source of bleeding is usually the inferior epigastric artery or one of its branches. The bleeding may be controlled by applying direct pressure with the operating port, open or laparoscopic suture ligation or tamponade with a Foley catheter inserted into the peritoneal cavity.

An innovative method to close fascial defects and/or control bleeding from an injured epigastric artery involves the use of an automatic fascial closure device or a suture passed percutaneously in around and back out through the peritoneal cavity, thereby ligating the injured vessel.

Several methods to control the bleeding are shown in Figure 25.3.

Major vascular injury

Major vascular injury occurs in less than 0.1% of cases and is the third leading cause of mortality during laparoscopy. The aorta, vena cava and iliac vessels are most often injured. Major vessel

Initial assessment of bleeding

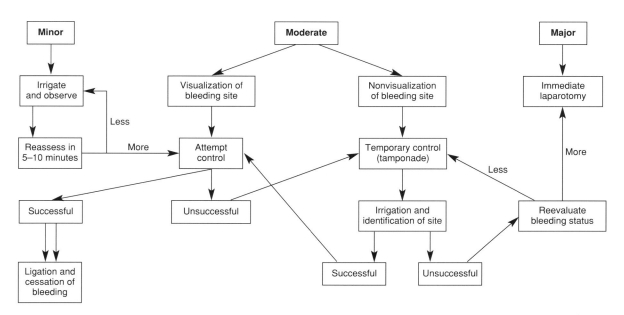

Figure 25.2 Management of bleeding.

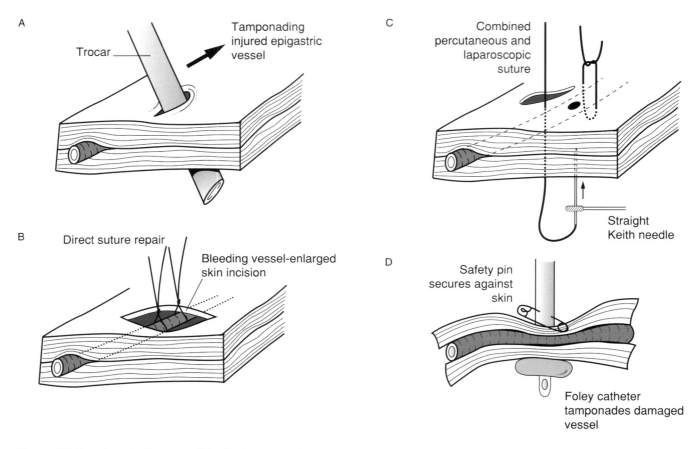

Figure 25.3 Techniques for the control of bleeding in laparoscopic surgery.

injury arising from a trocar or insufflation needle accounts for nearly one quarter of the patients requiring laparotomy for complications at laparoscopy. A Veress needle is responsible for the majority of injuries with a primary operating trocar and cannulas account for the majority of the remaining injuries. Delayed recognition of the injuries is common in fatalities. Major bleeding can be seen emanating either from the needle or operating port or there may be a sudden unexplained hypotension. Once the suspicion of vascular injury is verified immediate laparotomy should be performed. The Veress needle or operating port should not be removed because it will help locate the exact site of the injury and may help in tamponading the bleeding whilst performing the laparotomy.

Bleeding at specific operations

Laparoscopic cholecystectomy

The most common cause of bleeding during laparoscopic cholecystectomy is injury to the cystic artery and its branches. Other common sources of bleeding during the operation include haemorrhage from the gallbladder fossa itself or damage to the liver. Some surgeons do not dissect out the cystic artery and clip or ligate it, preferring to diathermy the smaller vessels on the

gallbladder wall. However, most surgeons prefer to dissect out the cystic artery and clip it or its branches. The clip should be properly spaced to allow division of the artery without the clips being flush with the cut end of the vessel. If the vessels are unusually large then loop ligatures should also be considered.

The cystic artery classically arises from the right hepatic artery and divides into anterior and posterior branches. However, there is a high degree of variation as to the point where the cystic artery branches. These may occur very close to the hepatic artery or very near to the gallbladder. An early branching anterior division may be mistaken for the main trunk of the cystic artery and following its ligation and division, the surgeon may not anticipate the presence of a large posterior branch, resulting in its division with subsequent haemorrhage.

It is often easier to dissect out the cystic artery once the cystic duct has been defined and divided. The surgeon must be aware of numerous aberrant or accessory branches of the cystic or hepatic arteries. If bleeding from the cystic artery occurs it is essential that the surgeon avoid dangerous blind diathermy or clipping into a pool of blood. This may increase the chance of injury to surrounding vascular and biliary structures. Usually a bleeding cystic artery can be grasped with forceps, the blood sucked out of the operative site and then a clip carefully placed under direct vision. If haemorrhage continues to be brisk despite all efforts, the procedure should be converted to an open laparotomy to avoid haemodynamic compromise or damage to surrounding structures.

Bleeding from the gallbladder fossa is also frequently encountered. Should this bleeding occur haemostasis should be achieved immediately. Further dissection without adequate control of bleeding would only lead to additional frustration and may increase the risk of gallbladder perforation. The bleeding can usually be controlled using diathermy, laser or argon beam (if available) or just pressure. If fibrin glue is available this may also be used. Prior to detaching the gallbladder from its liver bed the operative field should be carefully irrigated to ensure there has been adequate haemostasis.

Laparoscopic appendicectomy

Bleeding will occur from the appendicular artery or its branches in the appendix mesentery if these are not carefully controlled. They should be dissected out and clipped under direct vision. Often small vessels may be diathermied but in a fatty mesentery this can be difficult. If there is a shortened mesentery and the vessels cannot be located the vascular stapling device may be necessary.

Laparoscopic splenectomy

This is most likely to occur from direct splenic puncture when manipulating the spleen or from the short gastric vessels. The splenic artery and vein are usually clearly seen in the hilum and are easy to control. If there is brisk bleeding from a splenic puncture or from any of the vessels, early conversion is advisable.

Laparoscopic Nissen fundoplication

Bleeding from behind the oesophagus is usually easy to control. Most haemorrhage at this operation will occur when ligating and dividing the short gastric vessels. The use of the harmonic scalpel has proved very efficacious in this procedure. The only other vessel that could be damaged would be the left phrenic artery when mobilising the fundus of the stomach off the left crus. The anatomy and control of vessels during this operation are described later in the chapter.

Box 25.2 Bleeding

- Do not panic
- Take stock of situation
- Ensure good sucker and CO_2 flow
- Try and achieve temporary control
- Make plan to control bleeding point
- Identify site clearly
- Achieve permanent control

The old adage of 'prevention is better than cure' is definitely true of haemorrhage at laparoscopic surgery. Great care should be taken to dissect out the vessels and they should be carefully controlled with the correct placement of clips or ligatures.

Laparoscopic-assisted surgery

Definitions

In laparoscopic surgery all procedures are done through ports, the number being dictated by the complexity of the operation. If an organ or tissue needs to be removed, then it must be removed via one of these port sites without extension.

Laparoscopic-assisted surgery is an operation where the organ may be fully mobilised and then an incision made in the anatomical site most convenient for its removal. Examples include splenectomy and right hemicolectomy.

Use of retrieval bags

With the advent of video-assisted laparoscopic surgery, surgeons have started to perform all the operations that were performed during conventional surgery. One of the greatest problems encountered has been the difficulty of removing infected organs and bulky tissue. Laparoscopic surgery best lends itself to reparative operations such as Nissen fundoplication when there is no need to remove any tissue. The removal of small organs is also easily performed through the usual port incisions of 5 or 10 mm. However, the need to enlarge these incisions to remove more bulky tissue has not been popular with 'true laparoscopists' who feel 'cheated' that they have managed to perform the operation through tiny incisions, only to extend one of these to facilitate organ removal. Moreover, patients have come to expect that laparoscopic surgery means 'keyhole surgery' and dislike the idea of any enlargement of the port sites. However, there is no doubt that in some operations the surgery is best performed in what has become known as 'laparoscopic-assisted' operations. This is especially true in surgery of the large intestine where mobilisation of the colon and rectum can be performed laparoscopically, but then a small incision must be made to remove the tumour. This is not only necessary for most colectomies but also oncologically sound.

It is vital that attempting to remove organs through inadequate incisions does not compromise surgery for malignant conditions. There have been worrying reports of port site recurrences and, when removing left-sided colonic tumours through the rectum, of local seeding. However, it is possible to remove bulky tissue using retrieval systems, with or without morcellation.

Development of retrieval systems

When general surgeons took up laparoscopic surgery, the most commonly performed operations were cholecystectomy and appendicectomy. During the learning curve, many surgeons made holes in the gallbladder, with a resultant escape of calculi, and they found it tedious to remove these particles, singularly or by suction. Therefore, various retrieval systems were used such as a condom, a sterile glove or the finger of a sterile glove, the sterilised bag in which the cholangio-catheter was packaged and other available materials. The art of 'bagging' the gallbladder, in some hands, became routine. For others, placing the gallbladder into the bag was only used after a hole had been made or if the organ was rather bulky. The advantage of placing the gallbladder in a bag was that much more pull could be exerted on the bag without a rupture, when it was brought through the anterior abdominal wall. The use of a bag to retrieve the appendix became popular as surgeons found that if they could not pull the freed appendix out through a 10 mm cannula, they were faced with bringing it through the anterior abdominal wall and possibly causing infection. Therefore, many surgeons place the appendix into a retrieval bag before removing it.

Since those early days, many manufacturers have developed both small and large retrieval bags, with a variety of methods of closing them once the organ was placed inside. It is interesting that despite all these new retrieval systems on the market, there has been a recent article on the use of freezer bags. Dr Glasser has written about the use of everyday freezer bags; he uses them because condoms, and the special bags commonly used to remove gallbladders, were too small for large ovarian masses. Secondly, he found that freezer bags, even with the cost of sterilisation, were cheaper than manufactured bags. Dr Glasser pointed out that there was a specially designed net for removing a large ovarian mass laparoscopically, but its cost was about $105. Glad™ (or UK equivalent) freezer bags are not only much cheaper but they have a thick upper band that aids rolling for insertion into the laparoscope and a zipper seal that is blue on one side and yellow on the other. The colours make the clear bag easy to see in the abdomen and they are useful markings for the surgeon and the assistant. Gas sterilisation is effective and if done in large quantities, the cost is $1.35 per bag.

Present retrieval systems

There are many different types of retrieval bags produced by various companies in different sizes (Figure 25.4). Some bags are a simple open bag in different sizes, while others have a prestrung suture at the opening so that once the organ has been placed into the bag, it can be closed in the same manner as a pre-tied Endoloop. Many bags are made out of plastic and are not very strong, so that traction can cause the bag to burst. When dealing with malignant tissue, it is vital that the bag used is impervious. This is also important when removing splenic tissue that could exude through the bag and implant into the omentum.

The use of a large 33 mm port has been described for removing an adrenal gland. However, this organ can be dissected using the normal ports and placed into a bag as previously described. Ethicon has developed an 18 mm port with a plastic container and

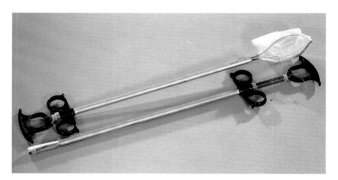

Figure 25.4 One of the currently available retrieval systems. Note the loop reinforcing the mouth of the bag to hold it open inside the pneumoperitoneum. (Picture courtesy of Ethicon Suture Ltd.)

flapper valve so that pneumoperitoneum is not lost when removing colons and other bulky tissue.

The modified sigmoidoscope with valve has been described by Carey and was first used for the easy removal of loose calculi, but can also be used for removing organs and bulky tissue.

Wolfe has manufactured a special operating rectoscope, with a large protuberant obturator, so that once the rectum has been cut across, this can be introduced without loss of pneumoperitoneum. The dissected free rectum and left-sided colon are brought down to the obturator, which is then removed. The specimen follows it out through this rectoscope. The obturator is replaced and the rectoscope withdrawn a little so that a staple can be placed across the rectum and an anastomosis effected.

Operations necessitating the use of a retrieval bag (Box 25.3)

Cholecystectomy

If the gallbladder is very inflamed or a hole has been made in it or if it is possible that there is a malignancy, then it should be placed in a retrieval bag prior to removal from the peritoneal cavity.

Appendicectomy

It is the policy of the authors to routinely place the appendix into a retrieval bag unless the appendix is thin enough to be extracted through a 10 mm port. The advantage of placing it in a bag is that wound infection should then not occur.

Splenectomy

A small spleen is not very common but can occur with idiopathic thrombocytopenic purpura. The organ can be placed in a bag and the bag removed with the spleen intact. Usually, the spleen is markedly enlarged and then an incision has to be made to remove it once it has been dissected free. It can also be placed in a large, impervious bag and the neck of the bag brought out to the abdominal surface. It is then possible to morcellate the spleen using forceps, a finger or the Cook morcellator. As the histology is not important, this is an acceptable practice. The surgeon must be extremely careful about spillage, as implanted splenic tissue can function later and cause subsequent problems.

Adrenalectomy

It is preferable to place the gland in a bag, even though they are rarely malignant. However, the gland is quite fragile and it is better preserved in a retrieval bag.

Liver resection

When performed laparoscopically, this procedure is usually for small peripheral metastases. The danger of seeding is very possible and therefore the tissue must be placed in a bag.

Laparoscopic nephrectomy

When this is done for benign disease, rather like splenectomy, the organ may be placed in a bag and the organ morcellated within the bag. If performed for malignancy (it is debatable as to whether this is an oncologically sound operation) then the kidney must be placed in an impervious bag and if large, the incision will have to be extended to facilitate its removal.

Ovaries

If removed as normal organs for the treatment of breast cancer, then they can be withdrawn through 10 mm ports. However, if there is any question as to whether there is malignant change, then they should be placed into an impervious bag and removed with the bag. If the ovary is cystic, once in the bag, the cyst may be punctured to facilitate removal.

Gastric resections

Whether for benign or malignant disease, the resected part of the stomach is best placed in the retrieval bag so that it can be examined histologically, even when a lesion is thought to be benign, as in the case of leiomyoma. There is always a possibility that there may be malignant change (see Complications).

Colectomies and anterior resection

We have changed our policy from performing these operations only by laparoscopy to performing laparoscopic-assisted resections. The real value of the laparoscopic approach for colonic surgery is mobilisation, especially mobilisation of the hepatic flexure in right hemicolectomies and the splenic flexure, when operating on the descending colon, sigmoid colon or rectum.

Occasionally, it is possible to do a colotomy for removal of a wide-based sessile polyp that cannot be removed colonoscopically. When this operation is performed, then it is possible to place the resected polyp into an impervious bag and remove it. The colotomy can be closed by either stapling or suturing laparoscopically.

During a right hemicolectomy, the surgeon has to make a small incision, either in the right iliac fossa or right hypochondrium, depending on the situation of the tumour. We feel it is best to perform the mobilisation laparoscopically and ligate the vessels if they are clearly seen. The division of the ileum and transverse colon and anastomosis is then performed extracorporeally, after the specimen has been removed. If the mesentery is very fatty and the vessels are not clearly seen, or it is difficult to tell if one is at the origin of the ileocolic and right colic vessels, then these vessels are also dealt with through the small incision.

When performing sigmoid colectomies and anterior resections, it is possible to bring the specimen out through the rectum. High ligation and division of the inferior mesenteric vessels is somewhat easier than vascular pedicles for right hemicolectomy. However, we do not feel it is oncologically sound to squeeze a malignant tumour out through the rectum and anus. For benign disease, it would be reasonable to remove the specimen through the anus but the common condition necessitating resection is diverticular disease and usually the bowel wall is thickened and the mesentery shortened. If the surgeon wishes to remove the specimen through the rectum and anus, it may be necessary to resect the sigmoid colon, then dissect it out to straighten it, so it can be passed out through the rectum and anus. We feel that a small incision adds little in the way of morbidity and is a much easier method of shortening the operating time needed.

Ilio-obturator lymph node clearance

This operation is performed as a staging procedure for prostatic carcinoma or as a clearance, for example for malignant melanoma. The dissected nodes are always placed in a bag prior to removal. A ligature should be placed at the proximal end to mark it for the pathologist.

Box 25.3   Retrieval bags

- Must be used for infected and malignant organs
- Should be impervious
- Large enough for specimen
- Incorporate ring to hold mouth open

Complications of laparoscopic surgery

Hernias

There have been an increasing number of papers reporting incidences of port site hernias. With the removal of bulky tissue through the port sites that are stretched and enlarged, especially in heavy people, it is difficult to close the fascia. If this can be done under direct vision, then port site hernias should not occur. The use of the Grice needle can make the placement of sutures under direct vision very much easier. It is our practice to use this method of placing the suture at the beginning of the procedure so that it can be ligated and ensure closure of the fascia at the end of the operation.

Spread of malignancy

Even more worrisome is the rising incidence of implantation of malignancy in port sites. There has always been implantation of malignancy into scars but these do not usually manifest themselves as quickly as malignancy within a small port site. We have had two port site malignancies: the first was following laparoscopic cholecystectomy, when 18 months later the female patient returned with a hard swelling in the epigastrium. When removed, it proved to be an ovarian cancer metastasis. The ovaries at operation had looked normal. The second case followed resection of a leiomyoma that histologically was found to be a leiomyosarcoma. The resected gastric specimen with the tumour was placed into a glove, which was then brought out through one of the 12 mm port sites. Unfortunately, with the tumour lodged in the port site, the glove burst. The gastric specimen with the tumour was retrieved with forceps but had been in contact with the abdominal wall. Seven months later, the patient re-presented with a large metastasis in that port site, which when resected was shown to be a leiomyosarcoma. It is imperative that when dealing with malignant tissue, the bags used are much stronger than those manufactured at the present time. It is vital that they be impervious. During this early phase of laparoscopic oncological surgery, there will probably be more cases of port site metastases.

Perforation

Perforation of the gallbladder usually occurs from one of two sources:

- excessive force applied to the gallbladder wall with grasping forceps or

- as a result of the energy source being used to dissect the gallbladder away from the liver.

If the gallbladder wall is injured this will lead to the escape of bile and/or calculi into the peritoneal cavity. Leakage of bile and calculi from the gallbladder occurs frequently during laparoscopic cholecystectomy, especially when a surgeon is inexperienced. It rarely leads to delayed postoperative sequelae such as intra-abdominal abscess formation or small bowel obstruction. In a very few cases when the bile is infected peritonitis can ensue if all the bile is not carefully removed.

Following perforation, attempts should be made to control any leakage immediately. The small opening in the gallbladder may be easily controlled by simply repositioning the grasping forceps to occlude it, though most defects, and especially large ones, will

require closure using either a loop or suture. Perforations are most likely to occur in the tensely distended oedematous or extremely thin-walled gallbladder. If the gallbladder is very distended it can be partially collapsed with controlled suction then closing the defect with a suture. If needle aspiration is used to decompress the gallbladder then often it is not necessary to close the gallbladder.

It is important to find and remove bile and calculi to minimise the recurrence of post operation collections or abscess formation.

If spilled calculi are clearly seen they should be removed either with grasping forceps or, if they are multiple and large, by placing them into a retrieval bag. If they are small then a large 10 mm sucker can be used to remove them (Box 25.4). Irrigation should not be carried out until the visible calculi are removed as it can cause displacement of calculi into places within the peritoneal cavity out of view. Once the calculi that are visible have been removed or collected in the bag then copious irrigation must be carried out to remove all the bile and, hopefully, all the calculi. The right subdiaphragmatic space must be carefully irrigated and fluid removed before completion of the operation to ensure that a subphrenic abscess, should the bile be infected, does not occur.

Even though a perforation has been closed the gallbladder should be placed into a retrieval bag to prevent further contamination of the fat and subcutaneous tissues. If a calculus escapes from the gallbladder and is larger than the port site it should be placed into a retrieval bag in which it may be crushed or shattered by some other means such as laser.

Migration of calculi left within the peritoneal cavity has been described and very occasionally has caused problems. One large calculus found in the pelvis was found on ultrasound and thought to be an ovarian tumour. Usually retained calculi become embedded in the omentum and do not cause future problems.

Box 25.4   Stone retrieval

- Prevention is easier – careful dissection
- If small, use large sucker
- If large, place in bag
- Attempt to remove all fragments

OPERATIVE SURGERY

Laparoscopy in acute emergencies

Laparoscopy in acute emergencies can be both diagnostic and therapeutic (Box 25.5). A diagnostic laparoscopy may proceed into a therapeutic procedure if the facilities are available and if it is appropriate to the experience of the operator.

Diagnostic laparoscopy has been performed since the 1960s, but its popularity has been delayed until recently due to limitations inherent in the actual procedure. It may be performed to aid diagnosis in acute abdominal pathology, ITU or trauma patients where physical signs may be obtunded or concealed.

Diagnostic laparoscopy as an emergency is most commonly performed for right iliac fossa pain. Whilst some of these patients have signs and symptoms which make the diagnosis clear, many cases may have other pathology which could account for their presentation. In these circumstances it is obviously advantageous to be able to view the right iliac fossa and pelvis in order to make a definitive diagnosis. In a large number of cases the condition can then continue to be managed laparoscopically, such as appendicitis or ovarian pathology.

Diagnostic laparoscopy is also a useful tool in cases where the history is vague and the symptoms equivocal, as is often the case with children. Here an early diagnosis and subsequent discharge home can avoid many days or weeks of expectant inpatient management.

Patients who have suffered multiple or localised abdominal trauma are often difficult to assess due to depressed levels of consciousness. They may be aggressive, confused, intoxicated, unconscious or anaesthetised, invalidating normal physical signs. Concomitant with initial resuscitation of these cases it is vitally important to assess the peritoneal cavity for concealed haemorrhage and intervene as appropriate.

Diagnostic peritoneal lavage is usually used as a first-line investigation and is extremely sensitive for haemorrhage in the peritoneal cavity. However, it has a low specificity and gives little idea of the severity of haemorrhage, which organ is bleeding and whether intervention is required. Radiological investigations such as ultrasound scanning and computed tomography are better at detailing the volume of intraabdominal fluids but do not generally differentiate between blood and other peritoneal fluids or localise and quantify the visceral injury.

If a department is appropriately supplied with personnel and equipment and the patient sufficiently stable to undergo investigation then needleoscopy with a 2 mm telescope can be performed. This procedure, possibly under local anaesthesia in the emergency department, can give valuable information regarding the nature and extent of visceral injury and enable appropriate treatment for these cases to be planned. The early use of laparoscopy in this subset of trauma patients should spare them the additional insult of an unnecessary laparotomy.

Evaluation of a potential acute abdomen in patients who require intensive care for concurrent medical/surgical problems is often difficult due to ambiguities in the physical diagnosis and ancillary diagnostic tests. The use of diagnostic laparoscopy in these cases is both highly sensitive and specific, with an extremely low procedure-related morbidity. It can help avoid non-therapeutic laparotomies or confirm the need for operative intervention in these complex cases.

Specific complications of performing laparoscopy in the acute setting include the risk of carbon dioxide embolism if the peritoneal cavity is insufflated in the presence of an open blood vessel. In trauma patients care must be taken to exclude diaphragmatic rupture before laparoscopy is performed and thus prevent respiratory embarrassment.

Box 25.5 Laparoscopy in emergency situations

- Diagnostic and therapeutic procedure
- Avoids insult of laparotomy in already sick patient
- Use in trauma

Laparoscopic appendicectomy

(See also Chapter 24)

This procedure is the most commonly practised example of a combined diagnostic and therapeutic procedure. The patient is prepared preoperatively in the usual way and prophylactic antibiotics are given on induction. As with all laparoscopic procedures, the patient is consented for conversion to an open operation.

Placement of operative ports

The patient is placed on the table in a supine position and the bladder catheterised if palpable. Port placement for this procedure has been covered earlier in the chapter.

Technique

The appendix is dissected free of any adhesions. The tip of the appendix is then grasped and drawn into the right-hand port. The appendicular mesentery and artery are divided and haemostasis achieved with diathermy, clips or ligatures. Two Roeder knots are placed around the base of the appendix and the lumen distal to this is occluded. There are different ways of securing the appendix base. Our preference is using a third loop or a clip if the lumen is narrow enough (Figure 25.5). Another method, more expensive, would be to use the Endo GIA stapler. Alternatively bipolar diathermy can be used. The appendix is divided at this site and removed through the right iliac fossa port in a retrieval bag. The peritoneal cavity is then aspirated and irrigated as required. If felt

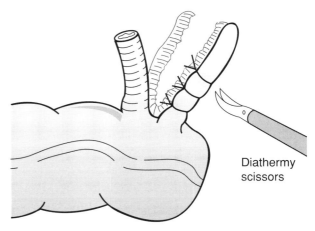
Diathermy scissors

Figure 25.5 Removal of appendix with stump secured.

necessary by the operator, a drain may be placed near the appendix stump. The ports are then removed and closed in a routine manner.

Postoperative management is as for open appendicectomies. Postoperative pain is reduced but timing of discharge and return to work are little different from open procedures. This is probably more determined by the disease process than the type of operative intervention.

Complications specific to laparoscopic appendicectomy are rare but an increase in reactionary haemorrhage has been reported in some series.

Laparoscopic management of perforated duodenal ulcer

At a diagnostic laparoscopy duodenal perforations can be easily visualised, as they are usually anterior. If appropriate then surgical repair of the perforation can be undertaken laparoscopically, either as a continuation of the diagnostic procedure or *de novo* if the diagnosis is confirmed preoperatively.

Placement of operative ports

The patient is prepared as for open surgery with preoperative resuscitation and a nasogastric tube inserted. In the emergency setting a urinary catheter should also be inserted. The patient is placed supine. The surgeon stands between the legs with an assistant on either side. The patient is prepared and draped in a routine manner. Instruments for conversion to laparotomy should also be available.

The pneumoperitoneum is established and maintained at a pressure of 14 mmHg. The first 10 mm trocar is inserted as usual subumbilically. A 0° laparoscope is inserted and the remaining three ports are inserted. A 10 mm port is inserted 5 cm above and to the left of the umbilicus and a 5 mm port is placed 5 cm above and to the right of the umbilicus. A further 5 mm port is placed in either the right subcostal or subxiphoid positions.

Operative technique

The peritoneal contaminant is aspirated and collected for microscopy and culture. The peritoneal cavity is then thoroughly cleaned using high-flow irrigation and aspiration. An omental plug is fashioned and the duodenal defect closed with interrupted monofilament absorbable sutures. The knots are tied inside the peritoneal cavity over the omental plug.

The decision whether or not to proceed at this stage with a surgical antiulcer procedure depends on the age of the patient, any associated medical diseases and time delay since perforation.

Postoperative management is as for an open procedure with the nasogastric tube usually being left *in situ* for 48 hours. Postoperative pain is usually minimal and the median time to

discharge is five days. Prolonged hospital stay is usually due to concomitant pathology.

Other emergency laparoscopic procedures

With the widespread uptake of laparoscopic surgery there are few emergency procedures that have not been performed laparoscopically. However, the instability of the emergency patient on the operating table together with the difficulty in controlling haemorrhage laparoscopically means that they are not widely practised at present.

Laparoscopy for intestinal obstruction is difficult because of bowel distension, but if the bowel can be adequately decompressed then it is relatively easy to divide an obstructing adhesion. Emergency laparoscopic small and large bowel resections are not commonly performed due to the reasons above. Emergency laparoscopic repair of incarcerated hernias has been reported and with further adoption of the technique of laparoscopic hernia repair, may be one area in which emergency laparoscopic surgery has a more extensive role to play.

Adhesiolysis

Introduction

Adhesions are the most common cause of small bowel obstruction and are usually the sequelae of surgical or gynaecological operations, pelvic inflammatory disease, appendicitis or endometriosis. Adhesions occur after abdominal surgery in over 60% of cases, although they are symptomatic in less than 30%.

Laparoscopic adhesiolysis has not been compared with classic laparotomy, but laparoscopy obviously diminishes peritoneal mesothelial cell ischaemic damage from trauma, drying, packs and delayed bleeding. It may also decrease the risk of new adhesion formation.

The use of laparoscopy for chronic adhesiolysis procedures has been accepted but its use in the acute abdomen with intestinal obstruction must only be undertaken by very experienced laparoscopic surgeons. The major difficulty that will be encountered would be the safe introduction of the pneumoperitoneum in somebody with distended intestines (Box 25.6).

Techniques

Adhesiolysis may be undertaken using scissor dissection, aqua dissection or lasers. The surgeon must be able to perform laparoscopic suturing prior to undertaking this type of procedure. The safest techniques are division of adhesions by scissors or aqua dissection.

Blunt or round-tipped scissors are used to divide thin and thick bowel adhesions sharply. Sharp dissection diminishes the potential for adhesion formation; electrolaser surgery is usually reserved for haemostatic dissection or where adhesions are very adherent.

Scissors are the best instrument to cut avascular or congenital adhesions and peritoneum. Pushing tissue with the partially open blunt tip of the scissors can develop natural planes.

Use of pressurised fluid to aid in the performance of surgical procedures has a definite place in liver surgery and also the division of adhesions. The use of a helicon-water jet with a suction device has proved to be very safe.

Monopolar diathermy should be avoided when working on the bowel and the use of a bipolar instrument is much safer. Monopolar cutting current is safe but the voltage must be kept low. One must be very careful that intestine beyond the field of view is not damaged, especially by electroinsulation defects or capacitance coupling.

Using a CO_2 laser gives the surgeon the ability to cut or ablate tissue. As this laser has only a 0.1 mm depth of penetration and its energy is absorbed by water it affords a margin of safety when working around the bowel, ureter and major vessels.

Classification

Peritoneal adhesiolysis procedures can be divided into enterolysis procedures and female reproductive system procedures. The extent, thickness and vascularity of adhesions vary widely.

Preoperative preparation

Patients must be informed preoperatively of the high risk of bowel injury. They should empty their bladders prior to arriving in the operating room and a catheter is only used if the bladder is distended or a long operation is anticipated. If the adhesions are in the pelvis then urinary catheterisation is mandatory. Perioperative antibiotics are routinely used and precautions to prevent deep vein thrombosis taken.

Incisions

When the procedure is being carried out for acute adhesiolysis then an open approach for the insertion of the first port must be undertaken. If there are extensive adhesions around the umbilicus or if a mid-line scar is present then the first port should be placed away from this site. Later the adhesions can be freed and an umbilical port then inserted safely. Other laparoscopic ports are placed as needed under direct vision.

Strategy for enterolysis

- Division of all adhesions to the anterior abdominal wall/parietal peritoneum: small bowel loops encountered during this process are freed from each other using the anterior attachment for countertraction.

- Division of all small bowel and omental adhesions in the pelvis: the rectosigmoid, caecum and appendix often are freed during this part of the procedure.

- Running of the small bowel. Using atraumatic grasping forceps and a suction irrigator for suction/traction, the bowel is 'run' starting at the caecum and terminal ileum and ending in the high upper abdomen at the ligament of Treitz, freeing loops and significant adhesions.

General adhesiolysis

The first adhesions that are encountered involve the anterior abdominal wall/parietal peritoneum. These consist of omentum and small bowel attachments with varying degrees of fibrosis and vascularity. Small bowel adhesions to the anterior abdominal wall are released. Adhesions are much easier to divide from above than from below, because the angle between the omentum or bowel and the parietal peritoneum is usually acute, which means gravity can help delineate the planes.

Initial adhesiolysis creates space that allows better access for further adhesiolysis. Safe entry sites for secondary ports become visible. The need for ongoing meticulous haemostasis is important.

Pelvic adhesiolysis

The next step is to free all bowel loops in the pelvis. When adhesion interfaces are obvious, scissors are used. When the adhesions blend in to one another aqua dissection distends the layers of adhesions, facilitating identification of the involved structures. It is not in the remit of this chapter to describe the treatment of endometriosis, the freeing of ovaries and/or tubes.

Bowel complications of adhesiolysis

Gastrointestinal injuries can occur during any laparoscopic procedure but they are of particular concern during adhesiolysis. The surgeon must be familiar with detection and management of these injuries. If necessary, conversion to a laparotomy should be undertaken.

Box 25.6 Laparoscopic adhesiolysis

- Extreme care if distended bowel
- Only divide if in full vision
- Minimal use of diathermy or other energy source
- Be prepared to convert to open procedure early

Unrecognised or delayed perforation

Delayed bowel injury can result from traumatic perforation not recognised during the procedure. Rarely, these delayed injuries are due to the perforation of mechanically devascularised bowel or to haemorrhagic ischaemic necrosis after mesenteric venous thrombosis. Bowel perforation due to thermal injury usually presents 4–10 days after the operation. With traumatic perforation symptoms of peritonitis usually occur within 24–48 hours.

The gross appearance of traumatic and energy injuries is similar. The perforation is usually surrounded by a white area of necrosis. A high index of suspicion must be maintained throughout the postoperative period.

Laparoscopic repair of a hiatus hernia with Nissen fundoplication

Introduction

Gastro-oesophageal reflux disease is one of the most common disorders affecting the gastrointestinal system. Conventional open surgery has been shown to be effective at curing reflux but is a major undertaking, which may be associated with considerable morbidity. Laparoscopic repair gives the potential to treat this common condition effectively whilst minimising the complications associated with large abdominal incisions.

Epidemiology

Gastro-oesophageal reflux disease accounts for approximately 75% of gastrointestinal pathology. Approximately one-third of the patients with heartburn who seek medical care have endoscopic evidence of oesophagitis and between 10% and 20% have severe complications of this oesophagitis.

Medical therapy

Conservative measures together with H_2 blockers or proton pump inhibitors are very effective in alleviating the symptoms of reflux. However, on stopping therapy up to 80% of patients with severe reflux will relapse within six months. Although a proton pump inhibitor may be used on a long-term basis to maintain remission there are fears that prolonged achlorhydria may cause neoplastic change of the enterochromaffin cells. In addition, studies have shown that the alkaline component of reflux may be responsible for some of the complications. Under these circumstances drugs aimed at reducing the exposure to acid will not prevent the damage caused by the reflux of biliary, duodenal and pancreatic secretions.

Indications for surgery

These include unresponsiveness to medical therapy, poor compliance, stricture, ulceration, Barrett's oesophagus and reflux-induced pulmonary disease. Preoperative assessment should include upper gastrointestinal endoscopy and biopsy, 24-hour oesophageal pH monitoring, oesophageal manometry and sometimes upper gastrointestinal radiographic studies. A significant proportion of people with reflux have hiatus hernia but many patients with hiatus hernia are asymptomatic. Only those with proven reflux with

evidence of oesophageal or bronchial symptoms or complications unresponsive to medical therapy and with a mechanically weak lower oesophageal sphincter, together with oesophageal body motor function, should be considered for surgery.

Patient selection

The choice of antireflux procedure is largely dependent on the surgeon's preference and any structural or functional anomalies associated with the reflux (Box 25.7). The importance of comprehensive preoperative assessment cannot be overemphasised, as this will allow accurate patient selection and use of the most appropriate procedure. It is important that patients with oesophageal motility disorders do not undergo fundoplication as the increase in lower oesophageal sphincter pressure may cause further dysphagia. A hiatal hernia, if present, should be reduced, the hiatal defect repaired and a total loose fundoplication performed to give added security.

Advantages

The advantages of the laparoscopic approach over open surgery in terms of postoperative pain, hospital stay, return to normal activity and cosmesis have led to the application of this approach to several gastrointestinal procedures. Whereas open antireflux surgery provides poor exposure using either abdominal or thoracic approaches, a laparoscopic approach provides an unparalleled view of the diaphragmatic hiatus. Indeed, the anatomical detail provided by this technique combined with the potential benefits of minimal access surgery have led to the reappraisal of several antireflux operations, including some that had been all but abandoned.

Consent

It is essential that all patients are conversant with the nature of the operation that has to be undertaken and understand that it may be necessary to convert to an open procedure, for instance because of haemorrhage. They should be advised preoperatively as to the likely length of hospital stay and time to return to work. They should also be told of any likely postoperative complications such as dysphagia, gas bloat, and postprandial fullness and reassured that these will be temporary.

Box 25.7 Laparoscopic antireflux procedures

Indications for surgery
- Failed medical treatment
- Volume regurgitation
- Recurrent chest infections
- Young patients requiring continuing acid blockade

Surgery
- Avoid sharp dissection around OG junction
- Avoid angulation of OG junction during passage of the bougie
- Use gentle movement to insert the bougie under direct vision
- Avoid high dissection in hiatus near pleura
- Be prepared to divide short gastric vessels if necessary
- Always repair crura

Setting up

The anaesthetised patient is placed in the modified Lloyd–Davis position with the legs apart and fairly straight so that the operating surgeon can stand between them. Two monitors should be used, one on each side of the patient's head so that all staff involved in the procedure can have an uninterrupted view. The operating surgeon stands between the legs, his first assistant with the camera stands on the patient's right and the second assistant/scrub nurse stands on the patient's left. The skin is prepared with an antiseptic solution and a laparoscopic drape applied. Sterile leggings should also be applied.

Incisions

A 1 cm incision is made in the mid-line 5–7 cm above the umbilicus and pneumoperitoneum introduced either using a Veress needle or by the open technique. It is usual to decompress the stomach with a nasogastric tube. The patient is then placed in a reverse Trendelenburg position with a considerable degree of tilt. The secondary port sites are shown in Figure 25.1.

When all five ports have been inserted and a full peritoneoscopy has been performed, the procedure commences. A liver retractor is used, either a fan retractor or a Nathanson retractor, under the left lobe of the liver. The area of the gastro-oesophageal junction is brought into view and the size of the hiatus assessed.

The stomach is grasped using Johann forceps just below the gastro-oesophageal junction, being careful not to include superficial blood vessels. The stomach is retracted inferiorly and to the left with a second pair of Johann forceps. Dissection can start either at the apex or on the right arms, the peritoneum being incised using scissors and gently swept inferiorly. When the left crus has been identified the forceps are placed on the medial aspect of the left crus using blunt dissection until the area between left crus and oesophagus is dissected out. However, dissection can start just above segment 1 of the liver on the right crus, dividing the lesser omentum above the vagal nerves to the liver. With this approach the right crus is dissected out first.

Full mobilisation of the abdominal oesophagus is facilitated by fully mobilising the stomach from the left crus, diaphragm and spleen. Occasionally there is a sizeable artery running over the inferior aspect of the left crus, which may need to be clipped and divided. Once the crura have been dissected out the peri-oesophageal tissue behind the oesophagus is dissected using a combination of blunt and sharp dissection. The oesophagus is lifted using the Johann forceps and this should bring the posterior vagus nerve into view. Dissection continues either between the vagus nerve and the oesophagus or posterior to the vagus nerve. Once a window has been made between the oesophagus and the crura, some surgeons insert a sling to help hold the oesophagus forward.

The fundus of the stomach is then mobilised by dissecting the greater omentum free from it and, if necessary, ligating and dividing the short gastric vessels. This can be performed by clipping the

vessels or using the harmonic scalpel. Occasionally three or four short gastric vessels have to be divided. Great care is needed to avoid damaging the spleen.

It is important always to close the crura, even if there is no obvious hiatus hernia. A non-absorbable suture is used and it is important not to close the crura too tightly. When the suture has been applied a large bougie (56 FG) is passed down the oesophagus through the oesophagogastric junction. The entry of the bougie into the stomach is observed under direct vision. Once in place the suture in the crura is then ligated, making sure that the closure is not too tight around the oesophagus. The bougie is then withdrawn into the oesophagus when it will be seen that the crural closure has left a space behind the oesophagus.

The oesophagus is now lifted anteriorly and the Johann forceps passed through the retro-oesophageal window. The fundus is then fed into the forceps and is gently drawn through the retro-oesophageal window to the right of the oesophagus. It should lie there without any tension. The bougie is pushed down through the oesophagogastric junction again, following which the left-hand side of the stomach is picked up with a suture as far laterally and superiorly as possible. The suture is passed through the muscular wall of the oesophagus and then through the fundus lying to the right of the oesophagus. The stomach has now been tented across the lower part of the oesophagus and the suture is tied and divided. One or two further sutures are placed below this first suture so that a full Nissen wrap is fashioned over approximately 5 cm. The bougie is withdrawn and the wrap tested by inserting an instrument between it and the oesophagus to ensure it is loose. Some surgeons place a final suture between the wrap and the apex of the crura or between the wrap and the right crus. This closes the gap between the wrap and diaphragm and fixes the wrap. Lavage is carried out to ensure haemostasis.

All 10 mm port sites are closed with a suture into the fascia and the skin wounds are closed with either sutures or Steristrips.

Postoperatively patients are allowed free fluids as soon as they are fully conscious and a light diet within 12 hours. They are advised to keep on soft foods for the first 2–3 weeks (Figures 25.6–25.10).

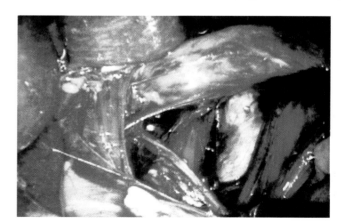

Figure 25.6 Hiatus fully dissected out exposing right and left pillars of crural sling. The abdominal oesophagus is mobilized and the posterior vagus nerve separated from it.

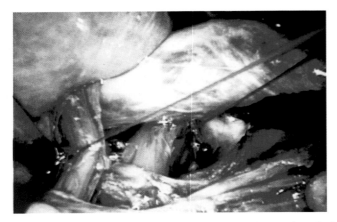

Figure 25.7 The crura are approximated having passed a bougie through the oesophago-gastric junction.

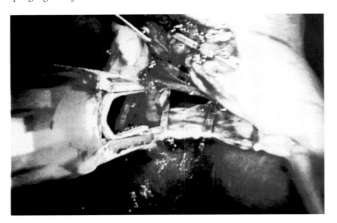

Figure 25.8 If necessary the short gastric vessels are controlled and divided.

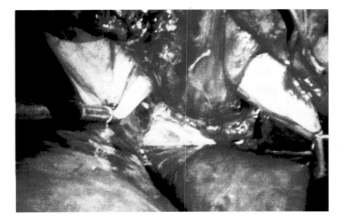

Figure 25.9 The mobilized fundus is brought through the retro-oesophageal window to the right side.

Specific complications

Haemorrhage

- Bleeding from port sites
- Bleeding from an aberrant branch of the right hepatic artery

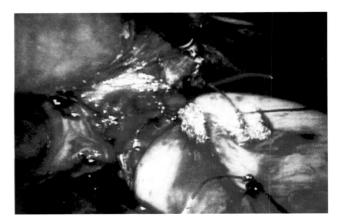

Figure 25.10 The loose wrap is completed.

- Bleeding from short gastric vessels
- Bleeding and injury to the spleen or liver
- Bleeding from major vessels

Pneumothorax

The pleura may be damaged while dissecting the lower oesophagus. It is nearly always the left pleura that is damaged. It occurs if a dissection is taken too extensively above the left crus. It is important to recognise that the pleura has been breached but apart from this it is of little consequence. If a large pneumothorax is present a chest drain will need to be inserted.

Injury to vagi

The posterior vagus is nearly always seen and easily recognised. It may be damaged while suturing the crura together and it is important to free the posterior vagus from the posterior aspect of the oesophagus in order to prevent this happening. The anterior vagus is rarely seen. The only time it is liable to damage is during suturing of the wrap, particularly the suture that incorporates the anterior wall of the oesophagus.

Gastric perforation

This can occur during the passage of the bougie which should be soft and malleable. A tapered soft tip bougie carefully passed should not cause perforation. Gastric perforation may also occur from instrumentation whilst dissecting out the retro-oesophageal window. If the stomach has been traumatised or if a perforation is present this area should be sutured.

Injury to oesophagus

This is potentially the most serious complication. The oesophagus should never be directly held with forceps. All dissection involving the oesophagus should be done by blunt dissection. If an injury occurs it is possible to close it with laparoscopic sutures and one must ensure that the wrap covers the sutured area.

Postoperative complications

Early wrap migration

This can occur after retching or vomiting forces the stomach and wrap into the lower chest. To prevent this complication it is important to always close the crura to minimise the defect of the hiatus and, if the patients are nauseated or vomiting, to withhold fluids and pass a nasogastric tube.

Dysphagia

Temporary dysphagia will occur in approximately one-third of patients. If patients are forewarned and keep to a soft food diet for the first 2–3 weeks, avoiding meat, bread and rice, no harm should come to them. If the dysphagia is more severe it will usually respond to the passage of an endoscope or, very rarely, gentle dilatation.

Postoperative management

In the early postoperative phase pain relief is important. Shoulder tip pain should not last for more than 24 hours and wound pain is unlikely if infiltration with bupivacaine has been used at the end of the procedure. The nasogastric tube is removed at the end of the procedure and only reinserted if the patient is retching or vomiting.

Patients are usually fully mobile on the first postoperative day and can be discharged home on the second or third postoperative day. The majority can return to work after two weeks.

FURTHER READING

Bailey RW, Flowers JL, eds. *Complications of Laparoscopic Surgery*. Missouri: Quality Medical Publishing, 1995

Cuschieri A, ed. *Laparoscopic Biliary Surgery*. Oxford: Blackwell Science, 1994

Meinero M, Melotti G, Mouret PH, eds. *Laparoscopic Surgery: The Nineties*. Masson, 1994

Rosin RD, ed. *Minimal Access General Surgery*. Oxford: Radcliffe Medical Press, 1994

Zucker KA, ed. *Surgical Laparoscopy*. Missouri: Quality Medical Publishing, 1991

Section 4

Breast surgery

26

Breast disease: diagnostic methods

J.M. Dixon

CLINICAL FEATURES

History

Details of the presenting complaint, length of symptoms, risk factors including family history and current medication should be obtained and recorded legibly in the patient's notes. The duration of symptoms can often give a clue to diagnosis – breast cancers usually grow slowly but cysts can appear overnight.

Clinical Examination

All patients should have careful inspection of both breasts and axillary regions performed in good light, first with the arms by the patient's side, then with the arms above the head and finally the hands pressing on the hips. Skin dimpling or change in breast contour is present in a high percentage of patients with breast cancer. Although the presence of skin dimpling is most commonly associated with breast cancer, it can follow surgery or trauma and be associated with benign conditions such as fat necrosis, infection or it can occur as part of breast involution.

Palpation of the breast is performed with the patient lying flat with her arms above her head and a pillow under her neck. The whole of the breast is gently palpated with the hand held flat. Any abnormality is then further assessed with the fingertips. To assess whether a mass is fixed to the underlying chest wall, the pectoralis major is tensed by asking the patient to press her hand on the hip of the affected side. All palpable lesions should be carefully measured in at least two planes with callipers. Exact details of size and location of the mass in the breast should be recorded with the location related to the clock face using figures 1–12 to represent the majority of the breast, with 13 being used when there is a central lesion and 14 denoting a lesion in the axillary tail or lower axilla.

Once the breasts have been palpated the regional nodal areas are checked. This is best performed with the patient sitting up. The right axilla is examined by supporting the right arm at the elbow in the examiner's right hand and assessing axillary nodes with the left hand and vice versa for the left axilla. Clinical assessment of axillary nodes is often inaccurate. Palpable nodes can be identified in up to 30% of patients with no clinically significant breast or other disease and approximately a third of patients subsequently identified to have lymph node metastases will not have palpable axillary nodes. Supraclavicular nodes should be assessed from behind with the patient seated.

Imaging

The modalities most commonly used to image the breast are mammography and ultrasonography.

Mammography requires compression of the breast between two plates and can be uncomfortable. The most commonly performed views are the oblique and craniocaudal views. With modern film screens, a dose of less than 1.5 mGy is standard. Mammography allows detection of mass lesions, areas of parenchymal distortion and microcalcifications. Because younger women's breasts are more dense, mammography is rarely of value in women under the age of 35.

Ultrasonography utilises high-frequency sound waves which are beamed through the breast. The reflections are detected and turned into images. Cysts show up as hypoechoic transparent objects, benign lesions tend to have well-demarcated edges and a homogenous echo pattern whereas cancers characteristically have indistinct outlines, are hyperechoic and have a posterior acoustic shadow.

Magnetic resonance imaging is an accurate way of imaging the breast. It may be valuable in demonstrating the extent of both invasive and non-invasive disease. Although it has a sensitivity over 95% for breast cancer, it has a lower specificity of approximately 80%. It is particularly useful in the conserved breast in determining whether a mammographic lesion at the site of surgery is due to scar tissue or cancer recurrence. It is currently being evaluated as a screening tool for high-risk women between the ages of 35 and 55. MRI is the optimum method for imaging breast implants.

Scintimammography and PET scanning can image breast lesions and ductography can identify pathological abnormalities in subareolar ducts but these imaging techniques have no role in the routine investigation or assessment of patients with breast problems.

Fine needle aspiration cytology

Needle aspiration can differentiate between solid and cystic lesions. Aspiration of solid lesions requires skill to obtain an adequate sample of cells and to prepare satisfactory smears and considerable expertise is required by the cytopathologist to interpret these smears.

Fine needle aspiration cytology (FNAC) of palpable lesions is usually performed freehand by a clinician or a cytopathologist. Impalpable lesions can be sampled by ultrasound, if visible on this modality, or by stereotactic guidance. Ultrasonography is more accurate, quicker, easier to perform, cheaper and associated with less patient discomfort. With newer high-frequency ultrasound, some microcalcifications are visible. Stereotaxis is the most accurate of the X-ray guided techniques.

To obtain a sample of cells from a palpable or impalpable lesion a 21 or 23 gauge needle is attached to a syringe. The needle is introduced into the lesion and suction is applied by withdrawing the plunger. The needle is then passed through the lesion at least 10–15 times following which suction is released, the needle withdrawn and aspirated material is spread on to microscope slides. These are then either air dried or sprayed with a fixative, depending on the cytologist's preference, and then stained. In some units these stained smears are examined immediately by the pathologist and a report is available within 30 minutes.

Core needle biopsy

This procedure is performed after infiltration of local anaesthetic. Ideally 10–20 ml of 1% lignocaine containing 1:200 000 adrenaline is infiltrated directly into the skin and around the lesion to be biopsied. A 14 gauge needle combined with a mechanical gun produces optimal samples and allows the procedure to be performed single handed. The point of entry of the needle through the skin should allow the core biopsy to be taken parallel to the chest wall. This ensures that when the gun is fired, the lesion does not penetrate structures deep to the breast. Providing sufficient anaesthetic is used, core biopsy is less painful than FNAC. Several cores can be removed from a mass lesion or an area of microcalcification by means of a cutting needle technique. By applying vacuum to the core biopsy needle and using a larger needle (11 gauge), multiple large cores can be obtained without withdrawing the needle from the breast, potentially improving the diagnostic yield compared to a 14 gauge device. Image-guided core biopsy of impalpable lesions using ultrasound or X-ray stereotaxis is highly accurate.

The advantage of core needle biopsy over FNAC is that it can differentiate invasive from *in situ* cancer. The disadvantage of core biopsy is that unlike FNAC, results are not available immediately but in many centres the result is available within 24 hours. New processing techniques will eventually allow diagnosis on core biopsy within 60 minutes.

Open biopsy

Open biopsy should be performed only in patients who have been appropriately investigated by clinical examination, imaging, FNAC and, if appropriate, core biopsy. It is rare that this combination of investigations does not establish a definitive diagnosis. Women who are told that investigations have demonstrated their lesion to be benign rarely request excision. Indications for excision of a breast lesion are:

- diagnosis of malignancy on cytology that is not supported by the results of other investigations when a mastectomy or axillary dissection is planned

- suspicion of malignancy on clinical examination or imaging when cytology indicates the lesion is probably benign and a core biopsy has failed to provide a definitive diagnosis

- request by patient for excision.

Impalpable lesions which need to be removed are marked by placing a hooked wire under image guidance in the tissues adjacent to the lesion. Lignocaine 1% with 1:200 000 adrenaline is infiltrated into the skin and down to the lesion before the wire is inserted. The wire is placed 1–2 hours before surgery and before the patient has had any premedication. Where an area of microcalcification is being localised, the use of multiple wires placed at the margins of the calcification can assist the surgeon in performing a complete excision. Following placement of the wire, it is secured in position by bending the wire and suturing it to the skin. Further films are then performed to demonstrate the relationship of the mammographic lesion to the wire and this allows the surgeon to identify the site of the abnormality in the breast and excise it. Accurate placement of the localising wire is essential. A variety of wire systems are available. Localisation biopsies are usually performed under general anaesthesia so following insertion of a wire, the patient returns to the ward and is given appropriate medication prior to surgery later in the day. A new technique using radio-isotope and a hand-held gamma camera to localise the lesion has recently been described and may have some advantages over the use of a localising wire.

If the procedure is being performed to establish a diagnosis, then a small representative portion of the lesion is excised through a cosmetically placed incision to ensure there is little cosmetic defect and a satisfactory cosmetic result is produced if the lesion is ultimately shown to be benign. The European Surgical Quality Assurance Guidelines require that such diagnostic surgical excision specimens performed in screen-detected lesions should weigh less than 30 g. Intraoperative specimen radiography is essential both to check that an impalpable lesion has been removed and if a cancer has been diagnosed and the procedure is therapeutic, this is performed to ensure that the whole of the mammographic lesion has been adequately excised.

Open biopsy is not without morbidity and in one series of patients who had breast biopsy for what turned out to be benign disease stimulated by breast screening, one in five developed a further lump under the scar or pain specifically related to the biopsy site.

Frozen section

Frozen section histopathological assessment should be used only in the following circumstances.

- To confirm a cytological diagnosis of malignancy before proceeding to definitive surgery (such patients should already have been told that the lesion in their breast is malignant and have been appropriately counselled and had time to consider treatment options).

- To assess excision margins to ensure complete excision of a palpable or impalpable abnormality. The accuracy of intraoperative assessment of margins by frozen section is not 100%.

- Assessment of axillary lymph nodes during operation to identify node-negative patients who do not require axillary dissection and node-positive patients who require a complete axillary dissection. The sensitivity of frozen section for nodal involvement is between 80% and 90%.

The routine use of frozen section to diagnose breast cancer is no longer acceptable.

Table 26.1 Accuracy of investigations in diagnosis of symptomatic breast disease in specialist breast clinics

	Clinical examination	Mammography	Ultrasonography	Fine needle aspiration cytology	Core biopsy
Sensitivity for cancers★	86%	86%	85%	95%	85–95%†
Specificity for benign disease#	90%	90%	88%	95%	95%
Positive predictive value for cancers≈	95%	95%	90%	99.8%	100%

★%   Of cancers detected by test as malignant or probably malignant (that is, complete sensitivity)
\# %   Of benign disease detected by test as benign
≈%   Of lesions diagnosed as malignant by test that are cancers (that is, absolute positive predictive value)
†   Sensitivity increases if core biopsy is image guided. Sensitivity can be as high as 98% when using image-guided 11 gauge assisted core biopsy (mammotome)

Accuracy of investigations

False-positive results occur with all diagnostic techniques (Table 26.1). Treatments can be planned on the basis of malignant cytology providing it is supported by diagnosis of malignancy on clinical examination and imaging. Cytology has a false-positive rate of about two per thousand and the lesions most likely to be misinterpreted are active fibroadenomas and areas of the breast that have been irradiated. The sensitivity of clinical examination and mammography varies with age and only two-thirds of cancers in women under the age of 50 are deemed suspicious or definitely malignant on clinical examination or mammography (Figure 26.1). In one study of 4000 patients, mammography had a sensitivity of 83%. When ultrasonography was added, the sensitivity of the two techniques increased to 94%. This 11% increase in sensitivity was mainly due to ultrasound either imaging mass lesions which were not visible on mammography or identifying malignant characteristic in lesions which were visible on mammography but which were deemed benign.

Triple assessment

Triple assessment is the combination of clinical examination, imaging (mammography ± ultrasonography of women aged over 35 and ultrasonography for women aged under 35) and FNAC and/or core biopsy. In one series of 1511 patients with breast cancer having triple assessment, only six patients (0.2%) had lesions which were considered to be benign on all three investigations.

INVESTIGATION OF BREAST SYMPTOMS

Breast mass

All patients with a discrete mass or a localised area of nodularity should be assessed by triple assessment. It is not necessary to excise all solid breast masses and a selective policy is recommended based on the results of triple assessment (Figure 26.2).

Nipple discharge

Physiological nipple discharge is common; two-thirds of pre-menopausal women can be made to produce nipple secretion by cleansing the nipple and applying suction. This physiological discharge varies in colour from white to yellow to green to blue-black. All discharge should be checked for the presence of blood by testing for haemoglobin.

Treatment depends on whether the discharge is spontaneous or whether it is from one or several ducts (Figure 26.3). The indications for surgery in a patient with a single duct spontaneous discharge are:

- bloodstained discharge or discharge which contains moderate or large amounts of blood on testing

- persistent discharge (occurs on at least two occasions per week)

- nipple discharge which is associated with a mass

- nipple discharge which is a new development in women over 50 years but is not thick or cheesy.

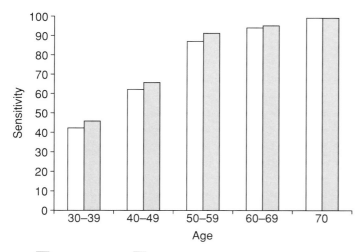

Key: ☐ = Clinical exam, ▨ = Mammography

Figure 26.1 Sensitivity of clinical examination and mammography by age in patients presenting with a breast mass (data from J.M. Dixon)

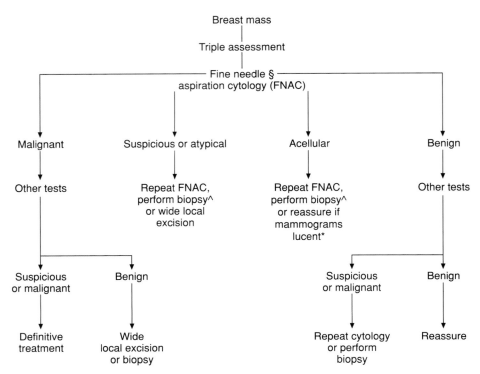

Figure 26.2 Investigation of a breast mass using cytology. § – some centres use core biopsy instead of or in combination with fine needle aspiration cytology. ^ – Biopsy – core biopsy freehand or preferably image guided.

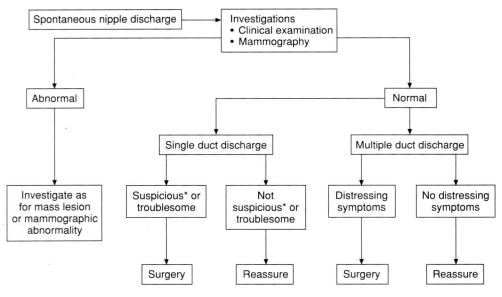

Figure 26.3 Investigation of nipple discharge. ★ Suspicious = discharge which is bloodstained or contains moderate or large amounts of blood on testing, is associated with a mass, is a new development in women over the age of 50 and the discharge is not thick or cheesy.

Multiple duct discharge normally requires surgery only when it causes distressing symptoms such as persistent staining of clothes.

Nipple retraction

Slit-like nipple retraction is characteristic of benign disease whereas nipple inversion, when the whole nipple is pulled in, can occur in association with both breast cancer and inflammatory breast conditions. The majority of women who present with nipple retraction or nipple inversion are older and in this age group, the sensitivity of clinical examination and mammography for malignancy is high. Patients with symmetrical slit-like retraction who have normal mammograms and no apparent clinical mass can be reassured that their symptoms are almost certainly benign (Figure 26.4).

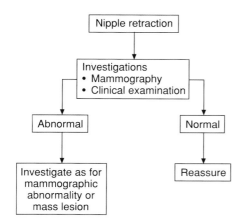

Figure 26.4 Investigation of nipple retraction.

FURTHER READING

BASO Breast Speciality Group. The British Association of Surgical Oncology Guidelines for surgeons in the management of symptomatic breast disease in the UK (1998 revision). *Eur J Surg Onco* 1998; **24**:464–476

Ciatto S, Rosselli Del Turco M, Catarzi S, Morrone D. The contribution of ultrasonography to the differential diagnosis of breast cancer. *Neoplasma* 1994; **41**:341–345

Confortini M, Minuti PA, Ciatto S. Fine needle aspiration cytology of the breast: improving the predictive value of equivocal cytologic reports by monoclonal antibody B72.3. *Breast* 1994; **3**:172–174

Dixon JM. Indications for and techniques of breast biopsy. *Curr Prac Surg* 1993; **5**:142–148

Dixon JM, Dobie V, Lamb J, Walsh JS, Chetty U. Assessment of the acceptability of conservative management of fibroadenoma of the breast. *Br J Surg* 1996; **83**:264–265

Dixon JM, Mansel RE. ABC of breast diseases: symptoms, assessment and guidelines for referral. *BMJ* 1994; **309**:722–726

Harris JR, Lippman ME, Morrow M, Hellman S. (eds). *Diseases of the Breast.* Philadelphia: Lippincott-Raven, 1996

Oellinger H, Heins S, Sander B et al. Gd-DTPA enhanced MR breast imaging: the most sensitive method for multicentric carcinomas of the female breast. *Eur Radio* 1993; **3**:223–226

Sacks NPM, Barr LC, Allan SM, Baum M. The role of axillary dissection in operable breast cancer. *Breast* 1992; **1**:41–49

Benign breast disorders

N.J. Bundred, A.D. Baildam

BENIGN BREAST PROBLEMS

Benign breast problems are common. Breast pain affects 40–60% of all women and it has been reported that 30% of all women visit a doctor with a breast problem in a 20-year period. Many breast problems are physiological rather than pathological and are related to normal cyclical, developmental and involutional changes which occur during the reproductive, perimenopausal and postmenopausal years. Confusion surrounding breast disorders is often caused by inadequate terminology and efforts have been made in recent years not to label women as having 'disease' but breast disorders. Autopsy studies show that most women have histological changes which correspond to benign breast features but a woman's symptoms do not always correlate with either signs or pathology. We therefore now use a symptom-based classification called ANDI or Aberrations of Normal Development and Involution. Stages of the classification are NORMAL → DISORDER → DISEASE.

For example, during normal breast development, new lobules develop. Failure of cells in the centre of a lobule to die back and canalise to produce a lumen leads to an aberration called a fibroadenoma (disorder). In contrast, at the menopause 30% of women have epithelial proliferation (disorder) while 1–5% have atypical epithelial hyperplasia or *in situ* cancer (disease). *In situ* cancer/atypical lobular hyperplasia is distinguished as a disease because follow-up of untreated patients reveals an excess risk of subsequent breast cancer whilst epithelial proliferation is a disorder because of a lack of association with subsequent cancer risk.

Cancer risk of benign breast disease

Detailed review of histological findings in a large series of women followed up for 10–20 years revealed that atypical ductal hyperplasia increased the risk of breast cancer (especially in the presence of a family history of breast cancer where risk is 7–9 times normal). Several recent studies suggest that aspiration of a breast macrocyst increases the risk of breast cancer over the next 10 years. Other pathological lesions or clinical features do not appear to have an increased risk of breast cancer.

Diagnosis of benign breast problems

All breast problems are diagnosed by a combination of:

- clinical history and examination
- radiological examination
- fine needle aspiration cytology

known as 'triple assessment'.

Clinical history is taken to elicit whether the patient has developed a lump, nipple discharge retraction or distortion. Breast pain is another common symptom.

Examination should be carried out in a good light to allow a detailed inspection, with arms both raised and by the patient's side. The patient is then reclined and with the hands behind the head, both breasts are palpated with the palms of the hand. The axilla is next examined to feel for lymphadenopathy and finally the supraclavicular fossa is palpated. Although clinical examination is important it needs to be carried out in parallel with both radiological and cytological assessment.

Radiological assessment should be by mammography in women over 35 years of age and ultrasound in younger women with a discrete lump. Mammography will detect 70% of cancers in women under 50 years of age and 90% in women after 50 years of age. Accordingly any discrete lump in a young woman (less than 50 years of age) requires ultrasound assessment as well as mammography.

Ultrasound will distinguish solid from cystic lesions and images the dense breast tissue in young women. If mammography fails to demonstrate a lesion in the presence of a clinically palpable mass, ultrasound is helpful. Ultrasound examination is highly operator dependent.

Fine needle aspiration cytology (FNAC) can be performed either freehand or under ultrasound/mammographic control. The FNAC is performed using a 10 ml syringe and 21 gauge needle. The needle is inserted into the palpable lump or nodularity and suction is applied to the syringe. The needle is passed through the lesion six or seven times in a range of directions with suction applied to obtain a representative sample of cells.

The suction is then released and the needle withdrawn from the breast. The syringe is disconnected from the needle and air sucked into the syringe which is then used to blow cells out of the needle onto microscope slides which are fixed according to the local protocol (i.e. air dried or alcohol/formalin fixative).

Most centres will now have a cytopathologist present in the breast clinic to provide immediate reporting of the slides. Cytology is coded from 1 (inadequate: insufficient cells detected) up to 5 (malignant). Benign lesions should produce benign epithelial cells (C2) and cytology has a sensitivity and specificity each in excess of 96%. Despite this it is normal to repeat the cytology on discrete benign lesions in the breast around 6–8 weeks later. FNAC should be carried out after radiological imaging since cytology may affect mammographic appearances. FNAC is extremely sensitive (98%: range 80–99%) and specific (98%: range 95–99%).

If cytology is inadequate or a tissue diagnosis is required prior to surgery, a core biopsy is performed. Core biopsy aims to remove a piece of breast tissue for histopathological examination. Most often a biopsy gun is used which allows one hand to fix the lesion and the other to fire the gun. In impalpable screen-detected lesions, stereotactic core biopsy (directed by ultrasound or mammography) is used to obtain a diagnosis.

Local anaesthesia is necessary (1% lignocaine with 1/250 000 adrenaline) and is infiltrated into the skin and down to and around the lesion. A small incision is made with a no. 15 blade and the lesion approached at an angle of approximately 45° to the breast to minimise the chance of damaging underlying structures in the chest. Once anaesthesia is established, the lesion is fixed between fingers and thumb and the needle is introduced through the skin and breast until its tip rests on the lesion. The gun is then fired and then withdrawn, allowing the core of tissue to be removed from the gun and placed in formalin. Usually this is repeated around four times. Following the procedure, firm pressure should be applied to prevent a haematoma developing.

A report on the core biopsy should be ready in 48–96 hours. If the biopsy is for microcalcification, the specimens can be subjected to radiological examination (prior to insertion in formalin) to confirm that representative microcalcification has been obtained.

If doubt still remains after triple assessment, formal diagnostic surgical biopsy may be necessary.

BREAST LUMPS/NODULARITY

Many women present with a breast lump which may be discrete or diffuse. Localised benign lumps require investigation by 'triple assessment'. This should exclude malignancy and also determine if the lump is localised radiologically.

Common causes of dominant lumps include fibroadenoma (15–35 years of age), breast macrocysts (30–60 years of age) and periductal mastitis (35–55 years of age).

If a lump is not visible by mammogram or ultrasound and benign cells are found on cytological examination it can be assumed the area is thickened nodular breast tissue. However, if the lump is discrete, cytology still needs to be repeated on at least two separate occasions and if any doubt remains, a thick needle (core cut) biopsy may be required.

Fibroadenoma (disorder)

There are four types of fibroadenoma:

● common

● juvenile

● giant (size greater than 5 cm) or

● phylloides.

Fibroadenomas develop from a lobule of the breast whereas cancers arise from a single cell, account for 10–12% of all palpable symptomatic lumps and show hormonal dependence like the rest of normal breast tissue, lactating during pregnancy and involuting during the perimenopausal period. Fibroadenomas are smooth, well-defined mobile lumps which predominantly occur in young, nulliparous women but can be induced in postmenopausal women by hormone replacement therapy.

A juvenile fibroadenoma occurs in teenage girls and tends to grow rapidly, often to a large size, whereas the majority of fibroadenomas grow to 2 cm in size and not beyond. Around 10% continue to enlarge and if they reach 5 cm or greater in size, they are classified as a giant fibroadenoma (disease). Such lesions occur more commonly in West Indian and Asian women. Phylloides tumours are distinct separate pathological entities which can behave in either a benign or malignant fashion. Only rarely does metastasis occur but frequently they recur locally which may necessitate a mastectomy.

Fibroadenomas present as a discrete palpable breast lump which is usually mobile, hence its alternative name of 'breast mouse'. Triple assessment is required to confirm the lesion is benign. Around 1% of clinical breast fibroadenomas at age 30 and 5% at age 40 are found to be a small carcinoma upon cytological assessment.

Mammograms may show characteristic coarse calcifications in a fibroadenoma.

Management

Large fibroadenomas over 4 cm in size are removed by surgical excision. However, in smaller lesions, once a definitive diagnosis is obtained, the patient may either have excision or follow-up at three months when cytology should be repeated. Provided cytology remains benign and the lump has not grown in size, it can be left alone. Any increase in size or failure to obtain benign cytology (C2) requires excision of the lump. Complex fibroadenomas which exhibit unusual pathological changes (e.g. cystic change or ductal hyperplasia) have a slightly increased risk of malignancy but otherwise breast cancer is not more likely to develop in a fibroadenoma or a breast containing a fibroadenoma.

Breast macrocysts

Around 7% of women in the Western world present with a breast cyst, usually between 35 and 50 years of age. Cysts present with a smooth discrete breast lump. Around half of the women have only one cyst in their lifetime, whereas the remainder develop recurrent cysts with 15% developing more than five.

All women over 35 years with cysts require a mammogram as 1–3% will have a coincidental cancer in one or other breast. Management of cysts is by aspiration of cyst fluid to dryness by a 21 gauge needle. Typically green or straw-coloured fluid is found on aspiration. Provided the cyst fluid is not bloodstained cytological assessment is unnecessary. Only four out of 10 000 cytological cyst smears will be graded malignant and three out of the four will be falsely positive! After the cyst has been aspirated the breast should be reexamined to ensure there is no residual mass. If a mass is present it requires investigation with cytology and ultrasound. Patients should be reviewed after 10–12 weeks to ensure the cyst has not refilled. Rapidly refilling cysts may require excision, as there is an association between repeated and rapidly refilling cysts and malignancy.

Women with breast cysts have an increased risk of breast cancer (2–4 times normal) and thus require careful assessment. They should be encouraged to have any breast lump assessed and aspirated. In addition, they should undergo mammography at presentation to exclude an underlying cancer.

BREAST INFECTION

A marked decline in lactational breast abscesses or infection means the most common cause is now periductal mastitis or non-lactating abscesses. In general, antibiotics should be given early in breast infections to prevent abscess formation. When abscess formation does occur, it is best dealt with by aspiration of pus and antibiotic therapy.

Lactating breast infection

Improved maternal and infant hygiene has decreased the incidence of this disorder, together with earlier treatment with appropriate antibiotics active against *Staphylococcus aureus*, so it is rarely seen nowadays.

Infection is believed to occur with a break in the skin (especially a cracked nipple) which allows bacteria to enter the breast through the nipple crack. Drainage of ducts in infection is poor and breast-feeding should be continued along with antibiotic therapy.

Women who are breast feeding present with pain, swelling and tenderness. There is usually erythema of the skin and in later stages a fluctuant mass with overlying, red skin is present. Systemic toxicity (e.g. pyrexia, tachycardia) is often present. Breast feeding can continue from the unaffected breast.

Lactating infection should be treated immediately with flucloxacillin 500 mg four times a day (erythromycin if penicillin allergy). Tetracycline and ciprofloxacin enter breast milk and may harm the child, so they should not be used. If fluctuation is present the lump/abscess should be aspirated to remove pus. Often 3–4 aspirations are needed to settle the abscess and antibiotics must be continued throughout until the abscess has settled. If the overlying skin is thinned or necrotic, the abscess can be drained by a stab incision under local anaesthetic (EMLA) cream applied for one hour. This allows the women to continue breast feeding whereas general anaesthetic drainage does not. If doubt exists about the presence of pus, ultrasound examination may help guide aspiration.

Non-lactating breast infection

Periareolar infection affects young women in the mid-30s age range and is more common in cigarette smokers. It is caused by periductal mastitis with underlying active inflammation around non-dilated ducts. Only later do the lactiferous ducts dilate. Smoking appears to induce damage to lactiferous ducts which allows bacteria (including anaerobes) to invade the damaged area and set up an infection/abscess.

Women may present with:

- a subareolar abscess
- periareolar tender mass (with or without inflammation) or
- mammillary fistulas.

The underlying bacterial cause is usually anaerobic or facultative anaerobes (e.g. bacteroides or enterococci) although occasionally *Staphylococcus aureus* is implicated.

Periareolar inflammation should be treated with antibiotics (co-amoxiclav or erythromycin and metronidazole) and aspiration (if a mass fails to resolve).

Antibiotics always relieve the erythema within seven days and if it persists, there may be an underlying inflammatory cancer. If the infection is recurrent, it may be necessary to excise the ducts beneath the nipple (total duct excision) under prophylactic antibiotic cover. Excision of the ducts prevents recurrent infections developing, presumably because the ducts harbour the bacteria responsible for the recurrent infections. Avoidance of incision and drainage of abscesses by early antibiotic therapy prevent the development of mammillary fistulas.

Recurrent abscesses can be managed by conservative aspiration but more often the pain and inflammation associated with the condition require surgical drainage under general anaesthesia.

Surgical management of breast abscesses

In many women who present early with erythema and pain in the breast (cellulitic phase), abscess formation can be prevented by antibiotic use. Often aspiration of small pockets of pus combined with antibiotic therapy will allow outpatient treatment of early abscess formation without the need for formal surgical drainage. Surgery in these early phases is unnecessary. Needle aspiration of the centre of the cellulitic area will determine whether pus has been formed and repeated needle aspiration together with prolonged (2–3 weeks) antibiotic therapy will resolve the infection.

In those abscesses where the overlying skin is normal EMLA cream should be left *in situ* for one hour. The abscess is then aspirated to dryness with a 19 gauge needle and syringe. Where the skin overlying the abscess is thinned or necrotic a small incision with a no. 15 blade is made over the point of maximum fluctuation or the necrotic skin excised and the abscess cavity irrigated, initially with anaesthetic solution and then with saline.

Very few abscesses now need drainage under general anaesthetic. Patients with recurrent periareolar sepsis require an operation to excise the diseased duct or ducts (i.e. microdochectomy or total duct excision) after settling any sepsis with antibiotics.

Mammillary fistulas

This usually presents as a discharging fistula at the skin junction of the areola and breast skin. There is a communication between the lactiferous ducts in the subareolar region and the areolar/breast skin junction. The underlying cause is periductal mastitis and the fistula is often preceded by incision and drainage of an abscess, spontaneous discharge of a periareolar inflammatory mass or biopsy of an area of periductal mastitis.

In around 50% of cases there is an associated transverse nipple retraction. The majority (90%) of women are heavy smokers and have usually had recurrent episodes of either abscess formation or periareolar inflammation.

The fistula is best treated by surgical excision through either a periareolar incision (to include the skin opening around the fistula) or a transverse radial incision which includes the nipple duct involved and the fistula. A periareolar incision requires sharp dissection of the underlying ducts from the back of the nipple, as in total duct excision, to prevent recurrent disease. If the operation is carried out under prophylactic antibiotic cover, primary closure can be performed but if not, the cavity should be left open to granulate.

Rare conditions: granulomatous mastitis

Some people consider this condition a variant of periductal mastitis. Young women (usually within two years of childbirth) are affected by either a hard breast mass (which mimics cancer) or recurrent breast abscesses. Bacteria are not found in the pus but histology shows granulomatous (non-caseating) change in lobules together with microabscesses. Once a diagnosis has been made conservative treatment is necessary, as the condition tends to recur aggressively over a period of approximately one year before it burns itself out. It is important to exclude tuberculosis (by culture and histopathology) and sarcoid (by Kveim test and serum ACE inhibitor levels). Corticosteroids have been advocated but are rarely necessary. In an exacerbation or during active disease a raised ESR, CRP or WBC may often be seen. When the presentation is with a hard mass, excision of the mass may be necessary to exclude carcinoma but the diagnosis can often be made by corecut biopsy under local anaesthetic in the outpatient department.

When abscesses occur they should be drained and packed. They are often acutely painful and require adequate draining and exploration under general anaesthetic to allow resolution. The condition resolves spontaneously in most cases.

FAT NECROSIS

Fat necrosis is generally thought to be secondary to trauma but a history of trauma is present in only about half of all patients. It commonly occurs after road traffic accidents as a result of seatbelt trauma to the breast or after a fall onto the breast. It is usually associated with bruising at the time of the injury.

It can be a clinical problem because it is difficult to distinguish between a cancer and fat necrosis on physical examination and mammography. There is often a mass in the breast which is firm, ill defined and poorly mobile, associated with skin retraction or thickening. It is most common in the subareolar region and diagnosis is made by cytological assessment, which often shows fatty granulomata. The patient seen late after traumatic fat necrosis may present with a fat cyst in the breast.

Management

One should be aware that fat necrosis does not resolve for up to three months in some cases and if suspicion of malignancy persists open surgical biopsy is required. In doubt, however, resolution can often be made by cytology or core biopsy of the lesion.

NIPPLE PROBLEMS

Discharge

Three questions need to be asked of patients who present with nipple discharge (see Figure 27.1).

- Is it spontaneous or expressed?
- Is it unilateral or bilateral?
- Is it single duct or multiple ducts?

The presence of expressed coloured multiple duct fluid is a manifestation of breast secretions which are physiological and occur in 70% of premenopausal and 40% of postmenopausal women. Moreover, nipple secretion is not associated with underlying breast cancer but is associated with cigarette smoking in parous women.

Bloody nipple discharge, which is single duct and spontaneous, or serosanguinous nipple discharge is often the manifestation of either an intraduct papilloma or epithelial hyperplasia in the breast.

Nipple discharge in women under 35 years of age needs to be investigated only if it is bloodstained or serosanguinous and this is usually best done by microdochectomy and removal of the affected duct.

In women over 35 years of age with bloody or serosanguinous discharge, mammography is the first investigation of choice. Either microdochectomy or total duct excision is indicated to relieve symptoms and produce a diagnosis.

Intraduct papillomas often present with a small palpable mass at the edge of the areola, which on pressure causes duct discharge. This is usually the papilloma itself which can in some cases be multiple. Although cytology has been used in the setting of bloody nipple discharge, it has a low diagnostic rate. Surgical excision of a duct can be performed through a very small circumareolar incision, as can total duct excision. These are very satisfactory operations but the patient needs to be warned of possible risks of loss of nipple sensation and on occasion some skin necrosis across the tip of the nipple.

Ductal carcinoma *in situ* is another potential cause of bloody nipple discharge but this is covered in the chapter on breast carcinoma.

Retraction

Nipple retraction is the description used when part of the nipple is pulled in, compared to nipple inversion when the whole of the nipple promontory is pulled in, as seen in duct ectasia.

Around 10–20% of women have some nipple inversion/retraction from the time of breast development (congenital). Retraction/inversion can also be acquired and the most common cause of acquired disease is duct ectasia/periductal mastitis, but malignancy needs to be excluded carefully.

If a woman over 35 years of age acquires nipple inversion/retraction she should be investigated by mammography. In the absence of a mass and normal mammograms, surgery is contraindicated. The management of a mass is as indicated previously by triple assessment.

Cosmetic operations to correct nipple inversions are problematic and best avoided.

Eczema/Paget's disease

Whereas nipple eczema is an eczematous change which involves the areola but does not spread onto the nipple promontory, Paget's disease always starts on the promontory and spreads outwards onto the areola.

Nipple eczema should be treated by 0.5–1% hydrocortisone cream under an occlusive dressing and care should be taken to wear cotton undergarments washed in hypoallergenic powder.

Paget's disease should be biopsied under local anaesthetic by either punch biopsy or excision of an elliptical portion of abnormal skin.

A mammogram is necessary in Paget's disease and in women with an accompanying mass lesion as underlying invasive cancer is found in over 80% of cases.

BREAST PAIN

Breast pain (mastalgia) is common, occurs in 70% of pre-menopausal women and can be divided into three groups:

- cyclical (70%),
- non-cyclical (15%) and
- chest wall pain (15%).

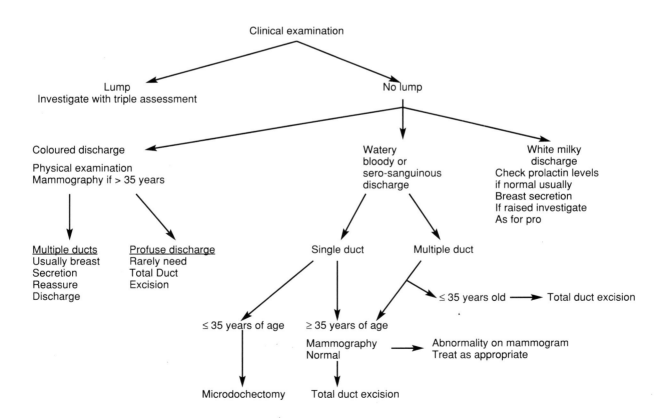

Figure 27.1 Management of nipple discharge.

Cyclical breast pain

Cyclical breast pain is worse before menstruation and is often associated with bilateral upper outer quadrant nodularity. In cases of doubt, the easiest way to determine whether or not the pain is cyclical is to ask the woman to fill out a breast pain chart, which on her return will allow cyclicity to be determined. Many women present with breast pain because they are worried about breast cancer and these women should be reassured, provided clinical examination is normal, and told that 30% of breast pain resolves spontaneously within three months of onset. Breast pain should be treated if it lasts for more than seven days of a month and is causing the woman distress or affects her lifestyle. Features such as being unable to hug her children or lie prone because of the pain warrant treatment. As 30% of breast pain settles spontaneously, she should be given a breast pain chart and encouraged to wear an exercise support bra. An explanation of how to fill out a breast pain chart should be given and the patient reviewed in two months. If she is over the age of 35 she should be sent for a mammogram at presentation. If the pain persists on review, consider instituting treatment.

In women with severe cyclical breast pain lasting for more than 14 days of the month, who have tried previous treatment, it may be necessary to institute treatment at the first clinic visit but this should be discussed with the patient herself. There is little point in giving a woman with severe breast pain evening primrose oil as first-line treatment, as it takes a minimum of four months to work and these women require quicker relief of pain. With this exception, the first-line treatment for the average woman with mild to moderate breast pain is evening primrose oil as it has low toxicity. A dose of Efamast 80 mg bd. (or evening primrose oil 3g/day) is used and the patient warned that 2% of women do get mild nausea, but otherwise there are few side effects. Other agents which can be used as second-line therapy include danazol, which should be used at a low dose, e.g. 200 mg a day for a month followed by 100 mg a day for two months. With a dose of 100 mg a day the side-effect profile of Danazol is low (14%). At 600 mg a day and above, there is weight gain, amenorrhoea, hirsutism and a reduction in breast size in up to 25% of women, which is dose related. Bromocriptine and tamoxifen are also useful agents, but they should only be prescribed after other agents have failed.

Non-cyclical mastalgia

Non-cyclical mastalgia is not associated with changes in pain intensity throughout the menstrual cycle and responds less well to drugs compared to cyclical mastalgia. It is often confused with chest wall pain and is important to differentiate between the two. Non-cyclical mastalgia tends to be in the upper outer quadrant or behind the nipple and is not associated with an obvious trigger spot. Treatment of non-cyclical mastalgia is the same as that of cyclical mastalgia, but women should be warned that the response rates are not as good.

Chest wall pain

Chest wall pain is associated with pain over the medial costal cartilages or the lateral ribs in the anterior axillary line. In the case of lateral rib pain, it is often best elicited by rolling the patient on to her side to drop the breast away from the point of the pain. It is best treated by either local injection with lignocaine and depomedrone (as two-thirds of patients get relief) or local NSAID ointment applied daily. Very rarely, women who have an area in the breast which causes pain on pressure may need excision of this area, but they should have had at least three repeat visits to the clinic and have seen a consultant before they are listed for excision of a trigger area.

Drug treatment for mastalgia should not last more than six months and the drug should then be discontinued to see if the symptoms recur. In 50% of patients the symptoms will recur, but some will not require further therapy as the pain is milder. The woman with severe recurrent mastalgia can be put back onto her original therapy or an alternative if the initial response has been poor. There is no evidence that diuretics, pyridoxine (vitamin B_6) or antibiotics benefit mastalgia.

GYNAECOMASTIA

The enlargement of the ductal and stromal tissue of the male breast is known as gynaecomastia and ranges from a palpable retroareolar nubbin of tissue to grade II gynaecomastia in which breast development is similar to that seen in a female breast. Clinically it presents at puberty and in old age.

At puberty some 30–70% boys develop some breast enlargement but the majority spontaneously resolve within two years. Occasionally the enlargement is sufficient to cause embarrassment in changing rooms and a mastectomy is indicated which can either be performed using liposuction or via a circumareolar incision. It is important to leave some tissue attached to the undersurface of the areola and some fat on the skin to prevent an unsightly depression in the anterior chest wall remaining. Excision of gynaecomastia is an entirely cosmetic operation and the possibility of a less than ideal end result should be clearly discussed and recorded in the patient notes.

Adult gynaecomastia

Around 50% of males aged 50 have adult gynaecomastia. Usually there is no endocrine abnormality although drugs, cirrhosis, lung and testicular tumours and hypogonadism (e.g. Klinefelter's syndrome) can all cause gynaecomastia. It is believed that an alteration in the circulating ratio of androgens to oestrogens leads to a relative increase in oestrogen, allowing breast development.

Usually breast development is soft, concentric and behind the nipple. If discrete lumps peripheral to the nipple develop, they should be investigated by FNAC and mammography.

Investigations of unilateral/bilateral gynaecomastia should include a careful drug history, liver, renal and thyroid function tests and serum prolactin levels.

The drugs that most commonly cause gynaecomastia are cimetidine, digoxin, oestrogens (stilboestrol) and spironolactone.

Treatment of an underlying cause (i.e. altering the drugs) will resolve the gynaecomastia.

In general bilateral gynaecomastia is best treated conservatively, although liposuction can be a useful alternative treatment.

OTHER BENIGN CONDITIONS

In breastfeeding women, a cystic lesion containing breast milk may present as a lump. It can be aspirated which provides a diagnosis and a cure.

Occasionally a firm subcutaneous band associated with skin changes and tenderness can occur, usually in the inframammary area. This is superficial thrombophlebitis (Mondor's disease). It usually resolves spontaneously.

OPERATIVE SURGERY

Drainage of a breast abscess

Indications

When the abscess does not respond to antibiotic therapy and aspiration surgical drainage is required.

Patient preparation

For lactating breast abscesses, flucloxacillin 500 mg qds is given to eradicate *Staphylococcus aureus*. For non-lactating breast abscesses, broad-spectrum antibiotics such as co-amoxiclav which cover *Staph. aureus* and anaerobe bacteria are necessary. Antibiotics help speed recovery after abscess drainage. The patient should be starved.

Anaesthesia and positioning

General anaesthetic is necessary for incision and drainage in view of the painful nature of a procedure where loculi in the breast need to be broken down. The patient is anaesthetised and laid supine on the operating table. The area is prepped with poridone-iodine.

Procedure (see Figure 27.2)

It is useful to aspirate the abscess over the area of maximum tenderness prior to making an incision. A transverse incision is made over the area of maximum tenderness if the lesion is peripheral in the breast but a circumareolar incision is used if the abscess is sub-areolar.

Most abscesses are multilocular and the loculi need to be ruptured with a finger to allow adequate drainage. Following drainage, the resultant cavity is packed with proflavine gauze and the wound left open. The packing is changed daily and the patient discharged home as soon as the packing can be changed under oral analgesia.

Healing usually occurs within four weeks and often produces little scarring.

An alternative approach is to pack the wound and place a subcuticular suture in the wound. The suture is left loose and packing carried out for 2–3 days. On the third or fourth day, under antibiotic cover, the pack is removed and the subcuticular suture pulled tight and tied. The wound will usually heal well by this stage.

Reduction mammoplasty

Indications

For some women, the size of their breasts, or their perception of the size of their breasts, makes them seek reduction mammoplasty. Reasons for requesting reduction mammoplasty are both physical and psychological. Large weighty breasts can cause physical discomfort, with back and neck pain and shoulder pain from the pressure of bra straps. The breasts may be uncomfortable or even painful, particularly on exercise, and the skin under the inframammary fold may be subject to chronic dampness and irritation. From a psychological standpoint, excessively large breasts can be socially troublesome as an unwelcome focus of attention and comment. The woman with very large breasts may be greatly embarrassed by her assumption that she is in this way abnormal.

Many patients request reduction mammoplasty for psychological as well as physical reasons. Preoperative psychological assessment can be an extremely useful procedure in which the patient's expectations of surgery and outcome can be investigated and if necessary re-set to reality. This assessment is particularly useful for women whose perception of their own breasts may be unrealistic or who for some reason may find their breasts unattractive or an irrelevant part of their own gender identity.

Surgical technique of reduction mammoplasty

Reduction mammoplasty involves the reduction of a hemispherical breast into a smaller hemisphere, whilst maintaining the proportionate position of the nipple, and resecting in such a way that bilateral symmetry is achieved. This is a complex and technically demanding procedure. Coupled with the goal of weight and volume reduction is the need to achieve aesthetic enhancement of the breasts. In recent years techniques of breast reduction have been refined and greater importance is now placed on aesthetic as

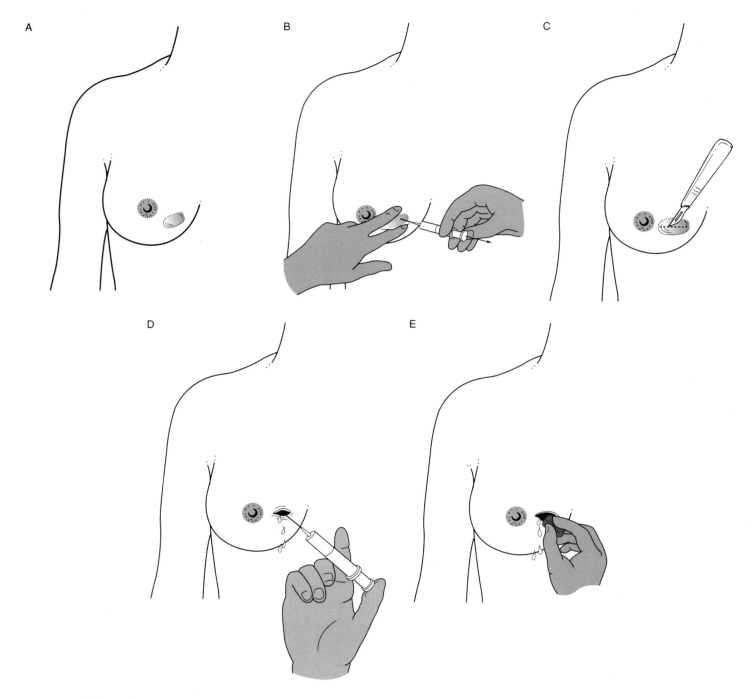

Figure 27.2 Drainage of a breast abscess.

well as physiological function than previously. A number of techniques has been developed to fill these demands, the two most difficult problems being the preservation of the blood supply to the nipple areola complex, which must be moved significant distances across the breast to a new position, and shaping of the new breast in a smaller, aesthetic and symmetrical way. Most modern techniques depend upon the concept of a deepithelialised dermal pedicle to maintain the blood supply to the nipple and a trilobed resection with a resulting T closure at the inframammary fold. Preoperative planning and marking is mandatory and unplanned resection to be avoided. Current developments are addressing efforts to limit the pattern and extent of scarring, to preserve sensation and enhance aesthetic shape and to preserve the physiological function of lactation.

The forerunner of most commonly used resections was the McKissock technique. The nipple is kept alive on a vertical pedicle acting as a bridge for the blood supply. Modifications and developments of this technique have been published.

All patients must undergo adequate preoperative counselling (Box 27.1).

Box 27.1 Counselling of patients

The following important points must be discussed with a patient as part of the information and consent process:

Technique and aims of surgery
Extent and placement of scars
Risk of poor scarring and possible keloid formation
Possible asymmetry
Positioning of the nipples
Sensory nipple loss
Infection, possible wound breakdown and prolonged time to heal
Use of drains and risk of haematoma
Risk of infection
Rare risk of perfusion failure to nipples
Subsequent change in shape of the breasts which may cause modest movement of the scars
Risk for further breast type surgery, for example, in subsequent pregnancy

---

Planning the operation is the most important step in the procedure. This is done with the patient standing or sitting up with markings using an indelible pen to precisely position the incisions on the breasts and chest wall.

A wide variety of techniques has been developed to achieve reduction mammoplasty but the most significant advances have been made in the last two decades. The choice of technique is determined by the extent of hypertrophy, the cosmetic goal desired and the presence of risk factors for complications, in particular whether the patient is a smoker or is morbidly obese. Overriding these factors are the skill and experience of the surgeon.

It is not the purpose of this description to provide a series of alternative procedures, each with its indications for technique and complications. One basic reliable technique will be described, but the surgeon must be aware that although this technique has a broad spectrum of application, it will not be the appropriate procedure in every case. Reduction mammoplasty is an operation which should be left in the hands of specialist breast surgeons and plastic surgeons and should not be undertaken infrequently or lightly by the general surgeon.

The vertical dermal pedicle technique for breast reduction was described by McKissock. In this method the nipple and areola are transposed superiorly on a vertical dermal pedicle, based superiorly and inferiorly. The modification of this technique, utilising the inferior pedicle, doing away with the superior pedicle and basing the nipple areola complex (NAC) on a central pyramidal breast mound, is in widespread use.

Patient preparation

Measurements are carried out with the patient in a standing position. The vertical lines of the keyhole should subtend an acute angle (Figure 27.3A). The planned new position of the NAC should be 20–22 cm from the sternal notch and similarly from the mid-clavicular line in the meridian of each breast. The pyramidal central and inferior pedicle encompasses a 2 cm circumferential area around the NAC and extends inferiorly, widening to a base on the inframammary fold.

Prophylactic pre- and postoperative antibiotics should be used to reduce the incidence of infection.

Anaesthesia and positioning

The patient is positioned under general anaesthesia slightly head elevated with the hands under the hips, elbows flexed and shoulders slightly abducted.

Procedure

- The skin is deepithelialised around the NAC and carried downwards over the pyramidal dermal flap, creating a wide-based pyramid (Figure 27.4).

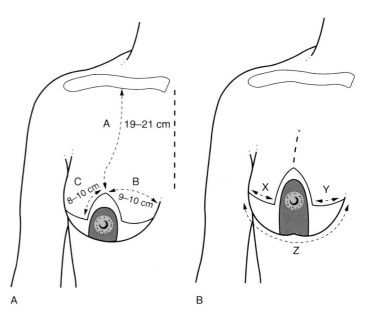

Figure 27.3A The patient is marked in the standing position. The meridian is drawn through the mid-clavicular line down to the position of the nipple and the upper margin of resection marked at a point 19–21 cm down the meridian (A). This should be at a point approximately 9–10 cm from the midline (B). Two equal sides of an open triangle are drawn, 8–10 cm long, which will become the vertical limb of the inverted T scar (C). **B.** The skin markings applied before reduction mammoplasty using an inferior central pedicle technique. The horizontal resection lines on the breast (X, Y) should be equal to the inframammary crease length (Z), as they will constitute the new inframammary fold scar. The area to be de-epitheliased from around and inferior to the nipple is marked with cross-hatching.

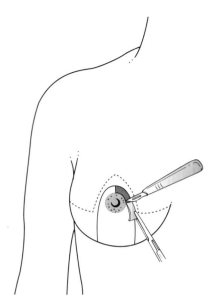

Figure 27.4 The operative sequence commences with the de epithelialisation of the pedicle bearing the NAC. Deepithelialisation carefully preserves all the marked skin of the nipple and areola, but removes the epithelium from around it and down to the inframammary fold.

- Following safe construction of the pyramid with the NAC perfused upon it, resection of lateral, medial and superior skin and glandular tissue is achieved by sharp or diathermy resection, leaving the upper skin flaps no less than 2 cm thick and taking care not to damage conserved skin (Figure 27.5).

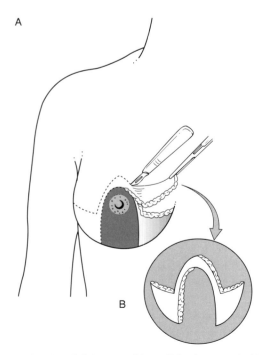

Figure 27.5 After deepithelialisation of the pedicle, the upper incision is taken through the marked skin lines and breast tissue and skin resected in a hoop shape. The resected tissue may be removed in one piece, as shown in the inset.

- Haemostasis must be meticulous, particularly as the redundant tissue is removed from the pectoralis fascia.

- The pyramidal mound is sutured into the medial half of the breast onto the pectoralis fascia, to fill the medial pole of the breast and to reconstitute the cleavage of the bustline. Once this is in position, the superior breast flaps are draped over the pyramid and sutured into position with Vicryl. A 14 French gauge drain is introduced on each side.

- The patient is now elevated head-up on the table and the final position for the NAC on each side can be determined by measuring and marking over the vertical scar upper position. The circle is cut and the NAC pulled through, to suture it into its new position using absorbable sutures such as 2/0 Vicryl (Figure 27.6).

- The skin is approximated using absorbable sutures such as 3/0 and 4/0 Monocryl and the wounds covered with tapes.

- If the measurement of the lines of resection preoperatively has been accurate, the incision, particularly at the T intersection, should not be under undue tension. Light dressings can be applied but it is not standard practice to use a bra for the first 48 hours, because of excessive pressure that it may exert upon the NAC and the skin flaps. A bra may be worn after 72 hours provided it is not constricting.

Postoperative care

Postoperatively the patient should be kept warm and well hydrated. The urine output should be measured and haemoglobin estimated the day following surgery. Blood transfusion is rarely required. Each NAC must be carefully observed to ensure perfusion by capillary refill. Any evidence of significant haematoma must be followed by a return to theatre and exploration of the breast. Pressure dressings should never be used as they will often lead to NAC or flap necrosis.

Complications

Preoperative and postoperative photographs of individual patients are essential. Breast reduction is associated with a number of complications which can be divided into errors of planning, errors of surgery and general postoperative complications. Imperative for a successful aesthetic outcome is accurate preoperative planning and marking to ensure adequate and symmetrical resection and planned placement of the nipple. The most common error of planning is to place the nipple too high. Inadequate skin or gland resection may result in a breast with a flattened inferior contour, whilst over-resection of skin or gland may make it difficult to produce a breast of appropriate size or shape. Excessive skin resection with skin tension on the wounds will result in breakdown of wounds and subsequent delayed scar healing. Disparate reduction of both breasts may result in asymmetry.

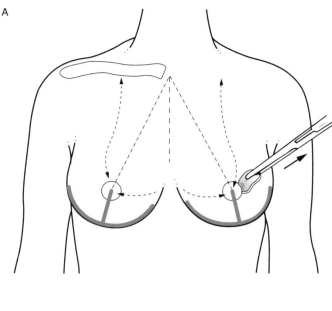

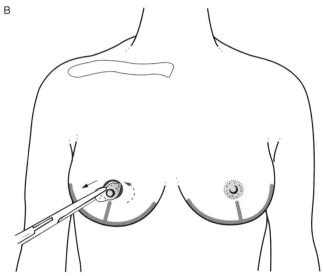

Figure 27.6 A After the upper skin flaps are joined together by layer suturing to create the inverted T scars, the patient is sat up on the operating table and the new position of the nipple areola complex (NAC) marked by a process of triangulation from the sternal notch of the manubrium and from the midline. On the left breast in **A**, the circular portion of skin overlying the new nipple areola position is shown having been circumcised and in the process of removal. **B.** The right NAC is brought through the excised skin disc and the left breast shows the NAC sutured into its new position. Great care must be taken whilst removing the skin disc not in any way to damage the underlying NAC or its pedicle.

Compromise of the NAC can occur from an overly narrow, inferiorly based dermoglandular pedicle or by pressure from haematoma or dressings. Devascularisation of skin through excessive resection or excessive skin tension may lead to ischaemia within the breast, skin flap necrosis and nipple areola loss or injury. Sinus formation may occur through the scars. It is important, however, to recognise that minor skin flap necrosis is not uncommon, particularly at the junction of skin closure of inverted T-shaped scars.

Infection after reduction mammoplasty is quite rare. Most surgeons do not generally employ prophylactic antibiotics. Postoperative bleeding or haematoma is also uncommon but is occasionally encountered. Drains are usually routinely employed, but this is not universally the case.

The most common postoperative complaint is of unfavourable or hypertrophic scarring. In most cases scarring generally fades with time but there are exceptions, especially where there has been marked tissue loss, where scars remain thick, wide, ugly and irregular. Tension on scars can be reduced by using a multilayered technique of suture closure. The application of dressing strips to the scars for several weeks can also reduce scar hypertrophy, in cases where healing proceeds easily and without complications. Most patients would expect to have well-healed breasts four weeks from the time of surgery with subsequent development of final shape within 2–3 months after surgery. Nipple sensation, if lost, may return slowly over several months. Gross breast tissue loss is extremely rare.

FURTHER READING

Breast Surgeons Group of the British Association of Surgical Oncology. Guidelines for surgeons in the management of symptomatic breast disease in the United Kingdom. *Eur J Surg Oncol* 1995; **21**(suppl A):1–13

Bundred NJ, Dixon JM, Chetty U, Forest APM. Mammillary fistula. *Br J Surg* 1987; **74**:466–468

Dixon JM. Breast infection. In: Dixon JM, Mansel RE, eds. *ABC of Breast Diseases*. London: BMJ Books, 1996

Hughes LE, Mansel RE, Webster DJT, eds. *Benign Disorders and Diseases of the Breast*. London: WB Saunders, 2000

McKissock PK. Reduction mammoplasty. *Ann Plast Surg* 1979; **2**:321

Ribiero L. A new technique for reduction mammoplasty. *Plast Reconst Surg* 1975; **55**(3):330–334

Robbins TH. A reduction mammoplasty with the areola-nipple based on an inferior dermal pedicle. *Plast Reconst Surg* 1977; **59**(1):64–67

Welch M, Durrant O, Gonzales J et al. Microdochectomy for discharge from a single lactiferous duct. *Br J Surg* 1996; **77**:1213–1214

Wilkinson S, Forrest APM. Fibroadenoma of the breast. *Br J Surg* 1985; **72**:838–840

28

Management of breast cancer

Steven D. Heys, Anthony K. Ah-See

SURGICAL MANAGEMENT

The surgical management of patients with breast cancer is a component of the multidisciplinary approach which is necessary to ensure that loco-regional recurrence is minimised and the best possible patient survival is achieved. Planning of definitive treatment for patients with breast cancer requires the expertise of the surgical oncologist, medical and clinical oncologists, together with contributions from all other contributing disciplines (e.g. cytologist, pathologist, radiographer, radiologist, reconstructive surgeon, nurse counsellor and psychologist). The patient (and their partner) require the provision of adequate information and the opportunity to take part in discussions about treatment options.

Surgical management, undertaken as part of this multidisciplinary approach to the treatment of patients with breast cancer, has the following aims:

- Firstly, to achieve local control of cancer in the breast, thus preventing local progression of disease and minimising the risk of local recurrence in the breast (after conservation) or chest wall (after mastectomy) to the minimum possible.

- Secondly, to achieve control of cancer in the regional tumour-draining lymph nodes in the axilla, infraclavicular and internal thoracic areas (either with surgery alone or in combination with radiotherapy).

- Thirdly, to gain prognostic information regarding the patient's likelihood of having micrometastatic disease which is based on the involvement of the axillary lymph nodes with tumour, and on the histological characteristics of the primary tumour in the breast). This information will influence the decisions as to whether adjuvant treatments are also required, which reduce the risk of subsequent disease relapse.

Surgical treatment of invasive operable breast cancer

Surgery to the primary tumour in the breast

Surgery is the oldest means of treating breast cancer and it is interesting to note that treatment for breast cancer dates back more than 3000 years. In 200 AD the Greek physician Galen, whose philosophy dominated medical practice at that time, recommended breast conservation surgery, believing that surgical removal of the tumour itself together with a healthy margin of normal breast tissue was adequate treatment. Over ensuing years medical knowledge suggested that cancer cells spread in a centrifugal pattern which was from the primary tumour to regional draining lymph nodes, and then to the vascular system and hence distant metastatic sites. This erroneous understanding of tumour biology influenced surgical practice for many years.

At the beginning of the 1900s, William Halsted (Johns Hopkins Medical School, Boston, MA, USA) recommended that a 'radical mastectomy', entailing removal of the breast, the underlying pectoral muscles and an axillary clearance, should be performed if adequate control of cancer was to be achieved. However, many other surgeons also reported that less radical surgery was associated with equally good results, in terms of control of the disease locally in the breast and overall patient survival. As a result of the many randomised controlled trials that have been carried out in recent years it is now accepted that patients with breast cancer who undergo breast-conserving surgery have as good a survival as those who undergo mastectomy.

Many operations have been devised, some discarded and others rediscovered. However, the surgical options (Table 28.1) for the treatment of the primary tumour in the breast are as follows:

- Breast Conservation – either lumpectomy (also called wide local excision), segmentectomy or quadrentectomy, all aiming to provide local control of disease but with a cosmetically acceptable residual breast, or

- Mastectomy.

Breast-conserving surgery

If breast conservation surgery is to be undertaken, a key issue to be considered is the concept of the *multifocality* and *multicentricity* of breast cancers. Although there are several definitions of these terms, it is commonly accepted that multifocality refers to the presence of multiple areas of malignancy in close proximity to, and in the same quadrant as, the primary tumour. In contrast, multicentricity refers to the presence of cancer in other quadrants of the same breast or at least 5 cm away from the primary tumour. Therefore, it is important to consider whether or not breast

Table 28.1 Operative procedures for breast conservation surgery

Type of surgery	Procedure
Lumpectomy (wide local excision)	Excision of the tumour with a clear margin of healthy tissue of greater than 1 mm
Segmentectomy	Excision of the tumour, including tissue from the nipple out to the periphery and with a 1 cm macroscopic clearance
Quadrantectomy	Excision of the tumour, including tissue from the nipple out to the periphery, with a 2–3 cm macroscopic clearance

(Adapted from Scottish Intercollegiate Guidelines Network, 1998; SIGN Publication Number 29, SIGN Secretariat, Royal College of Physicians, Edinburgh).

conservation will result in malignant disease (invasive or *in situ*) being left behind in the residual breast, which can result in local recurrence or a second primary appearing in the conserved breast.

In order to address the issue, several studies have examined how often multifocality and multicentricity can occur in a breast containing an invasive cancer. The following points should be considered:

- Multicentricity probably occurs in 25% of patients with breast cancer, with up to 10% of the second lesions being invasive cancers (the remainder being *in situ* cancer)

- Multicentricity is most likely to occur if the first tumour is in the retro-areolar region (occurring in up to 75% of cases)

- Multicentricity is more likely with larger primary tumours

- The risk of other cancer (invasive or non-invasive) at a distance of one cm or more away from the primary tumour may be as high as 40%

- At a distance of three cm or more away from the primary tumour, this risk is reduced to approximately 15%, and as the distance increases the risk decreases further.

Randomised controlled trials over the last 30 years, comparing the results of treatment with breast-conserving surgery or mastectomy, have been carried out in both Europe and North America. The two key outcome measures that they have focused on have been local recurrence of disease and overall patient survival. Patients included in these studies have usually had tumours up to four cm in clinical size and have undergone radiotherapy to the breast and tumour bed after breast-conservation surgery. The local recurrence rates and overall patient survivals has been comparable between the two groups of patients, and as a result, the generally accepted indications and contraindications for breast-conservation surgery are shown in Table 28.2.

There are also a number of relative contraindications to breast-conservation surgery because these features are associated with a much higher risk of local recurrence of disease if they are present. These conditions include, tumours with a clinical size of greater than four cm, incomplete excision of tumour, extensive associated ductal carcinoma *in situ* (DCIS), lymphatic and/or vascular invasion. Some have suggested that high histological tumour grade (e.g. Bloom and Richardson grade III) may be a relative contraindication to breast conservation although this is contentious. In addition, patients younger than 35 years of age have an increased risk of local recurrence if breast-conservation surgery

is undertaken, particularly if they have a strong family history with mutations in *BRCA1* and *BRCA2* genes.

ADJUVANT RADIOTHERAPY

If breast conservation surgery is undertaken, adjuvant radiotherapy to the breast, (4500 to 5000 cGy), will reduce significantly the risk of disease recurrence within the breast. This has been demonstrated by several randomised, controlled trials. Estimates of the effectiveness of radiotherapy indicate that the risk of local recurrence is reduced by up to 75% by giving radiotherapy in this adjuvant setting. This treatment is usually given as external beam irradiation to the whole breast. However, some trials have also suggested that a 'boost' to the site of the primary tumour (usually by external beam radiation or less commonly by using an interstitial implant) can reduce further the risk of local recurrence of disease in the breast.

The role of adjuvant radiotherapy to the breast, in reducing local recurrence, if the patient's tumour was small and well differentiated (e.g. less than two cm, grade I or II) is unclear and it has been suggested that radiotherapy may not be necessary for such patients. Currently, randomised, controlled trials are addressing this question and their results are awaited. However, at the present time it is generally recommended that such patients should receive adjuvant radiotherapy to the breast unless they are participating in these trials.

Mastectomy

A total mastectomy is now defined as an operation which results in excision of the whole breast including the overlying skin and nipple/aroela complex. The indications, and the categories of patients suitable for total mastectomy are inferred from Table 28.2.

ADJUVANT RADIOTHERAPY

The question of whether patients should receive adjuvant radiotherapy to the chest wall following total mastectomy in order to reduce the risk of local recurrence of disease is debatable. A recent overview of randomised studies of radiotherapy to the chest wall after mastectomy has been reported. This study concluded that radiotherapy to the chest wall did result in a lower risk of local recurrence in the chest wall by up to three-fold, and also a reduced risk of death from breast cancer (odds ratio for mortality

Table 28.2 Indications and contraindications for breast conservation

Indications	Contraindications
T_1 or T_2 (≤ 4 cm)	T_2 (≥ 4 cm), T_3, T_4
N_0 or N_1 nodal status	N_2 nodal status
Clinical tumour size >4 cm in a larger breast (dependent on breast: tumour ratio)	Central tumour in a small breast
Patient's desire for conservation	Multifocal or multicentric tumours
Patient must be fit for surgery and suitable for postoperative radiotherapy	Extensive *in situ* malignancy

was 0.94). However, it is important to note that there was found to be a significant increase in the risk of non-cancer deaths in patients receiving radiotherapy (odds ratio 1.24). This increased mortality was due to heart-related causes and was most likely to occur in women over the age of 60 years after 10 years, particularly when radiotherapy was given to the left side. In contrast, in women under 50 years of age there was little increased risk of death with radiotherapy.

In view of these facts, post-mastectomy radiotherapy has been recommended for selected patients who are most likely to experience chest wall recurrence. This includes patients with large tumours, lymphatic invasion, high histological grade and involvement of deep resection margins.

Surgery to the axillary lymph nodes

It is currently recommended that all patients with operable invasive breast cancer should undergo some form of axillary surgery as part of achieving regional disease control and also gaining prognostic information regarding the extent of tumour spread (nodal involvement) and to determine the need for adjuvant treatments. Indeed, axillary lymph node status is one of the most important prognostic indicators, for survival in patients with breast cancer. The greater the number of nodes that are involved with tumour, the poorer the prognosis.

However, at least 40% of patients with breast cancer will have no histological evidence of lymph node involvement with tumour at initial presentation. Moreover, in patients with tumours smaller than one cm in size, the incidence of lymph node involvement with tumour may be as low as 3%, although in some studies this may be up to 20% depending on tumour grade. More recently,

interest has focussed on the detection of malignant cells in the nodes using immunohistochemistry (e.g. using antibodies directed against the epithelial cell marker cytokeratin) but the prognostic significance of nodal metastases detected in this way remains to be clarified.

The second reason for undertaking surgical treatment of the axilla is that nodal metastases must be removed or this axillary disease will progress. Randomised clinical trials have revealed that if treatment is not given to the axilla, up to 20% of patients will subsequently experience progressive axillary disease. However, with appropriate treatment of the axilla (surgery and/or radiotherapy) axillary disease progression occurs in less than 3% of patients.

Anatomy of the axilla

The surgical anatomy of the axilla is important, in particular with respect to the lymphatic drainage of the breast. The axillary nodes that are located below the axillary vein can be classified into three levels, these being defined by their relationship to the pectoralis minor muscle (Figure 28.1). Although the number of lymph nodes in the axilla can range from as few as four to more than 50, most commonly there are in the region of 20 to 25 nodes present.

- Level 1 nodes are present below and lateral to the inferiolateral border of the pectoralis minor muscle (approximately 14 nodes).

- Level 2 nodes are behind the pectoralis minor muscle (approximately four to five nodes).

- Level 3 nodes are above the upper border of the pectoralis minor (two to three nodes).

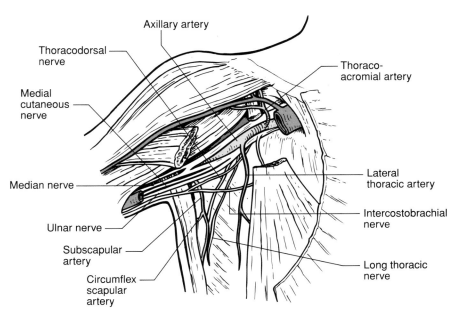

Figure 28.1 Anatomy of the axilla.

Surgical procedures to the axilla

The surgical treatment of the axilla is much discussed amongst clinicians but at present there are two main axillary surgical procedures which can be undertaken in order to gain information regarding the involvement of these nodes with tumour. These are as follows.

AXILLARY SAMPLING

This requires the removal of at least four lymph nodes from level 1 of the axilla. If lymph nodes are found to be involved with tumour then radiotherapy to the axilla and supraclavicular areas should be given to optimise regional control of disease. In addition, radiotherapy to the internal thoracic nodes should also be considered especially for tumours located in the medial aspect of the breast, where tumour spread to the internal thoracic nodes is likely.

The correlation between axillary and internal thoracic lymph node involvement is as follows:

- If axillary nodes are free of metastases, the internal thoracic nodes are involved in 4% of those with a lateral primary tumour and 13% of patients with a medial or central tumour

- If axillary nodes contain metastases, internal thoracic nodes are involved in 25% of patients with a lateral primary tumour and 50% of those with a central or medial tumour

- 90% of women with internal thoracic node involvement also have axillary node involvement with tumour.

AXILLARY DISSECTION

Axillary dissection is described as being performed to an 'anatomical level' (e.g. level 1, level 2 or level 3). If the dissection is carried out to level 3, all the axillary lymphatic tissue will have been removed and this is then termed an axillary clearance. If a level 1 or 2 dissection has been undertaken, radiotherapy to the axilla and supraclavicular nodes is also considered if the nodes are involved with tumour. However, a level 3 dissection (clearance) is also a therapeutic procedure for the axillary nodes and no radiotherapy is given even if the lymph nodes contain tumour. To do so would result in lymphoedema occurring in up to 30% of patients but does not improve regional control of disease or survival. Following axillary clearance alone, up to 5% of patients will experience chronic lymphoedema, but some studies have reported that this can be as high as 15%, depending on the severity of symptoms.

Controversies surrounding axillary surgery

The controversies surrounding axillary surgery focus on the question as to whether axillary sampling can stage the axilla accurately. Another frequently discussed problem concerns the possibility of 'skip metastases' in the axillary nodes. One study of more than 1000 patients demonstrated that in approximately 1.5% of patients there is no nodal involvement at level 1, but that there is nodal involvement at levels 2 or 3 in the axilla.

The most commonly quoted study to support the use of axillary sampling to stage the axilla is a randomised trial, carried out in Edinburgh, of 406 patients in which axillary sampling (four nodes, with radiotherapy given if tumour involvement was found) was compared with axillary clearance. There were no significant differences in the incidence of positive nodes in either group of patients (43% vs. 39%). Furthermore, after a follow-up period of more than 10 years, there were no differences in locoregional tumour recurrence and overall survival. Another important point to emerge from this study is that in the latter part of the trial the randomisation to sample or clearance was undertaken after an initial sample had been performed. It is interesting to note that in none of these patients, who had undergone axillary sampling and subsequently axillary clearance, did this change their axillary nodal status from that which had been determined by the axillary sample. Nevertheless, debate has still continued as to exactly how many axillary nodes should be removed in a 'sample' so as to be sure that the axilla has been adequately staged. The data discussed above does indicate that removing the four large nodes in the axillary sample is adequate to stage the axilla. However, data from some of the European studies has suggested that if a level 1 dissection is carried out (rather than 'picking out' the four largest nodes), then 10 lymph nodes should be removed to ensure that the axilla has been adequately staged.

There is no doubt, however, that axillary clearance does give a better quantitative assessment of the degree of axillary involvement with tumour but whether this additional information can be used and translates into a survival advantage for the patient is unclear. On the basis of previous studies this seems unlikely and this view has been reinforced by a study from the USA involving over 27 000 women. In this latter study it was found that there was only a 22% difference in survival rate between women with no axillary nodal involvement and those with more than 10 glands involved with tumour (see Table 28.3).

Table 28.3 Number of axillary nodes involved and survival rate

Number of involved nodes	5-year survival
0	85%
1	78%
4	65%
10	<55%

There is also controversy surrounding the morbidity which accompanies axillary sampling and clearance. Some studies have shown that more extensive axillary dissections are associated with a greater morbidity in the postoperative period (e.g. reduced range of shoulder movement, pain/paraesthesia in the arm, lymphoedema). However, it seems likely that the morbidity associated with axillary clearance and with axillary sample plus radiotherapy (if nodes were involved with tumour) is comparable and regional control of disease is also comparable with only 1–3% of patients experiencing axillary disease relapse.

Is it possible to select appropriate axillary surgery for an individual patient?

Considering the above facts regarding axillary surgery, the question which arises is whether it is possible to tailor the type of axillary surgery to the individual patient, with the aim of reducing post-operative morbidity? Some surgeons routinely carry out 'sampling' whereas others undertake 'clearance' in all patients. However, although approximately 40% of all patients with breast cancer (more for those with smaller tumours) will not have tumour in the axillary nodes, it is possible to identify those most likely to have tumour-containing axillary lymph nodes. For example, large tumours are more likely to be node positive and, therefore, undergo clearance. By contrast, patients with tumours smaller than one cm in diameter are only associated with involved lymph nodes in 3% to 20% of cases and such patients may undergo sampling. Similarly, the types of cancers detected in the breast screening situation are also likely not to have nodes involved with tumour. However, it is not yet possible to clearly define other possible subgroups of patients who are most likely to have axillary lymph nodes involved with tumour.

FUTURE DEVELOPMENTS IN STAGING THE AXILLA

Sentinel node biopsy

This new staging technique consists of excisional biopsy of the first lymph node which receives lymphatic drainage from a tumour. Initially, this concept was applied to the management of patients with penile cancer and malignant melanoma. However, it is now accepted that the concept of the sentinel node and tumour spread is also applicable to patients with breast cancer.

Theoretically, if the sentinel node were to be removed and examined histologically, this should correlate with the presence or absence of axillary lymph node disease. Thus, staging of the axilla could be simplified by removing only one node, minimising surgery to the axilla and reducing the postoperative complications that can occur when axillary samples or dissections are undertaken.

Preliminary studies have demonstrated that by using a combination of blue dye and a radionuclide (technetium[99] sulphur colloid), injected in close proximity to the primary breast cancer, the sentinel node can be identified in 90%–98% of cases. However, further studies are in progress to determine which technique is best for detecting sentinel nodes. Presently, a randomised, clinical trial (ALMANAC) is in progress to determine if sentinel node biopsy is indeed better than current axillary surgery in terms of staging the axilla and/or in reducing complications and morbidity. It will be important to determine whether patients who do not have detectable involvement of the sentinel node are

not compromised in terms of disease, free survival and overall survival when compared with patients undergoing the currently accepted procedures of axillary sample or clearance.

POSITRON EMISSION TOMOGRAPHY

It would be advantageous for the patient if there was a reliable non-invasive method of staging the axilla but this is not possible at the present time. One technique that is currently being investigated is positron emission tomography (PET). This technique involves the i.v. administration of a positron-labelled metabolic substrate (e.g. ^{18}F-fluoro-2-deoxy-D-glucose), which selectively accumulates in tumour cells when compared with normal non-malignant cells; the differential uptake by tumour can then be identified by scanning the patient's axilla in a PET scanner.

Preliminary studies have demonstrated that PET can stage the axilla with a sensitivity of 60 to 100% and a specificity of 66 to 100%. It has the greatest sensitivity with larger cancers and for these certain categories of patients, PET may have a role to play in staging the axilla. At present its role in routine clinical management is unclear and further studies are required to define the role of PET scanning in the management of patients with breast cancer.

Complications of radiotherapy

Radiotherapy given to a conserved breast, chest wall or axilla can be associated with complications that are listed in Table 28.4.

Table 28.4 Complications of radiotherapy	
Breast	Oedema, fibrosis, shrinkage, poorer cosmetic result, angiosarcoma
Lung	Irradiation pneumonitis, pulmonary fibrosis
Chest wall	Skin inflammation, telangiectasia, fat necrosis, rib fractures, angiosarcoma
Heart	Coronary artery damage
Axilla	Brachial plexus neuropathy, lymphoedema

Locoregional recurrence of disease following breast conservation and mastectomy: prognosis and treatment

Breast conservation

Following breast-conservation surgery and adjuvant radiotherapy, local recurrence of tumour can be defined as further breast cancer within the skin or parenchyma of the treated breast. Although recurrence rates of as high as 20% within five years of surgery have been reported, it is now generally accepted that local recurrence of disease occurs in up to 1% of patients per year and in each subsequent year.

The detection of recurrent disease currently depends on regular clinical examination and mammographic assessment of the breast.

Clinical examination can detect approximately two-thirds, and mammography up to 50%, of local disease recurrences. However, the results of these investigations can be difficult to interpret because mammographic examination may reveal abnormalities such as scar formation, fat necrosis, skin thickening, increased soft tissue density and microcalcification. These changes may represent benign disease, but could also be associated with malignancy. Nevertheless, mammography is recommended at regular intervals, but the optimal time intervals at which this should be carried out are unknown. Currently, there is a wide variation in clinical practice, with mammography being undertaken at intervals ranging from less than one year to more than two years in different centres.

The prognostic significance of a local recurrence of disease has been debated but although many studies have indicated that patient survival is not compromised if this recurrence is adequately treated, there is some evidence to suggest that these patients were at a higher risk of systemic disease relapse. Treatment of local recurrence is usually by mastectomy, but in selected patients further local excisions of the tumour recurrence in the breast may be undertaken. However, if breast conservation is carried out it is essential that the margins of the resected tissue are tumour-free to ensure that optimal local control of disease is obtained. In addition, systemic therapy should be considered in all patients because of the risk of systemic disease relapse.

Mastectomy and regional node recurrence

If mastectomy has been undertaken, local disease recurrence most commonly occurs in the chest wall, in or adjacent to the mastectomy scar. This may be clinically evident as an isolated nodule, or there may be an 'eczematous' appearance to the skin flap or a more diffuse nodularity, which makes diagnosis more difficult. If local recurrence occurs, approximately 20% of patients will have detectable metastatic disease simultaneously. Furthermore, almost 50% of women with local disease recurrence will have demonstrable metastatic disease within 5 to 10 years of the local recurrence occurring. Similarly, patients with regional recurrence in the axillary nodes also have a high risk of disseminated disease being present at this time.

The clinical diagnosis of local disease recurrence must be confirmed prior to treatment being instituted. It is important to remember that cytology taken from a possible local recurrence may be difficult to interpret, particularly if radiotherapy has already been given. Histological confirmation, therefore, is required. The treatment of locoregional disease recurrence is contentious but the following factors should be borne in mind when planning therapy:

- The size and extent of the tumour recurrence (those with multiple sites and larger lesions are more likely to have distant disease)

- Time from primary treatment to the disease relapse (the shorter the time the more likely there is to be distant disease)

- Previous locoregional treatment

- Previous systemic adjuvant treatment

- Hormone receptor status of the tumour (oestrogen receptor positive tumours have a better prognosis following recurrence)

- Presence or absence of detectable metastatic disease.

If there is an isolated nodule in the scar or mastectomy flap, this can be removed surgically and radiotherapy administered (if it has not already been administered at the time of treatment of the primary breast cancer).

Recurrence in the axillary node can be treated by surgical removal (and clearance if this was not previously performed) if this is technically feasible. If the node(s) cannot be removed, then radiotherapy is indicated.

It is important to try to achieve locoregional control of disease as it can lead to skin ulceration and infection, which is distressing to the patient and from which it is difficult to obtain relief.

Although the increased risk of disseminated disease in such patients is well recognised, the role of systemic therapy is unclear. In patients with aggressive recurrences (particularly if there is a short interval between primary treatment and recurrence) adjuvant systemic chemotherapy and/or hormone therapy should be considered. However, the beneficial effects in terms of prolongation of survival remain unclear.

Surgical treatment of *in situ* carcinoma of the breast

Carcinoma *in situ* can be categorised as either ductal carcinoma *in situ* (DCIS) or lobular carcinoma *in situ* (LCIS). The significance of these different types of cancers and the implications for management of the patient are outlined below.

Ductal carcinoma *in situ* (DCIS)

Ductal carcinoma *in situ* may present as either a nipple discharge, Paget's disease of nipple, a mass, or as an isolated mammographic abnormality without any clinical symptoms. There are a variety of histological types of DCIS; 25% of cases are the comedo type, which is the most aggressive type and is most likely to be associated with microinvasion and subsequent development of invasive cancer. The remaining 75% of cases of DCIS include the solid, cribriform, micropapillary and papillary variants. It is common to subdivide DCIS into high, intermediate or low grade, depending on the extent of necrosis and cytological atypia that is detected microscopically.

When considering the treatment of DCIS the following facts regarding its natural history and pathological features should be borne in mind as they have an important bearing on appropriate treatment:

- DCIS can be detected in 5% of women at postmortem examination

- It is estimated that the risk of subsequently developing invasive cancer is approximately 1 to 2% per annum

- Micropapillary, comedo and papillary types are most likely to be multicentric

- Microinvasion occurs in 15% of all cases of DCIS but this is related to tumour size. If the DCIS is less than 25 mm, less than 2% have microinvasion, but if larger than 26 mm, then up to 30% will have microinvasion. In addition, microinvasion is most likely to occur in the comedo type of DCIS

- 30% of all cases of DCIS are oestrogen receptor positive, but 80% of comedo DCIS do not express oestrogen receptors

- Lymph node involvement occurs in less than 1 to 2% of cases of DCIS.

The treatment of DCIS is contentious, with some authorities recommending mastectomy for all patients with DCIS, whilst others advocate breast conservation in selected patients. Following breast conservation, undertaken in patients who have DCIS localised to one area of the breast, tumour recurrence can occur in up to 20% of patients (although figures of 30% or even higher have been reported). In one-half of these patients the recurrence will be as an invasive breast carcinoma with or without lymph node involvement.

Patients most likely to experience local tumour recurrence are those with involved tumour margins and the presence of moderate to marked comedo-type necrosis. The role of radiotherapy following breast conservation for DCIS has also been debated but is now clearer. A randomised trial (NSABP-B17) has demonstrated that the addition of radiotherapy following breast conservation will reduce the risk of DCIS recurrence (13% to 8%) and also the risk of invasive tumour recurrence (13% to 3%). If such a recurrence is then treated with mastectomy, survival is comparable to patients who undergo mastectomy as their initial treatment.

By contrast if all patients with DCIS are treated by mastectomy, a recurrence rate of less than 2% will occur. However, mastectomy may be 'over-treatment' for many patients. In view of these facts, therefore, and in order to ensure adequate treatment, at the same time trying to avoid unnecessary mastectomies, a suggested treatment plan for DCIS is as follows.

- If there is extensive DCIS over an area of >four cm, or if the DCIS is multicentric, then mastectomy should be undertaken. This is because studies have suggested that if the DCIS is >four cm, incomplete excision of the tumour by breast conservation is likely to occur. However, some surgeons recommend mastectomy for DCIS lesions which are <two-and-a-half cm in size.

- If the DCIS is localised and confined to a smaller area than described above, breast conservation can be undertaken ensuring that the resection margins are clear of tumour. The extent of the resection margin is debated but a tumour clearance of >five mm is associated with a low risk of recurrence. Some suggest that the margin should be clear by at least 10 mm but this may be technically difficult to achieve and still preserve the breast with an acceptable cosmetic result.

- If breast conservation is undertaken, radiotherapy to the conserved breast is indicated if the resection margin is <1 cm, or if the DCIS is high grade.

- Axillary staging is not necessary. However, in those patients most likely to have microinvasion (comedo type, large tumours) some would recommend that axillary sampling be undertaken.

The role of tamoxifen as adjuvant treatment following surgery (and radiotherapy) for DCIS is unclear. Preliminary results from NSABP-24 have suggested that tamoxifen may reduce the risk of subsequent invasive and *in situ* cancer, but the magnitude of the benefit is small. However, the longer-term results of this study, and others, are awaited.

Paget's disease

Paget's disease of the nipple is characterised by changes in the nipple (reddening, excoriation, and/or scaling of the nipple, with or without a nipple discharge). Histologically, it is recognised by Paget's cells (large cells with a pale cytoplasm) in the epidermis of the nipple which signal the presence of invasive or *in situ* cancer within the breast.

In Paget's disease of the nipple 50% of patients will have a palpable mass in addition to the nipple/areola changes as described above and this will be an invasive carcinoma in approximately 90% of cases. In contrast, if there is no palpable lump, only one-third of patients will have an underlying invasive carcinoma.

The treatment of Paget's disease is also controversial. If mastectomy is undertaken the prognosis will depend on the presence or absence of an associated invasive carcinoma and its degree of spread. More recently, more limited surgical resections involving the nipple/areola complex and the underlying breast have been undertaken, followed with adjuvant radiotherapy to the breast. If breast conservation is undertaken and the resection margins are not clear of tumour, or if there is tumour multicentricity, mastectomy is then recommended. Axillary surgery and adjuvant treatment depend on the nature of any associated invasive component, as described previously.

Lobular carcinoma *in situ*

Lobular carcinoma *in situ* (LCIS) is less common than DCIS and is generally accepted to be an indicator for a risk of developing invasive cancer subsequently, rather than being a precursor of invasive cancer, as in the case of DCIS. LCIS lacks any distinguishing features on mammography and is not associated with microcalcification (unlike DCIS) and is usually diagnosed incidentally on a breast biopsy. The risks of further LCIS and invasive cancer in a patient with LCIS are as follows:

- In patients with an area of LCIS, up to two-thirds have further areas of LCIS in the same breast, and 30% have co-existing LCIS in the opposite breast

- There is a 1% per annum risk of developing an invasive cancer, which may be either infiltrating ductal (60%) or lobular cancer (40%), and the risk continues indefinitely as time progresses. The risk does not correlate with the size of the LCIS

- 50% of the invasive cancers that subsequently arise in patients with LCIS are in the opposite breast.

The treatment of LCIS remains controversial with a range of therapeutic options. The possible treatment options that are currently practised after a breast biopsy has shown LCIS to be present are:

(i) No further treatment, but careful clinical and mammographic long-term follow-up

(ii) Mastectomy

(iii) Bilateral prophylactic mastectomy, with or without breast reconstruction.

Axillary surgery is not required and the role of tamoxifen in the treatment of patients with LCIS is unknown at present.

Surgical treatment of impalpable invasive and *in situ* cancers

If an impalpable abnormality is detected in the breast by radiological imaging (mammography and/or ultrasound), which is shown to be malignant on fine-needle aspiration cytology (stereotactically, ultrasound guided) further treatment is undertaken. In the first instance, stereotactic core biopsy can be undertaken to determine if there is a detectable invasive component present. The lesion should then be removed in order to obtain a full and definitive histological diagnosis, in particular the extent of the *in situ* and/or invasive cancer. Preoperative localisation of the abnormality is carried out by inserting a needle localisation wire into the lesion under mammographic or ultrasound control. This will enable the lesion to be accurately found and removed surgically. The excised breast tissue is orientated and is then radiographed to ensure that the abnormality (usually either a soft tissue opacity, area of architectural distortion and/or microcalcification) has been removed completely.

If there is any doubt as to the completeness of excision, the cavity margins should also be excised. The breast specimen is then sent fresh to the Pathology department, and 'inked' to mark the margins of the specimen. Sections, three mm in thickness, are cut and are then radiographed again so that paraffin sections can be prepared for histopathological examination of the radiologically detected abnormal area.

The extent of the lesion and the necessity for further surgery will depend on the histological findings (e.g. tumour type, grade, size, resection margins) as described previously. All invasive lesions require axillary surgery but this is unnecessary if only DCIS is found. If the lesion is larger or there is multi-focal disease then consideration should be given to mastectomy (or re-excision in certain cases) because of the increased risk of recurrent malignancy or the subsequent development of further invasive cancers in the residual breast (see previous sections for full discussion of the treatment of invasive and *in situ* cancers).

NEOADJUVANT CHEMOTHERAPY

Neoadjuvant chemotherapy, also termed primary or induction chemotherapy, is defined as chemotherapy administered prior to any further treatment of the primary breast tumour being undertaken. The aims of neoadjuvant chemotherapy are to downstage the primary tumour in the breast and to destroy any existing micrometastatic disease. The rationale for this approach include the following:

- Micrometastases are exposed to chemotherapy at a time when their growth fraction is high

- There is less tumour cell heterogeneity at this time with less likelihood of drug-resistant cells

- Blood flow and oxygenation of the micrometastases is optimal thus allowing adequate delivery of chemotherapeutic agents

- The time delay to giving adjuvant chemotherapy after surgery (usually four to six weeks) is avoided by administering neoadjuvant chemotherapy.

Neoadjuvant chemotherapy is now generally accepted as the treatment of choice for patients with locally advanced breast cancer (LABC), which occurs in up to 15% of patients presenting with breast cancer. LABC can be defined using the following criteria:

- Presence of a large tumour (>five cm: T_3)

- Fixation of the tumour to the chest wall, skin oedema (peau d'orange) or infiltration, with or without ulceration (T_4)

- Large, fixed or matted axillary lymph nodes (N_2)

- Inflammatory carcinoma (localised or generalised induration of the breast, oedema and erythema of the skin, especially in the lower half of the breast [T_4d].)

If surgical resection of the tumour is undertaken in patients who have LABC, it has been shown that approximately 50% of them will develop a local recurrence of disease and the five-year survival is <10%, with most patients dying from metastatic disease.

A variety of combination chemotherapeutic regimens have been used, but most of these have contained doxorubicin (or other anthracyclins) as these have been shown to be the most effective cytotoxic drug against breast cancers. Examples of regimens that have been used include:

- Cyclophosphamide, vincristine, doxorubicin (given as an I.V. bolus) and oral prednisolone

- Epirubicin, cisplatin (I.V. bolus) and continuous I.V. infusional 5-fluorouracil

- 5-fluorouracil, adriamycin and cyclophosphamide (intravenous bolus)

- Doxorubicin and cyclophosphamide.

Such combination chemotherapeutic regimens can be effective in reducing the clinical size of the primary tumour and clinical complete and partial response rates of 75% or more have been reported.

Most commonly chemotherapy is administered as bolus injections at regular intervals (e.g. thrice weekly) and for a set number of cycles (usually six to eight), depending on the particular regimen used. The possibility of giving chemotherapeutic regimens using a continuous administration of certain drugs (e.g. 5-fluorouracil) has also been examined. However, the benefits of this approach in terms of disease control remain unclear.

Recent studies have suggested that the taxanes (e.g. taxotere), can be effective in up to one-half of patients with metastatic breast cancer which has failed to respond to anthracyclins. Taxanes may thus be added to doxorubicin-containing chemotherapeutic regimens with better results in terms of clinical and histological reductions in tumour size.

A clinical response (reduction in tumour size) does not always correlate with the findings on histopathology. In fact, a complete histopathological response, with destruction of all tumour cells, occurs in less than 20% of all patients treated with neoadjuvant chemotherapy. The remainder of patients have some evidence of residual tumour histologically, and in a small number of patients (less than 15%) no response at all to neoadjuvant treatment can be demonstrated.

At present, it is recommended that surgical resection of the residual tumour, (or the area of the breast where it was in patients with a complete clinical response), or mastectomy with appropriate axillary surgery should be undertaken after completion of neoadjuvant chemotherapy. However, if it were possible to identify those patients who have a complete histological response in the breast, these patients could then be managed differently – surgery might not be necessary for them. Preliminary studies have

suggested that magnetic resonance mammography (MRM) or PET scanning may allow such patients to be identified.

Using this combined approach, five-year survival rates of up to 65% or more have been reported, and local control of disease can be achieved in 85% of patients. A variety of factors which are associated with improved survival have been identified in patients undergoing neoadjuvant chemotherapy. These include a better clinical response, a complete histopathological response, a greater number of cycles of chemotherapy and the absence of tumour in the axillary nodes after neoadjuvant chemotherapy. If patients have a complete histological response, the five-year survival rate has been reported to be as high as 80% (Figure 28.2).

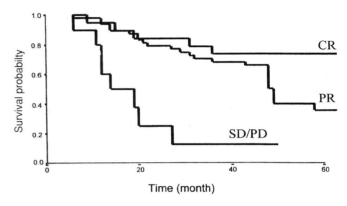

Figure 28.2 The effect of clinical response following neoadjuvant chemotherapy on overall survival. Key: CR – complete clinical response; PR – partial clinical response; SD – Satsis of disease clinically – PD – Progression of disease clinically.

Although neoadjuvant therapy was initially used for treating patients with LABC, in recent years there has been an increasing enthusiasm for its application to the treatment of patients with smaller tumours (e.g. as small as three cm in size as measured clinically). Using this approach, it is possible to undertake breast-conservation surgery more frequently (approximately a further 10% of patients do not require mastectomy). However, whether there is a prolongation of survival in patients receiving neoadjuvant chemotherapy remains unclear at the present time.

ADJUVANT CHEMOTHERAPY

The overall five-year survival for breast cancer is approximately 75%, with some variation between different countries, and different regions within those countries, being reported. However, this means that at least 25% of patients who undergo apparently 'curative' surgery for breast cancer and which is detectable only in the breast and regional areas, have micrometastatic disease at initial presentation. The most important risk factors for predicting disease recurrence are:

- Lymph node involvement with tumour

- Large primary tumour size

- High histological tumour grade (Bloom and Richardson, grade III).

Other indications of an increased risk of disease recurrence are well recognised and include lymphovascular invasion by tumour, oestrogen receptor negativity, increased rates of mitosis, and expression of growth factor receptors. It is possible to combine a number of prognostic factors to produce a prognostic index which predicts patient survival, and one such example is shown in Table 28.5.

Table 28.5 Nottingham prognostic index

Prognostic category	Index	10-year survival
Excellent	≤2.4	94
Good	≤3.4	83
Moderate I	≤4.4	70
Moderate II	<5.4	51
Poor	>5.4	19

(Adapted from: Blamey R.W. The design and clinical use of the Nottingham Prognostic Index. *The Breast* 1996; 156–157).

Over the last quarter of a century, randomised, controlled trials have evaluated the effects of a number of chemotherapeutic drugs in possibly prolonging survival when given to patients with breast cancer in the adjuvant setting. These have involved the administration of drugs (given singularly or as combinations), for varying periods of time, to women at different risks of disease recurrence, to patients of different ages, menopausal status, and of differing hormone receptor status. Although varying results have been obtained from the many studies, the Early Breast Cancer Triallists Collaborative Group (EBCTCG) has examined in detail 47 randomised, controlled clinical trials of over 18 000 women, which have evaluated the effects of adjuvant poly-chemotherapy on disease recurrence and overall survival in patients with breast cancer.

The EBCTCG considered the effects of all the studies combined together, and then subdivided the chemotherapeutic regimens into three groups for further statistical analysis:

- Trials of cyclophosphamide, methotrexate and 5-fluorouracil (CMF)

- Trials of CMF plus other cytotoxic drugs

- Other polychemotherapy regimens.

The overall results from this analysis are shown in Figure 28.3. It can be seen that the effects of polychemotherapy, given for several months, on disease recurrence and overall survival were:

- a 23.5% reduction in the annual hazard of disease recurrence

- a 15.3% reduction in the annual hazard of mortality.

These beneficial effects were similar when each of the three groups of trials were examined separately (see Figure 28.3 for analyses).

A further series of analyses for the effects of polychemotherapy on disease recurrence were undertaken based on the patient's age, nodal status and oestrogen receptor status. The effects of adjuvant polychemotherapy on overall survival according to age (younger than 50 years or age 50 to 69 years), and nodal status (node positive or negative) are shown in Figure 28.4. It can be seen that in all patients there was a significant reduction in mortality, but the effects were greatest in those patients who were younger than 50 years of age and whose axillary lymph nodes contained tumour. A similar pattern was also observed for disease recurrence in these patients. The majority of these benefits occurred in the first five years after randomisation into the study.

The effects of polychemotherapy on disease recurrence in women with either oestrogen receptor positive or oestrogen receptor negative tumours was also examined separately with respect to age. The results are shown in Table 28.6.

Table 28.6 Effects of chemotherapy on disease recurrence in patients according to age and oestrogen receptor status

Age	Oestrogen receptor status	
	Positive	Negative
<50 years	33% (8)	40% (7)
50–69 years	18% (4)	30% (5)

Values shown are proportional reductions in disease recurrence (SD) according to age and oestrogen receptor status. (Data from: Early Breast Cancer Trialists Collaborative Group. Polychemotherapy for early breast cancer: an overview of the randomised trials. *Lancet* 1998; **352**:930–941).

The other points that emerged from this analysis are summarised below:

- There were no significant differences in the effects between the three main groups of polychemotherapy studied

- There was no advantage to giving the chemotherapy for longer than six months

- There was a slightly better survival in patients treated with an anthracycline drug (e.g., doxorubicin) when compared with CMF (2.7%, but with a relatively large standard deviation of 1.4%).

These analyses have identified which patients are likely to benefit from adjuvant polychemotherapy in terms of reducing the risk of disease recurrence and increasing overall survival. However, the decision to proceed with such treatment requires full consideration of the patient's pre-existing physical state, their wishes, and the effects on quality of life. These all need to be taken into account, in full consultation with the multidisciplinary team managing the patient, so that an informed decision can be reached by the patient.

An alternative approach to polychemotherapy has been to give high-dose chemotherapy but at present there is no evidence to support such an approach.

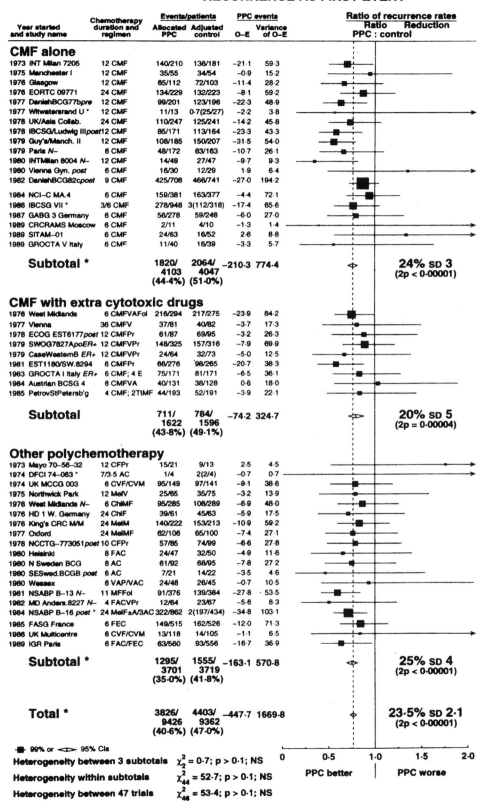

Figure 28.3 The effects of polychemotherapy on death in 47 trials of adjuvant chemotherapy. (Reproduced with permission from: Early Breast Cancer Trialists Collaborative Group. Polychemotherapy for early breast cancer: an overview of the randomised trials. *Lancet* 1998; 352:930–41).

MORTALITY (DEATH FROM ANY CAUSE)

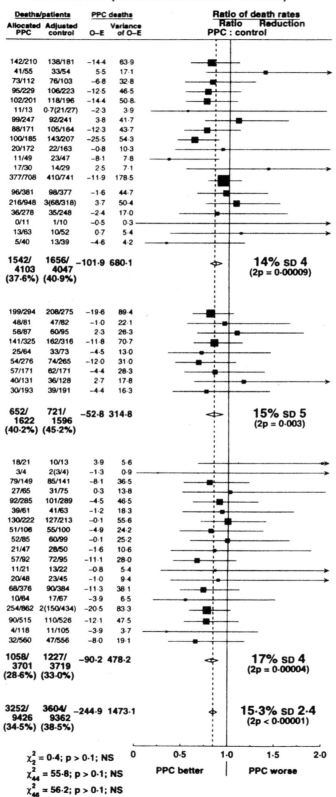

Figure 28.3 *continued*

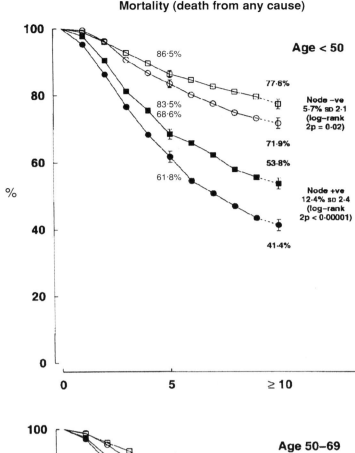

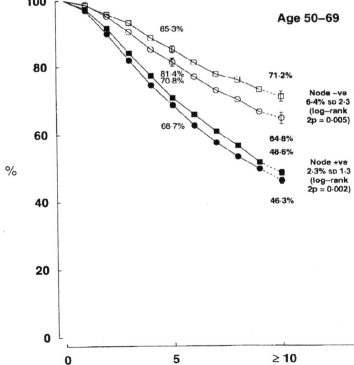

Figure 28.4 The effects of polychemotherapy on survival according to patients' age and lymph node status. (Reproduced with permission from: Early Breast Cancer Trialists Collaborative Group. Polychemotherapy for early breast cancer: an overview of the randomised trials. *Lancet* 1998; **352**:930–41).

HORMONE THERAPY

It has been more than 100 years since the association between breast cancer and oestrogens was recognised. Subsequently, *in vitro* and *in vivo* studies have demonstrated that oestrogen causes the production of a range of growth factors by, and proliferation of, breast cancer cells. Moreover, oestrogens are believed to be involved in the various stages of the carcinogenic process (induction, promotion and growth).

In premenopausal women, circulating oestrogens are produced by the ovaries, in a cyclical fashion and in response to stimulation by the pituitary gonadotrophins. Oestrogens are also synthesised by other peripheral tissues such as fat, muscle and the adrenal glands. The substrate for oestrogen synthesis in these peripheral tissues is androstenedione, which is converted into oestrone and then oestradiol by the aromatase enzyme system (hydroxylation reactions).

Following the menopause, the production of oestrogenic hormones by the ovaries reduces with advancing age and the circulating levels of oestrogens are then low. However, oestrogens are still synthesised in the peripheral tissues using the aromatase enzyme system as described above. It is interesting to note that more than one-half of breast cancers also contain aromatase and potentially, therefore, could synthesise oestrogens within the tumour itself.

Oestrogen receptors

These effects of oestrogens are mediated through the oestrogen receptor (OR), which is located in the cell nucleus and which, when bound to oestrogen, binds to DNA and then modulates expression of mRNA. It has been demonstrated that approximately 60 to 65% of all breast cancers are oestrogen receptor positive but this depends on the patient's age; in tumours in patients older than 70 years, 80% are positive, whereas in those younger than 40 years of age only approximately 40% are positive.

The oestrogen receptor status of the primary tumour correlates with the oestrogen receptor status of metastases in approximately 80% of all patients. However, this correlation is highest in lymph node metastases (90%), and least likely to correlate in bone metastases (less than 60%). In terms of tumour pathology, oestrogen receptors are most likely to be found in well-differentiated tumours, and in lobular or tubular cancers (i.e. those with a good prognosis).

Tamoxifen

Tamoxifen is a non-steroidal anti-oestrogenic compound, which was first introduced into clinical trials almost 30 years ago. It exerts its actions by blocking the binding of oestrogen to oestrogen receptors thus preventing the stimulatory effects of oestrogen on cell growth and proliferation. However, it can also act independently of the OR by increasing production of inhibitory growth factors (e.g. TGFβ). Cells treated with tamoxifen accumulate in the G0/G1 stage of the cell cycle and thus tamoxifen is cytostatic rather than cytocidal. It is important to remember that when tamoxifen is given orally it takes approximately four weeks for a steady-state serum level to be achieved and its active metabolite is N-desmethyltamoxifen.

Tamoxifen as primary treatment in elderly patients with breast cancer

Tamoxifen has been used as the primary treatment for breast cancer in elderly patients because of the increased chance that these tumours will be oestrogen receptor positive thus avoiding surgery. It has been shown that reduction in tumour size will occur in up to two-thirds of patients and in approximately one-third of patients over 70 years of age, a complete clinical response can occur. However, although the tumour may respond initially (median time to response is up to 20 weeks), relapse can subsequently occur in up to 40% of patients, and the disease progresses.

Three randomised, controlled trials, in patients 70 years and older, have evaluated the effects of primary treatment with tamoxifen compared with surgical resection of the primary tumour (either breast conservation or mastectomy). In the first of these trials, there was no significant difference in local disease relapse or progression between patients treated with surgery and those treated with tamoxifen alone. However, there was a high local recurrence rate (38%) following surgery, making interpretation of these results difficult. However, in the other two studies there was a significantly higher local disease relapse or progression rate in patients who were receiving tamoxifen, when compared with those who had undergone surgical resection of their primary tumour. In these latter two trials the local recurrence rates in patients undergoing surgical resection were 8% and 12%, respectively. In all studies there were no significant differences in time to distant recurrence or survival between patients in either of the study arms.

Primary tamoxifen therapy can bring about a tumour response in up to two-thirds of patients but there is a higher chance of local disease relapse/progression when compared with patients undergoing surgical removal of the cancer. Despite this increased recurrence in the breast, there is no difference in overall survival between patients treated either way.

Adjuvant tamoxifen therapy after surgery for operable breast cancer

Hormone therapy (usually tamoxifen) has been given to patients following surgery for breast cancer as adjuvant treatment with the intention of prolonging the disease-free interval and increasing overall survival.

The EBCTCG reported the results of an overview of 30 000 women with breast cancer who had participated in randomised, controlled trials comparing adjuvant tamoxifen versus placebo. The effects of tamoxifen on mortality for all patients and also according to their lymph node status are shown in Figure 28.5.

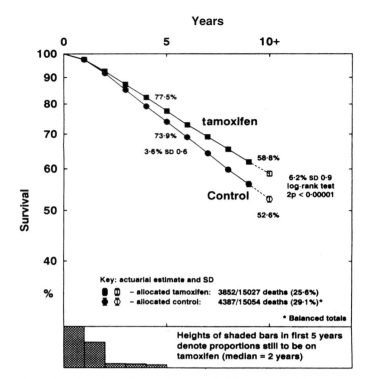

Figure 28.5 The effect of tamoxifen on survival in patients with breast cancer receiving adjuvant tamoxifen. (Reproduced with permission from: Early Breast Cancer Trialists Collaborative Group. Systemic treatment of early breast cancer by hormonal, cytotoxic or immune therapy. *Lancet* 1992; **339**:71–85).

These studies include patients who may also have received chemotherapy but were randomised to tamoxifen or no tamoxifen treatment. Patients receiving tamoxifen had a significantly reduced risk of mortality and by 10 years this was a 6.2% increase in survival. Similarly, there was a 5% reduction in the risk of disease recurrence in patients receiving tamoxifen.

When the data were examined according to lymph node status there was an 8.2% reduction in death in node-positive patients taking tamoxifen, and a 3.5% reduction in death in node-negative patients taking tamoxifen. Similarly, there were significant reductions is disease recurrence in node-negative and node-positive patients taking tamoxifen when compared with no tamoxifen treatment:

- There was a significant reduction in mortality in oestrogen receptor 'poor' patients (<10 fmol/mg), although the magnitude of this effect was less than those with oestrogen receptor positive (>10 fmol/mg) tumours

- Different doses of tamoxifen (20 to 40 mg/day) did not result in different effects on mortality

- Randomised trials of different tamoxifen durations demonstrated a non-significant trend towards a more favourable effect with longer treatment

- There was a 39% odds reduction in the risk of contralateral breast cancer, the benefit appearing to be greater from the trials of longer-term tamoxifen treatment.

Of concern has been the possible side effects of long-term tamoxifen use, in particular the risk of endometrial cancer which is up to twice the incidence found in the general population. However, this must be balanced against the possible protective effect of tamoxifen in postmenopausal women in reducing cardiovascular-associated disorders (e.g. strokes). Other side effects of tamoxifen include vaginal dryness, loss of libido, hot flushes and a small number of patients may develop retinal damage. Weight gain is often attributed to tamoxifen use but in placebo-controlled trials this has not been confirmed.

Ovarian ablation

Ovarian ablation can be carried out by either radiotherapeutic destruction or laparoscopic removal of the ovaries. Ovarian function can be suppressed by luteinizing hormone releasing hormone (LHRH) agonists. Eleven randomised trials of ovarian ablation alone or ovarian ablation in conjunction with chemotherapy versus no ovarian ablation have been examined (more than 1600 women) in patients aged younger than 50 at trial entry. The results demonstrated the benefits of ovarian ablation in reducing the risk of death and are shown in Table 28.7.

Table 28.7 The effects of ovarian ablation on the risk of death in patients with breast cancer

Trials	Annual odds of death reduction (SD)
Trials of ovarian ablation ($n = 878$ women)	28% (9)
Trials of ovarian ablation with cytotoxic treatment ($n = 5939$ women)	19% (11)
All trials combined	25% (7)

(Data from: Early Breast Cancer Trialists Collaborative Group. Systemic treatment of early breast cancer by hormonal, cytotoxic or immune therapy. *Lancet* 1992; **339**:71–85).

METASTATIC BREAST CANCER

Although five-year survival rates of up to 70% or more have been reported for all patients with breast cancer, this means that at least 30% of patients will have relapse with recurrent disease within this period of time. The distant spread is most commonly to bones, either alone or in conjunction with metastatic disease in the liver, lungs and soft tissues. Once metastatic breast cancer has been diagnosed, the mean survival of such patients is approximately 18 to 24 months. Thus, the aim of any treatment for metastatic breast cancer is to palliate, relieve symptoms and improve survival if possible. Quality should always be taken into consideration of life issues for patients who cannot be cured.

Treatments may include, therefore:

(i) general supportive care including relief of debilitating, disabling and distressing symptoms; management of pathological fractures; correction of disorders of body functions, etc. and

(ii) treatments specifically formulated to retard the growth of the tumour. These latter treatments include chemo- or hormonal therapies.

Chemotherapy for metastatic disease

Chemotherapy is associated with significant side effects which can impair the patient's quality of life. Thus only those patients who are likely to benefit in terms of symptomatic improvement and prolongation of life should be considered for chemotherapy. It has been demonstrated that those most likely to benefit include patients with:

● a good performance status

● visceral metastases

● metastatic disease in one or only a few sites.

A variety of chemotherapeutic agents, given either alone or in combination have been evaluated, but most benefit seems to accrue from the use of combination regimens, which usually contain one of the anthracycline group of drugs (e.g. doxorubicin, epirubicin). A recent meta-analysis of randomised controlled trials has examined what effects different chemotherapeutic regimens have on response rates (complete and partial) in terms of reduction in metastatic disease burden. The results are shown in Table 28.8.

Response rates were greater with combination chemotherapy than single-agent chemotherapy. Better response rates are obtained if an anthracycline was used in the combination regimen and there was also a suggestion that doxorubicin might be better than epirubicin. However, there was an increased risk of cardiac toxicity and bone marrow suppression with doxorubicin when compared with epirubicin. In terms of risk of death, there was a significant benefit with polychemotherapy and with doxorubicin-containing regimens. The median time to disease relapse was in the region of less than 12 months. Although other chemotherapeutic regimens

Table 28.8 Effects of chemotherapy given to patients with metastatic breast cancer

Comparison	Response rate	P
Combination chemotherapy vs single-agent chemotherapy (15 trials, $n=2442$)	48% vs 34%	<0.05
Combination chemotherapy with anthracycline vs combination chemotherapy without anthracycline (30 trials, $n=3756$)	51% vs 45%	<0.05
Epirubicin vs doxorubicin (10 trials, $n=1097$)	44% vs 47%	>0.05

(Data from: Fossati R, Confalonieri V, Ghislandi E, et al. Cytotoxic and hormonal treatment for metastatic breast cancer: a systematic review of published randomised trials involving 31 510 women. *J Clin Oncol* 1998; **16**:3439–60.

can then be tried, subsequent responses are in the region of 25% and often of shorter duration than those obtained with the first chemotherapy regimen used.

More recently, interest has focused on the use of taxanes (e.g. docetaxol), as second-line chemotherapeutic agents in the treatment of patients with metastatic breast cancer who have already been treated with an anthracycline-containing regimen. Responses to docetaxel treatment, with reductions in the extent of the tumour burden, have been reported to occur in 53% to 57% of patients who are resistant to anthracyclines, but the effects in terms of prolongation of survival remain unclear. Other drugs that have activity in relapsed metastatic breast cancer include capecitabine and vinorelibine.

Hormonal therapy for metastatic disease

Tamoxifen

In patients who have been pre-treated with tamoxifen (as adjuvant treatment before the development of metastatic disease), further tamoxifen treatment may produce a response in up to 50% of women with oestrogen receptor positive tumours and in 10% of those with oestrogen receptor negative tumours (median duration of response is approximately 20 months). Patients who are most likely to respond to hormonal treatment with tamoxifen include those that:

● have oestrogen receptor positive tumours

● have a longer disease-free interval after the initial treatment

● are older

● have disease in the soft tissues, bone and lung.

It is of note that tamoxifen may induce bone pain with or without hypercalcaemia within the first two weeks of use. This has been called the 'tamoxifen flare' and is thought to be due to the weakly oestrogenic effects that tamoxifen exerts. It is also important to remember that even if patients demonstrate no response to first-line hormonal therapy, 20% will respond to second-line hormonal treatment. A further 10 to 15% may show a response to third-line hormonal treatment. Therefore, several different hormone therapies may be given after each other because even when the response to one type fails, patients can then respond to the next hormonal agent that is tried. However, at any stage should hormonal manipulation fail, or should patients not be in the categories most likely to respond to hormone treatment, chemotherapy should be considered.

Other hormonal therapies

Other anti-oestrogens

Several new anti-oestrogenic compounds, some of which are pure anti-oestrogens, with no oestrogenic activity, have been synthesised and are being examined in clinical trials. One of these, toremifene has been licensed for use in the USA, but whether these drugs will prove to be of greater efficacy than tamoxifen, is as yet, unclear.

Aromatase Inhibitors

The first aromatase inhibitor used was aminoglutethamide, which was shown to be an effective hormonal therapy in some patients. However, not only did aminoglutethamide inhibit oestrogen synthesis, it also inhibited the production of glucocorticoids and mineralocorticoids by the adrenal cortex and thus, it was also necessary to administer hydrocortisone replacement therapy. In addition, side effects were significant. In view of these problems, new orally active, selective, competitive and non-competitive aromatase inhibitors have been developed which do not require corticosteroid replacement and have fewer side effects. These include anastrozole and letrozole, which are commercially available for use in clinical practice, and may also have a future use as adjuvant therapies.

Progestagens

Megesterol acetate (Megace) and medroxyprogesterone are less commonly used nowadays. Progestagens exert their actions by causing a down-regulation of the progesterone and oestrogen receptors with a resultant inhibition of cell growth. Other actions include binding to androgen and glucocorticoid receptors and reducing oestrogen production by inhibiting the hypothalamo-pituitary axis. The most notable side-effect is weight gain, which occurs in up to 20% of patients. Others include hypertension and cardiac failure. These are rarely used at present.

Luteinising Hormone-releasing Hormone (LHRH) Agonists

Luteinising hormone (LH) is produced by the hypothalamus and stimulates the pituitary gland to produce follicle-stimulating hormone (FSH) and LH. There is then a resultant stimulation of the ovary to produce oestrogens. A variety of LHRH agonists have been synthesised (e.g. goserelin and leuprolide) by replacing amino acids in the protein chain. The result of this is to produce a molecule, which has a longer duration of action than does LHRH.

If these compounds are given to pre-menopausal patients, there is an initial increase in FSH, LH and oestradiol levels. However, continued use results in a fall of oestradiol levels to those that would be expected if the ovaries had been removed. This effect is reversible with oestradiol levels returning to normal if the LHRH agonist is withdrawn. Of these agents, goserelin (Zoladex®) is commonly used in clinical practice and is administered in a depot form by a single monthly injection.

Anti-HER 2 therapy and treatment of metastatic disease

Human epidermal growth factor receptor-2 (HER 2) gene is a proto-oncogene which codes for the HER 2 receptor. This is a transmembrane glycoprotein which has tyrosine kinase activity and is involved in normal breast development and growth. Experimental studies *in vitro* with cancer cell lines have shown that stimulation of this receptor results in cell growth and proliferation. Studies in patients with breast cancer have shown that overexpression of the HER 2 receptor is associated with a poorer survival than that of patients who do not overexpress this receptor. Other studies have also shown that HER 2 positive tumours are more likely to be oestrogen receptor negative and that tumours overexpressing HER 2 are resistant to tamoxifen treatment.

It is also known that in approximately 25 to 30% of women with metastatic breast cancer there is an overexpression of the HER 2 gene with a resultant increased amount of the HER 2 receptor on the tumour cell surface. If this occurs, these tumours are known to be particularly aggressive.

Recently, a monoclonal antibody that selectively binds to the extracellular domain of the HER 2 receptor has become available and has been evaluated in preliminary clinical trials for patients with metastatic breast cancer. The data from these studies suggests that when the anti-HER 2 antibody is given in combination with chemotherapy, there is a prolonged time to disease progression and longer overall survival when compared with patients receiving chemotherapy alone. In addition, the effects of the HER 2 antibody were better when given with taxane chemotherapy than anthracycline-based chemotherapy.

OPERATIVE SURGERY

Mastectomy

Patient preparation

The patient (and partner) must receive appropriate information, counselling and psychosocial support. Reconstructive aspects of surgery should be discussed with the patient and immediate or delayed reconstruction considered if the patient wishes this, and if it is appropriate. This can be undertaken either by breast surgeons, reconstructive surgeons or a combined approach.

Informed consent must be obtained from the patient prior to surgery after a full discussion of treatment options and complications.

Antibiotic prophylaxis is not usually used. Prophylaxis against DVT with pneumatic compression stockings is used in all patients and pharmacological prophylaxis with a subcutaneous heparin may also be indicated.

Anaesthesia and positioning

General anaesthesia is used. The patient is placed in a supine position with the ipsilateral arm abducted and placed on a supporting board. The surgeon and 2nd assistant are on the ipsilateral side of the patient, the first assistant and scrub nurse on the contralateral side.

After preparation of the skin with chlorhexidene (the whole chest, upper abdomen, shoulder and arm to below the elbow), sterile drapes are applied (including wrapping the lower part of the arm) to allow full access to the breast and to permit full mobility of the arm.

Incision

The line of the incision is first marked on the skin. It usually takes the form of an ellipse located transversely across the chest wall and should surround the tumour, nipple/areolar complex, and any skin incisions from a previous biopsy or lumpectomy. The margin of skin to be removed around the tumour is variable and will depend on factors such as the size and location of the tumour, the size of the breast, skin laxity etc. but if possible should be more than 3 cm from the tumour. The upper and lower margins of the ellipse should be of similar length (Figure 28.6).

Procedure

- The upper skin flap is initially developed using argon-assisted diathermy (blood loss can be reduced to 75 ml or less), standard diathermy, or a scalpel, separating the skin and subcutaneous tissues from the underlying breast. To help in developing this plane, the assistants hold the cut edge of the skin with skin hooks at right angles to the plane of dissection (keeping the skin edge taut). The surgeon retracts the breast inferiorly with one hand over a gauze swab (thus maintaining

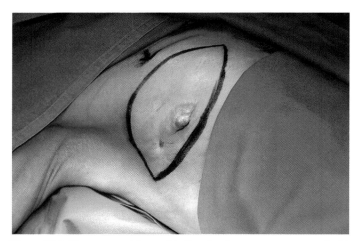

Figure 28.6 The upper and lower skin flaps for the mastectomy are marked in elliptical fashion to allow a resultant transverse scar. These flaps are of equal length so as to avoid 'dog ears' after skin closure.

counter-traction), allowing the upper skin flap to be cut with the other hand.

- This flap is continued superiorly until almost reaching below the clavicle, the upper limit of the breast tissue. The fascia overlying pectoralis major is now clearly identified.

- The lower flap is developed in a similar fashion and extends inferiorly until the anterior rectus sheath is reached (Figure 28.7).

- After both flaps have been developed, the breast is mobilised from the underlying pectoralis muscle usually removing the pectoral fascia with the breast major (some surgeons leave this fascia in place). The breast is removed from a superior to inferior, and a medial to lateral direction, continuing the dissection towards the lateral margin of the pectoralis major muscle. This can be achieved using diathermy or sharp dissection with a scalpel.

- Bleeding from small blood vessels passing from the muscle to the breast is controlled. The main arteries to be divided are the perforating branches of the internal thoracic artery passing through the 2nd, 3rd and 4th intercostal spaces extending into the deep surface of the breast.

- The medial border of the breast is carefully dissected away from the sternum and costal cartilages.

- The dissection extends to the lateral border of the pectoralis major muscle. The breast is then removed from the fascia overlying the serratus anterior muscle. As this is done, small vessels from the lateral thoracic artery and perforating branches of the intercostal arteries are also divided. Care is taken to identify and preserve the long thoracic nerve that supplies the serratus anterior muscle.

- A lateral plane of dissection is developed by pulling the breast medially and developing the place between the breast and skin, and subcutaneous tissues of the lateral chest wall. This plane is developed until the anterolateral border of the latissimus dorsi muscle is reached. Care is taken to identify the neurovascular bundle, containing thoracodorsal artery, vein and nerve, which are clearly identified and preserved.

- The breast is now completely mobilised except for the axillary tail (Figure 28.8).

- The axillary tail is now traced towards the axilla and separated from the pectoralis minor (anteriorly) and the latissimus dorsi (posteriorly). The axillary tail merges into the fat of the axilla and can be divided using diathermy or scissors. It is usual to find a relatively large vein entering into the axillary tail and this can be ligated and divided. The position of the intercostobrachial nerve should be noted as it often traverses the axilla in close proximity to the axillary tail of the breast.

- If axillary surgery is undertaken (sampling or clearance) this is performed as described below.

- Haemostasis is ensured, thoroughly checking the entire area.

- Two suction drains are inserted, with one positioned in the axilla and the other under the lower skin flap. These are brought out through stab incisions in the axilla below the skin incision.

- The subcutaneous fat is closed with interrupted absorbable sutures and the skin closed with a subcuticular (absorbable or non-absorbable) suture technique and steristrips are applied to ensure satisfactory skin apposition (Figure 28.9).

Postoperative management

Patients should be fully mobilised from the first postoperative day and shoulder exercises undertaken under the supervision of the physiotherapist.

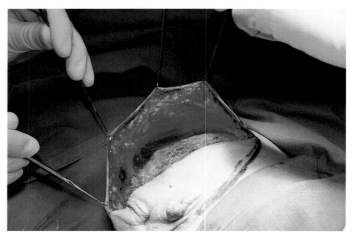

Figure 28.7 The upper skin flap is dissected and removed from the underlying breast and the lower flap is created in a similar fashion.

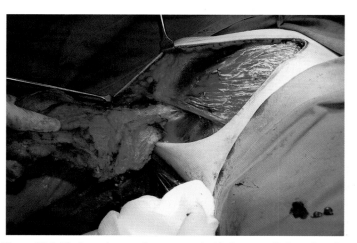

Figure 28.8 The breast has now been removed with the pectoralis fascia from the underlying pectoralis major muscle and the axillary tail of the breast is being defined as it passes into the axilla.

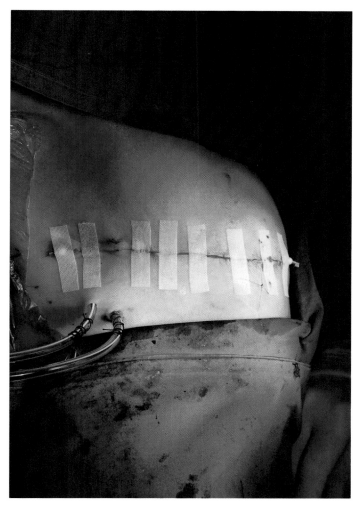

Figure 28.9 Skin closure following completion of the mastectomy with a transverse scar.

Drains are removed when the 24-hour volume is less than 30 ml. However, seromas (fluid transudates from the raw surface areas and lymphatics) can occur in up to one-third of patients after removal of the drains. These will require aspiration using a sterile technique at regular intervals until they settle. In some patients it is necessary to insert a suction drain under the skin flap if the seroma will not resolve with regular needle aspirations.

Other complications that can occur include infection and necrosis of the skin flap. The latter complication can occur if the skin flaps are too thin and if the skin is sutured together under tension. If necrosis does occur, it may heal spontaneously if a relatively small area is involved. However, if there is extensive skin flap necrosis, skin grafting may be necessary.

Patients may be discharged after the drains have been removed. However, selected patients may be allowed home at an earlier stage with the drains *in situ*, with the district nurse supervising the removal of these drains.

Wide local excision for breast cancer

Patient preparation

This is as described for patients undergoing mastectomy. However, reconstruction is not usually necessary, although in some situations a latissimus dorsi mini-flap may be used to reconstruct the breast if cosmetic deformity is likely. All patients should be counselled as to the possible cosmetic deformity that can arise following wide local excision, particularly if radiotherapy is given to the breast. The possibility that subsequent surgical correction may be necessary at a later date should be discussed.

Anaesthesia and positioning

As described above for mastectomy.

Incision

A circumferential incision centred on the palpable lesion, which is long enough to allow adequate access to the tumour, is made through the skin and subcutaneous tissues. If the tumour is lying too close to the skin and there is concern as to the proximity of the tumour to the overlying skin, then an ellipse of skin should also be removed.

Procedure

- Two skin hooks are used on either side of the incision to elevate the skin and subcutaneous fat. Skin flaps on either side of the incision are now elevated by sharp dissection trying to ensure that these extend to at least a two cm margin around the tumour.

- Langenbeck retractors can now be placed under the skin flaps. The area of the palpable tumour can now be seen with a margin of normal breast tissue around the tumour.

- The tumour and normal rim of breast tissue are removed by sharp dissection using a knife or cutting diathermy, incising down to the pectoral fascia. Some surgeons always remove this fascia with the specimen. The larger the margin of normal healthy breast tissue that is removed with the tumour, the better the chance of having margins free of tumour (see page 406). However, this also results in an increased likelihood of resultant cosmetic deformity of the breast.

- The specimen is now removed from the breast carefully and orientated for the pathologist; one suture is attached to the anterior border, two to the medial border and three sutures to the inferior border of the tumour specimen. This ensures that the pathologist can orientate the specimen and provide information regarding whether or not the margins of the tissue are clear of tumour.

- The margins of the cavity are also commonly excised and sent to the pathologist clearly labelled as to which part of the cavity they are taken from. A metal clip (or suture) can be placed on the side facing the original biopsy cavity so that the pathologist can orientate the specimen to determine whether or not the resection margins are free from tumour.

- Haemostasis must then be ensured, examining the cavity thoroughly, using diathermy or suture ligation where necessary. Some surgeons place metal clips in the cavity as an aid to planning of postoperative radiotherapy. However, as MRI is now an important technique in aiding the diagnosis of local recurrence of disease, metal clips will interfere with MRI and are not usually used.

- A closed low-suction drain is placed into the cavity and brought out through a stab incision in the skin of the breast (high suction is not used because the suction effect can result in distortion of the breast and a resultant poor cosmetic appearance.) Some surgeons do not use drains here.

- No attempt is made to obliterate the resulting cavity by suturing the breast tissue together as this will result in a cosmetic deformity. The subcutaneous fat is closed with interrupted sutures of an absorbable material. The skin is closed with a subcuticular technique of either absorbable or non-absorbable material, with steristrips to ensure accurate skin apposition. If the defect is large, then a small tissue flap e.g. breast tissue rotation or a latissimus dorsi miniflap may be used.

Postoperative management

Routine postoperative care following general anaesthetic and appropriate analgesia as required are essential.

If a drain has been inserted, this is usually removed after 24 hours unless drainage is excessive. If this is so, it can be left until the drainage is less than 30 ml in 24 hours.

If radiotherapy is indicated, this can be given after wound healing has occurred, usually four to six weeks later.

Wound infections occur in fewer than 1% of patients and are treated with antibiotics or incision and drainage if an abscess has formed.

Microdochectomy

Microdochectomy (excision of a single duct) is usually undertaken in patients presenting with a blood-stained nipple discharge (or discharge that is positive for blood on testing) and which comes from a single duct. This is most likely to be due to an intraduct papilloma or carcinoma, or duct ectasia. If the discharge comes from several ducts, excision of all the ducts (central duct excision) may be considered.

Patient preparation

Patients should be informed preoperatively of the possibility of cosmetic deformity of the nipple/areola and also of the possibility of impaired sensation in the nipple/areola complex. In addition, necrosis of the nipple can occur due to devascularisation. Informed consent is obtained after full discussion with the patient.

Pneumatic compression stockings are worn as prophylaxis against DVT.

Anaesthesia and positioning

The operation is performed under general anaesthesia.

The patient is placed in the supine position, with the ipsilateral arm abducted and placed on a supporting board. The surgeon and 2nd assistant are on the ipsilateral side of the patient, the first assistant is on the contralateral side, and the scrub nurse on the contralateral side.

After preparation of the skin of the breast and chest wall with chlorhexidene, sterile drapes are applied to allow full exposure of the breast that is being operated on.

Incision

A lacrimal probe can be inserted into the discharging duct from which the discharge is occurring, and carefully placed distally as far as possible (Figure 28.10). It is held in this position by the assistant and must not be moved. Alternatively, some surgeons insert a small plastic catheter into the discharging duct and through this inject a small amount of methylene blue dye into the duct system.

A periareolar incision is made along the edge of the nipple for up to one-third of its circumference on the same side as, and centred on, the discharging duct (recognised by the lacrimal probe). This allows adequate exposure for the operation to proceed.

Procedure

- The nipple/areola complex is retracted using two skin hooks and using sharp dissection, a flap comprising nipple/areola is elevated around the duct which is identified by the position of the probe (it can be swollen with blood-stained fluid) or visualised if methylene blue has been injected (Figures 28.11 and 28.12).

- The skin hooks are then repositioned under the skin of the breast and a flap of skin and subcutaneous tissue raised so that the duct can be traced out into the breast as it passes in a radial direction away from the nipple.

- Sharp dissection is then used to dissect the duct free from the surrounding breast tissue, extending from the undersurface of

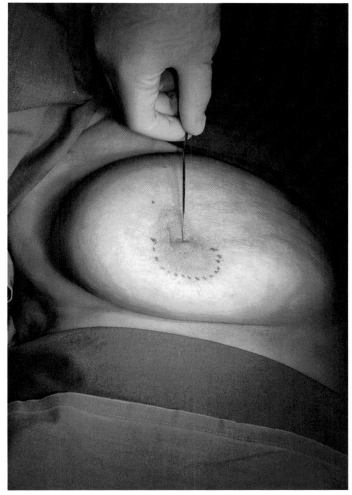

Figure 28.10 The circumareolar skin incision is shown by the dotted line and a lacrimal probe is placed into the discharging duct to define it. This probe passes distally towards the six o'clock position in the breast.

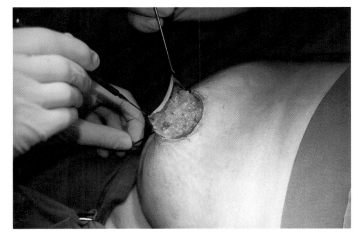

Figure 28.11 The skin and subcutaneous tissue are divided thus allowing the nipple to be retracted superiorly.

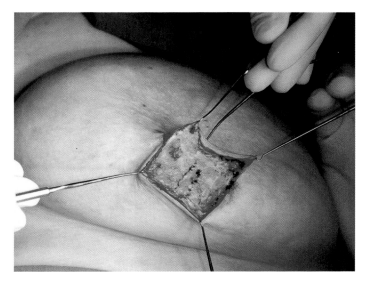

Figure 28.12 The nipple is being retracted superiorly and the lower margin of the incision is retracted inferiorly using skin hooks. This allows adequate exposure of the breast duct system. The duct to be removed is shown by the dotted line and this is identified by palpating the lacrimal probe as it passes distally into the breast.

the areola, distally into the breast tissue. The duct is then transected on the undersurface of the nipple.

- As the duct is then traced distally into the breast, the duct system will be seen to branch and so as to ensure that the duct system is removed, the excised tissue is removed as a wedge.

- Following removal of the tissue, the specimen is sent for histological examination. Haemostasis is secured within the cavity using diathermy, or suture ligation for larger vessels, and the cavity in the breast is irrigated.

- If there is any oozing from vessels within the cavity wall, a sealed drain can be inserted into the cavity and left for 24 hours prior to removal.

- The subcutaneous fat layer is closed with interrupted absorbable sutures and the skin incision can be closed using a subcuticular suture technique with an absorbable or non-absorbable material. Deep sutures to obliterate the cavity are not used as these can distort the appearance of the breast, resulting in cosmetic deformity (Figure 28.13).

Postoperative management

Oral analgesics may be required postoperatively and for a few days after surgery.

Postoperative haematomas can occur and if small will usually resorb without intervention. If the haematoma is of significant size but does not appear to be expanding, needle aspiration once the haematoma has liquefied, may be all that is necessary. If it is noted to be expanding, re-operation and exploration with ligation of the bleeding point is required. Postoperative wound infections occur in less than 1% of cases and are treated either with antibiotics or incision and drainage if an abscess has formed.

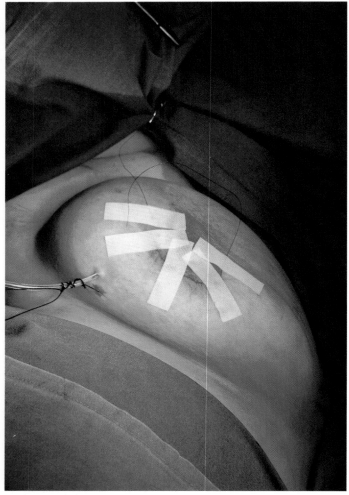

Figure 28.13 The circumareolar incision is closed using a subcuticular closure and steristrips, which gives an excellent cosmetic result.

Needle localisation biopsy

Patient preparation

Needle localisation biopsy for an impalpable lesion may be undertaken as a diagnostic procedure for a mammographically or ultrasonically detected lesion of unknown origin. Alternatively, then procedure may be a therapeutic excision of a mammographically or ultrasonically detected lesion, which has been confirmed to be malignant on a prior cytological and/or histological examination.

The investigations required preoperatively are those required for the breast lesion itself, and those required for anaesthetic assessment. The procedure is fully explained to the patient and informed consent is obtained. The patient must understand the reasons for the procedure that further surgery and other treatment may be necessary depending on the results. The patient must also understand the possible risks of cosmetic deformity in the appearance of the breast postoperatively.

A hooked needle is inserted by the radiologist into the lesion under stereotactic (or ultrasound) control prior to the patient proceeding to theatre for biopsy. A variety of needles exist for this and the choice of needle is determined by the preferences of the surgeon and radiologist.

Mammograms taken after insertion of the needle and with the abnormality marked by the radiologist (lateral and cranio-caudal views) must be available to the surgeon and must be brought along to the operating theatre with the patient. The surgeon can then determine the relationship of the abnormality to the needle and excision planned.

Anaesthesia and positioning

As for wide local excision for breast cancer.

Incision

A skin incision is made (if possible within the skin flaps that would be necessary if a mastectomy were to be required subsequently). The position of the incision will be determined by the site of the abnormality as seen on the mammograms (Figure 28.14).

Procedure

- After the skin incision has been made, skin hooks are used on either side of the incision to elevate the skin and subcutaneous fat. Skin flaps on either side of the incision are now elevated by sharp dissection to allow full access to this part of the breast (Figure 28.15).

- Langenbeck retractors can now be placed under the skin flaps and the needle localisation wire can then be sought by visualisation or by palpating with a finger. The needle may be

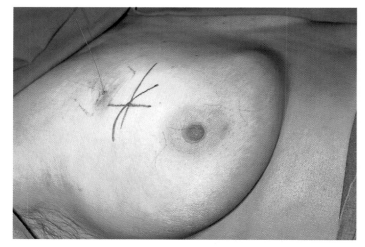

Figure 28.14 The needle localisation wire has been placed into the area to be removed. A skin incision is marked centred on the 'X', which is where the surgeon estimated that the abnormality would be on examining the mammograms.

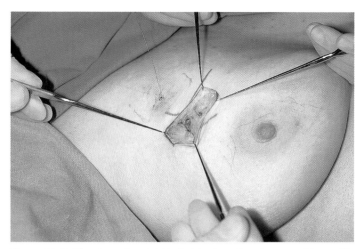

Figure 28.15 The circumferential skin incision is made and upper and lower skin flaps created and retracted using skin hooks.

• Care should be taken at all stages not to cut through the needle localisation wire. The extent of the resection has to be estimated and depends on the size of the lesion on mammography; the larger the resection the more likely the lesion is to be excised (Figures 28.17 and 28.18), but the greater the risk of cosmetic deformity of the breast.

• The tissue that has been removed is then sent to the radiologist for radiological examination to determine that it has been removed correctly by comparing with the original mammograms. If the lesion is not detected on the specimen radiograph, further excisions need to be undertaken. This can be done immediately and a radiograph of the specimen taken to determine if the lesion is present. However, this can be difficult for the surgeon because there is no guidance once the needle has been removed. If the lesion still cannot be found, no further procedure is undertaken at this stage. This must be

obvious, but sometimes a careful dissection is required to find exactly where it is. Different needles are available, some of which are easier to detect than others!

• The surgeon will already know where the abnormality is in relationship to the needle localisation wire. Often the needle used for localisation has marks/indentations on it, which can be seen on the mammogram. This is a useful guide to the position of the lesion in relationship to the needle localisation wire.

• Once the localisation wire has been found, the dissection is continued along the wire using scissors to cut the breast tissue along its surface to reach the particular mark on the wire (that is being used as a point of reference for the abnormality, Figure 28.16). Once found, the estimated area where the abnormality is can now be widely excised from the surrounding breast tissue.

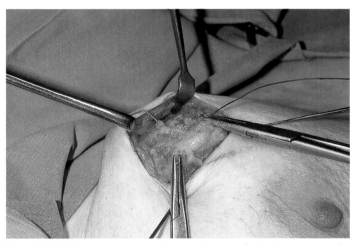

Figure 28.17 The area of suspicion has now been reached and a suture may be inserted into this area to identify this area clearly. The suspicious area is now removed, estimating how much breast tissue needs to be removed according to the mammographic appearances.

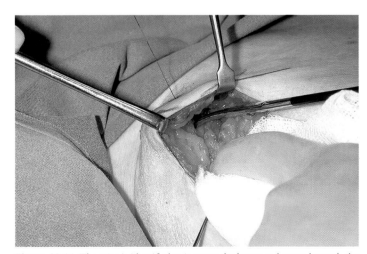

Figure 28.16 The wire is identified as it enters the breast and passes beneath the upper skin flap. The wire is then traced distally as it traverses towards the abnormality in the breast.

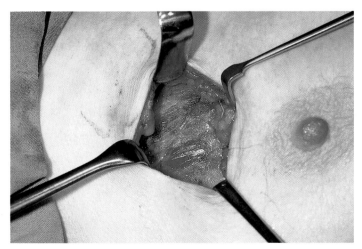

Figure 28.18 After removal of this area of breast tissue a cavity has been left, which in this case is down to the pectoralis major muscle. Closure is then as described in the text.

fully explained to the patient once they have recovered from anaesthesia and a decision to undertake a second needle localisation biopsy has to be considered.

- Following successful excision of the lesion, the cavity in the breast is carefully inspected to ensure haemostasis has been achieved. A closed drain is placed into the cavity and brought out through a stab incision in the skin of the breast (low suction drainage is used). Some surgeons do not, however, use drains in this situation.

- The subcutaneous fat is closed with interrupted sutures of an absorbable material. The skin is closed with a subcuticular technique of either absorbable or non-absorbable material with steristrips to ensure accurate skin apposition.

Postoperative management

As for wide local excision of breast cancer.

Axillary lymph node dissection

Axillary dissection is usually carried out at the same time as wide local excision or mastectomy, in patients with breast cancer.

Patient preparation

The risks of damage to the intercostobrachial nerve and subsequent sensory disturbances in its distribution should be explained to the patient. The small chance of arm swelling/lymphoedema, and the possible reduction in arm movements must also be discussed and explained.

Anaesthesia and positioning

As described earlier for mastectomy.

Incision

If axillary dissection is undertaken in conjunction with wide local excision (either at the same time or as a second procedure subsequently) a separate incision is used. This is made in the natural skin crease of the axilla, between the lateral margin of the pectoralis major and latissimus dorsi muscles over the lower part of the axilla (Figure 28.19).

The edges of the skin are retracted perpendicularly to the place of dissection and skin flaps are then raised superiorly and inferiorly by sharp dissection, to allow access to the axilla.

However, if axillary dissection is undertaken in conjunction with mastectomy, no separate incision is required. As described above, the breast is dissected into the axilla, towards the axillary fat and the dissection can be continued as described after.

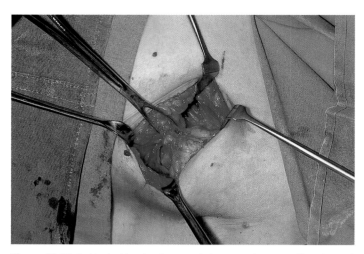

Figure 28.19 A skin incision has been made between the pectoralis major and latissimus dorsi muscles. The axillary tail of the breast has been identified and grasped by Littlewood's forceps. If an axillary sample is to be undertaken, four palpable nodes are removed from this lower part of the axilla.

Procedure

- Initially, the axilla is defined by identifying the borders of the pectoralis major and minor muscles. The posterior border is defined by the latissimus dorsi muscle and the upper border by the inferior surface of the axillary vein.

- Having defined the borders of the axillary fat/lymphatics, level 1 is dissected out by a combination of sharp and blunt dissection, from an inferior to a superior direction. Care is taken to ensure that the long thoracic nerve, the thoracodorsal artery, vein and nerve are preserved. Any small vessels are divided by metal clips or suture ligated as the dissection proceeds. The axillary contents are dissected off the chest wall medially and the skin and subcutaneous fat laterally.

- At all times the position of the axillary vein should be reviewed as any traction of the lower part of the axilla can displace the vein inferiorly. If major bleeding does occur this is likely to be due to avulsion of a branch of the axillary vein or possibly damage to the axillary vein itself.

- If this occurs, the area should be packed for five minutes. The packs are then carefully removed – it should be possible to see where the bleeding is coming from. If it is from a branch of the axillary vein this is clamped and tied. However, if it is coming directly from the axillary vein this can be more difficult to deal with. Using a sucker to identify the tear clearly, it may be possible to insert a prolene vascular suture to repair the damage. If it is still bleeding and difficult to identify, pressure on either side of the damaged area using a gauze swab or Cooley side clamp should be sufficient to allow the tear to be identified and repaired.

- The intercostobrachial nerve also crosses the axilla at this level and should be conserved, if possible, by dissecting it from axillary fat (Figure 28.20). However, even when it has been preserved, sensory disturbances can still occur.

- If a level 1 dissection is being performed, the dissection is continued superiorly until the axillary vein is reached (small veins entering the axillary vein will be identified, ligated and divided), and the infero-lateral border of the pectoralis minor is reached. Small lymphatic channels that are encountered should be ligated and divided.

- If a level 2 dissection is undertaken, the dissection is continued behind the pectoralis minor muscle (retracted with a Langenbeck retractor) and completed at the superio-medial border of pectoralis minor (Figure 28.21). The axillary vein forms the superior border.

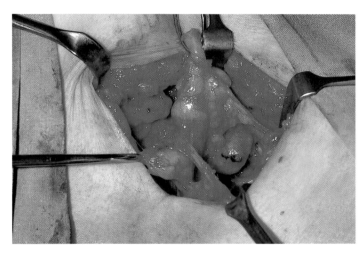

Figure 28.20 A palpable node is being removed here. The intercostobrachial nerve traverses the axilla and is preserved if possible.

- If a level 3 dissection (clearance) is being undertaken, further exposure is required to gain access to the axillary fat/lymphatics in this level. Although some surgeons just retract the pectoralis muscle, excellent exposure can be obtained by dividing the muscle. Improved exposure at this point may be obtained by abducting and moving the arm at the shoulder joint.

- The pectoralis minor is dissected free from the pectoralis major (Rotters' nodes and lymphatics can lie on the anterior surface of pectoralis minor). The next stage is to place an index finger along the inferior surface of the pectoralis minor, carefully passing the finger medially so that it then emerges anteriorly at the medial border of the muscle. This manoeuvre is completed by pushing the finger through the clavipectoral fascia, so that the muscle is encircled by the index finger. This muscle passes superiorly to its point of attachment to the corocoid process of the scapula. The finger is pushed along the muscle as far as possible and using diathermy the muscle can be cut as closely to its attachment as possible. It is important to remember the close proximity of the axillary vessels and the brachial plexus and it is important to protect these and ensure that they are not damaged.

- The pectoralis muscle can be dissected inferiorly to its attachments to the third, fourth and fifth ribs and removed from them and sent for histological examination (some surgeons, however, simply divide the muscle but do not remove it).

- Following this, the dissection is continued along the axillary vein superiorly to the outer border of the first rib at the apex of the axilla, thus removing all the axillary fat and lymphatics (Figure 28.22).

- After completion of the dissection, haemostasis is secured and a suction drain placed into the axilla, emerging through a stab incision below the main incision.

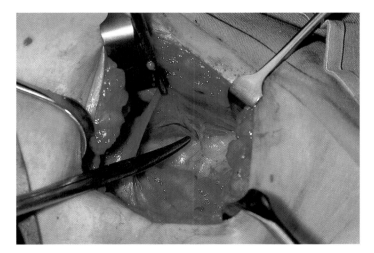

Figure 28.21 If a level I or II dissection is undertaken the axillary dissection is continued proximally to either the infero-lateral border of pectoralis minor or to behind the pectoralis minor, respectively. The lateral pectoral nerve and vessels are preserved during this dissection.

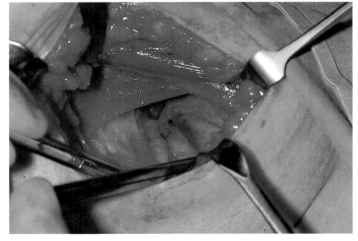

Figure 28.22 As the dissection continues proximally the axillary vein is identified and marks the upper limit of the dissection. If a level III dissection (clearance) is undertaken, the axillary fat is traced proximally to the outer border of the first rib where the axilla commences.

- The subcutaneous fat may be closed with interrupted absorbable sutures and the skin is closed with a subcuticular absorbable or non-absorbable suture and steristrips applied.

Postoperative management

The drain is removed when the 24-hourly drainage is less than approximately 30 ml.

Physiotherapy to the arm initially supervised by a physiotherapist, minimises any limitation of arm movements. Full instructions and an exercise protocol are given to the patient.

Wound infections occur in less than 1% of patients and are treated with antibiotics or incision and drainage as appropriate.

FURTHER READING

Blamey RW. The design and clinical use of the Nottingham Prognostic Index. *The Breast* 1996; 156–157

Early Breast Cancer Trialists Collaborative Group. Polychemotherapy for early breast cancer: an overview of the randomised trials. *Lancet* 1998; **352**:930–941

Early Breast Cancer Trialists Collaborative Group. Systemic treatment of early breast cancer by hormonal, cytotoxic or immune therapy. *Lancet* 1992; **339**:71–85

Fossati R, Confalonieri V, Ghislandi E, et al. Cytotoxic and hormonal treatment for metastatic breast cancer: a systematic review of published randomised trials involving 31 510 women. *J Clin Oncol* 1998; **16**:3439–3460

Scottish Intercollegiate Guidelines Network, 1998; SIGN Publication Number 29, SIGN Secretariat, Royal College of Physicians, Edinburgh

29

Advanced breast cancer

S.J. Leinster

INTRODUCTION

Advanced breast cancer is a vague term covering anything that is not early breast cancer. Conventionally, the latter is defined as localised disease T1–2 N0–1 M0. Overt metastases may be present at the time of diagnosis. Such cases are said to be 'advanced at presentation'. More commonly, metastases may occur some time after the original treatment and may be associated with locoregional recurrence. The median survival of patients with advanced breast cancer is said to be 18–24 months although some long-term survivors are reported; 1.5% of patients treated at the M D Anderson centre between 1973 and 1982 survived for 16 years. The currently accepted paradigm of breast cancer postulates the presence of micrometastases at the time of diagnosis in a significant number of women. It is the growth of these micrometastases that gives rise to advanced breast cancer.

The likelihood of recurrence can be calculated using formulae such as the Nottingham Prognostic Index. The predicted risk of recurrence varies from 10% to 60% at five years depending on the characteristics of the tumour. The Nottingham Index is based on the size of the primary tumour, the presence or absence of lymph node involvement and the histological grade of the tumour. Other features of the tumour, such as the absence of c-erbB2 or the presence of mutated p53, are associated with an increased risk of developing recurrent disease. These factors have not yet been incorporated into a coherent prognostic index.

The biological behaviour of metastases is unclear. A simplistic model regards the metastases as implanting at the distant site and growing there at a similar rate to the growth of the primary (Figure 29.1). Tumour growth is, however, unlikely to be linear, as most biological growth is Gompertzian (Figure 29.2). As the total tumour mass gets larger, the growth rate falls. It is a feature of Gompertzian systems that if the total biomass is reduced, rapid growth will again ensue. If the total tumour mass in the body (primary + micrometastases) is regarded as a single

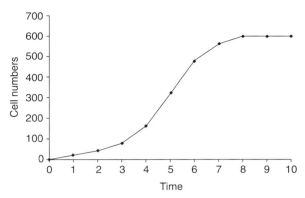

Figure 29.2 Gompertzian growth. The initial growth of the tumour is exponential but eventually the available nutrients become rate limiting and tumour growth slows and the tumour size reaches a plateau. If cell numbers are reduced, the tumour again enters an exponential growth phase.

biological entity, the micrometastases will start to grow rapidly when the primary is removed. This is one of the rationales for the use of adjuvant therapy. Both of these models account satisfactorily for the early appearance of metastases after initial treatment but it is a feature of breast cancer that metastases may appear many years after the primary has been treated. This cannot be explained by either of these models. It has been observed that late metastases may arise after a stressful life event or intercurrent illness. This has led to the hypothesis that the tumour lives in a steady state of symbiosis with the patient as a result of 'defence mechanisms' that balance the rate of tumour growth with an equal rate of tumour death until some external event leads to a reduction in the defence mechanisms, so allowing the tumour to grow. There is no experimental evidence to support this model.

Baum has called for a paradigm shift in our view of the process of metastatic spread. Based on the finding that macrophages in patients with breast cancer appear to contain retroviral-like DNA sequences, he suggests that genetic information from the breast cancer is transmitted in successive generations of macrophages. This information can then be passed to a somatic cell at a distant site, so transforming that cell and leading to the development of a metastasis. This does not answer the question of why the nucleic acid transfer should take place at a particular point in time, but does seek to explain the variable time for the appearance of metastases.

The whole question may seem irrelevant to the management of patients with breast cancer, but if we are going to improve our management we need to understand the basic mechanisms involved.

The molecular biology and histological type of the tumour may determine the site of recurrence. Tumours which express high levels of oestrogen receptors characteristically metastasise to bone, while those that are oestrogen receptor negative characteristically recur in soft tissue and viscera. Lobular tumours may give rise to diffuse intra- and retroperitoneal involvement and can cause intestinal obstruction or hydronephrosis.

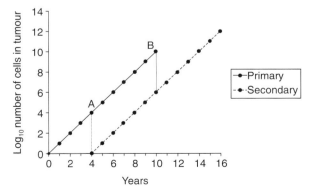

Figure 29.1 A simple model of metastic growth. The primary tumour begins growing. The example shown has a doubling time of approximately 100 days. At point A a metastasis implants at a distant site and begins to grow. It grows at the same rate as the primary tumour. At point B the primary is detected and removed but no adjuvant therapy is given. The metastasis continues to grow undisturbed until it reached 10^{12} cells and the patient dies.

PRESENTATION

The presentation of advanced breast cancer depends on the organ(s) involved.

The most common site of distant metastases is the skeleton. Metastatic disease tends to be 'centripetal' and to involve the spine, pelvis and the proximal ends of the long bones. It is rare for metastases to occur in the distal part of the limbs. Metastases are commonly multiple. The first indication of bone metastases may be pain, which is severe and progressive. Compression fractures of the spine are not uncommon and may be associated with compression of the spinal cord and neurological deficits. Metastases in the long bones may give rise to pathological fractures.

Widespread bony metastases may give rise to hypercalcaemia. Typically, the patient presents with drowsiness, confusion and vomiting. Thirst is sometimes a prominent feature. The differential diagnosis includes cerebral metastases and diabetic coma. Serum calcium levels must be measured in any breast cancer patient who develops these symptoms. Clinical examination is often unhelpful.

Lung metastases are often asymptomatic and are found during routine metastatic screening carried out because of the presence of other metastases. The common symptom of lung involvement is breathlessness. This may be associated with a dry, unproductive cough. There are two patterns of disease that may give rise to these symptoms. The first is pleural effusion and the second is lymphangitis carcinomatosis. In the latter case, the tumour cells have infiltrated the alveolar membranes and the breathlessness is a result of impaired diffusion of gases through the membrane.

The clinical findings of a pleural effusion are typical with decreased respiratory movement, dullness to percussion and decreased air entry on the affected side. In contrast, clinical examination may be entirely normal in lymphangitis carcinomatosis. A chest radiograph may show increased hilar shadowing and the presence of Kerley's 'A' and 'B' lines. The radiographic features are similar to those of acute left ventricular failure but lymphangitis is diagnosed because of the absence of clinical signs.

The prognosis of the two presentations is markedly different. After successful treatment, patients who have had a pleural effusion may live for several years. Long-term survivors do occur. Patients with lymphangitis have a median survival of three months if they do not respond to treatment and a median survival of nine months if they do. Parenchymal lung metastases occasionally occur. A solitary mass lesion on the chest radiograph is more likely to be a second (bronchogenic) primary than a metastasis.

Hepatic metastases may present with pain in the right hypochondrium. More commonly, they present with vague malaise and anorexia. Weight loss may be a prominent feature, as may nausea and vomiting. For symptoms to develop a large amount of the liver must be replaced by tumour. Hepatic enlargement is commonly detected clinically at this stage. The patient will eventually become jaundiced and ascites is likely to occur.

Ascites may also be a sign of peritoneal involvement, especially in lobular carcinoma.

Cerebral metastases usually occur as mass lesions which may be solitary or multiple. Much more rarely, the patient may develop meningitis carcinomatosis, with widespread small deposits affecting the meninges. The presentation of cerebral metastases is raised intracranial pressure. Typically, the patient will complain of headache which is worse in the morning and is often associated with nausea and vomiting. The latter may be the most prominent symptom. The patient will eventually become confused and drowsy and may lapse into coma. Focal neurological signs are usually a late manifestation but the patient may have papilloedema at an early stage. Often, however, clinical examination is unhelpful and the diagnosis can only be confirmed by CT or MR scanning. Neck stiffness may be a feature in meningitis carcinomatosis but the diagnosis is usually made because there is evidence of raised intracranial pressure but no mass lesion on scan. MR is better at demonstrating meningitis carcinomatosis than CT but it may be necessary to perform a lumbar puncture for confirmation.

Spinal cord metastases present with neurological symptoms and signs. The patient may have sensory loss or motor weakness, especially in the lower limbs. Bladder and / or bowel dysfunction may occur. These symptoms must be investigated urgently and an immediate MR scan is the method of choice. If cord compression is demonstrated, whether due to cord metastases or bony metastases, urgent treatment must be instituted.

Despite regular follow-up, metastatic or locally recurrent disease commonly presents symptomatically rather than being detected by the clinician in the preclinical phase. This failure of conventional measures to detect early metastatic disease has led to an increasing interest in tumour markers. The markers most commonly used are CEA and CA 15–3. Despite evidence that rising levels of the tumour markers do indicate the presence of clinically occult recurrent disease, the utility of these measures is still in doubt and they should only be used within the confines of a controlled study.

INVESTIGATION

When a patient presents with symptoms that might be due to recurrent disease, full investigation is essential.

The first requirement is confirmation of the diagnosis. Ideally, a tissue diagnosis should be obtained. Where the recurrence is accessible and the clinical appearances are typical, fine needle aspiration for cytology is useful. Pleural effusions and ascites may be aspirated for cytology. Cytology of solid lung and liver lesions may be carried out under imaging control. Some lung metastases may be accessible to assessment and biopsy by bronchoscopy. Where there is any doubt as to the nature of the tumour (is it a recurrence or a new primary?) a core needle biopsy may be needed. Locoregional recurrences may be excised in order to obtain definitive histology.

The biopsy of bony metastases is a more difficult procedure and it is customary, when the lesions are multiple, to rely on the imaging appearances for diagnosis. It is essential that a combination of isotope imaging and plain radiographs be used. In cases of doubt, a MR scan may be helpful. Failure to compare the appearances on all imaging modalities can lead to mistaken diagnosis and there is at least one case report of osteomalacia being mistaken for, and treated as, widespread bony metastases. When the correct diagnosis was eventually made, the patient was treated with vitamin D and calcium and made a dramatic recovery. Solitary metastases in bone should be biopsied if possible.

Similarly, the diagnosis of intracranial metastases is usually made on imaging.

SCREENING

Once the diagnosis has been established, the patient must be fully assessed.

Haematology

A full blood count will show evidence of any bone marrow involvement. The classic picture is of a leucoerythroblastic anaemia. Any diagnosis of marrow involvement should be confirmed by a marrow aspiration or preferably a trephine biopsy.

Biochemistry

The most subtle change suggestive of metastatic disease is a raised level of serum alkaline phosphatase activity. This will occur with hepatic and bony metastases. Isoenzymes can be measured to distinguish hepatic alkaline phosphatase from bony alkaline phosphatase but, in practice, this is seldom done as the diagnosis is usually made on imaging.

Plain radiographs

A chest radiograph is mandatory. A negative chest radiograph can usually be accepted as evidence that there is no significant disease in the lungs. Sometimes, the patient's symptoms suggest the presence of lung involvement but the chest radiograph is clear. Sometimes, there may be uncertainties in the interpretation of the chest radiograph. In either of these situations a CT scan of the chest is indicated.

Plain radiographs of the skeleton are indicated in the investigation of any painful area. It is also important to perform radiographs of any 'hotspots' detected on isotope bone scan to distinguish between metastases and other causes of increased bone turnover, such as Paget's disease, osteoarthritis and trauma.

Bronchoscopy

If the CT scan of the chest is clear and the patient continues to have respiratory symptoms, endobronchial metastases should be considered. These are rare but when they do occur are best detected by bronchoscopy.

Scan of liver

The liver should be scanned even if the biochemistry is normal. Note that this is different from the situation in early breast cancer. Ultrasound is effective and can reliably detect lesions over 1 cm in diameter. CT scan is also sensitive and can, in addition, give an accurate assessment of the retroperitoneal lymph nodes. However, the incidence of involvement of the retroperitoneal nodes is low and ultrasound of the liver is usually adequate.

Isotope bone scan

Technetium-99 is taken up by bone that is undergoing increased turnover. Following intravenous injection of technetium, the whole body can be scanned using a gamma camera. Areas of increased bone activity show up as 'hotspots'. Plain radiographs are necessary to distinguish metastases from other causes of hotspots such as Paget's disease, osteoarthritis and trauma. Isotope bone scans are more sensitive than plain radiographs and it is not uncommon to find completely normal radiographs at the site of a hotspot. If this area is symptomatic it is highly likely that there is early tumour development. When making the diagnosis is going to make a difference to management (for example, if there is no other evidence of metastatic disease), MR scanning may give a definitive answer.

The above tests should be carried out routinely in all cases of proven recurrent breast cancer. Other tests may be used in special circumstances.

CT scan

As indicated above, CT scan can be helpful in defining disease extent in the chest in cases where the chest radiograph is equivocal. If a solitary parenchymal lesion is being considered for resection, a CT scan should be done to exclude the presence of other small lesions throughout the remainder of the lung field.

CT scan of the abdomen is indicated especially in lobular breast cancer when intraperitoneal or retroperitoneal spread is suspected.

CT scan of the brain is indicated if there are symptoms or signs suggestive of intracranial metastases. It is not carried out as part of the routine assessment of a patient with recurrent disease.

MR scan

MR scan is useful because fibrosis can be distinguished from recurrent tumour by the characteristic uptake of gadolinium. This is particularly useful in diagnosing recurrence in a breast treated by breast conservation with wide local excision and radiotherapy. It can also be used in the diagnosis of lymphoedema of the arm when a distinction must be made between fibrosis and tumour in the axilla.

MR is also helpful in confirming the presence of bony metastases. It is now the investigation of choice when spinal cord compression as a result of metastases is suspected.

TREATMENT

All the common modalities of treatment may be appropriate in different cases of advanced breast cancer.

Surgery

The indications for surgery in advanced breast cancer are limited but real. It is important that surgeons remain involved in the multidisciplinary team discussions in all breast cancer patients.

The most obvious role for surgery is in the control of locally recurrent disease, especially if the area has been previously treated with radiotherapy. Wide excision of the area can be carried out and the defect repaired using a suitable flap. When the resection involves soft tissue and the underlying chest wall is intact, the thoracoepigastric or thoracoabdominal flap is a useful form of skin cover. When necessary, involved ribs and pleura can be resected and the defect repaired using a myocutaneous flap. The best flap for the purpose is the latissimus dorsi flap, which has a very dependable blood supply and a high success rate. When the resected area is very large an omental flap with skin grafting is a useful if somewhat unorthodox solution. The omental flap is particularly useful if the area is infected, as the omentum appears to have antibacterial properties.

There are anecdotal reports of benefit from resecting solitary metastases in a variety of viscera, including lung and brain. The presentation is so unusual that no proper study has been carried out. Nevertheless, the logic of the approach seems unassailable.

Surgery may also be needed in cases of GI tract obstruction due to metastatic lobular carcinoma.

Surgery has a long-established role in the management of bony metastases. Clearly internal fixation is necessary in the event of pathological fracture of the long bones. A pathological fracture of the hip may require a joint replacement. If the metastases are detected before fracture occurs, prophylactic surgery may be undertaken. The indication for this is thinning of the cortex, suggesting that the risk of fracture is high. More recently, surgery for spinal metastases has become feasible. Spinal surgery is indicated for localised metastatic disease, particularly when the major symptom is pain resulting from mechanical factors. Potential wedge fractures can be stabilised by posterior fixation. It is possible to resect vertebral bodies that are involved, with the remaining spine being stabilised by metal rods.

A less controversial indication for surgery is decompression of the spinal cord when compression develops. Evidence of developing cord compression is a surgical emergency. When the patient is fit for surgery and the compression is amenable to surgical decompression, this should be undertaken as soon as possible after confirmation with a MR scan.

In the past, surgical ablation of the adrenal glands or the pituitary gland played a major role in the management of advanced breast cancer. These operations have been superseded by drug therapy such as the aromatase inhibitors and goserelin.

Radiotherapy

Radiotherapy may be given in low dose to relieve the pain of bony metastases or in higher doses to control disease progression. In the latter case it is often combined with surgery.

Metastases in long bones

When metastases give rise to pathological fractures, the fracture should be fixed internally. When the fracture is in the neck of the femur it may be necessary to perform a total hip replacement. The area should be irradiated following surgery using doses of 30–50 Gy in 10–20 fractions. Similar doses may be given when the metastasis is detected before fracture. This may be preceded by prophylactic surgery if the cortex is thinned. When the cortex appears to be intact radiotherapy may be given without surgery. Since the objective is to prevent or treat a fracture, the local problem should be treated even when there are other metastases, especially when these are confined to the skeleton.

Spinal metastases

One or two fractions of radiotherapy (3–5 Gy) are often effective in controlling pain in the spine. It should always be considered when a proper analgesic regimen is failing to control the pain. Conventionally, it can only be used over a limited area and is focused on the most painful region. When the radiotherapy has been effective in controlling the pain but another area of the spine subsequently becomes painful, the treatment can be repeated.

When the pain is due to mechanical factors such as collapse, rather than active tumour, radiotherapy will not be effective. A careful history will distinguish the pain arising from mechanical causes from pain arising from active tumour. It is important to take a careful history to avoid inappropriate treatment. The radiological appearances will not diagnose the mechanism of the pain.

When spinal cord decompression has been carried out, the area should be irradiated to bring about regression or, at least, to delay progression of the tumour. If the patient is unfit for surgery, radiotherapy can be used as the primary treatment modality in spinal cord compression.

Cerebral metastases

Solitary cerebral metastases should be resected. The brain should then be irradiated to delay recurrence. When multiple metastases are present, control of symptoms may be achieved for up to one year by radiotherapy to the entire brain. Some reactive oedema occurs, which may result in a worsening of symptoms initially. This can be prevented by treatment with dexamethasone (12 mg daily in divided doses) prior to the radiotherapy. The dexamethasone often results in an initial improvement in the symptoms even before the definitive treatment starts. The dexamethasone should be reduced gradually over a period of several weeks to avoid the side effects of prolonged use. Too rapid a withdrawal could result in a rebound worsening of the raised intracranial pressure.

Visceral metastases

Radiotherapy has little role in the management of visceral metastases.

Locoregional recurrence

Radiotherapy is indicated in the management of soft tissue local recurrence if it has not been used previously. The outcome is likely to be better if it is possible to resect the lesion before treating with radiotherapy. When necessary soft tissue defects resulting from the debulking can be repaired using cutaneous or myocutaneous flaps.

Lymph node recurrences should be removed surgically where possible. Radiotherapy may improve the chance of preventing further recurrence but its use in this situation is associated with an increased incidence of lymphoedema of the arm. The contrasting risks of the two approaches must be carefully weighed and should be discussed with the patient before a decision is made.

Radio-isotopes

Strontium-89 has been shown to be effective as a palliative agent in widespread bony metastases from prostate cancer. On this basis, it has been suggested as a treatment for widespread painful bony metastases.

Hormone therapy

As everyone knows, the first reported use of hormone therapy in breast cancer was the use, by Beatson, of oophorectomy to treat advanced breast cancer. Since that time, hormone therapy has become established as a major treatment modality. Ablational hormonal therapy is effective in up to 30% of patients. Response is more likely if the interval from initial treatment to recurrence is long. Bony metastases are more likely to respond than soft tissue metastases, which in turn are more likely to respond than visceral metastases. Adrenalectomy and hypophysectomy became fashionable. If a patient

had had a response to oophorectomy and then relapsed, her chance of responding to second-line ablation was again of the order of 30%.

Curiously, although it was established that hormonal ablation resulted in tumour regression, some oncologists began to give exogenous hormones in the form of stilboestrol. This also produced a response rate of around 30%.

A well-recognised complication of hormonal treatment is tumour flare. In the early weeks of treatment the tumour may seem to grow more quickly or hypercalcaemia may develop. This can cause anxiety in the patient and the clinician but is usually associated with a subsequently good response.

Anti-oestrogens

In the mid 1970s, tamoxifen, an anti-oestrogen with partial agonist effects, was introduced. It had a response rate similar to oophorectomy but had the added advantage that, if it did not work, the patient had not undergone an operation.

The discovery of the oestrogen receptor led to an improved understanding of why some patients responded and others did not. When a tumour is oestrogen receptor positive, the response rate to hormone therapy is around 60% for bony metastases. If the tumour is oestrogen receptor negative, the response rate is around 10%. There is debate about the mechanism by which response occurs in oestrogen-negative tumours. Without doubt, some of the receptor-negative tumours that respond are false negatives as the result of laboratory or sampling error. It is postulated, however, that some oestrogen receptor-negative tumours respond because tamoxifen has actions that are independent of the oestrogen receptor.

A difference of approach developed in the UK and the USA. In the USA, reliance was placed on the oestrogen receptor result and patients were not given tamoxifen unless their tumour was oestrogen receptor positive. In the UK, many oncologists took the view that tamoxifen had such a mild side effect profile that it was worth trying it to see if there was any response even if the tumour was oestrogen receptor negative.

Many patients now will have had tamoxifen as adjuvant therapy. As long as there has been an interval of more than two years from the end of the adjuvant treatment till the recurrence, it is worthwhile trying tamoxifen again.

Tamoxifen is a partial oestrogen agonist. Pure anti-oestrogens have been produced and these are currently undergoing trials.

Other hormonal therapies are also effective. In general, they have not displaced tamoxifen as first-line therapy but they have a role in patients who relapse after an initial response.

Aromatase inhibitors

In postmenopausal women, the pathway of oestrogen production is dependent on the enzyme aromatase, which is found in the peripheral adipose tissue. Aromatase inhibitors lower the level of circulating oestrogen. The original member of the class, aminoglutethimide, also inhibits the production of cortisol in the adrenal gland but the newer members of the class are more specific and are better tolerated. The most widely used example in the UK is anastrazole (Arimidex, AstraZeneca). Recent trials have compared anastrazole with tamoxifen as first-line management for advanced breast cancer. Anastrazole appears to be equally effective in terms of response rate in oestrogen receptor-positive tumours but to have a longer time to first recurrence. There appears to be little difference in side effects. No data are available on overall survival rate and unless there is clear evidence in the future that the sequence anastrazole → tamoxifen is better than tamoxifen → anastrazole, there is really no reason to abandon tamoxifen as first-line hormonal therapy. Anastrazole is currently the preferred option as second-line therapy.

Progestogens

The progestogens are also active against breast cancer. The most commonly used progestogen is megesterol acetate. One of its side effects is increased appetite with consequent weight gain. This may be an advantage in patients with anorexia, particularly those with liver metastases.

LHRH agonists

When LHRH agonists are given in depot preparations, they produce a medical oophorectomy with complete obliteration of oestrogen production. There is evidence that treatment with goserelin produces responses comparable to oophorectomy.

Using hormonal therapy

When a patient responds to hormonal therapy and subsequently relapses, she should be prescribed another hormone therapy. A response rate of around 30% can be expected. If the patient does not respond to second-line therapy, chemotherapy will have to be considered. When there is a response to second-line therapy the patient should continue on it until relapse when third-line hormonal therapy can be tried. Again, 30% of patients can be expected to respond. At the point where no response is found, chemotherapy can be introduced if the patient is fit enough.

Chemotherapy

Breast cancer is comparatively sensitive to chemotherapy. The mainstay of treatment for many years has been the anthracyclines such as doxirubicin, epirubicin and mitoxantrone. They are often used in combination with alkylating agents, such as cyclophosphamide or with vinca alkaloids such as vincristine. In soft tissue disease these combinations will give response rates of up to 70%. The response rate in visceral disease is lower (around 40–50%) and

in bony disease is poor. Mitomycin C has also been used but has fallen out of favour because of a high incidence of serious side effects such as the haemolytic uraemic syndrome. There is no evidence at present that any one regimen is more effective than others.

Newer agents such as the taxanes show promise. At present, they are licensed for use in metastatic breast cancer where conventional chemotherapy with anthracyclines has failed. Clinical trials of docetaxel and paclitaxel show longer disease-free survival than standard control regimens. High-dose chemotherapy with stem cell rescue has also proved to be no more effective than conventional chemotherapy. At present, all patients regarded as suitable for chemotherapy should be offered the opportunity to enter clinical trials.

Other therapies

Herceptin (trastuzumab) is a monoclonal antibody to the HER2/neu receptor. This receptor is overexpressed in around 25% of all breast cancers and is a marker of poorer prognosis. Treatment of HER2 receptor-positive tumours, previously treated with chemotherapy, with herceptin produced a 21% response rate. When chemotherapy and herceptin are combined there is a prolonged survival compared to treatment with chemotherapy alone.

Bisphosphonates are useful in the control of hypercalcaemia and pain from bony metastases, but also have an antitumour effect. Pamidronate delays the development of complications in patients with known bony metastases.

SELECTION OF THERAPY

It is impossible to lay down clear protocols for the management of advanced breast cancer. The treatment must be tailored to the needs of the individual patient and the nature and extent of her disease. Nevertheless, there are certain principles that should be followed.

Since no form of treatment at present is curative, the main aim of therapy should be the relief of symptoms or the prevention of deterioration. The patient should be fully assessed to determine the extent of disease before a treatment plan is developed.

If the recurrence is localised, surgery or radiotherapy should be considered. When the disease is more widespread, systemic therapy is needed. If the tumour is known to be oestrogen receptor positive or, when the oestrogen receptor status is unknown, there has been a long disease-free interval, hormone therapies should be considered first. This is especially true in bony or soft tissue disease. In visceral disease, hormone therapy is less likely to be successful. However, if the patient is well and the disease does not appear to be progressing rapidly, a trial of hormone therapy may be made.

If the patient has a poor performance status, active treatment may not be of benefit and a regimen of palliative care may be more appropriate than aggressive chemotherapy. The patient should be fully engaged with a multidisciplinary team in making this sort of decision.

TREATMENT OF SPECIFIC PRESENTATIONS

Bony metastases

Solitary spinal metastases

The treatment of spinal metastases has become much more proactive. Patients with solitary spinal metastases should be discussed with a spinal surgeon as they may be suitable candidates for surgery. Minimal surgery would involve posterior stabilisation to prevent the development of mechanical instability, but it may be possible to resect the affected vertebra and replace it with a prosthesis. The area should then be irradiated.

If the patient is not already on hormonal therapy, this should be started. Patients who have had adjuvant tamoxifen can still experience benefit from its reintroduction. Alternatively, the patient could be started on anastrazole if postmenopausal. In premenopausal women, Zoladex should be considered. Monthly pamidronate has been shown to delay the onset of subsequent lesions.

Long bone metastases

The main consideration in metastases in the long bones is the likelihood of pathological fractures. When the cortex is preserved, the likelihood of fracture is low and full dose radiotherapy can be given for the local problem. If the cortex is eroded, surgical fixation should precede radiotherapy. When pathological fracture has already occurred at the time of detection of the metastases, internal fixation is again indicated but should be followed by radiotherapy. With adequate fixation and radiotherapy, the pathological fracture will heal. When the hip is involved, it may be technically more satisfactory to carry out a total hip replacement.

Systemic treatment should be started as above.

Multiple bony metastases

When metastases are widespread, the major consideration is pain control. Hormone therapy and bisphosphonates are helpful. Few centres will consider radio-isotope therapy or hemi-body irradiation.

Hypercalcaemia

When bony metastases are present, hypercalcaemia is a potential problem. The presentation may be subtle and it is necessary to maintain a high index of suspicion. Any patient who has breast cancer who presents with drowsiness, vomiting or vague malaise should be considered to have hypercalcaemia until proved otherwise. When the diagnosis is established, the patient should be rehydrated with intravenous saline. If the hypercalcaemia persists, the patient should be given an infusion of pamidronate. This will usually reduce the calcium level in 24–48 hours. Pamidronate has superseded other therapies such as high-dose steroids (which were found in properly controlled trials to be ineffective) and calcitonin.

Once the calcium level has been brought under control, consideration should be given to appropriate systemic therapy. This will usually be hormonal. The calcium level should be regularly monitored. It may be necessary to repeat the pamidronate infusion at intervals of 4–6 weeks, but long remissions do occur. There is some evidence that oral bisphosphonates such as clodrinate may be helpful in maintaining remission.

Spinal cord compression

It is important that spinal cord compression is treated as early as possible. Delay in diagnosis can occur because the patient does not recognise the problem as serious when it first appears. Minor difficulties with micturition or defaecation or minor neurological symptoms in the lower limbs may be dismissed as trivial. There is less excuse for medical and nursing staff failing to recognise the implications of these symptoms. Because of this, many oncologists warn patients who are diagnosed as having spinal metastases of the need to seek urgent medical attention if such symptoms appear. Early intervention may prevent the development of irreversible loss of function.

When a patient presents with suspicious symptoms, urgent MR scanning is indicated. This should be done within hours. If the scan confirms cord compression, the patient should be referred for urgent decompression of the cord with radiotherapy. If major neurological signs are already present, radiotherapy alone is the treatment of choice. There is little added gain from surgical decompression.

Breathlessness

There are two major metastatic causes of dyspnoea in patients with breast cancer. They are easily distinguished on clinical examination and radiography, although they may sometimes coexist. It is important to make the diagnosis, as the prognosis is very different for the two conditions.

Pleural effusion

The patient with pleural effusion will present with shortness of breath, initially on exertion, but progressing to dyspnoea at rest. There may be an associated dry cough. The diagnosis of malignant pleural effusion is confirmed by cytology of the aspirated fluid.

437

Once the diagnosis is made, a chest drain should be inserted. This will result in a rapid resolution of the symptoms. The effusion should be drained to dryness and pleurodesis carried out. Bleomycin (60 mg in 100 ml saline) is instilled through the drain and left in place for two hours. The patient is turned regularly during this time to distribute the solution over the whole of the pleural cavity. The bleomycin is then drained off. Alternatively, a solution of tetracycline can be used. If the effusion recurs rapidly, talc pleurodesis can be carried out under thoracoscopic control.

The patient's systemic treatment should be reviewed and hormone therapy or chemotherapy introduced. Long survivals are possible.

Lymphangitis carcinomatosis

Again, the presentation is with increasing breathlessness and a dry cough. The radiographic appearances are typical. The first aim of management is relief of the breathlessness. Although there may not be clinical signs to suggest airway obstruction, the patients often experience symptomatic relief from salbutamol nebulisers. Oral steroids should be prescribed. Prednisolone 20 mg daily is a useful starting dose. If the dyspnoea is severe and does not respond to these measures, the patient should be prescribed diazepam 2 mg three times a day. This will improve the subjective sensation of breathlessness although it will not improve the actual effectiveness of respiration. If this is ineffective, it may be necessary to prescribe morphine. The respiratory depression that may occur is accepted as an unavoidable concomitant of the symptomatic relief. By this stage, symptom relief takes precedence over other considerations. The risks should be fully discussed with the patient.

If the patient's performance status is reasonable active anticancer treatment can be considered. Because of the rapid progression of the disease and the likely poor response to hormone therapy, chemotherapy is indicated. The chemotherapy regimen should include one of the anthracyclines or the taxanes. The chance of response is not high, but some patients experience a useful response. Without a response to chemotherapy the median survival is three months. If there is a response, the median survival is nine months.

Cerebral metastases

Cerebral metastases present with headache, drowsiness, nausea and vomiting. Clinical examination will reveal papilloedema and may reveal focal neurological deficits. When cerebral metastases are suspected the patient should be treated with dexamethasone 12 mg daily in divided doses. This will result in the rapid relief of symptoms. An immediate CT scan of the brain should be ordered and further treatment planned on the basis of the results.

Mass lesions

The majority of the lesions will be mass lesions. When they are solitary, they can be treated by resection followed by radio-

therapy. Without treatment the median survival is three months. With radiotherapy alone the median survival is nine months but, if resection is carried out first, the median survival is extended to 14 months.

When the lesions are multiple, radiotherapy is the only useful option. The dexamethasone should be continued in full dose until the radiotherapy is completed when the dose can be tailed off.

Carcinomatosis meningitis

Rarely, there will be evidence of increased intracranial pressure without any evidence of mass lesion on the scan. In this case, carcinomatosis meningitis should be suspected. The diagnosis can be confirmed by lumbar puncture and cytology of the cerebrospinal fluid. Treatment consists of intrathecal methotrexate and radiotherapy to the brain and spinal cord.

Hepatic metastases

It is rare for the hepatic metastases from breast cancer to be solitary and resectable. When this does occur, resection should be considered. In cases of more diffuse disease, chemotherapy is the best option. Hormone therapy is unlikely to be effective. Many patients are not fit for chemotherapy by the time the diagnosis is made. Once again, anthracyclines or taxanes are the drugs of choice.

Patients with hepatic metastases may complain of anorexia. This is often a cause of major concern to the patient and her family. It may be associated with severe nausea and vomiting. These symptoms can be relieved by treatment with corticosteroids. Dexamethasone 2 mg three times a day or prednisolone 5 mg three times a day are both effective. Megestrol acetate can also be prescribed. While it is unlikely to be effective as an antitumour agent in this situation, it does improve the appetite and may give the patient an improved sense of general well-being.

If the liver is greatly enlarged, the patient may experience severe pain in the right hypochondrium. Morphine may be needed to control the pain. Dexamethasone may be useful as an adjuvant analgesic.

Soft tissue and lymph node metastases

Soft tissue metastases may be suitable for resection. Following resection, the area of the recurrence should be irradiated. When the area has previously been treated with radiotherapy, wide resection should be performed. If necessary, flaps can be used to cover the resulting defect. Such major surgery should only be carried out if there is no evidence of other active disease. The simplest option is the thoracoepigastric flap, which allows coverage of a large skin defect. When chest wall muscle or ribs have to be resected, it is better to use a latissimus dorsi flap. If the area is heavily infected, an omental flap with split skin grafting is a possible procedure.

In general, the long-term results are likely to be better if primary surgery is performed rather than treating the recurrence simply with radiotherapy or with chemotherapy followed by radiotherapy.

Metastases in the supraclavicular nodes are not suitable for resection. Axillary nodal recurrences may be irresectable because of local infiltration. In either case, the best approach is combination therapy with chemotherapy to debulk the disease followed by radiotherapy to consolidate the response.

Psychological support

The awareness that breast cancer has recurred is a major psychological challenge to the patient and to the family. It is important that a frank discussion of the nature of the problem and its implications takes place. The clinician must gain an understanding of the patient's expectations and wishes before embarking on a management plan.

For many patients, the support of the clinician and the specialist breast care nurses is sufficient to enable them to cope satisfactorily with the problem. This is especially the case if they have built up a high level of trust with the team during their period of follow-up. Clearly, the primary care team may also have a major role in supporting the patient and the family. Other patients will need more specialised help and should be referred to a clinical psychologist. Some patients will become clinically depressed and will need antidepressant therapy. It is important that this need is recognised and that the treatment is prescribed. It is useful to have a liaison psychiatrist and a clinical psychologist as associated members of the oncology team.

There is an intriguing suggestion that active management of the patient's psychological status can actually result in improved survival.

Symptom control

At some point the decision has to be taken that further attempts to control the cancer are no longer appropriate. At this point, symptom control is the major aim of therapy. The decision that this point has been reached must be made in discussion with the patient and her supporters. The multidisciplinary team should be involved and the decision should not be taken by a single clinician, however senior. Once the decision has been made the palliative care team should be involved in the management of the patient. Specialists in pain relief may also become involved.

Where should the patient be managed?

The patient should be treated in whichever setting is best for her. For some patients this will be in the acute hospital or oncology unit. For many more, a hospice will be the right place. Many patients can be managed in their own home providing appropriate community support services can be provided. No assumptions should be made about what is best for an individual patient. Each case must be carefully assessed.

Control of pain

The most important aspect for many patients is the control of pain. Everyone is familiar with the WHO analgesic ladder that starts with simple analgesics and gradually introduces more powerful drugs until pain relief is achieved. In practice, if a patient is suffering from severe cancer-related pain, it may be better to give them a powerful analgesic to break the pain cycle. Once the pain has been relieved, less powerful analgesics can then be tried. Commonly, patients will require morphine to control their symptoms. When the pain is the result of bony metastases, NSAIDs may be needed in addition. The morphine should initially be given by the oral route as required. Once the daily requirement has been determined, the morphine can be given in the form of slow-release tablets twice a day. The analgesic effect of morphine can be potentiated by the addition of corticosteroids and these should be prescribed if the pain is difficult to control. When the pain has a neuropathic element (recognised from the patient's description of it as burning) amitriptyline 25 mg at night may be helpful. Other adjuvant drugs, such as the anticonvulsants, may also be helpful.

Non-pharmacological treatments such as radiotherapy, acupuncture and transcutaneous electrical nerve stimulation (TENS) should also be considered.

Management of other symptoms

Opiate analgesia is associated with constipation, which can be very distressing to the patient. All patients who are taking regular opioids should be prescribed laxatives. Stool softeners such as lactulose may be added to bulking agents. In resistant cases, co-danthromer or senna can be added.

Nausea can be controlled with antiemetics such as cyclizine or prochlorperazine. Dexamethasone is useful in cases that are unresponsive to the standard antiemetics.

Emotional support

Patients by this stage of the disease will have an awareness that they are dying. It is important that this fact is acknowledged by the staff so that they can, if they wish, talk about it. The staff must be sensitive to the patient's wishes in this area. Some patients do not wish to talk while others wish to hold lengthy discussions. Many patients will wish to discuss spiritual matters and appropriate support must be provided. If the patient has regularly practised her faith, her usual spiritual advisor is likely to be the best person for this.

FURTHER READING

Breast Speciality Group. British Association of Surgical Oncology Guidelines. The management of metastatic bone disease in the United Kingdom. *Eur J Surg Oncol* 1999; **25**:3–23

Buzdar AU, Jones SE, Vogel CL et al. A phase III trial comparing anastrazole (1 and 10 milligrams), a potent and selective aromatase inhibitor, with megestrol acetate in postmenopausal women with advanced breast carcinoma. *Cancer* 1997; **79**(4):730–739

Clarysse A. Hormone-induced tumor flare. *Euro J Cancer Clinical Onco* 1985; **21**(5):545–547

Galea MH, Blamey RW, Elston CE, Ellis IO. The Nottingham Prognostic Index in primary breast cancer. *Breast Cancer Res Treat* 1992; **22**:207–219

Greenberg PA, Hortobaygi GN, Smith TL et al. Long-term follow up of patients with complete remission following combination chemotherapy for metastatic breast cancer. *J Clin Oncol* 1996; **14**:2197–2205

Hayes DF, van Zyl JA, Hacking A et al. Randomized comparison of tamoxifen and two separate doses of toremifene in postmenopausal patients with metastatic breast cancer. *J Clin Oncol* 1995; **13**:2556-2566

Hortobagyi GN, Theriault RL, Lipton A et al. Long-term prevention of skeletal complications of metastatic breast cancer with pamidronate. *J Clin Oncol* 1998; **16**(6):2038–2044

Leinster SJ. Rudland PS, Fernig DG, Leinster SJ, Lunt GG, eds. Impact of molecular biology on the clinical management of breast cancer. In: *Mammary Development and Cancer*. London: Portland Press, 1997

National Institute for Clinical Excellence. *Guidance on the Use of Taxanes for Breast Cancer*. Technology Appraisal Guidance No. 6. London: NICE, 2000

Norton L, Slamon D, Leyland-Jones B et al. Overall survival (OS) advantage to simultaneous chemotherapy (CRx) plus the humanized anti-HER2 monoclonal antibody Herceptin (H) in HER2-overexpression (HER2+) metastatic breast cancer (MBC). *Proc Am Soc Clin Oncol* 1999; **18**:483A, 127a

Perez EA. Current management of metastatic breast cancer. *Semin Oncol* 1999; **26**(4 Suppl 12): 1–10

Spiegel D, Bloom JR, Kraemer HC, Gottheil E. The effect of psychosocial treatment on survival of patients with metastatic breast cancer. *Lancet* 1989; **2**(8668):888–891

Taylor CW, Green S, Dalton WS et al. Multicenter randomized clinical trial of goserelin versus surgical ovariectomy in premenopausal patients with receptor-positive metastatic breast cancer: an intergroup study. *J Clin Oncol* 1998; **16**:994–999

30

Epidemiology, screening and clinical trials in breast cancer

S. Thrush, T. Bates

EPIDEMIOLOGY

The natural history of breast cancer is well described, but our understanding of the cause is still far from complete. Certain risk factors are well recognised and their clinical importance may be considered as high, intermediate or low risk (Box 30.1).

Box 30.1 Risk factors for breast cancer	
High risk	Age Family history Previous contralateral breast cancer Lobular carcinoma *in situ* Atypical ductal hyperplasia
Intermediate risk	Early menarche/late menopause Late first pregnancy Geography Benign breast disease Hormone replacement therapy >5 years Oral contraceptive pill
Low risk	Diet Alcohol Obesity

Geographical variation

There is a marked difference in the incidence of breast cancer between countries but the reason for this is unclear. In the United States and Europe breast cancer is the most common cancer in women but women who migrate from an area of low incidence such as Japan to an area of high incidence such as the USA develop a threefold increased risk of breast cancer. This increase in relative risk is only half that of the indigenous population but the risk does rise again in the second generation which underlines the importance of the environment in the aetiology of breast cancer.

Age

The risk of breast cancer increases with age and the age-specific incidence rises steadily from the age of 25. The overall mortality from breast cancer is higher in women under 35, which is associated with an increased rate of poorly differentiated grade 3 tumours, but the mortality rate rises with advancing age due to the greater number of deaths from intercurrent disease. Breast cancer is the most common cause of death in young women, between 44 and 50 years of age.

Gender

The incidence of male breast cancer is less than 1% that seen in females.

Family history

Genetic predisposition is related to only 5–10% of breast cancers but a woman's risk will depend on the number of relatives affected, how close they are in relation, at what age the disease developed and whether breast cancer was bilateral. A woman with one first-degree relative (mother, sister or daughter) who has developed breast cancer before the age of 50 has more than twice the population risk of breast cancer. If she has two first-degree relatives with breast cancer this risk increases to 4–6 times. For those at high risk this raises the possibility of benefit from early mammographic screening, chemoprevention or even prophylactic mastectomy. Guidelines for women with a family history of breast or ovarian cancer who might be considered for genetic screening are shown in Box 30.2.

Box 30.2   Management strategy for patients with a family history of breast cancer
Management of high–risk group ● Should be referred to a specialist cancer genetic consultation at a regional genetic cancer centre ● Gene testing may be appropriate if an infected relative is alive
Management of moderate–risk group ● Some visits after annual mammography from ten years before the age of the youngest affected relative, but in the absence of incidence there is no definitive advice
Management of low–risk group ● Explain to the patient the difference between familial and non-familial breast cancer ● Encourage participation in the National Breast Screening Programme at the appropriate age Adapted from British Association of Surgical Oncology 1998 Guidelines for surgeons in the management of symptomatic breast disease in the UK; BASO Breast Specialist Group 1998 European Journal of Surgical Oncology 464–476. Reprinted by permission of the publisher WB Saunders.

Several genes have been identified in breast cancer and they tend to be inherited in an autosomal dominant manner. The first gene to be identified was BRCA1 which was localised to the long arm of chromosome 17 in families with both breast and ovarian cancer. The BRCA1 gene has over 100 described mutations spread throughout its length and evidence now points to different susceptibility for ovarian and breast cancer in different sites, accounting for about 2% of all breast cancer and with 56% penetrance. A second gene, BRCA2, with a much higher penetrance of 80% has been identified on the chromosome 13q which is associated with families containing male breast cancer. Other genes have been described, such as the p53 gene, but this probably accounts for only a small proportion of familial breast cancer. The overall cumulative risk across all the linked families is 85% for breast and 60% for ovarian cancer. It is evident that further genes do exist that are yet to be identified since some clearly dominant breast cancer families are not linked to either BRCA1 or BRCA2.

The value of family history clinics is still controversial but there are a number of models for estimating the level of risk to an individual woman. Genetic testing is laborious and in practical terms is only available when a family member with breast cancer is still alive and prepared to give a blood sample. Preliminary counselling on the options to be considered in the face of a positive test is important.

Oestrogen

Prolonged exposure to oestrogen increases the incidence of breast cancer so that an early menarche and late menopause will increase the total number of menstrual cycles in a lifetime, which is associated with a greater risk. This risk decreases if the woman becomes pregnant, therefore interrupting the oestrogen cycle, especially if the pregnancy is at an early age. The relative risk of breast cancer in a woman having a first child after the age of 30 is 1.9 times that of someone who had their first child aged less than 20. Having a second child at a young age further reduces the risk. Nulliparity is a risk factor for breast cancer but an artificial menopause by oophorectomy or irradiation reduces the number of lifetime menstrual cycles and decreases the risk.

Exogenous oestrogens may also increase the risk of breast cancer. The oral contraceptive pill has a small effect during current use and for 10 years after exposure. This risk is very small with the low dose of hormones used in current contraceptives and in view of the major advantages, it is of no clinical significance to an individual woman.

Hormone replacement therapy (HRT) in postmenopausal women carries a slight increase in relative risk if taken for more than five years, rising to 1.5 after 10 years of use. However, the advantages of prophylaxis against osteoporosis may be considered to outweigh the potential risk of breast cancer. This increased risk returns to normal after five years from cessation of HRT. There is no evidence that HRT is a greater risk to women who are already at higher risk of breast cancer but the suggestion that oestrogen-related breast cancer carries a better prognosis has been discounted. The precise role of oestrogen in the aetiology of human breast cancer remains uncertain.

Previous breast cancer

The risk of developing a second (metachronous) cancer is increased especially in women when the first tumour is diagnosed before the age of 40, where the relative risk is in the range 1.2–1.5.

Benign breast disease

Most benign diseases of the breast do not have an effect on the risk of developing breast cancer. However, atypical ductal hyperplasia (ADH) carries a relative risk almost five times that of the population. Multiple ductal papillomas, breast cysts requiring intervention, ductal hyperplasia of usual type and complex fibroadenoma are less severe risk factors.

Obesity

Obesity is associated with a slightly increased risk of breast cancer in postmenopausal women. Fat cells are responsible for the production of small amounts of oestrogen by the metabolism of androstenedione from the adrenal gland. The levels of oestrone are higher in obese postmenopausal women and those with a body mass index greater than 35 have a relative risk twice that expected. Paradoxically obesity as a teenager seems to offer some protection to developing premenopausal breast cancer and tall girls may be at increased risk.

Diet and alcohol

Animal studies show that increased dietary fat may cause mammary tumours and the large variations in geographical incidence suggest that fat may be important in the aetiology of breast cancer. Correlation between per capita consumption of fat on a national basis and breast cancer mortality rates is convincing but it is difficult to find proof of this in the individual.

It has been suggested that a lack of food containing high levels of antioxidants (green vegetables and fruit) may be causally related to breast cancer.

A recent Italian study suggested that 12% of breast cancers can be attributed to alcohol consumption and although this finding was not supported by McPherson, the issue is well reviewed by Boyce. If there is an effect of alcohol this might be caused by increased circulating levels of oestrogens and oestradiols but the observed difference could be due to confounding factors. (A confounding factor is an alternative explanation for the observed facts.)

Smoking

Cigarettes have been linked to a number of cancers but do not appear to be a significant risk factor in breast cancer. Some studies even suggest they may have a protective effect in those who have smoked since a young age and are carrying the BRCA1 or 2 gene. Smoking has a slight anti-oestrogenic effect but if this is a real effect it might be a confounding factor in relation to social class since breast cancer is more common in women of higher socio-economic status.

Exercise

Physical activity, especially in teenage and young adult years, may have a protective effect in breast cancer which could be related to a reduction in the number of menstrual cycles. Athletes often develop amenorrhoea, which would reduce the cumulative exposure to oestrogen and progesterone, but whether physical activity has a role in primary prevention is still an open question.

Radiation

Women who have been previously exposed to high doses of radiation, such as the survivors of Hiroshima, Eskimos who received repeated chest radiographic screening for tuberculosis and women treated by radiation for postpartum mastitis, have a considerable close-related risk of developing breast cancer. This risk is greater in young women and becomes apparent after a latent period of many years.

SCREENING

Breast cancer is the most common cancer in women in the Western world, affecting approximately one in 12 women. The outcome in terms of survival directly depends on the stage and grade of the disease at presentation but there is some evidence that the identification and treatment of preclinical disease may reduce breast cancer mortality rates in the population. There has been a recent fall in the number of deaths from breast cancer in England and Wales but this trend was already apparent before screening, which started in 1988–9, could have taken much effect (Figure 30.1). It is likely that the effect is multifactorial.

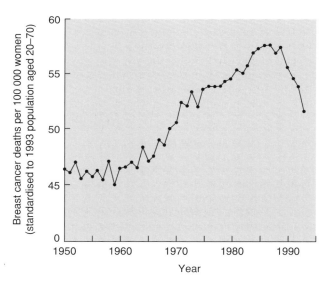

Figure 30.1 Breast cancer mortality in England and Wales, 1950–93. Reproduced with permission from Beral et al 1995.

Why breast cancer is suitable for screening

For a disease to be suitable for a screening programme it is important that a number of criteria are met. The natural history of the disease must be understood and treatment in the early stage of the disease should improve the prognosis. Breast cancer does have a recognised preclinical state, which can sometimes be detected by mammography and such tumours are more likely to be very small or *in situ* and to have negative axillary lymph nodes. The five-year survival of a patient with a tumour less than 1cm diameter without nodal involvement is >95% compared with 50–60% for the

overall population of patients with breast cancer. Screening has been shown to reduce the number of deaths from breast cancer in the screened population of randomised trials compared with the unscreened control groups and until a cure or preventive therapy becomes available, this appears to be the best way to reduce mortality.

Screening bias

The problem with generalising the outcome of patients with screen-detected tumours to those presenting symptomatically is that several biases may act to confound the results.

Lead time bias

Screen-detected tumours are usually identified at an earlier stage in the natural history of breast cancer than tumours which present symptomatically so that, even if there were no effect the eventual outcome, survival, which is taken as the interval between diagnosis and death, will be longer. Improved survival of patients with screen-detected breast cancer cannot therefore be taken as a surrogate marker of the success of a screening programme. If screening had no effect on the natural history of the disease the tumour would on average be detected about two years before it became symptomatic.

Length bias

Cancers grow at different rates, so that less aggressive cancers will spend longer in the preclinically detectable state (the sojourn time) than fast-growing tumours. Screening is therefore likely to detect a larger proportion of the slower growing tumours which have a better prognosis while aggressive tumours are more likely to present clinically in the interval between screens.

Selection bias

Screening depends on the cooperation of women to undertake a test and it is apparent that those who attend for an examination in response to postal invitation are more health conscious and probably have a better prognosis than non-attenders. This trend is apparent in screening programmes for most conditions. Opportunistic screening where women present themselves for mammography is very prone to selection bias since they may already have an unexpressed concern that something in the breast has changed. Opportunistic screening is more likely to be offered to women of higher socio-economic status.

The true effect of screening is best assessed by the comparison of a randomised screened population with a non-screened population or by monitoring the death rates from breast cancer in the population after the introduction of screening. However, this latter method may be confounded by other factors that affect breast

445

cancer mortality over the period of the study, such as the increased use of HRT.

Screening tests

Not only must the disease be suitable for screening but the available test should fulfil a number of requirements. The most important criteria are the sensitivity of the test (does it detect most of the cases, with few false negatives?) and the specificity (does it only detect the cancer patients, with few false positives?). It is also important that the test is acceptable to the population to be screened since the success of a programme will be directly related to compliance.

There are three main potential screening tools available in breast cancer:

- mammography
- physical examination by trained staff
- breast self-examination.

Of these, mammography is the only test that has been proven to reduce breast cancer mortality in randomised control trials.

The value of breast self-examination (BSE) as a screening method has proved difficult to assess. There has been no randomised clinical trial of BSE due to the difficulty of contamination (when women in the control group hear about the intervention from friends and family). In a study of eight UK towns, women in two towns who were recommended to perform monthly BSE were compared to women in two towns screened by annual mammography and those in four control towns. A greater number of breast cancer deaths occurred in the towns performing BSE and although this was a non-significant trend the unexpected finding caused great confusion and has not been satisfactorily explained (Figure 30.2). Women who perform regular BSE detect smaller tumours than those who do not but BSE has to be taught and this requires trained staff who are costly. Fewer than half the women invited for BSE training actually attended and for those that did there is no evidence to show that they continued to perform regular assessments.

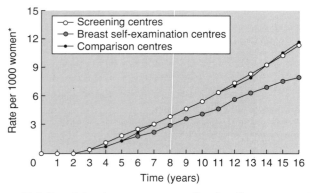

Figure 30.2 Cumulative breast cancer mortality for all age groups (non-randomised). Reproduced with permission from UK Trial of Early Detection of Breast Cancer Group 1999.

Whether a tumour has been detected by clinical examination or BSE, it is at least 10 mm in size by the time it is clinically palpable and the chance of detecting disease before dissemination is therefore much reduced. The current recommendations are for women to be breast aware, but there is no encouragement for BSE.

Other modalities

Ultrasound is increasingly useful as an adjunct to mammography and clinical examination as a result of improved image quality and radiological expertise. However, it is labour intensive and therefore expensive. The relatively high rate of both false-negative and false-positive examination has made ultrasound an unacceptable tool for population screening. Magnetic resonance imaging (MRI) has provided an additional screening modality, especially when there has been previous surgery to the breast. However, this technique may be associated with a reduced specificity and considerable expense which currently renders it unsuitable for population screening. There may be a place for screening with MRI in high-risk patients such as those with strong family history but this is currently under trial.

Evidence for mammography as a useful screening tool

Two randomised trials have been mainly responsible for the introduction of a national screening programme to the UK. The Health Insurance Plan study of New York (HIP) was the first trial of breast screening and the second was the Swedish Two-Counties Trial. The HIP study looked at 62 000 women aged between 40 and 64 years, who were randomly allocated either to screening by two-view yearly mammography and clinical examination or to a control group.

The study was performed between December 1963 and June 1966 and death from breast cancer was the end point. Initial attendance was 67% but only 40% attended all four screening examinations; 57% of cases diagnosed in the study group were without nodal involvement compared to 46% in the control group. In the 10 years after the closure of the trial there were 30% fewer breast cancer deaths in the study group.

In the Two-Counties Trial 163 000 women over 40 years of age were randomly allocated to a screened or a control group. The screened group were examined by single-view mammography on entry into the study and at intervals thereafter. The screening interval averaged 33 months in women aged 50–69 and 22 months in women 40–49. The ratio of screened women to controls was 2:1 in the Kopparberg population and 1:1 in Ostergotland County. Women were entered into the programme between 1977 and 1981 with 89% initial attendance in those between 40 and 74 years and 83% attendance at the second screen. Because the attendance was only 50% in women over 75 years the study only reported the outcome in 135 000 women younger than this. In the study group 61% of cancers were without nodal involvement compared to 37% in the control group. After the first seven years the trial showed a mortality reduction of 31% in the screened women compared to the control group. An update to the trial, which followed women up to 1990, showed that this mortality reduction was maintained at 30%.

Other trials have shown different degrees of reduction in mortality but an overview of these and other non-randomised studies shows that all report fewer deaths in the screened versus the non-screened population (Figure 30.3).

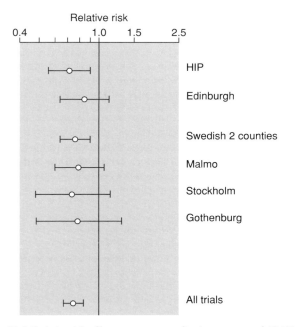

Figure 30.3 Relative risk of breast cancer mortality in women aged 40–74 years invited for screening compared with those not invited is shown for each trial together with the 95% confidence interval. The combined estimate is also shown for all trials: 0.78 (95% CI 0.7–0.87). Reproduced with permission from Wald et al 1993.

Controversies in mammographic screening

One or two views?

The UK Forrest Working Group on breast cancer screening in 1986 recommended single (oblique) view mammography for screening on the basis of the Swedish trials, where a single view was chosen to minimise the radiation dose. The radiation dose at mammography has been reduced considerably in recent years from 2–3 cGy to about 0.15 cGy. It has been calculated that a dose of 0.15 cGy may induce one breast cancer per two million women screened over the age of 50 after a latent period of 10 years. However, when this order of risk is compared to the natural incidence of 1400 breast cancers per million per year in women over 50 it puts into perspective the protective benefit of screening which far outweighs the theoretical risks of radiation.

The subsequent introduction of two-view (craniocaudal and mediolateral oblique) mammography at the initial (prevalent)

screen has improved the sensitivity from 94% to 96%. Although this difference may not appear impressive the number of cancers detected has increased by over 20%. Two-view mammography increases the cost of screening, but the number of women recalled for assessment decreased from 9% to 7% and this is now standard practice for the first round of the UK NHS breast screening programme (NHSBSP).

Double reading of the films by two radiologists also improves the sensitivity of mammography and may increase the yield of cancers detected by up to 15%. Screening radiologists with the highest detection rate (the highest sensitivity) also have the highest false-positive recall rate (the lowest specificity) and the opposite is true of radiologists with a low cancer detection rate. The recall rate of most screening units in the UK NHSBSP has increased due to the medicolegal threat of false-negative mammography and the corresponding delay in diagnosis. This risk is also threatening recruitment to the specialty.

Should the frequency of screening be one, two or three yearly?

In a screening programme cancers can be detected:

● at the first (prevalent) screen

● at subsequent (incident) screens

● in the interval between screens–interval cancers

● in non-attendees.

In the Two-Counties Trial the detection rate was highest in the prevalent screen but the reduction in mortality rate was greater than in subsequent screens due to the detection of slow-growing cancers at the first screen which produced length bias. The incidence of cancers in the follow-up screens rises with the increase in age of the population.

An interval cancer is a tumour that presents symptomatically between screens, following a negative mammogram. There are a number of studies showing that approximately 25% of tumours found on incident screens are retrospectively identifiable on the previous mammography. This delay in diagnosis has prognostic and medicolegal consequences but if these films are diluted to the screening situation most of these cancers are not detected on retest.

The frequency of screening will influence the rate of interval cancers but the NHSBSP adopted a three-yearly interval on the basis of the Two-Counties Trial. It was predicted that 74% of the expected incidence of breast cancers would be detected by screening at a 30-month interval among women aged 50–69 years. It has become evident that the incidence of interval cancers is higher than the targets which were set, especially in year 3, but this does not necessarily mean that more frequent screening would be more effective in reducing the number of breast cancer deaths. There is no proposal to increase the frequency of the NHSBSP but the interval is longer than other national screening programmes.

Age range

Age is also an important risk factor for breast cancer and there is general agreement that screening women between 50 and 64 years is beneficial. However, screening women between 40 and 49 years continues to be a controversial area since the increased density of the breast reduces the sensitivity and specificity of mammography. Most trials that have included this age group tend to show a small but delayed reduction in breast cancer mortality.

Data on screening women over 70 are scarce but compliance has proved better than expected and with an ageing population the political pressure to extend the screening age is considerable. The upper age of the NHSBSP is to be raised from 64 to 69.

Atypical ductal hyperplasia (ADH)

ADH found on breast biopsy is considered benign but is a significant risk factor for development of invasive carcinoma and patients with this condition may benefit from regular screening (see Chapter 27 Benign breast disorders).

Complications of screening

False positives

Although mammography is the best available screening tool it has a specificity of less than 100% and in consequence a significant proportion of the screened population without breast cancer will be recalled to undergo further imaging, biopsies or even an operation which subsequently prove unnecessary. Only one in 10 women recalled for further investigation will be found to have breast cancer and the recall rate is highest in younger women and those with dense breasts who may be on HRT. The recall rate in the NHSBSP has a target of 7%, but fear of litigation following a false-negative test has increased the recall rate to nearer 10%. A retrospective American study reported a 50% cumulative risk of a false-positive result following 10 mammograms, the economic consequences of which must be considerable.

Psychological morbidity

It would be expected that anxiety will increase on receiving a screening appointment but one study of women attending for screening compared to an age-matched sample showed no significant difference. The failure to show a difference in psychiatric morbidity between attendees and non-attendees was also unexpected.

Pain and discomfort

Mammography is not a pleasant investigation but less than 10% rate the discomfort as severe and for most it is bearable and short-lived.

Overdiagnosis of breast cancers

Approximately 20% of screen-detected cancers are ductal carcinoma *in situ* (DCIS) and although such tumours may become invasive, the proportion in which this occurs and the timescale are uncertain. It is probable that a number of low-grade *in situ* cancers would not develop into invasive cancer and therefore undergo unnecessary surgery. Furthermore, the borderline between ADH and DCIS is a difficult area for the pathologist, with a significant variation in opinion on the presence of malignancy.

Delay in diagnosis in screen-detected breast cancer

Legal liability for missing a cancer may be admitted if in the opinion of an expert it should have been detected by an ordinarily competent breast radiologist. The question of compensation may arise but the patient must then establish causation, that the delay in diagnosis has resulted in an injury in terms of more severe treatment, loss of life-years or, under some legal systems, the loss of the chance of a cure. In the screening situation the delay will usually be the same as the screening interval unless the cancer has presented in the interval between screens. Occasionally a cancer will be apparent with hindsight on two previous screens, which would indicate a six-year delay in diagnosis in the UK NHSBSP.

Does a delay of three years reduce the expectation of life? It is accepted that a screening programme for women over 50 will reduce the number of deaths from breast cancer by 25%. It therefore seems probable that delay in diagnosis of this order will reduce expectation of life by 25%. However, it is uncertain whether the reduction by 25% will affect all patients or whether 25% of patients have loss of a cure with no effect on the remainder.

Genetic screening

If there is a potential benefit from early detection of breast cancer this may also apply to patients with genetically determined tumours. Some units now offer regular mammographic screening to women on an annual basis starting at 5–10 years before the age at which the youngest first-degree relative developed cancer. At present this is usually offered to women with a relative risk of 2.5 compared with the general population but there is as yet no clear evidence of benefit.

It is also possible to test for the BRCA1 and BRCA2 genes in high-risk families but the mutation must first be identified in an affected relative to reduce the risk of a false-negative result.

Assessing the effectiveness of screening

Three main indicators are used to assess the success of a screening programme, of which a reduction in the number of breast cancer deaths in the population of screening age is the only valid outcome measure. Changes in the rate of advanced disease in the population and the parameters of the screening process are surrogate measures that may not represent a real effect. It was expected that the UK NHSBSP would lead to a 25% reduction in breast cancer mortality by the year 2000 as determined from the results of the Swedish trial.

There has been a reduction in mortality from breast cancer between 1985–9 compared to 1990–4 of about 10% that cannot be explained solely by screening. The largest effect appears in the younger women (25–49 years) with a reduction of 14%, whereas there is a decrease of 11% in women between 50 and 69 years and of only 5% in women between 70 and 79 years. This reduction appeared too early and across too wide an age range to be attributed to screening, which started in 1988–9, and the effect is probably due to the increased use of adjuvant treatment.

The future of screening by mammography

Screening by mammography continues to excite controversy and the validity of the randomisation in those screening trials which have shown a positive effect has recently been questioned.

The evidence of a major reduction in breast cancer deaths as a consequence of screening is still awaited and in the meantime the question of informed consent is pressing.

Implications of consent to mammographic screening

- Some women will be recalled unnecessarily (about 6%).

- Having been recalled, patients may be investigated/operated on unnecessarily (1%).

- Women may have a cancer detected earlier than they would have but with no difference in outcome.

- Women may receive treatment for a good prognosis cancer or in situ disease that would not have become apparent during their lifetime.

- Screening mammography only detects nine out of 10 breast cancers.

- If a breast cancer is present which is visible on mammography there is a one in four chance that it will not be apparent to the radiologist with the consequent loss of a chance of a cure.

CLINICAL TRIALS IN BREAST CANCER

Probably the first controlled trial was carried out in the British Navy in the 1740s when James Lind compared the effect of lemons for the treatment of scurvy with conventional treatment such as drinking seawater. There were only two sailors in each group but the effect was so strong that the benefit was obvious.

One of the first randomised control studies outside agriculture was conducted by Bradford Hill in the 1940s on the treatment of tuberculosis with streptomycin and again the treatment effect was so powerful that controversy arose over untreated control patients.

The randomised control trial (RCT) has been a great advance in providing robust evidence in order to determine best practice and must be regarded as the gold standard since observational studies are inevitably prone to bias. Although a randomised trial can be flawed by randomly occurring biases, these become increasingly less likely with large numbers. Increasing the size of an observational study does not necessarily reduce bias since if this is a systematic difference between the treatment groups, the size or effect of the bias will remain more or less constant. However, RCTs have been bedevilled by studies with small numbers which fail to show a statistical significance between the treatment groups. Many clinical trials have been undertaken which had little expectation of being able to recruit sufficient numbers from which to draw a valid conclusion. In this situation there is a risk of a type II error in drawing a conclusion that an intervention has no effect when one does in fact exist. The size of the 95% confidence intervals will give an indication of the size and the statistical power of a study (Figure 30.3).

There have also been problems with RCTs where the treatment groups have not been well designed. To a large extent these problems have been overcome by the introduction of sample size and power calculations to determine the numbers required in the control and treatment groups. This approach has had the following consequences:

- the need for multicentre trials in order to recruit a sufficient number of eligible patients

- the requirement for a data-monitoring committee and stopping rules for any RCT

- a reduction in the number of small RCTs

- the advent of metanalysis.

The practice of metanalysis where all published trials are considered has increased and the understanding of the potential pitfalls of this technique has improved considerably. However, publication bias against negative studies and the converse likelihood of a study with a significant treatment effect being accepted for publication may still be important.

The need for trials to be multicentre has also had a number of consequences:

- a need for central randomisation services: this has had the advantage of excluding ineligible patients from randomisation. It should also ensure allocation concealment (which may be more important than double blinding) in reducing allocation bias

- a need to recruit participating centres: this requires organisation and commitment

- *external supervision of each centre*: to ensure the entry of as many eligible patients as possible. It is also important that all participants have a clear understanding of the protocol and do not enter ineligible patients. This requires dedicated high-calibre personnel.

As a consequence of the need for multicentre recruitment most RCTs now need the support of a clinical trial organisation which will in turn require major funding. With regard to grant applications, the need to identify adequate funding and to seek ethical approval from regulatory authorities does cause considerable delay but peer review of the protocol does improve the prospect of a valid outcome to the proposed trial.

Scientific malpractice and fraud principally stem from the perceived need of academic workers to publish their results and this may lead to the entry of ineligible patients by the falsification of records. More serious irregularities have occurred where the outcome of high-dose chemotherapy appeared to give survival benefit.

Analysis of trials

Allowance must be made for the varying length of time each patient has spent in a study and life table analysis of patients in each treatment group is essential. Actuarial analysis of outcome by the Kaplan–Meir method with test of statistical significance by the log rank test is the current method of choice.

Difficulty with consent

Informed consent to randomisation has caused increasingly severe constraints to be applied to the conduct of clinical trials, especially when one treatment is obviously more severe than the other, e.g. for wide local excision for carcinoma of the breast versus a mastectomy.

Ethical committees now require that patients be given written information about the trial with the reassurance that if they decide against taking part, this will not affect their present or future treatment. It is also important that patients are given time to consider their decision. Ethical approval for the examination of retrospective data has also become a requirement for publication in some journals although the distinction between audit and research is often blurred.

The net result of this quite proper increase in the ethical constraints surrounding clinical trials is that it has become impossible to achieve ethical approval or to recruit sufficient patients to some studies. It is for this reason that some important questions are best assessed by observational studies although the conclusions to be drawn will be less robust than those from the gold standard, the randomised trial.

Observational studies

Cohort studies

All patients treated by mastectomy over a defined period of time might form a cohort and for example, if one was seeking risk factors for local recurrence their current status would be a cross-sectional study and the outcome over a period of time would be a longitudinal study. However, the cases with local recurrence may have been managed differently from those who are apparently free of disease or they may have been followed up more intensively and for a longer period.

Historical controls are particularly prone to biases, some of which can be predicted and therefore recognised and allowed for but there may be confounding factors which are not apparent which may lead to false conclusions. More severe disease will be treated by more severe treatment but the difference in severity may be too subtle to be apparent and may lead to an undetected systematic treatment bias. For example, the Intervention, Timing and Survival (ITS) Study is a current prospective cohort study of outcome related to the phase of the menstrual cycle in which primary breast cancer is operated on. This model has been used because it was not possible to randomise patients.

Case–control studies

A case–control study is one in which, for example, each case of local recurrence after mastectomy is matched with one or more controls who are nearest in age and had a mastectomy about the same time. This type of study is usually more robust than a cohort study but it is still prone to bias and any conclusions which are drawn will be less powerful than those from an RCT. In an observational study it is particularly important that the hypothesis to be tested is stated in advance of data analysis since the greater the number of comparisons made, the greater the risk that one will appear to be statistically significant by the play of chance.

The contribution of the Oxford Overviews of Randomised Controlled Trials (RCTs) in breast cancer has been immense since not only has this included all published work but, where necessary, it has defined the status of the treatment groups and has brought up-to-date the follow-up of previously published or incomplete studies.

Oxford Overviews

- More versus less surgery
- Radiotherapy versus no radiotherapy (Figure 30.4)
- Tamoxifen versus control, long versus short in duration (Figure 30.5)
- Oophorectomy versus nil (Figure 30.6)
- Chemotherapy versus no chemotherapy (Figure 30.7) Long versus short courses
- CMF versus anthracyclines

The above overviews are briefly described below.

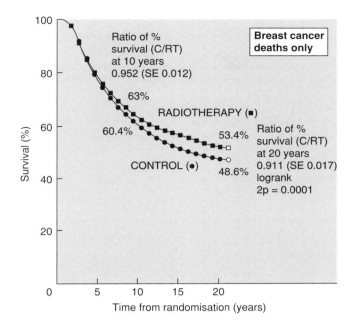

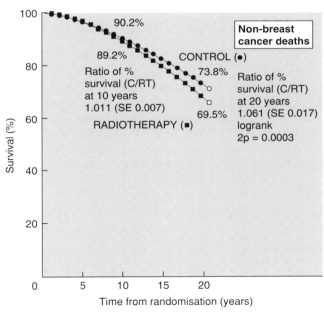

Figure 30.4 Absolute effects of radiotherapy on cause-specific survival. Reproduced with permission from Early Breast Cancer Trialists' Collaborative Group 2000.

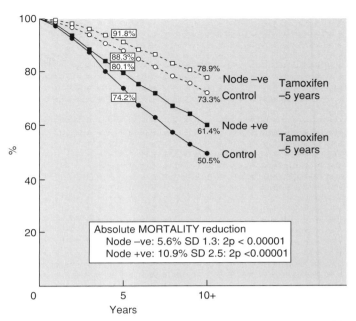

Figure 30.5 Absolute risk reductions during the first 10 years, subdivided by tamoxifen duration and by nodal status (after exclusion of women with ER-poor disease). Reproduced with permission from Early Breast Cancer Trialists' Collaborative Group 1998a.

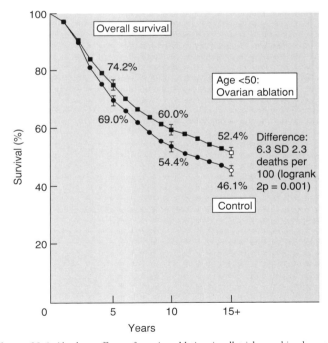

Figure 30.6 Absolute effects of ovarian ablation in all trials combined among women aged under 50 at entry. Reproduced with permission from Early Breast Cancer Trialists' Collaborative Group 1996.

Trials on the place of conservative surgery for early breast cancer

Up to the early 1970s the surgical procedure of choice for breast cancers was the radical mastectomy described by Halsted. This involved complete excision of the breast, pectoralis major and minor and the axillary contents up to the costoclavicular ligament. The procedure would often leave a poor cosmetic result and Crile in the United States campaigned for more conservative surgery. McWhirter from Edinburgh showed similar results from

radiotherapy (RT) after more conservative surgery although Keynes at Bart's had been using radium needles since the 1920s.

A randomised controlled trial from Manchester in 1981 comparing the radical to the modified radical operation showed in stage I and II breast cancer patients no significant overall or event-free

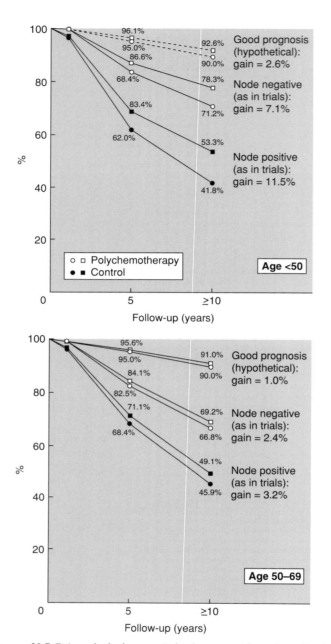

Figure 30.7 Estimated absolute survival advantage with prolonged poly-chemotherapy for populations of women with good, intermediate and poor prognosis (calculated by having the proportional risk reduction unaffected by prognosis). Reproduced with permission from Early Breast Cancer Trialists' Collaborative Group 1998b.

survival advantage to either procedure. However, there was significantly less morbidity in the group who underwent the modified radical mastectomy.

Several large randomised controlled trials subsequently compared breast conservation to mastectomy. The largest of these trials was the National Surgical Adjuvant Breast and Bowel Project (NSABP) B-06 which randomised over 1137 patients to either mastectomy, lumpectomy alone or lumpectomy plus postoperative breast irradiation. There was no difference in overall survival between the

mastectomy and the irradiated groups but locoregional recurrence was greater in the patients treated with breast-conserving surgery, especially in those who did not receive postoperative radiotherapy. The rate of the local recurrence after conservative surgery with postoperative RT was 10% versus 35% without RT.

This evidence is further supported by the Oxford Overview of all published RCTs which has enabled women with suitable tumours to be offered breast-conserving surgery with radiotherapy as an alternative to a mastectomy.

Adjuvant radiotherapy

There have been 46 trials including 20 000 patients. Overall they show a threefold reduction of local recurrence of 9% versus 27% at 10 years.

However, mortality benefit from reduction in breast cancer deaths has been offset by an increase in non-cancer death which were mostly cardiovascular following radiotherapy to the left chest wall. It is likely that the latter deaths will in the future be largely avoided by modern techniques for planning and delivery of radiotherapy. (see Figure 30.4).

Adjuvant tamoxifen in early breast cancer

The 1995 Oxford Overview reviewed 55 randomised trials of tamoxifen versus no tamoxifen including 37 000 women. In trials of about five years of tamoxifen the absolute improvement in 10-year survival was 10.9% in node-positive women and 5.6% in those who were node negative (see Figure 30.5). The absolute decrease in contralateral breast cancer was about twice that of the increase in endometrial cancer. Women who were ER negative had little benefit and those where the ER status was unknown had an intermediate response. For trials of one, two and five years of adjuvant tamoxifen there was a strong trend to greater effect with longer treatment.

Adjuvant oophorectomy

Sir George Beatson, a Glasgow surgeon, who noted that bilateral oophorectomy could lead to regression in metastatic breast cancer, first described the importance of hormonal stimulation on breast cancer. Before the introduction of tamoxifen, stilboestrol, oophorectomy and adrenalectomy were the available treatments for advanced breast cancer. Adjuvant oophorectomy has fallen into disuse but its survival advantage in premenopausal women with ER-positive tumours is comparable to the effect of adjuvant chemotherapy (see Figure 30.6).

Adjuvant chemotherapy

Cytotoxic chemotherapy, as an adjuvant to surgery, has been extensively investigated in the management of breast cancer following the impressive early result from Bonnadonna's group in Milan using cyclophosphamide, methotrexate and fluorouracil (CMF). The 1995 Oxford Overview analysed 47 trials of 18 000 patients who received prolonged chemotherapy versus no chemotherapy. There were 11 trials of longer versus shorter chemotherapy and 11 trials of routine CMF versus an anthracycline regime.

In women aged under 50, the absolute 10-year survival benefit for node-positive women was 11% versus 7% for those who were node negative. In women over 50 the corresponding benefit was only 3% for node positive versus 2% who were node negative (see Figure 30.7). Anthracyclines were marginally superior to CMF but were effective in a shorter course and may be better tolerated.

Ductal carcinoma in situ *(DCIS)*

Randomised trials on the best management of DCIS have been compromised to some extent by failure to record the adequacy of resection margins or the grade of cytology. Observational studies by Silverstein have contributed considerably to our knowledge of the best management of DCIS and although the early results of the UKCCCR DCIS trial support, the NSABP B24 and the EORTC trials which show that postoperative RT significantly reduces local recurrence in all but the best prognosis tumours. Small low-grade DCIS without comedonecrosis and a wide resection margin of 10 mm may not benefit from postoperative RT but in all other categories local recurrence is significantly reduced. This is particularly important since a proportion of local recurrence is invasive.

The place of adjuvant tamoxifen in the management of DCIS has been uncertain but early evidence from trials suggests that benefit is confined to a reduction in the incidence of contralateral tumours.

Prevention of breast cancer in women at high risk

Randomised placebo-controlled trials of tamoxifen in women with a strong family history of breast cancer or with atypical ductal hyperplasia have shown a reduction in the number of breast cancers in patients receiving tamoxifen. There is as yet no reduction in the number of deaths in the active treatment group which might be countered by the risks of endometrial cancer and thromboembolic disease. Controversy has arisen because the trial was stopped in America when the reduction of breast cancer risk became apparent but trials have continued elsewhere in order to answer the more important question as to whether prophylactic tamoxifen will avoid preventable death.

FURTHER READING

Andrews BT, Bates T. Delay in the diagnosis of breast cancer: medico-legal implications. *Breast* 2000; **9**:223–227

Bates T. Screening for surgical disease. In: Kirk RM, Mansfield AO, Cochrane J, eds. *RCS Course Manual*, 3rd edn. Edinburgh: Churchill Livingstone, 1996

Beral V, Hermon C, Reeves G, Peto R. Sudden fall in breast cancer death rates in England and Wales. *Lancet* 1995; **345**:1642–1643

Black N. Why we need observational studies to evaluate the effectiveness of health care. *BMJ* 1996; **312**:1215–1218

Bonadonna G, Valagussa P, Moliterni A, Zambetti M, Brambilla C. Adjuvant cyclophosphamide, methotrexate and fluorouracil in node-positive breast cancer: the results of 20 years of follow-up. *N Engl J Med* 1995; **332**:901–906

Daly CA, Apthorp L, Field S. Second round cancers: how many were visible on the first round of the UK National Breast Screening Programme, three years earlier? *Clin Radiol* 1998; **53**:25–28

Early Breast Cancer Trialists' Collaborative Group. Effects of radiotherapy and surgery in early breast cancer: an overview of the randomised trials. *Lancet* 1995; **333**:1444–1455

Early Breast Cancer Trialists' Collaborative Group. Favourable and unfavourable effects on long-term survival of radiotherapy for early breast cancer: an overview of the randomised trials. *Lancet* 2000; **355**:1757–1770

Early Breast Cancer Trialists' Collaborative Group. Ovarian ablation in early breast cancer: overview of the randomised trials. *Lancet* 1996; **348**:1189–1196

Early Breast Cancer Trialists' Collaborative Group. Tamoxifen for early breast cancer: an overview of the randomised trials. *Lancet* 1998a; **351**:1451–1467

Early Breast Cancer Trialists' Collaborative Group. Polychemotherapy for early breast cancer: an overview of the randomised trials. *Lancet* 1998b; **352**:930–942

Ellman R, Moss SM, Coleman D, Chamberlain J. Breast self-examination programmes in the trial of early detection of breast cancer: ten year findings. *Br J Cancer* 1993; **68**:208–212

Elmore JG, Barton MB, Moseri VM et al. Ten year risk of false positive screening mammograms and clinical breast examinations. *N Engl J Med* 1998; **338**:1089–1096

Fentiman IS, ed. *Challenges in Breast Cancer.* Oxford: Blackwell Science, 1999

Ferraroni M, Decarli A, Franceschi S, La Vecchia C. Alcohol consumption and risk of breast cancer: a multicentre Italian case-control study. *Eur J Cancer* 1998; **34**:1403–1409

Fisher B, Anderson S, Redmond CK, Wolmark N, Wickenham DL, Cronin WM. Reanalysis and results after 12 years of follow-up in a randomised clinical trial comparing mastectomy with lumpectomy with or without irradiation in the treatment of breast cancer. *N Engl J Med* 1995; **333**:1456–1461

Fisher B, Dignam J, Wolmark N et al. Tamoxifen in treatment of intraductal breast cancer: NASBP B-24 randomised controlled trial. *Lancet* 1999; **353**:1993–2000

Gail MH, Brinton LA, Byar DP et al. Projecting individualised probabilities of developing breast cancer for white females who are being examined annually. *J Natl Cancer Inst* 1989; **81**:1879–1886

Gotzsche PL, Olsen O. Is screening for breast cancer with mammography justifiable? *Lancet* 2000; **355**:129–134

Hartman LC, Schiad DJ, Woods JE et al. Efficacy of bilateral prophylactic mastectomy in women with a family history of breast cancer. *N Engl J Med* 1999; **340**:77–84

Julien J-P, Biker N, Fentiman IS, Peterse JL et al. Radiotherapy in breast-conserving treatment for ductal carcinoma in situ: first results of the EORTC randomised phase III trial 10853. *Lancet* 2000; **355**:528–533

Kopan S. Breast cancer screening with ultrasound. *Lancet* 2000; **354**:2096

McPherson K. Alcohol and breast cancer. *Eur J Cancer* 1998; **34**:1307–1308

Shapiro S, Venet W, Strax P, Venet L, Roser R. Ten year to fourteen year effect of screening on breast cancer mortality. *J Natl Cancer Inst* 1982; **69**:349–355

Silverstein MJ, Lagios MD, Gnoshen S et al. The influence of margin width on local control of ductal carcinoma in situ of the breast. *N Engl J Med* 1999; **340**:1455–1461

Steichen-Gesdorf E, Gallion HH, Ford D et al. Familial site-specific ovarian cancer is linked to BRCA1 on 17q 12–21. *Am J Hum Genet* 1994; **55**:870–875

Tabar L, Fagerberg CJ, Gad A et al. Reduction in mortality from breast cancer after mass screening with mammography. Randomised trial from the Breast Cancer Screening Working Group of the Swedish National Board of Health and Welfare. *Lancet* 1985; **1**:829–832

Turner L, Swindell R, Bell WGT et al. Radical versus modified radical for breast cancer. *Ann Roy Coll Surg Engl* 1981; **63**:239–243

UK Trial of Early Detection of Breast Cancer Group. 16 year mortality from breast cancer in the UK Trial of Early Detection of Breast Cancer. *Lancet* 1999; **353**:1909–1914

Wald NJ, Chamberlain J, Hackshaw A, on behalf of the Evaluation Committee. Consensus statement: report of the European Society for Mastology Breast Cancer Screening Evaluation Committee (1993). *Breast* 1993; **2**:209–216

Warren RM, Duffy SW, Bashir S. The value of a second view in screening mammography. *Br J Radiol* 1996; **69**:105–108

Wooster R, Bignell G, Lancaster J et al. Identification of the breast cancer gene BRCA2. *Nature* 1995; **378**:789–791

31

Breast reconstruction

Gavin M. Briggs, Christobel M. Saunders

INTRODUCTION

Body image is the second greatest concern, after cancer, of women undergoing breast surgery. Once the remit of plastic surgeons, breast reconstruction is today becoming ever more commonplace and, with increasing subspecialist training, is now performed by many general surgeons with an interest in breast disease. It includes postmastectomy and postconservative surgical reconstruction, contralateral surgery and nipple reconstruction as well as purely cosmetic augmentation, reduction and mastopexy. For the basis of this chapter we will describe reconstruction in the breast cancer setting which will incorporate the techniques for non-cancer aesthetic breast surgery.

History of breast reconstruction

The concept of breast reconstruction was first introduced around the time Halsted described his radical mastectomy in 1894. Initial attempts in the late 19th century using fat grafts failed due to lack of blood supply. In 1906 Tanzini performed the first autologous latissimus dorsi flap. This, however, did not gain acceptance nor did various other attempts using tubed pedicle flaps from the contralateral breast or other sites. This was mainly due to an insufficient volume of tissue to produce an adequate breast mound.

In the early 1960s, the first silicone implant was introduced by Cronin and Gerow. Due to lack of tissue coverage following radical mastectomy, this method was not totally successful until the popularisation of the modified radical mastectomy in the early 1970s. This allowed subpectoral insertion of the implant, which produced better coverage and lowered the risk of capsular contraction. Further improvement with implants came with the development of a chest wall tissue expander. This allowed for the subsequent placement of a larger implant which also gave the opportunity to produce ptosis of the reconstructed breast by initial overinflation. Radovan's technique was quickly superseded by Becker who introduced a permanent expandable implant which could be inflated after insertion (Figure 31.1). This one-stage technique is still commonplace today.

One of the major problems with the early implants was capsular contracture, leading to a painful, overly firm breast. This problem has to some extent been reduced by the use of textured implants.

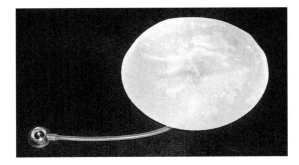

Figure 31.1 An example of an expandable prosthesis.

Latissimus dorsi (LD) flaps alone had been tried and largely abandoned during the first half of the 20th century but were reintroduced in the late 1970s used in combination with a silicon implant to achieve a breast mound. Interestingly, in some Third World countries, e.g. India, the LD flap is a popular 'stand-alone' reconstruction as it is relatively cheap compared to silicon. More recently, certain groups have employed fat-harvesting techniques to provide enough autologous tissue to reconstruct a breast of sufficient volume without the need for implants.

The transverse abdominis musculocutaneous (TRAM) flap was first introduced by Hartrampf in 1982 and has become the 'gold standard'. Debate remains as to the benefits of free flaps over pedicled rotation flaps but overall, the TRAM flap gives an adequate volume of tissue for most breast reconstructions and produces an aesthetically pleasing breast of the correct consistency.

Psychological considerations

There is no doubt that for women and men, the breast is one of the most important external features of femininity. Any surgery, from lumpectomy to mastectomy, therefore naturally raises great concern about body image to women with breast cancer. Common worries range from the ability to wear certain clothes, such as tight-fitting garments or swimwear, to fears about a change of attitude by partners, especially with regards to sexual appreciation of their body.

There has been a major shift in the last decade in the attitudes of both the surgeon and the patient towards breast reconstruction. This has been due to several factors including the greater availability of such procedures, increasing patient awareness and a rapidly expanding wealth of evidence showing the psychological benefits and improved quality of life following breast reconstruction.

Many studies have looked at patient satisfaction following breast surgery. The general consensus is that immediate reconstruction offers the best possible psychological outcome for the majority of patients. Unfortunately, however, not all patients are suitable for such surgery either due to physical reasons, e.g. coexisting medical disease, or psychological reasons. Also, those who are suitable do not necessarily receive consistent information from their carers. Morbidity from all breast reconstructive procedures is not insignificant and itself may have psychological repercussions.

Presurgery planning and patient counselling

A multidisciplinary team approach to breast cancer treatment is now standard practice. This team includes oncologic and reconstructive surgeons, medical and radiation oncologists, radiologists, pathologists and breast care nurses. In most breast units in the United Kingdom, this team meets once a week to discuss each new case individually. In this way, expert knowledge can be amalgamated in order to reach a treatment plan for each patient. Everyone involved in the care of the patient is therefore clear about what is considered to be the best option for each individual. This plan, however, is relatively flexible and is only ratified after a full discussion with the patient about the options available.

It is now accepted that to provide an adequate service to breast cancer patients, reconstruction should at the very least be discussed with every patient due to undergo mastectomy. This requires the breast surgeon either to be familiar with all the available reconstructive techniques or have a readily available plastic surgeon for reconstruction. The ideal is an 'onco-plastic' approach with expertise in both cancer and reconstructive surgery.

Oncologists have long been concerned that performing a breast reconstruction may delay detection of recurrence and may even compromise survival. There is little evidence that this occurs with a prosthetic reconstruction, not least because most recurrences occur in the skin or subdermal layers so placement of a sub-pectoral implant actually accentuates any recurrence by stretching the skin while still being remote from the recurrence. Noone et al diagnosed all recurrences at an early stage out of 185 patients undergoing immediate breast reconstruction and found that the presence of an implant did not interfere with detection of recurrence. Other studies in patients with autologous breast reconstruction did not find any evidence of delayed detection of recurrence or adverse effects on survival.

The underlying aim of any breast cancer surgery is local control of disease and in some cases, ultimately cure. Although extremely important, reconstruction should always take second place in the list of priorities. Any reconstructive procedure carries increased morbidity when compared to a mastectomy alone and this should be explained to the patient. This increase, however, depends on the type of reconstruction. With implants the main problems are infection, seroma, skin necrosis, capsular contraction and leakage. With autologous flaps, morbidity arises from donor site seroma, abdominal wall weakness or hernia, haematoma, infection and partial or total flap loss.

The role of breast care nurses in counselling is vital. Although an integral part of the multidisciplinary team, their role is very much that of 'patient's advocate'. They often maintain an informal contact with the patient throughout and spend many hours explaining the relative merits of the treatment options without undue bias. In many units they also provide a visible link to the patient between the various oncological disciplines. There is no doubt that the influence of the breast care nurse is a major factor in a patient's trust of the oncology team as a whole and as such they have become an important determinant in overall patient satisfaction.

It is evident that there is significant morbidity from all types of reconstruction. This, however, should not be an excuse for not offering every patient the options. Most patients are still happier following reconstruction even when complications have arisen.

This underlines the huge psychological importance of these procedures for women with breast cancer.

RECONSTRUCTION AFTER MASTECTOMY

It is following mastectomy that reconstruction is most commonly employed. With an increasingly recognised place for breast conservation surgery, mastectomy rates have decreased. Despite this, up to 50% of patients with breast cancer will still undergo mastectomy, either as a primary treatment or for recurrence. Post-mastectomy reconstruction can be either immediate or delayed and can generally be divided into prosthetic implants and myo-cutaneous flaps.

Patient selection

Most patients who are fit enough for mastectomy can also have breast reconstruction. The choice generally comes down to patient preference although in a few cases, some guidance is needed from the surgeon. Relative contraindications for the various types of autologous reconstruction include obesity, heavy smoking, increasing age, diabetes mellitus, abdominal scars and chest wall irradiation. For implants, the only strong contra-indication is radiotherapy to the chest wall. This has been found to greatly increase the overall rates of complication and failure. Abdominal scarring is a relative contraindication for a pedicled TRAM flap although a Pfannensteil incision is usually acceptable.

In general, autologous flaps give a better aesthetic result than implants as they often produce a more naturally contoured breast. This is particularly suitable for the younger patient who is worried about their 'naked' appearance with a partner. The downside, however, is greater chance of significant morbidity from a much more major operation. Implants, on the other hand, have less serious morbidity and involve less major surgery but tend to sit higher on the chest and are subsequently more asymmetrical in shape. This is particularly pronounced if the contra-lateral breast is ptotic. Correction for this can, however, be made by contra-lateral surgery (discussed below) and by a period of overexpansion of a prosthesis. Implants are particularly suitable therefore for the older patient who is less worried about her 'naked' appearance but simply wants an equal volume on each side which appears normal in clothes or a bathing costume and also for women with smaller, less ptotic breasts.

Implants

Implant technology has undoubtedly progressed since its intro-duction in the early 1960s. It remains a popular and important method of reconstruction despite the rapid increase in the number of autologous reconstructions which are being performed. This is mainly because it is relatively easy to perform by a non-plastic surgeon and is well tolerated by the patient due to a quick recovery and rehabilitation time. The early implants suffered from a high rate of complication and failure, principally from capsular contracture. This leads to difficulties with full expansion of the prosthesis, but, more distressingly for the patient, in its severest form often causes pain and deformity (Figure 31.2). Grading of this complication is according to Baker's classification (Table 31.1). Subpectoral placement and the use of textured implants have to some extent reduced this but it still remains a significant problem, with some series reporting rates of up to 29%. Perhaps a more important limitation is the final possible result both in terms of size and ptosis. Implants are therefore generally suitable for women with a breast cup size of B or less and only a mildly ptotic breast or for those who wish to achieve a breast mound which gives a good 'bra' appearance (Figure 31.3).

Choice of implant

Three broad techniques utilising different types of implant are currently employed, all of which have their relative merits.

Insertion of a simple prosthesis

This is suitable for women with very small, non–ptotic breasts.

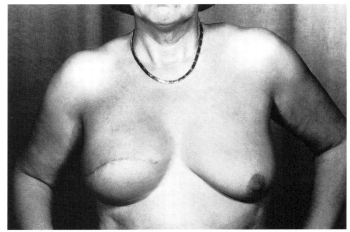

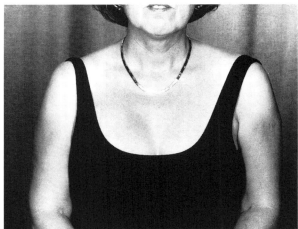

Figure 31.3 Patient undressed and dressed following implant reconstruction.

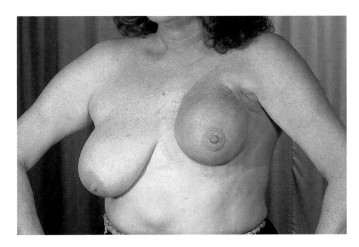

Figure 31.2 Severe capsular contracture.

Initial insertion of a tissue expander with secondary placement of a permanent prosthesis

This is believed to have two advantages. Firstly, overinflation allows for excess tissue to be gained allowing for a greater degree of ptosis and inframammary fold. Secondly, leaving the expander *in situ* for 2–3 months before definitive placement of a prosthesis may reduce the rates of capsular contracture although this has been questioned by some.

One-stage expander prosthesis reconstruction

This has the advantage of offering mastectomy and reconstruction at a single operation. Implants are either entirely saline filled or have two compartments: a small silicon-filled anterior cavity with an expandable saline-filled cavity posteriorly. After insertion, inflation is achieved by instilling sterile saline through a port and connection tube, which is sited subcutaneously. This can either be incorporated within the prosthesis or alternatively may be placed remotely in the inferior axilla. Purely saline-filled implants

Table 31.1 The Baker Scale as devised for augmentation mammoplasty	
Grade	**Description**
I	Absolutely natural: no-one could tell that the breast was augmented.
II	Minimal: Surgery is detectable but the patient has no complaint.
III	Moderate: the patient feels some firmness.
IV	Severe: the implant is obvious just on observation.

are liable to wrinkling which can produce an unsightly appearance of the breast. Most would therefore use a silicon/saline combination prosthesis to avoid this problem.

Surgical technique and positioning

Preoperative assessment for size of implant is obviously of the utmost importance. Whilst in the upright position, the width, projection and position of the breast are noted and the skin is marked to determine the correct position of the inframammary fold. This process also includes measurement and marking of the opposite side to achieve the best possible symmetry.

Standard practice today is to place any implant behind a muscular flap, usually pectoralis major. However, consideration must be made to allow for maximum expansion at the desired level. For breasts which are fuller in the lower pole, some advocate either detaching the inferior portion of pectoralis major and draping it over the prosthesis or use of a combination of flaps, including part of the anterior rectus sheath and serratus anterior. The former inevitably does not produce total muscle coverage but the proponents of this technique claim that this does not adversely affect outcome.

The second consideration is formation of the inframammary fold. This is achieved by undermining the inferior skin flap and suturing it tightly to the chest wall at the desired level. This allows for expansion above this level and therefore, with ptosis caused by the gravitational effects on the implant, an aesthetically pleasing breast can be produced.

With any operation, careful attention to sterility and haemostasis is important. This is especially true for implant surgery as infection can lead to the necessity for removal of the implant. All patients therefore should have drains inserted under and above the muscle flap. Prophylactic antibiotics are also administered perioperatively.

Complications

Morbidity from implant reconstruction, although significant in percentage terms, rarely leads to complete failure. Taking into account the precautions outlined above, this should be kept to a minimum. Complications are numerous and include haematoma, infection, skin necrosis, deflation or rupture, dislocation and

capsular contraction. Reports from various studies vary in the incidence of each and are outlined in Table 31.2. It is wise, therefore, to warn the patient before embarking on reconstructive surgery that there is a significant chance they will require corrective surgery at some point in the future.

Autologous myocutaneous flap reconstruction

Without doubt, the best possible aesthetic results can be obtained by flap reconstruction. The reasons for this are threefold. Firstly, there is usually ample tissue to produce a good volume breast and replace any skin deficit. Secondly, the consistency is more like that of a normal breast and lastly, a naturally shaped breast can be attained more easily with adequate ptosis and a good inframammary fold. The surgery, however, is much more complicated and time consuming, especially for free flaps, and complications when they arise can be more catastrophic. The recovery time for the patient is also longer, meaning a prolonged period off work and greater disability.

Latissimus dorsi reconstruction

Latissimus dorsi flaps were first introduced mainly when there was a large tissue defect following radiation necrosis or in cases of locally advanced cancer. For aesthetic reconstruction, they generally still require insertion of an implant to achieve adequate volume, especially if replacing a large ptotic breast, although for smaller breasts or with contralateral reduction this is not always necessary. Recent fat-harvesting techniques have further reduced the need for an implant. The real advantage over an expander implant technique is that skin defects can be replaced immediately and therefore some of the problems with expansion, such as capsular contracture, are eliminated (Figure 31.4).

Surgical technique involves first placing the patient in a lateral position. A slightly curved, transverse incision is made at the level of the tip of the scapula. A second incision is made below this to produce a skin island of the required size (Figure 31.5). The muscle is divided inferiorly to enable transposition to the anterior chest wall through a skin tunnel. Blood supply is usually from the thoracodorsal vessels which are branches of the axillary vein and artery. If these have been sacrificed during axillary surgery, a secondary blood supply is available from serratus anterior

Table 31.2 Complications following implant insertion in various studies (percentages in brackets)

Study	No. of prostheses	Infection	Leak/ deflation	Seroma/ haematoma	Capsular contracture*	Extrusion/ exposure	Skin necrosis/ Wound dehiscence
Mansel 1986	12	1(8)	2(16)	–	3(25)	–	
Dickson 1987	92	3(3)	15(16)	1(1)	12(13)	2(2)	5(5)
Slavin 1990	60	4(7)	3(5)	9(15)	–	5(8)	8(13)
Schuster 1990	56	3(5)	2(4)	6(11)	7(12)	2(4)	7(13)
Ramon 1997	52	5(10)	2(4)	3(6)	7(14)	3(6)	1(2)

* – Baker grade 3 or more

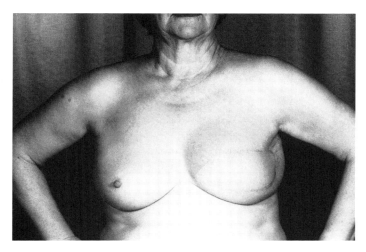

Figure 31.4 LD flap reconstruction.

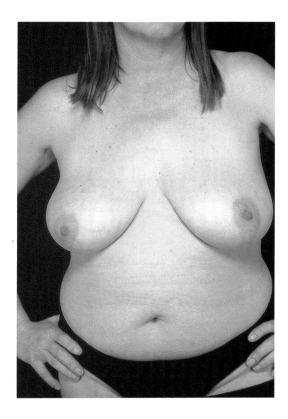

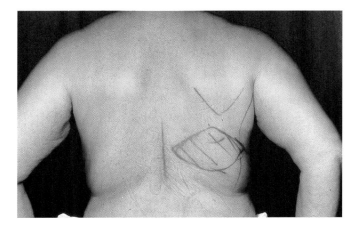

Figure 31.5 Preoperative marking of skin incision for a LD flap.

vasculature. Overlying skin is perfused via multiple musculo-cutaneous perforators. After harvesting, the flap is positioned to form the new breast mound and to replace any skin deficit. Usually too much skin is present so this can be deepithelialised and buried. If necessary a small implant can be placed behind the flap.

Transverse rectus abdominis musculocutaneous (TRAM) flap

This is the gold standard for breast reconstruction (Figure 31.6). It can either be pedicled, therefore retaining its original blood supply based on the superior epigastric vessels, or free, which requires microvascular anastomosis. The main advantage over latissimus dorsi flaps is that it is possible to harvest enough tissue to produce a good-sized breast mound without the need for an implant. It is not, however, suitable for obese patients, those with extensive abdominal scarring or those with compromised arterial vessels, e.g. smokers, diabetes or the elderly.

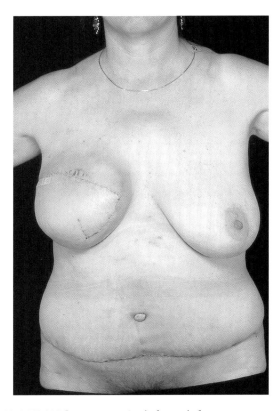

Figure 31.6 TRAM flap reconstruction before and after surgery.

Surgical procedures vary slightly for the pedicled and free flaps but the basic principle is to harvest an area of abdominal skin and fat based on a portion of the rectus muscle. Free flaps are usually based on the inferior epigastric artery. The incision is shown in Figure 31.7. This is bevelled to include as much fat as possible. The rectus muscle is next dissected, taking care to preserve the perforators. A portion of the medial and lateral edges is usually preserved to aid abdominal closure. For pedicled flaps, the muscle is divided inferiorly and the flap is then rotated up through a midline skin tunnel to the anterior chest wall. As with the latissimus dorsi flap, any skin loss is replaced and extra skin buried along with the rest of the flap after deepithelialisation. Any excess tissue is discarded, beginning with zone 4 which has the worst blood supply. For the free flap, the inferior epigastric pedicle is divided after dissection down to the iliac vessels. This is subsequently anastomosed to the thoracodorsal vessels.

Supercharging of a pedicled flap can also be achieved in this way if blood supply is poor. By using double pedicle flaps, enough tissue can be gained to reconstruct a large breast or for bilateral reconstruction. In this case abdominal closure usually requires prosthetic mesh. For single pedicle flaps, primary closure is usually achievable. There is much debate as to which technique is superior. Undoubtedly free flap reconstruction is considerably more time consuming and runs the risk of complete flap failure but some would argue that generally the blood supply is better, incidence of abdominal wall hernia is less and breast shaping can be achieved more easily.

Other flaps

Four other flaps have been described for breast reconstruction which all require microvascular anastomosis. These are the vertical rectus abdominis musculocutaneous (VRAM) flap, the superior and inferior gluteal flaps and the lateral thigh flap.

These tend to be second or third choice as the fat in these regions tends to be more rigid than that from the abdomen and therefore creates a breast of suboptimal consistency. As the names suggest, the VRAM flap is similar to the TRAM except that a vertical ellipse incision is made. The gluteal flaps are based on the vessels of the same name. With the inferior flap, exposure of the sciatic nerve inferior gluteal nerves during dissection can make sitting uncomfortable. The lateral thigh flap is perfused by the lateral femoral circumflex vessels.

Complications

Generally, overall complication rates from autologous reconstructions are less than from implants but when they do arise, they can be catastrophic, such as total or partial flap loss. More common problems are haematoma and seroma at the donor site. This can be reduced by meticulous haemostasis and insertion of subcutaneous drains. The other main problem is abdominal wall weakness or herniation following a TRAM flap. Careful patient selection is undoubtedly important as those who are obese or have risk factors for small vessel disease generally have the worst outcomes. For these patients, implant reconstruction is a better option. Table 31.3 below, gives complication rates for several different studies.

Contralateral surgery

For patients with extremely small or very large ptotic breasts, contralateral surgery is indicated to achieve symmetry. For small breasts, simple subpectoral or subglandular implant insertion can produce a normal volume breast to match that on the other side. For large or ptotic breasts, either reduction mammoplasty, mastopexy or a combination of the two is easier than trying to achieve a symmetrical match with unilateral reconstruction.

Reduction mammoplasty broadly involves removing wedges of breast tissue from the inferior part of the breast and then closing the defect. Mastopexy, which is usually performed at the same time as a reduction, moves the nipple and areola on a pedicle, higher up on the breast. This literally 'lifts' the breast surgically. This technique can also be used to effect a wide local excision of a breast carcinoma. This is particularly suitable for lower pole tumours which can often result in a pulled-down appearance of

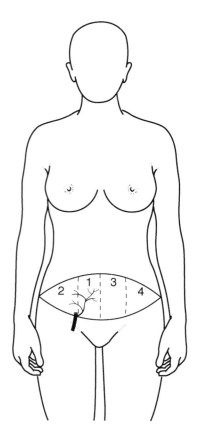

Figure 31.7 TRAM incision showing position of best to worst vascularised zones in order from 1 to 4.

Table 31.3 Complications following autologous flap reconstruction in various studies (percentages in brackets)

Study	Type of flap	Number performed	Infection	Partial flap loss	Total flap loss	Fat necrosis	Hernia	Haematoma	Seroma	Partial breast skin loss	Partial dorsal skin loss
Mansel 1986	LD	38	3(8)	1(3)	–	–	–	–	–	–	–
	TRAM	45	9(20)	10(22)	–	–	6(13)	–	–	–	–
Elliot 1993*	TRAM	190	(0–3)	(0–10)	(0.4–1)	–	(0–2.5)	(2.5–3.8)	–	(0.4–2)	–
Witterson 1995	TRAM	556	28(5)	28(5)	0(0)	59(11)	49(8.8)	7(1.3)	–	–	–
Delay 1998	LD#	100	2(2)	1(1)	1(1)	4 (4)	–	6(6)	79(79)	10(10)	3 (3)

LD, latissimus dorsi

TRAM, transverse rectus abdominis musculocutaneous

* Complication rates varied for free and pedicled flaps. Range in percentage terms is given

LD flap performed with fat harvesting. No implant was used

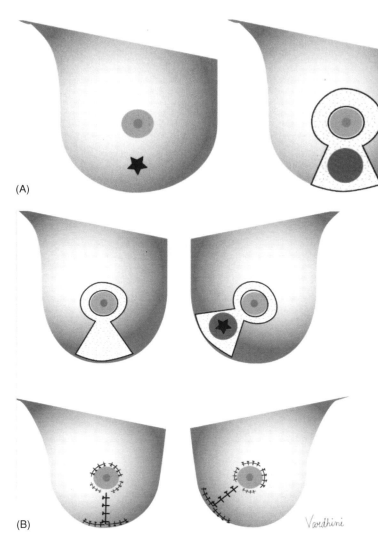

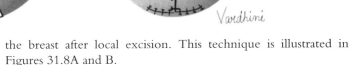

Figure 31.8 A Diagrammatic representation of incorporation of cancer resection within a reduction mammoplasty. **B** Bilateral reduction mammoplasty including wide local excision of a tumour in the lower inner quadrant.

the breast after local excision. This technique is illustrated in Figures 31.8A and B.

Nipple–areola reconstruction

Creation of a new nipple–areola complex is usually the final step in reconstruction. For some, it has great psychological importance and they do not feel completely symmetrical until it is achieved. Despite this, many women still decline this relatively simple operation. Timing of this procedure is important as the final shape and position of a reconstructed breast is not reached until about six months. Positioning of the new nipple at this stage is more reliable and usually involves input from the patient herself. Often a prosthetic nipple is worn for a while to ensure correct placement.

With regards to nipple reconstruction there are many different techniques described in the literature. Although a new nipple can be created using a donor graft from the opposite side, most surgeons employ one of the various types of local flap. A simple type is outlined in Figure 31.9. It is important to try and achieve projection of the nipple that is equal to the opposite side. With most local flaps, projection will decrease before becoming stable at about six months. The amount of shrinkage is variable but the

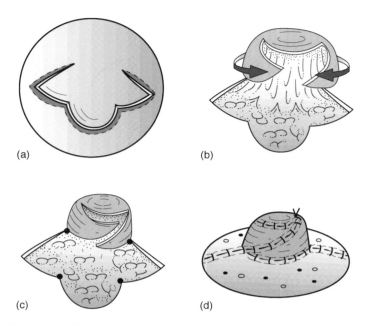

Figure 31.9 Diagrammatic representation of a local flap nipple reconstruction.

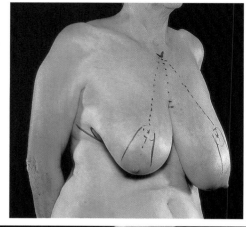

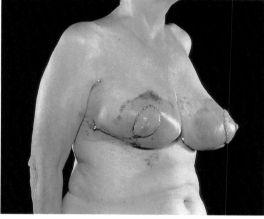

Figure 31.10 Postsurgical appearance following reduction mastopexy which incorporated a wide local excision of a primary breast cancer on the right side.

degree of initial overprojection can be calculated depending on the type of flap used.

The simplest method of areola reconstruction is tattooing of the skin. An accurate colour match is easily managed using charts. Tattooing of the new nipple can also be done. The other alternative is the use of a skin graft which can give a better texture to the skin. Also a small piece of cartilage can be placed subcutaneously to increase nipple projection.

Reconstruction after conservative surgery

With the increasing trend towards breast conservation surgery, due to good evidence of equivalent survival to mastectomy, the latter is becoming less common. The aim of wide local excision is to avoid the mutilating surgery of a mastectomy and so leave an aesthetically acceptable breast following breast cancer surgery. There are some patients who still end up with a poor cosmetic result following local excision and radiotherapy. This is particularly true for patients with large, inferiorly placed tumours in a small breast or for those who have a marked inflammatory response with subsequent scar contraction due to the radiotherapy. For these patients some form of reconstruction may be necessary either in the immediate setting or as a second procedure. Options for this, as with reconstruction after mastectomy, include local flaps, contralateral surgery or reduction mammoplasty incorporating the tumour in the resected tissue.

For large tumours in large breasts the best option is some form of breast reshaping similar to reduction mammoplasty. By carefully planning the surgery to remove breast tissue containing the

tumour and with contralateral reduction, a symmetrical, aesthetically pleasing result can be obtained. This works particularly well for tumours situated inferiorly or medially, as shown in Figure 31.10.

For moderate-sized tumours in smaller breasts, tissue transfer techniques are often required. The simplest way to achieve this is to move the defect to the axilla with the use of a local flap (Figure 31.11). Another technique to excise large, deeply seated tumours is to mobilise the breast through a lateral incision. The breast can then be reflected medially and the tumour removed from behind (Figure 31.12). For slightly larger tumours, however, it may be necessary to use a pedicled latissimus dorsi flap. This is particularly true if there is skin loss.

There is an increasing trend to try and anticipate these defects before oncological surgery and therefore to plan immediate reconstruction. There is no doubt that there are several advantages over mastectomy and reconstruction. Firstly, most of the breast is left behind, including the nipple–areola complex and inframammary fold; secondly, the time taken for these recon-

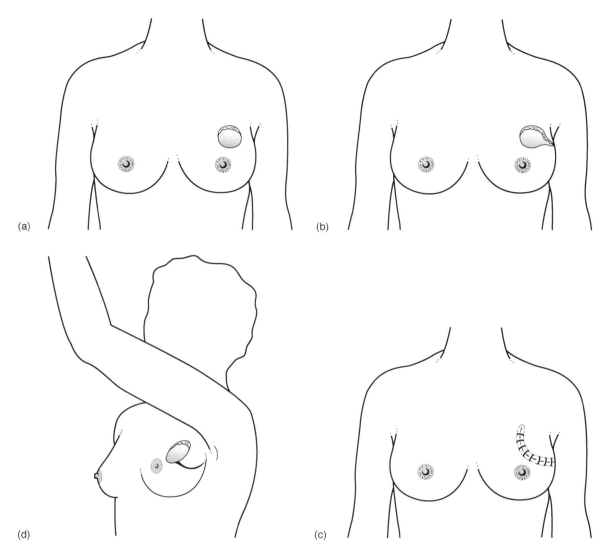

(a)

(b)

(d)

(c)

Figure 31.11 Diagram outlining the technique for local flap reconstruction of an upper breast defect following wide local excision.

structions is shorter and lastly, morbidity is much less than from a 'total' breast reconstruction.

Non-surgical options

Not all patients are either suitable for or desire breast reconstruction. For these women, the alternative is a prosthesis worn in the bra (Figure 31.13). In most clothes and even bathing costumes, these are invisible to the passer-by and most women are satisfied with their clothed appearance. This is especially true of older women who are not as worried about their naked appearance. Age alone, however, is not an absolute contraindication to surgical reconstruction and as mentioned above, all options should be discussed with every patient where appropriate.

For some women who have had surgical restoration of the breast mound but who decline the final nipple–areola reconstruction, prosthetic nipples can be used. These can be matched with the opposite side and can be particularly convincing under light clothing.

With changing attitudes, however, surgical breast reconstruction can only continue to become more commonplace.

Acknowledgements

Grateful thanks to Miss Josephine Woodhams and Miss Vardhini Vijay for their illustrations.

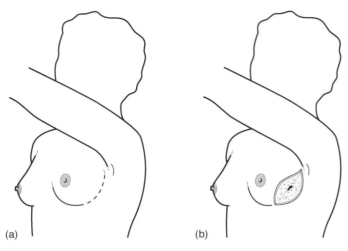

(a) (b)

Figure 31.12 Lateral approach to achieve wide local excision of a deeply seated tumour.

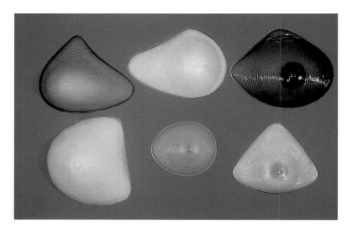

Figure 31.13 External breast prostheses.

FURTHER READING

Beasley ME. The pedicled TRAM as preference for immediate autogenous tissue breast reconstruction. *Clin Plastic Surg* 1994; **21**:191–205

Berry MG, al-Mufti RA, Jenkinson AD, et al. An audit of outcome including patient satisfaction with immediate breast reconstruction performed by breast surgeons. *Ann Roy Coll Surg Engl* 1998; **80**:173–177

Bhatty MA, Berry RB. Nipple–areola reconstruction by tattooing and nipple sharing. *Br J Plastic Surg* 1997; **50**:331–334

Clough KB, Kroll SS, Audretsch W. An approach to the repair of partial mastectomy defects. *Plastic and Reconstr Surg* 1999; **104**:409–420

Kat CC, Darcy CM, O'Donoghue JM, Taylor AR, Regan PJ. The use of the latissimus dorsi musculocutaneous flap for immediate correction of the deformity resulting from breast conservation surgery. *Br J Plastic Surg* 1999; **52**:99–103

Pusic A, Thompson TA, Kerrigan CL. Surgical options for the early-stage breast cancer: factors associated with patient choice and postoperative quality of life. *Plastic and Reconst Surg* 1999; **104**:1325–1333

Spyrou GE, Titley OG, Cerqueiro J, Fatah MF. A survey of general surgeons' attitudes towards breast reconstruction after mastectomy. *Ann Roy Coll Surg Engl* 1998; **80**:178–183

Section 5

Endocrine surgery

32

The pituitary

Ikram Shah Ismail

ANATOMY

The pituitary is a composite gland, the anterior lobe being derived from an evagination of the Rathke's pouch, while the posterior lobe is an extension of the forebrain. The weight of the adult human gland is approximately 620 mg. Nervous tissue is the principal component of the posterior pituitary and in women the posterior pituitary is 20% of the gland whilst in men it is 25%.

The gland lies in a bony fossa, and its stalk pierces the fibrous diaphragma sellae. The lateral wall of the sella is made up of the cavernous sinus in which lie the carotid siphon, and the cranial nerves III, IV and VI. The optic chiasm is situated immediately above the pituitary fossa, anterior to the pituitary stalk. The hypothalamus lies above the pituitary stalk, and extends to the lateral wall of the third ventricle. It is bounded anteriorly by the anterior commissure, posteriorly by the mammillary body, and is composed of many sets of nuclei and neuronal tracts, a number of which terminate in the median eminence.

Blood supply

The greater part of the arterial blood supply to the hypothalamus and pituitary gland is derived from the internal carotid artery and its branches (Figure 32.1). The posterior lobe is supplied by the inferior hypophyseal artery and the artery of the trabecula (a branch of the superior hypophyseal artery). There is no direct arterial supply to the anterior pituitary, and all of its blood supply comes from the long and short hypophyseal portal vessels that drain the median eminence. Branches from the Circle of Willis supply the hypothalamus, which is extremely well perfused. The

paraventricular and supraoptic nuclei receive blood from branches of the superior hypophyseal, anterior communicating, anterior cerebral, posterior communicating, and posterior cerebral arteries.

Venous blood from the anterior and posterior lobes of the pituitary enters the dural, cavernous, and inferior petrosal sinuses. Hypothalamic-releasing or hypothalamic-inhibiting hormones are secreted into the hypophyseal portal blood system and impinge on the anterior pituitary gland. Secretion of the pituitary trophic hormones is then regulated from specific cells that exhibit distinctive immunohistochemical characteristics (Figure 32.1). The clinical manifestations of hypopituitarism depend on the degree of pituitary hormone deficiency, which may be isolated or may occur as a combined multiple hormone deficiency. The spectrum of hormone loss resulting from a destructive pituitary lesion initially results in loss of growth hormone, followed by loss of gonadotrophin, thyroid-stimulating hormone, and finally corticotrophin secretion. Causes are outlined in Box 32.1.

Each anterior pituitary cell, either singly or in combination, may give rise to pituitary adenomas that express pituitary hormones. Most clinically non-functional tumours secrete gonadotrophins or their alpha-subunit. Prolactin, growth hormone, and pro-opiomelanocortin-expressing adenomas account for most clinically functional adenomas that are removed surgically.

PITUITARY DISEASE

The clinical features associated with hypo- or hyperfunction of the anterior pituitary gland depend on the specific trophic hormones whose secretion is disordered.

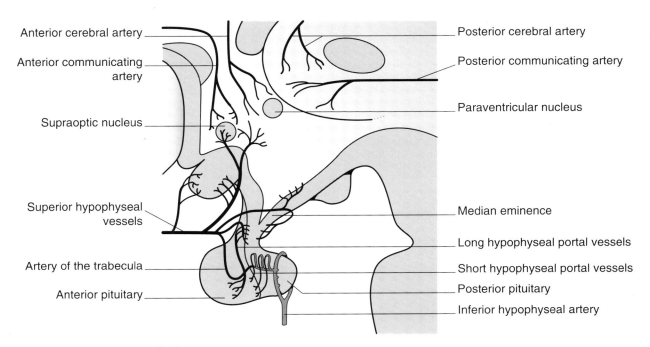

Figure 32.1 Blood supply to the pituitary gland.

> **Box 32.1**   Causes of hypopituitarism
>
> Congenital
> - Septo-optic dysplasia
> - Hypogonadotrophic hypogonadism
> - Prader-Willi syndrome
> - Laurence-Moon-Biedl syndrome
> - Isolated growth hormone deficiency
> - Basal encephalocoele
>
> Vascular
> - Pituitary apoplexy
> - Sheehan's syndrome
> - Arteritides and aneurysm
>
> Inflammatory
> - Lymphocytic hypophysitis
> - Histiocytosis
> - Sarcoidosis
> - Tuberculosis
>
> Physical agents
> - Trauma
> - Ionising radiation
> - Stalk section
> - Surgery
>
> Infiltrations
> - Haemochromatosis
> - Metastatic carcinoma
> - Amyloidosis
>
> Tumours
> - Hypothalamic
> - Craniopharyngioma
> - Glioma
> - Germinoma
> - Meningioma
> - Hamartoma
> - Leukemia and lymphoma
>
> Pituitary
> - Functioning or non-functioning macroadenomas
> - Empty sella

Hypopituitarism

Deficiency of growth hormone

Deficiency of growth hormone during infancy and childhood causes growth retardation with short stature, fasting hypoglycemia, and occasionally, delayed puberty. Adults may manifest central adiposity, muscle weakness, psychological depression, and hyperlipidaemia.

Deficiency of gonadotrophins

During childhood, central hypogonadism results in pubertal failure. Breast development is delayed, and pubic and axillary hair do not grow, although some sexual hair growth occurs if the corticotrophin-adrenal axis is intact and stimulates adrenal androgen production. In girls, primary amenorrhoea is present; in boys, small testes and phallus and sparse body hair are evident. Isolated

gonadotrophin deficiency results in tall adolescents with eunuchoid proportions (i.e. upper-to-lower segment ratio of less than 1). In postpubertal females, features of hypogonadism include secondary amenorrhoea, breast atrophy and loss of pubic and axillary hair. Men manifest testicular atrophy, decrease in body hair, decreased libido, impotence and infertility.

Thyroid-stimulating hormone deficiency

Deficiency of thyroid-stimulating hormone secretion causes thyroid failure. The lack of thyroid hormone secretion results in lethargy, cold intolerance, constipation, bradycardia and hoarseness. Low circulating levels of thyroid-stimulating hormone in the presence of low thyroid hormone levels distinguish thyroid-stimulating hormone deficient patients from those with primary hypothyroidism.

Corticotrophin deficiency

Corticotrophin deficiency causes adrenal failure with features including orthostatic hypotension, weakness, hypothermia, nausea, vomiting, dehydration, lethargy, coma and even death. Hypokalaemia is usually not present because of the maintenance of mineralocorticoid secretion by the intact renin-angiotensin system.

Vasopressin deficiency

Vasopressin deficiency occurs with posterior pituitary lesions, resulting in diminished release of vasopressin and resultant diabetes insipidus.

Diagnosis

Hypopituitarism should be suspected in all patients who have previously undergone pituitary surgery, irradiation, or recent pregnancy. Decreased pituitary reserves should also be suspected in patients with hypogonadism, infertility and unexplained hypothyroidism. The absence of an elevated pituitary trophic hormone in the face of adrenal, thyroid, or gonadal failure confirms the diagnosis. Biochemical testing for these patients involves dynamic assessment of growth hormone and gonadotrophin secretion. Attenuation of thyroid and adrenal pituitary reserves, however, usually only occurs later in the development of frank pituitary failure. Once the diagnosis has been confirmed, a magnetic resonance imaging (MRI) scan is helpful in excluding the presence of a pituitary or sellar mass that would impinge on normal pituitary tissue. Also, at least in patients with growth hormone deficiency, the morphologic appearance of the stalk and pituitary gland as determined by MR imaging may be useful in predicting the pattern and severity of the hypopituitarism.

Treatment of hypopituitarism is outlined in Box 32.2 later. Although growth hormone replacement in adult hypopituitary

<table>
<tr><td colspan="2">Box 32.2 Treatment of hypopituitarism</td></tr>
<tr><td>Trophic hormone
deficiency</td><td>Replacement</td></tr>
<tr><td>Corticotrophin</td><td>Hydrocortisone (20 mg am;
10 mg pm)
Cortisone acetate (25 mg am;
12.5 mg pm)</td></tr>
<tr><td>Thyroid-stimulating hormone</td><td>L-thyroxine (0.1–0.15 mg/day)</td></tr>
<tr><td>Follicle-stimulating hormone/
luteinising hormone</td><td>Males:
Testosterone enanthate (200 mg
intramuscularly every 2 weeks)

Females:

Ethinyl oestradiol (0.02–0.05 mgL
for 21 days)

Conjugated oestrogens
(0.625–1.25 mg day for 25 days)

Oestradiol skin patch (48 mg,
twice weekly) with progesterone
on days 16–25 to facilitate uterine
shedding

For fertility: Menopausal
gonadotrophins, human chorionic
gonadotrophins</td></tr>
<tr><td>Vasopressin</td><td>Intranasal desmopressin
(0.050.1 mL twice daily)</td></tr>
<tr><td>Growth hormone</td><td>Replacement is experimental in
adults</td></tr>
</table>

patients is experimental, its effects on body composition, muscle strength, exercise capacity and intermediary metabolism would be expected to improve quality of life.

Pituitary tumours

Patients with pituitary tumours may present with:

- Local neurologic effects
- Endocrine effects
- Hypopituitarism
- Pituitary hyperfunction.

Local neurologic effects of pituitary tumours

Most patients with pituitary tumours larger than 1 cm in diameter experience severe headache, probably as a result of pressure on the diaphragma sella by the tumour mass. The optic chiasm, which lies above the pituitary sella turcica, is frequently compressed by the encroaching tumour, causing loss of red perception, bitemporal hemianopia, or a superior bitemporal defect. Hypothalamic invasion by pituitary tumours can result in diabetes insipidus, sleep or appetite disorders and changes in autonomic function. Cavernous sinus invasion leads to cranial nerve palsies with ptosis, ophthalmoplegia, or diplopia; haemorrhage into the tumour may result in acute necrosis with severe headache, visual impairment, paralysis, lethargy and coma.

Diagnosis

Signs and symptoms of a pituitary tumour result from either the local effects of the pituitary mass or the hormonal abnormalities induced by adenomas. These may present initially with compression of adjacent neurologic structures with concurrent systemic effects resulting from excess peripheral hormonal action. Hypersecretion of a pituitary trophic hormone can cause acromegaly, amenorrhoea/galactorrhoea, impotence, or Cushing's disease (Box 32.3). Diagnosis of pituitary adenomas has been aided by sophisticated MR imaging procedures that detect microadenoma masses as small as 2 mm in diameter and provide the best visualisation of the hypothalamus. In doubtful cases, procedures such as inferior petrosal sinus sampling and cavernous sinus sampling can be used to distinguish pituitary Cushing's disease from occult ectopic adrenocorticotrophin syndrome and to predict the intrapituitary location of tumours.

<table>
<tr><td colspan="3">Box 32.3 Pituitary adenomas</td></tr>
<tr><td>Cell of origin</td><td>Product</td><td>Clinical syndrome</td></tr>
<tr><td>Lactotroph</td><td>prolactin</td><td>Hypogonadism,
galactorrhoea</td></tr>
<tr><td>Somatotroph</td><td>growth hormone</td><td>Acromegaly</td></tr>
<tr><td>Corticotroph</td><td>corticotrophin</td><td>Cushing's disease</td></tr>
<tr><td>Mixed GH
and PRL</td><td>growth hormone,
prolactin</td><td>Acromegaly,
hypogonadism</td></tr>
<tr><td>Plurihormona</td><td>Any</td><td>Varies</td></tr>
<tr><td>Gonadotroph</td><td>follicle-stimulating
hormone, luteinising
hormone, subunits</td><td>Hypogonadism or
no effect</td></tr>
<tr><td>Thyrotroph</td><td>thyroid-stimulating
hormone</td><td>Hyperthyroidism</td></tr>
<tr><td>Null cell; oncocyte</td><td>None</td><td>Pituitary failure</td></tr>
</table>

Growth hormone-secreting pituitary tumours

Increased growth hormone secretion may be caused by pituitary or extrapituitary tumours, and may manifest in different ways, depending on the age of the patient. In children or adolescents whose epiphyseal growth centres have yet to fuse, gigantism may occur. In adults, excessive secretion of growth hormone results in acromegaly in which clinical features occur slowly. The clinical presentation reflects the effects of local tumour growth, peripheral tissue changes, and the metabolic and systemic effects of continuous growth hormone and IGF-I hypersecretion.

Extrapituitary causes of acromegaly are rare and include pancreatic islet-cell, lung and intestinal carcinoid tumours. Regardless of the tumour location, patients with acromegaly present with the classical clinical features of acromegaly, along with elevated circulating levels of growth hormone and growth hormone-releasing hormone.

Clinical features of acromegaly include the following:

Local tumour effects
    Pituitary enlargement
    Visual field defects
    Cranial nerve palsy
    Headache

Somatic
    Acral enlargement
        Thickening of soft tissue of hands and feet
    Musculoskeletal
        Prognathism
        Malocclusion
        Arthralgias
        Carpal tunnel syndrome
        Proximal myopathy
        Hypertrophy of frontal bones
    Skin
        Hyperhydrosis
        Skin tags
    Colon
        Polyps
    Cardiovascular
        Left ventricular or septal hypertrophy
        Hypertension
        Congestive heart failure
    Sleep disturbances
        Sleep apnoea
        Narcolepsy
    Visceromegaly
        Tongue
        Thyroid
        Salivary gland

Endocrine/metabolic
    Reproduction
        Menstrual abnormalities
        Galactorrhoea
        Decreased libido, impotence
    Multiple endocrine neoplasia (type I)
        Hyperparathyroidism
        Pancreatic islet cell tumours
    Carbohydrate
        Impaired glucose tolerance
        Insulin resistance
    Lipids
        Hypertriglyceridaemia
    Mineral
        Hypercalciuria
        Urinary hydroxyproline

Diagnosis

Unrestrained growth hormone secretion is the hallmark of acromegaly. The best single test for acromegaly is measurement of serum insulin-like growth factor I IGF-I. Unlike growth hormone, serum IGF-I concentrations do not vary from hour to hour according to food intake, exercise or sleep, but instead reflect integrated GH secretion during the preceding day or longer. Serum IGF-I concentrations are elevated in virtually all patients with acromegaly and provide excellent discrimination from normal individuals. The results must be interpreted, however, according to the patient's age.

The most specific dynamic test for establishing the diagnosis of acromegaly is an oral glucose tolerance test. In normal subjects, serum GH concentrations fall to 2 ng/mL or less within two hours of ingestion of 50–100 g glucose. By contrast, the post-glucose values are greater than 2 ng/mL in over 85% of patients with acromegaly. Once GH hypersecretion has been confirmed, the next step is magnetic resonance imaging (MRI) of the pituitary, because a somatotroph adenoma of the pituitary is by far the most common cause of acromegaly. If no pituitary mass is detected, further imaging is performed to locate an ectopic tumour source of GH-releasing hormone (GH-RH) or GH. Measurements of immunoreactive serum GH-RH levels may distinguish between GH-RH and growth hormone sources.

Prolactin-secreting pituitary tumours

Prolactin-secreting pituitary tumours are diagnosed more often in women than in men, possibly as a result of the difference in clinical manifestations between women and men. Clinical features of prolactinoma in women include:

- Amenorrhea

- Oligomenorrhoea

- Galactorrhoea

- Headaches

- Infertility.

In men, the features more commonly include:

- Headaches

- Visual abnormalities

- Decreased libido

- Impotence

- Infertility.

Microadenomas are more common in women, and macroadenomas are more frequent in men, possibly reflecting a different natural history in men and women. Only a small percentage of microadenomas in women develop into macroadenomas. Prolactinomas frequently cause menstrual disturbances; therefore, tumours in women are generally discovered earlier than in men. In men, decreased libido, impotence and infertility are the presenting features. At diagnosis, macroadenomas may also have caused visual field abnormalities, hypothyroidism and adrenal insufficiency.

Approximately 15% of women with amenorrhoea have elevated levels of serum prolactin and approximately 33% of women with galactorrhoea without amenorrhoea have hyperprolactinaemia. Of women presenting with both signs, more than 75% have increased prolactin levels. Infertility occurs as the result of anovulation or an inadequate luteal phase in women and low sperm counts or impotence in men.

Elevated prolactin levels may suppress the cyclic release of gonadotrophins and may interrupt the peripheral action of gonadotrophins on the gonads. Women frequently present with oestrogen deficiency and decreased vaginal secretions, causing dyspareunia and osteopaenia.

Hyperprolactinaemia can also cause elevated androgen levels, leading to hirsutism and acne. In men, serum testosterone levels are depressed in at least 66% of patients with prolactinomas. When the tumour is detected and treated early, testosterone levels ultimately increase. Irreversible damage to the pituitary gonadotrophs by an expanding tumour may, however, prevent the normalization of testosterone levels. Elevated prolactin levels may also attenuate the peripheral action of testosterone, perhaps by interfering with the conversion of testosterone to dihydrotestosterone.

Diagnosis

Diagnosis of prolactin-secreting pituitary adenoma involves measuring basal serum prolactin concentrations. When levels exceed 4000 mU/L (upper limit of normal is 500), a pituitary tumour is likely to be present. Prolactin levels below 4000 mU/L may be caused by a variety of secondary conditions:

Physiologic

- Pregnancy and lactation
- Stress
- Exercise
- Chest wall trauma

Pathologic

- Hypothalamic
  Inflammation
  Tumour
- Pituitary
  Lactotroph microadenoma or macroadenoma
  Acromegaly
- Stalk section due to sellar mass
- Empty sella syndrome

- Peripheral
- Hypothyroidism
- Chronic renal failure

Pharmacologic

- Psychotropic agents
  Phenothiazines
  Tricyclic antidepressants
- Opiates
- Metoclopramide
- Cimetidine
- Antihypertensives
  Methyldopa
  Reserpine
- Hormones
  Oestrogens
  Thyrotrophin-releasing hormone

To confirm the presence of a tumour, MRI scanning of the pituitary region should be used when persistent hyperprolactinaemia is demonstrated. There is no definitive test to determine whether elevated prolactin levels result from pituitary tumours or from other causes.

Gonadotrophin-secreting pituitary tumours

Gonadotrophin-secreting pituitary tumours are usually non-functional and are associated with hypogonadism. Patients are usually asymptomatic or may seek care because of local pressure signs.

Most patients have increased circulating levels of glycoprotein hormone alpha-subunits, which may only be demonstrable after thyrotrophin-releasing hormone administration. Gonadal function is usually suppressed with low or normal testosterone levels, or low or normal sperm counts. Rarely, excess production of LH alone by a tumour may result in increased levels of testosterone.

Diagnosis

The diagnosis is difficult in women because of the associated high gonadotrophin levels usually found in postmenopausal women. Primary gonadal failure or menopause may cause secondary pituitary enlargement due to hyperplastic gonadotroph cells, further confounding the differential diagnosis.

Thyroid-stimulating hormone-secreting pituitary tumours

The thyroid-stimulating hormone secreting pituitary tumours are rare, often plurihormonal, and secrete growth hormone, prolactin, and glycoprotein subunits in addition to thyroid-stimulating hormone.

Thyroid-stimulating hormone secreting tumours present with signs and symptoms of hyperthyroidism, and features include thyroid-stimulating hormone levels inappropriate to the elevated thyroid hormone levels.

Approximately one-third of patients with thyroid-stimulating hormone secreting pituitary tumours have thyroid-stimulating hormone levels less than 10 U/L. Ultrasensitive thyroid-stimulating hormone radioimmunoassays should be used to discriminate between low and inappropriately normal circulating thyroid-stimulating hormone levels in patients with hyperthyroidism and suspected thyrotroph cell adenoma.

Treatment of pituitary tumours

The aims of treatment are suppression of unrestrained hormone secretion, reduction of tumour mass, correction of visual and neurologic defects, preservation of pituitary function, and prevention of tumour progression or recurrence. Generally, treatment options include surgery, irradiation and medical therapies.

Acromegaly

The primary treatment is transsphenoidal surgical resection of the GH-secreting adenoma. In some centres, the pituitary is also irradiated, resulting in hypopituitarism in 50% of patients within 10 years. A novel somatostatin analogue, octreotide, has been shown to effectively lower growth hormone and IGF-I levels when administered subcutaneously (100 µg three times daily). Tumours also shrink, and the soft tissue and metabolic sequelae of acromegaly are ameliorated. An important side effect of the drug is asymptomatic gallstone development. A long-acting form of octreotide and a long-acting somatostatin analogue (lanreotide), that require just one monthly i.m. injection, may soon replace regular octreotide for the medical treatment of acromegaly. Whether octreotide should replace transsphenoidal surgical resection as the primary treatment for selected patients with acromegaly is still undecided.

Prolactinoma

The outline of management is shown in Figure 32.2. Side effects of bromocriptine are nausea and anorexia, hypotension, peripheral vasospasm, headaches, nasal stuffiness and depression. Although bromocriptine is commonly accepted as primary therapy for microadenomas, its role in the primary treatment of macroadenomas is controversial.

Other tumours

All the other pituitary tumour types, including Cushing's disease should be managed by transsphenoidal surgical resection. Even elderly patients with coexisting medical disorders tolerate transsphenoidal surgical resection well and typically benefit from the procedure.

PITUITARY FUNCTION TESTS

The following is a description of some tests of pituitary function relevant to the practice of endocrine surgery.

Hypothalamic–pituitary thyroid system

In secondary hypothyroidism the basal level of T4 alone determines the need for replacement. The TRH test only assesses the 'readily releasable pool' of TSH and cannot be used to diagnose TSH deficiency. The TRH test is used in the differential diagnosis of pituitary TSH and hypothalamic TRH deficiency, diagnosis of Graves' disease and in hyperthyroidism. To test for pituitary thyroid-stimulating hormone reserve, thyrotrophin-releasing hormone (200 µg) is administered intravenously. TSH is measured basally and at 20 and 60-minutes. Normally, TSH rises by more than 2 mU/L to greater than 3.4 mU/L. The 20-minute value is higher than the 60 minute value. The TRH test does not diagnose secondary hypothyroidism; this diagnosis is made on the basis of a low T4 and a basal TSH, which is not raised. The TRH test response may be reduced, normal or delayed. A delayed TSH response to TRH (60 min value higher than 20 min value) is always abnormal; it is characteristic of hypothalamic disease but may sometimes be seen in pituitary disease or primary hypothyroidism.

In hyperthyroidism and in euthyroid ophthalmic Graves' disease, the basal TSH is suppressed and fails to respond to TRH. TRH tests are rarely required to diagnose hyperthyroidism as the sensitive immunoradiometric assays (IRMAs) for TSH give the same information from the basal level alone in thyrotoxicosis.

Hypothalamic–pituitary adrenal system

Testing for corticotrophin reserve should be carefully supervised because it is potentially hazardous in patients with compromised adrenal function.

Basal cortisol

To test basal ACTH secretion, serum cortisol should be measured at 8–9 am, the results being interpreted as follows:

- A serum cortisol value of = 100 nmol/L, confirmed by a second determination, is strong evidence of cortisol deficiency which, in a patient with a disorder known to cause hypopituitarism, is usually the result of the pituitary disease. In the absence of any known cause of hypopituitarism, this finding requires the measurement of serum ACTH. A serum ACTH value not higher

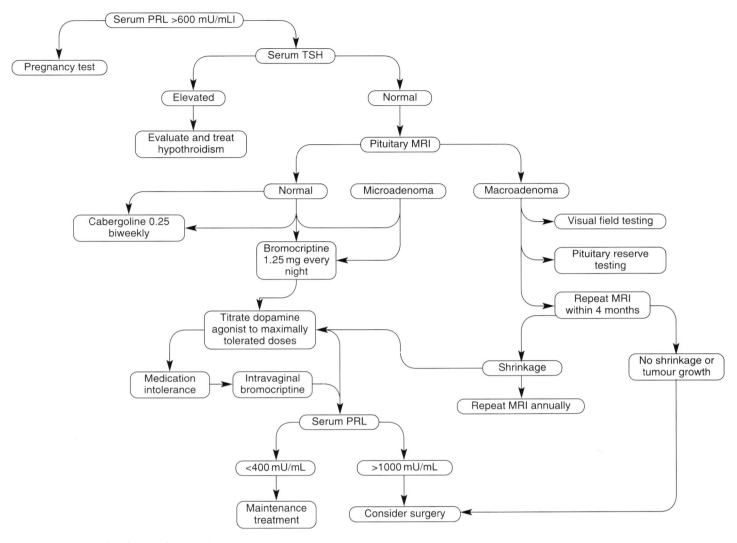

Figure 32.2 Approach to hyperprolactinaemia.

than normal is inappropriately low and establishes the diagnosis of secondary adrenal deficiency (i.e. pituitary or hypothalamic disease). A value higher than normal is consistent with primary adrenal insufficiency (i.e. adrenal disease).

● A serum cortisol value of 500 nmol/L or higher indicates that basal ACTH secretion is sufficient, and also that it is probably sufficient for times of physical stress.

● A serum cortisol value >100 nmol/L but <500 nmol/L that is persistent on repeat measurement is an indication to evaluate ACTH reserve.

Insulin-induced hypoglycaemia test

Indications:

● Assessment of ACTH/cortisol and GH reserve

● Diagnosis of Cushing's syndrome.

After i.v. insulin (0.05–0.1 U/kg) is administered, the blood sugar level should decrease to less than 2.2 mmol/L within 30–45 minutes. A plasma cortisol response of 170 nmol/L above the baseline, a doubling of the baseline cortisol, or a peak value of greater than 580 mmol/L indicates intact corticotrophin reserve. Cortisol peaks approximately 30–45 minutes after hypoglycaemia develops.

Insulin-induced hypoglycaemia is contraindicated in patients who have severe longstanding adrenal insufficiency or are elderly, suffer from ischaemic heart disease, or are prone to cerebral seizures. Before the procedure, make sure that the ECG is normal, and serum cortisol (09.00) must be above 100 nmol/l. Serum T4 must be normal (replace first if low). Dextrose 5% and 25% and i.v. hydrocortisone 100 mg ampoules should be available.

Synacthen stimulation test

As an indirect, but accurate, test of pituitary corticotrophin reserve, adrenal cortisol reserve is evaluated. Synthetic corticotrophin

(Synacthen 250 μg) given intravenously or intramuscularly results in a doubling of serum cortisol levels (i.e. an increase of at least 170 nmol/L) or peak levels of more than 580 nmol/L within 60 minutes. A blunted cortisol response indicates either impaired pituitary corticotrophin reserve or primary adrenal failure.

Corticotrophin-releasing hormone (CRH test)

Corticotrophin-releasing hormone administered intravenously (1 μg/kg) directly stimulates corticotrophin release. Subsequent serum cortisol responses are measured during the subsequent 60 minutes. A blunted response to CRH is indicative of pituitary failure, whereas patients with a corticotrophin cell adenoma causing Cushing's disease often have an exaggerated corticotrophin response to CRH. Patients with ectopic corticotrophin-secreting tumours do not usually demonstrate a further increase in corticotrophin levels in response to CRH.

Test for corticotrophin hypersecretion

At bedtime, 1 mg of dexamethasone is given and cortisol level is measured at 8 am to rule out corticotrophin hypersecretion associated with Cushing's disease. A normal response is a cortisol level less than 100 nmol/L.

Hypothalamic-pituitary gonadal system

Hypothalamic gonadotrophin-releasing hormone regulates the secretion of both pituitary luteinising hormone (LH) and follicle-stimulating hormone (FSH) and is secreted in pulses every 60–120 minutes. In women, LH regulates ovulation and maintenance of the corpus luteum; in men, LH controls testosterone synthesis and secretion by the testicular Leydig cell. FSH regulates ovarian follicular development and maturation and stimulates ovarian oestrogens in women. In men, FSH is responsible for development of seminiferous tubules and stimulates spermatogenesis.

Feedback regulation of gonadotrophin secretion is complex, with both positive and negative components mediated by steroids, polypeptide inhibitory hormones (inhibins), or stimulatory hormones (activins) of gonadal origin.

Gonadotrophins

Concurrent measurement of serum gonadotrophin and gonadal steroid concentrations provides an accurate assessment of gonadotrophins deficiency. In a man with hypopituitarism, LH deficiency can best be detected by measurement of the serum testosterone concentration. If it is low, LH secretion is subnormal and the patient has secondary hypogonadism. When the serum testosterone concentration is low, the serum LH concentration is usually within the normal range, but low as compared with elevated values in primary hypogonadism. If fertility is an issue,

the sperm count should be determined. In a woman who has pituitary or hypothalamic disease but normal menses, no tests of LH or FSH secretion are needed because a normal menstrual cycle is a more sensitive indicator of intact pituitary-gonadal function than any available biochemical test.

If the woman has oligomenorrhoea or amenorrhoea, serum LH or FSH should be measured, to be sure it is not high due to ovarian disease. In addition, at least two of the following three tests should be obtained:

- Measurement of serum oestradiol.
- Vaginal cytology for determination of the oestrogenisation index.
- Administration of medroxyprogesterone, 10 mg day for 10 days, to determine if vaginal bleeding occurs after the 10-day course, and, if so, if it is similar in amount and duration of flow to the patient's menses when they were normal.

Subnormal results for any two of these tests indicate oestradiol-deficiency as a consequence of gonadotrophin deficiency, and warrant prompt consideration of oestrogen treatment. Normal results, in association with oligomenorrhoea or amenorrhoea, could indicate sufficient gonadotrophin secretion to maintain normal basal oestradiol secretion but insufficient to cause ovulation and normal progesterone secretion.

Gonadotrophin-releasing hormone (Gn-RH) test

Administering 100 μg of Gn-RH results in LH levels peaking within 30 minutes and FSH levels plateauing after one hour. Normal responses vary according to stage of menstrual cycle, age and sex of the patient. LH levels usually increase about three-fold, whereas FSH increase is more blunted. The Gn-RH test does not diagnose gonadotrophin deficiency but rather the level of reserve of LH/FSH secretion. In the male this diagnosis is made on the basis of a low serum testosterone without elevation of basal gonadotrophins, and in the female on the basis of amenorrhoea, low serum oestradiol without elevated gonadotrophins and no LH/FSH response to clomiphene. In both cases the Gn-RH response may be subnormal (particularly in primary pituitary disease), normal or exaggerated (particularly with hypothalamic problems). The serum LH response to a single bolus dose of Gn-RH is not helpful in distinguishing secondary hypogonadism due to pituitary disease from that due to hypothalamic disease, because patients who have hypogonadism due to pituitary disease may have normal or subnormal serum LH responses to Gn-RH, as may those who have hypothalamic disease.

Hypothalamic pituitary growth hormone system

Somatostatin and GH-releasing hormone participate in a dual-control system. GH-releasing hormone stimulates the release of growth hormone from the somatotrophs, whereas somatostatin inhibits the secretion of pituitary growth hormone. Growth hormone, quantitatively the main hormone secreted by the pituitary, mediates linear growth. Peak secretory bursts occur between 11 pm and 2 am. Physical exercise, emotional stress and nutritional status regulate growth hormone secretion at the level of the hypothalamus. Growth hormone induces hepatic IGF-I production. IGF-I mediates most of the growth-promoting actions of growth hormone, and it suppresses growth hormone secretion. IGF-I is also produced by extrahepatic tissues and may play a role in local tissue growth. IGF-I is bound to several circulating binding proteins. Insulin-like growth factor binding protein (IGFBP)-3 is the main reservoir for circulating IGF-I, is growth hormone-dependent, and is, therefore, increased in acromegaly and decreased in hypopituitarism. Smaller IGFBPs may regulate IGF-I action by determining IGF-I access to tissues.

Testing for growth hormone reserve

The recent approval of growth hormone for treatment of abnormal body composition and serum lipid profile in adults who have growth hormone deficiency increases the interest in testing growth hormone secretion in patients who have hypothalamic or pituitary disease. I.v. administration of insulin (0.05–0.1 U/kg) should reduce blood glucose to at least 2.20 mmol/L, or to 50% of the patient's initial blood glucose levels. Growth hormone peak response (>40 mmol/L) occurs between 60 and 90 minutes afterward. For the GH-releasing hormone test, i.v. growth hormone-releasing hormone (1 µg/kg) directly tests somatotroph secretory capacity. Growth hormone levels peak within the first hour, and patients with hypopituitarism do not respond · to growth hormone-releasing hormone. A growth hormone response after repeated GH-releasing hormone stimulation may be indicative of a hypothalamic disorder, with defective synthesis of endogenous GH-releasing hormone. A blunted growth hormone response to GH-releasing hormone is also associated with obesity and type 2 diabetes. Arginine, L-dopa, and clonidine hydrochloride are additional pharmacologic stimuli of growth hormone.

Measurements of serum IGF-I or basal serum growth hormone do not distinguish reliably between normal and subnormal growth hormone secretion in adults. Furthermore, because a single test of growth hormone reserve may be subnormal in a normal person, a diagnosis of growth hormone deficiency should be made only if the patient has subnormal serum growth hormone responses to two provocative tests, each of which should be performed in the morning after an overnight fast.

Testing for growth hormone hypersecretion

Growth hormone normally is suppressed to less than 1 mU/L within 60 minutes of ingesting 75 g of oral glucose. Paradoxical growth hormone responses to glucose occur in approximately 75% of patients with acromegaly.

Measuring basal IGF-I levels is useful in screening growth hormone excess, because IGF-I levels do not fluctuate rapidly and reflect integrated growth hormone secretion over time. Levels above 2.2 U/mL usually indicate acromegaly or gigantism.

Hypothalamic-pituitary prolactin system

The primary hypothalamic prolactin inhibitory factor is dopamine. Dopamine antagonists, such as metoclopramide, enhance prolactin secretion, as do drugs that attenuate hypothalamic dopamine, including phenothiazines. Prolactin has a high degree of homology with growth hormone and placental lactogen, and prolactin secretion is stimulated by oestrogen, an important peripheral regulator of prolactin secretion.

Testing for prolactin reserve

I.v. administration of thyrotrophin-releasing hormone (200 µg) elicits a three-fold to five-fold peak prolactin response after 10–20 minutes.

Testing for prolactin hypersecretion

A basal prolactin level greater than 4000 mU/L strongly suggests the presence of a prolactin-secreting adenoma.

Quadruple bolus testing

An efficient and precise method to test anterior pituitary reserve is to administer all four hypothalamic-releasing hormones simultaneously (Box 32.4).

Box 32.4 Administration of hypothalamic-releasing hormones as a combined anterior pituitary function test

Hypothalamic hormone	Radioimmunoassay of pituitary hormone	Venous sampling time after infusion (minutes)
TRH 200 µg	TSH	15, 30
	PRL	10, 15
CRF 1 µg/kg	ACTH	10, 45, 60
GH-RH 1 µg/kg	GH	45, 60
Gn-RH 100 µg	FSH	45, 60, 90
	LH	15, 30

FURTHER READING

Abboud CF. Anterior Pituitary Failure. The Pituitary. Ed. Melmed S. Cambridge: Blackwell Scientific, 1995

Chrisoulidou A, Kousta E, Beshyah SA. et al. How much, and by what mechanisms, does growth hormone replacement improve the quality of life in GH-deficient adults? *Baillière's Clin Endocrinol* 1998; **12**:261–279

Cohen R, Bouquier D, Biot-Laporte S. et al. Pituitary stimulation by combined administration of four hypothalamic releasing hormones in normal men and patients. *J Clin Endocrinol Metab* 1986; **62**:892–898

Cunnah D, Besser M. Management of prolactinomas. *Clin Endocrinol* 1991; **34**:231–235

Graham KE, Samuels MH, Nesbit GM. et al. Cavernous sinus sampling is highly accurate in distinguishing Cushing's disease from the ectopic adrenocorticotrophin syndrome and in predicting intrapituitary tumour location. *J Clin Endocrinol Metab* 1999; **84**:1602–1610

Jorgensen JO, Vahl N, Hansen TB. et al. Determinants of serum insulin-like growth factor I in growth hormone deficient adults as compared to healthy subjects. *Clin Endocrinol (Oxf)* 1998; **48**:479–486

Maroldo TV, Dillon WP, Wilson CB. Advances in diagnostic techniques of pituitary tumours and prolactinomas. *Curr Opin Oncol* 1992; **4**:105–115

Molitch ME. Evaluation and treatment of the patient with a pituitary incidentaloma. *J Clin Endocrinol Metab* 1995; **80**:3–6

Turner HE, Adams CB, Wass JA. Pituitary tumours in the elderly: A 20-year experience. *Eur J Endocrinol* 1999; **140**:383–389

33

Surgical management of thyroid diseases

D. Lee, L.P. Marson

INTRODUCTION

The *Guidelines of Recommended Practice in Endocrine Surgery* produced by the British Association of Endocrine Surgeons (BAES) state that: 'All surgeons undertaking endocrine surgery should be able to demonstrate that they have been specifically trained in the subject'. This does not mean that all endocrine surgery must be performed by highly specialised endocrine surgeons but it is essential that all surgeons training in thyroid surgery should now be exposed to this in a properly structured endocrine unit. Many general surgeons with an endocrine interest will be able to perform routine thyroid and even parathyroid surgery to an acceptably high standard. This chapter is therefore aimed at those surgeons who wish to develop or who have an interest in thyroid surgery and outlines what can be regarded as an acceptable pattern of care for patients with thyroid disease requiring surgery, from time of referral and presentation to time of ultimate discharge.

There is now, however, little place for the 'occasional endocrine surgeon'. The BAES has indicated that only individuals who consistently have in excess of 50 thyroid cases per year should be regarded as suitable to be endocrine trainers and it is likely in future that only surgeons being exposed to this number of patients will be regarded as suitable to perform such surgery.

Since thyroid surgery, unlike many other areas of general surgery, will rarely need to be performed as an emergency, this is an ideal area for the development of the superspecialist.

Referral practice

Not all patients referred to a surgeon for assessment of thyroid disease will require surgery. Patients may be referred directly to the surgeon as their first referral and will therefore require full 'work-up'. Many may come via endocrine or general physicians, from other surgical colleagues or from other sources. It is important that all thyroid patients are fully assessed to decide whether surgery is necessary, required in the immediate future or whether such patients should be merely followed up.

It is essential that such patients are only referred to a surgeon who has access to appropriate support from an endocrinologist, a biochemistry department with access to endocrine facilities, a pathologist/cytologist experienced in endocrine diseases and an oncologist who can provide treatment by both radiotherapy and chemotherapy. It is important that the anaesthetist involved is experienced in goitre surgery, especially in patients who have airway obstruction or who are being treated for thyrotoxicosis.

It is hoped that this chapter will help to clarify the requirements needed for making the decisions about surgery in patients with thyroid disease; the investigations and what can be obtained from their use; the operative surgery, both the technical features and the hazards; and the essential features of aftercare required.

Disease spectrum

Most surgery for thyroid disease is performed either for diffuse toxic goitre or nodular goitre. It is not the purpose of this chapter to discuss these diseases in detail but rather to examine the management of these diseases from the surgical aspect. The features of thyroid diseases requiring surgery have been well described elsewhere.

CLINICAL FEATURES

History

Specific items to be highlighted from the presenting history of the patient with thyroid disease referred for possible surgery include the following.

Swelling

A clear indication of the duration of the goitre and its progression is important. Has the swelling remained static, increased or decreased in size or fluctuated since the time of first presentation? Have any other new swellings appeared? A progressive swelling may suggest malignancy. Fluctuation in a swelling is commonly associated with a thyroid cyst.

Pain

An indication of the severity of any pain should be obtained and also whether this has fluctuated. If the pain fluctuates, does this fluctuate with the goitre? Sudden onset of severe pain and a thyroid swelling is very typical of haemorrhage into a thyroid cyst. Pain from thyroid disease, especially from malignancy, may radiate towards the angle of the jaw and to the ear.

Obstructive symptoms

Cervical goitre *per se* rarely gives rise to obstructive symptoms. A patient may develop a huge cervical goitre with no obstructive features. There are three main situations where goitre is most likely to cause obstruction: malignancy, thyroiditis and retrosternal goitre. Of these, retrosternal goitre due to multinodular goitre is statistically the most common.

Dysphagia

When a patient presents with difficulty in swallowing and a goitre, it is very important to be certain that the complaint is one of food actually sticking. Patients frequently complain of difficulty in swallowing but this is more an awareness of swallowing due to the goitre moving rather than true dysphagia. Be certain that the dysphagia is obstructive in type and that the patient feels that the obstruction occurs at the level of the goitre.

Dyspnoea

Many patients with obstruction of the airway due to goitre present with a long history of 'asthma'. However, the problem of airway obstruction due to goitre tends to produce an inspiratory stridor rather than an expiratory wheeze, as in asthma or bronchitis. Careful observation of the patient to see at which phase of respiration the 'wheeze/stridor' occurs is most important. Inspiratory stridor is obstructive, expiratory wheeze could be either.

Patients may be wakened at night by respiratory obstruction due to retrosternal goitre and this symptom may therefore lead to the misdiagnosis of paroxysmal nocturnal dyspnoea. Dyspnoea suggests more severe obstruction than dysphagia because of the rigidity of the trachea due to the cartilage rings. The oesophagus, being soft, is easily compressible. Both symptoms can readily occur simultaneously and are frequently due to a retrosternal goitre at the level of, or just below, the thoracic inlet.

Venous congestion

Patients may present with the features of superior vena cava (SVC) obstruction with congested neck veins and a feeling of suffusion of the head and neck, especially on lying down. If compression is due to a retrosternal goitre, this is usually a very large intrathoracic goitre which splays and compresses the brachiocephalic veins. Since dysphagia and dyspnoea usually occur because of compression of the oesophagus or trachea at the thoracic inlet, the symptoms of venous congestion rarely occur with the other features of obstruction. Such a retrosternal goitre, being very large, is more likely to require thoracotomy for its removal.

Voice change

Voice change occurring at the time of detection of a goitre is very suspicious of malignancy. A thyroid surgeon should become aware of the typical features of the voice of a patient with recurrent laryngeal nerve palsy. Voice change, such as hoarseness, may be due to many other causes, especially cigarette smoking, but such a symptom demands urgent assessment and action.

Thyroid dysfunction

A clear history should be obtained to check whether the patient has features of hyper- or hypothyroidism. From the surgeon's point of view, it is important to check regarding cardiac symptoms such as any palpitations or angina, gastrointestinal symptoms such as weight gain or loss, diarrhoea or constipation and eye problems. It should not always be assumed that such symptoms are due to thyroid dysfunction, but these may also need to be investigated to exclude other pathologies.

Family history

Approximately 15% of patients seen with nodular goitre have a family history of thyroid disease of various forms. Although there is no direct pattern of inheritance, autoimmune (Hashimoto's) thyroiditis tends to be more common in patients with a family history of thyroid disease. Since this is associated with an increased incidence of hypothyroidism and of malignancy, such patients require thorough investigation.

A family history may also alert the surgeon to the possibility of a familial disorder and in this regard it is important to exclude a multiple endocrine neoplasia (MEN–2) syndrome.

Past history

A past history of neck pathology is most important (Box 33.1).

Has the patient had previous thyroid surgery? If so, it is very important to define the side on which the surgery has been performed, especially if further thyroid surgery is contemplated. Surgery on the same side of the thyroid as a previous operation is exceedingly difficult and should be referred to an experienced thyroid surgeon. The risk of recurrent nerve palsy is significantly increased in such patients, probably by a factor of about 10 times in inexperienced hands. Vocal cord check prior to surgery is vital to exclude previous recurrent laryngeal nerve damage so that the surgeon performing reoperation is not challenged at some future time with having been responsible for any nerve injury.

If surgery has been performed on the contralateral side of the thyroid, reexploration is not so hazardous. This depends on how extensively the previous surgeon has explored the neck. Where surgery has been performed on the opposite side, it is vital to try to find out whether one or more parathyroid glands have been identified and safeguarded. If there is doubt, it will be vital at reexploration to ensure that at least one parathyroid gland is protected.

Box 33.1	History taking		
Name *Address*	*D.O.B.*		*Unit No.*
History	Presenting problem		– pain – swelling
	Duration		
	Obstructive features		– dysphagia – dyspnoea – venous congestion
	Voice change		
	Symptoms of		– hyperfunction – hypofunction
	Family history		
	Past history		– endocrine problems – other
	Drug history		

A thyroid nodule appearing in a patient who has had previous radiotherapy to the neck is associated with a higher incidence of malignancy in the thyroid.

A history of other endocrine problems, such as disease of the parathyroid or adrenal, should alert one to the possibility of MEN-2 syndrome.

Drug history

If the patient is on antithyroid drugs and is for surgery, it is vital to ensure that the medication is continued until the time of operation. Beta-blocker drugs are contraindicated in patients with asthma/bronchospasm.

Some agents, such as lithium, may be goitrogenic and may cause abnormalities on histology which may make interpretation of cellular structure more difficult.

Examination

Clinical examination of the patient can be subdivided into three areas:

● general examination of the patient looking for features of thyroid disease

● local examination of the neck / thyroid

● eye examination.

General examination

Height and weight should be measured and can be used for future comparisons in patients after any treatment.

Patients should be examined to exclude the possibility of thyrotoxicosis. Pulse rate should be recorded and the presence of sweaty palms and fine finger tremor. Hyperexcitability and excess anxiety throughout the consultation should be recorded.

Contrary to this, features of hypothyroidism may be noted.

The skin changes of vitiligo may alert the clinician to the possibility of autoimmune thyroiditis.

Local examination of neck and thyroid

Positioning of the patient is important. The patient should sit in a good light with no shadows. Patients tend to raise their chin to assist with examination of the neck but this tightens the strap muscles, perhaps masking features detectable on inspection, and also makes swallowing difficult. The surgeon should therefore ensure that the patient sits with the head straight at equal eye level to that of the clinician.

Inspection should include a full look at the neck as well as the region of the thyroid. Deformity of the neck such as torticollis,

scars, skin changes, asymmetry, neck swellings, respiratory difficulty, including use of accessory muscles of respiration, and venous congestion should all be noted. The patient should then be asked to swallow and any movement of any neck swelling noted. If a mid-line swelling is noted, any movement on forward protrusion of the tongue may suggest a thyroglossal cyst. In this regard it is important that the patient be asked to hold the mouth open before protruding the tongue in order to see this sign clearly.

Palpation of the neck is performed both from in front and from behind. Initial examination from in front is performed to ensure that the trachea is central by palpation in the suprasternal notch. Palpation of the thyroid gland is best performed from behind. The surgeon should record whether the goitre is diffuse or nodular. If nodular, is the nodularity solitary or multinodular and are both lobes affected? If there is multinodularity present, is there a dominant nodule? Is there any tenderness? Is there retrosternal extension? This may be detected by careful palpation below the goitre, by percussion over the manubrium sternum and / or by observation of venous congestion on arm elevation. Is there any associated cervical lymphadenopathy? Finally the patient should be asked to swallow again during palpation of the thyroid. Fixity should be noted and again the opportunity taken to try to exclude a retrosternal extension of the goitre.

Final examination may include indirect laryngoscopy to exclude a vocal cord palsy. This is especially indicated if there is any voice change, if there has been previous thyroid surgery and if malignancy is suspected or proven.

Eye examination

Only patients with thyrotoxicosis develop the typical eye changes of thyroid disease, although this is not seen in those patients with toxic nodular goitre. Initial signs are lid retraction and lid lag. Exophthalmos is a more advanced sign and is best observed by standing behind the patient and inspecting the eyes from above for any forward protrusion. Ophthalmoplegia of the extraocular muscles is uncommon and most commonly affects the lateral rectus muscle although any can be involved. Lateral rectus palsy results in diplopia on looking to the affected side. Severe proptosis resulting in inability to close the eyelids tends to result in corneal abrasion and ulceration. Such patients may require treatment by lateral tarsorrhaphy or orbital decompression.

INVESTIGATIONS

Various investigations can be performed in the outpatient clinic depending on the structure of the clinic and the expertise available. Easily performed are blood samples for analysis, fine needle aspiration, indirect laryngoscopy and respiratory peak flow measurements. If the expertise is available, it may be possible to perform cytological examination at the clinic.

Box 33.2 lists a comprehensive range of investigations performed for patients with thyroid disease. Not all investigations are required in all patients. Some investigations, however, are essential. Of all the investigations, probably only thyroid function tests are essential in all patients. If thyroid-stimulating hormone (TSH) is abnormal, thyroxine (T4) is required. If this is normal, triiodothyronine (T3) must be performed.

Box 33.2 Investigations

Blood analysis	– haematology
	– biochemistry
	– thyroid function tests★: TSH, T4, T3
	– calcium/albumen★
	– thyroid antibodies
X-rays	– chest★
	– thoracic inlet
	– soft tissues of neck
Fine needle aspiration	
Scanning	– ultrasound
	– isotope
	– CT/MRI
Pulmonary function tests	

(★ = investigations regarded as essential prior to thyroid surgery)

It is also recommended that calcium be estimated prior to any neck exploration (either ionised calcium or total calcium with albumen estimation to allow correction). Associated hyperparathyroidism must be treated at the same time as thyroid surgery and not left to a future neck exploration.

In any patient with nodular goitre, a chest radiograph is essential to exclude radiological evidence of a retrosternal goitre or any metastases from thyroid malignancy. In such a patient, a radiograph of the thoracic inlet may alert the anaesthetist to an airway compression problem which might complicate endotracheal intubation.

In a patient with a solitary nodule, fine needle aspiration is considered important. Cytology of a papillary carcinoma is usually diagnostic and treatment can then be planned accordingly. Diagnosis of a follicular lesion gives a clear indication that surgery is essential. However, both these lesions can be confirmed on frozen section analysis if this is more readily available or a skilled cytologist is not available. However, the diagnosis of a suspected medullary carcinoma on cytology may result in a different line of management. In this situation, a serum calcitonin is required and if this is high, it is essential to exclude MEN-2 syndrome before proceeding to surgery. Such a diagnosis dictates the exclusion of a phaeochromocytoma before any thyroid surgery is performed since this would require treatment first.

Isotope scanning is now thought to be only essential in a patient with thyrotoxicosis and a solitary thyroid nodule. In this situation, an isotope scan will inform the surgeon whether this is a non-functioning nodule in a diffuse thyrotoxic gland or a toxic 'hot' nodule. The treatment of the former will be total lobectomy of the side with the nodule and subtotal lobectomy of the contra-lateral side, while treatment of the latter can be either by radio-iodine therapy or total lobectomy of the affected side only.

Ultrasound scanning affords good visualisation of the nodular gland with resolution down to 1 mm. It will confirm whether a nodule is solid or cystic and whether solitary or multinodular. In a patient with a solitary thyroid cyst, ultrasound scanning may show thickening of the cyst wall, alerting the clinician to the possibility of tumour.

It may also suggest whether the gland may have a retrosternal extension if the lower end cannot be seen. It is, however, not possible to see the retrosternal component, if present, on an ultrasound scan because of the sternum which deflects the sound waves. In this instance, a CT or MRI scan may be indicated to observe the extent of the lesion in the chest. Despite various attempts to describe 'typical' features, scans are unable to differentiate between benign or malignant lesions.

The detection of thyroid autoantibodies, which are present in approximately 25% of patients with nodular goitre, is of value in the prediction of post-thyroid lobectomy hypothyroidism. Over 60% of those patients who are strongly antibody positive will become hypothyroid after surgery and they will require close prolonged follow-up, whereas patients who are antibody negative rarely need any treatment. Serum autoantibodies are also recommended in thyrotoxic patients.

Pulmonary function tests are of value in predicting the presence of a retrosternal goitre and may alert the anaesthetist to significant airway compression problems.

INDICATIONS FOR SURGERY

Primary thyrotoxicosis

Patients with primary thyrotoxicosis can be treated either by drugs (e.g. carbimazole, propylthiouracil), radio-iodine or surgery. By tradition, drugs have been used in the young patient (<45 years) and radio-iodine reserved for the older patient.

Drug treatment may fail for a number of reasons. Patients may not be compliant with taking their medication, may develop an allergic reaction such as skin rash, requiring the drug to be stopped, or may not be well controlled by the drug. Prolonged usage also may result in marrow aplasia and treatment therefore rarely progresses beyond 18 months. Over 50% of patients relapse after cessation of drug therapy and will require some other form of treatment.

Radio-iodine ablation is now being increasingly used in younger patients. The concerns about risks of thyroid malignancy or ovarian damage seem not to have been justified to any marked degree. However, many clinicians still worry about treating young people with radiation therapy.

Surgery is indicated in those patients who have relapsed after, or been non-compliant with, medical treatment, who are young, who have severe eye problems or who have a large goitre cosmetically.

The options for treatment and any potential complications must be discussed with the patient. The role of surgery should be clearly explained and the decision to treat this way must be made jointly with the endocrine physician and the patient.

Multinodular goitre

Multinodular goitre (MNG) is a very common condition world-wide. It is estimated that 4% of the world's population have a multinodular goitre and the incidence is relatively high even in areas of non-endemic goitre and non-iodine deficiency. Treatment by thyroxine suppression has been unsuccessful in controlling the autonomous nodules. Although radio-iodine therapy is effective in reducing individual nodule and overall gland size, after two years the gland will start to increase again. The only option for permanent cure is by surgery.

However, the risk of malignancy developing in MNG is very low (1–2%) and this is not therefore an indication for surgery. The main indications are if:

- the gland is cosmetically very large
- the gland is increasing in size
- there is a large dominant nodule in the background of a mild multinodularity
- one of the nodules is steadily increasing in size
- there are compression symptoms
- there is retrosternal extension, even if not causing compression, as this will eventually cause a problem
- fine needle aspiration of a nodule is 'suspicious'
- the gland is hyperthyroid either clinically or biochemically (MNG has a tendency in time to become overactive).

It is now accepted that surgery by subtotal thyroidectomy or subtotal lobectomy results in an unacceptably high recurrence rate (up to 15%) in the subtotal remnant. In these patients, treatment is by reoperation and completion thyroidectomy, with its attendant risks of recurrent laryngeal nerve damage (up to 5%) and permanent hypoparathyroidism (up to 4%). Most endocrine surgeons now favour a total or near total thyroidectomy/lobectomy with thyroxine replacement therapy for MNG. Nerve damage rate should be zero but hypoparathyroidism still runs at just over 1%.

Solitary thyroid cyst

Thyroid cysts are normally treated by simple aspiration. The risk of malignancy in a thyroid cyst is low but, of cysts referred to the surgeon for excision, over 10% are associated with malignancy by the time of removal. The indications for thyroid cyst excision are:

- recurrent cyst after needle aspiration
- fluid aspirated is frankly bloodstained
- persistent swelling after cyst aspiration
- ultrasound scan of the cyst prior to aspiration confirms (suggests) a nodule in the wall of the cyst
- haemorrhage into a cyst causing compression problems.

Cytology of the fluid is unhelpful in excluding malignancy. Surgery is by total lobectomy and not simple cyst excision. This affords the ability to visualise the surrounding thyroid tissue microscopically.

Solitary solid thyroid nodule

Approximately 80% of solitary solid thyroid lesions are benign follicular adenomata. In the 20% related to malignancy, approximately two-thirds are papillary carcinomata.

Ultrasound scanning will help to decide whether the lesion is truly solitary.

Fine needle aspiration may assist the decision regarding treatment of the solitary nodule. The cytology of papillary carcinoma is specific showing cells with optically clear nuclei and nuclear grooves. An aspirate showing follicular cells is unable to differentiate benign adenoma from malignant adenocarcinoma, the cell cytology being identical. Diagnosis depends on capsular invasion or penetration and for this, the nodule has to be examined microscopically after removal by thyroid lobectomy. In this situation, frozen section analysis may be helpful. Medullary carcinoma may be suspected from an aspirate and lead to a diagnosis of MEN-2 before surgery.

Adenoma

Treatment of a benign follicular adenoma is by total lobectomy.

Carcinoma

If the lesion is a papillary carcinoma, the surgical treatment is by total thyroidectomy and 'cherry picking' of enlarged glands. Block neck dissection is of no proven value with this type of lesion. Subsequent treatment may include radio-iodine treatment. All cases require thyroxine therapy long term at a dosage to suppress TSH completely.

If the lesion is a 'microinvasive follicular carcinoma' with capsular invasion but no penetration, treatment is by total lobectomy and TSH suppression by thyroxine.

If the lesion is a frankly invasive follicular carcinoma, the surgical treatment is by total thyroidectomy, central block node clearance out to the carotid sheath on both sides and lateral block neck dissection if nodes lateral to the carotid are affected. Subsequent treatment is by radio-iodine therapy and thyroxine to suppress TSH completely.

Anaplastic carcinoma may require formal biopsy to confirm diagnosis prior to treatment by external radiotherapy.

Thyroiditis and lymphoma

Autoimmune thyroiditis has a tendency to hypothyroidism and this is not therefore an indication for surgery *per se*. However, this condition predisposes to nodule formation and a higher incidence of malignancy, especially lymphoma but also carcinoma. By FNA, it may prove difficult to differentiate lymphoma from lymphocytic thyroiditis. Surgery may therefore be required to obtain tissue for formal histology. Treatment of lymphoma, however, is not primarily by surgery, but by external radio-therapy.

ASSESSMENT FOR SURGERY

The decision having been made that surgery is required and the above investigations having been performed, the patient will then require formal assessment for fitness for surgery.

In addition to the above, routine haematology and biochemistry should be performed. All thyrotoxic patients and those over the age of 50 should have a routine ECG. Diabetes should be excluded. A coagulation screen should be performed especially if there has been any previous worry about a bleeding tendency, either with the patient or with relatives.

It is important to ensure that all thyrotoxic patients continue to take their medication till the time of surgery and that they are clinically and biochemically euthyroid at the time of operation. This can be achieved by either a titrated dose of an antithyroid drug or by a large dose of an antithyroid drug combined with thyroxine replacement. There is good evidence that oral iodine, either as Lugol's iodine or as iodide or iodate tablets, significantly reduces the blood flow through the thyroid and thus reduces operative blood loss.

It is important to note the patient's current medication and to consider whether this can safely be stopped or must continue. In particular, patients on steroid therapy should have a boost over the operative period. Patients should be discouraged from smoking for at least 24 hours prior to surgery.

Informed consent

The patient should be aware of the indications for surgery and all the results of the investigations performed.

In thyrotoxic patients, the various options for treatment should be discussed together with their effectiveness and their complications. If surgery is recommended, it is very important that the patient understands the reasons for surgery being the preferred choice and why the other options are not.

In patients with multinodular goitre, the reason for recommending surgery should be made clear. It is also very important to discuss with the patient if the recommendation is not to operate. Many non-operated patients may require follow-up and the reasons for this should also be discussed.

In patients with solitary nodules of unproven nature, the risks of malignancy must be discussed and the various forms of therapy which will be required depending on the nature of the lump. If frozen section is to be performed, this must also be explained and what action may be taken consequent on the result. The risks of hypothyroidism in a unilateral lobectomy should also be discussed.

In patients with proven malignancy, the treatment required must be defined for the patient. The patient must be aware if total thyroidectomy is to be performed and the chances of thyroxine therapy being required. The method of management of the cervical lymph nodes must also be discussed. Depending on the patient and the clinical situation, it may also be appropriate to discuss the success of the proposed treatment.

Postoperative complications must also be discussed in detail, especially voice problems and hypoparathyroidism.

OPERATIVE TECHNIQUES

Total lobectomy/thyroidectomy and subtotal thyroidectomy

Position of the patient

Surgery will be facilitated with the use of a north-facing endotracheal tube (Figure 33.1). After induction of anaesthesia, it is

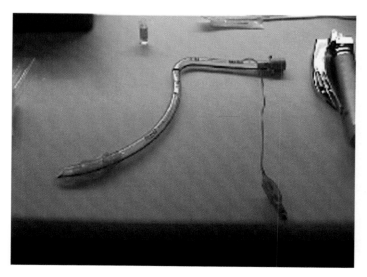

Figure 33.1 North-facing endotracheal tube.

important that the patient be correctly positioned for surgery. It is normal to place a sandbag under the shoulders and position the head on a ring. However, the degree of extension of the neck should be only that necessary to allow for easy access for surgery. Marked hyperextension of the neck will result in unnecessary discomfort for the patient for 24–48 hours after surgery.

Incision

The skin incision should be placed transversely about two finger-breadths above the sternal notch. Many textbooks advise that the incision be placed to the lateral borders of the sternomastoid muscle on each side but this is rarely necessary. An incision placed at the medial borders of sternomastoid suffices in the majority of cases. If the goitre is too large to remove through this size of incision, the wound can be easily extended on either side. Accurate placing of the line of the incision can be facilitated by marking the patient's neck with a waterproof marker before preparing and draping the patient (Figure 33.2). There is normally a skin crease in the neck which forms a good line for incision. Some surgeons prefer to mark the site of incision using a silk thread.

The incision is made in the line of the mark through skin, sub-cutaneous fat and platysma (Figure 33.3) down to but not through the deep cervical fascia.

Skin flaps

Following this, skin flaps can be raised to the thyroid notch superiorly and the sternal notch inferiorly, taking care to remain superficial to the deep fascia. The flaps can then be held by a self-retaining retractor such as a Joll's retractor.

Using a medium-sized Kocher's retractor, the superior flap is retracted upwards and a vertical incision made through the deep fascia between the strap muscles (Figure 33.4). This extends from the thyroid notch down to the sternal notch. Small inter-

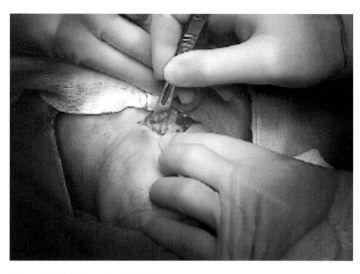

Figure 33.3 Performing the incision.

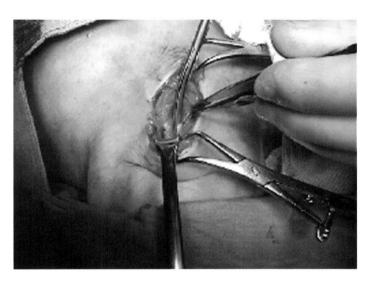

Figure 33.4 The mid-line incision between strap muscles.

communicating vessels between the anterior jugular veins may need to be diathermied or ligated.

Elevation of strap muscles

Tissue forceps are placed on the edge of the strap muscles and these are elevated (Figure 33.5). Initially the sternohyoid is raised until the free edge of the sternothyroid is reached and this is then grasped and elevated. Dissection of the strap muscles from the thyroid gland should be done under direct vision and any small intercommunicating vessels diathermied and divided. Failure to do so may result in quite brisk haemorrhage. Dissection should continue over the gland until the carotid sheath is visualised. The tissue forceps are now removed and the Kocher's retractor inserted to allow lateral retraction.

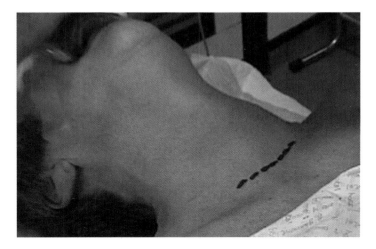

Figure 33.2 Incision site marked.

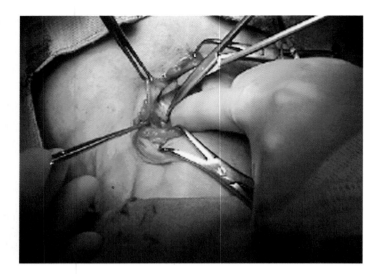

Figure 33.5 Elevation of the sternohyoid.

Middle thyroid vein

The middle thyroid vein is a tributary of the internal jugular vein and is very variable both in size and number. It is commonly absent. Frequently there are two or three small branches. Each needs division after ligation or diathermy depending on the size of the vein. This should be performed well lateral to the thyroid gland to avoid any potential damage to the recurrent laryngeal nerve.

Superior thyroid vessels

The superior thyroid artery (Figure 33.6) arises as one of the first branches of the external carotid artery. It is large and, if divided, it bleeds freely. The superior thyroid vein(s) drain into the internal jugular vein.

Care must be taken when dividing the superior vessels (Figure 33.7) to try to avoid damage to the external branch of the superior laryngeal nerve. It is recommended therefore that these vessels be divided individually which will reduce the chance of nerve damage. Alternatively, the use of a nerve stimulator with an audible signal may allow the surgeon to map the course of the nerve and thus avoid any injury.

Superior laryngeal nerve

The superior laryngeal nerve arises as a branch of the vagus nerve soon after it emerges from the base of the skull. It quickly divides into an internal and an external branch.

The internal branch enters the pharynx/larynx and runs submucosally to supply the mucosa down to the level of the vocal cords. Division of this branch will result in dryness of the throat which will be permanent. This branch runs into the larynx well superior to the site of dissection and therefore is rarely damaged.

The external branch runs down over the side wall of the larynx in very close proximity to the superior thyroid vessels where it is very susceptible to injury. It enters the larynx at a variable level to supply the cricothyroid muscle and this is therefore the only internal muscle in the larynx which is not supplied by the recurrent laryngeal nerve. When the cricothyroid muscle contracts, this gives extra tightening to the vocal cords. Damage to this branch therefore does not affect normal speech but will affect the power of the voice on shouting and singing high notes and will result in easy voice tiredness such as speaking in a crowd or talking for long periods on a telephone.

Inferior thyroid artery

The thyroid gland can now be rolled medially to allow dissection on the posterolateral side. The first structure to easily identify is

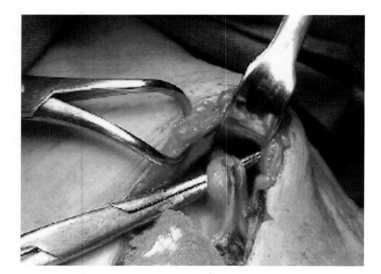

Figure 33.6 The superior thyroid pedicle.

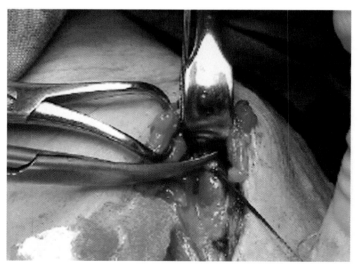

Figure 33.7 Division of the superior thyroid pedicle.

the inferior thyroid artery (Figure 33.8). This is a branch of the thyrocervical trunk which comes from the first part of the subclavian artery. The artery emerges from behind the carotid sheath and runs transversely. It then divides into several branches before entering the thyroid gland. It can be located at approximately the level of the junction between the upper two-thirds and lower one-third of the gland.

Some surgeons now ligate this vessel out laterally near the carotid sheath without division (ligation in continuity). However, ligation at this point not only ligates the vessel before supplying the thyroid, but also before it supplies branches to the parathyroid glands. Most endocrine surgeons therefore ligate the branches of the inferior thyroid artery adjacent to the thyroid capsule after careful identification of the parathyroids and the recurrent laryngeal nerve. This preserves the blood supply to the parathyroid glands. Beware that the recurrent laryngeal nerve, which normally runs posterior to the artery, may in fact run anterior or even through the branches of the artery.

Recurrent laryngeal nerve

The recurrent laryngeal nerve is a branch of the vagus nerve and is the main nerve supply to the larynx, supplying all the internal muscles of the larynx apart from cricothyroid. Rarely the nerve is non-recurrent but this occurs only in about one in 6000 people and only on the right side. It is associated with an anatomical variation of the branches of the aortic arch in which the right subclavian and right carotid arteries arise as separate branches from the aortic arch and the innominate artery is absent. Damage to the recurrent laryngeal nerve results in major voice change due to paralysis of the vocal cord on the side of the injury.

On the right side the nerve recurs round the subclavian artery while on the left side, it recurs around the aortic arch. On both sides the nerve then runs in the tracheo-oesophageal groove immediately behind the thyroid to enter the larynx below cricothyroid. At this point it is normally in immediate contact with the thyroid gland and is therefore prone to damage at this site if care is not taken to identify it clearly.

The nerve is identified by first locating the inferior thyroid artery. Again it should be noted at this time that care must be taken to ensure that the nerve does not run in front of the artery. The nerve is then normally seen behind the artery (Figure 33.9). Its presence can be confirmed by the direction in which it lies and also by the fact that a tiny capillary vessel tends to run over its surface.

When performing subtotal lobectomy or thyroidectomy, some surgeons try to stay well anteriorly without visualising the nerve throughout the procedure. Such a practice will result in a recurrent nerve damage rate of about one in 400. Most experienced endocrine surgeons would therefore dissect along the nerve and visualise it clearly throughout its course in the neck to avoid any damage.

The position of the recurrent laryngeal nerve is normally very constant. However, in patients who require reoperation or who have a large retrosternal goitre, the nerve may be displaced. The main danger here is that the nerve runs anterior to the gland or to a recurrent or retrosternal nodule and is therefore very easily damaged. Exceptional care must be taken when performing such surgery.

Parathyroid glands

There are normally four parathyroid glands although this is variable. It is vital during thyroid surgery that parathyroid tissue is left *in situ* in the neck. The visualisation of one gland may be all that is necessary. When performing a unilateral thyroid lobectomy, the presence of the parathyroid glands must be documented.

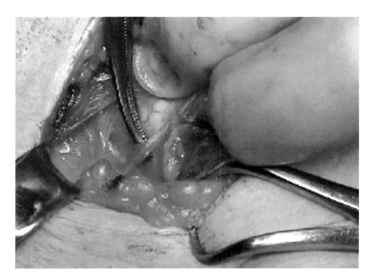

Figure 33.8 The inferior thyroid artery.

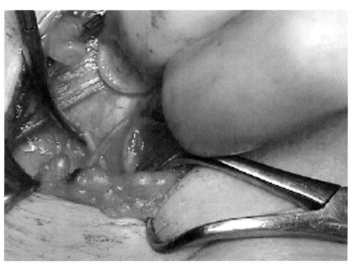

Figure 33.9 The recurrent laryngeal nerve.

Failure to attempt to see the parathyroid glands may result in their removal. If subsequent surgery is required on the opposite side and neither parathyroid gland can be found on that side, the opportunity to preserve parathyroid tissue may have been lost.

The superior parathyroid gland is quite constant in position. It normally sits in a pad of fat adjacent to where the inferior thyroid artery and the recurrent laryngeal nerve cross (Figure 33.10). The parathyroid has a brownish colour compared to the normal yellow fat. To find this gland, therefore, identify the artery and the nerve first (Figure 33.11). Exploration in the immediate vicinity should locate the parathyroid. Occasionally the gland may be on the surface of the thyroid capsule. It is rarely distant from this site.

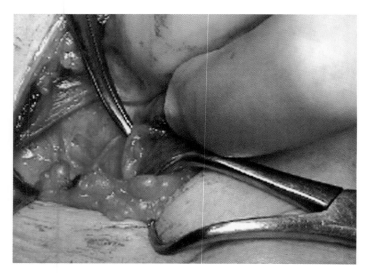

Figure 33.10 The superior parathyroid gland.

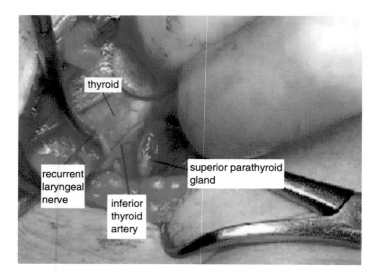

Figure 33.11 Location of the superior parathyroid gland.

The inferior parathyroid gland is variable in position. In approximately 90% of people, the inferior gland is situated either at the lower pole of thyroid, in the upper cornua of thymus or in the intervening thyrothymic tract. Failure to locate the parathyroid here may involve a very extensive search.

If the inferior parathyroid is not located, the problem may be one of non-descent, overdescent or ectopic descent. The inferior gland develops with the thymus and follows its track in the neck. An inferior gland may therefore lie above the upper pole of thyroid, behind the thyroid, down in its normal position from thyroid to thymus or may have descended further into the chest with the thymus and be in the superior mediastinum.

An ectopic gland may lie between the trachea and oesophagus, behind the oesophagus, laterally in the fat of the neck from the thyroid, especially lateral to the lower pole, be within the carotid sheath or even be located within the thyroid gland.

Normal practice therefore is to try to identify the superior parathyroid, which is the easier, and if this is seen, the thyroid lobe is removed, staying very close to the gland. If a parathyroid is seen, this should be preserved. If no inferior parathyroid is seen, this must be in another location. If no superior gland can be found, dissection should continue to try to locate the inferior gland in the sites documented above.

Inferior thyroid veins

The inferior thyroid veins come from the lower pole of the thyroid as a leash and quickly coalesce to form a single trunk on each side. These run into the thorax and enter the brachiocephalic veins just before they unite to form the superior vena cava. The veins should be divided as the tributaries on the thyroid capsule.

The next stage depends on which operation is being performed.

Total lobectomy/thyroidectomy

The thyroid gland is now rolled over and dissected from the trachea to which it is loosely attached. Any small vessels can be diathermied, preferably using bipolar diathermy. Dissection is continued across the mid-line to the junction of isthmus and opposite lobe. Clamps are applied at the site and the lobe and isthmus removed. Any pyramidal lobe is dissected upwards to its superior limit and removed with the specimen. The opposite lobe is oversewn in two layers to ensure haemostasis. The strap muscles overlying the other side are now elevated and the opposite side inspected to ensure no pathology is present.

Subtotal thyroidectomy

This is performed for thyrotoxicosis and, now rarely, for nodular goitre.

After the vessels have been ligated on one side and the nerves and parathyroids identified and safeguarded, the isthmus is elevated by passing a clamp behind. The isthmus is now divided and the dissected lobe is mobilised. A radical subtotal lobectomy is performed leaving a remnant of approximately 3 gm (approximately 3×1×1 cm). A set of Crile's artery forceps are clipped around the lobe at the level at which the removal will occur (Figure 33.12).

When these are in place, the gland is excised above the clamps using a scalpel. Because the inferior artery has not been formally divided, there may be some active bleeding but this will be controlled when the gland remnant is oversewn in two layers.

Attention is now turned to the opposite side. The lobe is oversewn in two layers to ensure haemostasis and then formally dissected and resected in the same way as the first lobe.

Current practice is to make this resection radical. The aim is to control hyperfunction. Radical removal leaves a small remnant which becomes hypothyroid and is easily treated with thyroxine. Insufficient removal of tissue may result in recurrent hyperthyroidism which may prove exceedingly difficult to control and may necessitate radio-iodine treatment. The purpose of the surgery was obviously to avoid this and in this situation the operation has therefore failed.

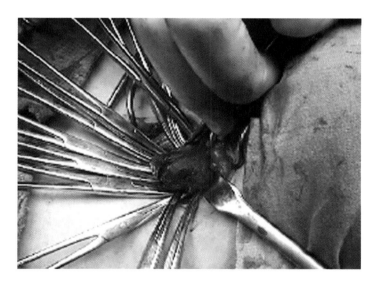

Figure 33.12 Subtotal thyroidectomy

Closure

Haemostasis is ensured. The bed of the removed gland should be completely dry before closure.

The strap muscles are reopposed in the mid-line. The flaps are then brought back in place after removal of the self-retaining clamp. Platysma is now sutured and the wound is closed either with clips or a subcuticular suture.

Drainage

Use of drains is controversial. The insertion of a suction drain always produces some fluid. This accumulates usually for no more than about four hours and therefore the author's practice is to insert a suction drain brought through one end of the wound. If there is minimal drainage at four hours post-operation, the drain is simply removed. If more than 25 ml accumulates in this time, the drain is usually left *in situ* overnight and removed the following morning. No complications have occurred as a result of drain usage.

Suture materials

The use of non-absorbable sutures in the neck should be avoided. Any suture sepsis will clear if absorbable sutures are used throughout. Infected non-absorbable sutures may result in suture sinus formation. Exploration of the neck to try to locate any infected non-absorbable suture is usually unsuccessful.

POSTOPERATIVE CARE

Position

The position adopted by the patient should be the one of most comfort. It is unnecessary to sit patients upright for several hours after thyroid surgery. This does not reduce the incidence of wound haemorrhage or haematoma formation.

Analgesia

The incision used for thyroid surgery is rarely severely painful. Strong analgesia can therefore be avoided in the majority of cases, thus avoiding side effects such as nausea and vomiting. If the patient has been positioned for surgery with the neck hyper-extended, this frequently causes troublesome neck pain for several days. Cervical nerve blocks are unnecessary and may predispose to increased neck swelling. Many patients complain of a sensation of swelling in their throat which can be improved by drinking iced water.

Drainage

If a drain has been inserted, a record should be made of the amount of drainage at approximately four hours post operation. If this is minimal, the drain can be removed at this stage. If the drain is to remain overnight, measurement should be taken in the late evening to allow a comparison next morning so that the drain can then be removed.

Postoperative problems and their management

Immediate postoperative problems

Hypocalcaemia

The serum calcium level always drops after thyroid surgery, even after single lobectomy. The degree of drop is greater with bilateral surgery and particularly if this has been for thyrotoxicosis. Serum calcium should therefore be checked on the evening after surgery for patients who have had bilateral resection and the following morning for all cases.

Where the level of total serum calcium falls below 2 mmol/l (corrected for albumen) or the patient develops symptoms of hypocalcaemia, such as tingling around the lips or in the fingers, oral calcium medication should be prescribed.

Where the level drops below 1.8 mml/l or if the patient develops muscle contractions, intravenous calcium should be administered very slowly. If the drop is profound, patients should also be prescribed vitamin D.

Patients should not be discharged home until the calcium level has been stable or is rising over a 24-hour period without any intravenous calcium injection. Patients discharged on calcium and/or vitamin D must continue their oral medication until review and recheck at the outpatient clinic.

Although approximately 25% of patients will require some supplementation in the immediate postoperative period, only 1–2% of patients ultimately require long-term calcium or vitamin D therapy.

Wound haematoma formation

Wound haematoma causing respiratory compression is very rare. However, because this is an unexpected and immediately life-threatening complication, it is important that all thyroidectomy patients remain in hospital overnight after surgery. The equipment required to remove sutures/clips should be immediately available at ward level in case it is necessary to open a wound. It is vital that the staff know that they should open all layers of the wound, including the deep fascia.

The indications that a patient may be developing a subfascial wound haematoma include undue restlessness, marked neck swelling and/or bruising, excess drainage from the suction drain and/or increasing difficulty in breathing. These signs require very urgent management at ward level by releasing all the skin suturing or staples and dividing all the sutures in the subcutaneous/platysma layer, followed by division of the sutures in the vertical fascial layer. Only when this layer has been opened can the clinician guarantee that tracheal compression is no longer a problem.

Long-term problems

Hypoparathyroidism

Hypoparathyroidism is rare as a long-term problem. Approximately 25–30% of patients undergoing bilateral thyroid surgery will experience hypocalcaemia immediately postoperatively, but only 1–4% will go on to experience this as a long-term problem requiring treatment. Identification of parathyroid glands and preservation of blood supply should reduce the chances of this complication but despite this, permanent problems will still occur. Treatment with calcium replacement is unlikely to control hypoparathyroidism and patients should be commenced on vitamin D supplements. Frequently, vitamin D alone will suffice to control this. Treatment will be lifelong.

Voice problems

It is almost impossible to operate on the thyroid gland and not have subtle voice changes in all cases.

Damage to a recurrent laryngeal nerve is very uncommon but will obviously have a profound effect on the voice. Temporary neuropraxia of the nerve is not common but may result in early temporary cord weakness with a typical voice. Although nerve damage may be due to poor surgical technique, this is by no means always the case and a very difficult thyroidectomy may prove very taxing to ensure no damage occurs. An incidence of recurrent nerve damage of over 0.25% in thyroidectomy patients who have had no previous neck surgery is unacceptable. It is important therefore that surgeons audit their results in this regard. The paralysed cord will tend to adopt a neutral position and the patient will develop a very typical voice with a 'bovine' cough. Although in some cases, after several months, the functioning cord may overcompensate and eventually be able to come in contact with the palsied cord, this is by no means guaranteed. Even if this occurs, the patient may still have a marked air escape on talking and exercise. If the voice does not recover after a reasonable length of time, a thyroplasty may be required.

More common is damage to the external branch of the superior laryngeal nerve as outlined above. In this situation, patients will have a normal voice during normal speech, but will complain of difficulty in shouting, singing high notes and having lengthy conversations. Occasionally the patient may also complain of a very dry throat, indicating the possibility of internal branch damage. These symptoms tend to improve in time but again this is not guaranteed.

A surgeon should always warn patients of the possibility of voice change due to potential nerve damage. This may play a major factor in the decision to operate and patients should be aware of this. This is especially the case in patients who are professional singers or depend on their voice for their occupation, e.g. clergy.

Wound problems

Infection of a thyroidectomy wound is rare. This is a 'clean' operation and an incidence of infection of over 1% requires a critical analysis, with the aid of a bacteriologist, to try to identify the source of the problem. Haematoma formation in a wound will increase the risks of sepsis and a suction drain should therefore be inserted in all cases where haemostasis is not absolute.

Hypertrophic and even keloid scars do occur and can be very distressing to the patient, especially if young and female. Good surgical technique with careful placing of the incision transversely, combined with meticulous wound closure, may reduce this complication but not in all cases. Although the reaction in the wound may be treated by intra-wound injection of triamcinolone, it will still unfortunately result in a broad and obvious scar in many cases. Careful placing of the scar is therefore very important. A scar which can be hidden behind a normal collar or which sits such that a necklace will cover it will be much appreciated by the majority of patients.

Scars which have been infected or become hypertrophic or keloid tend to tether to the deeper layers and therefore tend to raise on swallowing. Surgical release of this is unlikely to result in any good improvement and this should be explained to the patient if this is contemplated. Patients normally are very aware of this complication and feel the structures in the neck raise whenever they swallow. It may settle to some degree over the year after operation.

Hypertrophic and keloid scars which settle after treatment may remain persistently discoloured. Laser treatment to such a scar may improve the appearance immensely.

Management protocols

Thyroid surgery lends itself well to the production of protocols and guidelines. The surgery is repetitive and the immediate post-operative management is similar in all cases. Specific potential problems can be clearly defined and flowcharts for their management easily developed and produced for use at ward/outpatient level.

In an endocrine surgical unit, protocols and database sheets should be produced for the following.

Outpatient clinic

- History and clinical examination data
- Investigations to be performed
- 'Results of investigations sheets' to ensure that all data are collated prior to any planned admission
- Management of non-operated cases

Inpatient

- Drain management protocols
- Flowcharts for the management of hypocalcaemia

Follow-up

- protocols should be put in place for the management of malignancy, thyrotoxic patients and those with benign nodules

Early follow-up

Many surgeons will see their thyroidectomy patients within one week of discharge from hospital. This allows the following aspects to be covered.

Wound inspection and dealing with any possible problems

At this stage, there is usually a degree of wound oedema, especially of the upper flap, and the patient can be reassured that this will subside over the next month or so.

Discussion of final histology results with the patient

Final results of paraffin histology will now be available. If benign, the patient can be immediately reassured. If malignant, the diagnosis can be discussed and any further therapy required can be outlined to the patient. If relevant at this stage, the prognosis of the problem after treatment can also be discussed with the patient and relatives.

Decisions regarding further management

Whether this is simply for further follow-up or further treatment, a combined or parallel running clinic with an endocrine physician may allow easy and definitive decisions to be made at this time.

Management of any immediate postoperative problems

In particular, this will allow blood samples to be obtained, e.g. for serum calcium if the patient had any immediate postoperative hypocalcaemic problem.

Medication

Follow-up at one week allows the clinician to ensure that the patient is receiving the correct medications as prescribed on discharge from hospital. Some patients fail to continue therapy as was outlined to them in hospital, some may have continued on the wrong dosage of a drug, while some patients may need a change of medication at this stage. More than most other surgical specialties, it is vital to ensure that patients who have undergone thyroid surgery receive the correct postoperative medication.

A careful reappraisal of medication at this time, with clear guidance to the patient, may prevent any future potential problems and will clarify for the patient the importance of any therapy which may have been started.

Long-term follow-up

The frequency of follow-up and its duration depend on the primary problem. In many instances, the patient may be returned to the care of the referring endocrine physician.

Thyrotoxicosis

In patients who have been treated by bilateral subtotal thyroidectomy, there will be an immediate drop in thyroid function, which in the early stages may drop to hypothyroid levels. Over the following 3–6 months, the thyroid remnant will regain some of its function under the stimulation of elevated TSH. By six months, maximal recovery will have taken place and no further improvement in thyroid function can be expected.

In the initial period, therefore, it is normal to find that blood levels of TSH will be high and T4 will be low. Unless the levels are profound or the patient is very symptomatic, this does not require treatment.

However, if by 3 months the blood levels are not heading back towards the normal range, it may be appropriate to start therapy. Certainly if levels are not normal by six months, treatment with thyroxine should be instituted.

It is normal to commence therapy with a small dose of thyroxine, e.g. 0.5 mg daily, and to increase this as necessary. The dose should be adjusted according to blood levels and also according to the patient's symptoms.

In view of the small number of patients who develop recurrent hyperthyroidism after subtotal thyroidectomy for thyrotoxicosis (<1%), many surgeons are becoming more radical with the thyroidectomy performed, carrying out near total excision. Although such an approach results in a reduction of recurrent disease to nil, it is associated with an increase in permanent hypoparathyroidism.

In view of the fact that the majority of these patients have been followed and treated by an endocrine physician for a number of years, and that the surgery is merely being seen as an extension to the physician's line of therapy, it is important that these patients be referred back to the physician for further assessment and follow-up.

Once the patient's thyroid function is stable, either at six months post surgery or after commencing replacement thyroxine, no further long-term follow-up should be necessary.

Thyroid lobectomy for benign disease

In patients who have been treated by hemithyroidectomy for solitary nodule, the incidence of hypothyroidism in the long term is approximately 3%. This incidence, however, is markedly elevated in patients who have a background auto-immune thyroiditis, detected either by histology of the thyroid surrounding the nodule showing lymphocytic infiltration or by autoantibody estimation. In this case, over 60% of patients may require treatment by thyroxine. Therefore those patients with thyroiditis require a longer term follow-up of their thyroid function.

In patients treated by hemithyroidectomy who have no evidence of thyroiditis, if thyroid function is normal at three months, no further review is necessary. If, however, there is evidence of thyroiditis, such patients require follow-up of thyroid function for at least two years.

Hemithyroidectomy for minimally invasive follicular thyroid carcinoma

Although the prognosis for this group is outstandingly good, long-term follow-up is recommended.

These patients should receive thyroxine to suppress TSH. Regular blood checks are necessary initially with adjustments of oral thyroxine to achieve this.

Eventual follow-up by annual review is adequate with good clinical examination of the neck, TSH estimation to confirm suppression and thyroglobulin assay.

Hemithyroidectomy for multinodular goitre

Follow-up depends on the contralateral lobe. If this is minimally affected at the time of surgery, it is recommended that an ultrasound scan be performed at one year post surgery to confirm that no change is occurring. If this is the case, the patient can be discharged from follow-up, to return if any swelling appears clinically. The chance of malignancy developing in the remaining lobe is negligible.

Some surgeons prescribe thyroxine in an attempt to suppress the contralateral lobe, but there is no evidence that this is of value, the nodules in a multinodular goitre being autonomous and independent of TSH stimulation.

Approximately 15% of patients undergoing hemithyroidectomy for multinodular goitre will return with contralateral swelling requiring surgery.

Thyroid carcinoma

In view of the further treatment which may be required, particularly by radio-iodine therapy, these patients should be referred to an endocrine physician for consideration of further medical management and follow-up.

Management of the non-operated case

Since the patients referred to the endocrine surgeon have normally been preselected, it is unusual for a surgeon to see a patient with thyroid disease and not to recommend surgery. Most patients will have been seen and investigated by an endocrinologist and referred accordingly. However, even if referred directly to the endocrine surgeon from another source, these patients have usually been identified by a clinician as having a particular surgical problem.

The commonest reason for referral to an endocrine surgeon and surgery not to be recommended occurs with patients with multinodular goitre. In this situation, the patient is referred for an opinion and it may be that the surgeon feels that there are no clear indications for surgery as outlined above.

In this situation, follow-up, perhaps on a six-monthly or annual basis with ultrasound scanning and thyroid function tests, may be appropriate.

All patients referred directly to the surgeon for treatment of thyrotoxicosis and who have not been seen by an endocrine physician must be referred for a medical opinion.

In all instances where a patient has been referred for surgery and the surgeon feels surgery is inappropriate, this decision must be jointly taken by the surgeon and his endocrine physician colleague.

OUTPATIENT CLINIC

Most thyroid patients will receive all their work-up and assessment as an outpatient.

Structure

Although many surgeons will see thyroid patients during their general surgical clinic, many ideas for improvement may come from the examination of the layout of a specialist surgical endocrine clinic.

Ideally such a clinic should be run with an endocrine physician either as a combined clinic or in parallel, thus allowing easy inter-communication and transfer of patients. In particular, this would allow the surgeon to discuss the management of any thyrotoxic or malignant patient and the physician may be able to discuss more easily the management of a patient with a nodular goitre, compression problems or also with malignancy.

Ideally, a cytologist should be immediately available to examine fine needle aspirations. This may allow early diagnosis with immediate decisions about treatment and may also allow feedback if further slides are desired, which can then be obtained immediately.

A designated session in the imaging department for this clinic may allow the possibility of running a 'one-stop clinic' with the patient's future care being outlined at the time of their first consultation.

Analysis of thyroid function and other biochemistry such as serum calcium should also be rapidly available.

Such a clinic should be designed such that trainee surgeons and undergraduate medical students have the maximum opportunity to examine patients and to be involved in the discussion of the patient's future care and management. The trainee would then benefit from discussions with the endocrine physician, the pathologist/cytologist, the radiologist and the biochemist as well as with the endocrine surgeon and would be able to observe and examine directly all the specimens/scans/results obtained.

INTERDEPARTMENTAL MEETINGS

Interdepartmental meetings are an essential part of a specialist unit. These meetings should include case presentations, journal club, research presentations and problem sessions and these should occur on a very regular basis. In an endocrine unit, it is essential to have endocrine surgeons, physicians, pathologists, biochemists, trainees and students present at all meetings for an interchange of thoughts about the management of interesting or difficult patients.

FURTHER READING

Bramley MD, Harrison BJ. Papillary microcarcinoma of the thyroid gland. *Br J Surg* 1996; **83**(12):1674–1683

Buchanan MA, Lee D. Thyroid auto-antibodies, lymphocytic infiltration and the development of post-operative hypothyroidism following hemithyroidectomy for non-toxic nodular goitre. *J R Coll Surg Edinb* 2001; **46**(2):86–90

Walsh RM, Watkinson JC, Franklyn J. The management of the solitary thyroid nodule: a review. *Clin Otolaryngol Allied Sci* 1999; **24**(5):388–397

Weetman AP. Medical progress: Graves' disease. *N Eng J Med* 2000; **343**(17):1236–1248

Woeber KA. Update on the management of hyperthyroidism and hypothyroidism. *Arch Int Med* 2000; **160**(8):1067–1071

Parathyroid glands

David Smith, Graham Leese

PARATHYROID ANATOMY AND EMBRYOLOGY

In a normal individual, there are four parathyroids (two superior, two inferior) although the number may vary between two and six in total. A normal gland weighs about 50 mg and is usually tan in colour and oval in shape. They are supplied mainly by the inferior thyroid artery, although there is some collateral from the superior thyroid artery and branches from the oesophagus and trachea. The superior and inferior parathyroids are derived separately embryologically and the embryology and the potential variations are important to understand when approaching parathyroidectomy.

The superior glands are derived from the dorsal tip of the fourth pharyngeal pouch, and in association with the ultimobranchial body (which gives rise to the parafollicular calcitonin-secreting cells of the thyroid), migrate a short distance to the posterior part of the middle third of the thyroid lobes. This relatively short migration means that the superior parathyroids are usually consistent in their position – 90% of them are located in a 2 cm circle, centred 1 cm above the junction of the recurrent laryngeal nerve and the inferior thyroid artery. There is only rarely a failure of the migration of the superior parathyroid glands, although occasionally they may be located in an intrathyroidal position. About 1% of superior glands may be located either para-oesophageal or retro-oesophageal and in these instances, if enlarged, may be pulled down into the posterior mediastinum by a combination of swallowing, gravity and negative intrathoracic pressure. In this instance, the superior gland may be found inferior to the inferior parathyroid gland.

The inferior parathyroid glands are derived from the dorsal aspect of the third pharyngeal pouch, in conjunction with the thymus from its ventral aspect. The third pouch descends ventral to the fourth pouch, and hence the inferior parathyroids are more anterior in their final position than the superior parathyroids. The longer migration path of the third pouch means that the inferior parathyroids are less consistent in their position than the superior parathyroids. 50% of the inferior parathyroids are located at the level of the inferior thyroid pole, with a further 25% located in the thyrothymic ligament. In addition they may fail to migrate distally and in these instances are located above the superior gland. Occasionally the inferior parathyroids may fail to dislocate from the thymus and may then be pulled down into the superior or anterior mediastinum.

In summary (Figure 34.1):

- 90% of superior parathyroids are located in a 2 cm radius above the junction of the recurrent laryngeal nerve and the inferior thyroid artery.

- 50% of inferior parathyroids are located at the level of the inferior pole of the thyroid.

- Either gland may be located within the thyroid.

- If the superior parathyroid cannot be located, search below the inferior parathyroid.

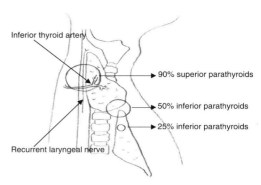

Figure 34.1 Position of normal parathyroid glands.

- If the inferior parathyroid cannot be located, search above the superior parathyroid.

- The inferior may be pulled down into the superior mediastinum or the anterior mediastinum (the aortopulmonary window).

- The inferior parathyroid may be located on the carotid sheath.

PHYSIOLOGY OF CALCIUM METABOLISM

Functions of calcium and phosphorus

Calcium and phosphorus are essential elements involved in many intracellular and extracellular functions. Calcium and phosphorus constitute 65% of bone mass and 99% of calcium is found in bone. In blood the total calcium concentration is about 2.2–2.6 mmol/l and 45% is ionised, which is metabolically active, whilst 45% is protein bound and the remaining 10% is bound to anions such as bicarbonate and phosphate. Phosphorus concentrations are usually 0.8–1.45 mmol/l and half is free and half protein bound.

Calcium is an essential cation, and fundamental to many physiological processes. It is integral in bone mineralisation and remodelling, and at a cellular level is essential for exocytosis (secretion), stabilisation of membranes and excitation–contraction coupling, e.g. in muscle. Calcium is also an enzyme cofactor and acts as a secondary messenger. Phosphate is also a major component of bone and is found in DNA, RNA and membranes. It is an essential part of intracellular phosphorylation processes and cAMP, which are important in pathways of intracellular signalling and metabolic control. Phosphorus is also a component of high-energy intermediates such as ATP and creatinine phosphate.

Control of calcium homeostasis

Calcium homeostasis is regulated by the interaction of parathyroid hormone (PTH) and vitamin D metabolites. PTH increases serum calcium rapidly by promoting renal tubular *reabsorption* of calcium and osteoclastic bone *resorption* with a slower increase in calcium *absorption* from the intestine (Figure 34.2). PTH also acts to lower

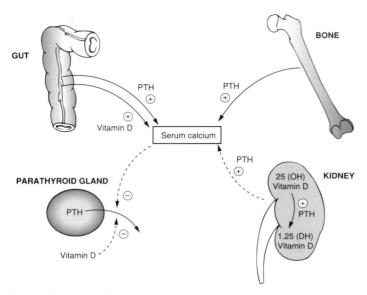

Figure 34.2 Calcium homeostasis.

serum phosphate, and exerts its actions by binding to specific receptors. At least two distinct receptor types have been identified 1: type 1 in bone, kidney and intestine, and type 2 receptors in intestine and brain. Receptor binding results in activation of membrane-bound G proteins and causes an increase in cyclic AMP production initiating a cascade of intracellular phosphorylations, which result in increased flux of calcium into the blood through calcium channels in the membrane.

Vitamin D is a fat-soluble vitamin and is an important mediator of calcium homeostasis. It is available from a diet, including fatty fish, liver, eggs and milk. Vitamin D is also transformed from 7-dehydrocholesterol in the skin when exposed to ultraviolet B light (UVB). Vitamin D is hydroxylated in the kidney and liver to produce 1,25 dihydroxy-vitamin D, which in turn acts on the intestine to promote calcium and phosphate absorption. Vitamin D metabolites also act on bone in a subtle way which is thought to help promote bone mineralisation. The rate-limiting step is 1-alpha hydroxylation in the kidney which is stimulated by low concentrations of $1,25(OH)_2D$, PTH and low phosphorus concentrations. Hence there is a complex interaction between vitamin D and PTH.

Parathyroid gland activity is inversely proportional to concentrations of serum ionised calcium. Serum calcium acts on specific membrane-bound calcium-sensing receptors, which influence parathyroid mRNA production. In addition vitamin D can bind to parathyroid glands to decrease the production of parathyroid mRNA.

Parathyroid-related peptide and calcitonin

Parathyroid hormone is only produced in the parathyroid gland. Parathyroid hormone-related peptide (PTHrp) is a similar homologue which is produced by many tissues including cartilage, but

is normally found in very low concentrations. PTHrp has similar activity to PTH and is commonly a cause of hypercalcaemia of malignancy when secreted by malignant tissues in sufficient quantities. Rarely, PTHrp can be elevated in renal disease or pregnancy.

Calcitonin is produced from the parafollicular C-cells of the thyroid, and acts to suppress osteoclastic action in the bone, and thus inhibits bone resorption. Calcitonin works in opposition to PTH, but the exact role of calcitonin in human physiology is unclear. It is not an important mediator of calcium homeostasis in people, reflected by the observation that post-thyroidectomy patients do not develop hypercalcaemia.

HYPERPARATHYROIDISM

Primary hyperparathyroidism (PHP)

Clinical aspects of PHP

In the 1970s there was a surge of PHP diagnoses after the introduction of widespread biochemical assays, which were more straightforward to perform. The incidence of PHP is now thought to be about eight per 100 000 people per year. The majority of patients have asymptomatic disease with non-progressive serum calcium concentrations. Early manifestations may include non-specific neuromuscular, gastrointestinal and psychiatric symptoms. These may be anorexia, nausea, vague abdominal pains, constipation, muscle aches and weakness, fatigue and behavioural changes. More classic symptoms tend to present later with renal stones or bony involvement. Osteoporosis may result in fractures and bone pain. The bone loss in PHP is classically cortical rather than trabecular, which is the opposite of that observed in post-menopausal conditions. In the past, classic bone changes of PHP resulted in subperiosteal resorption of middle phalanges, cystic changes and occasionally the 'brown tumour' of PHP (Figure 34.3). PHP is associated with cardiac calcification and left ventricular hypertrophy, even in the absence of hypertension in some patients. However, hypertension is present in 50% of patients with PHP, but rarely reverses after surgery.

In a 'crisis' patients may become very dehydrated and develop symptoms of thirst and renal impairment.

The diagnosis is likely if there is a raised serum parathyroid hormone in the presence of raised serum calcium, or more accurately an ionised calcium. Identifying an elevated urinary calcium excretion will help confirm the diagnosis. Inactive forms of PTH can interact with the assay and produce misleading results, especially in renal failure.

Causes of PHP

In at least 85% of cases PHP is due to a parathyroid adenoma, 15% due to parathyroid hyperplasia and less than 1% parathyroid

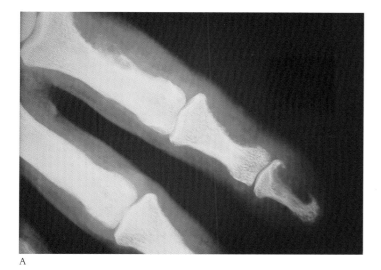

A

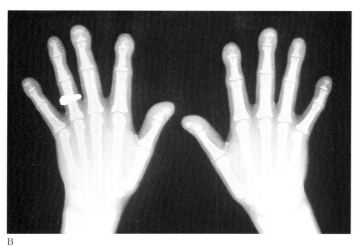

B

Figure 34.3 X-ray appearances of the hand in severe hyperparathyroidism.

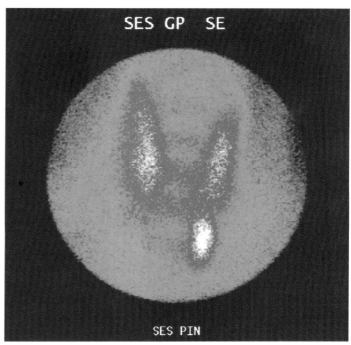

Figure 34.4 Technecium-Sestamibi isotope scan, showing left inferior parathyroid adenoma.

carcinoma. Adenomas can be identified by ultrasound CT-scan, or by subtraction scintigraphy, such as Technetium Sestamibi scans (Figure 34.4). Around half of patients with four-gland hyperplasia will have a hereditary form of PHP, due to either multiple endocrine neoplasia (MEN – see below) or familial non-MEN-PHP.

Important differential diagnoses include sporadic PHP secondary to neck irradiation or lithium therapy. The latter stimulates parathyroid cells. One important differential diagnosis is familial hypocalciuric hypercalcaemia. This autosomal dominant condition results in a mutation in the calcium sensing receptor. This results in the parathyroid glands and peripheral tissues being insensitive to the high serum calcium concentrations. Due to renal calcium insensitivity, the urine calcium excretion is normal, which is the hallmark of this condition. Familial hypocalciuric hypercalcaemia is not thought to be associated with any adverse outcome. Due to this and the fact that surgery does not lower the serum calcium, parathyroidectomy is <u>not</u> advised.

Management of PHP

The definitive treatment for PHP is parathyroidectomy. Many patients are asymptomatic and the disease may not progress such that they do not warrant surgery and can be managed conservatively. There is published evidence that the life expectancy of patients under 70 years with asymptomatic hyperparathyroidism may be reduced, mainly as a result of cardiovascular and cerebrovascular disease. As yet, however, there is no evidence that parathyroidectomy improves outcome and there are no prospective randomised trials comparing conservative therapy with surgical intervention. In 1990, the National Institute of Health (NIH) developed criteria to identify patients who should normally be referred for surgery, and these are still helpful. These include:

- Serum calcium of >3 mmol/L

- Patients with symptoms (including renal stones)

- Asymptomatic patients <50 years old

- Presence of osteoporosis (bone density <2 SD of age matched controls)

- Creatinine clearance <70% expected

- Calcium excretion >10 mmol/day.

Patients not going for surgery should be encouraged to maintain a high fluid intake to avoid dehydration. Potent diuretics should be avoided. The role of diet is not clear. High calcium intake may aggravate the hypercalcaemia, but low calcium intake could stimulate the parathyroid glands further. Medical treatment is generally ineffective. Bisphosphonates can be helpful, but only in the short term, whilst oral phosphates can lower calcium by up 0.25 mmol/L. In women, oestrogen therapy has been advocated for bone protection. New calcimimetic compounds, which stimulate calcium-sensing receptors on the parathyroid glands, are under clinical trial and look promising.

SECONDARY AND TERTIARY HYPERPARATHYROIDISM

Secondary hyperparathyroidism

Secondary hyperparathyroidism occurs in patients with prolonged negative flux of calcium, which may or may not be associated with hypocalcaemia. It usually develops in patients with renal failure, or occasionally with vitamin D deficiency or gluten enteropathy. The negative flux of calcium in renal failure is caused by an inability to excrete phosphate, leading to relative hyperphosphataemia with resultant hypocalcaemia. In addition, there is a reduction in the 1-hydrolase activity within the kidney, leading to a decrease in 1,25 DHCC (dehydroxycholecalciferol) and consequent decrease in calcium absorption from the gut. This difficulty in maintaining normal serum calcium concentrations stimulates the parathyroid glands to secrete PTH, leading to hyperplasia of all the parathyroid glands. In renal patients with normal calcium concentrations, raised alkaline phosphatase concentrations is a clue, but even before this, raised PTH concentrations indicate the presence of secondary hyperparathyroidism and risk of renal osteodystrophy.

The medical treatment of secondary hyperparathyroidism consists of initially reducing the serum phosphate (if >1.7 mmol/L) by dietary restriction of phosphate-containing food products and oral phosphate-binding agents such as calcium carbonate, which inhibits phosphate absorption by binding to the phosphate within the gut. If the serum-corrected calcium rises, non-calcium-containing phosphate binders such as sevelamer (renagel) may be used. Vitamin D supplements, such as 1-alphacalcidol, can also be used, and the dose titrated until the serum-corrected calcium and PTH concentrations are normal. 95% of patients with secondary hyperparathyroidism can be treated medically in this way, but if the patient develops significant symptoms, such as intractable pruritus, severe ectopic calcification or significant bone pain (a raised alkaline phosphatase may be an indicator of bone destruction), or ischaemic necrosis of the skin (calciphylaxis), then surgery is required, either as a total parathyroidectomy with autotransplantation of one gland, or subtotal parathyroidectomy (removal of 3½ glands). In both total and subtotal parathyroidectomy, a bilateral cervical thymectomy is required, to remove potential parathyroid rest cells, or supernumerary parathyroid glands, which may be found within the thymus.

Tertiary hyperparathyroidism

Tertiary hyperparathyroidism is an autonomous condition, which occurs in patients with longstanding secondary hyperparathyroidism. It can also occur in patients following renal transplantation, when despite the removal of the cause of relative hypocalcaemia and hyperphosphataemia, the hyperparathyroidism persists and is usually associated with hypercalcaemia. Tertiary hyperparathyroidism is best treated by either total parathyroidectomy with autotransplantation or subtotal parathyroidectomy.

HYPOPARATHYROIDISM

In the vast majority of cases, hypoparathyroidism is caused by inadvertent damage to the parathyroids during thyroidectomy or occasionally other head and neck operations such as laryngectomy. 5% of patients undergoing thyroidectomy may develop hypoparathyroidism and, if the hypocalcaemia persists for more than a year, then it is defined as permanent hypoparathyroidism (about 2–3% of patients). The patient may develop symptoms of hypocalcaemia, which include circumoral tingling, digital and facial paraesthesia and in extreme cases, hyperventilation, convulsions and frank tetany. Examination may reveal two signs:

- a hyperexcitable facial nerve (tapping over the facial nerve inducing spasm of the ipsilateral facial muscles (**Chvostek's sign**)
- inflating a cuff to above systolic pressure on the arm may induce carpopedal spasm, with classically main d'accoucheur – thumb opposition, wrist flexion and extension at the metacarpo-phalangeal joints (**Trousseau's sign**).

The serum calcium should be measured in all patients following total thyroidectomy, as asymptomatic hypocalcaemia may occur. Blood investigations may reveal low serum-corrected calcium, raised serum phosphate and a low serum PTH. The treatment of acute symptomatic hypocalcaemia consists of giving 10 ml of 10% calcium gluconate or chloride as a slow bolus intravenously over 10 minutes with the patient on an ECG monitor (patients with hypocalcaemia may have a prolonged QT interval). This may need to be repeated every four to six hours depending on symptoms. If the patient is asymptomatic and the corrected calcium is <2 mmols/l, then the patient is treated with oral calcium tablets initially, or if the corrected calcium is <1.8 mmol/L, then i.v. calcium gluconate is required. Oral vitamin D (1-alphacalcidol) may be required if the patient remains hypocalcaemic, despite oral calcium supplementation. Patients should not be discharged until the corrected calcium level is stable for 24 hours. Permanent hypoparathyroidism is treated with vitamin D.

Occasionally, patients may become hypocalcaemic following thyroidectomy for thyrotoxicosis. This may be due to longstanding thyroid osteodystrophy and a reverse flux of calcium ions into the bone occurs rapidly after surgery ('hungry bones'). In this instance the hypocalcaemia is transient and not caused by damage to the parathyroids. Other rare causes of hypocalcaemia include hypomagnesaemia and other causes of hypoparathyroidism, including autoimmune conditions and congenital absence. Pseudohypoparathyroidism is a condition in which there is a resistance to the action of PTH in the target tissues (bone and kidney), due to defects in the PTH receptor; this may be associated with short stature, obesity, and brachydactly – Albright's hereditary osteodystrophy. Pseudo-pseudo hypoparathyroidism occurs in patients with the same phenotypic characteristics of Albright's but not the resistance to PTH.

MULTIPLE ENDOCRINE NEOPLASIA (MEN)

These are rare, interesting syndromes involving associated disorders of the endocrine glands, including the pituitary, pancreas, adrenal, thyroid and the parathyroids.

Multiple endocrine neoplasia type I (MEN I)

This is an autosomal dominant disorder affecting the parathyroids, pancreas and pituitary. MEN I is due to an inactivating mutation in the tumour suppressor MEN I gene, located on chromosome 11q13. MEN I is characterised by:

- Hyperparathyroidism – in 95% of cases
- Multiple endocrine adenomas of the pancreas – usually gastrinomas but occasionally insulinomas, in 75% of cases
- Pituitary adenoma – usually a prolactinoma – in 30% of cases

In MEN I hyperparathyroidism, the commonest cause is 4-gland parathyroid hyperplasia, and there may be marked hypercalcaemia. Supernumerary parathyroid rest cells or glands may coexist in up to 20% of these patients and the surgical treatment therefore consists of subtotal parathyroidectomy and cervical thymectomy as a minimum, otherwise the hyperparathyroidism may recur. Rarely, there may be an associated phaeochromocytoma, although this is more common with MEN II.

Multiple endocrine neoplasia type II (MEN IIa and MEN IIb)

This is also an autosomal dominant disorder, due to an activating mutation in RET proto-oncogene located to chromosome 10q, and affects the thyroid, adrenal and parathyroid glands. It is characterised by:

- Medullary thyroid carcinoma – in 100% of cases
- Phaeochromocytoma – in 50% of cases
- Hyperparathyroidism – in 25% of cases

MEN IIb patients have a Marfanoid habitus, and also have characteristic ganglioneuromas of the lips and tongue. Hyperparathyroidism is uncommon in MEN IIb. They have a far worse prognosis than MEN IIa, with an aggressive form of medullary thyroid carcinoma. Family members should be screened in both MEN I and MEN II, as they are both autosomal dominant disorders.

OPERATIVE SURGERY

PARATHYROIDECTOMY

Pre-operation and consent

Prior to the operation, the patient notes should be checked to confirm the diagnosis of hyperparathyroidism. The preoperative corrected calcium should be checked and electrolytes and CXR carried out as for anaesthetic requirements. It is not necessary to determine the patient's blood group and save a blood sample (group and save). When obtaining consent from the patient it is important to highlight the risk of damage to the recurrent laryngeal nerve (leading to hoarseness) in less than 1% of operations (there is a higher risk if the patient has undergone previous local neck surgery). It is not usually necessary to check the vocal cords pre-operatively, unless the patient has had previous thyroid or parathyroid surgery carried out. In addition, the possibility of temporary hypocalcaemia should be explained, as the normal parathyroid glands may have been suppressed for some time. If a subtotal or total parathyroidectomy is to be performed (for parathyroid hyperplasia), the risks of hypocalcaemia are greater.

Type of anaesthesia

Parathyroidectomy is generally performed under general anaesthetic, although it may be done under either a regional cervical plexus block or direct infiltration with local anaesthetic. Hypnotherapy also has been used. Antibiotic prophylaxis is not usually indicated.

Positioning of the patient

The patient is placed with a head ring to stabilise the head and a sand bag placed under the scapulae to help extend the neck. The patient is then prepped from the chin down to the manubrium sternum.

Lateral approach

A lateral approach may be used in patients with primary hyperparathyroidism who have had a parathyroid adenoma localised, either by ultrasound or by Sestamibi scanning:

- A 4 cm incision is made along the skin creases, centred over the medial border of sternocleidomastoid. The platysma is divided in the line of the incision and the medial border of sternocleidomastoid reached.
- The space between the strap muscles and sternocleidomastoid is opened (Figure 34.5) and the lateral border of the thyroid is

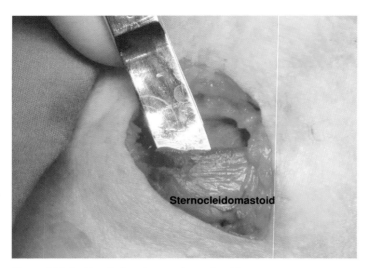

Figure 34.5 Incision for lateral approach parathyroidectomy.

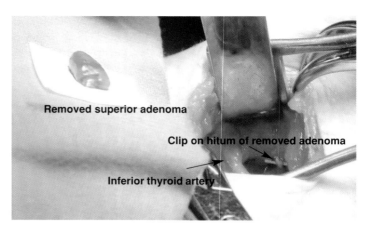

Figure 34.6 Excision of left superior adenoma.

reached. At this point it is important to identify the inferior thyroid artery and then identify the recurrent laryngeal nerve, which is usually just medial to the artery. This junction of the nerve and artery is an extremely important landmark in then identifying the parathyroids (see Parathyroid anatomy and embryology section).

- A search is then made for the superior parathyroid gland, which is usually located 1–2 cm above the junction of the nerve and the artery.

- The inferior gland is usually found at the lower pole of the thyroid or at the apex of the thyrothymic ligament. Occasionally it can migrate down to be within the thymus itself or separate within the superior mediastinum.

- An adenoma will appear enlarged, and of a more ruddy colour. Care must be taken on handling the adenoma, as it is vascular. The vascular hilum of the adenoma should be divided and the adenoma excised and sent for frozen section, to confirm parathyroid tissue. It can, however, be difficult to differentiate between adenoma and hyperplasia on frozen section.

- Both the site of the parathyroid adenoma and the normal parathyroid should be marked with a titanium ligaclip, in case future surgical exploration is required (Figure 34.6). Care must be taken when applying the clips so as not to catch the recurrent laryngeal nerve or the blood supply to the normal parathyroid. If both the parathyroids appear enlarged, the patient may have either parathyroid hyperplasia or multiple adenomas, in which case a bilateral approach is mandatory. 5–10% of parathyroid adenomas are multiple.

Other possible intraoperative adjuncts

- Rapid assay intact PTH assay may be carried out, due to the short half-life of PTH. This is a carried out 5–10 minutes following removal of the adenoma, and the PTH level should fall by at least 50% of the preoperative value. If the PTH level does not drop, then a bilateral approach should be carried out to look for a further adenoma.

- Some surgeons prefer the use of intraoperative methylene blue, which is taken up by the parathyroid glands and aids their identification. A quantity of 5 mg/kg methylene blue in 500 ml of crystalloid is infused intravenously one hour before the operation and selectively stains parathyroid tissue. It should be explained to the patient that the dye will cause their urine to turn green and their face blue!

Bilateral approach

This should be undertaken for all patients with secondary and tertiary hyperparathyroidism requiring surgery, and patients with primary hyperparathyroidism in whom localisation studies have not demonstrated an adenoma:

- Through a standard transverse cervical incision, the strap muscles are divided in the midline, and the strap muscles elevated from the thyroid on both sides.

- The junction of the inferior thyroid artery and the recurrent laryngeal nerve is again identified and the parathyroids looked for in a similar fashion to the lateral approach.

- In patients undergoing a subtotal parathyroidectomy with cervical thymectomy for secondary or tertiary hyperparathyroidism, it is important to identify one parathyroid (usually an inferior) that may be halved to leave half the gland *in situ*. Should the patient require a further exploration of the neck for recurrent hyperparathyroidism, it is generally easier to find the inferior parathyroid rather than the superior.

- The resected parathyroids may be cryopreserved for later reimplantation, in case of resistant postoperative hypocalcaemia.

Other techniques

Minimally invasive parathyroidectomy procedures are now being carried out, using either helium or carbon dioxide and 5 mm ports (minimally invasive video-assisted parathyroidectomy – MIVAP). Although there are many proponents of this approach, there is no significant benefit to the patient over a lateral approach.

FURTHER READING

Marx SJ. Hyperparathyroid and hypoparathyroid disorders. *N Engl J Med* 2000; **343**(25):1863–1875

NIH Consensus development conference statement. *J Bone Miner Res* 1991; **6**:59–63

Reeve TS, Babidge WJ, Parkyn RF et al. Minimally invasive surgery for primary hyperparathyroidism: a systematic review. *Aust N Z J Surg* 2000; **70**(4):244–250

See ACH, Soo KC. Hypocalcaemia following thyroidectomy for thyrotoxicosis. *Br J Surg* 1997; **84**:95–97

35

The adrenal gland

Paul Atkins, David Cave-Bigley

THE ADRENAL GLAND

Disorders of the adrenal gland present as a functional abnormality, a benign or malignant enlargement, or as an incidental finding on imaging the abdomen.

Anatomy

The adrenals, each weighing about 5 g, are paired yellow retroperitoneal glands lying close to the upper poles of the kidneys (Figure 35.1). The adrenal consists of a cortex and a medulla, which though structurally one are developmentally and functionally separate. Approximately 90% of the gland is formed by the cortex derived from coelomic endoderm and 10% by the medulla, derived from the neural crest. The cortex consists of three layers; an outer zona glomerulosa, a much wider middle zona fasciculata (75% of the cortex) and an inner zona reticularis. The medulla consists of chromaffin cells and preganglionic autonomic nerve fibres from the renal and coeliac plexuses which synapse with chromaffin and ganglion cells. Neuroendocrine fibres are also found in the cortex. Numerous arterioles enter the periphery from the aorta, inferior phrenic and renal arteries. Venous drainage on the right is by a short wide vein into the vena cava, whilst the left adrenal vein usually joins the inferior phrenic to form a longer vessel before entering the left renal vein. Lymphatic drainage is to the lateral para-aortic nodes.

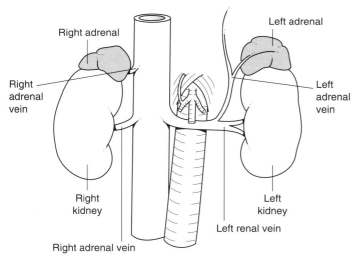

Figure 35.1 The adrenal gland.

Physiology

Cortex

Three classes of corticosteroids are produced (Figure 35.2): mineralocorticoids from the zona glomerulosa, glucocorticoids from the zona fasciculata and zona reticularis and androgens from the zona fasciculata and reticularis. Aldosterone is the principal mineralocorticoid, cortisol the main glucocorticoid and dehydroepiandrosterone the main androgen. Dehydroepiandrosterone sulphate is formed only in the zona reticularis.

Glucocorticoids

The main effect of cortisol is on the metabolism of carbohydrates, protein and fat, overall increasing blood glucose concentration. Under physiological conditions glucocorticoids have only a minor mineralocorticoid effect. They maintain blood pressure by potentiating vasoactive substances, e.g. catecholamines and vasopressin, increase glomerular filtration rate and are important in resistance to stress.

Mineralocorticoids

Aldosterone acts principally on the distal convoluted tubules to cause sodium reabsorption with potassium and hydrogen excretion so that excess alkalosis occurs. Increased plasma sodium stimulates hypothalamic osmoreceptors causing release of vasopressin from the neurohypophysis. This in turn stimulates water reabsorption from the collecting ducts to increase plasma volume.

Adrenal androgens

Adrenal androgens are relatively weak and their effect only becomes apparent with cortical hyperactivity. Dehydroepiandrosterone is secreted in the largest quantity together with androstenedione, dehydroepiandrosterone sulphate and testosterone. Small quantities of progesterone and oestrogens are secreted, though the conversion of androstenedione to oestrone occurs principally in fat, liver and pancreas.

Regulation

Corticotrophin (ACTH) from the anterior pituitary stimulates the structure, growth and secretions of the zona fasciculata and zona reticularis but has only a minor role in aldosterone synthesis and secretion. Free cortisol exerts a negative feedback control on corticotrophin-releasing hormone (CRH) from the hypothalamus and on ACTH from the anterior pituitary.

Mineralocorticoid control. Decrease in renal perfusion, plasma volume and sodium, or an increase in plasma potassium stimulate juxtaglomerular cells to release renin. Renin acts on the plasma protein angiotensinogen to form angiotensin I, which in turn is converted to angiotensin II. The octapeptide angiotensin II stimulates the formation of aldosterone.

Androgen secretion is stimulated by ACTH but androgens do not affect the feedback mechanism.

Medulla

Chromaffin cells of the adrenal medulla synthesise, store and secrete catecholamines in response to stimuli from sympathetic preganglionic nerve fibres. Catecholamines are metabolised from dietary tyrosine with a small amount from hepatic conversion of phenylalanine to tyrosine (Figure 35.2).

Basal secretion of catecholamines is low but is greatly increased in stress and exercise. The principal catecholamines adrenaline, noradrenaline and dopamine exert profound effects on metabolism of all organs and tissues. Noradrenaline is a neurotransmitter for the autonomic nervous system and is synthesised at all sympathetic nerve endings as well as in the adrenal medulla. Adrenaline is produced only in the medulla and the organ of Zuckerkandl as methyl transferase is necessary for conversion of noradrenaline to adrenaline. Adrenaline and noradrenaline are present in the adrenal in a ratio of 4:1 but overall less than 2% of noradrenaline is of adrenal origin.

Adrenaline and noradrenaline have a half-life of only one to two minutes. Their excretory metabolites, metanephrines and VMA, are found in the urine.

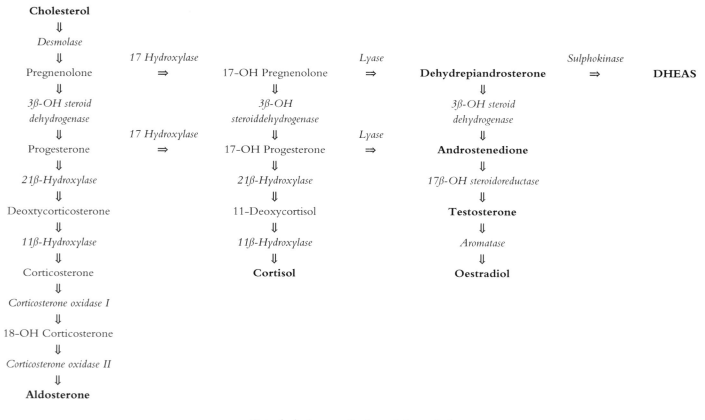

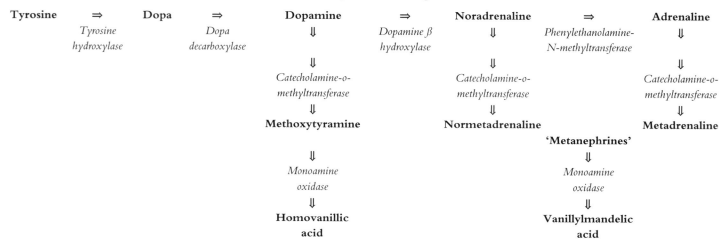

Figure 35.2 Outline of pathways concerned in corticosteroid synthesis and catecholamine synthesis and degradation.

Cushing's syndrome (hypercortisolism)

In 1932 Cushing described the clinical features of the syndrome that bears his name. He believed that the condition, subsequently shown to be due to hypercortisolism was caused by pituitary basophilism. The term Cushing's disease is therefore reserved for pituitary-dependent adrenal hyperplasia.

In clinical practice, treatment with glucocorticoids or their analogues is the commonest cause of Cushing's syndrome.

Pathogenesis

Spontaneously occurring Cushing's syndrome is either ACTH dependent, or is due to autonomous adrenal hypersecretion (Table 35.1).

ACTH-dependent Cushing's syndrome

Cushing's disease forms 65–80% of adult cases. Adrenal hyperplasia is stimulated by increased ACTH levels from a usually benign microadenoma or occasionally macroadenoma (>10 mm) in the anterior pituitary. In a small number (5%) the increased ACTH is due to excess hypothalamic CRH.

Ectopic ACTH syndrome is seen in 10–15% of adult cases. Adrenal hyperplasia results from an ectopic source of ACTH and rarely from an ectopic source of CRH. The commonest cause is an oat cell carcinoma of bronchus or a carcinoid. Rare possibilities include islet cell tumour, medullary thyroid carcinoma, thymoma and an ovarian tumour.

Autonomous adrenal hypersecretion

Autonomous adrenal tumours Most are benign and account for 15–20% of adult patients with Cushing's syndrome in the United Kingdom, but up to 50% in Japan. Adrenal tumours form a larger proportion of cases in children and pregnancy.

Macronodular hyperplasia and primary pigmented nodular hyperplasia are very rare causes of autonomous adrenal hyper function. The latter condition may be part of Carney's syndrome in which mesenchymal tumours e.g. cardiac myxoma, skin pigmentation, peripheral nerve tumours, and other endocrine abnormalities occur.

Clinical presentation

Spontaneous Cushing's syndrome occurs in all races with an incidence of 1–3 per million of the population. It can occur at any age although it is most common in the fourth and fifth decades. There is a female preponderance with a ratio of 3:1, which is less pronounced in cases of Ectopic ACTH syndrome. Patients may have had symptoms that have waxed and waned for many years, a condition called cyclical Cushing's syndrome.

Clinical features of Cushing's syndrome (Table 35.2) are similar irrespective of the cause (Orth 1995). They are due to the effect of hypercortisolism on carbohydrate, protein and fat metabolism and on electrolyte balance. Minor differences depend on the rapidity of development and the varying extent of androgen and mineralocorticoid secretion – features which may help to suggest the underlying pathology.

A striking feature is weight gain and many obese patients are referred for an endocrine opinion to exclude Cushing's syndrome. The typical body configuration however is truncal, neck and facial obesity producing a plethoric 'moon face' and 'buffalo hump' with increased intraabdominal fat. Increased protein catabolism causes muscle wasting, especially of the limbs, giving a 'lemon on matchsticks' appearance. The skin becomes thin, bruises easily and purple striae may occur on the abdominal wall, breasts and in lines of stress. Osteoporosis produces kyphosis with fractures particularly of the vertebrae and ribs. Polyuria, hypercalcuria and renal stones may occur and impairment of glucose tolerance may produce frank diabetes.

Androgen excess results in acne, hirsutism, frontal balding and amenorrhoea. These features are more common in Cushing's disease than in Cushing's syndrome due to adrenal adenoma. However, in adrenal carcinoma there is often overt virilisation, hypertension and hypokalaemic alkalosis.

The Ectopic ACTH syndrome invariably develops rapidly, with less change in body configuration, but proximal myopathy, hypokalaemic alkalosis, skin pigmentation and oedema are pronounced.

Table 35.1 Cushing's syndrome – pathogenesis

ACTH dependent

- Pituitary/hypothalamus dependent – Cushing's disease
- Ectopic ACTH and rarely ectopic secreting CRH tumours
- Formerly therapeutic excess with ACTH or analogue

Non-ACTH dependent

- Adrenal tumour benign and malignant
- Macronodular cortical hyperplasia
- Primary pigmented nodular cortical disease
- Glucocorticoids or analogues

Table 35.2 Clinical features of Cushing's syndrome

- Weight gain and change in body configuration
- Moon face and high colour
- Skin pigmentation
- Limbs thin with muscle wasting
- Bruising and striae, poor wound healing
- Hypertension
- Osteoporosis and fractures
- Polyuria
- Impaired glucose tolerance
- Amenorrhoea, hirsutism, frontal balding, acne
- Growth retardation
- Depression
- Venous thrombosis

Profound depression or agitated psychoses occur in 60–70% of patients. Other well-recognised features include chemosis, poor wound healing, increased susceptibility to infection and deep venous thrombosis and there is probably a higher incidence of peptic ulceration than normal. In childhood, Cushing's syndrome may cause impaired development.

Prognosis

Untreated 50% of patients will die within five years of the first symptom. Treatment usually produces marked improvement but compared with the general population, an increased mortality persists, mainly from cardiovascular disease.

Investigations

There are three stages:

- Confirmation of hypercortisolism

- Determination of whether it is ACTH dependent

- Imaging to localise the anatomical and pathological abnormality.

Biochemical investigations are listed in Table 35.3. Individual laboratory results vary and interpretation of tests should be based on local values.

Pulses of ACTH and cortisol occur throughout the 24-hour period, with levels highest at 8 am (Plasma cortison 100–500 nmol/L) and lowest at midnight (Plasma cortison <150 nmol/l). Plasma cortisol may be raised in stress, depression, obesity and chronic alcoholism while a random cortisol may be normal in Cushing's syndrome. Consequently a random cortisol is an unsatisfactory investigation, though loss of diurnal rhythm is frequently the earliest indication of Cushing's syndrome.

Confirmation of hypercortisolism

- Overnight dexamethasone suppression test

The simplest outpatient test is to prescribe 1 mg of oral dexamethasone to be taken at midnight measuring plasma cortisol at 9 am the following morning. Failure to suppress basal cortisol levels by 50% or a level >120 nmol/L suggests Cushing's syndrome, although false-positives can occur in the elderly and depressed.

Table 35.3 Biochemical investigation of Cushing's syndrome

Test	Normal	Cushing's disease	Adrenocortical tumour	Ectopic ACTH syndrome
Confirmation of hypercortisolism				
Plasma cortisol	08.00 hr 100–500 nmol/L 24.00 hr <150 nmol/L	Loss of diurnal rhythm	Loss of diurnal rhythm	Loss of diurnal rhythm
Overnight dexamethasone 1 mg at 24.00 hr	08.00 hr <50% of midnight value & <120 nmol/L	↑	↑	↑
24 hr urine collection for cortisol	100–350 nmol/24 hr	↑	↑	↑
Low dose dexamethasone 0.5 mg 6 hourly for 48 hr	Plasma cortisol <120 nmol/L Urine free cortisol <100 nmol/24 hr	↑	↑	↑
Determination of cause				
Plasma ACTH	09.00 hr <25 ng/L 24.00 hr <10 ng/L	↑	↓	↑↑
High dose dexamethasone 2 mg 6-hourly	Plasma and urine cortisol ↓	↓	↑	↑
Metyrapone 6 doses 750 mg 6 hourly	Plasma ACTH and Urine 17-hydroxysteroids ↑	↑↑	↔	↔
CRH 100 μg	Plasma ACTH and cortisol ↑	↑	↔	↔
Bilateral inferior petrosal sinus sampling	Normal ACTH	1.5–3 × > caval value	Sinus:Cava 1:1	Sinus:Cava 1:1

NB: Local laboratory must be consulted for normal ranges

● Urinary free cortisol

An accurate 24-hour urine collection measuring free cortisol (normal 100–350 nmol/24 hr) reflects total cortisol production. It is raised in Cushing's syndrome. This investigation has been claimed to have a diagnostic accuracy of 95%.

● Low-dose dexamethasone suppression test

On each day of the test a 24-hour urinary free cortisol is collected and plasma cortisol measured at 8 am and midnight. Basal levels are determined over the first 48 hr. Dexamethasone 0.5 mg is given six-hourly for 48 hr. In the normal person, plasma cortisol is suppressed to <120 nmol/L and urinary cortisol to <100 nmol/24 hr. All forms of Cushing's syndrome fail to suppress.

Tests to determine whether hypercortisolism is ACTH dependent

ACTH ASSAY

Plasma ACTH measurement is the most direct way to differentiate the cause of Cushing's syndrome; normal levels are <25 ng/L at 9 am and <10 ng/L at midnight.

Plasma ACTH is normal or moderately raised in Cushing's disease, often grossly raised in the ectopic ACTH syndrome (>200 pg/ml) and low or even undetectable in adrenal tumours. Levels tend to be variable in adrenal nodular hyperplasia.

HIGH-DOSE DEXAMETHASONE SUPPRESSION TEST

The low-dose test is repeated but with 2 mg of dexamethasone six-hourly. Cortisol levels are suppressed in pituitary-dependent Cushing's disease but not usually with adrenal tumour, the ectopic ACTH syndrome or the majority of patients with primary nodular hyperplasia – the non pituitary causes.

Assay of ACTH and dynamic testing of the hypothalamic pituitary adrenal axis by dexamethasone tests clarify the diagnosis in most cases; when doubt remains other tests may be employed.

METYRAPONE

Metyrapone is an inhibitor of 11β-hydroxylase, an enzyme involved in the final stage of cortisol synthesis. Six doses of 750 mg are administered four-hourly. ACTH levels rise with an increase in 11-deoxycortisol, the immediate cortisol precursor. This rise is reflected by an increase in urinary 17-hydroxy steroids in the normal person but a two-fold rise suggests Cushing's disease. Adrenal tumours, ectopic ACTH syndrome and nodular hyperplasia are generally reported as not producing a rise although doubts have been expressed on the reliability of the test.

The situation most likely to cause difficulty is distinguishing between Cushing's disease and a low-grade ectopic source of ACTH. In this dilemma CRH stimulation of ACTH and inferior petrosal sinus sampling for ACTH may be helpful.

CRH STIMULATION OF ACTH

In the normal person 100 μg of CRH produces an increase in plasma ACTH and cortisol. In Cushing's disease there is a normal or exaggerated response. In autonomous adrenal disease and the ectopic ACTH syndrome there is no response.

BILATERAL INFERIOR PETROSAL SINUS SAMPLING FOR ACTH

Comparison of ACTH levels from the inferior petrosal sinuses with that of the vena cava at adrenal level allows pituitary or adrenal origin of the syndrome to be determined. In Cushing's disease a gradient of 1.5–3 is expected. The concentration ratio of the two sinuses may help to lateralise a microadenoma. A refinement is to stimulate ACTH with CRH (Padayatty et al. 1998).

Imaging techniques

Biochemical results will suggest the most appropriate imaging methods to be used (Table 35.8).

A chest radiograph is always necessary. It may reveal rib fractures in all forms of Cushing's syndrome and a bronchial tumour in ectopic ACTH syndrome.

THE PITUITARY

A skull radiograph only rarely shows sella enlargement or erosion of the anterior clinoid processes.

Computed tomography (CT) will reveal a microadenoma in 50 % of Cushing's disease while magnetic resonance imaging (MRI) is claimed to detect two-thirds of microadenomas. Non-functioning microadenomas may cause confusion.

THE ADRENALS

CT: A small well-encapsulated mass in one adrenal suggests an adenoma whilst a carcinoma is usually larger, often irregular, and non-homogenous with low-density areas from necrosis. Both adrenals are enlarged in Cushing's disease and ectopic ACTH syndrome, although the enlargement may be only moderate in Cushing's disease and difficult to distinguish from normal glands.

MRI: Tissue planes and in particular invasion of the vena cava from an adrenal tumour are best shown on MRI. A higher signal intensity with T2 weighted images is seen in malignancy.

Nodular hyperplasia may be distinguished from ACTH-dependent hyperplasia with either CT or MRI.

Isotope scanning: ^{131}I-iodomethyl-19 norcholesterol (NP59) usually clarifies the diagnosis. There is unilateral uptake on the side of an adenoma with suppression of the normal gland. In carcinoma there is no uptake either by the malignant tissue or normal adrenal, which is suppressed because of hypercortisolism. The uptake is bilateral and uniform in hyperplasia but asymmetric in nodular hyperplasia. A disadvantage of the technique is high radiation exposure.

IMAGING IN THE ECTOPIC ACTH SYNDROME

CT and MRI are used to demonstrate carcinoid, thymic, bronchial and islet cell tumours.

Treatment

Treatment aims to normalise cortisol levels and ideally return pituitary and adrenal function to physiological control. This is best achieved by transsphenoidal microadenectomy in Cushing's disease and by unilateral adrenalectomy where Cushing's syndrome is due to an adrenal tumour.

Bilateral adrenalectomy is no longer the treatment of choice for Cushing's disease. Although hypercortisolism was cured and two-thirds of patients had a satisfactory quality of life there was lifelong steroid dependence and a third, particularly younger patients developed Nelson's syndrome – an invasive pituitary tumour with melanocyte-stimulating hormone-induced skin pigmentation.

Patients with Cushing's disease are particularly prone to poor wound healing, infection, venous thrombosis and vascular accidents. Overall, the mortality and morbidity following bilateral adrenalectomy exceeds that following transsphenoidal microadenectomy. Bilateral adrenalectomy is therefore reserved for recurrence after pituitary surgery, for some instances of ectopic ACTH syndrome and for cases of nodular hyperplasia and pigmented nodular disease.

Preoperative preparation

Metyrapone alleviates the symptoms of Cushing's syndrome. A daily dose of 250 mg to 6 g is given in six-hourly divided doses until plasma cortisol is restored to the 300 nmol/L level. Hypertension and cardiac failure are controlled and hypokalaemia and hyperglycaemia corrected.

Peri- and postoperative medication

Steroids are essential throughout the perioperative period. Hydrocortisone 100 mg I.M. is administered one hour prior to surgery and continued as 100 mg I.V. eight-hourly. Provided progress is satisfactory the dose is halved every 24 hr postoperatively with oral substitution once intestinal absorption is re-established. The usual maintenance dose is 20 mg in the morning and 10 mg at night. Fludrocortisone 100 μg is introduced on the third day in patients who have undergone adrenalectomy; adjusting the dose according to electrolyte values. It is not required after pituitary surgery but patients who have undergone total hypophysectomy require full hormone replacement with hydrocortisone, thyroxine, testosterone or oestrogens.

Adrenalectomy for tumour

An *adenoma* is removed by unilateral adrenalectomy, tumours <5 cm by a posterior or laparoscopic approach. This invariably cures the syndrome. Steroids must be continued until the remaining suppressed gland resumes normal function after six months or longer. The synacthen test can be used to indicate return to pituitary control.

An *adrenal carcinoma* is often large with metastatic spread at presentation. Less than half are amenable to radical *en bloc* removal but debulking may be worthwhile. Radiotherapy is used in some centres but chemotherapy, using mitotane alone or with streptozotocin, is commonly preferred. Its use has been advocated for all malignant tumours, even those confined to the adrenal. Steroid replacement must accompany treatment with mitotane, as it destroys all adrenal tissue. Worthwhile palliation can be achieved if the patient is able to tolerate the side effects produced by the optimal 8 g/day.

MANAGEMENT OF THE ECTOPIC ACTH SYNDROME

Logically, the tumour producing ACTH or CRH should be identified and removed, a feasible proposition if the tumour is benign or is a slow growing carcinoid. Unfortunately the tumour is usually malignant with the most common being a small cell carcinoma of the bronchus (oat cell) – a particularly aggressive tumour. Successful removal of an ectopic tumour should produce remission of Cushing's syndrome but recurrence of symptoms is indicative of metastatic disease.

Bilateral adrenalectomy should be considered when the primary tumour is unresectable and in patients where the ectopic source defies identification. It may occasionally be appropriate in the patient with stable recurrent disease.

Other options, which have been used with varying success, are somatostatin, which can inhibit release of ACTH from ectopic tumours, metyrapone, aminoglutethamide and mitotane.

Adrenocortical insufficiency

This may be acute or chronic (Addison's disease). Lack of glucocorticoids and mineralocorticoids are responsible for the clinical features (Table 35.4).

Acute adrenocortical failure

The most important causes are iatrogenic. Bilateral adrenalectomy and hypophysectomy render patients dependent on prescribed glucocorticoids, and after adrenalectomy, mineralocorticoids for the rest of their lives. Patients having unilateral adrenalectomy and pituitary microadenectomy may well need glucocorticoids during the first postoperative year and the former may also require mineralocorticoids.

Table 35.4 Adrenocortical insufficiency, aetiology of acute and chronic adrenal insufficiency and treatment essentials

Adrenocortical insufficiency

Acute
- Iatrogenic – Bilateral adrenalectomy, Variable period after unilateral adrenalectomy
- Iatrogenic stress and infection in patient on glucocorticoids or analogues Sudden withdrawal
- Waterhouse-Friderichsen syndrome – septicaemia usually meningococcal
- Adrenal haemorrhage due to anticoagulants
- Adrenal venography

Chronic
- Autoimmune disease
- Tuberculosis
- Secondary tumour
- Sarcoidosis
- Amyloidosis
- Histoplasmosis
- Haemochromatosis
- Congenital adrenal hyperplasia

Secondary adrenocortical failure occurs in hypopituitarism treatment Essentials

I.V. fluids particularly normal saline	Hydrocortisone 20 mg in morning 10 mg at night
I.V. hydrocortisone 100 mg 6-hourly	Fludrocortisone 50–300 mg/day
In septicaemia I.V. antibiotics	

Prescribed glucocorticoids and their analogues suppress cortical function and cause adrenal atrophy. Insufficiency can persist for years after treatment has stopped. Sudden withdrawal of glucocorticoids leads to adrenocortical failure while stress and intercurrent infection increase the need for glucocorticoids.

Patients taking steroids should carry a 'steroid card' or 'medic-alert bracelet/necklace' with information about the drug, dosage and possible complications.

Acute adrenocortical failure may occur with septicaemia, usually meningococcal in children – the Waterhouse-Frederichsen syndrome and with endotoxic shock, post-partum haemorrhage, intraadrenal haemorrhage from anticoagulants and adrenal venography,

Clinical features

Acute adrenocortical failure is characterized by very severe hypotension and drowsiness lapsing into coma as well as manifestations of the precipitating disorder.

Treatment of acute adrenocortical failure

This is best managed in an ITU. Resuscitation is with large volumes of I.V. saline and I.V. hydrocortisone 100 mg six-hourly.

This is guided by careful monitoring of BP, CVP and urine output and subsequently by serum electrolytes. Other measures will depend on the cause e.g. in septicaemia appropriate antibiotics will be given intravenously.

Chronic adrenocortical failure – Addison's disease

Autoimmune disease is today the commonest cause of chronic adrenocortical failure. Secondary tumour deposits especially oat cell tumours of the bronchus and tuberculosis remain important causes – the latter particularly in the Third World. Rare causes are amyloidosis, sarcoidosis, fungal disease and congenital adrenal hyperplasia.

Reduced aldosterone secretion leads to hyponatraemia, hyperkalaemia and dehydration. Lack of glucocorticoids depresses gluconeogenesis with resulting hypoglycaemia. Vomiting increases the fluid and electrolyte disturbance.

Clinical features of chronic adrenocortical failure

Addison's disease has an equal sex ratio and usually presents in the third and fourth decades. The condition may present as an acute crisis but is usually characterised by gradually increasing lassitude, anorexia, weight loss, muscle weakness and particularly hypotension; spontaneous hypoglycaemia may occur. Skin pigmentation (at points of pressure and flexion creases particularly the base of the terminal phalanges) and mucosal pigmentation feature as does vitiligo and loss of body hair.

Investigations

SHORT SYNACTHEN TEST

Tetracosatrin (analogue of ACTH) – 250 μg I.M. is given as a single dose and plasma cortisol measured at 30 minutes.

LONG SYNACTHEN TEST

1 mg of tetracosatrin in depot form is given I.M. and plasma cortisol measured at five hr.

The normal rise in cortisol in both synacthen tests is impaired in Addison's disease.

ADDITIONAL INVESTIGATIONS

These are performed to determine the aetiology and include detection of autoantibodies, chest and abdominal radiographs and CT scans of the adrenals.

Treatment

Acute crises require urgent resuscitation. Chronic impairment is treated with regular steroid replacement. Clinical assessment and electrolyte estimates determine the maintenance dose, typically hydrocortisone 20 mg in the morning and 10 mg at night with fludrocortisone 50–300 micrograms/day.

Aldosteronism

Excessive and persistent secretion of aldosterone is classified as primary or secondary. In primary aldosteronism secretion from the zona glomerulosa is autonomous. In secondary aldosteronism it results from prolonged and excessive stimulation of the adrenal through the physiological renin angiotensin aldosterone mechanism. In both instances sodium and water are retained, potassium and hydrogen ions are lost.

Pathology

Primary aldosteronism (Conn's Syndrome)

In 1955, Conn described the physiology, pathology and clinical features of mineralocorticoid excess due to adenoma or hyperplasia of the zona glomerulosa. Originally thought to be responsible for 20% of a hypertensive population it is now believed to occur in only 1–2% of unselected hypertensive patients. Furthermore 80–90% of primary aldosteronism was initially ascribed to an adenoma but it is now suggested that as many as 50% are due to hyperplasia.

AETIOLOGY

Aldosterone-secreting adenomas

These are usually single but may rarely be multiple in the same gland or bilateral. 60% arise on the left. An adenoma is usually between 8–20 mm in diameter, commonly projects from the cortical surface and is yellow in colour.

Bilateral cortical hyperplasia (micro and macronodular)

Nodules (hypertensive) often occur in hyperplasiai when present they do not secrete aldosterone but may secrete glucocorticoids.

Familial hyperplasia

This is rare. A glucocorticoid suppressible form occurs which is inherited as an autosomal dominant disorders. A non-glucosteroid suppressible form is also recognised.

Carcinoma of the adrenal and ovary

These have also been recorded as causing aldosteronism.

Secondary aldosteronism

This is much more commonly seen than primary aldosteronism. Excess renin produced by decreases in plasma volume, plasma sodium and renal perfusion leads to increased aldosterone secretion. This occurs in conditions such as congestive cardiac failure, cirrhosis, the nephrotic syndrome, accelerated hypertension, renal artery stenosis and very rarely a renin-secreting tumour and juxtaglomerular hyperplasia. The most common cause is treatment with diuretics.

Other hypermineralocorticoid states

Hypokalaemia and hypernatraemia may be seen from consumption of liquorice, therapy with carbenoxolone, Cushing's syndrome especially ectopic ACTH syndrome and deoxycorticosterone-secreting adrenocortical carcinoma.

Clinical features

Primary aldosteronism

This has a sex ratio of women : men of 2:1 and usually presents in the fourth and fifth decades. Hypertension, often severe, is sustained and headache common. Hypokalaemia causes weak muscles, increased thirst, polyuria and nocturia. Paraesthesia, tetany and cramps may also feature, especially in women. Hypokalaemia suppresses insulin secretion producing carbohydrate intolerance in 50% of patients. Hypokalaemia <3.5 mmol/L found repeatedly in a hypertensive patient should raise the possibility of 1° aldosteronism although medication with thiazide diuretics is much the more likely cause of hypokalaemia. Primary aldosteronism may rarely be seen with normokalaemia (Edwards 1992).

Secondary aldosteronism

This has an equal sex ratio and patients are older. Unlike the primary form oedema is often a prominent feature. The clinical picture is dominated not by aldosteronism but the underlying cause, e.g. hypertensive cardiovascular disease and cardiac failure.

Investigations

It is important to withdraw thiazides, loop diuretics, potassium supplements and spironolactone for three weeks prior to investigation (Table 35.5). Anti-hypertensive treatment is continued only if the blood pressure exceeds 170/100.

Screening tests

Aldosteronism is first suspected if plasma potassium is repeatedly below 3.5 mmol/L and urinary potassium >30 mmol/24 hr (normal 35–90 mmol/24 hr). Often present although frequently missed, is a slight hypernatraemia and an alkalosis in primary aldosteronism contrasting with hyponatraemia in secondary

Table 35.5 Primary aldosteronism–screening and confirmation, differentiating adenoma from hyperplasia

Primary aldosteronism

Screening

- Plasma potassium <3.5 mmol/L in hypertensive patient
- Inappropriate urine potassium >30 mmol/24 hr

Confirmation

- **Correct hypokalaemia**
- 24-hour urinary aldosterone after 3 days' salt loading 9 g/day is raised (normal 10–25 nmol on unrestricted salt diet)

Resting

- Plasma aldosterone (80–300 pmol/L)
- Plasma renin (0.2–2.8 ng/ml/hr)

Physiological tests

Primary aldosteronism, adenoma and hyperplasia

Normal	Aldosterone	Renin Activity
Resting 08.00 hr	80–300 pmol/L	0.2–2.8 ng/ml/hr
Ambulant for 4 hr 12.00 hr	140–850 pmol/L	1.5–5.7 ng/ml/hr

Primary aldosteronism

Resting		
Adenoma	Raised	Near zero
Hyperplasia	Raised	Near zero
Ambulant		
Adenoma	< Resting value	Near zero
Hyperplasia	> Resting value	Renin detectable

NB: Local laboratory must be consulted as normal ranges vary from laboratory to laboratory

aldosteronism. Adenomas tend to have a lower plasma potassium, higher sodium and higher aldosterone than is seen in hyperplasia.

Confirmation of aldosteronism

Hypokalaemia is corrected and adequate salt intake ensured. Plasma aldosterone and renin levels are measured after the patient has been resting for 15 minutes.

In primary aldosteronism aldosterone (80–300 pmol/L) is raised and renin (0.2–2.8 ng/ml/hr) suppressed to near zero. In secondary aldosteronism aldosterone is increased but so also is renin.

Physiological tests to differentiate the cause of primary aldosteronism

Normal individuals show an increase in both aldosterone and renin activity with ambulation. In primary aldosteronism the raised aldosterone level seen at rest falls after four hr ambulation in the case of an adenoma and rises in hyperplasia. Renin remains near zero with an adenoma and becomes detectable in hyperplasia.

Dexamethasone suppression of aldosterone

Dexamethasone 0.5 mg six-hourly is administered for five days and either plasma or urinary aldosterone measured. A transient suppression is seen with adenoma but persists in glucocorticoid suppressible aldosteronism.

Imaging

Most aldosterone-secreting adenomas are small but will be detected on **CT** or **MRI** unless they are <10 mm diameter. Small non-functioning cortical adenomas are common however and the biochemical diagnosis must be certain before a visualised adenoma is assumed to be responsible for aldosteronism (see Table 35.8).

An isotope scan with 131-I-iodomethyl-19 norcholesterol (NP 59) after five days of dexamethasone to suppress normal cortical tissue will differentiate an adenoma; which alone takes up the isotope, from the symmetrical but less brisk uptake of hyperplasia. The test can be misleading if the patient has been on long-term spironolactone as reactivation of the renin angiotensin mechanism will have occurred. Bilateral uptake is then seen in the presence of an adenoma.

Selenomethyl cholesterol may be preferred to NP59 because of lower radiation levels.

Venous sampling for aldosterone

Cannulation of adrenal veins is difficult, particularly on the right. Use of the technique is limited by risks of extravasation, bleeding within the adrenal and subsequent necrosis. Venous sampling is therefore confined to two instances:

- The biochemical diagnosis is secure but imaging has failed to reveal an adenoma
- An adenoma has been shown but is non-functioning.

Simultaneous assay of cortisol is used as a correction factor to adjust for positional errors of the catheter. Aldosterone levels on the side of an adenoma are high, while those from the contralateral suppressed side are low. High levels are found on both sides in hyperplasia. The technique establishes the cause of primary aldosteronism and localises 90% of adenomas.

Treatment

Adenoma

Preoperative preparation consists of salt restriction, potassium supplements of 50 mmol/day and spironolactone in doses of 100 g–400 mg/day to block the renal action of aldosterone. There is a rapid return to normokalaemia, but three months may elapse before hypertension is controlled and the renin angiotensin system recovers. Spironolactone is discontinued 48 hr prior to surgery.

A posterior or laparoscopic approach is used to accomplish adrenalectomy. Removal of the adenoma preserving the rest of the adrenal has been advocated as an alternative. Bilateral adenomas arguably are best managed with spironolactone and this is also the management adopted when the patient's general condition precludes surgery.

Postoperatively hypoaldosteronism is rarely seen despite suppression of aldosterone secretion in the remaining adrenal. Function quickly returns but fludrocortisone 0.100mg/day may be temporarily required.

Adrenalectomy cures the metabolic defect. Approximately 75% of patients are rendered normotensive and the remainder require less medication (Young et al. 1990).

Hyperplasia

There is no place for bilateral adrenalectomy which invariably fails to correct hypertension and renders the patient steroid dependent. Life-long spironolactone, 50–400 mg/day, is prescribed along with an ACE inhibitor if blood pressure remains uncontrolled. Amiloride should be substituted if gastrointestinal disturbance, impotence, gynaecomastia or menstrual irregularity complicate the use of spironolactone.

Glucocorticoid suppressible aldosteronism

Prednisolone or dexamethasone is given in the smallest dose which will control hypokalaemia and aldosterone levels.

Congenital adrenal hyperplasia

This rare condition, also known as the adrenogenital syndrome, results from a defect in one of the enzymes concerned with cortisol synthesis (see Figure 35.2). Six types have been described, but more than 90% are due to a defect in the 21-hydroxylase enzyme, the next most common is a defect in 11β-hydroxylase (White et al. 1987). The enzymes are encoded by single genes and a defect is inherited as an autosomal recessive trait. The prevalence of a 21-hydoxylase defect has been calculated as 1 in 10 000 births.

21-hydroxylase defect

Synthesis of cortisol is reduced as is aldosterone in two-thirds of patients. The resulting ACTH stimulus to the adrenal causes hyperplasia of the cortex and is sufficient to achieve near normal levels of cortisol but accumulated precursors follow the synthetic pathway to form excess androgens.

11β-hydroxylase defect

Androgen precursors and deoxycorticosterone accumulate, the latter causing hypertension and hypokalaemia. Hypertension distinguishes this defect from 21-hydroxylase deficiency.

Clinical features

The features seen depend on the genetic sex, age at presentation and severity of the enzyme defect.

Fetus and infancy

During fetal life the female develops pseudohermaphrodite characteristics which at birth may lead to incorrect gender assignment. The infant has clitoral hypertrophy, labial fusion, first-degree hypospadias, absent testes, a uterus, fallopian tubes, ovaries and enlarged adrenals. In male infants, the condition is commonly unrecognised at birth, unless they are salt losers and present with an adrenal crisis. Diagnosis is usually delayed until pseudopuberty develops between the ages of two and four years. Rapid growth occurs with premature closure of the epiphyses eventually resulting in short stature.

Children

In children late onset of hyperplasia, or an adrenal carcinoma from which it must be differentiated, results in precocious puberty in boys and male secondary sexual characteristics in girls.

Adults

Virilism in adults can result from late-onset hyperplasia but is usually due to an adrenal or ovarian tumour. In the female masculinisation may be recognised. In males clinical features of increased masculinisation are easily overlooked but infertility is likely from excess androgens inhibiting the hypothalamic/ pituitary drive to the testis.

Biochemical investigations

21-hydroxylase defect

At birth plasma 17-hydroxyprogesterone remains grossly elevated (normal 100–200 ng/L). Urinary pregnanetriol, a metabolite of 17-hydroxyprogesterone and 17 ketosteroids, is also raised.

11β-hydroxylase defect

Plasma 11-deoxycortisol and 11-deoxycorticosterone levels are raised as are their urinary metabolites particularly tetrahydro-11-deoxycortisol. Differentiation of the syndrome from adrenal and ovarian tumours is determined by biochemical investigation.

Treatment of congenital adrenal hyperplasia

In infancy urgent treatment is commenced immediately after the diagnosis is established. In 21-hydroxylase deficiency hydrocortisone 5 mg/day is given to suppress ACTH. I.v. saline in severe cases and later fludrocortisone 0.05–0.1 mg/day are required if aldosterone is low or renin activity raised. In childhood, hydrocortisone 10–50 mg/day and after puberty, dexamethasone 0.25–0.75 mg are prescribed. The effectiveness of glucocorticoids is monitored by measuring plasma 17-hydroxyprogesterone or urinary pregnanetriol. 11β-hydroxylase defect is similarly treated with hydrocortisone.

Prompt glucocorticoid therapy ensures fertility in both sexes and restores feminisation in the female, although plastic reconstruction may be necessary.

Genetic counselling should be advised as one in four members of a family may be affected.

Phaeochromocytoma

This is a tumour of chromaffin cells which secretes catecholamines. It is a correctable cause of hypertension but untreated it is a lethal condition.

Incidence and pathology

It accounts for between one and five per 1000 new cases of hypertension. The sex distribution is equal and although it may occur at any age it is most often seen in the fourth and fifth decades.

Most arise from the adrenal medulla (90%). Others are extraadrenal arising from chromaffin cells in paraganglionic tissue of the sympathetic chain and the organ of Zuckerkandl. Approximately 10% of tumours are bilateral, extraadrenal, multiple, familial and malignant. Phaeochromocytomas in childhood account for about 20% of cases. Bilateral disease, extra-adrenal tumours and malignancy are more common than in the adult. Malignancy approaches 60% in patients under the age of 18. The majority of extraadrenal tumours are intraabdominal but rarely are found in the mediastinum, heart, neck and bladder.

Most phaeochromocytomas are about 5 cm in diameter, encapsulated, vascular, haemorrhagic and often necrotic. On microscopy solid masses of 'tawny-coloured' polyhedral cells which stain yellow/brown with chromium salts are seen. Malignancy, more common in extraadrenal tumours, may not be recognised until metastases have occurred, as the only specific feature on histology is extra-capsular vascular invasion. Phaeochromocytoma is an important feature of MEN IIa and IIb and also occurs in other genetically determined neuroectodermal disease such as von Recklinghausen's disease, von Hippel–Lindau disease, Sturge–Weber disease, tuberose sclerosis and acromegaly. Familial phaeochromocytoma can also occur without these associations. In all these syndromes multiple tumours are frequent.

Clinical features

The biological action of the predominant catecholamine secreted determines the symptoms and signs.

- *Adrenaline-secreting tumours* (adrenal) stimulate both alpha and beta receptors. During pressor crises patients exhibit tachycardia and hyperglycaemia.

- *Noradrenaline-secreting tumours* (extraadrenal) activate peripheral alpha1 and alpha2 receptors which results in widespread cutaneous pallor and splanchnic vasoconstriction. Pressor crises may be accompanied by baroreceptor-mediated bradycardia overcoming initial tachycardia.

- *Dopamine and dopa-secreting tumours* are very rare and invariably malignant. They are associated with hypotensive attacks.

Because of its varied clinical presentation phaeochromocytoma has aptly been named 'the great mimic' and also 'the panic syndrome' (Table 35.6).

Hypertension is the principal feature. It may occur as a classical paroxysm, as sustained hypertension occurring in at least 40% or as persistent hypertension with superimposed paroxysms.

During a paroxysm, of which there is often a premonition, headache, anxiety with a conviction of impending doom, arrhythmia recognised by the patient, a pounding sensation and pain in the chest or abdomen occur. Patients appear pale and sweaty with a tachycardia, although bradycardia occurs if noradrenaline predominates. Myocardial infarction, pulmonary oedema, hypertensive encephalopathy and stroke may result.

The attack usually lasts less than 15 minutes and for less than one hour in 80% of patients. Postural hypotension may follow the attack.

Paroxysms can be provoked by various stimuli including emotion, exercise, certain postures, the Valsalva manoeuvre, micturition if a tumour is situated in the bladder, pressure from the palpating hand and invasive diagnostic investigation.

Drugs may have profound effects on blood pressure. Hypertension can follow use of beta-blocking agents such as propranolol, due to an unopposed alpha-adrenergic drive while hypotension may be precipitated by the alpha-blocker phenothiazine. Morphine, ACTH and guanethidine also promote hypertension by stimulating release of stored catecholamines.

Physical signs are often sparse, the patient is usually thin and there may be neuroectodermal dysplasias but rarely is a tumour palpable. Overzealous abdominal palpation should be actively discouraged due to the risk of provoking a crisis. Nonetheless the blood pressure may not be elevated until there is a stressful event such as induction of anaesthesia or surgical stimulation.

Hypertension in a child is uncommon while it is a frequent finding in pregnancy, but in both instances a phaeochromocytoma must be excluded.

Table 35.6 Clinical presentations of phaeochromcytoma

1	**Asymptomatic**	Discovered incidentally
2	**Classical paroxysms**	Headache, sweating, tachycardia, pallor, anxiety, sense of impending doom
3	**Sustained hypertension**	Simulating essential hypertension
4	**Hypertension with paroxysms**	As above with extreme fluctuations and paroxysms
5	**Anaesthesia/surgery**	Unexplained arrhythmia, tachycardia, hypo- or hypertension
6	**Sudden death**	After exercise or minor injury
7	**Diabetes simulation**	Polydipsia, polyuria, glucose elevation, abnormal glucose tolerance test
8	**Thyrotoxic simulation**	Weight loss, tachypnoea, tremulousness, increased metabolic rate
9	**Anxiety state**	Nervousness, tremor, tachypnoea
10	**Psychotic state**	Nervousness, personality change, psychotic reaction
11	**Septic state**	Fever, hypotension, leucocytosis
12	**Shock state**	Acute heart failure, collapse, unrecordable BP. BP>300 requires arterial line for diagnosis – easily missed
13	**Congestive cardiac failure**	Catecholamine myocarditis
14	**Retroperitoneal haemorrhage**	Haemorrhagic necrosis, rupture, massive retroperitoneal bleed

Adapted from Scott HW: The Panic syndrome: phaeochromocytoma. In Friesen SR and Thompson NW (Eds) *Surgical Endocrinology* Philadelphia. Lippincott 1990 p 165

Investigations

The diagnosis of phaeochromocytoma is established by measurement of catecholamines or their metabolites (Table 35.7).

Biochemical screening

This should be undertaken in three circumstances:

Table 35.7 Normal urine and plasma catecholamine values, pre- and intraoperative medication

Phaeochromocytoma

24-hour urine screening normal values

VMA 0–35 μmol
Metanephrines <7 μmol
HVA 0–82 μmol
Adrenaline 30–190 nmol
Noradrenaline 120–590 nmol
Dopamine 650–3270 nmol

Plasma values resting

Adrenaline 0.1–0.3 nmol/L
Noradrenaline 0.5–3.0 nmol/L
Dopamine < 0.1 nmol/L

NB: Local laboratory must be consulted as normal ranges vary from laboratory to laboratory

Preoperative Medication
- Phenoxybenzamine 10 mg b.d. $\longrightarrow$ until slight hypotension
- Propranolol 40 mg/day $\longrightarrow$ only after alpha blockade
- Metirosine 250 mg q.d.s. $\longrightarrow$ 4 g/day

Intraoperative Medication

- **Hypertension**

Sodium nitroprusside 0.3–1.5 μg/kg/min infusion
Phentolame 1 mg/min infusion

- **Hypotension**

Fluid replacement
Dopamine 2–5 μg/kg/min infusion
Noradrenaline 6.4–13.2 μg base/min infusion

- Hypertensives who have clinical features suggestive of phaeochromocytoma

- Patients with conditions known to be associated with phaeochromocytoma

- Unexplained hypertension in young and when severe in pregnant patients.

24-HOUR URINE COLLECTION FOR CATECHOLAMINES OR METABOLITES

The mainstay of investigation until recent years has been measurement of VMA, i.e. 4-hydroxy-3-methoxy mandelic acid (normal <35 μmol/24 hr) and if raised metanephrines (normal <7 μmol/24 hr) and homovanillic (normal 0–82 μmol/24 hr) from an acidified 24 hour urine collection. The greater sensitivity afforded by measurement of adrenaline (normal 30–190 nmol/24 hr) and noradrenaline (normal 120–590 nmol/24 hr) has led to many centres adopting this as their screening investigation. Dopamine (650–3270 nmol/24 hr) is assayed if hypotensive episodes have occurred. High levels of this or homovanillic acid raises the possibility of malignancy.

PLASMA CATECHOLAMINES

Adrenaline (0.1–0.3 nmol/L) and noradrenaline (0.5–3.0 nmol/L) may be measured by radioimmunoassay. Samples are taken from an indwelling cannula after the patient has been recumbent for 30 minutes in a stress-free environment. A single specimen may be less representative than a 24-hour urine sample if the patient is normotensive between crises and is ideally repeated on three occasions.

Imaging

This is undertaken once a biochemical diagnosis is certain (Table 35.8).

Table 35.8 Biochemically established imaging techniques for cushing's syndrome, primary aldosteronism and phaeochromocytoma

| | **Cushing's syndrome** | | | |
	CT/MRI pituitary	CT/MRI adrenal	Idocholesterol scan adrenal	Bilateral petrosal sinus sampling
Cushing's disease	Microadenoma in 50/75%	Bilateral enlargement/normal	Bilateral uptake	Gradient of 1.5–3.0 × cava sample
Ectopic ACTH syndrome		Bilateral enlargement/normal	Bilateral uptake	
Adrenal adenoma		Unilateral mass	Unilateral uptake in adenoma	
Adrenal carcinoma		>5 cm ? carcinoma	No uptake in carcinoma	
Macronodular cortical hyperplasia		Bilateral enlargement knobbly/normal	Variable uptake	
Primary pigmented nodular cortical disease		Often normal	Variable uptake	

Primary aldosteronism

- **CT and MRI** Adenomas <10 mm may not be detected

- **19 – iodocholesterol** after 5 days of dexamethasone suppression – adenoma takes up isotope with other gland suppressed. Hyperplasia bilateral but less brisk uptake

- **Venous sampling** from adrenal veins. Aldosterone high on side of adenoma. High on both sides in hyperplasia Assay cortisol and use as correction factor

Phaeochromocytoma

- **CT and MRI** MRI better in case of extraadrenal tumour

- **MIBG scan** detects extraadrenal tumours and metastases

CT and *MRI* are both satisfactory in demonstrating phaeochromocytomas of the adrenal but CT is less reliable when the tumour is extraadrenal. CT demonstrates up to 96% of adrenal phaeochromocytomas.

MIBG scan
The radionuclide ^{131}I-meta-iodobenzylguanadine is concentrated in adrenergic vesicles and is particularly useful for detection of extraadrenal lesions and metastases. Sensitivity has been reported as 90%.

Selective venous sampling for plasma catecholamines risks provoking a hypertensive crisis and has been superseded by non-invasive measures.

Treatment (Table 35.7)

Excision is indicated unless there is evidence of extensive malignant disease or serious medical contraindications to surgery. If a clinical diagnosis of phaeochromocytoma has been made, measures to control hypertension must be instituted without delay. Untreated patients with phaeochromocytoma exhibit an overall vasoconstriction and reduced plasma volume. At least two weeks should be spent in preoperative preparation to correct this.

- α adrenergic receptors are blocked with oral phenoxybenzamine. Starting with 10 mg b.d. the dose is increased to the point where there is slight postural hypotension. Dizziness, compensatory tachycardia, lassitude and nasal congestion may be side effects. A high fluid intake is encouraged thereby 'topping up' the increased plasma volume; this can unmask anaemia, which may warrant blood transfusion.

- When effective alpha blockade has been established, beta blockade is added should there be persistent tachycardia, arrhythmia or the catecholamine secreted is predominantly adrenaline. Beta-blockers should not be used until alpha blockade has been obtained as this may precipitate a hypertensive crisis. They are also contraindicated in bronchial asthma, obstructive airways disease and uncontrolled heart failure. Propranolol is used in a divided dose of 40–60 mg/day as judged by control of tachycardia.

- Alpha Methyl tyrosine (metirosine) may be used to suppress catecholamine production. Its side effects particularly in the elderly have limited its use.

Phaeochromocytoma in pregnancy

An untreated phaeochromocytoma risks maternal death and fetal abortion. In the first and second trimesters the patient is managed in similar fashion to the non-pregnant patient though imaging should be limited to the use of US and MRI. Termination as an alternative may be considered for those in the first trimester. Those in the third trimester must have a caesarean section and not a vaginal delivery. Ideally the phaeochromocytoma should be removed at the same time. If delayed for two to three weeks alpha blockade must be continued until surgery, as half the maternal deaths have been reported as occurring in the postpartum period.

Undiagnosed phaeochromocytoma and surgery

A patient may unexpectedly present with a hypertensive crisis, tachycardia or arrhythmia during induction of an anaesthetic or during the course of unrelated surgery such as a cholecystectomy. Immediate treatment of hypertension is instituted with infusion by either nitroprusside 0.3–1.5 μg/Kg/min or phentolamine 1 mg/min. Alternatively phentlamine 2–5 mg may be given by I.V. injection repeated if necessary. The operation must be postponed or rapidly curtailed. Only when the patient has been investigated and prepared should surgery for the phaeochromocytoma be undertaken.

Surgery for phaeochromocytoma

Despite preoperative preparation the possibility of a hypertensive crisis and profound hypotension after removal of a phaeochromocytoma must always be borne in mind. Central venous pressure, arterial pressure, urine output and ECG should be monitored. A Swann-Ganz catheter helps prevent fluid overload and pulmonary oedema and is used routinely in some centres.

Anaesthetic agents and techniques should be selected to lessen stimulation of catecholamine release and minimise their effects. Enflurane or isoflurane are used rather than halothane as they are associated with less sensitisation of the myocardium to the arrhythmic effects of catecholamines than halothane. Pancuronium or vecuronium are suitable relaxants as they do not elicit histamine release.

Hypertension during the procedure is best controlled with infusions of sodium nitroprusside 0.3–1.5 μg/kg/min or phentolamine 1 mg/min. Hypotension on removal of the tumour will usually be controlled by fluid replacement but may require infusions of dopamine 2–5 μg/kg/min or noradrenaline (Levophed) at an initial rate of 6.4–13.2 μg base/min.

Arrhythmias may be controlled with propranolol 1 mg or lignocaine 50–100 mg given intravenously. Electrocardioversion may rarely be necessary.

APPROACH

Improved imaging has led some centres to recommend a posterior (Geoghegan et al. 1998) or laparoscopic approach for tumours of <5 cm or so. The alternative of an anterior abdominal approach remains popular. The most important considerations in surgical technique are non-manipulative dissection of the tumour, early control of adrenal vessels, avoidance of capsular rupture and clearance of the adrenal fossa in case there is malignancy. With the anterior approach both adrenal glands can be examined and possible sites of intraabdominal extraadrenal phaeochromocytomas explored. If there is not an appreciable fall in blood pressure when a tumour has been removed every effort to find multiple tumours should be made. If the tumour is obviously malignant it should be removed in its entirety if possible but failing this careful debulking is of benefit. Rarely in association with MEN II hyperplasia of the adrenal medulla is found and bilateral adrenalectomy with steroid cover is then appropriate.

POSTOPERATIVE CARE

In the immediate postoperative period monitoring, started in theatre, is continued in an ITU. Particular care is required with fluid replacement, blood glucose is monitored hourly and hypoglycaemia, which may result from withdrawal of catecholamines, corrected. Steroid medication is continued should bilateral adrenalectomy have been necessary.

ADJUNCTS TO SURGERY

Useful adjuncts in malignancy are radiotherapy and ^{131}I-MIBG. Symptomatic treatment may require continuation of alpha and beta blockade or the use of methyltyrosine.

FOLLOW-UP

Follow-up is life long. Urinary catecholamines are assayed after recovery from surgery and are then repeated annually. Hypertension, requiring continued medication, may persist in some patients as a result of renal damage and a minority of patients will declare an initially unsuspected malignancy.

Multiple endocrine neoplasia (MEN) type II – Sipple's syndrome

MEN has been described as 'a genetically inherited multifocal tumour formation of the polypeptide APUD system'.

MEN II patients have one of two syndromes both characterised by medullary thyroid cancer and phaeochromocytoma.

Group IIa exhibits hyperparathyroidism.

Group IIb patients rarely have hyperparathyroidism but often Marfanoid features, thick lips, lax ligaments and multiple mucosal neuromata. Hypertrophied corneal nerves, skeletal defects and alimentary abnormalities including diffuse ganglioneuromatas have also been described (O'Riordan et al. 1995).

MEN II is inherited as an autosomal dominant disorder with varying but high penetrance. Mutations of the Ret-proto-oncogene, responsible for the syndrome have been identified at codon 634 in MEN IIa and 918 in IIb.

Children with phaeochromocytomas and adults with bilateral or multiple tumours should be carefully investigated for evidence of MEN II. If positive, first-degree relatives should be screened. Urinary adrenaline is the best indicator of adrenal hyperplasia, which is the forerunner of phaeochromocytoma in these familial syndromes. Identification of the germ line mutations in the Ret-proto-oncogene now allows a DNA-based diagnosis.

Neuroblastoma and ganglioneuroma

These are ganglion cell tumours which arise from the adrenal, sympathetic chain or occasionally the parasympathetic system. They may occur in the posterior mediastinum, cervical region, pelvis and as a retroperitoneal mass. Neuroblastoma and ganglioneuroma represent opposite ends of a spectrum in which the former is highly malignant, the latter usually benign.

Neuroblastoma

Incidence and pathology

Neuroblastoma is the most common solid tumour of childhood with an equal sex distribution. It develops from immature nerve cells with 50–80% arising within the abdomen – most commonly from the adrenal medulla but also from along the sympathetic chain. They are usually massive, nodular, haemorrhagic and necrotic tumours. Spread is rapid with local extension, involvement of lymph nodes and haematogenous spread to liver and bones. Their characteristic microscopic appearance is of small round cells arranged in rosettes in the centre of which are large numbers of fine nerve fibrils.

Clinical features

Neuroblastoma presents in infancy and early childhood usually with a large mass which must be differentiated from a Wilms' tumour. Pain, hypertension, pressure-induced gastrointestinal symptoms and cachexia may feature. Two eponymous modes of spread are recognised; Pepper's type characterised by a right-sided abdominal tumour with liver metastases and Hutchison's type consisting of a left-sided tumour with secondaries in the orbit, skull and long bones. Recognised associations with neuroblastoma are Hirschprung's disease, Klippel-Feil syndrome and Beckwith-Wiedermann syndrome.

Investigations

These aim to confirm the diagnosis and stage the tumour.

BIOCHEMICAL INVESTIGATIONS

VMA, metanephrines and vasoactive peptide are frequently raised, although clinical features of catecholamine excess are rare.

IMAGING

Chest radiographs, CT, skeletal survey and MIBG scan can be used to determine the extent of the tumour.

BONE MARROW ASPIRATION

May indicate evidence of secondary spread.

Staging

I   Localised tumour

II   Local extension beyond organ from which it arises but not beyond midline

III   Tumour extension beyond midline

IV   Distant metastases

IVs   Small primary with metastases confined to liver, skin or bone marrow but without cortical bone involvement.

Treatment

STAGES I AND II

Surgical excision with adjuvant chemotherapy in Stage II.

STAGE III

Attempted excision followed by chemotherapy and radiotherapy to which the tumour is sensitive. Alternatively preoperative radiotherapy may be given to downsize an irremovable tumour. Tumour debulking may be of benefit in an irremovable tumour before continuing radiotherapy and chemotherapy.

STAGE IV

Combination chemotherapy in advanced disease is of benefit. Cyclophosphamide, vincristine, and cisplatin have all found a place in different protocols (Leung 1998).

STAGE IVs

Attempted excision before chemotherapy is probably worthwhile.

Prognosis

Spontaneous regression of the tumour with maturation of cells towards those of a ganglioneuroma has been reported in 5% of children under the age of two but in the majority the prognosis is dismal.

Ganglioneuroma

Incidence and pathology

Ganglioneuromas occur in an older age group than neuroblastomas. They are usually benign, and most often arise from the sympathetic trunk in the posterior mediastinum. They are firm, encapsulated and consist of mature ganglion cells and nerve fibres both myelinated and non-myelinated.

Clinical features

Although they may secrete catecholamines they usually present with a mass, its pressure effects or as an incidental finding on imaging.

Investigation

Investigation is as described for neuroblastoma.

Treatment

The tumour should be excised and in general the prognosis is good.

Non-functioning adrenal tumours and incidentaloma

Non-functioning adrenal tumours have no clinical features of hormone excess. Nonetheless biochemical investigations will show hormone abnormalities in many. Some patients present with a mass but increasingly do so because of an incidental finding on imaging for an unrelated condition. About 2% of patients undergoing abdominal CT for unrelated conditions will be found to have an unsuspected adrenal lesion (Ross and Avon 1990). Adrenal and retroperitoneal masses were discovered in 0.1% of 41 357 healthy subjects using less sensitive ultrasound screening (Masumori et al. 1998).

- *Adrenal cortical adenomas:* are found in 5% of autopsies. Most are between 2 and 5 cm diameter.
- *Adrenal cortical carcinomas:* are usually large, have imaging features to suggest malignancy and all too often have metastasised.
- *Secondary adrenal tumours* are frequent and often bilateral. Lung, breast, the gastrointestinal tract and melanoma are common primaries. Rarely functioning tissue is so reduced by tumour or haemorrhage that a steroid crisis occurs.
- *Other non-functioning tumours*: Neurogenic tumours such as neurilemmoma and ganglioneuromas, cysts, myelolipoma, tuberculoma and haematoma may all present as non-functioning adrenal tumours.

The patient with an adrenal mass or incidentaloma presents the clinician with the problem of determining whether the tumour is functioning and/or malignant.

Investigations

Biochemical investigations

All patients require biochemical assessment. If, for example, subclinical Cushing's syndrome due to an adrenal adenoma with suppression of the contralateral adrenal is not diagnosed, the serious potential problems are obvious. 50% of adrenal cortical carcinomas will have abnormalities. Excessive synthesis of glucocorticoids, mineralocorticoids and androgens may all be seen. Raised urinary 17-ketosteroids are very suggestive of adrenal malignancy.

Imaging

CT is the most commonly used imaging modality. MRI has some advantages as it allows determination of operative planes and the T_2-weighted image helps to characterise the lesion; this can be improved by perfusion with gadolinium diethylene triamenepentacetic acid (Gd-DTPA). The spin-echo images of the tumour are compared with liver and fat; the ratio is <1.4 in cortical adenoma, >3 with phaeochromocytoma and between these two values in primary and secondary malignancies.

Adrenal cortical adenomas are 'small' (2–5 cm), homogeneous, have a regular outline and have a low uptake of contrast on dynamic CT. Adrenal cortical carcinomas on the other hand are usually 'large' (>6 cm), heterogeneous, irregular in outline with variable uptake of contrast due to necrosis and varying vascularity. The other tumours mentioned are well shown on CT and have a smooth outline. Calcification may be seen with ganglioneuromas and tuberculosis, whilst myelolipoma has a similar density to surrounding fat on CT, as well as being echogenic on ultrasound.

Fine-needle aspiration

Use of CT-guided FNA or cyst aspiration must not be considered before biochemical assessment has excluded a phaeochromocytoma. FNA has probably been overused in the recent past. Interpretation of cytology is particularly difficult in endocrine tumours and definitive diagnosis by this means is uncommon. Potential spillage of malignant cells may compromise the chance of cure. FNA is best reserved to confirm lesions that are almost certainly secondaries or to aspirate tuberculous pus for culture and sensitivity.

Management

The indications for surgery in non-functioning tumours and incidentalomas are:

- Evidence that the lesion is hormonally active

- Risk of malignancy from the imaging appearance

- Lesions of 5 cm diameter or larger in patients under the age of 50. This figure is variously quoted as between 4 and 6 cm

- Increase in size of incidentaloma during follow-up.

Non-functioning apparently benign lesions of <4–5 cm are followed up with regular CT and biochemical investigation if appropriate. Increase in size is an indication for surgery.

It should be recalled that although large tumours are more likely to be malignant than small lesions the risk of malignancy in a 'small' tumour is greater in the young than the old. The opportunity to resect a small early cortical carcinoma should not be missed as the five-year survival is of the order of 90%; once the tumour exceeds 6 cm survival plummets to 10%.

OPERATIVE SURGERY

Adrenalectomy

Adrenalectomy has traditionally been achieved by open operation but in 1992 Gagner and co-workers advocated a laparoscopic approach. 100 consecutive procedures were reported in 1997 (Gagner et al 1997). This technique for some adrenalectomies has been taken up in many centres. A study of laparoscopic compared with open adrenalectomy has been reported (Imai et al. 1999). Fundamental to its success have been improvements in imaging and laparoscopic equipment. Enthusiasts claim a lower morbidity and shorter hospital stay to set against the learning curve of a demanding technique.

Adrenalectomy is performed under a general anaesthetic with controlled respiration and precautions taken as noted in earlier sections (Figures 35.2 and 35.3).

Approaches

Currently the adrenal may be removed by an open operation, with the incision placed anteriorly, laterally or posteriorly (Wellbourn 1982) or the procedure may be laparoscopic (Marescaux et al. 1996).

An anterior approach gives the greatest freedom to deal with the unexpected be it multiple phaeochromocytomas, malignancy or unrelated pathology.

A lateral incision, which may have a thoracic extension, is reserved for large tumours or 'redo' surgery.

A posterior approach is popular with many surgeons, although anaesthetists do not always share this enthusiasm. It is generally well tolerated and convalescence is rapid. It is applicable in hyperplasia causing Cushing's syndrome, and unilateral benign tumours of 5 cm or less whatever their aetiology.

The laparoscopic approach may be recommended for the same group with most surgeons resorting to an open approach above 5/6 cm. Gagner et al. with their great experience suggest benign lesions <15 cm may be removed laparoscopically (1997).

Common to all approaches is non-manipulative dissection of the adrenal, early control of adrenal vessels and careful haemostasis accompanying dissection around the periphery of the gland. The plane between adrenal and kidney is separated last as downward traction of the kidney improves adrenal exposure.

Anterior approach

Patient lies supine. Depending on the patient's build and expected pathology a mid-line (thin adults and children) or subcostal incision (the adult of moderate build) is chosen. This may be bilateral (Figure 35.3A).

Left adrenal exposure

Different methods are available:

- 30° tilt to right. Peritoneum lateral to spleen incised. Spleen and tail of pancreas mobilised medially. (Figure 35.3 B and C).

- Peritoneum lateral to descending colon incised. Colon swept medially to expose kidney, adrenal and pancreas. Exerting gentle traction on kidney in downward and forward direction helps to expose adrenal.

- Incision through transverse mesocolon lateral to inferior mesenteric vein.

- Incisions through gastro colic omentum and then along inferior or superior pancreatic margin to reveal adrenal depending on its position. Care must be exercised to avoid inadvertent ligation of a superior pole renal artery.

Right adrenal exposure

With a 30° tilt to the left, the duodenum is 'Kocherised'. Hepatic flexure of the colon is retracted downwards and the liver upwards. The inferior vena cava is exposed down to the right renal vein and upwards to above the entry of the short adrenal vein.

Lateral approach

The patient is lying on their side, uppermost, with the table 'broken' just above the costal margin (Figure 35.4A).

Left adrenal exposure

The 11th rib is retracted or resected, with the pleura pushed upwards and the diaphragm divided in the line of the wound.

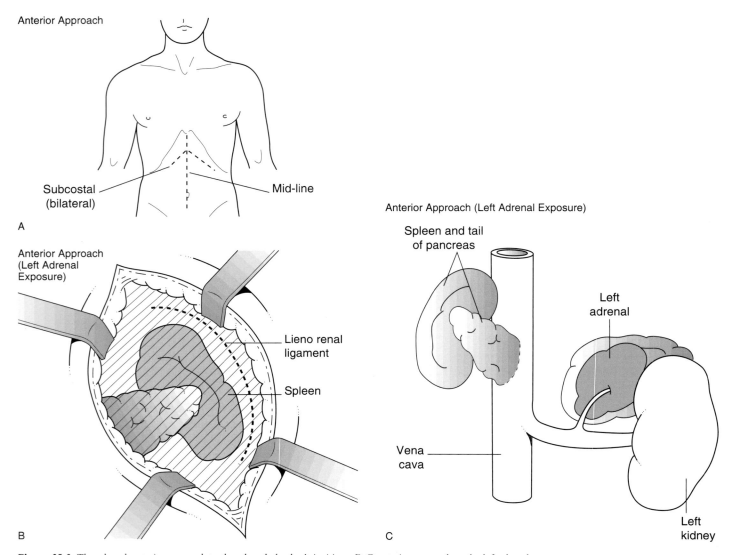

Figure 35.3 The adrenal–anterior approach to the adrenal glands. A-incisions; B-C-anterior approach to the left adrenal.

RIGHT ADRENAL EXPOSURE

The 10th rib is retracted or resected, the diaphragm incised posteriorly and at right angles to the main incision over the upper pole of the kidney. The renal fascia is opened.

Closure is accompanied by an intercostal tube.

ALTERNATIVE EXPOSURE

Flank incision either below or through the bed of the 12th rib is made but remaining extrapleural is an alternative. The choice depends on the disease and size of the adrenal.

Posterior approach (Hockey stick)

The patient is prone with the table broken (Figure 35.4B). Careful support is essential to prevent damage to skin and bone. Land-marks

are then marked. A vertical incision from the 9th to 12th ribs, 5 cm from the spine on the affected side (Figure 35.4C). At the 12th rib, incision follows the line of the rib which is resected.

EXPOSURE

The deep layer of periosteum andrenal fascia are opened. The pleura is pushed upwards and the diaphragm opened vertically. If the exposure is inadequate, it is necessary to resect a segment of the 11th rib. Alternatively carry the incision down to the posterior superior iliac spine. Closure is best achieved with the patient lying flat.

Laparoscopic approach (transabdominal)

Two television monitors are located at the head end of the table. The patient is initially placed in the supine position. The penumoperitoneum is established with CO_2 at a maximum pressure of

15 mm Hg via a Veress needle placed through small subumbilical stab incision (Figure 35.4D) (Alternatives are a subcostal site and an open Hassan technique). A full lateral position is adopted, allowing the weight of organs anterior to the adrenal to 'fall away'. Four 10 mm trocars are placed 2 cm below the costal margin at the mid-clavicular anterior, mid and posterior axillary lines.

Readiness by the surgeon to convert to an open procedure is essential if difficulty is experienced in visualisation or with bleeding not readily controlled by tamponade.

renal veins – the key to orientation. Dissect the adjacent tissue from the adrenal and tumour not the adrenal from related tissues. Identify the inferior phrenic vein to expose the adrenal vein, adrenal, superior aspect and hilum of left kidney. The left adrenal vein is double clipped in continuity before division. Dissect around the periphery of the adrenal with diathermy coagulation of small vessels; larger vessels are clipped. Place freed gland securely in a collection bag to avoid cell spillage and remove it through the subumbilical incision, which is widened to 3–5 cm. Careful haemostasis is obtained before closing port sites.

LEFT ADRENALECTOMY

Incise the peritoneum along the lateral aspect of the spleen and splenic flexure. The splenic flexure is mobilised and retracted inferiorly and medially, the spleen and pancreas superiorly enabling dissection behind the pancreatic tail. Identify the splenic and left

RIGHT ADRENALECTOMY

The operating table is in position 15–20 reverse Trendelenberg position. Expose triangular ligament and bare area of liver. Retract the liver superiorly and medially to expose the right adrenal. Dissect along the medial border of the adrenal, exposing

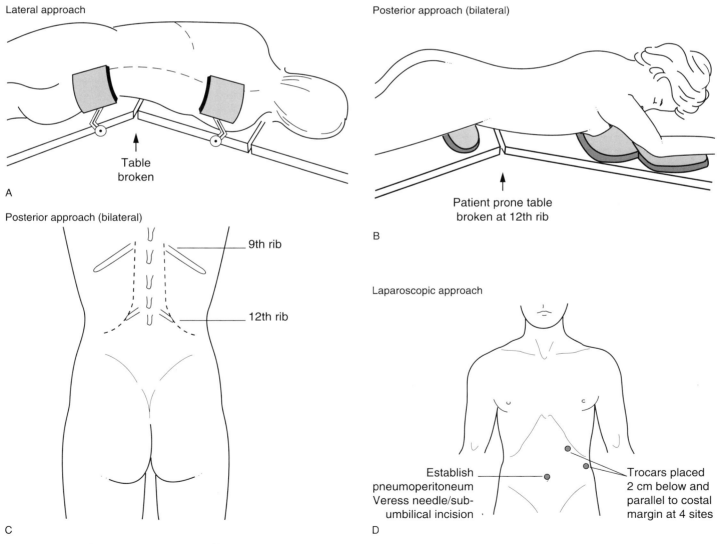

Figure 35.4 Lateral (A), posterior (B and C) and laparscopic approaches (D) to the adrenal glands.

the lateral border of the inferior vena cava. The short right adrenal vein is identified and doubly clipped in continuity before division. Seek an occasional accessory vein superior to this. The procedure continues as on the left.

Complications of adrenalectomy

Complications specific to adrenal surgery have been outlined but as with any major surgery haemorrhage and infection may occur. Patients with Cushing's syndrome are particularly susceptible to venous thrombosis, infection and poor healing of wounds. Low-dose heparin is given for prophylaxis of venous thrombosis and early mobilisation and breathing exercises encouraged. In surgery for Cushing's syndrome or prolonged operations antibiotics are given. Pneumothorax, bleeding and pancreatitis resulting from damage to closely related structures, respectively the pleura, spleen and pancreas, should be borne in mind. Complications after the laparoscopic approach include port site incisional hernias, bowel injury from trocar insertion and hypercapnoea induced by CO_2 pneumoperitoneum.

FURTHER READING

Edwards CRW. Disorders of mineralocorticoid hormone secretion. In Ed. Grossman A Clinical Endocrinology. Oxford: Blackwell Scientific Publications, 1992: 405–420

Gagner M, Pomp A, Heniford BT et al. Laparoscopic adrenalectomy: Lessons learned from 100 consecutive procedures. *Ann Surg* 1997; **226**:238–246

Geoghegan JG, Emberton M, Bloom SR, Lynn JA. Changing trends in the management of phaeochromocytoma. *Br J Surg* 1998; **85**:117–120

Imai T, Kikumori T, Ohiwa M, et al. A case controlled study of laparoscopic compared with open lateral adrenalectomy *Am J Surg* 1999; **178**:50–53.

Leung CK. Fifteen years' review of advanced childhood neuroblastoma from a single institution in Hong Kong. *Chin Med J* 1998; **111**:466–469

Marescaux J, Mutter D, Wheeler MH. Laparoscopic right and left adrenalectomies. Surgical procedures. *Surg Endosc* 1996; **10**:912–915

Masumori N, Adachi H, Noda Y, Tsukamoto T. Detection of adrenal and retroperitoneal masses in a general health examination system. *Urology* 1998; **52**:572–576

O'Riordan DS, O'Brien T, Crotty TB et al. Multiple endocrine neoplasia Type IIb: More than an endocrine disorder. *Surgery* 1995; **118**:926–942

Orth DN. Cushing's syndrome. *New Engl J Med* 1995; **332**:791–803

Padayatty SJ, Orme SM, Nelson M et al. Bilateral sequential inferior petrosal sinus sampling with corticotrophin–releasing hormone stimulation in the diagnosis of Cushing's disease. *Eur J Endocrinol* 1998; **139**:161–166

Ross NC, Avon DC. Hormonal evaluation of the patient with an incidentally discovered adrenal mass. *N Engl J Med* 1990; **323**:1401–1405

Wellbourn RB. Operations on the adrenal glands. In Eds. Dudley H, Pories W. Rob and Smith's Operative Surgery 4th Edn. London: Butterworth 1982: 397–414

White PC, New MI, Dupont B. Congenital adrenal hyperplasia. *N Engl J Med* 1987; **316**:1519–1524

Young WF, Hogan MJ, Klee GG et al. Primary aldosteronism diagnosis and treatment. *Mayo Clin Proc* 1990; **65**:96–110

Section 6

Vascular surgery

36

Diagnostic techniques in vascular surgery

Roderick T.A. Chalmers, C. Vaughan Ruckley

ARTERIAL DISEASE

Introduction

In this era of rapid advances in imaging technology, it is tempting to think that the clinical assessment of patients with vascular disease is largely a thing of the past. This is not the case. In many ways, well-developed clinical acumen is more important than ever in order to avoid the modern tendency to perform a needless battery of sometimes harmful and increasingly expensive investigations. Many of the tests available today have superseded their traditional predecessors (duplex scanning commonly replacing arteriography is a good example) but in some settings, investigations can be complementary.

A key advance in the investigation of the vascular patient has been the evolution of the vascular laboratory. This concept has progressed from the original idea of providing a facility for the assessment of ankle pressures and exercise tolerance treadmill tests into a resource capable of providing a wide range of investigations, integrated into a vascular service in such a way as to answer specific clinical questions at every stage of vascular care from primary care to long-term postintervention surveillance. Ideally, the vascular laboratory runs in parallel with outpatient clinics so that patients can be screened, clinically assessed, investigated non-invasively and a treatment plan prepared all in the same visit.

Clinical features

History

For many of the common conditions presenting to a vascular specialist the identifying characteristics are relatively specific if the clinical history is taken with care.

Intermittent claudication

Patients describe a tightness or cramping pain that comes on after walking a typical distance on the flat. Rest for a few minutes leads to complete resolution of the pain. Symptoms limited to the calf are usually attributable to femoral artery disease, whilst more proximal thigh pain is due to iliofemoral occlusion and buttock pain to aortoiliac level disease.

If, instead of describing a cramping pain localised to specific muscle groups, the patient describes a generalised dead or weak feeling in the leg, suspect spinal cord ischaemia or arterial occlusion at aortic level. If the pain corresponds to sciatic distribution, suspect cauda equina or sciatic root compression and such patients virtually always have a history of 'back trouble' such as prolapsed disc, injury or spinal osteo-arthritis. If the exercise-related pain is generalised and associated with swelling or feelings of bursting and not relieved by rest until the patient sits or elevates the leg, suspect venous claudication. Such a patient will have a history consistent with iliac deep vein thrombosis. Pain present at rest, standing and/or when the patient first starts walking is usually arthritic. A burning pain, constantly present, is likely to indicate peripheral neuropathy. Also bear in mind the possibility that atherosclerotic and neurogenic claudication may co-exist.

Although the most common cause of claudication is occlusive atheromatous disease other pathologies such as popliteal aneurysm, entrapment syndromes and cystic disease must not be forgotten.

Ischaemic rest pain

This compelling pain is experienced when the patient has been lying flat for some time. The only relief is obtained by placing the affected limb in a dependent position or sitting up in a chair. Patients have a typical look of complete exhaustion often due to the loss of many nights' sleep. Even opiates may be ineffective in relieving the pain. The history is usually unmistakable but differential diagnoses include peripheral neuropathy, night cramps/restless legs and gout/other arthropathies.

Abdominal pain

Mesenteric ischaemia is often only diagnosed too late as the presentation is confused with other more common causes of abdominal pain, such as diverticulitis or constipation. Typically the patient with chronic visceral ischaemia has other manifestations of occlusive arterial disease such as angina, a history of myocardial infarction or claudication. Typically there is post-prandial pain so severe that patients acquire a fear of food and lose weight. Bloating and watery diarrhoea shortly after eating are common. Frank steatorrhoea is unusual.

Aortic aneurysm may present with abdominal pain but more often the pain is localised to the back or loins, occasionally the groin or genitalia. The differential diagnosis includes pancreatitis, peptic ulcer disease, renal colic and arthritic back pain.

Cerebral ischaemia

Although many patients with atherosclerosis have carotid artery stenosis, not all will have symptoms related to the carotid arteries. Ipsilateral amaurosis fugax due to retinal artery embolisation and ipsilateral hemispheric (contralateral body) symptoms (transient cerebral ischaemic attack or stroke) are highly suggestive of symptomatic carotid disease.

A tumour of the carotid body presents as a mass in the carotid triangle which may appear pulsatile. The differential diagnosis lies between carotid aneurysm (rare), tortuosity of the carotid arteries (common in elderly patients) and the transmitted pulsation of normal carotid vessels through overlying masses affecting other tissues such as lymph nodes, parotid or submandibular gland tumours, laterally placed thyroid masses. Clearly, further appropriate investigations are crucial to accurate diagnosis in this instance.

Examination

The basics of clinical examination for vascular disease should include the following.

- Inspection for signs indicative of peripheral arterial disease (nicotine staining of the fingers, xanthelasma, Buerger's test, venous guttering, capillary refill, skin nutrition, etc.). Palpation of all limb pulses and measurement of blood pressure in both arms.

- Auscultation over the carotid and subclavian arteries, aorta, iliac and femoral regions for bruits.

- Abdominal palpation for aortic aneurysm.

- Simple neurological tests should also be routine, such as straight leg raising with passive ankle dorsiflexion when spinal claudication is a possibility and tests of cutaneous sensation in diabetics.

Investigations

Blood tests

The assessment of a patient presenting with peripheral vascular disease includes a number of routine blood tests. Clinically inapparent abnormalities will often be discovered which could indicate fairly significant disease. Secondary prevention by risk factor assessment and control is an important, but often neglected part of the work of a vascular service. Urea and electrolyte levels could reveal renal insufficiency indicative of disease of either renal artery or parenchyma. Many patients who present to vascular clinics are found to have an abnormal random plasma glucose and this should be measured routinely. If abnormal, a formal glucose tolerance test should be arranged. In recent years, risk factor assessment and control has become standard practice in patients with vascular disease. Cholesterol and triglyceride levels should be measured in all patients and actively treated. In patients who have had a proven 'vascular event' (myocardial infarction, stroke), including all patients with established arterial claudication, the aim is to get the cholesterol level below 5 mmol/l (using a statin agent) and to normalise the triglycerides.

A full haematological profile should be measured. Patients with arterial insufficiency who are also anaemic will often note a marked improvement in their symptoms when this is corrected. Needless to say, a cause for such an anaemia must be found. Most patients with arterial disease also smoke and a proportion suffer from polycythaemia. Pathologically high haemoglobin levels and haematocrit can contribute to small vessel thrombosis in patients with critical limb ischaemia. The erythrocyte sedimentation rate is often elevated but this finding may be a useful indicator where graft infection, inflammatory aneurysm or a connective tissue disorder is suspected. Patients who present with symptoms suggestive of a vasospastic or vasculitic problem may require more extensive autoantibody screening tests as dictated by the individual patient's presentation.

Other more specific investigations that can be helpful in certain clinical settings include the measurement of urinary myoglobin and serum creatinine kinase in skeletal muscle infarction and elevation of serum lactate in (suspected) infarction of the intestine.

Clinical tests using continuous-wave Doppler

Systolic blood pressure at the ankle, using the hand-held continuous-wave (CW) Doppler ultrasound probe, is measured by noting the pressure at which the Doppler signal returns when deflating a blood pressure cuff placed around the calf. This figure can be related to the systolic pressure at the brachial level, which should also be measured by Doppler, giving the so-called ankle: brachial pressure index (ABPI). Typically, a claudicant will have an ABPI of 0.6–0.9. More severe ischaemia will usually be manifested by lower indices or even absent audible signals. The European Consensus stated that an absolute pressure of 50 mmHg or less in the presence of rest pain or tissue loss was indicative of critical ischaemia.

It should be remembered that calcified vessels are relatively incompressible (especially in diabetic patients) and so care must be taken in the interpretation of ABPI measurements in such individuals. In these circumstances the pole test may be employed. With the Doppler probe placed over an ankle artery, the height that the foot is elevated to above the horizontal, as measured on a calibrated pole, at which the Doppler signal disappears is equal to the perfusion pressure.

In patients with critical ischaemia in whom revascularisation is planned, hand-held Doppler can tell the examiner whether any distal arteries are patent. This is best assessed with the limb dependent. Often this will indicate whether or not distal reconstruction is an option. Some authors have recommended a modification of this technique. With a tourniquet around the thigh or proximal calf, the tibial arteries are insonated with the hand-held Doppler probe. By rapid inflation of the cuff to several hundred millimetres of mercury and deflation, a pulse is produced in the distal calf vessels if they are patent. This so-called 'pulse-generated' assessment of the run-off (PGR) is said to be a more sensitive guide to distal artery patency and utility for distal bypass.

Exercise test

Even after careful history and examination, it is sometimes difficult to be sure about the cause of exertional leg pain. Equally, in the setting of true vascular claudication, patients often underestimate the distance they can walk both before the onset of pain and before they have to stop. Therefore, it is desirable to have some form of objective assessment of the severity of disease. Some practitioners recommend taking the patient for a walk along the hospital corridor (the so-called 'corridor test').

A more accurate means of documenting the severity of claudication and, in difficult cases, excluding a vascular cause for the symptoms is the exercise test. The basic premise is that exercise leads to vasodilatation of the lower extremities and if there is a compromise to the arterial inflow of the limb, the measured pressure will drop after exercise and take some minutes to recover. The standard test involves measuring the ABPI, exercise on a treadmill at 3.5 km/hour at a 10° slope for three minutes or until symptoms preclude walking further. Sometimes, because of other problems (cardiac disease, arthropathy) patients cannot tolerate this test and various modifications have been developed. Suffice to say, a completely normal exercise test more or less rules out a vascular cause of leg pain. The same caveats apply to calcified, incompressible vessels as apply to resting ankle pressure measurements.

Hand-held Doppler and monitoring patients after treatment

Many surgeons use the hand-held Doppler to document patency during arterial operations. The waveform detected will alert the operator to the presence of turbulent or obstructed outflow. Also, during *in situ* vein bypass, the Doppler can be used to identify arteriovenous fistulae.

After intervention for lower limb ischaemia, either via percutaneous means or open surgery, it is important to monitor patients carefully. If the expected increase in ABPI is not observed immediately after surgical arterial reconstruction or endovascular therapy, the possibility of early failure should be suspected and investigated. Postoperative graft surveillance is a standard part of vascular practice. During follow-up, if disease recurs prior to vessel or graft occlusion, repeat intervention to maintain patency is often reasonably straightforward. As well as clinical parameters of recurrent stenosis (return of claudication or night pain), a drop in the ABPI may indicate incipient occlusion. However, it is not wise to rely upon this means of surveillance alone, as it is not sufficiently sensitive. As will be seen, the use of colour-flow Doppler ultrasound has revolutionised the surveillance of vascular reconstructions.

Toe pressures

One way of avoiding the spurious high ankle pressures encountered in diabetics and in patients with extensive vascular calcification and at the same time obtain an objective measure of distal perfusion is to measure the toe pressures. This technique utilises the same method as standard ABPI measurement, but with a small, specially designed cuff that fits around the digit (usually the hallux). This can be very helpful in deciding which diabetic patients with digital ulceration or gangrene will benefit from a revascularisation procedure. As a rule, in the normal subject, toe pressures are approximately two-thirds of ankle systolic pressure.

Transcutaneous oxygen saturation

By using an electrode applied directly to the skin surface, it is possible to obtain information on cutaneous oxygen tension, which in turn gives an indication of skin blood supply. In daily

clinical practice, the most frequent use of this device has been to determine the level of limb amputation that will achieve healing. However, the method does not appear to have been widely adopted.

Plethysmography

In the field of arterial surgery plethysmography has largely been used as a research tool. The technique measures the changes in limb volume that are attributable to changes in the circulation. There are different methods described, including volume plethysmography (still used in the technique of segmental pulse volume measurement), impedance plethysmography (which depends on the fact that the impedance to electrical conduction in a limb is related to the volume of blood 'the conductor' contained in the leg at the time) and photoplethysmography (which assesses skin blood flow in relation to the amount of light reflected). The use of plethysmography is more applicable to patients with venous disease, not least because it can be a cumbersome technique to perform and reproduce and also because much of the information yielded can be obtained from colour-flow Doppler ultrasound.

Ultrasound scanning

In arterial surgery, standard B-mode ultrasound is used to study the morphological features of arteries. One of the commonest uses of ultrasound is in the diagnosis and measurement of arterial aneurysms. Most vascular surgeons monitor small abdominal aneurysms with serial ultrasound scanning. This modality has been the investigation of choice for screening programmes and in the recently completed UK Small Aneurysm Trial. The machine is small and easily transported and it is relatively easy to acquire adequate skills to perform accurate scans. However, it should be appreciated that interobserver variability exists. The angle of insonation is very important in establishing the true anteroposterior diameter of an aortic aneurysm. A small variation between observers could lead to up to 20% difference in measured dimensions. In the UK Small Aneurysm Trial the repeatability of measurement of aneurysm diameter was ± 2 mm. The same limitation applies to the use of ultrasound in determining the level of the aneurysm neck in relation to the renal arteries.

More recently, it has become apparent that with ever-improving technology and image resolution, it is now possible to evaluate vessel wall morphology. Atheromatous plaques can be characterised according to their calcium content, their homogeneity, stability and the presence of surface ulceration and thrombus. This information is of particular use in the field of carotid artery surgery, where duplex scanning has largely replaced arteriography.

Combined B-mode and Doppler (duplex) ultrasound scanning

The investigation and management of arterial disease has been revolutionised by the advent of duplex ultrasound. It provides the

537

investigator with the morphological information of B-mode ultrasound together with the flow and velocity data obtained from spectral analysis of the entire arterial waveform. (Figure 36.1). Thus it is possible to insonate an artery, detect areas of abnormal flow and assess the region of abnormal and neighbouring normal flow in order to quantify the degree of stenosis.

Probes of differing frequencies are used according to the depth beneath the skin of the artery in question. For a superficial vessel such as the carotid artery, a 7.5 MHz probe is suitable, whereas a 3.5 MHz probe may be required to insonate the renal arteries.

It is a technology that is very observer dependent. Small variations in the angle at which the ultrasound probe is applied to the patient's skin can alter significantly the clarity of image obtained and, more importantly, the accuracy of the resulting velocity data. Experienced operators switch frequently between the B-mode and Doppler function (which shows colour flow within the vessel, red for one direction, blue for the opposite and increasingly lighter and brighter for regions of stenosis). By so doing, the Doppler function can be applied to the centre of the flow lumen to obtain the most accurate velocity data. The maximum blood velocity is seen at the highest point of the systolic waveform and this 'peak systolic velocity' increases with increasing degrees of stenosis.

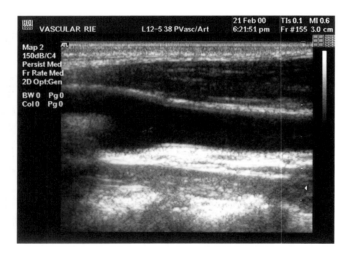

Figure 36.1 Duplex ultrasound scan of normal carotid bifurcation.

Clinical applications of arterial duplex scanning

CAROTID ARTERY DISEASE

Carotid endarterectomy (CEA) is one of the most frequently performed peripheral arterial operations. The initial investigation of choice for patients with unilateral cerebral hemispheric symptoms, amaurosis fugax or stroke with good recovery is duplex scanning of the carotid arteries. The clinician is provided

with information on the degree of stenosis, the status of the contralateral carotid artery (often diseased) and on the vertebral arteries. Damped signals in the common carotid artery raise the possibility of proximal or aortic arch disease, the presence of which could change the management of the patient. Accurate assessment of the morphology of the atherosclerotic plaque and the extent of disease is also obtained and from a practical point of view, as far as planning surgery is concerned, the level of the carotid bifurcation in relation to the mandible can be determined. As high-quality duplex scanning can provide so much information on carotid artery structure and function, many vascular surgeons now proceed to carotid endarterectomy on the strength of duplex alone and have largely abandoned conventional arteriography in this clinical setting. This creates a problem in relation to the indications for intervention since the internationally agreed criteria are based on the findings of multicentre trials, the European Carotid Surgery Trial (ECST) and the North American Symptomatic Carotid Endarterectomy Trial (NASCET), whose protocols were founded on the arteriographic estimation of stenosis. This is important in an operation carrying risk of serious morbidity and where the balance between risk and benefit is so finely poised. Clinicians relying on duplex scanning should validate its accuracy against arteriography if inappropriate interventions are to be avoided.

After many vascular surgical operations, some form of quality control study is performed before the patient leaves the operating room. After carotid surgery, some surgeons perform routine completion duplex scans prior to wound closure. The dual benefits of morphological and flow data guarantee as good a technical result as possible.

Transcranial Doppler (TCD) ultrasound is a further development that is being used increasingly for the intraoperative monitoring of CEA. A 2 MHz probe insonates the ipsilateral middle cerebral artery transcutaneously via the thinnest part of the petrous temporal bone. Microembolisation during dissection and after removal of clamps can be detected and minimised. Also, flow within the middle cerebral artery before and after clamping can be measured. If collateralisation from the vertebrobasilar and contralateral carotid systems is inadequate, flow will decrease significantly, indicating the need for shunt insertion. The patency of the shunt can be continuously monitored. Postoperatively, the TCD is often left *in situ* for a period during early recovery. It can detect occult emboli and indicate early problems (such as the development of thrombus at the endarterectomy site) and cerebral hyperperfusion syndrome which, if left untreated, could result in life-threatening neurological damage.

Duplex scanning is also the investigation of choice for patients suspected clinically of suffering from symptoms attributable to occlusive disease of the vertebral, subclavian and more distal upper limb arteries. Although often difficult to image the vessel in question directly (for example, the retroclavicular subclavian artery, the origin of the vertebral artery), the velocities obtained and the distal waveform can often detect significant stenoses and occlusions, various forms of compression (for example by cervical rib or anomalous fibrous band) and even differentiate between atherosclerotic disease and other forms of stenosis such as arteritis and radiation injury.

LOWER EXTREMITY ISCHAEMIA

As with carotid artery disease, in many centres, the initial investigation of patients presenting with lower limb ischaemia, especially those with intermittent claudication, is by means of duplex scanning. The information obtained determines which patients should proceed to invasive investigation and/or treatment. The precise location of disease, the degree of stenosis, the length of stenoses or occlusions and the status of the distal run-off can all be documented accurately. In obese subjects and in patients with a lot of intraluminal bowel gas, accurate visualisation of the aorta and iliac arteries is sometimes not possible but in experienced hands, this only happens in about 25% of such patients. This non-invasive and easily repeatable imaging technique avoids the potential complications of arteriography (see below) and other invasive means of visualising the arterial tree. Even if the patient is treated subsequently by percutaneous transluminal balloon angioplasty, the initial assessment with duplex will reduce significantly the number of arteriograms performed and identify the exact location and nature of the treatable lesion(s).

In the setting of surgical reconstruction, duplex scanning has a number of important roles to play. It has been used by some authors to identify the optimal tibial vessel for use as the run-off in femoro-distal bypass. More subtly, stenoses of the common femoral and profunda femoris arteries can be quantified using duplex-derived velocity criteria. This can often influence the planned reconstruction. Preoperative duplex mapping of the proposed vein conduit (ipsilateral/contralateral long saphenous vein, short saphenous vein, arm vein) obviates the need for fruitless blind vein exploration with all the associated wound-healing problems. Some surgeons use intraoperative duplex scanning to assess the completed graft on-table.

Postoperative vein graft surveillance constitutes a considerable part of the routine work of a vascular laboratory. Approximately 30% of infrainguinal vein bypass grafts develop haemodynamically significant stenoses as a direct consequence of their placement into the arterial circulation. The vast majority of these lesions occur in the first 12 months after graft placement and therefore the most intensive period of surveillance is during this early post-bypass period (Figure 36.2). Intervention to correct haemodynamically significant stenoses (usually where the velocity within the stenotic segment is three times or greater than that in the normal neighbouring graft) greatly enhances long-term patency. The patency of such grafts when a thrombectomy or thrombolysis has been required to recanalise them after occlusion is poor and more or less condemns the patient to repeat bypass or amputation if no other bypass option is available.

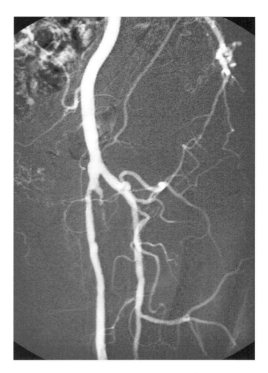

Figure 36.2 IADSA of arm vein femoro-popliteal graft in which duplex surveillance had identified a significant proximal graft stenosis. This was repaired with a vein patch.

RENAL AND MESENTERIC VASCULAR DISEASE

Although attractive in concept, the use of duplex scanning to image the renal and visceral arteries, as the primary imaging technique, has not gained widespread favour. Consistent and reproducible scans of the arteries are difficult to obtain owing to body habitus, the presence of bowel gas and the variation in angulation of the vessel origins. Thus in routine clinical practice, arteriography remains the preferred diagnostic tool. Nevertheless, there are proponents of the use of duplex scanning to monitor these vessels after intervention.

INTRAVASCULAR ULTRASOUND

In recent years, with the expansion of endovascular techniques, including angioplasty, stenting, atherectomy and endoluminal stent grafting, the use of intravascular ultrasound (IVUS) to image the vessel after intervention has been introduced. This sophisticated technology enables the operator to visualise both the vessel lumen and its wall in cross-section. Computer technology can be used to assess the efficacy of treatment. It is possible to obtain this analysis during treatment and, if necessary, perform secondary interventions based upon the result. This is largely a research tool at present.

Arteriography

The standard against which all the newer imaging techniques are compared is arteriography. Arteriographic technology has also advanced such that high-quality images can be obtained in multiple planes with minimal morbidity. Nowadays, the contrast agents used are usually non-thrombogenic, non-ionic and non-iodine based. The most common route for gaining access to the arterial tree is via the femoral artery. A catheter (3 or 4 French gauge) is passed into the infrarenal aorta by the Seldinger technique and, using an injection pump system, 10–15 ml boluses of contrast are injected as the images are taken. If the infrarenal aorta or iliac arteries are occluded or not accessible for other reasons (for example, previous surgery in the groins, infection), the radial or brachial arteries can be utilised. Translumbar arteriography is no longer performed. In certain circumstances, the injection of contrast into the venous system will give adequate arteriograms.

Modern arteriography is performed using digital subtraction technology which produces superior images. First an image of the area of interest is taken without any contrast, after which a bolus of contrast agent is given and a further image taken with the original background subtracted by computer. This gives clear definition of vessels, especially smaller, distal arteries in low-flow situations, which were notoriously difficult to image using conventional, non-subtracted images. Another feature of contemporary arteriography is the ability to produce images in multiple planes. More often than not, atherosclerotic stenoses are eccentric. In extreme cases, depending on the angle from which the arteriogram is taken, such a lesion may not be apparent or at least, the degree of stenosis may be underestimated (Figure 36.3). Under such circumstances, a combination of biplanar arteriography and duplex scanning can be complementary, both in determining the severity of disease and in aiding the plan for treatment. Digital subtraction arteriography can provide excellent

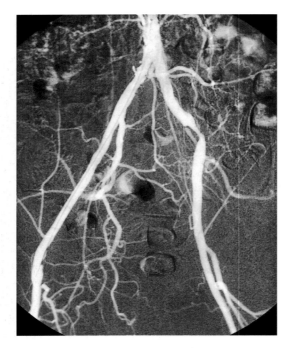

Figure 36.3 IADSA of tight, eccentric left common iliac artery stenosis.

images of the entire peripheral arterial tree including the pedal and carpal circulations. Compared to traditional arteriography, the dose of radiation and contrast is significantly less. It is also possible to quantify the degree of stenosis during arteriography by measuring the pressure gradient across it. This is particularly helpful in the aortoiliac segment when endovascular therapy is proposed.

The complications of intraarterial arteriography are related to the procedure itself and to the side effects of the contrast agent used. Puncture site bleeding and haematoma are not uncommon but usually relatively minor, especially with modern fine-gauge catheters. However, false aneurysms are still encountered, especially when arteriography has been combined with endovascular manipulations, such as angioplasty or stenting involving larger catheters. Iatrogenic false aneurysms of the femoral artery present to the vascular surgeon on a fairly regular basis. Generally speaking, those lesions measuring less than 2 cm in diameter tend to close off spontaneously. Some radiologists and surgeons practise the technique of duplex-directed manual compression to seal the defect in the femoral artery. Recently, this approach has been supplemented with the local injection of thrombin. This is an uncomfortable experience for the patient. The indications for surgical repair of an arterial false aneurysm include size greater than 3 cm, symptomatic expansion, evidence of compression of neighbouring structures (for example, the femoral vein or nerve) and incipient skin ulceration. Occasionally, distal embolisation can occur. Catheter-induced intimal dissection and athero-embolisation are seen occasionally.

Contrast-related complications are a not infrequent occurrence. Iodine sensitivity, if not previously noted, can lead to anaphylactic reactions of variable severity. Patients with peripheral arterial disease often suffer from cardiac and renal insufficiency and a significant proportion are diabetic. In these patients, the potential for contrast-induced pulmonary oedema and acute-on-chronic renal failure should be appreciated. In recent years, it has become apparent that non-insulin dependent diabetic patients taking metformin can be at risk of lactic acidosis and renal failure after the administration of iodine-containing contrast agents. It is now advised that such patients do not take metformin for two days prior to arteriography and that this medication is only recommenced when the renal function is normal or at least restored to pre-arteriographic levels.

As mentioned above, in some circumstances, where intraarterial arteriography is not available, adequate images can be provided by an intravenous injection of contrast. One advantage of this approach is the avoidance of the complications of arterial puncture. Some clinicians prefer this approach for the investigation of patients with localised aortoiliac disease, carotid artery disease and the assessment of the proximal neck of aortic aneurysms. However, intravenous digital subtraction arteriography (IVDSA) has a number of problems associated with it. A far larger dose of contrast agent is required in order to obtain clear images and even then, patient movement can lead to blurring of images and the consequent loss of definition. In addition, good cardiac function is necessary to allow adequate contrast to reach the femoral and more distal vessels. Therefore, poor cardiac function and renal impairment are two major contraindications to the use of IVDSA. In most centres duplex ultrasound scanning has largely replaced IVDSA.

In recent years, some authors have suggested that the complications associated with iodine-based contrast can be overcome by using alternative agents. Carbon dioxide arteriography has been described and literally involves direct intraarterial injection of carbon dioxide. Blood is displaced by the gas and images obtained. In expert hands, the images obtained seem to be of reasonable quality, but this technique has not really been widely adopted. Because carbon dioxide is very soluble in blood, detail of long arterial segments and distal vascular beds is not easy to visualise. The use of magnetic resonance without contrast (see below) is another innovation that obviates the need to use iodine-based agents.

Although much of the initial screening of patients can be performed using non-invasive tests such as ABPI measurement, exercise testing and duplex scanning, arteriography remains the mainstay of imaging prior to arterial intervention, most surgeons feeling more comfortable with a map of their target area. Decisions whether to operate can be taken on the basis of duplex scanning, leaving arteriography if required to be performed on the operating table. Even in carotid surgery, where many vascular surgeons readily perform endarterectomy on the strength of duplex scan information alone, there is still a place for arteriography. Patients with hemispheric symptoms in whom the duplex scan fails to define the extent of disease in the internal carotid artery are best investigated with selective carotid arteriography, albeit at the risk of a quoted procedure-related stroke rate of 0.5–1%. Patients with extremely calcified vessels and those with multilevel, arch, carotid and possible siphon disease are often best investigated with intraarterial arteriography.

Patients who require intervention for lower limb ischaemia can mostly be identified using duplex. Percutaneous interventions and operative reconstruction require accurate, detailed arteriograms and only a few surgeons with access to the highest quality non-invasive studies operate for lower limb ischaemia on the strength of duplex alone. For post-reconstruction intraoperative quality control the completion arteriogram is the preferred option. After endovascular intervention (angioplasty, stenting) this is naturally the most obvious and readily performed study. With catheters *in situ*, it is possible to assess objectively whether the pressure gradient across a stenosis has been successfully eradicated. During open bypass operations, it is very easy to obtain views of the entire graft and run-off vessels. After vein bypass, a fine-gauge cannula can be introduced via a tributary and on-table arteriograms obtained. Abnormalities of the conduit and anastomosis (residual valve cusps, intraluminal thrombus, extrinsic compression) can be identified and thus guide immediate corrective intervention. Intraoperative arteriography is also an important quality check during embolectomy or thrombectomy.

Intraarterial arteriography is the investigation of choice for renovascular disease and mesenteric vascular disease. In the investigation of aortic aneurysms, patients with involvement of the renal or visceral arteries often have occlusive lesions affecting these vessels, anatomic variants are not uncommon and surgery is aided by the use of preoperative arteriography. This is undoubtedly the case for thoracoabdominal aneurysms where arteriography is one of a number of complementary investigations performed as a matter of routine. Other clinical situations where intraarterial arteriography is still important include: the thoracic outlet syndrome, with arterial symptoms as the presenting feature, vascular trauma, carotid body tumour assessment (now being replaced by magnetic resonance imaging (MRI) and arteriography (MRA) in some centres) and the preintervention imaging of arteriovenous malformations which have a significant arterial component.

Computed tomography

The investigation of many conditions has been greatly enhanced by the accuracy and level of detail offered by modern computed tomography (CT). Nowhere is this more true than in the investigation of patients with aortic aneurysms (Figure 36.4) One of the problems with ultrasound scanning is the potential for variability between observers in determining the true anteroposterior diameter of the aneurysm. Although this problem can still exist with CT scans if the cuts are in any way oblique, in practice, this is not a major problem and probably only accounts for at most a few millimetres of variation. The introduction of spiral CT scans minimises this problem, allows for easy assessment of the relationship of the renal arteries to the aneurysm neck and enables a three-dimensional image of the aortic aneurysm to be reconstructed. This has potential benefits for planning endovascular

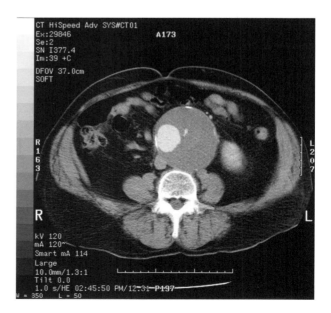

Figure 36.4 Computed tomogram of infrarenal abdominal aortic aneurysm.

541

stent graft repair. Indeed, CT scan is one of the means used to monitor stent grafts post insertion. Most surgeons use CT scanning as the primary investigation for aortic aneurysms, whether infrarenal, visceral or thoracoabdominal. Contrast medium is injected intravenously and the scans timed to coincide with maximum concentration within the arterial circulation. Standard scans are performed with either 5 or 10 mm intervals between cuts. With modern spiral CT it is possible to perform much narrower cuts than this. In areas of specific interest, for example at the level of the renal arteries, to establish the exact level of the proximal aortic aneurysm neck, cuts 1 mm apart can be produced.

CT scanning confers the bonus of identifying co-existent pathology that is clinically inapparent. In our experience, the identification of tumours of the pancreas, liver and bladder detected during the work-up of patients with aortic aneurysms has radically influenced the subsequent clinical management.

The value of CT scanning in the management of patients with AAA presenting as an emergency is debatable. Delay is seldom justified and it has been demonstrated that CT is not a particularly sensitive or reliable imaging modality for the detection of small leaks. The role of CT in this setting is probably to give information about the proximal extent of aneurysmal disease in those patients who are stable and in whom an urgent suprarenal or thoracoabdominal repair would not be contemplated.

CT scanning is also the investigation of choice for patients suspected of having an acute aortic dissection. Valuable information can be obtained about the proximal and distal extent of the dissection, the presence of co-existing aneurysmal disease and the status of the visceral and renal arteries in relation to the true and false lumina.

Finally, in relation to aortic surgery, if a patient is suspected of having an infected aortic prosthesis, CT scan is again the first-line investigation of choice. The presence of fluid and, more particularly, gas around an aortic graft is diagnostic of graft infection although it is not unusual to see air within the closed sac around the graft for several days after insertion. Anastomotic false aneurysms will also be demonstrated by CT.

In the field of extracranial carotid artery disease, CT scanning is used to image the brain of patients being considered for carotid endarterectomy. Some authors question the worth of this investigation as a matter of routine and argue that rarely do the findings on CT scan of the brain influence the clinical decision to operate on patients with hemispheric symptoms or amaurosis fugax who have severe carotid artery stenosis. However, the presence of preoperative CT scan infarcts is a surgical risk factor. In many patients thought to have sustained only transient cerebral ischaemia, areas of infarction can be found. The presence of haemorrhagic infarction is of major significance both in terms of the decision to operate and also in relation to the use of systemic anticoagulation. Occasionally, some other form of intracranial pathology will be encountered. For these reasons, many clinicians perform routine CT scanning of the brain prior to carotid

endarterectomy. When stroke occurs as a postoperative event CT scanning is employed to distinguish between intracranial haemorrhage and infarction.

Magnetic resonance imaging (MRI)

In the investigation of patients with vascular disease, this technology offers the dual advantages of avoiding ionising radiation and iodine-containing contrast agents. MRI depends on high-powered magnetic fields and their effect on the protons in the body tissues. After computer processing the images obtained are similar in appearance to CT scans. If required, reconstructions can be created in the sagittal and coronal planes. Because of its ability to focus on tissues of one density, MRI provides excellent discrimination between a lesion and the surrounding tissues.

The indications for and uses of MRI in vascular surgery are expanding all the time. Reconstructed images in different planes are helpful in determining the morphology of aortic aneurysms and in particular the relationship of the aneurysm to the renal arteries.

The imaging of arteriovenous malformations and vascular tumours has been greatly improved by the ability of MR to distinguish these lesions from surrounding muscle and connective tissues. This unique attribute makes MRI extremely useful in the investigation of carotid body tumours.

Because of its ability to distinguish between connective tissues and fluid/solid interfaces, MRI has proved useful in determining the extent of soft tissue and bone involvement in sepsis associated with the diabetic foot. Several authors have compared conventional plain radiology, bone scans with radioisotopes and MRI and the latter has proved the most sensitive and specific. MRI studies have shown that in foot sepsis, bony involvement is usually to one level more proximal than indicated by the other two imaging techniques.

Non-iodine containing contrast agents have been developed for use in conjunction with MRI. As a result, magnetic resonance angiography (MRA) is now being used increasingly in some centres (Figure 36.5). Although an exciting prospect, MRA is not yet at the stage of superseding conventional digital subtraction arteriography.

Radio-isotope scans

In vascular surgery, infection is one of the clinician's greatest enemies. The accurate detection and delineation of the extent of infection is crucial to the optimum treatment of the patient.

Prosthetic graft infection is an insidious entity and, especially when aortic grafts are involved, may not be obvious at initial presentation. Patients are often non-specifically unwell with malaise, weight loss, night sweats, etc. but have no clear clinical signs of graft sepsis. As mentioned previously, CT scanning may

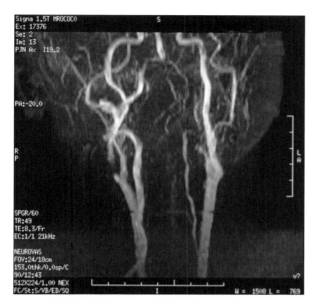

Figure 36.5 Magnetic resonance angiogram of a high-grade right internal carotid artery stenosis.

demonstrate the presence of gas around the prosthesis, which is pathognomonic of infection. However, sometimes the CT scan is unhelpful or at most demonstrates the presence of perigraft fluid, which is not necessarily diagnostic of infection, particularly if the graft has only been *in situ* for a short period of time. In these circumstances, the use of a labelled white cell scan can prove very helpful. The technique involves taking 60–100 ml of blood, spinning the sample to separate out the white blood cells, labelling these white cells with a radio-isotope (usually indium-111 or technetium-99) and then reinjecting the labelled cells back into the patient. The patients are scanned with a gamma camera 1–2 hours later and then again after a few more hours (exact times vary according to the isotope used and departmental practice). A positive scan shows a 'hot spot' in the region of the vascular prosthesis where the labelled white cells have migrated. The specificity of this test in the investigation of graft infection has been estimated at 90%.

Plain radiographic studies

It should not be forgotten in these days of advanced technology that conventional investigations still have an occasional part to play in patient assessment. Plain radiographs of the chest are performed as part of routine preoperative work-up of many patients. The possibility of the co-existence of lung malignancy and other diseases should always be borne in mind. Chest radiographs and specific thoracic outlet views demonstrate cervical ribs and notching of the ribs in coarctation of the aorta. Asymptomatic aortic aneurysms are diagnosed quite frequently by specialists in other disciplines on plain radiographs. Although inferior to MRI, plain radiographs will identify osteomyelitis of the foot in the majority of cases.

VENOUS SYSTEM

Introduction

Increasing specialisation means that venous disease has become largely the province of the specialist rather than the general surgeon. Its management requires in-depth knowledge of epidemiology, pathology, haemodynamics, haemostasis fibrinolysis and venous anatomy and its variations. Regular access to a vascular laboratory is essential. Testimonies to the need for such specialisation are the high recurrence rates after varicose vein surgery and the poor healing rates and high recurrence rates for chronic leg ulcer whether treated conservatively or by surgery.

Congenital venous malformations and venous tumours are rare. The bulk of phlebological practice arises from valvular dysfunction (varicose veins, chronic venous insufficiency and venous ulcer) together with venous thromboembolic disease both acute and chronic.

One of the impediments to research and quality assurance in phlebology has been the proliferation of definitions, terminology and eponymous nomenclature. Various classifications have been proposed, the most recent being the CEAP classification in which disease is scored according to **C**linical signs, (**A**)**E**tiology, **A**natomic distribution and **P**athophysiological dysfunction.

Clinical history

Chronic venous disease

It is important when taking a history from a patient with varicose veins to detect any unusual aetiology such as prior deep venous thrombosis (DVT) or congenital anomaly. Careful enquiry about possible previous DVT is essential for several reasons: it highlights the need for antithrombotic precautions in 'at-risk' situations; postthrombotic varicose veins may represent the development of collateral channels bypassing occluded deep segments; and postthrombotic damage to deep veins is a major risk factor for poor prognosis in the conservative or surgical treatment of venous ulceration. Operative intervention in such a case, without taking into account the presence of postthrombotic disease, may be harmful to the patient. Although many venous thromboses are never diagnosed, DVT sufficient to lead to secondary varicose veins will usually have been a clinically obvious event known to the patient, such as peripartum leg swelling, major trauma or an acute hospital episode. Venous anomalies are usually apparent in childhood, with varicose veins appearing at an unusual site and commonly associated with venous capillary angioma.

A history of leg swelling should raise warning flags. The most common cause of leg swelling is posture, dependency or prolonged standing giving rise to unremitting high venous pressure. This may occur in an otherwise normal leg. It is aggravated by immobility, occupations involving a lot of standing, obesity, pregnancy or varicose veins. Postural causes give rise to foot swelling and puffiness at the ankles but more extensive oedema affecting the upper calf or thigh indicates DVT, lymph-oedema or systemic disease, usually cardiac or renal. The significance of the location of the swelling, especially at time of onset, is critical to correct diagnosis and is discussed below in relation to DVT.

In distinguishing venous ulceration from other causes of chronic leg ulceration a history of varicose veins and/or deep vein thrombosis is obviously central. Other important associated diseases include arterial disease, diabetes and rheumatoid disease. The chronicity of leg ulcer and whether the patient has had multiple episodes provide important clues to its likelihood of responding to conservative therapy. The prevalence of chronic leg ulcer peaks in the eighth decade and in that age group approximately 20% of the general population will be found to have arterial insufficiency. This is an important condition to recognise, regardless of whether it is responsible for the ulceration since, if severe, it will impair healing and prevent the application of compression therapy.

Many chronic ulcers are relatively pain free. The complaint of excessive pain especially at night should raise the possibility that the ulcer is arterial in type. Sometimes even a small venous ulcer can be very painful especially if it is inflamed, exudate is causing skin maceration or if it overlies a sensitive structure such as the malleolar periosteum. Rest with elevation will normally provide relief. If it aggravates the pain an arterial cause is likely.

DVT in the great majority of cases occurs in a predisposing context such as trauma, pregnancy, acute illness, malignant disease, surgery, immobility or travel. When it occurs without any such predisposing event consider occult malignant disease. A history of repeated thrombotic episodes should suggest thrombo-philia, especially when occurring at an unusually young age or when there is a positive family history. Most early DVTs are non-occlusive and occult and are therefore not diagnosed by either history or examination. The first indication may be pulmonary embolism. The cardinal presenting leg symptoms are pain localised to the affected venous segment and swelling. Both are late symptoms in the thrombotic process, the pain being due to a periphlebitic inflammatory response and swelling the manifestation of extensive occlusive thrombus possibly aggravated by lymphatic compromise.

A key question in relation to new swelling in the limb is 'Where did the swelling begin?'. The common variety of DVT commences in the calf veins and may or may not progress proximally. If swelling occurs at all it will be maximal in the foot and ankle. Swelling which begins in mid-calf or around the knee and only later extends to the ankle and foot is not typical of DVT and is much more likely to be due to other pathology such as ruptured Baker's cyst or calf haematoma. In venous thrombosis affecting the iliac segment, as for example when associated with pregnancy or hip surgery, the swelling commences in the thigh, extending later and in lesser degree to the lower leg.

Examination

Varicose veins

There are two distinct circumstances in which varicose veins are examined in detail and different techniques are employed. The first is the assessment of the patient in the outpatient clinic. Here the questions are:

- What type of varicose veins are we dealing with?

- Is there anything to suggest venous anomaly or arteriovenous malformation?

- Is treatment indicated and if so, what type of intervention would be appropriate?

- What are the probable sites of deep to superficial reflux?

- If intervention is planned, what prior investigation is required?

- Are the varices (and the patient) suitable for day surgery?

The second circumstance is immediately before surgical intervention. The assessment must be made by the surgeon who is to operate. Here the questions are:

- What are the anatomical connections between the veins to be removed and the known sites of deep to superficial reflux?

- Where exactly do I need to place my incisions to give optimal access to sites of deep to superficial reflux?

- Which varices are to be removed?

The patient stands on an elevated surface, in a good light, in a warm environment. The surgeon should be seated so that the examination can be comfortable and unhurried. Inspection, if carefully done, will take the clinician a long way towards correct assessment of the nature of the problem, especially in primary varicose veins. This may not be the case, however, in the obese or swollen leg, nor in recurrent varices or chronic venous insufficiency. By and large, in the primary condition, varices will be in the distribution of the known tributaries of the saphenous stems. The distribution of varicose veins gives a strong indication as to the likely location of deep to superficial reflux, as does the distribution of lipodermatosclerosis. The surgeon may be misled by variations in the termination of the short saphenous vein and its connections with the long saphenous. Varices which are most prominent on the posterolateral aspect of the thigh or upper calf should raise suspicion of a congenital abnormality such as the Klippel–Trenaunay syndrome (Figure 36.6). Capillary angioma is part of the syndrome but may not always be conspicuous.

Poor results of surgery can to a large extent be attributed to inadequate preoperative assessment and marking. Palpation and percussion over dilated venous segments assist the delineation of incompetent channels. Insonation with a CW Doppler may indicate sites of deep to superficial reflux, but generally if surgery is planned the anatomy should be checked with duplex ultra-sonography, especially when a reflux signal is heard over the popliteal fossa. Preoperatively the varices should be mapped out in full with an indelible marker so that during operation, when the veins are empty in the supine position, the anatomy of the incompetent system is still explicit (Figure 36.7).

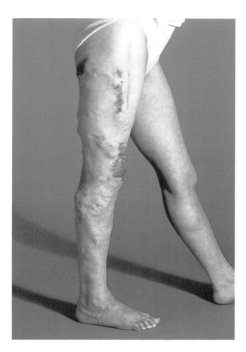

Figure 36.6 Klippel–Trenaunay syndrome. Note the lateral distribution of the varicose veins and the presence of capillary angioma.

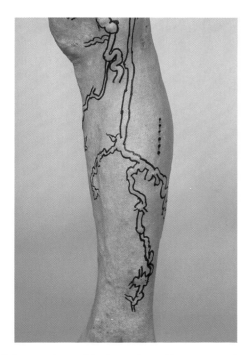

Figure 36.7 Preoperative marking in a patient with recurrent varicose veins.

Chronic leg ulcer

The aetiology of most leg ulcers can be diagnosed simply by inspection. The site is important, as is the condition of the surrounding skin. Venous ulcers are typically located in the ankle 'gaiter' area but may extend on to the foot and/or up the calf (Figure 36.8). The skin changes of lipodermatosclerosis (pigmentation, induration, atrophy blanche, dermatitis) will be present. Not every venous ulcer is associated with visible varicose veins, especially in the obese, oedematous or postphlebitic leg. A venous ulcer is most commonly located on the medial side, related to long saphenous incompetence and overlying or just below one or more incompetent perforators. An ulcer originating on the posterolateral aspect of the ankle is commonly associated with short saphenous incompetence. Venous ulcers are typically single, oval in shape and relatively shallow with a shelving margin, although with chronicity the appearances may change. A heaped-up margin and/or a bleeding tendency suggests malignancy. The presence of tendon in the bed of an ulcer indicates arterial insufficiency or occasionally an acute vasculitis.

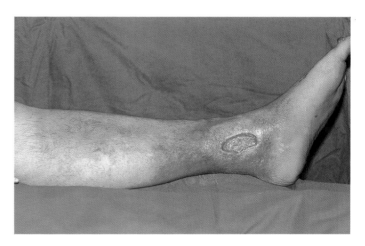

Figure 36.8 A typical venous ulcer with extensive lipodermatosclerosis.

DVT

Examination of the leg for DVT is performed with the patient supine. Early signs often quoted are the warm limb due to opening of collateral circulation and distended superficial veins. These are seldom seen. Homan's sign, calf discomfort on passive dorsiflexion, is non-specific and unhelpful. The two cardinal signs are oedema and local tenderness. They are usually relatively late signs in the pathological process and diagnostic errors are common. The level and degree of swelling provide important clues as to the location of the thrombus. Any degree of swelling suggests a serious, occlusive thrombosis. Swelling affecting the ankle region is likely to be associated with a thrombus extending at least into the popliteal vein. Swelling extending up to the knee suggests occlusive thrombosis involving at least the common femoral vein and swelling in the thigh points to iliofemoral or even caval thrombus. If both legs are swollen caval thrombus becomes highly probable. Iliofemoral thrombosis with occlusion of the major stem veins (but not of all collaterals) results in swelling and pallor of the limb – phlegmasia alba dolens. If both the stem veins and collateral channels including the micro-circulation are affected by the thrombotic process such that the outflow to the limb is seriously impeded the limb becomes both grossly swollen and blue – phlegmasia caerulea dolens. This is a pregangrenous condition and most commonly associated with disseminated malignant disease.

The differential diagnosis includes trauma, lymphoedema, ruptured Baker's cyst, acute arterial occlusion, infection, dependent oedema and various systemic causes of chronic swelling.

Hand-held continuous-wave Doppler (CWD)

The development of this simple tool in the 1970s made possible for the first time a discriminating non-invasive assessment of the venous system. Although overtaken by duplex, CWD is still useful and is best regarded as a routine component of physical examination rather than a formal laboratory investigation. The patient is examined standing in the same way as described for physical examination. Muscles and fascia should be relaxed by slight flexion of the knee. Reflux is elicited by a calf squeeze followed by release. Reflux through a perforator can be distinguished from a superficial vein by placing a venous tourniquet above the suspected perforator. CWD requires considerable practice and experience, however, and cannot be relied upon as an infallible guide upon which targeted surgical intervention can be based.

The main difficulty is the distinction between deep and superficial reflux, especially in the popliteal fossa. If the incompetent stem or varix is tracked up the limb from a lower level with the Doppler probe, the experienced observer can usually resolve the difficulty but in the case of complex veins such as anatomical anomalies or recurrent varicose veins, more discriminating investigation is essential. To further complicate the situation, duplex ultrasonography has brought with it the recognition that the demonstration of valvular competence at the saphenofemoral or saphenopopliteal junction does not exclude the need for surgery to the saphenous stem at a lower level. Segmental reflux in a saphenous stem, fed for example from a thigh perforator, can commonly be detected by means of duplex below a competent junction.

Investigations

The investigation of venous disease comes under two headings: imaging and tests of venous function. Imaging tests are an indispensable part of everyday clinical practice whereas venous function tests are mainly employed in specialised centres and are largely the province of the research laboratory. For detailed

discussion of the investigation of venous disease, the reader is referred to specialist texts.

Imaging tests

Conventional contrast phlebography, ultrasonography, CT and MRI may all play a part in the management of venous disorders. In routine practice the dominant role of phlebography has been taken over by ultrasonography.

Duplex Scanning

CHRONIC VENOUS DISEASE

Duplex scanning offers, for the first time in the history of venous surgery, the opportunity for the surgeon to tailor the intervention with precision to the pattern of valvular reflux by means of a non-invasive investigation. A considerable level of skill on the part of the sonographer combined with sound anatomical knowledge is required for venous scanning which means that there is a long learning curve.

Duplex scanning is a test of both image and function. Colour coding assists rapid vessel localisation and vessel morphology can be examined. Imaging provides the map to guide the surgeon. The improved definition offered by the latest generation of scanners is making it possible to assess the competence even of tibial veins and individual calf perforators so that the haemodynamic abnormalities which underlie clinical patterns of disease and which determine clinical outcomes are now being unravelled. Reflux in the popliteal segment, for example, is associated with poor ulcer healing rates and a liability to recurrence. Duplex scanning has also been used to guide sclerotherapy.

The patient is examined standing or, if this is difficult for the patient, semi-supported at a 30° angle. Reflux is elicited by Valsalva or more reliably by release of a calf squeeze. The latter can be standardised by use of a pneumatic compression device but most experts prefer to use a manual squeeze. The quantification of reflux on duplex has presented an unresolved problem. Even normal valves will reflux to some degree in normal physiological circumstances. The duration of reflux which is pathologically significant is generally taken to be >0.5 s.

The duplex scan is utilised prior to surgery. The sonographer should provide information on both the superficial and deep systems, in terms of incompetence and patency. In the case of short saphenous incompetence the site of the saphenopopliteal junction should be precisely and indelibly marked to facilitate accurate placement of the incision. The same applies to localisation of perforators. The sonographer should provide a detailed map of the findings.

Patients with complex varices should be assessed with duplex prior to surgery. Many argue a convincing case that all patients with varicose veins should be scanned given the high levels of recurrence and increasing litigation, but limited resources are a countervailing consideration in most UK centres. Certainly, where there is any difficulty in deciphering the anatomy by physical examination with CWD, as for example in the obese leg, duplex should be undertaken. In the case of primary varices in experienced hands CW Doppler will usually clarify the presence and location of saphenofemoral reflux. However, in the popliteal fossa the detection with CWD of any reflux is an indication for a duplex scan both to confirm short saphenous incompetence and to define the anatomy in an area where there are many variations, recurrence is common and dissection carries a risk of nerve damage.

DEEP VENOUS THROMBOSIS

Duplex scanning has also transformed the clinical management of suspected DVT while at the same time posing considerable logistical and staffing problems for sonography services in many institutions phlebography being performed by radiologists and ultrasonography in the main by technologists. The availability of a non-invasive method attracts increased referrals.

It is important to understand the limitations of duplex diagnosis of DVT. The detection of DVT by duplex scans depends on a combination of the observation of intraluminal thrombus, compromised flow and non-compressibility of the target vein by the examining probe. Early non-occlusive thrombus which does not limit flow and in which the process of organisation has not stiffened the vein is therefore difficult to detect. As noted earlier, when DVT presents with leg symptoms of pain, tenderness or swelling the inflammatory process of organisation is well advanced, the thrombus will almost invariably have become occlusive and will thus be detected by duplex assuming that the target vein is sonographically accessible. Thrombus in cava, iliac veins or tibial veins may not be detected, especially if non-occlusive.

Recent studies have shown that a systematic approach to the diagnosis of DVT and pulmonary embolism by means of a protocol involving plasma D-dimer measurement by rapid ELISA, duplex ultrasonography and lung scan can reduce the need for pulmonary angiography to as little as 5% and phlebography to <1% in patients presenting with suspected venous thromboembolism.

PULMONARY EMBOLISM

The majority of patients who die of embolism have had one or more prior embolic events. Therefore, in the patient presenting with suspected pulmonary embolism, provided that life is not immediately threatened, the top priority is the identification and definition of the source of the embolism. Duplex scanning is a reasonable first line of attack and, if clearly positive and the extent of the thrombus effectively defined, can provide the basis for therapy. However, if the scan is negative or equivocal bilateral ascending phlebography should be performed.

In summary, symptomatic thrombus in femoral or popliteal veins can be diagnosed with confidence by duplex ultrasonography. A

high diagnostic accuracy can also be achieved for symptomatic calf vein thrombosis, given high-resolution colour flow equipment and a high level of sonographic skill. However, scanning at calf level may be difficult and time consuming. Difficulties may be encountered in the iliac veins and cava and also in the shoulder region. In addition, duplex cannot be depended upon as the sole diagnostic modality in patients without leg symptoms who present with suspected pulmonary embolism nor can it be recommended as a screening tool for DVT which has not yet manifested clinical symptoms in the limb.

It follows that a protocol employing duplex scanning as the prime diagnostic tool for suspected DVT should involve early repetition of the examination, say within 2–3 days, in any patient in whom there is remaining diagnostic doubt, especially if it is not planned to treat the patient with a full course of anticoagulation. The alternative is phlebography.

Phlebography

This time-honoured method has underpinned much of what we know about the pathology and natural history of venous disease and remains the reference standard. It has been partially eclipsed by duplex scanning, but does still have an occasional place in a range of venous disorders and clinical circumstances.

CHRONIC VENOUS DISEASE

For patients in whom there is a strong suspicion that chronic venous insufficiency is postphlebitic in nature, especially where there is doubt as to the advisability of operating on the superficial veins, an ascending phlebogram provides more useful information than a duplex scan. Whenever reconstruction or bypass of the deep veins is contemplated the surgeon will usually require the detailed anatomical definition provided by ascending or occasionally descending (per-femoral) phlebography.

VENOUS THROMBOSIS

In DVT, as outlined above, phlebography may be required to confirm or supplement duplex scanning, especially in locations less readily defined by ultrasound such as the iliac veins, vena cava, shoulder region or mediastinum. Phlebography may also be required in conjunction with thrombolytic therapy. Non-thrombogenic contrast medium is employed. In the case of suspected lower limb DVT, ascending phlebography is the method of choice and should generally be done bilaterally even when the symptoms are entirely unilateral. There are two reasons for this. The first is that unsuspected but clinically important DVT may be present in the asymptomatic limb and secondly that unless there is a sufficient volume of contrast ascending from both limbs adequate, visualisation of the inferior vena cava, into which life-threatening iliac thrombus commonly extends, is seldom achieved. A phlebogram which fails fully to visualise the entire venous pathway from the site of injection to the inferior vena cava may be seriously misleading. If the policy of routinely employing bilateral ascending phlebography is followed perfemoral phlebography should seldom be needed. Ascending phlebography should not be attempted in patients who have a major degree of outflow obstruction from the limb, i.e. plegmasia alba or caerulea dolens, because aggravation of the condition may occur or damaging extravasation of injected contrast.

Upper limb phlebography has an important place in venous thoracic outlet syndrome, axillary or subclavian thrombosis both for initial diagnosis and for monitoring the response to thrombolytic therapy, which is often more successful in lysing DVT in the upper limb than it is in the lower.

Phlebography by direct venous injection or by visualisation of the venous phase of an arteriogram is utilised in the investigation of vascular tumours. Phlebography is also employed in centres where venous valve reconstruction is undertaken.

Computed tomography

CT has a limited place in the assessment of venous pathology. However, one example of its value is the diagnosis, using contrast enhancement, of iliac thrombosis during pregnancy. Spiral CT with the injection of contrast may be used for the diagnosis of pulmonary embolism.

Magnetic resonance imaging

The main indication for MRI in the investigation of patients with venous pathology is in defining the extent and anatomical relationships of vascular malformations and tumours. It can also be used to diagnose venous thrombosis in the abdomen and pelvis. It is, however, a more expensive method than ultrasound or CT.

Tests of venous function

As stated earlier, tests of venous function are seldom utilised in routine clinical practice outside specialist centres. In patients with chronic venous insufficiency, including venous ulcer, surgical correction of the imaged abnormality is unlikely to result in a satisfactory clinical outcome unless the haemodynamic abnormality is also corrected. Ideally, therefore, pre- and postoperative tests of venous function should be integral to protocols for the management of complex venous disease.

Venous function tests may be divided into those which measure venous insufficiency or calf pump dysfunction and those which measure outflow obstruction. The term, 'venous insufficiency', implies venous reflux due to valve dysfunction. Although often used synonymously, venous insufficiency and calf pump dysfunction are not quite the same thing. For example, a fixed ankle joint will completely inactivate the calf pump although the venous valves may be intact.

Evaluation of calf pump function and valvular insufficiency

Common to this group of tests is the principle that exercise, by emptying lower leg veins, results in a decrease in limb volume and superficial venous pressure. When the exercise is stopped, in the normal leg the volume is replaced and the pressure restored by arterial inflow but in the pathological state by vein valve reflux. Thus each test of venous function, whether it involves direct pressure measurement, volume change or reflected infra-red light, produces a typical 'venous curve' in response to a standard exercise (Figure 36.9). From such a curve two standard measurements are derived: the change in pressure (or expelled volume) and the return to baseline pressure (or refilling time). The former is a measure of the pump's ability to expel venous blood from the lower leg while the latter is an index of valvular incompetence.

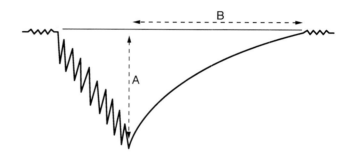

Figure 36.9 A standard venous function curve. In an ambulatory venous pressure test the distance 'A' represents the fall in pressure with exercise. In plethysmographic tests the curve represents the fall in limb volume. In both types of test the distance 'B' represents the refilling time. Since the point at which the curve rejoins the baseline is often indistinct this value is usually expressed as RT50 or RT90.

AMBULATORY VENOUS PRESSURE (AVP)

Although seldom used in routine clinical practice, this test remains the reference standard for measurement of the severity of venous valvular insufficiency and of calf pump function. Cannulation of a dorsal foot vein, connected to a pressure transducer, an amplifier and a pen recorder allows measurement of venous pressure while standing and during a standard exercise of 10 tip-toe movements of one second each. The patient stands holding on to an orthopaedic frame so that the calf muscles are relaxed during measurement of resting pressure. Application of a 2.5 cm venous tourniquet below the knee allows the test to be repeated with occlusion of the saphenous systems, thus simulating the effects of saphenous surgery.

Measurements made on the standard curve are the fall in pressure below baseline, a measure of overall pump function, and the time in seconds for the peak to return to baseline, i.e. the refilling time (usually expressed as 90% RT), a measure of valve reflux. Correlations of AVP in patients with a range of venous conditions have been well documented.

PHOTOPLETHYSMOGRAPHY (PPG) AND LIGHT REFLECTION RHEOGRAPHY (LRR)

Similar principles govern these two non-invasive techniques which measure refilling time by producing a curve similar in shape (although inverted) to that produced by AVP. Reflected infra-red light, which is influenced by cutaneous blood flow, is detected by a photodetector applied to the foot or ankle. This test can be performed with the patient standing as with AVP or alternatively with the patient sitting with the lower leg dependent. A timed sequence of flexion/extension movements at the ankle is performed, with and without a below-knee tourniquet. The only parameter which can be quantified is the refilling time (RT90). This is a useful screening technique for the detection of venous insufficiency but insufficiently precise for measuring the effects of therapy such as, for example, the effects of varicose vein surgery or valve reconstruction.

AIR PLETHYSMOGRAPHY (APG)

This non-invasive technique depends on the measurement of limb volume changes in response to exercise and postural change. The lower leg is encased in a calibrated air chamber. The patient is examined first supine with the leg elevated, then standing followed by a single step movement followed by a 10 tip-toe sequence. Parameters measured include the increase in leg volume on standing or functional venous volume (VV), the venous refilling time (VRT90), the decrease in leg volume as the result of one tip-toe movement or ejected volume (EV) and the volume of blood left in the veins after 10 tip-toe movements or residual volume (RV). This test has considerable theoretical advantages although not all workers have been able to confirm its practical value.

Evaluation of venous outflow obstruction

An obstruction to venous outflow can be demonstrated by duplex scan or by ascending phlebography. In patients with venous outflow obstruction there may be a place for some form of venous repair or bypass such as the Palma femoro-femoral crossover transposition. Such a bypass is unlikely to work unless the outflow obstruction gives rise to a substantial pressure differential. There are various methods of quantifying such an obstruction.

During ambulatory venous pressure measurement a rise in pressure in response to exercise is indicative of outflow obstruction. Alternatively, in the supine patient, by simultaneously cannulating a brachial vein the arm/foot pressure differential can be measured and repeated after reactive hyperaemia. Using this technique limbs with outflow obstruction have been classified into four grades. Venous outflow resistance can also be measured with strain gauge plethysmography or with APG.

Synopsis of investigation of specific venous conditions

Uncomplicated varicose veins

This category is made up of patients with primary varicose veins who have had no previous surgery, no history suggesting previous DVT and whose pattern of varices indicates typical saphenous stem incompetence. Ideally all patients undergoing varicose vein surgery should undergo preoperative duplex scanning of the deep and superficial systems. Where resources are limited scanning may be reserved for patients who are difficult to assess, those in whom hand-held CWD gives equivocal results and any patient with reflux in the popliteal fossa.

Complex varicose veins

This category comprises patients with recurrent varicose veins, the skin manifestations of chronic venous insufficiency (lipodermatosclerosis or ulcer), the postphlebitic syndrome, primary or secondary varices of atypical distribution and congenital vascular anomalies. Duplex ultrasonography is the principal diagnostic tool but phlebography may also be required as a guide to surgery, particularly in the case of recurrent varices and venous reconstruction.

Chronic leg ulcer

All patients with chronic leg ulcer, even though clinically diagnosed as principally venous in type, should have their ABPI recorded. When ulcer patients have mixed arterial and venous disease an ABPI of 0.6–0.9 will allow compression bandaging provided that pressure points are carefully protected with padding. In an ulcerated leg with an ABPI <0.6 treatment of the arterial disease should take priority.

All patients with chronic leg ulcer of whatever apparent 'clinical' aetiology should be investigated with duplex ultrasonography and the treatment tailored accordingly.

Deep vein thrombosis and pulmonary embolism

The first line of diagnostic attack in the patient presenting with symptomatic DVT or non life-threatening PE is duplex ultrasonography. The aim is not merely to confirm or exclude a diagnosis of DVT but also to define its location, extent and whether it is likely to give rise to further emboli. For example, an iliac thrombus which does not extend beyond the iliac confluence is less of a threat to life than one from which propagating non-occlusive thrombus extends into the inferior vena cava. The latter may be an indication for caval filtration. In a minority of cases, for the reasons outlined earlier in this chapter, bilateral ascending phlebography is indicated.

549

Pelvic congestion syndrome

Pelvic venous congestion due to ovarian vein incompetence is a well-recognised cause of chronic pelvic pain. The pain is worse premenstrually and aggravated by standing, fatigue and coitus. There may be perineal heaviness and urgency of micturition. As a prerequisite to intervention, whether by catheter embolisation techniques, laparoscopic venous interruption or open operation, the diagnosis can be made by duplex scan or by selective catheter phlebography.

Thoracic outlet venous compression

Venous compression at the thoracic outlet presents either with features of chronic intermittent venous congestion in the limb or, more commonly, with acute venous thrombosis, sometimes termed 'effort' thrombosis because it may be precipitated by exercise such as weight training. External compression of the vein is caused either by downward depression of the clavicle, as in the 'military position', or by hyperabduction and external rotation of the arm. MRI can be used to clarify whether the vein is being compressed between the costo-coracoid ligament and the first rib, the subclavius muscle and the first rib, the clavicle and the first rib or the clavicle and the anterior scalene muscle.

Phlebography, via an antecubital vein, is much the most useful and accurate method of defining both the obstruction and the collateral circulation. In the chronic intermittent variety or after the thrombus has been cleared by lytic therapy (more effective in acute DVT of the upper limb than the lower) serial films should be taken with the limb in standard position, hyperabducted and in the exaggerated military position in order to demonstrate the effect of the external compression and to determine the need for surgical intervention such as first rib resection.

Venous malformations and tumours

Most vascular malformations are treated conservatively whenever possible. Active investigations are only recommended if some form of intervention is being contemplated. In the case of malformations which present as atypical varicose veins, such as the Klippel–Trenaunay syndrome, duplex ultrasonography may be helpful in defining the deep to superficial connections. Normally, however, both arteriography and phlebography will be required. Where the soft tissue extent of a vascular mass needs to be defined, MRI will provide the best images.

FURTHER READING

Adam DJ, Bradbury AW, Stuart WP et al. The value of computed tomography in the assessment of suspected ruptured abdominal aortic aneurysm. *J Vasc Surg* 1998; **27**:431–437

Beard JD, Scott DJA, Evans JM, Skidmore R, Horrocks M. Pulse-generated run-off: a new method of determining calf vessel patency. *Br J Surg* 1988; **75**:361–364

Bradbury AW, Ruckley CV. Foot volumetry can predict recurrent ulceration after subfascial ligation of perforators and saphenous ligation. *J Vasc Surg* 1993; **18**:789–795

Brittenden J, Bradbury AW, Allan PL, Prescott RJ, Harper DR, Ruckley CV. Popliteal vein reflux reduces the healing of chronic venous ulcer. *Br J Surg* 1998; **85**:60–62

Burnand KG, Lea Thomas M, O'Donnell TE, Browse NL. The relationship between post–phlebitic changes in the deep veins and results of surgical treatment of venous ulcers. *Lancet* 1976; **1**:936-938

Chalmers RTA, Kresowik TF, Sharp WJ et al. The impact of color duplex surveillance on the outcome of lower limb bypass with segments of arm veins. *J Vasc Surg* 1994; **19**:279–289

Christopoulos D, Nicolaides AN, Szendro G. Venous reflux: quantification and correlation with the clinical severity of venous disease. *Br J Surg* 1988; **75**:352–356

European Carotid Surgery Trialists Collaborative Study. MRC European Carotid Surgery Trial: Interim results for symptomatic patients with severe (70–99%) or mild (0–29%) carotid stenosis. *Lancet* 1991; **337**:1235–1241

Fowkes FGR, Callam MJ. Is arterial disease a risk factor for chronic leg ulceration? *Phlebology* 1994; **9**:87–90

North American Symptomatic Carotid Endarterectomy Trial Collaborators. Beneficial effect of carotid endarterectomy in symptomatic patients with high-grade carotid stenosis. *N Engl J Med* 1991; **325**:445–453

Porter JM, Moneta JL and an International Consensus Committee on Chronic Venous Disease. Reporting standards on venous disease: an update. *J Vasc Surg* 1995; **21**:635–645

Raju S. A pressure based technique for the detection of acute and chronic venous obstruction. *Phlebology* 1988; **3**:207-216

Scandinavian Simvastatin Survival Study Group. Randomised trial of cholesterol-lowering in 4444 patients with coronary heart disease: the Scandinavian Simvastatin Survival Study. *Lancet* 1994; **344**:1383–1389

Second European Consensus Document on Chronic Critical Limb Ischaemia. *Eur J Vasc Surg* 1992; **6**(suppl A):1–32

Smith FCT, Shearman CP, Simons MH, Gwynn BR. Falsely elevated ankle pressures in severe limb ischaemia: the pole test: an alternative approach. *Eur J Vasc Surg* 1994; **13**:296–300

UK Small Aneurysm Trial Participants. Mortality results for the randomised controlled trial of early elective surgery or ultrasonic surveillance for small abdominal aortic aneurysms. *Lancet* 1999; **352**:1649–1655

VEINES International Task Force. The management of chronic venous disorders of the leg. *Phlebology* 1999; **14**(Suppl 1)

Vascular trauma

Frank C. T. Smith, Roger N. Baird

INTRODUCTION

Injuries to major blood vessels rarely occur in isolation. Significant arterial and venous trauma is often associated with other major injuries which must be diagnosed and treated in order of priority. Catastrophic disruption of the great vessels may be rapidly fatal, frequently at the scene of the accident. For lesser injuries, assessment and appropriate treatment may prevent early death from haemorrhage and hypoxia. Basic resuscitative measures prior to retrieval of a patient from the scene of injury include securing a patent airway with stabilisation of the cervical spine, preservation of the mechanisms of breathing and direct control of external haemorrhage. Subsequent definitive management is best undertaken in a hospital setting by a trauma team working to defined principles such as those described by the Advanced Trauma Life Support (ATLS) system.

The initial management phase for the acutely injured patient has been described as 'the golden hour'. During this period early diagnosis and appropriate treatment of injuries according to clinical priorities has the greatest impact on favourable outcome in terms of morbidity and mortality. Maintenance of an airway and preservation of the mechanisms of breathing and respiratory function remain priorities during management of the critically injured patient. After securing the airway, control of haemorrhage, circulatory support and early vascular repair are vital to ensure adequate organ perfusion and tissue oxygenation. This chapter reviews the epidemiology, diagnosis, investigation and management of vascular injuries.

EPIDEMIOLOGY AND CLASSIFICATION OF VASCULAR TRAUMA

Epidemiological variation in the causes of vascular trauma occurs between rural and urban areas and according to geographical locality. Military and civilian injuries tend to have separate characteristics. Lower limb extremity injuries account for 50–60% of vascular injuries in war and 25% of those in civilian life. Abdominal vascular injuries are unusual in battle but may account for up to 25% of civilian vascular injuries in urban areas. In those areas of the world subject to urban strife and easy access to firearms, gunshot and stab wounds are common causes of penetrating vascular trauma. Penetrating injuries may also be caused by glass and industrial accidents. Severe vascular injury as a result of blunt trauma occurs most commonly due to road traffic accidents but may also occur following falls. In the United Kingdom the vascular surgeon is most likely to encounter vascular trauma in the form of iatrogenic complications arising from diagnostic or interventional cardiological and radiological procedures.

Vascular trauma tends to spare the very young and the elderly. The highest incidence of injury occurs during the second and third decades of life when the victim's energies are not always tempered by experience. A secondary smaller peak occurs between 50 and 70 years due to iatrogenic injuries incurred during invasive clinical investigations or therapeutic interventions.

Arterial obstruction may be classified as intrinsic or extrinsic. Intrinsic causes of obstruction include invasive intraluminal catheters introduced for monitoring or radiological purposes or the use of cardiac-assist devices such as intra-aortic balloon pumps. These invasive techniques may cause arterial rupture, intimal damage, embolus, dissection with local thrombosis, clot propagation and arterial occlusion. A false aneurysm may occur at the site of arterial puncture when the intravascular catheter is withdrawn. Arteriovenous fistula may be a late complication. Inadvertent intraarterial injection of foreign substances, for instance as a result of drug abuse, may cause infection, peripheral arterial occlusion, ischaemia, pain and extensive tissue loss. Therapeutic irradiation is a rare iatrogenic cause of arterial injury. This causes an arteritis resulting in eventual fibrosis and stenosis or occlusion. The neck vessels, subclavian and axillary arteries are most commonly affected, following radiotherapy to the thyroid or to the breast and axilla.

Extrinsic arterial injuries may be blunt or penetrating. Examples of penetrating injuries include gunshot and stab wounds or lacerations from broken glass. Stab wounds are more common than gunshot wounds in the UK and throughout most of Europe and involve the extremities more frequently than the trunk. In the USA gunshot wounds predominate. In a low-velocity gunshot wound where the projectile has a velocity of less than 1200 feet per second, the extent of damage is principally limited to its track. High-velocity gunshot wounds (2000–3000 fps) may be accompanied by extensive tissue damage despite a deceptively small entry wound, due to the cavitational effects of pressure waves generated by the projectile.

Arterial damage may present as a puncture wound, laceration, transection, contusion or gross obliteration of the vessel. Where mural contusion occurs, arterial wall smooth muscle spasm may contribute to arterial insufficiency but clinical findings of distal ischaemia should never be ascribed solely to arterial spasm unless proven directly. Blunt trauma as a result of road traffic accidents frequently involves severe acceleration/deceleration forces which apply shearing stresses to major vessels. In this situation mural disruption may occur at junctions where one component of the arterial system is comparatively tethered compared to the adjacent artery.

Fractures and joint dislocations may affect vessels in their vicinity. Fracture of a long bone requires great force and can result in significant soft tissue injury with contusion to local vessels. Alternatively arteries and veins may be pinched or kinked between fractured bone fragments. Bone shards may lacerate or puncture vessels resulting in haemorrhage or thrombosis. Dislocation of a joint implies powerful distraction forces which may be sufficient to avulse or tear vessels, particularly where they lie closely tethered to a joint. Complications of vascular injuries are listed in Box 37.1.

Box 37.1 Complications of vascular injury

Early	*Late*
Haemorrhage	Infection and secondary haemorrhage
Coagulopathy	Arteriovenous fistula
Thrombosis	False aneurysm
Embolus	Mycotic aneurysm
Infarction	Deep vein thrombosis
Compartment syndrome	Chronic arterial insufficiency
False aneurysm	Volkmann's ischaemic contracture

PATIENT ASSESSMENT

After preliminary resuscitation has been carried out, a history of the mechanism of injury and of any preexisting relevant medical conditions should be obtained. Thorough examination of the patient is undertaken. The following signs and symptoms should alert the examining clinician to the likelihood of vascular injury and the probable need for operative intervention.

- History of arterial bleeding or major haemorrhage

- Persistent hypotension or shock

- Expanding or pulsatile haematoma

- Absent or diminished peripheral pulses

- Distal ischaemia

- Bruit at or beyond the site of injury

- Injury to anatomically associated nerves

Penetrating injury or a fracture along the anatomical line of an artery may suggest vascular trauma. Where the major artery to a limb has been severely damaged or occluded distal ischaemia is often apparent. The limb will appear cool and pale, venous filling and capillary refill are diminished and pulses will be absent. However, these signs may also occur with systemic hypotension. Paraesthesia, anaesthesia and paralysis are late features of acute limb ischaemia but may also occur with concomitant nerve damage. Conversely the presence of a distal pulse and absence of obvious ischaemia, implying arterial continuity, may reassure the unwary. A pulse may persist in the presence of significant arterial injury, particularly if the arterial wall is only partially breached, and arteriography should be undertaken whenever suggested on grounds of clinical suspicion to prevent significant injury escaping detection.

Use of a hand-held continuous-wave Doppler may provide confirmation of distal perfusion but a Doppler signal can be falsely reassuring if the peripheral circulation is maintained by collateral vessels. Continuous-wave Doppler will rarely demonstrate intimal defects or small false aneurysms. Comparison of pulses and Doppler signals in a traumatised limb with its contralateral un-injured counterpart usually provides valuable information. Diminished Doppler pressures are an indication for angiography. Reduction of a fracture or dislocation may restore a pulse but if any doubt of arterial integrity exists angiography should be performed. In the elderly and in diabetics and smokers, pre-existing peripheral vascular disease may sometimes confuse the issue. Again diagnostic angiography should be considered. Duplex Doppler has a limited role in rapid non-invasive assessment of limb vessel trauma and of the extracranial arterial circulation. This modality may be useful in detecting the presence of false aneurysms, arteriovenous fistulas and intraluminal defects but it is extremely operator dependent and does not have the resolution of angiography.

Contrast spiral CT scanning and magnetic resonance imaging (MRI) are useful screening tools for injuries to the major vessels of thorax and abdomen when extravasation of contrast, mural damage or vessel dissection may be apparent. However, if haemorrhage or vessel disruption is suspected an angiogram should be obtained, particularly to check for aortic rupture.

Arteriography remains the gold standard for assessment of arterial trauma. Development of low osmolar contrast media, smaller catheters and high-resolution digital subtraction imaging techniques (DSA) have facilitated performance of emergency angiography. However, movement artefacts degrade image resolution and the patient must be capable of keeping still and suspending respiration whilst images are obtained. Intraarterial DSA requires significantly smaller volumes of contrast than intravenous DSA and is more useful in the emergency situation. The majority of essential angiograms in arterial trauma can be undertaken under local anaesthesia by percutaneous retrograde femoral or brachial approaches. Arteriography should not delay urgent operative intervention where indicated on clinical grounds. The investigation should therefore be reserved for stable patients in whom the results may avert the necessity for surgery or for whom planning of a surgical procedure is dependent on preoperative imaging. Urgent surgery should not be delayed where clinical signs are unequivocal. In such patients early exploration and vascular control allow the presence of suspected vessel injury to be confirmed by subsequent on-table angiography.

GENERAL PRINCIPLES OF RESUSCITATION AND MANAGEMENT

Circulating blood volume in a 70 kg adult is approximately 5 litres. Loss of 15–30% (750–1500 ml) may provoke tachycardia but compensatory physiological mechanisms may prevent decompensation and hypotension until the loss of 30–40% blood volume (1500–2000 ml). External haemorrhage should be controlled by direct pressure and intravenous access for fluid replacement obtained by placement of at least two large-bore intravenous catheters. Blood samples should be taken for typing and cross-matching and assessment of baseline haematological parameters. A pregnancy test should be undertaken for all females of child-bearing age.

Oxygen should be provided and resuscitation with an isotonic salt solution, such as Ringer's lactate or Hartmann's solution, commenced. Up to 2–3 litres of crystalloid solution warmed to 37°C may be administered rapidly as an initial bolus infusion to elicit an appropriate haemodynamic response in the adult patient. Subsequent administration of type-specific blood or, if unavailable, low-titre type O or O-negative blood may be necessary. Many patients are hypothermic and attempts should be made to restore normothermia. Urine output is a sensitive indicator of renal perfusion and should be regularly assessed in the severely injured patient along with pulse and blood pressure. Adequate volume replacement should produce a urine output of at least 0.5 ml/kg/h in the adult patient. Central venous pressure provides an index of filling pressure although direct assessment of cardiac function via a Swan–Ganz catheter may be indicated, especially if cardiac injury is suspected. Constant re-evaluation is necessary to avoid excessive or inadequate fluid administration. Continued blood loss should be controlled by urgent operative intervention in addition to restoration and maintenance of intravascular volume.

Tourniquets should be avoided because of the risks of perpetuating limb ischaemia, unless released intermittently, and because they may occlude important collaterals and initiate venous thrombosis. Puncture wounds should not be probed but explored under direct vision with adequate exposure. Blind application of haemostatic forceps is usually inappropriate and more likely to cause injury than to control haemorrhage.

Arterial injuries often occur in conjunction with contamination from penetrating or open wounds and early broad-spectrum antibiotic prophylaxis is appropriate. Tetanus prophylaxis should be considered for patients with open or penetrating wounds. Where a patient has previously been adequately immunised a booster dose of 0.5 ml of adsorbed tetanus toxoid should be given intramuscularly for tetanus prone wounds but may otherwise be omitted. In the non-immunised patient 250 units of human tetanus immune globulin (TIG) should be administered by IM injection together with 0.5 ml of toxoid given at a separate site. The immunisation course should subsequently be completed.

Arterial wounds should be repaired as expeditiously as possible. Significant haemorrhage may also occur from venous wounds. In the limbs, where feasible, large veins should be repaired in conjunction with arteries but in the arm and neck, venous injuries may sometimes be treated by oversewing or ligation without incurring significant morbidity.

General anaesthesia is preferable to regional techniques in the treatment of major vascular trauma. Patient positioning and skin preparation should take into account the need for adequate exposure of the injury and the possible necessity for harvesting vein grafts. Control of damaged vessels proximal and distal to the site of the injury is obtained using encircling Silastic loops or vascular clamps. Where a laceration or tear of a large artery or vein exists and initial control is difficult to achieve, introduction of appropriately sized Fogarty or Foley balloon catheters through the tear, with proximal and distal luminal balloon inflation, facilitates temporary control of haemorrhage. This provides a period of respite during which further dissection may allow more formal control with vascular clamps.

Once bleeding at the site of injury has been controlled the injury is assessed prior to formal repair. Ragged lacerations should be debrided. It may be necessary to evacuate clot or thrombus at the site of injury and in the proximal and distal vessels using a gently manipulated Fogarty catheter. Frequent repeated catheter passages are rarely productive and intimal damage should be avoided. Irrigation of the injured vessels with physiological heparinised Hartmann's solution (5000 IU in 500 ml) reduces the risk of further thrombosis at the site of injury but systemic heparinisation is usually contraindicated in the multiply injured patient.

Simple puncture wounds and small clean arterial lacerations can often be repaired by lateral suture. Where debridement is necessary or large lacerations occur, direct closure is likely to cause stenosis. This can be avoided by using autogenous vein to create a patch angioplasty. Rarely it may be possible to excise a short segment of a damaged vessel and to carry out a direct end-to-end anastomosis of the remaining two ends of healthy vessel using interrupted sutures. A basic tenet of repair in this situation is that the limb should be in a neutral position and that the anastomosis is tension free. This may require extensive mobilisation of healthy vessel ends.

Occasionally arterial spasm will compromise a favourable anastomotic outcome, especially in small low-flow vessels. Local infusion of 15–60 mg of papaverine will produce a temporary vasodilatory response. Longer term beneficial vasodilatation can be achieved by allowing a small vascular swab soaked in papaverine to lie in direct contact with the constricted vessel.

Mural contusions are often associated with separation of the media and intima of an artery. Vessel continuity may be maintained only by the adventitia. If left unrepaired, likely sequelae include thrombosis, dissection or development of false aneurysms. In these cases the damaged section of vessel should be excised and repair undertaken using a reversed vein interposition graft. The long saphenous and cephalic veins provide convenient sources of conduit. The ends of the vein graft and recipient vessel should be spatulated to enlarge the anastomotic area, to reduce the risk of stenosis. Meticulous repair ensuring intimal apposition and eversion of the edges of the anastomosis is carried out using non-absorbable polypropylene sutures. In children, use of interrupted sutures will allow for future vessel growth. Where there is disparity in size between a small vein graft and a larger vessel to be repaired, for instance in the iliac veins or the IVC, opening the vein graft along its length, dividing it into two and sewing the pieces together side by side will provide a graft of half the length but double the circumference (Figure 37.1A,B). Incising a vein along its length and constructing a continuous spiral graft around an appropriately sized rigid support produces a similar effect (Figure 37.1C). In larger vessels such as the aorta and iliac arteries, if the wound is relatively clean then it may be feasible to repair the injury with a prosthetic graft. However, if there is gross contamination of the operative field, use of an extraanatomic (axillo-

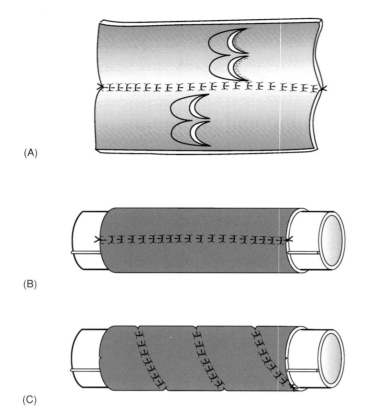

(A)

(B)

(C)

Figure 37.1 Construction of cylindrical (**A**,**B**) and spiral (**C**) vein grafts to compensate for size mismatch between a small vein graft and a larger damaged vessel.

femoral or femorofemoral) bypass graft, avoiding the site of contamination, combined with oversewing of the damaged vessels may be more appropriate.

Reperfusion injury and compartment syndrome

Significant limb swelling may occur as a result of reperfusion injury following successful revascularisation of the extremities. During a period of acute ischaemia tissue PO_2 falls and noxious vasoactive metabolites can cause muscle damage. Myonecrosis may occur in striated muscle after 4–8 hours of warm ischaemia. Acute ischaemia lasting for more than eight hours results in high amputation rates and ischaemia lasting for more than 12 hours frequently results in an unsalvageable limb. However, the reintroduction of oxygenated blood after lesser periods of ischaemia causes considerably more damage than that induced by ischaemia alone.

A variety of factors are implicated in reperfusion injury. During ischaemia xanthine oxidase and hypoxanthine accumulate in ischaemic tissue. When reperfusion occurs xanthine oxidase converts hypoxanthine to xanthine, generating superoxide and initiating the release of oxygen free radicals and hydrogen peroxide within endothelial cells. These initiate lipid peroxidation, causing

structural and functional endothelial damage. Platelet-activating factor (PAF) is released, as are the breakdown products of arachidonic acid, particularly thromboxane A2 and leukotriene LTB4 which are potent chemoattractants for neutrophils. Neutrophil activation and adhesion to vascular endothelium is induced. Release of lysosomal proteolytic enzymes and oxygen free radicals, including the superoxide and hydroxyl radicals, and hydrogen peroxide causes further damage to the endothelium, resulting in increased intracellular calcium accumulation and increased microvascular permeability with resultant cell swelling. Ultrastructural changes result in increased neutrophil cytoskeletal rigidity which causes capillary plugging, further impairing reflow. This may be compounded by microcirculatory thrombosis after long periods of ischaemia.

In experimental situations neutrophil depletion, the use of monoclonal antibodies to the neutrophil adhesion glycoprotein (CD18 integrin) or its endothelial determinant the intercellular adhesion molecule (ICAM-1) and free radical scavenging agents have all been shown to be effective in preventing reperfusion injury.

The outcome of reperfusion injury is an increase in striated muscle capillary permeability which allows the development of significant muscle oedema. The extent of this injury is proportional to the duration of warm ischaemic time. The muscles of the leg are bounded by taut inelastic fascial envelopes. As blood flow is restored to the now highly permeable muscular capillary network, muscle compartment pressures rise due to capillary leakage, to the extent where there may be injurious compression of nerves travelling within these compartments. Increased pressures impede venous drainage, compounding compartment swelling. Compartment pressures may even rise to the extent where they become great enough to overcome arterial perfusion pressure, obliterating inflow vessels.

Clinical features of a compartment syndrome are those of tense swelling of the compartment accompanied by acute pain on passive muscle stretching. During the early period of development of a compartment syndrome the presence of pulses and adequate skin perfusion presents a trap for the unwary. Late features are loss of sensation and motor function by which time irreversible muscle necrosis and neurovascular damage may have already occurred. Significant muscle necrosis may result in myoglobinaemia and hyperkalaemia which in turn may cause renal and metabolic problems. A disabling and distressing long-term outcome is the development of Volkmann's ischaemic muscle contracture with fibrosis and shortening of paralysed muscles within the compartment.

The necessity for recognising potential development of a compartment syndrome cannot be overemphasised. It is good practice to carry out fasciotomies, at the time of limb revascularisation after a period of profound ischaemia, whenever the prospect of a compartment syndrome is even considered (Figure 37.2). Whilst it is possible to measure compartment pressures by introducing a sterile needle, attached to manometer tubing and a pressure transducer, into each muscle compartment (pressures of greater than 30–40 mmHg below mean arterial pressure carry diagnostic significance), the clinical suspicion of compartment syndrome is justification enough for timely fasciotomies.

In the lower limb it is important to carry out adequate decompression of all four fascial compartments in the calf which can be achieved by posteromedial and anterolateral incisions, (Figure 37.3). Decompression can be carried out blindly by a 'closed' technique through small incisions with long scissors, but the authors favour longer incisions which allow visualisation of adequate fascial division and muscle decompression. Inadvertent damage to tibial arteries is more easily avoided using the latter technique (Figure 37.4).

Forearm decompression is occasionally required. It is achieved through a long skin incision from proximal to the antecubital fossa, extending into the palm, through which the fascial compartments are lysed. Care must be taken to avoid damage to the recurrent branch of the median nerve. It is seldom possible to close skin incisions at the time of fasciotomy and open wounds are temporarily dressed with occlusive antiseptic Betadine-soaked dressings. It may be necessary to reassess the wounds at 24 hours

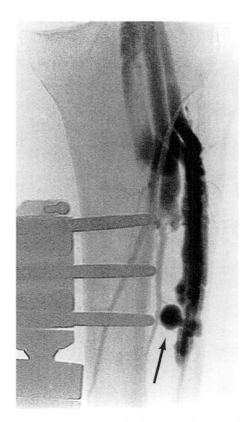

Figure 37.4 Iatrogenic arteriovenous fistula (arrowed) between tibial artery and vein following external fixation of tibial fracture.

by which time demarcation of necrotic muscle has usually occurred, allowing debridement of grey non-viable muscle back to pink, adequately perfused tissue. Placement of a loose running nylon or polypropylene subcuticular suture in the skin at the time of the fasciotomy allows delayed primary closure of the wound, achieved by simply tightening the suture when the limb swelling has settled. This averts the necessity for a further trip to the operating theatre. Placement of the lower limb in a temporary plaster backslab with the foot dorsiflexed to 90° combats an early postoperative tendency towards foot drop.

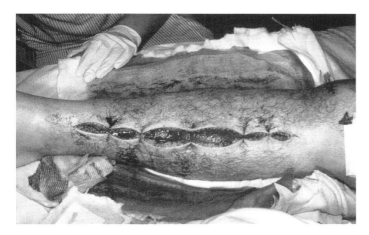

Figure 37.2 Tibial fasciotomies following repair of a vascular injury.

TREATMENT OF SPECIFIC VASCULAR INJURIES

Carotid trauma

The majority of injuries to the carotid artery occur as a result of penetrating trauma. The wound is usually of low velocity and damage is confined to the tract. In patients with a potential penetrating carotid injury, associated nerve damage and trauma to the oesophagus, trachea and larynx should also be considered. Clinical signs arousing suspicion of carotid injury are:

- penetrating wound or haematoma in the lateral side of the neck

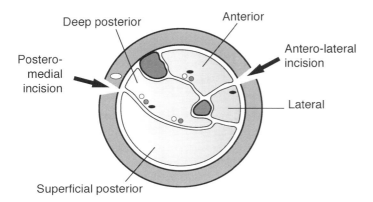

Figure 37.3 The four lower leg fascial compartments and sites for fasciotomy incisions.

- transient ischaemic attacks

- Horner's syndrome

- hemiparesis or hemiplegia

- lucid interval after injury

- monocular visual field defects.

Only 3–5% of carotid injuries are caused by blunt trauma. However, hyperextension injuries of the neck may cause contusion and intimal damage. A tear of the intima where the carotid passes over the transverse processes at the level of C2–3 may result in arterial dissection. The damage is suspected on carotid duplex scanning and confirmed by contrast or magnetic resonance angiography. Approximately 60% of patients with carotid arterial dissection present clinically with transient ischaemic attacks occurring within hours or days. Fifty percent of patients complain of severe headaches and amaurosis fugax may be present in up to 35% of cases.

Patients with a penetrating carotid injury may be divided into three groups.

Group I   No neurological deficit
Group II   Mild to moderate neurological deficit
Group III Severe neurological deficit with hemiparesis or hemi-
           plegia

Group III patients with an occlusion of the internal carotid artery have a poor prognosis. Surgery is rarely beneficial in this group and revascularisation may convert an ischaemic cerebral infarct into a haemorrhagic infarct. In patients with penetrating injuries piercing the platysma muscle or anterior triangles of the neck, with neurological status in groups I or II, surgical repair should be undertaken.

In patients with a carotid occlusion secondary to blunt trauma, in the absence of neurological symptoms, it is rational to avoid surgical repair although there is little evidence to support this approach unequivocally.

For acute carotid dissections in isolation, conservative management with early anticoagulation and subsequent medium-term warfarinisation is currently the preferred method of treatment. Follow-up duplex studies will confirm recanalisation in approximately 50% of these cases. Subadventitial dissection or false aneurysm formation, however, are best treated by surgical repair with resection of the injured segment of artery and replacement with an interposition graft.

Although non-invasive duplex and MRA scans may be useful when positive, the gold standard for diagnosis of carotid injury in a stable patient remains intraarterial contrast angiography.

Prior to carotid surgery for trauma, cranial nerve function, the integrity of the brachial plexus and vocal cord function should be carefully assessed and documented. An oblique neck incision is placed along the anterior border of the sternomastoid muscle but can be extended into the chest via a median sternotomy if intrathoracic control of proximal vessels is required. Control of the common, external and internal carotid arteries is achieved with loops or tapes. Small puncture wounds or lacerations may be repaired directly. If more extensive repair is required the vessels may be clamped and a shunt inserted between the common carotid and distal internal carotid artery, maintaining cerebral perfusion.

A proximal internal carotid wound may sometimes be dealt with by using the external carotid as a source of inflow. The distal external carotid artery and its proximal side branches are ligated and divided. The proximal external carotid artery is then mobilised and swung across, anastomosing it end to end to the healthy distal internal carotid artery after resection of the injured proximal portion of this vessel. A satisfactory alternative is the use of a reversed vein interposition graft after resection of the damaged portion of the internal carotid artery. The vein is mounted over a shunt and sewn into position, removing the shunt prior to completion of the second anastomosis. In a few patients damage may be so extensive that carotid repair is not feasible and ligation of a bleeding internal carotid may be required. Even in patients with an adequate stump pressure, stroke rates of up to 50% may be expected following this manoeuvre.

Thoracic vascular injuries

Vascular injuries in the chest account for 9–12% of all vascular trauma. Most injuries are caused by penetrating trauma although blunt and deceleration injuries are also seen. Intrathoracic vascular injuries are responsible for 10–15% of deaths from road traffic accidents and the incidence of aortic rupture may be up to 25% in patients ejected from vehicles. Injuries to the intrathoracic aorta and great vessels result in the highest mortality of all arterial wounds. Many patients are dead on arrival at hospital or in haemorrhagic shock and co-existing major injuries are common. Associated nerve injuries occur frequently in conjunction with vascular thoracic outlet injuries. In blunt deceleration trauma the thoracic aorta is prone to injury at several specific sites. The highest prevalence of injury occurs between the left subclavian artery and the ligamentum arteriosum at the aortic isthmus. This is due to the relative mobility of the heart, ascending and transverse aorta which continue to move forwards during deceleration whilst the descending thoracic aorta remains relatively fixed. Avulsion of the relatively fixed origin of the innominate artery may occur by the same mechanism (Figure 37.6). Major disruptions of the pulmonary vessels are usually rapidly fatal.

Diagnosis of injuries to intrathoracic vessels and the heart may present difficulties due to their relative inaccessibility during examination. Suspicion of these injuries may be aroused by knowledge of the mechanism of trauma and by the following findings.

- Cardiac arrest

- Persistent shock

- Recurrent haemothorax
- Chest X-ray findings:
  - widened mediastinum (>8 cm)
  - blunting of the aortic knuckle
  - loss of the radiolucent aortopulmonary window.

Arteriography remains the definitive modality of investigation for intrathoracic arterial injuries although spiral CT and trans-oesophageal ultrasound are useful non-invasive investigations for suspected aortic isthmus damage in the stable patient.

Great vessel exposure is best achieved by thoracotomy or median sternotomy (Figure 37.5). For the left subclavian artery an antero-lateral fourth or fifth space thoracotomy may be carried out. Access to a disrupted innominate artery is achieved via a median sternotomy which can be extended to the right subclavian region. The origin of the innominate artery may be controlled with a Wylie-J clamp or a Satinsky vascular clamp. Distal control of the innominate is obtained proximal to the bifurcation of the carotid and right subclavian arteries and an 8–12 mm interposition Dacron graft is anastomosed end to side to the proximal ascending aorta and distally end to end to the innominate artery (Figure 37.6). The innominate stump on the aortic arch is then oversewn. Options for repair of the intrathoracic aorta include interposition grafting, sutureless grafts and more recently the deployment of endovascular covered stent grafts.

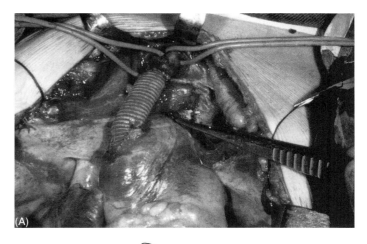
(A)

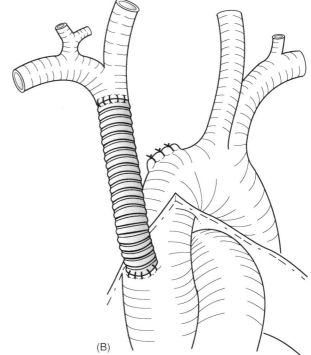
(B)

Figure 37.6 A,B Repair of aorto-innominate artery disruption by interposition Dacron graft following deceleration injury.

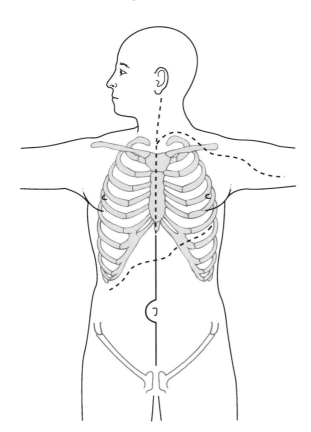

Figure 37.5 Incisions giving access to vessels of neck, chest, upper limb and abdomen.

Cardiac tamponade

Cardiac tamponade presents an immediately life-threatening situation and merits discussion. Tamponade most commonly occurs as a consequence of penetrating cardiac injury but may arise as a result of blunt trauma to the thorax. Classic findings include tachycardia, engorged neck veins due to venous pressure elevation, hypotension resistant to fluid resuscitation and muffled heart sounds. In a deteriorating patient who fails to respond to resuscitation, prompt pericardiocentesis should not be delayed for further investigations.

Needle pericardiocentesis may be performed by the subxiphoid approach. The patient's vital signs and ECG should be monitored throughout the procedure. Using aseptic technique, a six-inch 18 gauge over-the-needle catheter attached to a three-way tap and syringe is passed through a skin puncture placed 1 cm beneath and to the left of the xiphisternal junction. The needle is advanced in a cephalad direction at 45° to the chest wall, aiming towards the tip of the left scapula and maintaining suction. As the needle tip passes into the pericardial sac fresh blood may be withdrawn into the syringe and expelled through the three-way tap. Removal of even small amounts, as little as 15–20 ml of blood, may immediately relieve the haemodynamic effects of tamponade. If the needle is advanced too far, coming into contact with the myocardium, dysrhythmias may be observed on the ECG and the needle should be gently withdrawn back into the pericardial sac. Positive pericardiocentesis should be followed up by formal pericardiotomy and inspection of the myocardium via a median sternotomy or thoracotomy carried out in an operating theatre setting by a qualified surgeon.

Cardiac tamponade may occasionally be confused with the other critical condition of tension pneumothorax. In the latter, unilateral absent breath sounds and hyperresonance to percussion over the affected hemithorax, with mediastinal shift away from the mid-line, may help to differentiate between the two diagnoses. Prompt decompression by placement of a large-gauge needle over the rib in the second intercostal space in the midclavicular line on the affected side will treat the latter problem and resolve the immediate diagnostic dilemma. Reassessment and placement of a formal chest drain may subsequently be necessary.

Upper limb vascular injuries

Vascular injuries to the upper limb represent up to 50% of all vascular trauma and include injuries to the subclavian, axillary, brachial, radial and ulnar arteries. Penetrating injuries are more common than blunt injuries and stab wounds are more frequent among civilians than military personnel. Iatrogenic brachial artery injuries due to invasive radiological procedures have become progressively more common, as have injuries caused by inadvertent intraarterial drug abuse (Figures 37.7, 37.8).

Because of an extensive upper limb collateral blood supply even major arterial injury in the upper limb rarely results in limb loss. However, the close proximity of major nerves in the neurovascular bundles means that nerve damage frequently accompanies arterial trauma and is often the cause of persisting morbidity following adequate arterial repair. Blunt trauma to the upper limb may also result in brachial plexus disruption accompanying arterial damage which may lead to catastrophic loss of limb function. Early rehabilitation to ensure optimal functional outcome is essential but occasionally amputation may be necessary when a functionless limb causes gross physical hindrance. This difficult decision should only be undertaken after full efforts have been made to provide adequate rehabilitation.

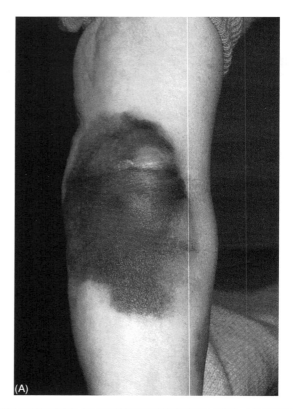

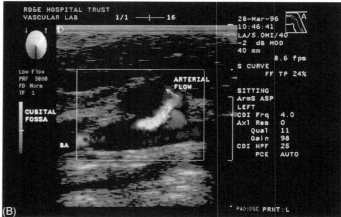

Figure 37.7 Antecubital fossa haematoma following diagnostic brachial artery catheterisation (**A**). Duplex ultrasound illustrates a false aneurysm of the brachial artery (**B**).

The principles of arterial repair described earlier in this chapter should be followed for most upper limb vascular injuries. In contrast to the leg, venous repair is not required in most upper limb trauma and damaged veins may usually be ligated. Soft tissue coverage of vascular repairs is mandatory.

Upper limb arteries are prone to injuries due to bone fractures and dislocations at several specific sites. Severe clavicular fractures or traction injuries may injure the subclavian artery. Fracture through the surgical neck of the humerus may disrupt the axillary artery (Figure 37.9), as may shoulder dislocation and subsequent

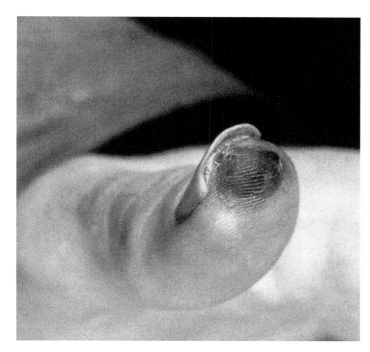

Figure 37.8 Embolic digital ischaemia following intraarterial drug abuse.

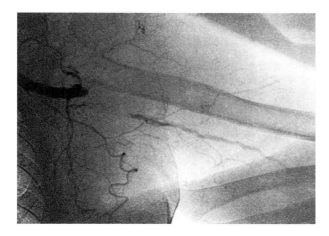

Figure 37.9 Arteriogram showing occlusion of the axillary artery caused by fracture of the neck of the humerus.

reduction. The brachial artery is vulnerable where it lies in proximity to the humeral shaft and in 20–30% of children there may be brachial artery injury following supracondylar fractures of the humerus. Primary reduction of the fracture often restores the circulation. If in doubt, arteriography must be performed to exclude arterial damage and to reduce the late risks of Volkmann's ischaemic contracture. Radial and ulnar arterial injuries in isolation rarely compromise the hand circulation. Repair requires meticulous small vessel techniques but in the emergency setting simple ligation of the damaged artery usually suffices.

Upper limb arterial exposure

Proximal control of the left and right subclavian arteries can be achieved through a median sternotomy. The first part of the subclavian artery on the left side may be accessed via an antero-lateral thoracotomy through the fourth intercostal space. Penetrating injuries to the subclavian artery in the thoracic outlet can be exposed via an incision over the clavicle, if necessary excising the medial portion of this bone (see Figure 37.5). The second part of the subclavian artery lies behind the scalenus anterior muscle which can be detached from its insertion on the first rib, taking care first to identify and retract the phrenic nerve which lies on the anterior surface of the muscle. Reversed cephalic, basilic and long saphenous veins provide excellent interposition grafts if primary arterial repair is not feasible. If such reconstruction is not possible, extra anatomic bypass by axillo-axillo or femoro-axillo bypass using ring reinforced PTFE or Dacron grafts may comprise suitable alternatives. Injuries to the jugular and subclavian veins can usually be dealt with by simple ligation in the multiply injured patient.

The proximal axillary artery is best exposed via an infraclavicular incision, splitting the fibres of the pectoralis major muscle and dividing the clavipectoral fascia and pectoralis minor. The distal axillary artery is exposed by a medial incision behind pectoralis major in the arm. This can be extended from the axilla to the antecubital fossa to allow exposure of the brachial artery but if continued into the forearm, the incision should be converted into an 'S' shape as it crosses the antecubital fossa to prevent the effects of subsequent scar contracture and tethering.

Abdominal vascular injuries

Abdominal vascular injury may present as a haematoma or as acute haemorrhage mandating early laparotomy. The indications for laparotomy following penetrating wounds to the abdomen are not absolute. A percentage of wounds in which minor penetrating injuries have occurred and in which the patient remains haemo-dynamically stable during close observation can be managed conservatively. Likewise, a retroperitoneal haematoma incurred by blunt injury may be dealt with expectantly if the patient remains stable during serial observations. Gunshot wounds and stab wounds that penetrate the peritoneum should be explored. After initial evaluation a plain abdominal radiograph following administration of contrast for an IVU should be performed. Contrast-enhanced CT scans and arteriography are valuable diagnostic adjuncts but should not delay urgent laparotomy if clinically indicated. Alternatively, in the multiply injured patient undergoing resuscitation in the accident and emergency department, early diagnostic peritoneal lavage (DPL) may help to confirm suspected intraabdominal bleeding. However, a negative DPL does not rule out retroperitoneal haemorrhage.

In the United Kingdom road traffic accidents cause the majority of blunt abdominal vascular trauma. The vessels of the upper abdomen or pelvis are often involved. Injuries occur due to avulsion of a vessel at a site of fixation or due to deceleration forces which may result in mural injury, for instance to the mesenteric or renal vessels, with haematoma formation or thrombosis. The presence of 'seatbelt' bruising of the abdomen and chest gives a clue as to the severity of the injury. Laparotomy for blunt trauma will frequently reveal a damaged liver or spleen as a source of intraabdominal bleeding. Pelvic fractures may disrupt presacral venous plexi with massive internal blood loss and are best dealt with by external pelvic fixation or selective embolisation. Open pelvic repair in the presence of venous bleeding is likely to release tamponade and carries high mortality, morbidity and infection rates.

The concept of dealing with abdominal vascular injuries according to anatomical zones ensures a systematic approach to repair and reduces the likelihood of missed injuries. The areas in which surgical assessment should be concentrated include the supra- and inframesocolic zones, the lateral pelvic, perirenal, portal and retrohepatic regions.

A mid-line incision allows rapid exposure of all areas of the abdomen and can easily be extended to a thoracolaparotomy or to a rooftop incision (see Figure 37.5). Control of the sub-diaphragmatic aorta approached through the lesser sac or at the diaphragmatic crura is an essential prerequisite to exploring an expanding or pulsatile retroperitoneal haematoma. The presence of a retroperitoneal haematoma without these features is not necessarily justification for surgical exploration since this may disturb clot and increases potential for infection.

Exposure of the upper abdominal aorta may be achieved by reflecting the intraabdominal viscera, left colon, spleen, kidney, tail of pancreas and fundus of stomach towards the mid-line. Division of the left crus of the diaphragm improves access to the aorta at this level, allowing proximal control. Kocher's manoeuvre of duodenal mobilisation and medial reflection of the ascending colon allows access to the inferior vena cava (IVC) and can be extended proximally to expose the suprarenal aorta.

The mortality rate due to aortic trauma is between one-half and two-thirds. Aortic injuries are repaired either by direct suture, patch or by interposition grafting. In life-threatening situations it is reasonable to ligate a haemorrhaging coeliac axis branch. If possible, however, these wounds and injuries to the superior mesenteric artery should be repaired. A posterior penetrating wound of the aorta may be closed from within the aorta via an anterior aortotomy and a similar technique used to deal with posterior penetrating wounds of the IVC.

Where infracolic repair of an abdominal aortic wound is necessary, the surgical approach is similar to that for infrarenal aortic aneurysm repair (Figure 37.10). In the trauma situation mesenteric closure over a graft is not always possible. Graft coverage with omentum reduces the risk of late aortoenteric fistula and omentum can be brought down posteriorly through a defect developed in the transverse mesocolon and tacked into place to cover the suture line and graft.

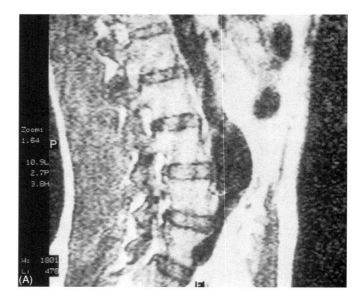

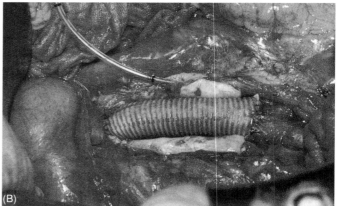

Figure 37.10 MRI scan showing abdominal aortic dissection caused by a seatbelt-type deceleration injury incurred in a road traffic accident (**A**). Operative repair was undertaken with a Dacron tube graft. The plastic catheter demonstrates the site of dissection (**B**).

In the presence of overwhelming peritoneal contamination it may be necessary to oversew a damaged aorta and to carry out extraanatomic bypass. Where lesser soiling has occurred prosthetic grafting may still be feasible after copious washouts. Although little hard evidence exists to support the practice, some surgeons soak Dacron grafts in rifampicin or employ juxtaprosthetic gentamicin beads, powder or impregnated felt in attempts to reduce the incidence of the late complications of graft infection and aortoenteric fistula. It has been suggested that PTFE grafts may be less susceptible than Dacron to infection in the presence of contamination, because of the smaller graft interstices in the former material, but again there is little prospective evidence to vindicate this stance.

The majority of IVC injuries are penetrating. Caval trauma carries a mortality of approximately 50% and in three-quarters of cases another retroperitoneal injury is also present. Temporary control of bleeding from lacerations of large veins or the IVC can some-times be achieved by simple pressure using swabs mounted in sponge-holding forceps applied firmly to either side of the injury. Use of a Satinsky side-biting vascular clamp to exclude a laceration allows caval flow to be maintained whilst repair is undertaken. Swift primary closure of such wounds should be undertaken with interrupted polypropylene sutures. Occasionally a vein patch or prosthetic patch will be necessary to replace a large caval wall defect. Large defects may be repaired with spiral vein grafts but constructing these is time consuming and when fatal exsanguination due to distal caval damage threatens, simple infrarenal ligation of the IVC may be indicated.

Iliac arterial wounds can usually be controlled directly, allowing repair or interposition grafting. A bleeding internal iliac artery can be dealt with by simple ligation in most cases without adverse outcome. Iliac vein wounds are often much more difficult to isolate because of their anatomical position behind the arteries. Insidious large-volume blood loss can occur from a damaged iliac vein and it is occasionally necessary to divide the overlying iliac artery to gain access to repair the damaged vein, following which the artery is reconstituted.

Perirenal haematomas should not be explored following blunt injury if an IVU confirms that the renal collecting system is intact and a normal renal shadow and function are noted. However, if active bleeding occurs, particularly in the presence of a penetrat-ing injury, surgical intervention may be necessary. The renal vessels are best controlled at their origins at the aorta and IVC on each side. A healthy kidney may tolerate normothermic ischaemia for 30–45 minutes. Local infusion with heparinised Hartmann's solution at 4°C induces a degree of renal hypothermia and reduces the risk of microvascular thrombosis where surgery is likely to be prolonged. Papaverine and the prostacyclin analogue iloprost have also been employed for their vasodilatory and reno-protective pharmacological properties.

Before operating on either kidney an IVU is mandatory so that the functional status of the contralateral kidney is known. A damaged left renal vein may be ligated proximal to the gonadal and adrenal veins if necessary. On the right side ligation of the renal vein may necessitate nephrectomy which should only be undertaken if the functional status of the contralateral kidney is assured. As a rule, nephrectomy should rarely be undertaken unless the architectural damage is so great that function cannot be restored. Renal artery injuries may be dealt with by direct repair, patching, interposition grafting or by autotransplantation to the iliac fossa. The mobilised splenic artery can be swung down to replace a damaged left renal artery, offering a further potential source of revascularisation for the left kidney.

Injuries to the retrohepatic IVC carry a high mortality because of their inaccessibility. Various methods have been described to control high IVC injuries. Principles of management include early tamponade of bleeding with abdominal packs; reduction of inflow by aortic clamping at the diaphragm; and extensive exposure, usually necessitating right thoracolaparotomy or combining a mid-line incision with a median sternotomy. Atriocaval shunts have been used to isolate perihepatic caval injuries. Control may also be improved by passing occluding tapes around the supra- and infrahepatic cava after hepatic mobilisation and reflection by division of the falciform and left and right triangular ligaments. Simultaneously the portal vein and hepatic arteries are occluded using Pringle's manoeuvre.

Catastrophic blood loss from abdominal vascular trauma is often complicated by coagulopathy due to massive transfusion, metabolic acidosis and hypothermia at surgery. Early volume resuscitation, use of autologous salvaged blood and administration of fresh frozen plasma, platelets and clotting factors with correction of acidosis and patient warming may help to stave off the frequently lethal outcome from this combination of adverse factors.

Vascular trauma in the lower limb

Proximal vessel control may be necessary prior to repair of injuries to lower limb arteries. The external iliac artery is controlled by a muscle-splitting incision above and parallel to the inguinal ligament. The femoral artery is exposed via a vertical groin incision. The superficial femoral artery can be approached by an anteromedial thigh incision to expose it in the subsartorial canal. Penetrating popliteal artery injuries are accompanied by high subsequent amputation rates. Early repair is indicated and systemic heparinisation and intraoperative thrombolysis can be valuable therapeutic adjuncts. The best exposure of this vessel is achieved by an 'S'-shaped incision placed over the popliteal fossa with the patient prone, although proximal and distal popliteal vessels can be approached by medial incisions placed above and below the knee in the supine patient. Popliteal artery and vein occlusions in knee dislocations and tibial plateau fractures are best immediately revascularised with temporary shunts to preserve the circulation to the extremity. Once the bony injuries have been stabilised, definitive vascular repairs are undertaken. Fasciotomies are often required (Figure 37.2). In severe crush and open tibial fractures with bone loss and tibial vessel disruption, arterial repair is some-times not feasible and in these cases expectant management may be appropriate. Occasionally early amputation will be the only surgical option, but the vascular injury itself is rarely the deciding factor.

Fractures of long bones with associated vascular injuries present a problem of clinical priorities. Ideally arterial and venous repair should be attempted as expeditiously as possible to prevent the deleterious effects of prolonged ischaemia and subsequent reperfusion injury. However, fixation of long bone fractures involves distraction of the bony fragments, often requiring a degree of force, and considerable manipulation may be necessary before achieving a satisfactory position for internal or external fixation. During this period the newly constructed and fragile vascular repair may be at risk. A compromise allowing early reperfusion and optimal conditions for vascular repair is to place vascular shunts as temporary bridges across damaged arteries and veins prior to fracture fixation (Figure 37.11).

Several types of Silastic shunts are available. Before shunt deployment the damaged vessel ends are carefully controlled proximal and distal to the site of injury. Any necessary debridement of the injured vessel can be carried out at this time. Proximal and distal thromboembolectomy with appropriately sized Fogarty balloon catheters may be necessary to reestablish adequate inflow and run-off patency and irrigation of the prepared vessels with heparinised Hartmann's solution should be undertaken. An appropriately sized shunt can then be used to bridge the damaged segment. In the authors' experience the simplicity of the Javid shunt is favoured where feasible, although the Brener shunt, which has a side-arm enabling intraoperative irrigation, and the Pruitt-Inihara shunt, which features balloon occlusion, provide satisfactory alternatives. The shunt is secured into healthy proximal and distal vessels by means of Silastic loops passed around the vessels. This avoids the use of the standard Javid ring clamps which can get in the way during fracture fixation.

Attempts should be made to restore both arterial and venous continuity so that venous outflow obstruction does not exacerbate limb swelling, increasing postoperative morbidity. On restoration of vascular flow, the fracture can be carefully reduced and fixed. Formal vascular repair by end-to-end anastomosis or, more frequently, employing an interposition graft is then carried out (Figure 37.12). In the latter case, the graft, usually a segment of reversed vein, is 'loaded' onto the shunt which remains *in situ* during the repair. It is a simple procedure to remove the shunt prior to completing the final few sutures of the last anastomosis. Any further wound debridement and identification of associated nerve injuries are carried out. Severed nerves can be tagged for later repair.

It is essential that the site of the vascular repair has adequate tissue cover to reduce the risks of infection and secondary haemorrhage. It may be necessary to mobilise a muscle flap to cover the repair. Once this has been carried out the wound may be either closed or left open for delayed primary closure. In cases of extensive skin loss or debridement, split-skin grafting may be indicated. Fasciotomies should be carried out where necessary. The best results from repair of long bone fractures with associated vascular injuries are obtained when there is close communication and cooperation between the orthopaedic surgeons fixing the fractures and the vascular surgeons repairing the damaged blood vessels.

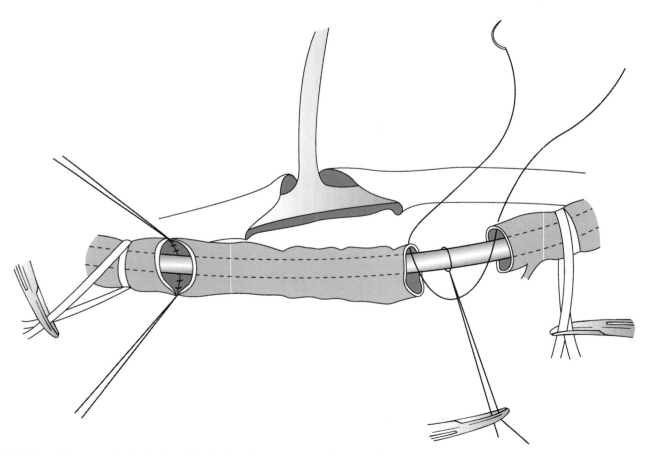

Figure 37.11 Use of shunts to maintain distal arterial perfusion and venous drainage during vascular repair.

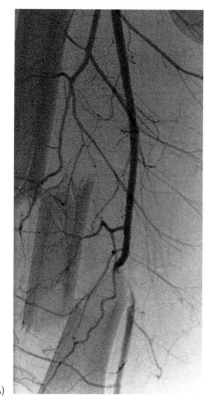

(A)

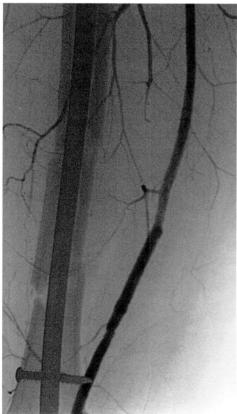

(B)

Figure 37.12 Femoral shaft fracture with damage to the superficial femoral artery (**A**). Arteriogram showing repair by interposition vein graft following shunting and internal fixation of the fracture (**B**).

RECENT DEVELOPMENTS

The advent of endovascular surgery and improvements in imaging techniques enlarge the vascular surgeon's armamentarium of procedures to treat vascular trauma. Growth in the numbers of therapeutic and diagnostic radiological procedures performed has resulted in a parallel increase in the incidence of false femoral aneurysms. Duplex-guided localisation and compression techniques promote aneurysm thrombosis and have been used to treat false aneurysms non-invasively with success, although they have proved largely ineffective in the anticoagulated patient. Duplex-guided false aneurysm thrombin injections have also been described and provide a further alternative to surgical repair, whilst deployment of a collagen plug to seal the artery on completion of angiography may be a useful preventive measure against initial false aneurysm formation.

Recent series have described the use of covered stents to treat traumatic false aneurysms and arteriovenous fistulas in aortic, iliac, subclavian, axillary and carotid arteries. Uncovered stents may be deployed to secure intimal flaps and dissections. Where intra-operative fluoroscopic facilities are available, early control of aortic and caval injuries can be achieved by retrograde femoral passage and proximal inflation of balloon catheters. Similar techniques to obtain temporary control of aortoduodenal and aortocaval fistulas prior to definitive surgery have also been reported. Selective embolisation of pelvic and visceral arteries may be useful in helping to control haemorrhage, for instance with pelvic fractures.

The development of similar endovascular techniques to treat vascular trauma is likely to increase in the future as the available technology improves.

FURTHER READING

Feliciano D, Burch J, Graham J. Abdominal vascular injury. In: Moore E, Mattox K, Feliciano D, eds. *Trauma*, 2nd edn. Norwalk: Appleton and Lange, 1991

Greenhalgh RM, Hollier LH, eds. *Emergency Vascular Surgery*. Philadelphia: WB Saunders, 1992

Johansen KH. Vascular Trauma. In Rutherford RD, ed *Vascular Surgery* Philadelphia: WB Saunders, 2000.

Perry MO. Arterial injuries. In: Bell P, Jamieson C, Ruckley C, eds. *Surgical Management of Vascular Disease*. Philadelphia: WB Saunders, 1992

38

Abdominal aortic aneurysms and aortic dissection

A.A. Majid

ABDOMINAL AORTIC ANEURYSMS

Anatomy of the abdominal aorta

The normal adult infrarenal aorta is approximately 20 mm in diameter. The diameter varies with age and in adult males it increases in size from a mean diameter of 17 mm at the age of 25 to about 21 mm at the age of 70. There is also a direct relationship to body size. Thus in a small-sized Body Surface Area (BSA 1.7 m²) 25-year-old man the aortic diameter is just under 14 mm, whereas in a well-built (BSA 2.3 m²) man of 75 years the aortic diameter is about 22 mm. There is also an apparent sex difference (males appear to have larger aortic diameters) but once correction for body size has been made this apparent difference disappears. The above data are based on information obtained at post mortem and dimensions are slightly smaller than the diameters obtained in life by ultrasound, computed tomography (CT) or other imaging techniques because of the lack of distending forces from the intra-aortic blood pressure.

With regard to its shape, the infrarenal aorta is not completely cylindrical but tapers slightly as it reaches the aortic bifurcation.

Histology of the abdominal aorta

The aorta is an elastic artery and consists of three layers – the adventitia, the media and the intima. Some features of the adventitia and media relevant to abdominal aortic aneurysms (AAAs) are briefly mentioned below.

The adventitia is made up largely of elastin and collagen fibres with a few cells interspersed between the fibres. The amount of elastin and collagen fibres is not evenly distributed throughout the adventitia: there are equal amounts of elastin and collagen fibres in the inner third, whereas in the outer third there are more collagen fibres than elastin fibres. Elastin provides elasticity to the adventitia whilst collagen provides its strength. The adventitia is much tougher than the media because of its collagen content, even though it is a much thinner layer.

The media is the thickest layer of the aorta. It consists of a cellular component, mainly made up of smooth muscle cells, and a very specialised extracellular matrix.

The extracellular matrix is made up of a number of proteins and glycoproteins:

- Elastin is an important component of the aortic media. It is a protein that is able to stretch and recoil due to the random coil conformation of its molecules. It has a long half-life (about 70 years) and once it has been laid down it is not usually replaced. A single gene, the elastin gene, codes for it. This gene is located at 7q11.23.

- Collagen, unlike elastin, is coded for by about 30 different genes. To date, 19 different types of collagen have been discovered. Some, such as types I, III and V, which have a

continuous triple helical structure, form fibrils. Type I collagen is made up of two α1 chains and one α2 chain whilst type III collagen consists of three α1 chains. Type I collagen is thicker and has more tensile strength than type III collagen. Both types I and III collagen are found in the aortic media. Other types of collagen such as type IV and type VIII have a different structure in which the triple helices are separated by globular segments, so that types IV and VIII collagen do not form fibrils but instead form a network.

- Fibrillin, which is a large glycoprotein, forms microfibrils that provide a framework for the deposition of elastin.

- Fibronectin, which is also a large glycoprotein, is involved in the adhesion of cells to the extracellular matrix.

The cellular and extracellular matrix of the aortic media is arranged in a special way so that the media consists of layers of concentric lamellae made of elastin interconnected by elastin fibrils. The structural and functional unit of the media is the lamellar unit, which consists of two elastic lamellae and the contents of the interlamellar space. The interlamellar space contains the collagen fibres and smooth muscle cells. Thick collagen fibres containing types I, III and V collagen with interspersed clumps of type IV collagen, are circumferentially arranged between the elastic lamellae. They act to limit the extent of aortic distension when the blood pressure rises above physiological levels.

Definition

An abdominal aortic aneurysm (AAA) has been defined as 'an abnormal localised dilatation of the aorta'. This definition, which was sufficient for clinicians and pathologists prior to the introduction and widespread use of non-invasive imaging techniques, is now in need of improvement. Techniques such as ultrasound, computed tomography and magnetic resonance imaging (MRI), are able to provide very precise images of the aorta, and as a result smaller aneurysms can now be detected and their diameters measured with great accuracy. It has been necessary to improve the definition to provide criteria to distinguish a normal aorta from an AAA because of the implications with regard to surgical management of AAAs, in particular small AAAs. This has not been easy; a number of definitions have been proposed, but none has been found to be totally satisfactory, mainly because of the wide variation in size of the normal aorta related to age, body size and sex.

The following are some of the physical criteria that have been forwarded to attempt to define the cut-point between the upper limit of the normal abdominal aorta and an AAA.

- *Arbitrary absolute values.* An arbitrary value of 3 cm or greater has been proposed as the cut-point since this diameter is much larger than the upper limit of normal, regardless of age, sex and body size (BSE). However, a diameter of 3 cm is considered by many to be too small to be of clinical significance and others have proposed a diameter of 4 cm. Thus the ADAM

(Aneurysm Detection and Management) Study included two definitions of the cut-point: 3 cm as well as 4 cm.

- *Ratio of the infrarenal/suprarenal aortic diameter.* Since the infrarenal aorta is normally smaller than the suprarenal aorta, the suprarenal aorta provides a convenient reference measurement whatever the individual's age, size or sex. Thus it has been suggested that an AAA can be said to be present when the diameter of the infrarenal aorta is larger than that of the suprarenal aorta by at least 1.5 times. This definition is only useful if the suprarenal aorta is normal and not itself dilated or narrowed. It also cannot be used reliably with ultrasound since the suprarenal aorta is not always easily measured by ultrasound. It is useful, however, when CT or MRI is used since the suprarenal aortic diameter can be obtained very precisely with these methods.

- *Ratio of infrarenal–suprarenal aortic diameter combined with an absolute value.* Since the infrarenal aorta normally has a smaller diameter than the suprarenal aorta, the infrarenal–suprarenal ratio should be less than 1. Thus an infrarenal–suprarenal aorta ratio greater than 1.2 (provided that the infrarenal aorta is less than 3 cm in diameter) represents an AAA.

- *Absolute value together with a difference in size between suprarenal and infrarenal aorta.* A diameter of at least 4 cm or a difference in size of at least 5 mm between infrarenal and suprarenal aortic diameter, the rationale being that risk of rupture is very low when the aortic diameter is less than 4 cm.

- *Ratio of aorta to the predicted normal diameter.* The Society for Vascular Surgery/International Society for Cardiovascular Surgery (SVS/ISCS) definition is 'A permanent localised (i.e. focal) dilatation of an artery having at least a 50% increase in diameter compared to the expected normal diameter of the artery in question'. It is difficult to use this definition because normal values of the aorta that take into account age, sex, body size and race are not yet available. In addition, for smaller individuals whose expected aortic diameter might be, say, 16 mm, an aneurysm would then be defined as a dilatation greater than 24 mm, a figure which might be considered by some to be too small to be labelled an AAA.

- *Relative ratio of the aorta to a body structure.* The ratio of aortic diameter to the third lumbar vertebra on CT measurements has also been used.

The terms 'ectasia' and 'arteriomegaly' need also to be defined. The SVS/ISCS have defined these terms as follows:

- Ectasia is dilatation of less than 50% of the normal aortic diameter.

- Arteriomegaly (aortomegaly) is diffuse arterial enlargement involving several arterial segments (i.e. non-focal) with increase in diameter of more than 50% by comparison to the expected normal diameter.

It is now becoming apparent that by basing the definition of an aneurysm purely on its physical features alone, insufficient attention is being given to the disease process or processes that affect the aortic wall and cause it to dilate. Perhaps a definition is needed which emphasises the disease process that leads to localised weakening of the aortic wall rather than the physical end result of the disease (dilatation). With a better understanding of its pathogenesis it may be possible to use enzyme or genetic markers of the disease process in combination with measurements of aortic dilatation to provide a better definition of aneurysm disease. This will be more useful in managing patients with AAAs, especially in identifying those patients whose AAAs are at risk of rupture.

Aneurysms have been classified according to shape as fusiform or saccular. Fusiform aneurysms are not only wider in diameter but are also elongated compared to the normal aorta. So-called 'false aneurysms' do not involve all three layers of the aortic wall and are caused by an intramural haematoma.

The natural history of an AAA varies considerably; AAAs enlarge at different rates, some very rapidly, others very slowly, although in general it is more rapid the larger the aneurysm. The expansion rate is generally of the order of 10% of the diameter of the aneurysm, i.e. from 0.25 to 0.5 cm per year. Complications of AAA include rupture, infection, embolisation and rarely (<2%) dissection. Some AAAs grow to a very large size before rupturing whilst others may rupture at a very small size. Others may be completely asymptomatic and never rupture during the lifetime of the patient.

Epidemiology

Prevalence

It is difficult to obtain precise data on the prevalence of AAAs since aneurysms are generally asymptomatic. Prior to the introduction of non-invasive techniques epidemiological information obtained from autopsy studies provided a rate of 1–4% in men and a rate half of that (0.5–2%) in women. It also revealed prevalence rates of less than 1% in patients less than 60 years old and increasing with age to a peak of 6% at the age of 80 in men and 4.5% at the age of 90 in women.

Data from screening studies reveal prevalence rates ranging from about 1% to 9%. This wide range in prevalence rates is related to differing definitions of aneurysms as well as the age and sex mix of the populations in the studies, and thus depends on the techniques of study (such as whether they are population studies, case-control studies or cross-sectional studies). The following are data from some important studies:

- The Cardiovascular Health Study reported a prevalence rate of 8.8% in subjects who were more than 65 years old, mostly females (60%), and included small and large aneurysms (defined by an infrarenal aortic diameter of >3 cm, or an infrarenal–suprarenal ratio of >1.2).

- Oxford Screening Programme – 6.3%.

- British Practitioners – 4%.

- RCS England – 6.8% in men and 1% in women aged 65–79 years (AAAs >3 cm in diameter).

- In the ADAM (Aneurysm Detection and Management) Study (1997 and 2000) the ages of subjects ranged from 50 to 79 years; they were mostly males (97%). Prevalence rates for small aortic aneurysms were reported using two criteria:
  (i) 1.2–1.4% for aneurysms 4–4.5 cm in diameter
  (ii) 3.6% for aneurysms 3–4.5 cm in diameter.

Ultrasound screening studies confirm the previous data obtained from post mortem studies, i.e. that prevalence increases with age and, in a cohort which includes men and women, rises from 2.7% in the 65–69 year age group to 4.4% in the 75–79 year age group (RCS England – Vardulaki).

Incidence

A wide range in incidence of asymptomatic AAA has been reported, from as low as 3 to as high as 117 per 100 000 person years. This apparent wide range in incidence can be accounted for by the differences in criteria utilised to identify AAAs. The incidence has been noted to rise with age and has been reported to be rising in many Western countries. Two reports from the Mayo Clinic record a threefold increase in incidence from 12.2% to 36.2% per 100 000 over the three decades from 1951 to 1980. To some extent this is an apparent increase due to the better detection methods currently available (such as the increased use of ultrasound) as well as greater awareness of the condition. However, there is also a true increase in incidence related to factors such as the ageing population in Western countries as well as the late effect of the higher rate of smoking prevalent in the 1950s and 1960s.

Hospital admissions

Abdominal aortic aneurysms account for 53 000 hospital admissions in the USA and 5638 hospital admissions in Canada annually. Approximately 40 000 operations for AAA are performed in the USA each year.

Mortality rate

Ruptured AAAs account for 1–2% of all male deaths in Western countries. In England and Wales in 1995 they accounted for 1.8% of all deaths in men (4907 men) and 0.7% of all deaths in women (1991 women). Ruptured AAAs account for 1000 deaths annually in Canada and 12 000–13 000 deaths annually in the USA. The incidence of rupture is 1–21 per 100 000 person-years, and the overall annual rupture rate is 2.5–10%. Besides rupture, patients with AAAs also have a higher rate of mortality from other cardio-vascular diseases, and the overall rate of mortality from other cardiovascular diseases in patients with AAAs is double that of subjects who do not have an AAA.

The mortality rate of ruptured AAAs is more than 80%. Most patients (60–80%) die before they can reach a hospital. For those patients who then undergo surgery, the operative mortality is high (50–70%) and the overall survival is only of the order of 10%.

Most AAAs (about 55%) rupture posteriorly into the retroperitoneal space, usually on the left side. If the tear is not too large haemorrhage may be contained in the retroperitoneal space and the amount of blood lost limited to some extent. This, together with the ensuing hypotension, may provide sufficient time for the patient to be brought to a hospital. Large tears, particularly those that rupture anteriorly into the peritoneal cavity, usually result in catastrophic haemorrhage, shock and death.

The following are associated with a mortality rate approaching 100%:

- Age greater than 80 years.

- Loss of consciousness.

- Low haemoglobin level.

- Cardiac arrest.

- Respiratory disease.

Recognised risk factors for rupture include:

- Large initial diameter.

- Elevated mean blood pressure.

- Chronic obstructive airways disease.

- Female sex.

- Smoking.

- Decreased FEV_1.

- Elevated levels of collagenase.

- Presence of a mural thrombus: a rapidly growing thrombus within the aneurysm is associated with rupture; mural thrombus is not a protective factor.

- An increase in MMP-9.

- Age greater than 60.

By far the most important risk factor for rupture identified so far is the initial size of the aneurysm at the time of detection. This was first clearly shown by Szilagyi, who found that large AAAs (diameter >6 cm) had a five-year survival of 6% whereas smaller AAAs (diameter <6 cm) had a five-year survival of 50%. As a guide, a patient with a AAA with a diameter of 3 cm has a 3% chance of rupture in five years, but the risk of rupture increases rapidly with increasing size so that AAAs of 5 cm, 6 cm and 7 cm have a 50%, 60% and 70% chance of rupture respectively.

This relationship between diameter and risk of rupture is related to Laplace's Law. Thus, the larger the aneurysm, the greater the wall tension and hence the greater the likelihood of rupture. Laplace's Law:

$$\text{wall tension } T = \frac{P \times R}{W}$$

where P = mean arterial pressure, R = radius, W = wall thickness of the vessel.

Besides diameter, the importance of other factors is being appreciated as important in causing rupture of AAAs, for example enzymic activity in the aortic wall, particularly MMP-9, leading to focal areas of weakness.

Aetiology

Abdominal aortic aneurysms are classified on the basis of aetiology into non-specific, mycotic (infective) and inflammatory causes. The term 'non-specific' has been used for AAAs which were previously thought to be caused by atherosclerosis although the term 'idiopathic' may be just as appropriate since the aetiology has yet to be determined.

A number of risk factors have been identified and are discussed below.

Risk factors

Sex

Males have a six times higher risk of developing an AAA than females. Whether this is due to genetic or hormonal factors, or whether it is because of increased exposure to other risk factors such as smoking has yet to be determined.

Age

The prevalence of AAAs in the under-60s is less than 1% but rises steeply in the 60–75 year age group before reaching a plateau above the age of 80. A decrease in the number of lamellae in the aortic wall with age has been observed and may be related to degradation or degeneration of elastin with age – the half-life of elastin is of the order of 60 years and the adult aorta appears to be incapable of producing much elastin.

Smoking

Death rates from AAA are greater in smokers than in non-smokers and increase with the amount smoked. Smokers who smoke one or two packets a day are eight times more likely to have an AAA than non-smokers. In addition, AAAs grow faster in smokers. The ADAM Study showed a strong association between smoking and AAAs. However, the effect of smoking is reversible to some extent. The risk of having an AAA decreases from eight times to three times on cessation of smoking, and the rate of aneurysm growth also decreases on cessation of smoking.

Smoking may be an initiator of mechanisms that operate at cellular level. Human polymorphs are known to release elastase when exposed to cigarette smoke. Studies of granular elastolytic activity have demonstrated that smoking causes an imbalance between proteolytic and antiproteolytic activity which may be related to development of AAAs. Smoking may also be related to activity of matrix metalloproteinases.

Family history of abdominal aortic aneurysm

Between 10% and 20% of patients with AAA have at least one first-degree relative who has an AAA. This may be due to underlying genetic factors or may simply represent familial clustering of other risk factors such as smoking.

Hypertension

Epidemiological studies have yielded conflicting results: some types of studies (prospective and case-control studies) suggest that hypertension is a risk factor, whereas screening studies do not give much support for this view.

This may be attributed, to an extent, to selection bias in the prospective and case-control studies or alternatively cross-sectional biases in the screening studies. The different inclusion criteria for hypertension may be partly responsible for the confusion as some studies have used systolic BP, others mean BP, or diastolic BP as well as including patients on antihypertensive medication. Despite this, if diastolic blood pressure is used there appears to be some correlation with risk of AAA formation.

Race

Studies from the USA have revealed that AAAs are more common in Caucasian men than in men of African origin.

Serum cholesterol and lipids, chronic obstructive pulmonary disease

The relationship between AAA and serum cholesterol and serum lipids has been the subject of case-control, prospective and screening studies; so far, these have not yet clearly established a relationship between the two.

Although there have been reports of an association between chronic obstructive pulmonary disease and AAAs, recent studies such as the ADAM Study have not found such an association.

Diabetes

There appears to be an inverse relationship between diabetes and AAAs. Screening studies have found that diabetics are less likely to develop AAAs and also that patients with AAAs are less likely to have diabetes.

Pathogenesis

A number of interrelated processes occur which lead to weakening of the aortic wall and result in AAAs:

- Atherosclerosis.
- Proteolytic destruction of the connective tissue matrix.
- Abnormal collagen formation.
- Chronic inflammation.
- Structural and functional predisposing factors.

Atherosclerosis

Abdominal aortic aneurysms were previously thought to occur as a complication of atherosclerosis and there are many risk factors common to both AAAs and atherosclerosis. These include male gender, smoking, age and hypertension. However, there are also differences. The peak age distribution of AAAs is between the ages of 65 and 75 years, whereas occlusive atherosclerotic disease occurs in younger patients (55–65 years of age). The prevalence of AAAs also appears to be rising in Western countries, whereas the clinical manifestations of atherosclerosis, such as coronary artery disease and stroke, appear to be declining. The observation that diabetes, a well-established risk factor for atherosclerosis, has an inverse association with AAAs also does not support the idea that AAAs occur as a complication of atherosclerosis. In addition, atherosclerosis is primarily a disease of the intima, whereas aneurysms result from weakness of the media and adventitia.

In spite of the above observations atherosclerosis may still play a role in the pathogenesis of AAAs. One hypothesis proposes that, as a result of atherosclerosis, oxidised lipid leaches into the aortic wall from the intima and excites an inflammatory response. Proteolytic enzymes (MMPs) released as a result of this inflammatory response damage the connective tissue matrix, particularly the elastin and collagen. The weakened media then stretches to produce the AAA. Another hypothesis is based on the observation that the media of the abdominal aorta is deficient in vasa vasorum and is dependent to some extent on diffusion from the lumen for its nutrition. Atherosclerosis of the intima and overlying thrombus interfere with the diffusion of nutrients to the aorta, resulting eventually in weakening of the media and formation of an aneurysm.

Proteolytic destruction of the connective tissue matrix

It has been proposed that destruction of the elastin and collagen components of the connective tissue matrix is important in the development of an AAA.

Proteinases

The following proteinases have been implicated in the development of AAAs:

- Metalloproteinases.
- Serine proteinases.
- Cysteine proteinases.

METALLOPROTEINASES

The matrix metalloproteinases (MMPs) are a group of proteolytic enzymes produced by a variety of cells in the body. The number of types of MMPs that have been identified has been increasing rapidly: to date, more than 20 have been identified. They include the interstitial collagenases, gelatinases and stromelysins, which act to degrade collagen, gelatin and elastin and other matrix components (Table 38.1).

Table 38.1 Matrix metalloproteinases and their substrates

Matrix metalloproteinase	Substrate(s)
MMP-1 interstitial collagenase	Collagen I, III
MMP-2 gelatinase-a	Type IV, type I collagens, fibronectin
MMP-3 stromelysin 1	Elastin, collagen
MMP-7 matrilysin	Laminin, fibronectin, proteoglycans
MMP-9 gelatinase-b	Collagen IV
MMP-12 metalloelastase	Elastin
MMP-14 MT-1-MMP	Pro-MMP 2

In the aortic wall, metalloproteinases are mostly secreted by the macrophages, with lesser amounts from the smooth muscle cells (Table 38.2). They are dependent on zinc and calcium ions and are released from the cells in an inactive form as a proenzyme. They are subsequently activated by plasmin in the tissues which exposes the active (Zn binding) site. A subgroup of MMPs are closely associated with the cell membrane and are known as the membrane type of MMPs (MTMMPs).

Table 38.2 Sources of matrix metalloproteinases

Source	Matrix metalloproteinase
Vascular smooth muscle cells	MMP-1, -2 and -3
Vascular endothelial cells	MMP-1, -2, -3, and -9
Mononuclear phagocytes, macrophages	MMP-9
Lymphocytes stimulate macrophages to release	MMP-9

MMP-1, MMP-2, MMP-3 and MMP-9 have been shown to be important in the pathogenesis of aneurysms.

- MMP-1 (interstitial collagenase) is responsible for the initiation of the breakdown of type I collagen.

- MMP-2 is thought to be responsible for initiating aneurysm formation. MMP-2 is secreted by the smooth muscle cells of the media in an inactive form and needs to be activated. Membrane type 1 MMP (MT-1-MMP) has been found to activate MMP-2 to initiate the process of elastolysis. Elastin-derived peptides then attract leucocytes which cause further damage (see below). Besides MT-1-MMP, homocysteine has been shown experimentally to activate MMP-2 and induce elastinolytic activity. Mild hyperhomocysteinaemia has been found in patients with AAAs.

- MMP-3 (stromelysin-1) digests collagen as well as other matrix proteins. MMP-3 is found in large quantities in the aneurysm wall. It has been suggested that upregulation of this enzyme may have a role in the formation of an AAA.

- MMP-9 is associated with an increase in size of the aneurysm and has been found to be overexpressed ten times in AAA tissues.

Detailed knowledge of the local regulation of the MMPs is not yet available but it has been shown that their activity is inhibited by:

- α_1-antitrypsin and α_2-macroglobulins, which inhibit the MMPs through their effect on plasmin.

- Specific tissue inhibitors of metalloproteinases (TIMPs) from the mesenchymal cells, which block the MMPs by competitive inhibition.

- Binding to cell membranes.

It has been suggested that a predominance of activators over inhibitors of MMPs results in increased MMP activity leading to a breakdown of the protein matrix and AAA formation.

SERINE PROTEINASES

Serine proteinases such as plasminogen and its activators u-PA and t-PA are indirectly involved in the breakdown of the matrix. As mentioned above, they activate prometalloproteinases to form the active MMPs resulting in matrix degradation.

CYSTEINE PROTEINASES

The cathepsins are a group of cysteine proteinases with elastolytic and collagenolytic activity.

- Cathepsin S is a potent elastase. Interferon gamma, which has been found in the wall of AAAs, is known to stimulate smooth muscle cells to secrete cathepsin S.

- Cathepsin K is a collagenase active on types I and III collagen.

- Procathepsin L binds with proteoglycans from the media of the aorta and catalyses matrix proteins.

Inhibitors of cathepsins include the cystatin family, of which cystatin C is the most abundant. There is a significant inverse relationship between blood levels of cystatin C and aortic dilatation, suggesting that cystatin C has a protective role against the effects of the cathepsins.

Abnormal collagen formation

As a result of elastolysis and breakdown of the elastic lamella, the mechanical load in the aortic media has to be borne by the collagen fibres. Production of collagen is increased and new collagen is laid down but it has been found that these collagen fibres are not properly formed – there is impaired fibril formation of the type III collagen fibres that may result in decreased tensile strength.

Chronic inflammation

Features of inflammation often seen in patients with AAA include:

- The presence of leucocytes in the media and adventitia.

- Elevated circulating levels of cytokines – interleukins (IL) 1 and 6, and tumour necrosis factor (TNF) α.

Leucocytes are a major source of MMPs and serine proteases (e.g. tissue plasminogen activator). These enzymes are able to degrade the structural proteins (elastin, collagen, laminin, etc.) and weaken the aorta. Besides producing proteolytic enzymes, infiltrating leucocytes can induce apoptosis of vascular smooth muscle cells with decreased production of matrix proteins. What it is that initiates the inflammatory response has yet to be determined – elastin fragments and oxidised low-density lipoproteins are currently being investigated.

Structural and functional predisposing factors

The infrarenal aorta has fewer lamellae than more proximal parts of the aorta. The infrarenal aorta also may be the site of turbulence and wall stress.

Clinical features

Most AAAs are asymptomatic and are often only discovered on routine abdominal examination for other conditions. An expansile mass in the abdomen is the best clinical sign. A large AAA in a thin patient is easy to palpate; however, the sensitivity of abdominal examination decreases when the AAA diameter is smaller than 5 cm and when the abdominal girth is more than 100 cm (40 inches). Thus AAAs in such patients are often missed.

Flexing the hips and knees helps to relax the abdominal muscles, and combined with careful deep palpation helps reduce the chance of missing such an AAA. Besides technique, intention is important. Studies have revealed that if a clinician does not have a specific intention to palpate the aorta to look for an AAA, even large AAAs can be missed.

An infrarenal AAA can be distinguished from a suprarenal AAA clinically: 'if you can get above the aneurysm' (i.e. insinuate the examining hand between the aneurysm and the xiphisternum) it is most likely to be an infrarenal AAA.

Expansion of the AAA can cause abdominal or back pain. Complications of AAAs such as embolisation, leaks and rupture also cause symptoms. Microemboli to the lower limb cause multiple infarcts, especially in the feet (trash foot). In these patients the peripheral pulses are usually good, in contrast to patients with arterial insufficiency.

Leaking and ruptured aneurysms

Three scenarios are commonly seen:

- A large tear in the aortic wall. This causes exsanguination into the peritoneal cavity resulting in death within minutes to a few hours.

- A medium-sized tear which ruptures into the peritoneal cavity or into the retroperitoneal para-aortic tissues. In these patients the clinical features of hypovolaemic shock (hypotension, tachycardia, sweating,) back pain, abdominal distension and tenderness, as well as a pulsatile abdominal mass are seen. Left untreated, circulatory collapse and death occur within 24 hours.

- Leaking AAAs are caused by a small tear in the aortic wall. The leak may be sealed temporarily by an intraluminal thrombus on the aneurysm wall or by the haematoma surrounding the leak within the posterior peritoneum. These patients often complain of back pain caused by the retroperitoneal bleeding. When the blood leaks into the peritoneal cavity it causes abdominal pain. These patients are often slightly hypotensive due to the retroperitoneal haemorrhage but can remain haemodynamically stable for a few days.

Other presentations such as rupture into a viscus occur less commonly and present with features of haemorrhage into the viscus, e.g. rupture into the duodenum results in massive upper gastrointestinal haemorrhage.

Investigations

Plain abdominal radiographs

Approximately 25% of AAAs have some amount of wall calcification and can be visualised on plain abdominal radiographs.

Ultrasound

Ultrasound has a high sensitivity (95%) and specificity (100%). It is non-invasive and as such it is useful for screening and monitoring of AAA size. It does have some important limitations, however: the acoustic window is affected by superimposed bowel gas and the patient's anatomy. In addition, only the anteroposterior (AP) diameter can be relied on to give consistent readings. Interobserver as well as intraobserver variability is greater when the transverse diameter is measured. Since the widest diameter of the AAA may not be the AP diameter, the AAA size may be underestimated. Furthermore, it can be difficult to visualise the cranial extent of the AAA, the relationship of the renal arteries to the AAA, and the extent of involvement of the iliac vessels. Thus, although it is useful for screening, ultrasound does not provide sufficient information for preoperative evaluation.

Computed tomography

Computed tomography is widely available and provides detailed information, particularly when used with contrast media (Figure 38.1). It is very useful in the preoperative workup of the patient and provides information on the proximal and distal extent of the AAA, involvement or otherwise of the renal arteries, extent of surrounding fibrosis, and location of other structures such as adherent bowel. When contrast is used it shows not only the renal vessels but also the size of the kidney, as well as to some extent its excretory function. In cases of leaking or ruptured AAAs (Figure 38.2) CT not only reveals the size and extent of the aneurysm but also the site of the leak and the extent of the retroperitoneal haematoma surrounding the AAA as well as free fluid in the peritoneal cavity.

Helical CT is an improvement on conventional CT. It is much faster and provides more detailed images, allowing for a better

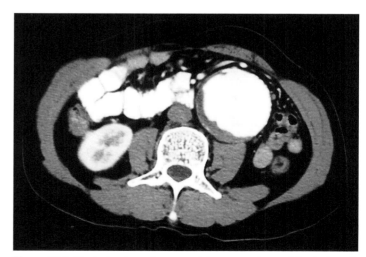

Figure 38.1 Contrast-enhanced computed tomogram shows abdominal aortic aneurysm extending anteriorly to just below the rectus muscle. Note the presence of intraluminal thrombus.

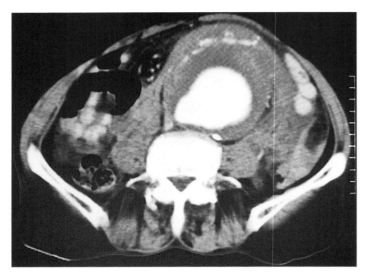

Figure 38.2 This computed tomogram shows a leaking abdominal aortic aneurysm. Extensive retroperitoneal haematoma surrounds the aneurysm.

preoperative assessment. It is also becoming widely available. In CT angiography, three-dimensional reconstructions of the AAA are made (Figure 38.3).

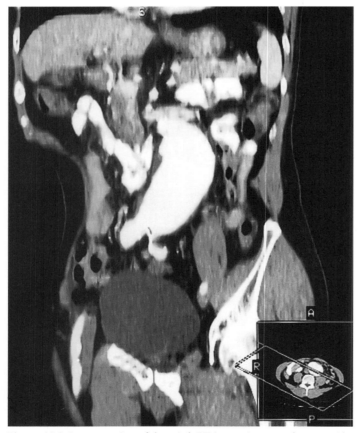

Figure 38.3 Reconstruction of the spiral CT images in many planes provides detailed information regarding the extent of the AAA and its relationship to surrounding structures.

Magnetic resonance imaging

Magnetic resonance imaging is non-invasive and provides images that are useful in the preoperative evaluation of the patient. Iodinated contrast is not needed and the patient is not exposed to ionising radiation. It is more expensive than CT, however, and not as readily available.

Aortography

Aortography (Figure 38.4) allows the abdominal aorta as well as its branches to be visualised and provides information on the relationship of the renal arteries, coeliac and mesenteric arteries to the AAA as well as the presence of disease in these vessels. This helps in planning the surgical procedure. However, the presence of intraluminal clot may cause the size of the aneurysm to be underestimated. In addition, since aortography is an invasive procedure and exposes the patient to irradiation it has largely been replaced by CT and MRI in the preoperative workup. Aortography and fluoroscopy are also now used for placement of endovascular stents in the AAA.

Management

Elective management

There are two management groups based on the size of the AAA:

- Patients with small AAAs (<5.5 cm in diameter) are managed by ultrasonographic surveillance and elective surgery on enlargement or development of symptoms.

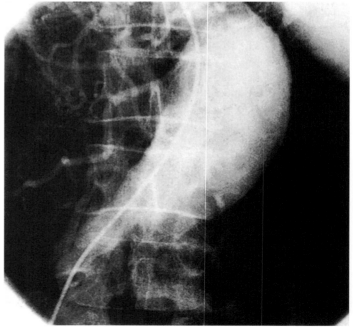

Figure 38.4 This aortogram reveals the tortuous course and extent of this AAA.

- Patients with AAAs greater than 5.5 cm in diameter are offered early elective surgery.

Small abdominal aortic aneurysms (i.e. diameter <5.5 cm)

Small aneurysms enlarge at a rate of 2–4 mm per year and there is a small but significant risk of rupture (1–5% per year or 5–23% over five years). The UK Small Aneurysm Trial was thus set up to study whether patients with small AAAs would benefit from early elective surgery. It found that early surgery for aneurysms did not confer a survival advantage compared to a policy of ultrasonic surveillance and elective surgery. The operative mortality rate was 5.8% (which was higher than the expected 2%) and was due to underlying renal and respiratory disease.

Thus, based on information from the UK Small Aneurysm Trial (UKSAT), small asymptomatic AAAs less than 5.5 cm in diameter which are limited to the infrarenal abdominal aorta (i.e. not involving the iliac vessels) are best managed by ultrasonographic surveillance (six-monthly if the diameter is <5 cm, or three-monthly if the diameter is 5–5.5 cm). Surgical intervention is indicated if:

- The diameter exceeds 5.5 cm.
- There is pain or tenderness.
- There is an increase in size of more than 1 cm diameter per year.
- Iliac or thoracic repair is needed.

In the UKSAT, patients under ultrasound surveillance and elective surgery carried a 2.2% risk of rupture with a risk of mortality 1% per year. For patients kept under ultrasound surveillance the risk factors for rupture were:

- Female sex.
- Larger initial diameter.
- A decrease in FEV_1.
- Smoking.
- Increased mean blood pressure.

Over a five-year period more than half (about 60%) of the patients under observation will require operation.

Abdominal aortic aneurysms with a diameter greater than 5.5 cm

Patients with AAAs greater than 5.5 cm in diameter are offered early elective surgery because of the risk of rupture in aneurysms of this size. In the preoperative evaluation the size and proximal and distal extent of the AAA are assessed. Preoperative evaluation also assesses the general condition of the patient and any illnesses. Elective surgery carries an operative mortality of 3–5% in the absence of comorbid illnesses but this rises to 8–12% in the

presence of ischaemic heart disease, chronic renal failure, chronic lung disease, and liver cirrhosis with portal hypertension. When these comorbid illnesses are severe, as listed below, elective aortic reconstruction is contraindicated:

- Ischaemic heart disease, especially myocardial infarction in the preceding 6 months, intractable angina and heart failure.
- Pulmonary insufficiency causing dyspnoea at rest, or FEV less than 1 litre.
- Severe chronic renal failure (serum creatinine >400 μmol/L, or requiring dialysis).
- Stroke with significant residual effects.
- Short life expectancy.

Endoaneurysmorrhaphy involves the insertion of a tube or bifurcated graft to act as a conduit connecting the aorta above to the aorta or distal vessels below the AAA. The details of the procedure are provided in the Operative Surgery section below.

Results of surgery

The operative mortality rate for elective aortic repair of AAA ranges from 4% to 12%. The one-year survival is in the region of 90% and the five-year survival is about 67%.

Early complications after elective surgery include:

- Cardiac complications such as myocardial ischaemia, cardiac arrhythmia, heart failure.
- Respiratory complications.
- Acute tubular necrosis.
- Haemorrhage.
- Lower limb embolism.
- Wound infection.
- Ischaemic colitis.

Late complications include:

- Graft infection.
- Aortoenteric fistulas.
- Graft occlusion.
- Anastomotic aneurysms.

Emergency management of leaking or ruptured abdominal aortic aneurysms

Again, there are two management groups:
- Patients who are haemodynamically stable.
- Patients who are haemodynamically unstable.

For patients who are mildly distressed but haemodynamically stable there is time for fluid resuscitation and imaging prior to transfer to theatre. Peripheral and central venous cannulae are inserted and fluids or blood are transfused to maintain blood pressure (BP) at approximately 80–90 mmHg. If necessary, inotropes are started. Imaging by bedside ultrasonography or preferably by CT scan (with a spiral CT if available) gives valuable information regarding the site and extent of the aneurysm, the retroperitoneal haematoma, site of rupture, and the length of normal aorta above the AAA, which can be helpful during the operation.

Patients who are haemodynamically unstable need to have large-bore peripheral and central venous cannulae inserted and be rapidly transferred to the operating theatre. There is often no time for imaging. Ten pints of blood and 4–6 units of fresh frozen plasma are requested from the blood bank.

Measures which may help control bleeding include:

- Pneumatic abdominal compression with a medical anti-shock trouser suit (MAST).

- Induction of anaesthesia and intubation only after skin preparation and draping the patient. There is often a fall in BP on induction of anaesthesia due directly to the vasodilator effect of the anaesthetic agents as well as indirectly through relaxation of the abdominal muscles; this decreases the abdominal tamponade and allows further intra-abdominal bleeding.

- Thoracotomy to cross-clamp the aorta and control bleeding; use two teams – one abdominal team and one thoracic team. The thoracic team can perform internal cardiac massage and defibrillation if necessary.

- Insertion of a balloon catheter into the AAA through the site of rupture or through an aneurysmotomy and inflation of the balloon to occlude the aorta proximal to the AAA.

- Occlusion of the aortic tear with a large Satinsky side clamp.

- Insertion of a finger into the tear in the aorta to prevent bleeding.

- Compression of the aorta above the AAA with an occluder or with a vascular clamp.

Results of surgery

There is a 50% mortality associated with leaking and ruptured AAAs. Five factors have been found to be important in predicting the outcome and form the basis for the Hardman score:

- Age greater than 76 years.
- ECG features of ischaemia.
- Loss of consciousness.
- Haemoglobin less than 9 g/dL.
- Serum creatinine greater than 190 μmol/L.

If any one of the above is present preoperatively the survival falls to around 65%; this decreases to 25% if any two are present. The presence of three or more of the above factors is associated with a survival of close to 0% with surgery. Thus, although there are no absolute contraindications to surgery, patients with a Hardman score of 3 or more should be very carefully evaluated prior to offering surgery.

Data from the USA reveal that, despite the many improvements in diagnostic imaging and intensive care over the last 20 years, the rate of elective repair and the mortality rates for elective AAA surgery and emergency surgery for ruptured AAA remain unchanged.

Other techniques

The following approaches are currently being evaluated:

- Endovascular grafting.
- Minimal access approaches.

Endovascular grafting

Endovascular grafting of AAAs was introduced by Parodi and colleagues in 1991 and is still being evaluated. A variety of devices have been devised which are:

- Fully or partially stented.

- Self-expanding or requiring balloon expansion.

- Tube grafts, bifurcated grafts, tapered aortouni-iliac grafts, or modular grafts. Tapered aortouni-iliac grafts are often used in conjunction with a femoro-femoral crossover graft. Modular bifurcated grafts consist of two parts, which are inserted separately and then joined intraluminally.

The advantages of endovascular grafting over open surgery are that it is less invasive, and that the postoperative morbidity and mortality are lower. Patients are thus sooner able to resume oral intake and return to normal activities.

Contrast enhanced spiral CT with 3D reconstruction of images and angiography to visualise the blood supply to the bowel and the presence of accessory renal arteries are used to assess whether endovascular grafting is feasible. The AAAs may be classified on the basis of morphology for purposes of assessment for endovascular repair. The Allenberg and Schumacher classification is based on the length of the proximal neck and the site and size of the distal cuff:

Type I   Proximal neck 1.5 cm, distal cuff 2 cm.

Type II   Proximal neck 1.5 cm, short distal cuff (<2 cm).

Type III Short proximal neck (<1.5 cm) and short distal cuff (<2 cm).

The Dorros classification is based on the length of the proximal neck, the length of the distal cuff, and the state of the iliac vessels:

Type I Confined to the aorta (subgroups A, B, C used to describe length of neck and distal cuff).

Type II Neck greater than 1.5 cm, normal iliacs.

Type III Neck greater than 1.5cm, diseased iliacs.

Type IV Short neck (<1.5 cm), both iliac aneurysms.

Type V(ABC) Ilio/iliofemoral disease.

Technique of deployment of endovascular stents

The procedure is performed under general anaesthetic, or more recently under local anaesthetic, with angiographic imaging via a C-arm. An on-table angiogram is performed and an assessment made. If suitable for endovascular grafting, one or both femoral arteries are dissected or cannulated, and guide wires and sheaths introduced. Self-expanding devices are inserted through a sheath. Grafts that require balloon inflation to expand the stent cause aortic occlusion and require some form of controlled hypotension or asystole, since occlusion may be needed for up to a minute. Controlled hypotension prevents hypertension proximal to the occluding balloon, cardiac failure or graft migration. Short-acting hypotensive drugs (e.g. propofol, SNP or nitroglycerin) or high doses of inhalational anaesthetics are used to induce hypotension whilst adenosine is used to induce controlled asystole.

Complications of endovascular stenting

The mortality rate is 2.6% (i.e. lower than open surgery, which has a mortality of around 7%). This is related to:

● ASA class III and IV.

● Learning curve.

● Adjuvant procedures.

The complication rate is 18% (compared to 23% for open surgery) and is related to:

● Age greater than 75 years.

● Depressed cardiac status.

● The patient being considered unfit for an open procedure.

Major intraprocedural and early complications include:

● Rupture of the aneurysm or iliac artery.

● Embolic graft occlusion.

● Myocardial infarction.

● Endoleaks.

● Occlusion of one or both renal arteries.

● Embolisation of the mesenteric arteries.

ENDOLEAKS

An endoleak is leakage of blood between the endovascular graft and the aneurysm wall. It is referred to as primary if it occurs less than 30 days after graft deployment, or secondary if it occurs more than 30 days after graft deployment.

Endoleaks are more common in females and in patients over 75 years of age. They are divided into four groups according to their aetiology:

I Located at the proximal or distal attachment zones and occurring when there is an incomplete seal.

II Occurring as a result of patent vessels, e.g. lumbar, inferior mesenteric vessels which allow backfilling of the aneurysm sac.

III Occurring as a result of tears in the graft fabric.

IV Leakage through a porous graft or suture line.

All endoleaks can lead to graft compression as well as the persistence of expansile forces on the aortic wall with the risk of rupture. Some endoleaks may seal spontaneously. If the endoleak persists for three months or the AAA increases in size, it should be treated.

LATE COMPLICATIONS

Data from the Eurostar Study reveal that there is a late failure rate for first- and second-generation devices of 3% per year. This is made up of a rupture rate of 1% per year (which carries a mortality rate of 65%) and graft-related complications (2% per year). The latter comprise endoleaks (proximal, midgraft and distal) as well as graft migration and graft kinking. These complications can be diagnosed on a plain abdominal radiograph, which may show movement or rotation. They are more accurately visualised on spiral contrast CT. Management of endoleaks, migration and kinking is by open repair, and has a mortality rate of about 25%.

The above data apply to elective endovascular grafting of AAAs in patients fit for anaesthesia and surgery. Endovascular grafting in patients who are unfit for anaesthesia or surgery is associated with a poor outcome. Initial results on endovascular grafting for ruptured AAAs are encouraging.

Minimal access approaches

Minimal access approaches have the potential for decreasing postoperative pain, a shorter intensive care unit and hospital stay, and earlier return to normal activities. Laparoscopic, video-assisted and minilaparotomy techniques have been described and are currently under evaluation. In the laparoscopic and video-assisted techniques, a retroperitoneal approach via the left loin is used and a retroperitoneal tunnel created using balloons and insufflation. In the minilaparotomy approach a periumbilical midline incision is used.

Medical treatment

Cessation of smoking decreases the rate of enlargement of AAAs. However, no other medical therapy is available for management of AAAs. A number of types of drugs are being evaluated and they include the following:

- Beta-blockers to lower the blood pressure with the aim of reducing the growth rate of the AAA.

- Tetracycline-based drugs such as doxycycline. These drugs block MMP-9 and may be able to reduce the rate of AAA growth.

Prevention

Primary prevention refers to the measures that are taken to prevent the development of a condition. In the case of AAAs the only preventable risk factor is smoking. Secondary prevention involves early detection and surgical treatment. Early detection in the population requires some form of screening programme and it is generally accepted that to start a screening programme the condition must be quite prevalent, should be detectable by tests that are inexpensive, accurate and acceptable, and should be treatable with low risk. The method of screening must be effective, do more good than harm (including psychological trauma), and be cost-effective.

At present there is debate about whether screening can save lives. There is evidence from screening programmes such as the Gloucestershire Aneurysm Screening Programme to show that they can reduce the rate of AAA rupture. Another issue being debated concerns the best method for screening the population and relative costs and potential detection rates:

- Mass screening: the capital costs are high and the detection rate low, but the benefits to the low-risk individuals saved are likely to be great.

- Selective screening: the screening of that section of the population likely to have a high risk (e.g. smokers) where the detection rate is likely to be higher.

- Opportunistic screening: there are no start-up costs and the detection rate may be sufficiently high.

Inflammatory aneurysms

It is not clear whether an inflammatory aneurysm represents a separate disease entity or merely a variant of non-specific AAA with a particularly marked inflammatory component. It accounts for 3–10% of all AAAs and occurs predominantly in males in their early 60s. In this condition there is thickening of the aorta and a periaortic inflammatory reaction extending to the surrounding retroperitoneal area. This causes dense adhesions, which can involve the duodenum, inferior vena cava, left renal vein, ureters and small bowel. If the triad of abdominal or back pain, weight

loss and a raised erythrocyte sedimentation rate (ESR) is present in a patient with an AAA, the possibility of AAA should be entertained. A very thick walled AAA is often revealed on CT. With regard to medical management, the role of corticosteroids is controversial. Surgery is often hazardous: where possible, avoid dissecting the duodenum or small bowel off the aorta since bowel perforations are potentially lethal. Ureteric obstruction by adhesions can be relieved by lysis; however, the place of lysis of these adhesions in the absence of overt ureteric obstruction remains unclear.

Saccular aneurysms

Saccular aneurysms are thought to arise as a result of a focal aortic wall infection. Ulceration and subsequent penetration of the internal elastic lamina and media by the haematoma leads to a localised dissection. The weakened media and adventitia balloon out to form the aneurysm. Surgical treatment is by insertion of a tube graft.

Thoracoabdominal aneurysms

Crawford has classified thoracoabdominal aneurysms into four types:

Type I   From the proximal half of the descending thoracic aorta to the abdominal aorta above the level of the renal artery.

Type II   From the proximal half of the descending thoracic aorta to the abdominal aorta below the level of the renal artery.

Type III   From the distal half of the descending thoracic aorta to the abdominal aorta.

Type IV   The entire abdominal aorta.

The indications for surgery include aneurysms greater than 5.5–6 cm in diameter. Surgery is technically demanding and the risk of complications is high. There is a particular risk of spinal cord injury due to ischaemia from interruption of the blood supply to the spinal cord. There is also a risk of visceral injury, particularly to the kidneys and bowel.

Mycotic aneurysms of the aorta

Mycotic aneurysms are more correctly referred to as infected aneurysms and are found to occur in patients who have undergone gastrectomy or who are being treated with antacids. Salmonella is the most common organism found in these aneurysms. The reservoir is thought to be the gall bladder. The presence of fever in a patient with abdominal pain and an expansile abdominal mass may point to the diagnosis but in many cases the features may be non-specific. Management can be difficult since the diagnosis is not often made preoperatively, and the appropriate antibiotics may not have been administered at the time of operation for insertion of the prosthesis. If frank pus is seen at the time of insertion of the prosthesis, an arterial allograft (if available) may be the prosthesis of choice since they have been shown to be less vulnerable to infection. Once sensitivities are available, antibiotics should be continued for at least six weeks. There is some evidence to suggest that, if oral medication is available, the antibiotics should be continued for the duration of the lifetime of the patient. Cholecystectomy should be routinely performed to eliminate the possible reservoir of bacteria. At one time extra anatomic reconstruction was thought to be the best approach but it is now indicated only if the CT scan shows retroperitoneal infection or spondylitis.

AORTIC DISSECTION

Terminology

Although the terms 'aortic dissection' and 'dissecting aneurysm' are both commonly used, it has been pointed out that 'aortic dissection' is more precise than 'dissecting aneurysm' since many, if not most, cases of dissection of the aorta arise in aortas where no aneurysm is present. 'Dissecting aneurysm', derived from Laennec's 'aneurysm dissequant', is really only appropriate when a dissection occurs in an already established aneurysm (such as may occur in Marfan's syndrome).

Pathology

Aortic dissection, which occurs as a result of a split in the aortic wall, is a disease that can have acute and catastrophic consequences for the patient. Most aortic dissections occur in the thoracic aorta; only 2% of all aortic dissections arise from the abdominal aorta.

The process of aortic dissection can be divided into two phases – the initial phase and the propagation phase. In the initial phase a split occurs between the inner and outer two thirds of the media of the aorta. This split may occur in one of two ways:

- Most commonly, an intimal tear usually occurs as the primary event. This allows blood under pressure to enter the aortic wall and results in a split in the media. The intimal tear usually occurs at the site of greatest wall stress, such as the ascending aorta or at a point of fixation along the aorta.

- Less commonly, rupture of the vasa vasorum within the aortic media itself results in a haematoma which causes the media to split. The haematoma then expands and ruptures through the intima to cause the intimal tear, allowing blood from the aortic lumen to enter the aortic wall.

In the propagation phase, once blood under pressure enters the aortic wall, the intramural haematoma so formed continues to split the layers of the media, and then swiftly dissects through the aorta. The dissection may proceed in an antegrade or retrograde direction, or both. The extent of dissection is quite variable and may be limited to one segment of the aorta, where it may terminate at one of the aortic branches, or it may extend throughout the length of the aorta to reach the iliac arteries or beyond.

In most cases the intimal tear occurs transversely and in many cases it may enlarge to form an intimal flap. The dissected aorta has two lumens – the original 'true' lumen and the newly dissected 'false' lumen. These two lumens are separated by a septum consisting of the endothelium and part of the media.

Once aortic dissection occurs, a number of serious and potentially lethal complications may ensue. It is estimated that approximately 10–15% of patients die within the first 15 minutes of the dissection. The complications include:

- *Rupture*. Massive rupture of the false lumen into the thorax or abdomen results in instantaneous death. Leakage of the false lumen into the thorax results in haemorrhagic shock. This occurs in about 45% of patients with dissections involving the descending aorta.

- *Re-entry*. The false lumen may rupture distally into the true lumen – re-entry. The false lumen then cannot thrombose.

- *Thrombosis of the false lumen*. This may be a good thing as it may limit further dissection. If this occurs in a leaking dissecting aneurysm, the site of leakage may seal off.

- *Occlusion of the aorta and/or its major branches*. This will cause ischaemia of vital organs: stroke from involvement of the arch vessels, renal infarction, mesenteric ischaemia, paraplegia from occlusion of the blood supply to the spinal cord.

- *Retrograde dissection*. This will cause acute aortic regurgitation, coronary artery occlusion, or rupture into the pericardium to cause cardiac tamponade. Cardiac tamponade occurs in 70% of cases of dissections involving the ascending aorta.

Classification

A number of pathological classification systems for dissecting aneurysms are available. Some of these are briefly mentioned below.

The DeBakey classification is based on the site of origin and extent of the dissection and consists of three types:

Type I   starts in the ascending aorta and involves the entire length of the aorta.

Type II   starts in the ascending aorta and is limited to the ascending aorta.

Type III   starts in the descending aorta but spares the ascending aorta and arch.

The Stanford classification is based primarily on whether the ascending aorta is involved, and consists of:

Type A, which involves the ascending aorta.

Type B, which involves the aorta distal to the left subclavian artery.

The Lansman modification of the Stanford classification includes aortic arch dissection. The Guilmet classification includes the whole of the aorta, i.e. intrathoracic as well as intra-abdominal aorta. The classification is based on:

1. Site of intimal tear:

   A – ascending aorta

   B – transverse aortic arch

   C – descending aorta

   D – abdominal aorta.

2. Extension – the most distal segment of the aorta involved:

   I   ascending aorta

   II   transverse arch

   III thoracic descending aorta

   IV   abdominal aorta and iliac arteries.

Aetiology

Causes of aortic dissection can be grouped under the following categories:

- Congenital: congenital defects in the formation of the connective tissue matrix of the aorta.

- Acquired: degeneration of the aortic matrix, acute hypertension, trauma.

Congenital defects in the formation of the connective tissue matrix of the aorta

Marfan's syndrome

Fibrillin, together with other proteins, forms a meshwork of microfibrils on which elastin is deposited. Together with other components (lysyl oxidase, proteoglycans) they form elastic fibres. Marfan's syndrome has been shown to be caused by mutations in the *FBN1* gene that encodes the glycoprotein fibrillin-1. These mutations result in defective fibrillin-1 being produced. Fibrillin monomers polymerise in a parallel head to tail conformation with lateral cross-links. The available evidence suggests that the abnormal fibrillin associated with the *FBN1* gene is deficient in cross-links, ultimately resulting in abnormalities in elastin deposition. In the aorta this results in a weakened aortic wall and predisposes to aneurysm formation and aortic dissection.

Ehlers–Danlos syndrome type IV

In Ehlers–Danlos type IV the gene *COL3A1*, located on chromosome 2, codes for an abnormal type III procollagen and results in weakened type III collagen being produced. In the aorta this (weaker) abnormal type III collagen predisposes to dissection.

Familial causes

A gene mutation on *COL3A1* on chromosome 2 can also cause abnormal type III procollagen and hence abnormal type III collagen to be produced.

Acquired causes

Degeneration of the extracellular matrix of the aorta

- *Hypertension.* This is present in 75% of patients with aortic dissection. The ascending aorta and the upper descending aorta are subjected to torsion and flexion with each ventricular contraction. The pulsatile forces are accentuated in patients with hypertension.

- *Collagen and elastin degradation by MMPs.* Segments of the aorta subjected to haemodynamic stress are associated with changes in the smooth muscle cells, which may be responsible for alterations in the extracellular matrix. The stresses are greatest in the ascending aorta: smooth muscle cells in the region of the greatest wall stresses produce MMPs, resulting in degradation of the surrounding collagen and elastin fibres. This weakens the aortic wall.

- *Cystic medial degeneration.* Necrosis of smooth muscle cells and degeneration of elastin and collagen used to be accepted as the cause of aortic dissection but the features described are now regarded as simply being a part of the ageing process in the aorta.

- *Age.*

- *Bicuspid aortic valves.* Aortic dissection is nine times more common in patients with bicuspid (bileaflet) aortic valves compared to those with trileaflet aortic valves.

- *Coarctation.* Aortic dissection occurs secondary to hypertension proximal to the coarctation as well as related to the increased incidence of bicuspid aortic valves in patients with coarctation.

- *Turner's syndrome.* This is associated with bicuspid aortic valves and coarctation of the aorta.

- *Pregnancy.* Aortic dissection usually occurs in the third trimester as a result of an increase in relaxin. Oestrogen may also have a role through inhibition of collagen and elastin deposition, thus weakening the aorta.

Acute hypertension

The acute hypertension and tachycardia associated with cocaine abuse may predispose to dissection. In weight lifting, acute and severe hypertension and straining may be associated with the Valsalva manoeuvre. In these situations, seen more often in young people, the acute hypertension reaches very high levels, with the systolic pressure approaching 400 mmHg. This acute hypertension causes acute distension of the aorta and results in a split in the intima. This allows blood under pressure to enter the aortic wall to cause the dissection.

Trauma

IATROGENIC

Cardiac catheterisation and balloon angioplasty for coarctation of the aorta may cause intimal tears. Dissection may also arise after aortic cannulation (cannula inserted into the media) or aortic cross-clamping (damage caused by local compression of the aortic wall, often on a diseased aorta).

MOTOR VEHICLE ACCIDENTS

The shearing forces associated with high-speed acceleration or deceleration injuries in motor vehicle accidents cause either an intimal tear or rupture of the vasa vasorum and may result in dissection. Traumatic dissection usually occurs between the media and adventitia, unlike all the other mentioned causes of dissection in which the dissection occurs within the aortic media.

Clinical features

Clinically, aortic dissection is classified into two groups according to time of presentation:

- Acute dissections – those that present early, i.e. less than two weeks after the onset of symptoms.

- Chronic dissections – those that present more than two weeks after the onset of symptoms.

Patients may present with a tearing pain in the chest and features of :

- Haemorrhagic shock secondary to rupture into the thoracic cavity, presenting with hypotension, tachycardia and sweating.

- Cardiogenic shock: retrograde dissection may cause acute aortic regurgitation or cardiac tamponade.

- Occlusion of major branches of the aorta:

  - occlusion of the coronary arteries causing myocardial ischaemia or infarction

  - occlusion of cerebral vessels or spinal arteries causing neurological disorders

- occlusion of visceral arteries – kidney, coeliac, superior mesenteric – causing acute renal failure, mesenteric ischaemia and ischaemic colitis respectively

- occlusion of iliac arteries, causing acute ischaemia of the limb.

Diagnosis and assessment

The electrocardiogram may reveal features of myocardial ischaemia and left heart strain. The chest radiograph in the early stages of aortic dissection may show widening of the superior mediastinum. Once intrathoracic leakage occurs, a small effusion or an obvious haemothorax may be seen.

Transthoracic echocardiography is used to visualise the aorta to look for a double lumen and an intimal flap. It is also used to look for a pericardial effusion as well as to assess aortic valve competence. Whilst it is good for assessing the ascending aorta, it is less good for assessing the arch and not very useful for assessing the descending thoracic aorta. Single plane and multiplane transoesophageal echocardiography allow more detailed visualisation of the arch and descending thoracic aorta.

Computed tomography (Figures 38.5 and 38.6) is available in most hospitals. It is non-invasive and useful for identifying the true and false lumens, the extent of the dissection, and the involvement or otherwise of important branches of the aorta. Spiral CT with contrast provides images very rapidly and allows 3D reconstruction of the images to be performed. Magnetic resonance imaging provides very detailed images of the dissection and its extent. However, it takes longer to perform compared to spiral CT and is not as widely available.

Angiography carries a risk and may cause some delay besides being difficult to perform in these cases. Aortography may show

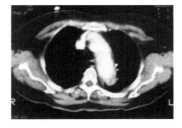 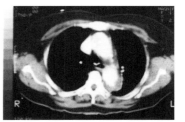
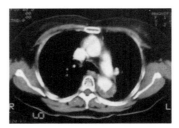 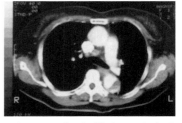

Figure 38.5 Stanford type A aortic dissection; note the double lumen in both ascending and descending aorta.

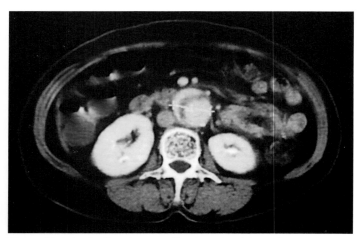

Figure 38.6 Aortic dissection extending into the abdominal aorta; note the double lumen.

the intimal flap, and true and false lumens. However, once thrombosis of the false lumen occurs none of these features may be visualised. Coronary angiography allows the coronary ostia to be visualised and also reveals the presence of concomitant coronary disease. Since coronary artery disease is an important cause of early and late mortality after repair of aortic dissection, it is indicated if there is a history of angina, myocardial infarction, in a known case of coronary artery disease, previous coronary artery bypass graft, or if acute ECG changes are present.

Rapid biochemical tests such as assays of smooth muscle myosin heavy chain are also under investigation and look promising.

Management

Emergency management in acute dissection

The aim of initial emergency management is to prevent further extension of the dissection, limit the amount of leakage, and prevent rupture by some degree of controlled hypotension. This involves:

- *Rapid initial assessment.*

- *Continuous monitoring* of the ECG, BP (preferably by intra-arterial cannula), central venous pressure (CVP) and hourly urine output.

- *Control of the blood pressure.* Vasodilators are used to control hypertension and reduce the wall stress to decrease the chance of rupture and rate of leakage. Sodium nitroprusside (SNP) by infusion is easy to use for titration against the blood pressure because of its rapid response and short half-life. Although it is possible to control the hypertension with vasodilators alone, they are often used in combination with beta-blockers. This is because vasodilators such as SNP cause a decrease in afterload, which causes the diastolic pressure to fall and the pulse pressure to widen, causing an increase in dP/dt and thus an increase in wall stress. In addition, there is often a compensatory

tachycardia that increases the number of impulses on the aortic wall per minute. Beta-blockers are thus added to decrease the force of contraction and to reduce the heart rate in order further to reduce shear stresses on the aortic wall.

- *Stabilisation* by blood transfusion to maintain the pressure (if the patient is hypotensive), sedation and pain relief, and respiratory support.

Ascending aortic dissection (Stanford type A)

Emergency surgery is indicated in Stanford type A patients because of the high risk of rupture, acute aortic insufficiency, cardiac tamponade and risk of occlusion of cephalic vessels. Surgery is performed using cardiopulmonary bypass. It involves resection of the segment of the ascending aorta that includes the entry site and replacement of the resected aorta with a graft. If the aortic valve is incompetent, the Bentall procedure is performed. This involves the replacement of the aortic valve and ascending aorta with a valved conduit and implantation of the coronary arteries onto the graft. Surgery carries a mortality rate of 10–25%.

Descending aortic dissection (Stanford type B)

Surgery carries a high mortality (5–30%) and also a high morbidity. The morbidity is related to the need for aortic cross-clamping, which carries the risk of causing paraplegia and renal failure. It is thus indicated only for special situations such as leakage, impending rupture, malperfusion of a distal vessel, and persistent pain. Medical treatment with control of blood pressure provides results comparable to surgery and is the preferred method of treatment. Stenting with a stent graft across the descending aortic dissection is under evaluation and initial results look promising.

Prognosis after emergency treatment

Patients who are successfully managed in hospital have a five-year survival rate of 80% and a ten-year survival rate of 40%.

Long-term management

Patients with aortic dissection should be kept under life-long review. Hypertension needs to be well controlled and, in the case of type A dissections where the aortic valve was preserved, the aortic valve should be regularly assessed echocardiographically for features of incompetence. The whole of the aorta should be imaged using CT or MRI.

Prevention

Patients with Marfan's syndrome should have their blood pressure closely monitored and controlled with beta-blockers. Surgery is indicated if the diameter of the ascending aorta exceeds 6 cm, if there is significant aortic regurgitation, or if a female patient is considering pregnancy.

OPERATIVE SURGERY

Elective repair of an abdominal aortic aneurysm

Tube graft (aneurysm confined to the aorta) or bifurcated graft

Indications for elective repair

- Abdominal aortic aneurysms with a diameter greater than 5.5 cm.

- Small aneurysms (<5.5 cm diameter) which are complicated by pain, emboli or a rapid increase in size.

Preoperative evaluation

The presence and severity of other illnesses, particularly coronary artery disease, needs to be assessed; a cardiologist should see patients with a history of angina or previous myocardial infarction. Non-invasive tests such as resting and exercise (stress) electrocardiograms, echocardiography and coronary angiography (Figure 38.7) may be needed. If significant disease is found, cardiological intervention (with angioplasty or stenting) or surgery for myocardial revascularisation may be required.

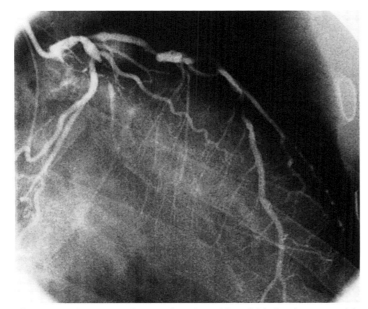

Figure 38.7 Coronary angiogram of a patient with an AAA showing severe triple vessel disease. Myocardial revascularisation with coronary artery bypass grafting was performed initially, followed by repair of the AAA some months later.

Patient preparation

- Bowel preparation.

- Prophylactic antibiotics.

- Cross-match 2–4 units of blood.

Anaesthesia

Large-bore peripheral and central venous cannulas are inserted. Full monitoring is required; this includes the ECG, pulse oximetry, continuous monitoring of intra-arterial pressure and central venous pressure, as well as bladder catheterisation to monitor urine output. General anaesthesia is used and an epidural catheter inserted for management of postoperative pain.

Position

The patient lies supine on the operating table with a sandbag positioned behind the lumbar spine to cause some hyperextension. The surgeon stands on the patient's right side.

Incision

A long midline incision is used.

The procedure

- A Balfour or similar self-retaining abdominal retractor, and Deaver retractors are used to retract the wound edges. A Harrington retractor is useful for the upper (xiphisternal) end of the wound. The abdominal viscera are carefully examined.

- The small bowel is exteriorised and packed in a plastic bag to one side of the abdominal wound. Free the small bowel mesentery from the anterior of the aorta, taking care to avoid damaging the inferior mesenteric artery.

- Identify the normal aorta above the aneurysm and encircle it with a tape. The renal vein may have to be retracted with an encircling tape or even divided in order to get above the aneurysm. Another encircling tape may be passed around the aorta distal to the aneurysm or around the common iliac arteries, taking care to avoid damage to the common iliac veins and ureter (Figure 38.8).

- Request the anaesthetist to first provide 5–10 mL of the patient's blood for the purposes of preclotting the prosthesis (see below) and then to administer heparin 2 mg/kg to the patient. Request also that the blood pressure be reduced to around 100 mmHg. The aorta is then cross-clamped proximal to the aneurysm. A distal clamp is then applied on the lower end of the aorta or on the common iliac arteries, depending on the distal extent of the aneurysm.

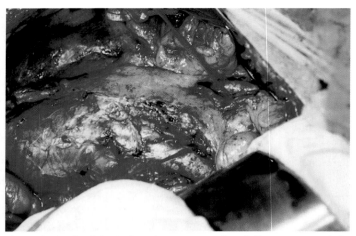

Figure 38.8 The abdominal aortic aneurysm and encircling tapes around the common iliac arteries.

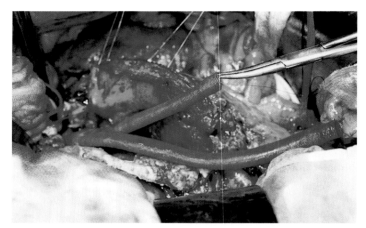

Figure 38.9 The preclotted bifurcated prosthesis within the aneurysm sac – the proximal anastomosis has been performed.

- Open the aneurysm with a longitudinal aortotomy. Evacuate the blood and mural thrombi. The aortic wall is often heavily atheromatous (handle it with care!) and ensure that all debris is removed. The inferior mesenteric artery is looped with a fine silk tie. Back-bleeding from the lumbar arteries can be quite vigorous. These vessels are oversewn with 4 'O' pledgetted Prolene sutures.

- Measure the internal diameter of the aorta and choose a suitable prosthesis. Prostheses of woven or knitted Dacron or polytetrafluoroethylene are available. Knitted Dacron grafts are very porous and, if they are not already gelatin impregnated, should be preclotted prior to use. Suture the graft in position using a 3 'O' Prolene continuous suture. The aortic wall is often fragile so take good, deep full-thickness 'bites', especially posteriorly to take some of the lumbar prevertebral fascia. Use a 'parachute' technique to bring the graft down and ensure that it sits snugly within the aorta. It is now a good time to check if the anastomosis is watertight. Clamp the graft with another cross-clamp and carefully release the proximal aortic cross-clamp. If there are leaks on the lateral or posterior aspects of the anastomosis they are controlled at this time, i.e. before performing the distal anastomosis. Perform the distal anastomosis – either to the aorta in the case of a tube graft, or to the common iliacs or femoral arteries in the case of bifurcated grafts (Figures 38.9 and 38.10).

- Prior to removal of the aortic cross-clamp ensure that the patient is not hypovolaemic by checking the CVP or pulmonary artery wedge pressure (PAWP) and transfuse blood if necessary. Since the vascular tree in the lower limb is likely to be empty it is important to fill it gradually to avoid sudden hypotension on releasing the cross-clamp since acute hypotension can have disastrous consequences. Release the cross-clamp slowly whilst watching the blood pressure on the monitor – there is usually a momentary fall in pressure. This can usually be managed by rapid transfusion, and by reducing the flow through the graft by intermittently and gently

occluding it by compressing the graft between thumb and forefinger.

- The distal anastomosis is then inspected and any leaks over-sewn. The colon is inspected: if there is any doubt about its blood supply, the inferior mesenteric artery, together with a cuff of aortic wall, is anastomosed to the graft.

- Close the aneurysmal sac over the graft. Return the abdominal contents (small bowel, omentum, etc.) to the abdomen. Secure haemostasis and use a mass closure technique for the abdominal wall.

Complications

Myocardial infarction may occur as a result of acute hypertension or acute hypotension. Acute hypertension may occur because of the sudden increase in afterload on application of the aortic cross-clamp. This may cause acute myocardial strain, resulting in myocardial infarction/injury. It may be prevented by the infusion of short-acting vasodilators such as sodium nitroprusside to

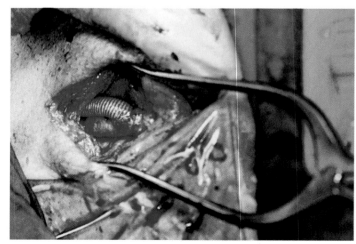

Figure 38.10 The completed distal anastomosis of the bifurcated graft to the femoral artery.

decrease the afterload prior to aortic cross-clamping. Acute hypotension secondary to blood loss is a cause of myocardial infarction. As mentioned above, another cause of acute hypotension is the release of the aortic cross-clamp on completion of the procedure.

Return of metabolites and ions, particularly K+ and H+ ions, from ischaemic tissues distal to the cross-clamp may provoke a cardiac arrest. Careful monitoring of the pH and K+ ions and treatment is needed.

Renal failure secondary to intraoperative blood loss is a well-recognised complication and is difficult to manage.

Transfusion-related complications such as hypothermia and hyperkalaemia may occur if large volumes of blood need to be transfused.

Bacterial translocation may occur during AAA repair and is associated with an increase in septic morbidity. This may be a mechanism for infection of aortic prosthetic grafts. Bacterial translocation may also be involved in the pathogenesis of multiorgan dysfunction, which occurs in a proportion of patients.

Postoperative management

Patients are best managed in an intensive care unit with full continuous monitoring of ECG, BP, CVP, PAWP, blood gases and urine output. ·The patient is usually sedated and ventilated overnight. The systolic arterial blood pressure is maintained at around 140 mmHg using short-acting vasodilators to control hypertension and blood transfusion to manage hypovolaemic hypotension. Antibiotics are continued for at least three days. Oral fluids are commenced once bowel function returns.

FURTHER READING

Alcorn HG, Wolfson SK, Sutton-Tyrrell K, Kuller LH, O'Leary D. Risk factors for abdominal aortic aneurysms in older adults enrolled in the Cardiovascular Health Study. *Arteriosclerosis, Thrombosis, and Vascular Biology* 1996; **16**:963–970

Bengtsson H, Nilsson P, Bergqvist D. Natural history of abdominal aortic aneurysm detected by screening. *British Journal of Surgery* 1993; **80**:718–720

Bengtsson H, Sonesson B, Lanne T et al. Prevalence of abdominal aortic aneurysm in the offspring of patients dying from aneurysm rupture. *British Journal of Surgery* 1992; **79**:1142–1143

Blanchard JF, Armenian HK, Friesen PP. Risk factors for abdominal aortic aneurysm: results of a case-control study. *American Journal of Epidemiology* 2000; **151**:575–583

Bode MK, Soini Y, Melkko J et al. Increased amount of type III pN-collagen in human abdominal aortic aneurysms; evidence for impaired type III collagen fibrillogenesis. *Journal of Vascular Surgery* 2000; **32**:1201–1207

Collin J. A proposal for a precise definition of abdominal aortic aneurysm: a personal view. *Journal of Cardiovascular Surgery (Torino)* 1990; **31**:168–169

Collin J, Walton J, Araujo L, Lindsell D. Oxford screening programme for abdominal aortic aneurysms in men aged 65 to 74 years. *Lancet* 1988; **ii**:613–615

Crowther M, Goodall S, Jones JL, Bell PRF, Thompson MM. Localization of matrix metalloproteinase 2 within the aneurysmal and normal aortic wall. *British Journal of Surgery* 2000; **87**:1391–1400

Fowkes F, Macintyre C, Ruckley C. Increasing incidence of aortic aneurysms in England and Wales. *British Medical Journal* 1989; **298**:33–35

Gillum R. Epidemiology of aortic aneurysms in the United States. *Journal of Clinical Epidemiology* 1995; **48**:1289–1298

Guilmet D, Bachet B, Goudot J, Dreyfus G, Martinelli GL. Aortic dissection: anatomic types and surgical approaches. *Cardiovascular Surgery* 1993; **34**:23–32

Hallett JW. Management of abdominal aortic aneurysms. *Mayo Clinic Proceedings* 2000; **75**:395–399

Harris PL, Vallabhaneni SR, Desgranges P, et al. Incidence and risk factors of late rupture, conversion and death after endovascular repair of infrarenal aortic aneurysms: the EUROSTAR experience. *Journal of Vascular Surgery* 2000; **32**:739–749

Johansson G, Swedenborg J. Ruptured abdominal aortic aneurysms: a study of incidence and mortality. *British Journal of Surgery* 1986; **73**:101–103

Johnstone KW, Rutherford RB, Tilson MD, Shah DM, Hollier L, Stanley JC. Suggested standards for reporting on arterial aneurysms. *Journal of Vascular Surgery* 1991; **13**:444–450

Lederle FA, Johnson GR, Wilson SE et al. Prevalence and associations of abdominal aortic aneurysm detected through screening. *Annals of Internal Medicine* 1997; **126**:441–449

Lederle FA, Johnson GR, Wilson SE et al. The Aneurysm Detection and Management Study screening program: validation cohort and final results. *Archives of Internal Medicine* 2000; **160**:1425–1430

MacSweeney ST, Ellis M, Worrell PC, Greenhalgh RM, Powell JT. Smoking and growth rate of small abdominal aortic aneurysms. *Lancet* 1994; **344**:651–652

MacSweeney ST, Powell JT, Greenhalgh RM. Pathogenesis of abdominal aortic aneurysm. *British Journal of Surgery* 1994; **81**:935–941

Miller JS, Lemaire SA, Coselli JS. Evaluating aortic dissection: when is coronary angiography indicated? *Heart* 2000; **83**:615–616

Moher D, Cole CW, Hill GB. Epidemiology of abdominal aortic aneurysm: the effect of differing definitions. *European Journal of Vascular Surgery* 1992; **6**:647–650

Office for National Statistics. *Mortality Statistics: Cause*. London: HMSO, 1995

Parodi JC, Palmaz JC, Barone HD. Transfemoral Intraluminal graft implantation for abdominal aortic aneurysms. *Annual of Vascular Surgery* 1991; **5**:491–499

Petersen E, Gineitis A, Wagberg F, Angquist K. Activity of matrix metalloproteinase-2 and -9 in abdominal aortic aneurysms. Relation to size and rupture. *European Journal of Vascular and Endovascular Surgery* 2000; **20**:457–461

Powell JT, Adamson J, MacSweeney ST, Greenhalgh RM, Humphries SE, Henney AM. Influence of type III collagen genotype on aortic diameter and disease. *British Journal of Surgery* 1993; **80**:1246–1248

Powell JT, Brady AR, Brown LC et al. Mortality results for randomised controlled trial of early elective surgery or ultrasonographic surveillance for small abdominal aortic aneurysms. *Lancet* 1998; **352**:1649–1655

Pretre R, Von Segesser LK. Aortic dissection. *Lancet* 1997; **349**:1461–1464

Reed D, Reed C, Stemmerman G, Hayashi T. Are aortic aneurysms caused by atherosclerosis? *Circulation* 1992; **85**:205–211

Salim M, Alpert B, Ward J, Pyeritz R. Effect of betaadrenergic blockade on aortic root dilatation in the Marfan syndrome. *American Journal of Cardiology* 1994; **74**:629–633

Strachan DP. Predictors of death from aortic aneurysms among middle-aged men: the Whitehall study. *British Journal of Surgery* 1991; **78**:401–404

Szilagyi DE, Smith RF, De Russo FJ et al. Contribution of abdominal aortic aneurysmectomy to prolongation of life. *Annual of Surgery* 1966; **164**:678–699

Vardulaki KA, Walker NM, Day NE et al. Quantifying risks of hypertensions, age, sex and smoking in patients with abdominal aortic aneurysms. *British Journal of Surgery* 2000; **87**:195–200

Wolinsky H, Glagov S. A lamellar unit of aortic medial structure and function in mammals. *Circulation Research* 1967; **20**:99–111

39

Management of peripheral arterial disease

Rob Smith

INTRODUCTION

General surgeons, particularly those working in general hospitals, will inevitably have to manage patients with vascular disease. The patient may present as an emergency with an arterial problem and there may not be a vascular surgeon available. However, the patients may also present with pathologies requiring surgery which may be affected by peripheral arterial disease (such as an ingrowing toenail); symptoms due to arterial disease mimicking another pathology (such as chronic intestinal ischaemia mimicking peptic ulceration); trauma involving vessels; or another pathology which happens to involve major vessels. It is, therefore, important for all surgeons to have a basic knowledge of the aetiology, pathology, clinical presentation, investigation and treatment of patients with arterial disease. They must also have a basic knowledge of the principles of the various surgical techniques employed by the vascular surgeon.

ACUTE ARTERIAL OCCLUSION

Acute arterial occlusion may occur as a result of four separate pathological processes.

- Embolism
- Thrombosis
- Vasospastic and microocclusive diseases
- Trauma

Aetiology

Embolism

Embolism results from a variety of sources.

Cardiac

- Atrial thrombus (atrial fibrillation)
- Ventricular thrombus (subendocardial infarction)
- Atrial tumours (myxoma)

Arterial

- Aneurysms
- Atherosclerotic ulcers (thrombus and cholesterol emboli)
- Arterial wall following angioplasty or reconstructive surgery ('trash foot')

Other

- Paradoxical embolism (from the venous circulation through a patent atrial septal defect)
- Catheter embolism (materials from catheters or thrombus from their surface)
- Air embolism
- Therapeutic materials (sponges and coils used in interventional radiology)
- Fat embolism, usually following long bone fractures

Thrombosis

Thrombosis may result from alterations in any of three factors: blood flow, arterial wall and blood constituents.

Flow

- Reduced cardiac output (cardiac failure, shock)
- Arterial stenoses (atherosclerosis)
- Turbulence (aneurysms, arterial anastomoses)
- Vasospasm (cold injury)

Arterial wall

- Atherosclerosis (stenosis and ulceration)
- Infection
- Inflammation (e.g. Buerger's disease or Takayasu's arteritis)
- Trauma

Blood constituents

- Increased thrombogenicity (activated clotting factors, thrombocytosis)
- Increased viscosity (dehydration, increased plasma fibrinogen concentration, cold agglutinins and polycythaemia)

Vasospastic and microocclusive diseases

Conditions which cause vasospasm or occlusion of small vessels may also cause thrombosis.

Small vessel occlusive disease

- Diabetic microangiopathy
- Buerger's disease
- Connective tissue disorders (scleroderma, polyarteritis)

Vasospastic disorders

● Primary Raynaud's disease

● Secondary Raynaud's phenomenon (vibration white finger)

● Cold injury

Trauma

Trauma may cause arterial occlusion in a number of ways.

● Complete or partial transection of the artery

● Contusion with intimal damage

● Compression from without

Pathology

Emboli passing through the arterial circulation will lodge at sites of narrowing (bifurcations or atherosclerotic stenoses). There are therefore a number of obvious sites of lodgement (e.g. aortic and femoral bifurcations or the superficial femoral artery in the adductor hiatus).

Sites of thrombosis, however, depend on the aetiology. Atherosclerotic disease tends to result in occlusion of large and medium-sized vessels whereas those with diabetic vascular disease will have occlusions of the microcirculation. In Buerger's disease the medium-sized vessels in the calves and forearms are affected.

Vasospastic disorders may cause thrombosis by reducing arterial flow or may be associated with inflammation of the vessel wall, causing intimal damage.

Trauma may cause extensive full-thickness damage of the arterial wall or may result in intimal damage alone which causes thrombosis without complete arterial disruption.

Clinical presentation

The effect of the occlusion depends upon the extent and the site. Certain areas have a good collateral circulation and so the clinical effects are minimised (such as the superficial femoral artery in the adductor hiatus) but other areas (such as the popliteal bifurcation) have a poor collateral and the effects are acute and serious. The clinical features as shown in Table 39.1 may indicate the severity of the ischaemia.

It is essential to recognise peripheral ischaemia rapidly in order to prevent progression from the 'threatened' category to the 'irreversible category'. Failure to recognise ischaemia is a potentially litigious mistake.

Following thrombosis or lodgement of an embolus, the circulation distally and proximally (as far as the next proximal tributary) ceases and the stasis may result in propagated thrombosis. This occurs more rapidly in diseased than in normal arteries. The thrombus may propagate into the small tributaries, resulting in further ischaemia and also the occlusion of vessels too small to be cleared by surgery. As time progresses ischaemic damage to the tissues occurs with anaerobic respiration, damage to cell membranes, increased vascular permeability and release of oxygen free radicals, potassium, hydrogen ions and myoglobin.

Investigation

Careful clinical assessment is the most important aspect of the assessment of limb ischaemia and the categorisation according to the features in Table 39.1 gives an indication of the urgency and necessity for further investigations.

● *Doppler assessment:* this is used to measure the pressure at the ankle (or wrist) and also to detect arterial and venous flow.

● *Duplex scan:* this is of value for identifying areas of diminished flow but is not sufficiently comprehensive to be useful in planning therapy. It does identify venous thrombosis which, if extensive ('white leg'), may be clinically confused with arterial occlusive disease.

● *Angiography:* of value in identifying the extent of the disease, particularly in cases of thrombosis, and in planning treatment. It is not essential in all cases of embolism. During operation on-table angiography or angioscopy may be carried out to assess completeness of clearance.

Table 39.1 Clinical presentation of ischaemia

Category	Description	Capillary return	Muscle weakness	Sensory loss	Arterial Doppler	Venous Doppler
Viable	Not threatened	Intact	None	None	Audible >30 mmHg	Audible
Threatened	Salvageable if treated	Intact Slow	Mild Partial	Mild Incomplete	Inaudible	Audible
Irreversible	Tissue loss even if treated	Absent (marbling)	Paralysis Rigor	Anaesthetic	Inaudible	Inaudible

Non-surgical treatment

The two established forms of non-surgical treatment for major arterial occlusions are anticoagulation with heparin and thrombolytic therapy. Other techniques in development but as yet unproven include various techniques of mechanical disruption of the clot, with or without thrombolysis, and extraction of the effluent. Angioscopy has also been used as an adjunct to graft clearance.

Patients who have haematological conditions, such as polycythaemia, should be treated appropriately.

For patients with vasospastic disease the treatment is largely medical and depends on the cause. Surgery is only rarely indicated for severe disease.

Anticoagulation

Anticoagulation with heparin alone was initially popularised by Blaisdell who demonstrated that simple heparinisation resulted in a lower mortality than surgery (which may be 10–20%) but a higher rate of limb loss (20–40%).

However, unless there are specific contraindications, it is essential to heparinise the patient systemically immediately a diagnosis of acute limb ischaemia is made. This helps to prevent propagation into the microcirculation while investigating and preparing for alternative therapies.

Thrombolytic therapy

The principle of thrombolytic therapy is the activation of the intrinsic thrombolytic system (plasmin) by a variety of activators. The activators usually used are streptokinase (produced by streptococci), urokinase (extracted from human urine) and tissue plasminogen activator (tPA) (produced by recombinant DNA technology). Streptokinase is the cheapest, least effective and most antigenic. Tissue plasminogen activator is the most expensive, most effective and least antigenic.

Early attempts at systemic thrombolysis resulted in a high rate of haemorrhagic complications and so the technique of local intra-arterial thrombolysis was developed in which a catheter is inserted into the thrombus by the Seldinger technique and the activator is slowly infused. Much smaller doses are required than with systemic thrombolysis. It may be combined with a hydraulic disruption technique called 'pulsed spray' which breaks up the thrombus and exposes more of the thrombus to the activator.

The advantages of thrombolysis over surgery are:

- it is less traumatic and has a lower mortality and morbidity

- it is less likely to result in damage to the artery

- clearance of small arteries that are too small to allow access by thrombectomy catheters may be achieved

- neo-intima in arterial grafts may be better preserved.

Successful clearance may reveal the underlying cause of the occlusion and therefore early intervention to correct the abnormality may be required. This could involve transluminal angioplasty, stenting, open patch angioplasty or bypass.

The results of thrombolysis have been compared in a number of trials. In general, the mortality is lower with thrombolysis but the limb salvage rate is equivalent. The following list shows the criteria, which indicate a better prognosis for success of thrombolysis.

- Duration of occlusion less than seven days.

- Occlusion less than 10 cm long.

- Occluded graft rather than native artery.

- Embolus rather than thrombus.

- Suprainguinal occlusion rather than infrainguinal.

- Good run-off vessels.

Contraindications to thrombolysis include:

- critical ischaemia with neurological defect (insufficient time for thrombolysis)

- recent surgery (danger of haemorrhage)

- irreversible ischaemia

- potential source of haemorrhage (peptic ulcer, recent haemorhagic stroke, etc.).

Treatment of vasospastic disorders

Firstline treatment usually involves the use of calcium channel blockers such as nifedipine, amlodipine or diltiazem. Others include ACE inhibitors, vasodilators (naftidrofuryl), alpha-2 adrenoceptor blockers and parenteral prostacyclin analogues. Conservative medical measures include cold avoidance, avoiding smoking and cessation of potentially harmful drugs. Newer, unproven techniques include the use of tPA, eradication of *Helicobacter pylori* infection, antioxidants, serotonin antagonists and iontophoresis.

REPERFUSION INJURY

When the circulation is reestablished after a period of ischaemia there are a number of pathophysiological processes which occur in the reperfused area which can result in further damage. This damage is called 'reperfusion injury' and is due to a large number of complex phenomena which interact to cause local and distant tissue injury and even death.

Reperfusion injury does not occur if there has never been any loss of circulation and therefore it holds that prevention of ischaemia or reducing the duration of ischaemia to a minimum will prevent or significantly reduce the adverse effects.

Reperfusion injury occurs in the following situations:

- following successful embolectomy
- following arterial reconstruction in a chronically ischaemic limb
- after prolonged arterial clamping with a poor collateral circulation
- after the use of an arterial tourniquet
- after transplantation of an organ
- after cardiopulmonary bypass with cardioplegia
- following successful thrombolysis for myocardial infarction.

Ischaemia

When the blood supply to a tissue is interrupted a sequence of events takes place which may ultimately lead to cell death. The reduction in oxygen delivery causes the metabolic processes to become anaerobic which results in the production of lactic acid. The acidosis interferes with normal enzymatic function and there is a loss of production of the high-energy phosphate bonds which are essential for normal cellular function. Lack of energy prevents normal homeostasis and the normal transmembrane ionic gradients are lost. This results in sodium and water passing into the cell and potassium passing out. The net result is intracellular oedema and loss of function. Further damage caused by calcium overload leads to mitochondrial malfunction and further loss of energy production. Eventually loss of intracellular compartmentalisation with swelling of lysosomes and the endoplasmic reticulum leads to leakage of intracellular enzymes, loss of membrane integrity and eventually autolysis and cell death.

Reperfusion

The restoration of circulation has two beneficial effects: the restoration of an energy supply and the removal of toxic metabolites. However, reperfusion also has two adverse effects: the return of toxic metabolites may have serious systemic ill effects and further local damage may be produced.

Systemic effects

Restoration of perfusion causes hydrogen ions, potassium, myoglobin and activated leucocytes to be returned to the systemic circulation. The combination of a metabolic acidosis and hyperkalaemia may result in cardiac arrhythmias (even sudden death). Myoglobinaemia may result in acute renal failure due to deposition of myoglobin in renal collecting tubules and this will further compound the problem of hyperkalaemia. Non-cardiogenic pulmonary oedema develops due to a combination of increased permeability (thought to be due to a complement-mediated

effect) and the accumulation of leucocytes activated by various agents released from ischaemic tissue. There is also some evidence for neurally mediated effects, particularly in cases of intestinal ischaemia.

Local effects

The return of circulation to an ischaemic vascular bed results in a burst of oxygen free radical release. Free radicals cause lipid peroxidation which further damages cell membranes as well as damaging DNA and extracellular components such as collagen and hyaluronic acid.

Leucocytes are activated by platelet-activating factor (PAF), leukotriene B4 (LTB4) and free radicals. These activated leucocytes adhere to and migrate across the endothelium and then cause further tissue damage by the release of proteolytic enzymes and peroxidase. Activated leucocytes have an important role in the development of multiorgan failure.

Vascular endothelium modulates vascular tone by the secretion of a wide variety of agents such as PAF, nitric oxide and endothelin. In addition, a number of other factors such as the leucocyte adhesion molecules and the cytokines (Il-1, Il-6 and TNF-α) also contribute to tissue damage.

Clinical consequences

Local

The various agents and mechanisms described above produce oedema, tissue necrosis and neurological malfunction. The microcirculation may fail due to capillary occlusion following activation of platelets and clotting factors (no-reflow phenomenon).

The oedema may result in increased tissue pressure (compartment syndrome). This is diagnosed clinically by characteristic features:

- pain and tenderness in the compartment
- muscle pain on passive dorsiflexion
- hardness of the compartment
- loss of sensation in the distribution of the deep peroneal nerve
- loss of neuromuscular function
- a compartment pressure >30–40 mmHg or <40 mmHg below diastolic pressure.

Systemic

The systemic effects include cardiac arrhythmias and failure, non-cardiogenic pulmonary oedema and renal failure ultimately resulting in the multiple organ dysfunction syndrome.

Treatment

The treatment of reperfusion injury must commence before the ischaemic tissue is reperfused. Despite the evidence of the multitude of factors involved there is little evidence for the effects of any specific intervention. Currently accepted treatments include the following.

- Fluid therapy to ensure a high CVP as the reperfused vascular bed is maximally vasodilated. It is also important to help maintain urine flow.

- Intravenous mannitol to act as a free radical scavenger and to ensure a high urine output to prevent myoglobin deposition in the tubules.

- Thrombolytic therapy to lyse capillary thrombi.

- Limb cooling to reduce ischaemic damage.

- Elevation of the limb to reduce venous pressure.

- Fasciotomy should be carried out if compartment pressure rises. (Many surgeons believe that if you think of the possibility of compartment syndrome you should perform a fasciotomy.)

The most important aspect of management is the prevention of prolonged ischaemia by prompt management of acutely ischaemic limbs and reducing tourniquet times to a minimum.

CHRONIC ISCHAEMIA

Definition and classification (Tables 39.2 and 39.3)

Chronic ischaemia may present clinically in two stages:

- intermittent claudication
- critical ischaemia (rest pain or gangrene).

There are six principal groups of pathology which cause chronic ischaemia:

- atherosclerosis
- arterial aneurysm
- diabetes mellitus
- arteritis
- trauma
- miscellaneous (embolism, entrapment, cystic degeneration, fibromuscular hyperplasia, dissection)

Epidemiology and natural history

By far the most common cause of chronic ischaemia is atherosclerosis. Atheroma is found almost universally in autopsies in the over-40 year old group in Western cultures.

Prognosis for a patient presenting with recent onset of claudication is good with regard to the limb but poor with regard to life. Claudication is a marker of generalised vascular disease (Table 39.4).

Seventy-five percent of claudicating patients will either show improvement in their symptoms (due to collateral development) or remain unchanged. The risk of major limb-threatening ischaemia is about 10% after 15 years but in diabetics this risk is increased fivefold. The risk of death (from cardiac and

Table 39.2 Clinical grades and categories of limb ischaemia:

Grade	Category	Clinical description	Objective criteria
0	0	Asymptomatic	Normal exercise test
0	1	Mild claudication	Complete treadmill exercise Postexercise ankle pressure >50 mmHg but >25 mmHg below brachial
I	2	Moderate claudication	Postexercise pressure >50 mmHg but >50 mmHg below brachial
I	3	Severe claudication	Fails to complete exercise test Postexercise pressure <50 mmHg
II	4	Ischaemic rest pain	Resting ankle pressure <40 mmHg Toe pressure <30 mmHg
II	5	Ischaemic ulceration or gangrene of toes	As for 4
III	6	Gangrene extending to mid-foot no longer suitable for salvage	As for 4

Table 39.3 Prevalence of ischaemic symptoms in three age groups

Age	Claudication males %	Claudication females %	Ischaemic heart disease %	Ischaemic stroke %
40–49	1	0.5	4	0.5
50–59	3	2	10	2
60–69	5	3	20	3

Table 39.4 The incidence of complications for a patient with recent-onset claudication

Outcome	5 years %	10 years %	15 years %
Critical ischaemia	3	6	10
Critical ischaemia (diabetic patients)	15	30	50
Death	30	50	70

cerebrovascular disease) is seven times the risk of developing critical ischaemia. Claudication is therefore a marker for widespread vascular disease.

Pathology

Atherosclerosis

The typical atheromatous arterial wall lesion consists of a plaque containing variable amounts of lipid, complex carbohydrates, blood and blood products, fibrous tissue and calcium. The lesion initially involves only the intima but with progression of the disease the media becomes involved as well.

The aetiology of atheroma is poorly understood but the two principal theories are:

- the proliferation of smooth muscle cells is followed by lipid accumulation

- endothelial damage results in the deposition of fibrin and platelets that undergo metamorphosis into atheromatous plaques. Substances released from platelets or the vessel wall cause smooth muscle proliferation.

Aneurysms

The causes of aneurysmal disease of arteries are as follows.

- Degenerative disease (arteriosclerosis)

- Congenital anomaly (berry aneurysms, Marfan's syndrome)

- Inflammation (syphilitic)

- Infection (mycotic aneurysms)

- Arteritis (polyarteritis nodosa, Behçet's disease)

- Traumatic (false aneurysm and arteriovenous fistula)

- Anastomotic

Aneurysmal disease occurs most commonly in the elderly who also suffer from atherosclerosis but its role in the development of aneurysms is uncertain. The current theories regarding the aetiology of aneurysmal disease include:

- a hydraulic distending effect due to reflected pressure waves from distal bifurcations

- vibratory forces from turbulent flow induced by proximal run-off vessels

- reduced arterial wall collagen and elastin content

- increased arterial wall collagenase and elastase activity

- a genetic predisposition: first-degree male relatives of patients with abdominal aortic aneurysms have a relative risk of up to 10.

Examination

The examination of the patient with peripheral arterial disease should include assessment of:

- peripheral cutaneous lesions (ulcers, gangrene, etc.)

- peripheral temperature

- skin colour and capillary refill time

- palpable pulses

- arterial bruits

- presence of abnormally dilated arteries (aorta, femoral, popliteal)

- blood pressure in both arms.

Investigation

A variety of invasive and non-invasive techniques of investigation can be used.

Ankle pressures

The pressure in the arteries at various points in the limb may be measured using a blood pressure cuff and an ultrasonic Doppler flow detector. In practice, the only measurement of value is the tibial or digital pressure with the flow detector applied to the arteries at the ankle or in the digits. The measurement of segmental pressures does not contribute significantly to management. The technique may be used for diagnosis, monitoring progress of disease and following progress after arterial reconstruction.

The pressure is converted into an index in relation to the brachial pressure (ankle brachial pressure index or ABPI). The ABPI results are fairly consistently related to the severity of symptoms:

1.0–1.2	normal
0.5–0.9	claudication
<0.4	rest pain
<0.15	threatened limb loss.

The ankle pressure measurement may be inaccurate in patients with arterial calcification (especially in diabetics).

Exercise test

In some patients the ABPI may be normal in the presence of arterial disease (especially with iliac disease). On exercise, with vasodilatation, the pressure will fall initially and recover again on resting. This is a useful test to discriminate between arterial and non-arterial causes of claudication.

Duplex scanning

The duplex scanner combines a system which produces an anatomical image of the artery with a Doppler system that detects velocity and direction of blood flow. It is useful in the assessment of occlusive disease of the carotid bifurcation and aneurysmal disease of most extracranial arteries. It can also be used as an initial screening test of patients with occlusive disease of the limbs but is time consuming to perform and does not produce the 'road map' of the circulation that most surgeons prefer to plan intervention. The technique is, however, useful in screening reconstructions. (See Surveillance below.)

The velocity of blood flow increases within a stenosis and the measurement of the peak systolic velocity ratio (PSVR = PSV in the stenosis / PSV proximal or distal to the stenosis) gives an indication of the severity of the stenosis. A PSVR of 2.0–2.5 indicates a stenosis of approximately 50% of luminal area.

Transoesophageal scanning (TOE) is useful for assessing the aortic arch in cases of traumatic rupture or dissection.

False aneurysms of the femoral artery may be treated using prolonged compression by a duplex scanning head which enables the aneurysm to be occluded while maintaining flow in the underlying artery.

Angiography

This remains the standard technique in most hospitals for the assessment of occlusive disease but is being superseded by other techniques. It is used by most interventionists for angioplasty and thrombolysis. Most angiography is performed by the Seldinger technique using digital subtraction processing (DSA). It is important to remember that single-plane views may not give a good impression of the degree of stenosis. When assessing the iliac arteries and the origin of the profunda femoris, oblique views are of value. Occasionally it is impossible to achieve arterial access for technical reasons. A catheter may be inserted transvenously to the right atrium and digital images of the arterial circulation may be obtained following injection of a bolus of contrast.

Complications of angiography (<2%) include thrombosis, embolism and false aneurysm.

Angiography may also be carried out during operation. Excellent single-shot images may be obtained by direct injection into the artery after crossclamping the inflow. This may be used to assess run-off, the adequacy of embolectomy and the quality of an arterial anastomosis or to monitor intraoperative thrombolysis.

CT angiography

The development of spiral CT has dramatically reduced the acquisition time and hence enables high-quality images of segments of the body during a single breath hold. The digital images may be processed to produce single collapsed views of the vessels (iliac and femoral vessels) or three-dimensional reconstructions (particularly useful for aneurysms).

The technique requires a large amount of data (thin sections) and hence with a limited acquisition time (one breath hold) it is only useful for imaging localised sections of the arterial tree.

MR angiography

This describes a variety of techniques used to visualise the vascular tree. The advantage of MRI is that it detects flowing blood without the need for contrast material. It has been shown to be as good as angiography in the assessment of the aortoiliac segment and has recently been shown to be even more accurate at identifying patent tibial vessels than DSA.

Other techniques

There are a number of additional investigative techniques available but these are not routinely used in clinical practice. These include plethysmography, isotope clearance, pulse volume recording, thermography and transcutaneous oxygen tension monitoring.

Treatment

The indications for treatment of patients with chronic arterial disease vary considerably and are affected by:

- severity of symptoms
- site and extent of vascular disease
- age and mobility of the patient
- co-morbidity of the patient
- availability of resources for intervention
- expectations of the patient
- attitude of the surgeon.

Surgical treatment

Few surgeons would disagree that patients with rest pain or gangrene require consideration for intervention but the main controversy arises from the attitude of individual surgeons to intervention for claudication alone. In general, intervention for infrainguinal disease in claudicants is not usually considered unless the claudication is interfering with their ability to work or has a major effect on their life. Patients with diabetes mellitus are at greater risk of complications and therefore less likely to have interventions for claudication alone. As with most specialties, younger surgeons tend to be more interventional than older ones!

The techniques of surgical treatment are covered below.

Non-surgical treatment

Non-surgical treatment of chronic ischaemia involves the use of four modalities.

Pharmacological

ANTIPLATELET AGENTS

- Aspirin (75 mg daily)
- Dipyridamole (100–200 mg three times daily)
- Clopidogrel (75 mg daily)

ANTICOAGULANTS

- Unfractionated heparin
- Low molecular weight heparin
- Warfarin

LIPID-LOWERING AGENTS

- Statins
- Fibrates

FIBRINOGEN-LOWERING AGENTS

- Clofibrate

VASODILATORS

- Naftidrofuryl
- Nifedipine
- Thymoxamine

OTHERS

The pharmacological control of other diseases related to periph-eral ischaemia is also of importance. Included in this category is the control of diabetes mellitus, hypertension, arteritis and heart failure. Beta blockers, however, may cause deterioration of peripheral vascular disease symptoms.

Long-term control of peripheral vascular disease is dependent on lipid-lowering and antiplatelet agents. Anticoagulants are used in hypercoagulable states and following embolic episodes. Vasodilators such as nifedipine and thymoxamine are of limited value in Raynaud's disease and naftidrofuryl is of minimal benefit in claudication.

Haematological techniques

The main aim of haematological techniques is to reduce viscosity and hypercoagulable states. Whole-blood viscosity is related to cellular content and plasma viscosity. The cellular content may be reduced by treatment of polycythaemia or leukaemia and plasma viscosity may be reduced by lowering fibrinogen concentrations. Dextran solutions given intravenously will also reduce plasma vis-cosity. Hypercoagulable states may be helped by anticoagulation, defibrination and antiplatelet agents.

Sympathetic blockade

Sympathetic blockade in the lower limb is carried out by phenol injection under radiological control and in the upper limb by a thoracoscopic technique. Destruction of the sympathetic chain results in vasodilatation, predominantly in the skin vessels, and cessation of eccrine sweating. The effect on blood vessels only lasts for about 2–3 years before the vessels become sensitised to circulating adrenal medullary hormones. Sympathetic stimulation of arteries in muscle causes vasodilatation and, hence, sympathetic blockade is contraindicated in claudication.

The indications for sympathectomy include:

- control of pain from ischaemic tissue
- assists in healing ischaemic skin lesions
- occasional use in severe vasospastic disease
- treatment of hyperhidrosis.

Transluminal angioplasty

Using the Seldinger technique, a balloon catheter may be directed into a diseased artery and a stenosis or short occlusion may be dilated by inflation of the balloon. The indications for this technique are still controversial. The dilatation of iliac stenoses is perhaps the most universally accepted indication but it can be used in arteries below the inguinal ligament, in visceral arteries, coronary arteries and recently in the carotid arteries.

The effect of forcible dilatation of the stenosis results in rupture and fissuring of the plaque and dilatation of the vessel. A new technique has recently been reported whereby a false passage is made with the balloon catheter in the subintimal plane (subinti-mal angioplasty). This creates a much smoother and, theoretically, less thrombogenic passage.

Implanted metal mesh stents have been employed to try and prevent embolisation of the loose atheromatous debris and restenosis. These stents may be self-expanding (using memory metal or thermal expansion) or require dilatation with a balloon.

Relative contraindications to angioplasty are:

- eccentric stenoses (balloon stretches normal wall without compressing plaque)
- multiple stenoses (multiple areas of damaged vessel wall increase the risk of thrombosis)
- calcification (wall is too rigid to dilate)
- occlusions >10 cm (too extensive an area of abnormal vessel wall leads to postangioplasty thrombosis).

At the time of angioplasty some aspirin, heparin or vasodilators may be used singly or in combination. Aspirin should be continued long term.

DIABETIC VASCULAR DISEASE

Patients with both type 1 and type 2 diabetes mellitus are at increased risk of vascular disease. They have a twofold increased risk of stroke, a two- to threefold increase in risk of myocardial infarction and a fivefold increase in the risk of major limb amputation.

Aetiology

The reasons for the increased risk of major limb (usually lower limb) amputation are as follows.

- Increased risk of developing atheroma which tends to be worse in the more peripheral vessels (tibials) than the larger proximal vessels.
- Disease of the microvasculature which is characterised by thickening of the capillary basement membrane which acts as a diffusion barrier.
- Peripheral neuropathy, both autonomic and somatic.
- Reduced resistance to infection due to raised tissue glucose levels and reduced local immune competence.

The neuropathy leads to unrecognised trauma (such as chafing from new footwear), that in turn leads to infection due to the reduced resistance to infecting organisms. The neuropathy may also lead to Charcot-type changes that result in disintegration of the skeleton of the foot and consequent gross deformity. The ischaemia prevents adequate repair and the subsequent tissue damage causes swelling which in turn leads to further ischaemia and spread of the infection.

The neuropathy may also lead to loss of the normal foot mechanics and the altered posture of the foot (particularly clawed toes and Charcot changes) causes the development of callosities which may become infected and lead to deep penetrating ulcers.

Simple infective lesions (such as tinea pedis or an ingrowing toenail) may lead to spreading infection due to the lack of an adequate local response. This may progress to gangrene.

Management

The management of diabetic foot disease has four components:

- prevention of complications
- local treatment of complications
- amputation
- rehabilitation.

Prevention of complications

- Regular foot inspections
- Regular chiropody to deal with callosities and toenails
- Moulded soles and special footwear for neuropathic feet
- Pamidronate for developing Charcot changes
- Early antibiotic therapy for infections
- Control of tinea pedis
- Careful foot hygiene
- Care of pressure areas when confined to bed
- Good diabetic control
- No smoking

Local treatment of complications

Ulcers

The aim of treatment is twofold.

- Promote healing in those in whom healing is possible.
- Prevent further complications in those in whom healing is unlikely. (A limb with an unhealing painless ulcer may be of more use to a patient, whose expectation of life may be limited, than a healed amputation stump.)

ANTIBIOTICS

Long-term antibiotics should be given until the ulcer is healed. This helps to prevent further spread of infection. A broad-spectrum antibiotic such as co-amoxiclav is useful and if bone is involved clindamycin should be used.

DEBRIDEMENT (WHICH MAY HAVE TO BE REPEATED SEVERAL TIMES)

- Mechanical with a blade (dead tissue is insensitive)

- Lavage of all loose tissue

- Desloughing agents including weak acids, enzymes (varidase), hydrogen peroxide cream, hydrocolloid dressings

CLEANING

- Soak in water with salt or povidone iodine added

- Irrigate wound

- Gentle cleansing with swabs

APPLICATIONS

- Alginate dressings (encourages collagen production) – particularly good for deep wounds

- Growth factor applications (PDGF)

- Tissue engineering using dermal fibroblast cultures

- Encourage skin growth (sharp debridement)

- Prevent overgranulation with ischaemic granulation tissue (silver nitrate, copper sulphate, light abrasion of wound)

DRESSINGS

- Keep moist

- Protect from trauma

- Keep out bacteria

- Non-adherent

- Hide wound and prevent odour

Dry gangrene

- Prevent wet gangrene.

- Encourage mummification and spontaneous separation (try to avoid amputation).

- Consider reconstruction after angiography. Angiography is usually not worthwhile if the popliteal pulse is palpable, gangrene extends to the mid-foot or the foot has gross sepsis.

Wet gangrene

- Broad-spectrum antibiotics (especially covering anaerobes).

- Repeated debridement to drain infected areas.

- Desloughing agents.

Amputation

Amputation for diabetic vascular disease may be feasible at a more distal level than in patients with purely atheromatous major vessel disease. Digital amputations may be feasible for patients with palpable ankle pulses or even with absent ankle pulses but a palpable popliteal pulse. Clearly the amputation must be carried out through healthy vascularised tissue and frequently the subcutaneous spread of necrosis may be much further than expected. Digital gangrene may be associated with spreading necrosis in the intermetatarsal spaces and in this situation excision of the metatarsal along with the toe may be necessary. This creates a 'cleft foot' which, if it heals, gives a remarkably functional result. It is pointless trying to save a foot which has lost large areas of plantar skin.

Gangrene extending to the mid-foot almost always requires below-knee amputation.

Rehabilitation

Rehabilitation must commence as soon as possible as the earlier it starts, the better the outcome. The use of a rigid dressing has considerable advantages in that it protects the stump, gives uniform compression to prevent oedema and encourage venous return, prevents the development of flexion contracture of the knee and allows early ambulation in a temporary prosthesis. The main disadvantage is that it is more difficult to ensure that the quadriceps muscle tone is being maintained. However, if a window is created in the plaster over the patella the physiotherapist may check the function of the quadriceps.

Of patients with a unilateral below-knee amputation, 70% should walk satisfactorily with a prosthesis and even 30% of bilateral amputees should have a useful walking ability.

Patients with partial foot amputations must be fitted with appropriate insoles and inserts for their footwear to prevent further trauma due to the altered foot dynamics.

ARTERIAL SURGERY

Refer to the Operative Surgery section below for details of specific operations.

Vascular sutures

Arterial anastomoses are dependent on sutures for variable periods of time. The closure of an arteriotomy results in a sound natural union within about two weeks and therefore does not require prolonged suture support. A vein-to-arterial anastomosis forms a similar sound union but it is not complete until about eight weeks. In contrast, the anastomosis between a prosthetic graft and an artery never achieves compete healing and the anastomosis is therefore dependent on the sutures for life.

Vascular sutures need to have the following properties:

- non-absorbable
- non-thrombogenic
- durable
- low coefficient of friction
- form safe knots.

They may be either braided or monofilament but monofilament sutures tend to have less thrombogenic potential and greater resistance to infection.

The principal materials used for vascular sutures are:

- polypropylene
- expanded polytetrafluoroethylene
- braided polyester.

Polypropylene is a synthetic monofilament suture with a degree of elasticity. It has a low coefficient of friction and therefore slides through tissues very easily. This is useful when using the 'parachuting' technique of anastomosis. It has a 'memory' which some surgeons regard as a disadvantage and needs to be carefully knotted to prevent slippage. In general, five throws are required and the excess material should be cut at about 3–4 mm. It must not be grasped by metal instruments, as this will alter its surface structure and may lead to late failure. The needles are of a larger diameter than the material and this leads to excess suture hole bleeding when used with PTFE grafts due to the lack of 'memory' of the PTFE.

Expanded polytetrafluoroethylene (PTFE) is a synthetic monofilament suture with a soft texture. It does not have a memory but also requires multiple throws to ensure safe knots. It has a higher coefficient of friction than polypropylene. The needle-to-suture diameter ratio is closer than with polypropylene and therefore it is better for use on PTFE grafts.

Coated polyester is a synthetic braided suture without a memory. It has quite a high coefficient of friction despite the coating and is therefore less useful when using the parachuting technique. It retains its strength permanently but is less resistant to infection than monofilament sutures.

Arterial grafts

Some arterial reconstructions may be carried out without the use of grafts (such as endarterectomy) but most reconstructions for aneurysmal or occlusive disease require some form of graft of natural or synthetic origin. All grafts have inherent advantages and disadvantages. The closer a graft is to the normal artery in structure and physical characteristics, the better the long-term patency. It is important that the graft material should become endothelialised and that it should have a similar compliance to the native artery. No prosthetic grafts yet fulfil this ideal.

Grafts may be classified as follows:

Natural

- Vein autograft:
  - reversed
  - in situ
- Umbilical vein allograft
- Arterial autograft
- Arterial allograft

Synthetic

- Dacron:
  - Knitted
  - Woven
  - Velour
  - Sealed knitted
- Expanded polytetrafluoroethylene (ePTFE)
  - Standard
  - Reinforced
  - Carbon bonded
- Macroporous fluoropolymer

Natural graft materials

Autogenous vein

The long saphenous vein is the most widely used autograft for arterial reconstruction. If long saphenous vein is unavailable short saphenous or cephalic vein may be used. The superficial femoral vein may also be used but available length is short.

Veins are of small calibre and are unsuitable for the reconstruction of large-diameter vessels such as the aorta or iliac arteries. Short segments of wider diameter conduit may be constructed by sewing strips of vein together longitudinally. The superficial femoral vein may also be used as this is about twice the diameter of the saphenous; however, only short lengths are available. These are useful techniques for the repair of short segments of vein (such as a damaged common femoral vein) but are not suitable for longer arterial reconstructions.

The long saphenous vein may be completely removed after ligation of the tributaries, reversed to prevent valve function and then implanted. Alternatively the vein may be left *in situ*, the tributaries ligated and the valves destroyed with a valvulotome. The vein is mobilised sufficiently at both ends to swing it across and anastomose it to the arteries. See p. 612 for techniques of saphenous vein harvesting.

Vein is more resistant to infection than prosthesis and for femorodistal reconstructions has a higher patency rate. It is easier to suture, is more haemostatic at the anastomoses and costs nothing.

The disadvantages of vein are that it may be of insufficient calibre, quality and length. The wound created by removal of the vein often suffers delayed healing. It is prone to a variety of pathological processes which may cause narrowing, including:

- fibrous stricture following damage from the dissection or clamping
- stricturing due to ligation of tributaries too close to the vessel
- fibrotic valves
- myointimal hyperplasia
- atherosclerosis.

The first two causes may be prevented by a careful technique. Fibrotic valves may not be detected at implantation unless angiography or angioscopy is performed.

Myointimal hyperplasia occurs as a result of proliferation of myointimal cells in areas denuded of endothelium under the influence of platelet-derived growth factor (PDGF). The myointimal cells begin to proliferate during the period of endothelial loss and will then continue to do so at a slower rate even after reendothelialisation. Attempts to prevent it have not been successful. Prevention of endothelial loss is probably the most important factor but the use of antiplatelet agents, which does increase graft survival, has not been shown to significantly reduce myointimal hyperplasia.

Atherosclerosis does not normally involve veins but when veins are transplanted into the arterial circulation, they become susceptible. The same factors that are responsible for myointimal hyperplasia are also thought to be responsible for atherosclerosis. Atherosclerotic plaques are found in about 10–15% of femoropopliteal vein grafts after 3–5 years. Atherosclerosis is associated with the development of vein graft aneurysms.

Umbilical vein allografts

Human umbilical veins may be rendered non-antigenic and strengthened by tanning with glutaraldehyde. The problem of aneurysm development which bedevilled early grafts has been solved by using an external support of Dacron mesh. The graft is available in different diameters and lengths but is thick walled and requires careful preparation before implantation. Longer grafts are prepared at the time of manufacture by suturing two lengths together. The graft is easily damaged by rough handling and is difficult to stitch due to the varying thickness of the wall. It

becomes soundly incorporated because of the reaction caused by the Dacron sheath and is more resistant to infection than prosthetic grafts.

Arterial autografts

There are sections of the arterial tree that may be used as autografts. These include the internal iliac, the internal thoracic and external carotid arteries. These may be either completely removed and reimplanted or mobilised distally and reanastomosed to another organ. Arterial homografts are of limited length but are the graft of choice in infants as they will grow in proportion to the growth of the rest of the arterial tree. Internal thoracic artery bypass for coronary revascularisation is probably the most common role for this type of graft.

Arterial allografts

Arterial allografts are difficult to harvest and require complex preparation. They have been used in the past but proved unsuccessful due to a high incidence of early occlusion and aneurysm formation. Interest is redeveloping in view of the successful preparation of umbilical veins but inevitably there will be problems of supply and processing and at present there is no commercially available arterial allograft.

Prosthetic grafts

Prosthetic tubes implanted into the circulation remain permanently thrombogenic and in order to overcome this problem arterial grafts are designed to allow the ingrowth of connective tissue which coats the prosthetic material. The lumen is lined by fibroblasts but never develops an endothelial layer except close to the anastomoses.

As well as reducing their thrombogenicity the tissue ingrowth also reduces the risk of infection.

Dacron

Dacron is a braided polyester which can be machine woven or knitted into seamless tubes. It is most suitable for the replacement of large-calibre arteries such as the aorta or iliac arteries and is not usually regarded as being suitable for infrainguinal reconstruction. It is porous and therefore allows tissue ingrowth that ultimately seals all of the prosthetic material. The material is prepared in three different ways: woven, knitted and knitted velour. There is little to choose between the various forms with regard to long-term performance. The woven graft is less porous and does not require preclotting, it is more rigid and less easy to stitch and is less resistant to infection. The knitted versions are porous and must be carefully preclotted, they are softer and easier to stitch and are slightly less prone to infection.

To avoid the problems of preclotting the knitted grafts and to reduce their thrombogenicity, they may be impregnated with collagen or gelatin which renders them waterproof. The impregnated material is gradually removed with connective tissue ingrowth. A recent study has shown that Dacron impregnated with collagen has an equivalent performance to PTFE in infrainguinal reconstruction.

The grafts may also be further impregnated with rifampicin (60 mg/ml) for use in situations with a high risk of infection. The collagen or gelatin may retain the rifampicin in useful concentrations for up to 48–72 hours.

Expanded polytetrafluoroethylene (ePTFE)

PTFE is a polymer which is highly hydrophobic. It is chemically inert and does not activate platelets as much as Dacron. It is manufactured by extrusion which creates a material with fibrils joining lines of nodules and is therefore not a textile. It is used widely as a small-diameter conduit but has not displaced Dacron from its role in large-diameter arterial replacements. It is less compliant than knitted Dacron.

It does tend to kink on crossing joints and so a system of reinforcement using a helical wrap of polypropylene bonded to the outside has been developed. There is some evidence that coating the inside of the graft with carbon may reduce its thrombogenicity.

Macroporous fluoropolymer

This is a recently developed material which may be an advance on PTFE. The graft is composed of fluoropolymer molecules bonded onto a macroporous substrate which combines an antithrombogenic capacity with good handling characteristics and good tissue ingrowth. Long-term results are not yet available.

REVISIONAL SURGERY

Revision of a vascular reconstruction may be required as an acute event in the immediate post-operative period or as an emergency or elective procedure at a later date.

Immediate revision

Immediate revisions are required for two main reasons:

- haemorrhage
- thrombosis.

Haemorrhage

Haemorrhage following arterial reconstruction or embolectomy may occur from vessels damaged during dissection, from the anastomosis or from bypassed vessels which have been ligated or sutured. The haemorrhage may result in hypovolaemia and its associated complications or haematoma formation which may compromise wound healing.

Haemorrhage from intraabdominal reconstructions may be occult and usually presents with hypovolaemia whereas bleeding from peripheral reconstructions is usually less in volume and presents with swelling in the wound and external bleeding.

Minor bleeding and bruising are of no great significance but major haemorrhage and accumulation of haematoma is an indication for reexploration. Compression of oozing wounds over arterial reconstructions in an attempt to control bleeding is dangerous as it may result in graft thrombosis.

Hypovolaemia after major reconstruction may be due to inadequate replacement of fluid during operation but clearly ongoing haemorrhage requires reoperation.

Management of postoperative haemorrhage

- Check coagulation profile and haemoglobin and correct anomalies.
- Ensure crossmatched blood is available.
- Fully resuscitate with blood, colloid and electrolyte solutions.
- Give a further dose of prophylactic antibiotic.
- Reopen wound under general anaesthesia.
- Evacuate all haematoma and control haemorrhage from surrounding tissues.
- Inspect all anastomoses and apply further sutures if necessary, taking care not to cause stenosis. If haemorrahge is due to previously inserted sutures cutting out, the anastomosis may need to be completely resutured using buttressed sutures.
- Inspect ligated arteries and religate or suture if necessary. Back bleeding from the ligated or sutured iliac arteries after end-to-end aortic anastomosis is not uncommon.
- Inspect sites of possible venous bleeding. These include lumbar renal and iliac veins in the abdomen and femoral and popliteal veins in the femorodistal reconstructions. Ligation, clipping or suturing may be required.
- The most troublesome site of bleeding is that in a tunnel through which a graft has been inserted. This may require radical exposure of the whole tunnel.

Thrombosis

Early detection of postoperative graft occlusion is essential to prevent irreversible occlusion. Evidence of acute ischaemia is usually provided by pallor of the limb and low ankle pressures. Even limbs which remain pink despite graft occlusion may blanch on elevation.

603

Reexploration as soon as possible is indicated as success is more likely if propagation of thrombus is limited.

Management of graft occlusion

- Ensure that the patient is fully resuscitated.

- Give a further dose of prophylactic antibiotic.

- Reopen wound under general anaesthetic.

- Give systemic heparin.

- Expose proximal anastomosis. If the graft is empty it implies a problem with run-in; if dilated and thrombosed, it implies an outflow problem.

- Make an axial arteriotomy in the proximal graft hood and clear the graft and inflow with a Fogarty catheter. If good inflow cannot be obtained by this technique a more proximal reconstruction may be required. This could include the addition of an aortofemoral or crossover bypass.

- The distal anastomosis may now be assessed by on-table angiography or angioscopy. If neither technique is available the hood of the graft at the distal anastomosis may be opened and the anastomosis directly inspected. The most common distal problem is that of a raised intimal flap. Disconnection of the graft and resuturing may be required or, if the anastomosis is stenosed, a patch may be used to widen the outflow. If the problem is a poor distal run-off the graft may be extended to a healthier area more distally by adding another piece of graft material. Alternatively if there is a short distal stenosis in the native vessel, angioplasty may employed.

- Increasing the flow through a graft will help to reduce the risk of rethrombosis and this may be achieved by reducing the peripheral resistance by warming the patient and by ensuring a good cardiac output.

Late revisions

Late revisions are required for three principal reasons:

- graft sepsis
- thrombosis
- anastomotic aneurysms.

Graft sepsis

This is covered on p. 606.

Thrombosis

Thrombosis may occur at a late stage due to:

- progression of occlusive disease in native arteries proximal or distal to the reconstruction

- graft stenosis due to deposition of thrombus in the graft or the development of atherosclerosis or myointimal hyperplasia in vein grafts or at anastomoses

- compression and occlusion of the graft, particularly in those placed in a subcutaneous position

- hypercoagulable states such as polycythaemia

- hypotension (e.g. following myocardial infarction)

- graft sepsis

- anastomotic aneurysm formation (see below).

Late thrombosis may present as an episode of acute ischaemia (see p. 591) or as a redevelopment of chronic symptoms. When the presentation is acute there is a potential for graft salvage if investigation and treatment are carried out expeditiously. However, the presentation is often delayed by which time the graft may no longer be cleared.

Acute presentation

There are four options for treatment.

- *Thrombolysis followed by correction of underlying abnormality.* Immediate angiography is carried out and intraarterial thrombolytic therapy commenced. Repeat angiography is used to monitor lysis. If and when the lysis is complete, identification of the underlying cause of the thrombosis may be possible and this must be treated immediately to prevent rethrombosis. Treatment may include transluminal angioplasty, patch angioplasty or graft extension.

- *Thrombectomy and correction of underlying abnormality.* Under general anaesthetic the graft is cleared and on-table angiography or angioscopy is used to identify the cause. This is then corrected by the techniques described above. Thrombectomy is less successful than thrombolysis in clearing the graft and propagated thrombus. Complete graft replacement is often required.

- *Anticoagulation with a view to urgent investigation and regrafting.* Anticoagulation with heparin is used to prevent further propagation of thrombus. Angiography and further urgent reconstruction are carried out as detailed below for late presentation.

- *Amputation.* In patients who have had a reconstruction for end-stage vascular disease the graft may have occluded because of lack of run-off. Attempted clearance may be pointless and amputation after allowing the limb to demarcate may be in the best interests of the patient rather than embarking on a fruitless attempt at further reconstruction.

Chronic presentation

When the patient presents with a recurrence of the chronic symptoms due to graft occlusion, the urgency of investigation is dictated by the severity of symptoms. It may be that the symptoms are not sufficiently severe to warrant further reconstruction as repeated reconstructions have an ever-diminishing chance of long-term success. Alternatively further reconstruction may be deemed impossible due to progression of native arterial disease or the presence of significant co-morbidity.

If further reconstruction is thought to be possible full angiography should be carried out. In the case of patients with no palpable femoral pulses transvenous digital subtraction angiography may be employed. The criteria for considering further reconstruction include:

- symptoms sufficiently severe to warrant a procedure with a higher than usual risk of failure
- a limb with a potential for useful function if revascularised
- a suitable high-pressure arterial inflow
- a suitable low-resistance arterial outflow
- adequate cardiorespiratory function.

Repeated reconstruction has much greater technical difficulty than primary reconstruction. The difficulties are due to:

- scarring causing loss of tissue planes
- scarring causing devascularisation of overlying soft tissue (especially in the groin)
- fibrous incorporation of prosthetic grafts
- adhesion of adjacent structures (veins, ureters, gut, etc.) to arteries and grafts
- presence of anastomotic aneurysms
- further deterioration of the native circulation
- the requirement for a more distal site for the outflow anastomosis
- further deterioration of the patient's general cardiorespiratory fitness.

TECHNICAL ASPECTS

Approach

In certain circumstances, particularly if the graft is being extended to a more distal implant site, it may be possible to avoid dissection of the same area as on the previous occasion. An approach through unoperated tissue is much simpler and safer.

Incision

In the groin particularly, it is wise to reexcise the old scar if it is broad and avascular but sufficient soft tissue must be retained to cover the graft. The incision should follow the same direct route to the artery as on the previous dissection to prevent additional soft tissue devascularisation or lymphatic damage. It should, however, be longer to enable an approach to the previously undissected artery above and below.

Arterial dissection

The area of the previous anastomosis is likely to be fibrotic, with adjacent organs (particularly veins) adherent.

Distally it is simpler to identify the native artery above and below the site of previous dissection. The periarterial plane is then entered and followed towards the anastomosis from each end. In circumstances where the adjacent veins are densely adherent it may be simpler to avoid the risk of trying to separate them and simply clamp the veins along with the artery.

At the aortic anastomosis there may be insufficient space below the renal arteries to dissect out a fresh segment of aorta and therefore the previous anastomosis may have to be mobilised. This can be particularly hazardous as the inferior vena cava may be adherent on the right, as well as the lumbar vessels on the posterior aspect. It is feasible to clamp the IVC along with the aorta to avoid damage and clamping in the sagittal plane avoids the need for a posterior dissection. IVC clamping time should be kept to a minimum due to the effect on venous return.

If the duodenum is adherent, the aorta should be clamped before attempting to dissect it off. It is better to remove a disc of aorta and leave it adherent to the duodenum than to make a hole in the duodenum.

Graft tunnel

It is safer to place the graft in a new route than to try to follow a previous tunnel. Creating a blunt tunnel in an area where a graft has been placed previously has a major risk of producing venous bleeding which may be difficult to control. If a femoropopliteal graft has been routed orthotopically on the first occasion it is safer to place it subcutaneously at the time of replacement to avoid the danger of retunnelling the popliteal fossa.

Anastomotic aneurysms

Aneurysms developing at the anastomosis may be due to infection, poor suture material, poor arterial quality or inadequate suturing. Anastomotic aneurysms will develop in 1–4% of bypass grafts.

Graft infections are covered in the following section.

Current suture materials are non-absorbable and retain their strength indefinitely. It is therefore unusual for suture failure to be a cause of aneurysm formation unless the suture has been damaged.

Poor arterial quality in association with poor anastomotic techniques are the commonest causes. Patients operated on for aneurysmal disease are more likely than patients with occlusive disease to develop anastomotic aneurysms. Patients with Behçet's disease are particularly at risk. The commonest site is in the femoral artery.

There are techniques which may help to prevent aneurysm development and these are covered elsewhere (p. 614). The techniques used to treat anastomotic aneurysms are as follows.

- *Reanastomosis at the original site.* The anastomosis is dissected out and the artery and graft are clamped. The graft is cut off the artery and the aneurysm is resected back to healthy arterial wall. The graft is then resutured to the original site using a buttressed suture technique.

- *Reanastomosis more distally to healthy artery.* The graft is separated from the original artery and the artery ligated. The graft is then extended and resutured to a more distal healthy arterial segment using buttressed sutures.

- *Ligation and extraanatomic bypass.* Aneurysms at the proximal end of an aortic graft are particularly difficult to deal with, especially if they are close to the renal arteries. It may be possible to insert an extended thoracoabdominal graft if the aorta proximally is aneurysmal but this has a high morbidity and mortality. If the proximal aorta is healthy the aorta may be oversewn with buttressed sutures and an extraanatomic axillobifemoral bypass inserted.

- *Triple ligation.* The artery above and below and the graft are all ligated. This is only indicated in cases of major haemorrhage in patients unfit for reconstruction.

GRAFT INFECTION

Infection in any arterial reconstruction is a disaster that risks the life and limb of the patient.

Aetiology and prevention

The incidence of graft infection is very low, being approximately 2–3% for aortic grafts and 3–4% for femorodistal grafts. Graft infection may become manifest soon after implantation or may not appear for many years. It is thought that most infections are due to contamination at the time of operation or in the immediate post-operative period and that relatively few are due to secondary infection. There are, however, a number of case reports which show a relation between an episode of bacteraemia and subsequent graft infection. Antibiotic prophylaxis before anticipated episodes of bacteraemia in patients with arterial implants is not yet routine and there is no good evidence for it but it may be a wise precaution.

The factors associated with an increased incidence of arterial graft infection are difficult to assess, due to the low incidence of the complication and the fact that the infection may not become apparent for many years, but include the following.

- Incisions involving the groin crease
- Operations complicated by wound infection
- Emergency operations and reoperations
- Operations with a large blood loss
- Operations on patients who are diabetic, nutritionally compromised or immunosuppressed
- Use of artificial as opposed to natural graft materials
- Operations on patients with infected distal lesions
- Failure to use prophylactic antibiotics at the time of implantation.

Prevention is dependent on a number of factors for which it is difficult to produce evidence but there are some standard surgical practices that it would seem prudent to use. Avoidance of incisions in the groin is difficult as both proximal and distal reconstructions often require access to the common femoral artery. Careful skin preparation is a prerequisite of all surgery and antibiotic prophylaxis has been shown to reduce the incidence of wound and graft infections. The duration of antibiotic prophylaxis is undetermined but most vascular surgeons will use at least three doses and there is some evidence to support a more prolonged course for patients with infected peripheral lesions. The presence of organisms in the aortic wall or in thrombus from the lumen of an aneurysm is of uncertain significance. Careful surgery with minimal dissection and avoidance of tissue ischaemia and haematoma will all contribute to the avoidance of wound problems. However, the use of a suction drain in groin wounds has not been shown to reduce the risk of infection in wound or graft. Avoidance of synchronous operations on the gastrointestinal tract is probably prudent although there is some evidence that it is not hazardous. The choice of graft is of some significance in experimental situations but it is difficult to show an effect in clinical practice. It appears that saphenous vein has a lower incidence of infection than prosthetic grafts and, of the prosthetics, the PTFE graft seems more resistant to infection than Dacron. A recently described technique of bonding antibiotics to impregnated grafts may hold promise for the future but the evidence of success is not yet available.

Diagnosis

The diagnosis of graft infection is difficult as the onset may be very insidious and produce few symptoms or signs. The early infection may have a typical septic presentation with a septicaemia, septic emboli and discharge of pus from the wound. Late graft infection may present with swelling in the groin, a sinus, graft thrombosis or false aneurysm. Occasionally major gastrointestinal bleeding may occur with aortoenteric fistula.

Confirmatory tests include the following.

- *Bacteriology*: blood culture is positive in only about 50% and even culture of the fluid from sinuses may be negative. Culture of fluid aspirated from around the graft under imaging may be useful.

The most common five infecting organisms are: *Staphylococcus epidermidis* and *aureus*, *Streptococccus faecalis*, *Escherichia coli* and Klebsiella.

- *Sinogram*: injection of contrast into a sinus may outline the graft.

- *Ultrasound scan*: this will show large amounts of fluid and false aneurysms but is less useful than CT and MRI.

- A*ngiography*: infection will not be specifically diagnosed by angiography but it is useful in defining the state of adjacent vessels and will show false aneurysms.

- *Gallium scanning*: this is not of much use due to the uptake in other abdominal organs and in any other areas of inflammation.

- *CT scanning*: the identification of perigraft gas or fluid is indicative of infection at a late stage but similar appearances may be present with uninfected grafts up to two months after implantation. The diagnostic accuracy has been variably quoted at 45–100%.

- *Indium-labelled leucocyte scans*: this technique detects inflammation around the graft and has an accuracy varying from 60% to 85%. It may give false-positive results following replacement of inflammatory aneurysms.

- *MRI*: this is probably the investigation of choice as it will detect much smaller quantities of perigraft fluid than CT scanning and will differentiate between fluid and oedema. Sensitivity and specificity of 100% have been reported in one series.

Treatment

It is important to consider the risks of attempting to save a limb when the surgery may result in the loss of a life. Sometimes it is more appropriate to sacrifice the limb.

The fundamental principle regardless of the approach is to use high doses of appropriate antibiotics before, during and for a prolonged period after surgery.

The method of treatment of an infected prosthesis is dependent on a number of factors.

- *The general physical state of the patient*: all vascular patients have diffuse vascular disease and therefore are poor-risk patients. Chronic sepsis may cause further morbidity and major reconstructive surgery in these patients is particularly hazardous.

- *The site of the infection*: the centre of the graft or the anastomosis. Infections of the anastomosis are much more critical as there is a major risk of secondary haemorrhage.

- *The site of the graft*: aortic or distal. An infected aortic graft has a high mortality whereas an infected distal graft rarely causes death but may result in limb loss.

- *The organism involved*: *Staphylococcus epidermidis* produces a very slowly progressive infection with serous fluid and not much reaction whereas *Staph. aureus* is much more aggressive, producing frank pus and necrotic material.

- *The state of the collateral circulation*.

- *The presence of an aortointestinal fistula*: this is a major complication with a very high mortality.

There are a number of approaches to graft infection which all have advantages and disadvantages.

Complete excision of graft and arterial ligation

This is appropriate for patients in whom there is a good collateral circulation, where the patient is unfit for major surgery or where the distal end of the graft is near the ankle, precluding a more distal anastomosis. This is the simplest and safest technique but has the highest rate of limb loss.

Complete excision and extraanatomic revascularisation

This is appropriate for grafts at any level provided that there is healthy artery above and below and there is an infection-free route between the two. Examples of this would include the excision of an infected aortic graft and insertion of an axillobifemoral graft or the removal of a femoropopliteal graft and insertion of an iliopopliteal graft through the obturator foramen. With excision of an aortic graft there is a risk of subsequent breakdown of the aortic stump due to continuing infection.

Partial excision and bypass

This is appropriate for infection in one limb of an aortobifemoral graft as long as the infection has not progressed as far as the bifurcation. Revascularisation is carried out via the obturator foramen to a thigh vessel distal to the infected groin.

Complete excision and in situ replacement

Patients who have a graft with infection confined to the central part, particularly if due to *staph. epidermidis*, may be treated by graft excision and insertion of an antibiotic bonded graft resutured to the healthy artery above and below.

In situ debridement and irrigation

In high-risk patients debridement and irrigation with povidone iodine or antibiotics has occasionally been successful. In a few patients with central graft infection in a superficially placed graft, the graft has been exposed and subsequently granulated over and reincorporated.

Of the above techniques, the complete excision and extraanatomic bypass has the best chance of complete cure and limb salvage but the highest mortality. *In situ* replacement is useful in central graft infections and excision with arterial ligation will resolve the infection but with a high risk of limb loss.

SURVEILLANCE IN ARTERIAL SURGERY

The aim of a surveillance programme is to detect new vascular lesions or to monitor progression or relapse of existing lesions. At present there are five potential areas for surveillance.

- Follow-up of femoropopliteal grafts to detect stenosis
- Follow-up of lesions treated by angioplasty
- Follow-up of carotid endarterectomy
- Monitoring of abdominal aortic aneurysms
- Follow-up of aneurysms treated by endovascular stenting

Femoropopliteal graft surveillance

Vein grafts (the material of choice for femoropopliteal bypass) are susceptible to the development of stenotic lesions in the first year which may lead to graft occlusion. It has been postulated that early detection and treatment of developing stenotic lesions may result in a 10–20% improvement in long-term outcome.

The stenoses may be detected by duplex scanning which detects an increase in velocity in the region of the stenosis. The first year is the period during which these remediable lesions are most likely to appear and therefore screening by duplex scan has become a routine for the first year's follow-up in many units.

Some doubt has been cast on the value of this procedure as some trials have shown that although patency may be improved, the long-term limb salvage was unchanged. At present there is no definitive evidence for the cost effectiveness of a screening programme for vein grafts but a European trial is currently under way. There may be a role for selective screening of grafts with high output resistance or poor flow.

Screening of prosthetic grafts has no value.

Post angioplasty

Balloon angioplasty is still a controversial treatment as the long-term results have not been fully assessed and the indications are still a subject of debate. It has been postulated that routine surveillance by duplex may be of value in improving long-term patency but as yet there is no evidence to support a costly surveillance programme.

Postcarotid endarterectomy

Carotid endarterectomy is complicated by restenosis in 8–15% of cases although restenosis was not inevitably associated with a further stroke. In a recent trial only 40% of patients who had a further stroke had a restenosis. At present there is no evidence to support routine screening following carotid endarterectomy.

Monitoring of abdominal aortic aneurysms

There are two roles for duplex scanning in the management of abdominal aortic aneurysms:

- screening of a healthy population – aimed at high-risk groups
- monitoring known aneurysms to detect an increase in size.

Rupture is a complication of abdominal aortic aneurysms with a high mortality (well over 70% including out-of-hospital deaths). Elective surgery for aneurysms is associated with a mortality less than 5% and therefore elective replacement is recommended. A recent trial has shown that there is no survival advantage in operating on aneurysms less than 5.5 cm in AP diameter.

Surveillance of endovascular stents

The technique of endovascular repair of abdominal aortic aneurysms is still undergoing assessment and during the development stage there is a fairly high incidence of complications. It is mandatory during development to carry out regular surveillance to detect complications such as endoleaks which may result in aneurysm rupture. When the technique is fully and widely established the requirement for surveillance will be rationalised.

Summary of indications for surveillance

PROVEN

- Abdominal aneurysm monitoring

CONTROVERSIAL

- Follow-up of vein grafts
- Population screening for aneurysms

CONTRAINDICATED

- Follow-up of carotid endarterectomy
- Follow-up of angioplasty
- Follow-up of prosthetic grafts

Patients with aneurysms of 4.0 cm or more should be screened by duplex on a six-monthly basis until the aneurysm reaches 5.5 cm, when it should be repaired if the patient is fit.

Screening for asymptomatic aneurysms is still controversial but there is some evidence to support the screening of first-degree relatives of patients with abdominal aortic aneurysms and the screening of men over the age of 50 (3% incidence of AAA).

OPERATIVE SURGERY

Anastomotic Techniques

A number of principles are essential in the formation of a vascular anastomosis.

- It must be performed under strictly aseptic conditions.

- There must be an adequate inflow pressure.

- There must be a low-resistance outflow.

- The suture line should not produce any stenosis of the origin or recipient vessels or of the graft.

- With an end-to-side anastomosis the cross-sectional area of the anastomosis should be about 1.5 times that of the graft.

- The suture line should be everted to ensure an intima-to-intima anastomosis as the adventitia is highly thrombogenic.

- The anastomosis should be smooth and generate a minimum of turbulence.

- The intima must not be grasped with forceps as this may cause corrugations, which encourage thrombosis. The artery should be grasped by the adventitial layers only.

- The suture should be non-thrombogenic and permanent.

- Care must be taken to ensure that the intima is sutured to prevent flaps being raised when blood flow is restored.

- The suture should pass from within to without on the artery to prevent dissection of the inner layers of atherosclerotic arteries.

- If the suture must pass from without to within (such as when closing an arteriotomy) gentle counterpressure on the intima with a blunt instrument may prevent dissection.

The anastomosis may be completed with either a continuous or interrupted technique. A continuous stitch is more haemostatic but runs the risk of producing a stenosis by the 'pursestring' effect. When suturing small vessels or creating an end-to-end anastomosis an interrupted suture technique is safer.

Closure of an arteriotomy

A polypropylene suture is used (3/0 or 4/0 for aorta, 4/0 or 5/0 for iliac or common femoral, 5/0 or 6/0 for popliteal or brachial and 6/0 or 7/0 for tibial or radial). The suture is inserted just beyond the end of the arteriotomy and tied. It is then continued with a simple continuous suture to just beyond the opposite end of the

arteriotomy and tied, again taking care to pull it tight enough to approximate the edges without inversion. When passing the suture from without to within, gentle counterpressure with a smooth instrument may prevent separation of atheromatous plaques.

With small vessels it may be necessary to close the arteriotomy with a patch to prevent stenosis.

End-to-end anastomosis

It is important to ensure that the two vessels to be joined in an end-to-end fashion have a similar diameter. Cutting the smaller vessel obliquely, thereby increasing its cross-sectional area may compensate for minor discrepancies in diameter. With small-diameter vessels, if both are cut diagonally there is less chance of stenosing the anastomosis (Figure 39.1).

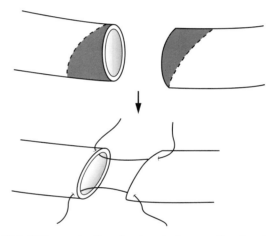

Figure 39.1 Oblique cut of small artery to increase the diameter of the anastomosis.

Small vessels

The main difficulty with small vessels (e.g. popliteal artery) is to avoid picking up the opposite wall with the suture. Inserting stay sutures can prevent this. The technique is as follows (Figure 39.2).

- Insert a double-needled suture in the middle of the deep aspect of the anastomosis, tie it in the middle of the suture and leave both needles attached.

- Insert another suture in the middle of the superficial aspect. This may be tied or left loose. With very small vessels it is easier if an additional stay suture is inserted such that the stays are 120° apart (Figure 39.3).

- Complete each side from deep to superficial with the double-needled suture and tie both ends to the superficial stay(s).

- With very small vessels interrupted sutures are less likely to cause stenosis.

The technique for large vessels (e.g. aorta) is described in the section below on aortofemoral grafting.

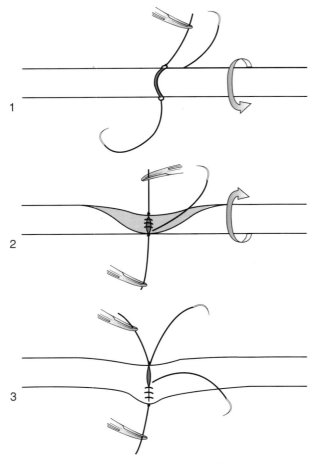

Figure 39.2 Technique of end-to-end anastomosis with two stays.

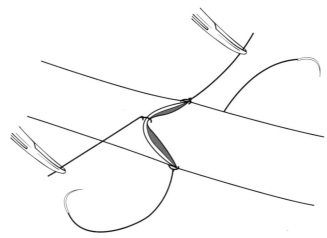

Figure 39.3 Three-stay technique for end-to-end anastomosis.

End-to-side anastomosis

This is the simplest anastomosis to create if there is a discrepancy in size between the two vessels. It also increases run-off as the blood may flow both proximally and distally in the recipient artery. The technique is as follows (Figures 39.4, 39.5).

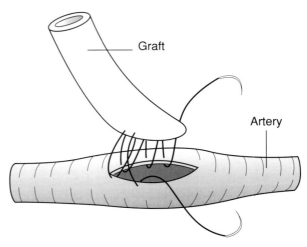

Figure 39.4 Parachuting technique for end-to-side anastomosis.

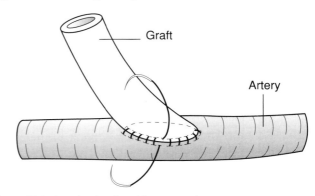

Figure 39.5 Completed end-to-side anastomosis.

- A longitudinal arteriotomy is made in the recipient artery.

- The end of the graft is cut with an S-shaped cut to produce a circumference which is twice the length of the arteriotomy. The S-shape produces a transverse cut proximally and distally which helps to keep the inflow and outflow sites from being stenosed.

- A double-needled suture is then inserted into the heel of the graft and four or five sutures are then inserted around the heel with the graft held up and away from the artery. This enables the heel to be sutured carefully under good vision.

- The sutures are then pulled tight to approximate the heel of the graft to the artery.

- Using one needle, the anastomosis is then completed by suturing down one side, around the toe and back up to meet the other end of the suture in the middle of the side of the anastomosis. The knot should not be formed at the toe as this may narrow the outflow or inflow. At the proximal and distal ends of the arteriotomy the sutures must be placed in the axis of the artery to prevent stenosis.

- If the cut end of the graft appears to be too long for the arteriotomy, it may be trimmed to size when a side has been almost completed.

- When suturing very small arteries it may be easier to insert at least some of the sutures (especially at the toe) as interrupted sutures that are tied when all the sutures have been inserted.

Patch angioplasty

In patch angioplasty a patch is applied to a vessel to widen the lumen. It is a useful technique with which trainees should be familiar as it is a simple method of great value in situations where the only alternative may be a more extensive and complex bypass procedure.

The uses of patch angioplasty are as follows:

- to close an axial arteriotomy in a small vessel to prevent stenosis
- to widen a stenotic artery
- to repair a traumatised artery.

Examples of the use of patch angioplasty include:

- closure of an arteriotomy after brachial or popliteal embolectomy or after femoral embolectomy in a small-diameter femoral artery
- closure of the arteriotomy after carotid or iliac endarterectomy
- widening of a stenotic vessel which cannot be achieved by transluminal angioplasty such as the origin of the profunda femoris artery (profundaplasty)
- widening of a stenosis at the outflow of a bypass graft by either a separate patch or an extension of the hood of the graft. Extension of the hood of the limb of an aortofemoral graft down the profunda as a profundaplasty is a common use of this technique
- repair of an artery where part of the wall has been irreparably damaged.

The materials used for patch angioplasty are:

- vein
- PTFE
- Dacron
- artery.

Technique

The technique of patch angioplasty will be described here using profundaplasty as the example (Figure 39.6).

The operation may be carried out under a general anaesthetic, regional or local anaesthesia.

The common and superficial femoral arteries are dissected out through a vertical incision from the mid-inguinal point distally for about 7 cm. The junction between the common and superficial femoral arteries is identified by the reduction in diameter at this point. Slings are passed round the common and superficial femoral arteries and both are retracted medially. The profunda femoris artery is then identified usually arising from the postero-lateral aspect of the common femoral artery. Care must be exercised in mobilising the profunda as it is a fragile vessel and may be easily torn. About 0.5 cm from the origin of the profunda, at or just above the first bifurcation, a small vein runs anterior to the profunda artery but posterior to the superficial femoral artery. This vein is easily damaged and should be identified, ligated and divided. The superficial femoral artery is retracted medially, allowing the dissection to be continued along the profunda as far as necessary. All branches and the main vessel are controlled with Silastic slings.

The long saphenous vein is identified in front of the medial malleolus and a segment about 1 cm longer than required is dissected out and the tributaries ligated. The vein is opened longitudinally, creating an oblong patch, and the corners of one end of the patch

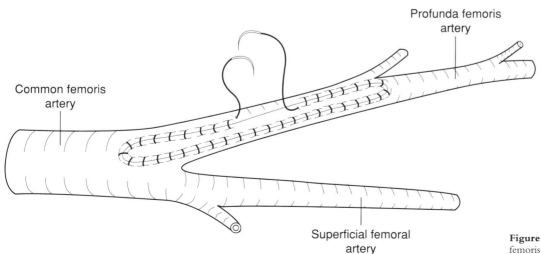

Common femoris artery

Profunda femoris artery

Superficial femoral artery

Figure 39.6 Patch angioplasty of the profunda femoris artery.

are cut off, producing a rounded end. The patch is grasped across the other end with a pair of small artery forceps.

The patient is then systemically heparinised (70–100 units/kg intravenously) and the common, superficial and profunda femoral arteries and the relevant branches are all clamped.

A long arteriotomy is made from the common femoral artery down the anterior aspect of the profunda for about 1 cm beyond the distal end of the stenosis. If the stenosis is very irregular or ulcerated it may be necessary to carry out a local endarterectomy. Care must be taken to ensure the distal leading edge is sutured down to prevent dissection.

Most short vein patches from this source do not have valves and therefore may be applied either way; however, if there are valves they must be orientated in the correct direction. The apex of the curved end of the vein patch is then sutured to the apex of the proximal end of the arteriotomy using a 5/0 double-ended vascular suture. The assistant holds the patch with the artery forceps under slight tension and about 75% of each side of the suture line is completed. The distal end of the patch is then cut to length and tailored to fit the distal end of the arteriotomy. One suture is then used to suture round the end of the patch and tied to the other suture on one side of the patch.

The clamps are then released and haemostasis ensured before closing the wound without a drain.

Saphenous vein harvesting

The saphenous vein is used for a variety of purposes, including vein patching and bypass grafts. The commonest uses are for femoropopliteal bypass and aortocoronary bypass.

There are four techniques for harvesting the saphenous vein.

- Open dissection for reversed vein
- Open dissection for *in situ* grafting
- Keyhole dissection for *in situ* grafting using an arterioscope
- Endoscopic dissection

Open dissection for reversed vein grafting

This technique is used for femoropopliteal bypass, aortocoronary bypass and vein patching.

The vein is dissected out at the appropriate level for the diameter required. Usually the below-knee vein is used for aortocoronary bypass and the above knee for femoropopliteal bypass. The vein is identified at one end of the desired segment and the incision is made in short lengths sequentially to ensure that the incision is kept strictly in line with the vein because if the skin has to be undermined it may result in necrosis of the skin edge. Alternatively the incision may be made in short discontinuous lengths but this makes the dissection more difficult. The tribu-

taries are ligated or clipped and divided. Care must be taken to ensure that any clips or ligatures are accurately applied to the saphenous vein side to ensure that the vein is not narrowed. It is always safer to harvest a longer length than appears necessary.

After removal the vein should be gently distended with heparinised blood to ensure that there are no divided tributaries which have not been ligated. It is better to use blood than saline to avoid osmotic damage to the endothelium. It is also important to avoid overdistension as pressures in excess of 400 mmHg may be readily achieved and a pressure in excess of 200 mmHg may damage the vessel wall. The vein is then reversed before use.

Open dissection for in situ grafting

The proximal end of the vein is fully mobilised and the vein is swung laterally and anastomosed to the common or superficial femoral arteries. The vein is then fully exposed as described as above. The distal end of the vein is divided and a valvulotome is inserted. After release of the clamps the vein graft will distend down to the first valve. This is then divided with the valvulotome and the vein then distends down to the next valve. The process is then repeated until all the valves have been divided and there is a good flow of blood out of the distal end. The side branches are clipped flush with the main vein. The distal end of the vein is mobilised sufficiently to allow it to be passed into the popliteal fossa and anastomosed to the popliteal artery. After release of all the clamps it is important to ensure that the tributaries have all been ligated. A Doppler flow detector in a sterile plastic sheath is applied to the vein near its proximal anastomosis and the vein graft is occluded near to the distal anastomosis. If flow is detected there is a persisting tributary. The occluding finger is then moved up the graft until the flow ceases and this identifies the level of the persisting tributary.

Keyhole dissection using the arterioscope

In patients undergoing *in situ* vein bypass it is possible to prepare the vein using an arterioscope.

The vein is mobilised at the saphenofemoral junction and distally at the most distal part required. A valvulotome is inserted in the distal end and passed up to the proximal end. An arterioscope is then inserted into the proximal end of the vein. All valves are identified and divided under direct vision. The side tributaries are identified and the site is located by the light of the arterioscope seen through the skin. A small incision is made at the site and the tributary is clipped flush with the vein. This procedure is continued as far distally as necessary. A length of distal vein must be fully mobilised to enable the vein to be passed into the popliteal fossa.

Endoscopic dissection

A device has been developed through which the saphenous vein may be dissected through incisions at the proximal and distal ends.

The device resembles a long proctoscope. The upper end of the vein is divided and pulled into the end of the instrument. The instrument is then advanced down the thigh around the vein and the tributaries are identified, clipped and divided. The procedure is continued as far as the distal end and the vein is then divided and removed. The advantage of this technique is that the vein may be completely dissected and removed with only two small incisions. The disadvantages are that it takes considerably longer than open dissection and the equipment costs are greater. The technique is still being evaluated.

Aortofemoral grafting

Aortofemoral grafts may be used for both aneurysmal and occlusive disease. For occlusive disease it may be unilateral or, more commonly, bilateral and the proximal anastomosis may be either end to end or end to side. The techniques used are as follows.

Incisions

The abdominal incision may be transverse (supraumbilical for aneurysms and supra- or infraumbilical for occlusive disease), vertical mid-line or a long left paramedian curving medially at its lower end for an extraperitoneal approach. The author's preference is for a transverse as this is less likely to produce an incisional hernia and is more comfortable in the immediate postoperative period.

Dissection of the aorta

The aorta is exposed through a long vertical incision in the posterior peritoneum that is kept to the right of the aorta distally to avoid the inferior mesenteric vessels and to the left proximally to avoid the duodenum. For aneurysmal disease the aorta has to be dissected just below the renal vessels but for occlusive disease the aorta may be dissected at any convenient point above the area to be bypassed. If necessary the inferior mesenteric vein and the renal vein may be divided to improve access. The renal vein must be divided near to the inferior vena cava and the left inferior adrenal and gonadal veins should be preserved to maintain collateral circulation. A segment of aorta can be mobilised completely to gain adequate control. This involves dissecting around the aorta and passing a nylon tape. This must be done carefully with the finger to ensure that lumbar arteries and veins are not damaged. Some surgeons prefer to avoid the posterior dissection and simply mobilise the sides of the aorta to enable it to be clamped in the sagittal plain. This gives less adequate control and the clamp is more readily displaced.

Dissection of the femoral arteries

The femoral arteries are dissected out through vertical incisions commencing about 2 cm above the inguinal ligament so that the common femoral artery is exposed just below the inguinal ligament (Figure 39.7). The length of incision depends on the size of the patient and whether the profunda has to be dissected out for the distal anastomosis. The common femoral and, if necessary, the profunda and superficial femoral arteries are mobilised and Silastic slings passed around them.

Insertion of graft

The patient is systemically heparinised (100 units per kg) and the aorta is clamped in the coronal plain with a suitable clamp (Satinsky) above and below the site of anastomosis. For an end-to-end anastomosis the aorta is transected and the distal end is oversewn with a continuous 3/0 polypropylene suture. This must be carefully carried out, as it is liable to bleed after insertion of the graft when the distal circulation is repressurised. A suitable sized impregnated knitted Dacron graft is trimmed to size (grafts usually lie better if the bifurcation is placed slightly higher than the natural bifurcation). It is then sutured end to end as described below (Figure 39.8).

- Use a 000 polypropylene suture or occasionally, if the vessel is very calcified, a braided polyester, as it is less likely to be damaged by calcified plaques.

- Insert a suture in the left lateral position and leave it loose.

- Suture towards you along the posterior wall until about four or five sutures have been inserted. (It is a good idea to alter the distance of each suture from the edge of the vessel so you do not create a line of perforations, which may tear. Large

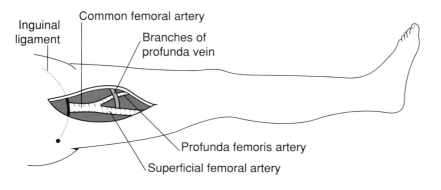

Figure 39.7 Anatomy of the common femoral artery dissection.

Inguinal ligament
Common femoral artery
Branches of profunda vein
Profunda femoris artery
Superficial femoral artery

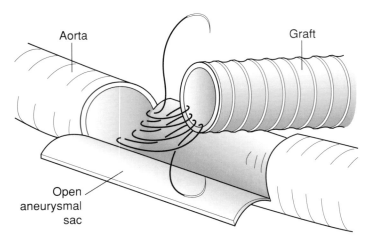

Figure 39.8 Technique of end-to-end aortic anastomosis for an aneurysm replacement.

calcified plaques may be sutured around or perforated with a towel clip to create a hole for the suture.)

- Pull the suture tight and slide the graft down to the aorta.

- Complete the posterior wall as far as the right anterior aspect.

- Change to the other end and complete the anastomosis, again stitching towards you along the anterior wall, and tie the two ends together with a reef knot with five throws.

- The graft should be occluded just below the anastomosis and the clamp is released. This will identify any major leaks that may be oversewn with additional sutures.

The anastomosis can be reinforced with a sleeve of Dacron graft (Figure 39.9).

For an end-to-side anastomosis the graft is sutured to the front of the aorta as described above.

Tunnels are developed from the retroperitoneum to the groins by blunt finger dissection. The tunnel should be generated along the anterior surface of the iliac arteries and posterior to the ureters. Care should be taken just above the inguinal ligament to avoid the inferior epigastric arteries that run upwards and medially from the distal external iliac arteries. After testing the anastomosis the limbs of the graft are passed into the groins, taking care to avoid kinking or rotation.

The graft is then trimmed to size and anastomosed end to side to the femoral arteries. If the common femoral is occluded the graft may be sutured to the profunda alone or if the common femoral is patent and the profunda stenosed, the graft may be sutured to both the common and profunda arteries as a long patch angioplasty. Before the distal anastomosis is completed it is wise to transiently release the proximal clamp to ensure there is no thrombus in the aorta. The graft is then flushed out with heparinised saline. For patients with aortic and iliac aneurysms, Fogarty catheters are also usually passed distally to ensure any emboli are cleared.

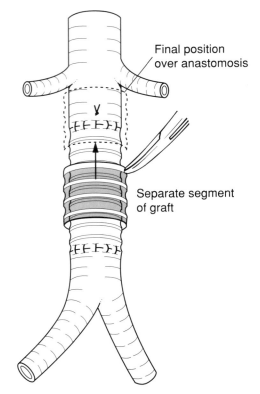

Figure 39.9 External reinforcement of an aortic anastomosis.

The proximal aortic clamp is released first to fill the graft and remove the air. The proximal femoral clamp is then removed to pass any thrombus into the bypassed pelvic circulation before releasing the clamps distally.

Haemostasis is ensured best by gentle pressure on the bleeding points. Additional sutures are only needed for major leaks. It may be necessary to reverse the heparin with protamine.

Closure of the retroperitoneum

It is essential to close the retroperitoneum over the graft to prevent bowel becoming adherent. This may be difficult if there is considerable bulk with an end-to-side anastomosis. If necessary, a pedicled segment of omentum can be mobilised and sutured over the graft.

The wounds are closed without drainage using a mass polydioxanone continuous suture to close the abdomen. It is probably better to close the groin with absorbable sutures in the superficial fascia but excessive suturing may cause damage to the lymphatics. The skin wounds are closed with a nylon or a subcuticular absorbable suture.

Inferior mesenteric artery

Patients who have a patent inferior mesenteric artery and have the iliac arteries bypassed or occluded are at risk of intestinal ischaemia. If in doubt, it is better to reimplant the inferior mesenteric artery into the main stem of the graft or its left limb or to carry out an end-to-side aortic anastomosis with preservation of the IMA origin from the aorta.

Extraanatomic bypass

An extraanatomic bypass is one which follows a route not normally followed by a blood vessel. The reasons for using an extraanatomic route are as follows.

- To avoid a more major procedure in a patient with significant co-morbidity (such as an aortofemoral graft in a patient with serious respiratory problems).

- To avoid placing the graft in an area of sepsis (e.g. with an infected aortic prosthesis).

- To avoid risky surgery in a previously damaged area (such as a 'hostile abdomen').

Grafts may be placed from virtually any artery to any other artery provided there is a high-pressure inflow and a low-resistance outflow. The principal disadvantages of extra anatomic bypasses include risk of compression, if they are placed subcutaneously, risk of kinking when crossing joints and risk of thrombosis because of their length. Examples include:

- femorofemoral bypass (usually used in unilateral iliac occlusions in high-risk patients)

- axillofemoral bypass (used in patients with aortic graft infection and in patients with occlusive aortoiliac disease who are very high risk)

- obturator bypass (used for patients with infected arterial reconstructions in the groin)

- bypasses between the supra-aortic trunks (used to avoid entering the chest for patients with supra-aortic trunk disease).

Femorofemoral bypass

Both femoral arteries are exposed through vertical incisions in the groin and the arteries are fully dissected out. If the common femoral artery is occluded on the recipient side the dissection is continued down onto the profunda or superficial femoral artery. An 8 or 10 mm impregnated knitted Dacron graft is placed in a subcutaneous tunnel from one groin to the other. Some surgeons place the graft under the abdominal wall, especially in thin people, but this is more technically difficult and may result in the graft being compressed by the inguinal ligament. The graft is cut to size and anastomosed end to side to both femoral arteries using 4/0 or 5/0 polypropylene. The graft lies more comfortably if the arteriotomy is placed obliquely from proximal and medial to distal and lateral. It is important to put the graft under some tension to prevent radial movement with the pulse that may cause skin erosion. The wounds are closed in the usual way using an

absorbable suture to close some soft tissue over the graft before suturing the skin.

For patients who have concomitant femoropopliteal occlusion it may be necessary to continue the graft down to the popliteal artery. In that case a 6 or 8 mm PTFE graft may be used.

Axillofemoral bypass

This may take the form of an axillounifemoral or an axillobifemoral graft. The evidence suggests that axillobifemoral grafts have a better long-term patency.

The inflow is taken from the first part of the axillary artery as this is the least mobile part and the easiest to dissect.

The artery is approached through an incision from the clavicle down along the line between the pectoralis major and deltoid muscles. The clavipectoral fascia is divided after mobilising the cephalic vein and the first part of the artery is dissected out from within the axillary sheath. The axillary vein lies anteromedial and the cords of the brachial plexus lie posterior to the vessels. Some small branches of the vein require division.

The femoral arteries are dissected out and the appropriate tunnels are developed. A tunnel is fashioned subcutaneously from the groin on the donor side to a small incision in the mid-axillary line about the level of the eighth rib. A further tunnel is made from there to the axillary artery between the pectoralis minor and major muscles. A further tunnel is created from the other groin to join the vertical tunnel about 8–10 cm above the inguinal ligament.

A spirally reinforced PTFE graft is preferred as this is more resistant to occlusion by compression at the costal margin. The crossover part of the graft is sutured to the side of the distal vertical part before implantation and the graft is pulled into the tunnel, taking care not to twist the graft or to kink the crossover component. Ready-made crossover grafts are available commercially.

After clamping the appropriate arteries, the graft is anastomosed using an end-to-side technique with 4/0 or 5/0 PTFE sutures. The wounds are closed without drains using an absorbable subcutaneous suture as well as a skin suture.

Obturator bypass

The common or external iliac arteries are dissected out through the extraperitoneal route and a tunnel is developed, taking care to avoid the obturator vessels, through the obturator canal using a tunnelling device. The tunnel is developed as far distally in the medial aspect of the thigh as necessary to reach a healthy segment of artery. A reinforced PTFE graft is passed through the tunnel and anastomosed in end-to-side fashion at both ends. The infected graft in the groin may then be removed and the arteries ligated.

Supra-aortic trunk bypass

In patients who have occlusive disease of a single supra-aortic trunk, a bypass may be inserted from any single trunk to the diseased trunk distal to the occlusion. The commonest example is that of the common carotid to subclavian bypass for occlusions of the first part of the subclavian artery.

Femorodistal bypass

Femorodistal bypass is usually carried out for occlusive disease but may occasionally be necessary for aneurysmal disease of the popliteal artery. The proximal origin of the bypass is usually the common femoral and the distal insertion is the popliteal either above or below the knee. For patients with more extensive disease it may be necessary to continue the graft down to the tibial arteries or even the dorsalis pedis. In general the long-term patency rates are worse with the more distal grafts.

The techniques used are as follows.

The femoral artery is dissected out and mobilised down to its bifurcation. The anastomosis is usually fashioned as far distally on the common femoral as possible to allow preservation of a length more proximally in case of a need for revision at a later date.

The popliteal artery is then dissected out through a medial approach either above or below the knee (above-knee bypasses have a marginally better long-term patency). For the above-knee popliteal artery the incision is made along the anterior border of sartorius (care being taken to avoid damage to the saphenous vein). Sartorius is displaced posteriorly and the fascia deep to it is incised to open the popliteal fossa. The vessels are identified in the flat lying close to the posterior aspect of the femur.

Exposure of the below-knee popliteal is made through an incision along the posterior border of the upper quarter of the tibia. Care should be taken to avoid dividing the main trunk of the saphenous vein. It is often better to dissect out the distal part of the vein at this stage to ensure that the branch with the largest lumen is preserved. The deep fascia is incised as far as the tendons of sartorius, gracilis and semitendinosus. The fat in the popliteal fossa is separated with blunt dissection and the artery is found in a fascial sheath with one or more veins which have to be separated. The anterior tibial artery usually lies just above the origin of soleus and tethers the artery anteriorly at this level.

The vein is mobilised by one of the techniques described above. For a reversed bypass the graft may be placed orthotopically. The tunnel behind the knee is carefully dissected by passing a finger from above and below. It is essential to pass the graft between the heads of gastrocnemius and not through one of the heads. The author also dissects the proximal tunnel by finger dissection deep to sartorius to ensure a wide and unconstricted tunnel.

When inserting an *in situ* graft, the lower end of the vein must be fully mobilised and passed through the deep fascia into the popliteal fossa. This forms a right-angled bend which is a potential source of constriction. Some surgeons mobilise a long length of vein for below-knee grafts and lead the graft into the proximal popliteal fossa with an orthotopic course from there to the distal popliteal fossa.

The vein is then anastomosed at both ends in end-to-side fashion using polypropylene sutures. With *in situ* grafts there is sometimes insufficient proximal length even after mobilisation to reach the common femoral artery. In such situations the proximal superficial femoral artery is used as the origin. This may be either an end-to-side anastomosis if the artery is patent or an end-to-end anastomosis after local thromboendarterectomy if the artery is occluded.

SUMMARY

There are a number of rules to remember in vascular surgery:

- Always ensure a high-pressure inflow and low-resistance outflow.
- Avoid creating irregularities or stenoses where thrombus may accumulate.
- Do not be afraid to use heparin before, during and after operation but ensure your anastomoses are watertight.
- Be scrupulously careful about asepsis as graft infection is a disaster.
- Amputation may be more appropriate than reconstruction for some patients.
- Patients with atherosclerosis have a limited life expectancy.

FURTHER READING

Belli AM. Thrombolysis in the peripheral vascular system. *Cardiovasc Intervent Radiol* 1998; **21**: 95–101

Blaisdell FW, Steele M, Alien RF. Management of acute lower extremity arterial ischaemia due to embolism and thrombosis. *Surgery* 1978; **84**: 822–834

Brewster DC. The role of angioplasty to improve inflow for infra-inguinal bypasses. *Eur J Vasc Endovasc Surg* 1995; **9**: 262–266

Dormandy JA, Loh A. The management of the unreconstructable limb. *Curr Pract Surg* 1992; **4**: 81–89

Grace PA. Ischaemia-reperfusion injury. *Br J Surg* 1994; **81**: 637–647

Ihiberg L, Luther M, Tierala E et al. The utility of Duplex scanning in infra-inguinal vein graft surveillance: results from a randomised controlled study. *Eur J Vasc Endovasc Surg* 1998; **16**: 19–27

Lorentzen JE, Nielsen OM, Arendrup H et al. Vascular graft infection: an analysis of sixty two infections in 2411 consecutively implanted synthetic vascular grafts. *Surgery* 1985; **98**: 81–86

Pell JP, Fowkes FGR, Lee AJ. Indications for arterial reconstruction and major amputation in the management of chronic critical limb ischaemia. *Eur J Vasc Endovasc Surg* 1997; **13**: 315–321

Scott RAP, Wilson NM, Ashton HA et al. Influence of screening on the incidence of ruptured abdominal aortic aneurysms: 5 year results of a randomised controlled study. *Br J Surg* 1995; **82**: 1066–1070

STILE investigators. Results of a prospective randomised controlled trial evaluating surgery versus thrombolysis for ischaemia of the lower extremity. The STILE Trial. *Ann Surg* 1994; **220**: 251–268

UK Small Aneurysm Trial Participants. Mortality results for randomised controlled trial of early elective surgery or ultrasonographic surveillance for small abdominal aortic aneurysms. *Lancet* 1998; **352**: 1649–1655

Varty K, Nydahl S, Nasim A, Bolia A, Bell PRF, London NJM. Results of surgery and angioplasty for the treatment of chronic severe lower limb ischaemia. *Eur J Vasc Endovasc Surg* 1998; **16**: 159–161

40

Extracranial carotid and vertebral artery disease

J. Brittenden, John McCormick

STROKE AND TRANSIENT ISCHAEMIC ATTACKS: DEFINITION AND INCIDENCE

A stroke is defined as an acute loss of cerebral function of greater than 24 hours duration, with no apparent cause other than that of a vascular origin. Worldwide, strokes are the third most common cause of death. The annual UK incidence is two per thousand of the population. This figure is set to increase, with the projected increase in the elderly population. Over half of strokes occur in patients older than 75 years, but 25% do occur in patients younger than 65.

A transient ischaemic (TIA) attack is defined as an acute loss of focal cerebral function or monocular vision loss with symptoms lasting less than 24 hours, with no apparent cause other than vascular origin. Transient ischaemic attacks may in some cases be preceded by straining, bending or sneezing but in the majority of cases occur randomly. TIAs are a warning of possible future stroke, which may be severe or disabling. It is difficult to assess the incidence of TIAs as many episodes go unreported or are not referred or investigated appropriately. The estimated UK annual incidence of TIAs is five per thousand of the population.

Anatomy

Collateral pathways can protect brain perfusion in the presence of severe carotid disease. The circle of Willis at the base of the brain allows flow between the right and left carotid territories via the anterior communicating artery and between the basilar and carotid circulation via the posterior communicating artery. An incomplete circle of Willis, estimated to occur in 35% of patients, theoretically may lead to an increased risk of stroke in patients with carotid disease and an increased risk of intraoperative stroke without cerebral protection.

Pathology

The Oxford study found that the pathological causes of stroke were: 80% cerebral infarction, 10% primary intracerebral haemorrhage, 5% subarachnoid, 5% uncertain type. Cerebral infarction, so-called ischaemic strokes, are thromboembolic in origin. Up to 80% of these occur within the carotid territory. The aetiology of carotid territory infarction is shown in Table 40.1.

Outcome of stroke and transient ischaemic attack

The 30-day mortality rate for patients with cerebral infarction is 10%, which is lower than that for haemorrhage. In the Oxford study, at one year post stroke 23% of patients with cerebral infarction were dead and 65% were functionally dependent. The stroke recurrence rate is 5% per annum, but is higher in the early recovery period and in patients with severe carotid stenosis. Stroke patients have a high incidence of medical complications, which

Table 40.1 Aetiology of carotid territory infarction

Aetiology	Notes
Carotid emboli	Most common
Cardiac emboli	5%
Focal thrombotic occlusion of intracranial artery	Elderly patients, lacunar infarction
Hypoperfusion	Rare – watershed infarct
Hypercoagulable states	Thrombocytosis, polycythaemia
	Protein C and S deficiency, activated protein C resistance, antiphospholipid syndrome, homocystinuria
Haematological	Sickle cell, myeloma
Vasculitis/vasculopathy	Giant cell arteritis, SLE, fibromuscular dysplasia
Amyloid	Elderly, affects small vessels

may be reduced by proper stroke unit care. Indeed, in the Western world the stroke mortality has reduced by 20% over the past two decades. TIAs are a warning of future stroke, with a risk of 10% per year.

Stroke: risk factors and prevention

Risk factors for stroke which have been shown to be causal are hypertension, cigarette smoking, atrial fibrillation and diabetes mellitus. Both systolic and diastolic pressures are important in the development of stroke and the aim of treatment is to reduce levels to less than 140 mmHg and 90 mmHg respectively. Cigarette smoking has been shown to increase the risk of stroke by 50%. However, the Framingham study has shown that after five years of cessation the risk of stroke is equivalent to that of non-smokers. In patients with atrial fibrillation, anticoagulation with warfarin has been shown to significantly reduce the rate of stroke. Other possible causal factors of stroke are raised plasma cholesterol, fibrinogen and homocysteine. The lowering of plasma cholesterol in patients who have not yet had a stroke appears to reduce stroke risk. Indeed, it has been suggested that RMG Co-A reductase inhibitors may help stabilise the plaque in addition to reducing LDL-cholesterol levels.

In patients with a history of stroke or TIA, low-dose aspirin has been shown to significantly reduce the risk of further stroke, myocardial infarction or vascular death. Clopidogrel has been shown to be equally effective. Prevention of stroke, in addition to treating the above risk factors, should include exercise. Increased physical activity has been linked to lower incidence of stroke and ischaemic heart disease. It should be noted that one-third of patients with ischaemic stroke already have a history of angina or prior myocardial infarction. Exercise may act by reducing raised blood pressure, increasing HDL-cholesterol, lowering LDL-cholesterol and improving glucose tolerance. The heart protection study has shown that all patients who have had a neurological event should be prescribed a statin if their cholesterol is greater than 3.5 mmol/L

Clinical presentation

Carotid territory symptoms are listed in Box 40.1. Ischaemic infarction of the brain supplied by the internal carotid artery and middle cerebral artery results in contralateral hemiplegia and sensory loss mainly of the face and arm. Dysphasia may also be present, especially if the dominant hemisphere is affected. Patients with total anterior circulation infarction present with the triad of:

- contralateral hemiplegia and sensory loss of the face, arm and leg
- higher cortical dysfunction such as dysphasia and visuospatial neglect
- homonymous hemianopia.

Transient ischaemic attacks present with similar symptoms and signs, which resolve within 24 hours. Patients may also experience amaurosis fugax, which is transient blindness occurring in the ipsilateral eye described as a grey mist or curtain coming down. Features suggestive of a haemorrhagic stroke are coma, vomiting, severe headache, meningism and a systolic blood pressure greater than 220 mmHg.

The differential diagnoses include vasculitis (polyarteritis nodosa, systemic lupus erythematosus and giant cell arteritis), haematological diseases (sickle cell anaemia, myeloma, polycythaemia and thrombocytopenia), migraine, Todd's transient paralysis following focal partial seizure, space-occupying lesions, arteriovenous malformations, multiple sclerosis and peripheral nerve lesions.

Box 40.1   Clinical presentation

Carotid territory	*Vertebrobasilar*
Contralateral hemiplegia	Dizziness, vertigo, nystagmus
Contralateral sensory loss	Impaired balance
Dysphasia, special neglect	Dysarthria
Homonymous hemianopia	Bilateral blindness
Amaurosis fugax	

Patient assessment

Patients presenting with TIAs or stroke require a full history and examination. It is important to confirm the diagnosis, identify risk factors and patient co-morbidity. Physical examination involves assessment of residual neurological deficit and the detection of vascular signs. Ausculation should include the carotid and subclavian regions as well as the heart. The presence of a bruit indicates turbulence in the underlying vessel which may be the external carotid. However, a carotid bruit is only present in 40% of patients with greater than 50% stenosis of the internal carotid and may be present in patients with minor stenosis only. Blood pressure in both arms should also be compared.

General investigations including full blood count, ESR and ECG should be performed. Patients with carotid territory symptoms should undergo non-invasive imaging of their carotid arteries.

Treatment involves risk factor management and surgery is indicated for patients with greater than 70% stenosis of the internal carotid artery.

Investigations

Duplex ultrasonography

This non-invasive test combines B-mode ultrasound (Figure 40.1) and colour Doppler flowmeter. It was originally used as a screening method to detect patients with carotid disease, before proceeding to angiography. However, with improved techniques and machines, the sensitivity and specificity have improved to such a degree that in many centres the findings on duplex are thought to be sufficient to allow planning of surgery without the

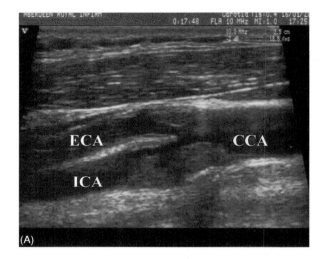

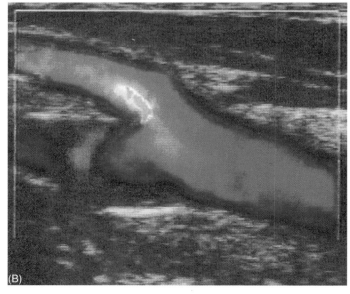

Figure 40.1 A. B-mode ultrasound and (**B**) colour Doppler of a stenosed (>70%) internal carotid artery. CCA, common carotid artery, ECA, external carotid artery, ICA, internal carotid artery.

need for further imaging of the carotid bifurcation. Duplex scanning is able to assess the site and extent of disease, the course and diameter of the internal carotid artery, the anatomical level of the bifurcation and dampened flow suggestive of proximal disease. It is non-invasive and painless.

The main limitations are the inter- and intraobserver variability and differences in the criteria used to assess stenosis. In each vascular laboratory duplex scanning should be validated against angiography which is considered to be the current gold standard. Duplex scanning may be of limited value in heavily calcified vessels and in determining true from subtotal occlusions. However, the recent availability of ultrasound contrast agents using stabilised microbubbles allows improved detection of true occlusions. In patients with contralateral disease, duplex scanning may overestimate the degree of stenosis.

In addition to flow dynamics, it is possible to assess the type of plaque present using B-mode. Plaques may be echolucent or echogenic. Echolucent plaques appear to be more common in patients with symptomatic high-grade stenosis compared to asymptomatic patients, suggesting that this plaque is unstable and tends to embolise.

In summary, carotid endarterectomy can be performed safely based on the duplex scan alone in the majority of patients, but in a select number angiography may be required.

Angiography

This is regarded as the current gold standard (Figure 40.2). However, it is invasive and carries a risk of stroke of approximately 1.2–2% due to disruption of emboli by the catheter tip. In addition, there is the risk of an adverse reaction to contrast. Angiography has been used in most of the major carotid endarterectomy trials. There are two main techniques for measuring the degree of stenosis (Figure 40.3). In North America, the diameter of the diseased internal carotid artery (3) is compared to the diameter of the distal internal carotid artery (2). In Europe, it is compared to the carotid bulb diameter (1). Angiography, like duplex scanning, is subjected to inter- and intraobserver variability. However, it can detect plaque surface irregularity and ulceration, which has been shown to be associated with an increased risk of ipsilateral ischaemic stroke, but is not able to quantify the type of plaque present.

Magnetic resonance angiography

This technique is non-invasive and shows considerable promise as a routine screening investigation. Initial techniques known as 'time-of-flight' were associated with long imaging times and artefactual signal losses. The recent development of rapid imaging sequences combined with contrast enhancement has now increased the clinical applications of this technique. It can be used

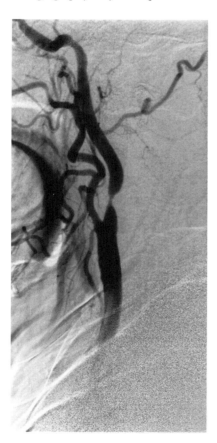

Figure 40.2 Angiogram of severely stenosed internal carotid artery.

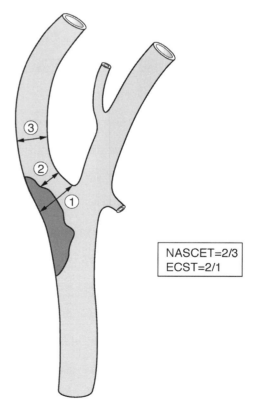

NASCET=2/3
ECST=2/1

Figure 40.3 The European and North American methods of measuring carotid stenosis.

623

to assess the entire circulation from the aortic arch through to the circle of Willis. In addition to detecting stenosis, it can also provide information on flow dynamics and plaque morphology.

Spiral CT angiography

This technique is now becoming more widely available. The arteries are enhanced with venous contrast and three-dimensional and multiplanar reconstructions are produced. Studies to date have shown that spiral CT angiography is able to reliably quantify degree of stenosis and detect true occlusions.

CT scan

There is an increased tendency to perform CT scans within the first three hours of development of symptoms so that haemor-

rhagic lesions can be excluded and thrombolytic therapy instituted if appropriate. At this stage acute ischaemic lesions may appear as dense areas with blurred margins, but complete infarction is not present until after 24 hours (Figure 40.4). Patients with cortical infarcts are more likely to have severe ipsilateral carotid stenosis or atrial fibrillation than those with lacunar infarct.

Preoperative CT findings in some studies have been shown to predict outcome from carotid surgery, with an increased complication rate in patients with proven infarct. CT evidence of cerebral infarction has also been shown to be present in a significant proportion of patients with apparently asymptomatic carotid artery stenosis.

SURGICAL TREATMENT OF CAROTID TERRITORY SYMPTOMS

Carotid surgery in order to prevent stroke was first performed by Eascott in 1954 in the UK. De Bakey carried out the first carotid endarterectomy in 1953 on an occluded carotid. The use of carotid endarterectomy in the prevention of strokes increased until the mid-1980s and then declined following adverse publicity regarding inappropriate patient selection and adverse outcomes. In addition, there were no clear guidelines as to which patients should undergo CEA. This led to the undertaking of two large randomised controlled trials, the European Carotid Trial (ECST) and the North American Symptomatic Carotid Trial (NASCET).

Carotid endarterectomy for symptomatic >70% stenosis

In 1991, the ECST and NASCET clearly demonstrated that CEA was beneficial in patients with high-grade (>70%) symptomatic stenosis. CEA in addition to best medical therapy significantly reduced the rate of ipsilateral stroke and major stroke and fatality compared to best medical therapy alone (Table 40.2). In contrast, CEA for stenosis less than 70% had no proven benefit. In the European trial at three-year follow-up the risk of ipsilateral ischaemic stroke was reduced sixfold in patients undergoing surgery compared to best medical therapy alone.

The NASCET has shown that the degree of benefit from CEA varies according to the severity of stenosis. Patients with stenosis greater than 90% have an absolute reduction in the rate of

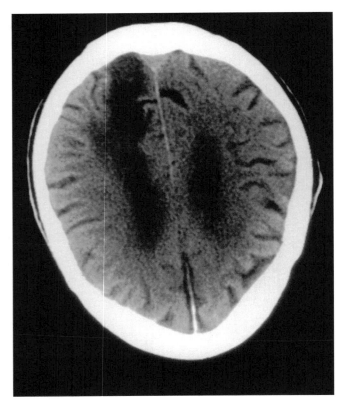

Figure 40.4 CT scan demonstrating large left cerebral infarct.

Table 40.2 RCT of carotid endarterectomy for severe (>70%) symptomatiac stenosis

Trial	Patient numbers	Isilateral stroke rate~	Major stroke/death★
European (ECST)	778	16% in BMT group 10.4% in surgical at 3 year follow-up	8.4% in BMT group 4.8% in surgical
North American (NASCET)	663	26% in BMT group 9% in surgical at 2 year follow-up	13.1% in BMT group 2.5% in surgical

★ Includes perioperative 30-day complications
BMT, best medical therapy

ipsilateral stroke twice that of patients with 70–79% stenosis. More recently, the final report of the ECST has stated that the decision to perform CEA in patients with symptomatic severe stenosis should be based on a model comparing age, sex and degree of stenosis. Use of this model now implies that CEA should be performed in symptomatic patients if their stenosis is greater than or equal to 80%. Despite the proven benefit of CEA, epidemiological studies have shown that it remains an under-utilised means of stroke prevention.

Outcome of CEA

The 30-day major stroke and fatality rate in the ECST was 3.7% and in the NASCET 3%. The total neurological event rate, including minor strokes and TIA, was 7.5% and 5.5% respectively. For centres to be able to reproduce the beneficial results of these trials it is important that the complication rates are carefully monitored and are equivalent or less than the trials. Clearly, with this type of prophylactic operation, designed to prevent further strokes, the risk/benefit equation is very important.

Studies have shown that the long-term benefit of surgery is greater and the risk of stroke with medical treatment is higher for men than woman, patients who have had strokes rather than TIAs and for patients with hemispheric compared with ocular symptoms.

RISK FACTORS FOR PERIOPERATIVE STROKE

A recent metaanalysis has shown that the risk of developing a peri-operative stroke is increased in women, patients aged greater than 75 years, with systolic blood pressure >180 mmHg and a history of peripheral vascular disease. The perioperative stroke and mortality rate was also increased in patients with contralateral internal artery occlusion. Presenting symptoms were also shown to influence outcome, such that patients with ocular symptoms only had a significantly lower complication rate compared to those with TIAs and CVAs. No difference in outcome was noted between patients who had presented with strokes compared to TIAs. It is questionable whether patients with diabetes have poorer outcomes.

RECURRENT STENOSIS POST CEA

The incidence of recurrent stenosis (>50%) reported in the literature varies from 4% to 16%. it is generally accepted to have a benign course with a stroke incidence less than 0.5%. Due to this low risk many centres do not now follow up patients post CEA with duplex scans.

THE OCCLUDED INTERNAL CAROTID ARTERY

Patients who have presented with symptoms of carotid territory ischaemia may on subsequent investigation be found to have a totally occluded internal carotid artery. Occlusion may also occur without symptoms. In these patients it is essential to ensure that there is a true rather than subtotal occlusion, especially if duplex scanning is used. Sensitivity may be increased by the use of ultrasound contrast agents but if doubt persists an angiogram should be performed. Generally speaking, if the internal carotid artery is occluded it should not give rise to further symptoms and the patient is no longer at risk. However, a small proportion of patients do have symptoms due to the so-called carotid stump syndrome. The stump of the occluded internal carotid artery may act as a source of emboli to the external carotid artery, which may then pass by the ophthalmic artery to the carotid syphon. Another cause for recurrent symptoms may be reduced flow in the watershed areas distal to an occlusion, which may occur following a period of hypotension.

Carotid endarterectomy for asymptomatic severe stenosis

This is currently being investigated in a large multicentre randomised European trial. Data from two American trials suggest that CEA is beneficial in asymptomatic patients with severe stenosis, but it is estimated that 30 CEAs would have to be performed to prevent one stroke (VA/ACAS). It is estimated that 5–10% of patients over 65 years have asymptomatic carotid disease amenable to surgery. There are resource implications involved in operating on asymptomatic patients, especially as CEA remains an underutilised means of stroke prevention in symptomatic patients.

Carotid angioplasty

In the CAVATAS trial, 504 patients were randomised to surgery or carotid angioplasty. The rates of non-disabling and disabling strokes were similar in both groups, but much higher than would be expected from the ECST and NASCET trials and subsequent publications on CEA outcome. A further trial is under way evaluating the use of stents. At present the technique of carotid angioplasty and stenting is still evolving and patients should only undergo this treatment as part of a randomised controlled trial.

Other carotid disease

Internal carotid artery dissection

This is a serious and undiagnosed condition, which is the cause of stroke in 20% of younger patients. The mean age of patients is 40–46 years, although children may also be affected. Bilateral carotid artery dissections may occur in 9–21% of cases. It can occur following minor trauma or physical effort, such as prolonged telephone calls with the neck flexed. There is a break in the intima and blood tracks into the wall, causing a haematoma or false passage. Cerebral ischaemia occurs as a result of reduced blood flow or from emboli from the damaged arterial wall.

Patients classically present with ipsilateral headache, neck pain and Horner's syndrome with the later development of cerebral ischaemic symptoms. Dissections can be detected by angiography or MPA. Duplex scanning is less specific and may not demonstrate the distal extent. There are no randomised controlled trials to guide treatment but anticoagulation is often used. The role of surgery is limited and endovascular treatment with the use of stents has been described. The prognosis is generally good, but depends on the distal extent of the dissection. Recanalisation may occur and the risk of recurrence is low.

Carotid body tumours

These are rare tumours of chemoreceptor tissue located at the carotid bifurcation. It tends to occur in patients living at high altitude and presents as a slowly enlarging asymptomatic mass. There are two forms – sporadic and familial – which are bilateral in 5% and 32% of cases, respectively. The features on angiogram are of a highly vascular tumour with spraying of the internal and external carotid arteries.

These lesions should be treated with surgery if possible. Although only 10% are frankly malignant, they may be locally invasive.

Carotid aneurysms

These are rare and present as swellings in the neck or as recurrent TIAs. The most common cause is atherosclerosis and, more rarely, trauma or fibromuscular dysplasia.

Arteritis

Arteritis that may rarely affect the carotid arteries includes giant cell, Takayasu and fibromuscular dysplasia.

VERTEBROBASILAR DISEASE

Vertebrobasilar symptoms include bilateral blindness, impaired balance, dysarthria, homonymous hemianopia, dizziness, vertigo or diplopia (see Box 40.1). Blackouts and isolated symptoms of dizziness, vertigo or diplopia are common and should not be attributed to vertebrobasilar disease. If the patient has classic symptoms and greater than 75% stenosis of both or of a dominant artery then surgery may be considered. This is difficult due to the anatomy and location of the veretebral artery and is infrequently performed. Surgery consists of dividing the artery above the stenosis and connecting it to the carotid artery. However, angioplasty alone or with a stent is increasingly being used to treat this condition.

OPERATIVE SURGERY

Carotid endarterectomy

Indications

Symptomatic high-grade stenosis. Patients should receive optimal medical therapy prior to proceeding to carotid endarterectomy.

Medical therapy involves risk factor management.

- Stop smoking
- Antiplatelet therapy: aspirin (75–300 mg), clopidogrel (75 mg)
- Check and treat elevated cholesterol
- Stabilise blood pressure
- Optimise cardiac function

Preoperative investigations

- Duplex scan
- Selective use of angiography
- Others: MRA, CT, angiography

Surgery

The current standard procedure used in the management of symptomatic high-grade stenosis is carotid endarterectomy and this is described below. Other techniques that may be employed are eversion endarterectomy and interposition vein grafting with more extensive lesions. Eversion endarterectomy, performed in some areas of Europe, involves dividing the internal carotid artery at the carotid bifurcation, everting the advential and outer medial layers of the artery and removal of the plaque. The internal carotid artery is then reimplanted to the carotid bifurcation.

TIMING OF SURGERY

CEA should be performed in patients who have had symptoms within the past six months. A delay in surgery may reduce the benefits of carotid endarterectomy. The European trial has shown that the main benefit from surgery is in the first year or so, whereas this extends to two years for non-disabling strokes.

Within a few days of an ischaemic stroke the safety and effectiveness of CEA are unknown. CEA can be performed safely six weeks following a stroke. Earlier series have shown a high morbidity and mortality for surgery performed within six weeks of a stroke, but recent studies suggest that this may be outdated.

CEA may have a role in patients with crescendo TIAs.

CONSENT

Emphasise that this is a prophylactic procedure. Discuss the likelihood of a further ischaemic event despite treatment with best medical therapy. A rough estimate is a 10% risk per year (26% risk of ipsilateral stroke at two years in the North American trial, 21% at three years in the European).

Explain fully the risks from the procedure.

PATIENT PREPARATION

Antibiotic prophylaxis – one dose, broad spectrum, especially if a patch is to be used.

ANAESTHETIC: GENERAL VERSUS LOCAL

A recent metaanalysis of non-randomised trials suggests that the neurological, cardiac and pulmonary complication rate and mortality are reduced by 50% when local anaesthetic is used. The three randomised trials to date have involved small numbers and have been unable to confirm these findings. A further large trial designed to address this issue is currently under way. The benefit of local anaesthetic may be due to its ability to preserve auto-regulation. This procedure may not be suitable in all patients, especially those who are very anxious, have difficulty communicating due to expressive dysphasia or have challenging anatomy.

PATIENT POSITIONING

Supine with the head turned to the opposite side (Figure 40.5). Avoid excessive rotation or extension, which may compromise cerebral blood flow.

INCISION

Upper two-thirds of the anterior border of the sternocleido-mastoid.

PROCEDURE

- The carotid bifurcation is exposed and the common, internal and external arteries slung (Figure 40.6).

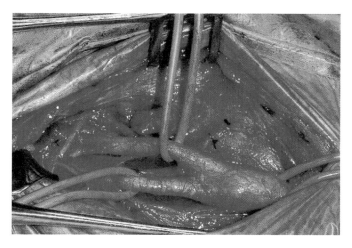

Figure 40.6 Exposure of carotid bifurcation.

- There should be minimal manipulation of the carotid arteries in order to avoid emboli.

- Heparinisation prior to clamping, longitudinal arteriotomy of the carotid bifurcation.

- Endarterectomy is performed and the entire stenotic lesion cored out (Figure 40.7).

- Magnifying loops may be used to ensure a clean endarterectomy site is obtained.

- Selective versus routine use of a shunt – there remains considerable controversy with regards to the use of shunts. Some surgeons routinely shunt in order to prevent cerebral ischaemia, while others pursue a selective policy and rely on intraoperative monitoring to detect signs of ischaemia. This is due to the associated morbidity of shunts which may kink, occlude or cause intimal damage. A recent Cochrane Review

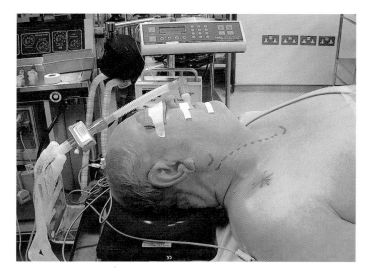

Figure 40.5 Correct patient positioning.

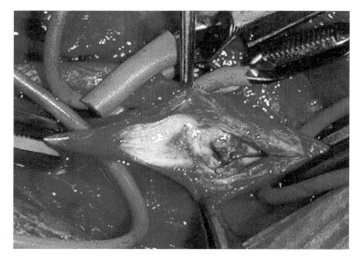

Figure 40.7 Internal carotid artery following arteriotomy, ulcerated plaque visible.

found that the current data available are too limited to either support or refute the use of routine or selective shunting in carotid endarterectomy. In addition, for selective shunting there are no clear guidelines as to which monitoring should be performed.

- Distal intimal flap is secured with tacking sutures where necessary to prevent dissection.

- Primary closure versus patch angioplasty – there remains debate about the indications and routine use of patch angioplasty. Many surgeons may use it selectively in patients with internal carotid diameters less than 5 mm in diameter. However, a recent metaanalysis performed by the Cochrane group found that patch angioplasty is associated with lower risks of perioperative arterial occlusions and restenosis, with an associated reduction in the number of strokes.

- Quality control – intraoperative assessment of technical perfection is monitored by angioscopy. Duplex scanning is best practice but is not universally used. Generally, the incidence of major technical defects during CEA is low, but completion angiography, angioscopy and Doppler may allow detection and possible correction of these defects. Due to the low complication rates now experienced in many centres it is difficult to prove that these techniques can further improve outcomes.

- Drain – risk of haematoma in confined space.

INTRAOPERATIVE MONITORING

Intraoperative ischaemia may occur in up to one-third of patients and may be assessed by:

- cerebral blood flow

- cerebral perfusion – somatosensory evoked potentials. This technique is less commonly used

- direct neurological examination – awake testing under local anaesthetic is reliable.

Cerebral blood flow

- *Transcranial Doppler* (Figures 40.8, 40.9). Possible in the 90% of patients who have an 'acoustic window'. It requires the availability of a technician and provides continuous monitoring of middle cerebral arterial velocity and allows detection of emboli. A decrease in middle cerebral artery velocity of greater than 50% is considered to indicate the need for a shunt.

- *Stump measurement.* Allows a single measurement of the degree of backflow and the collateral circulation. A mean stump pressure less than 50 mmHg indicates the need for a shunt.

- *Cerebral oximetry*, near infra-red spectroscopy with the probe positioned on the forehead. A decrease in cerebral oxygen saturation of greater than 10% is thought to indicate cerebral ischaemia. It is difficult to determine exactly what blood

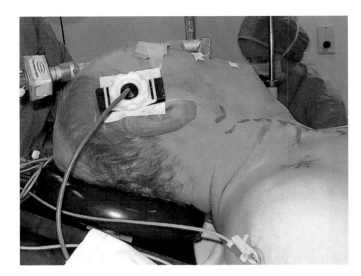

Figure 40.8 Transcranial Doppler positioned over acoustic window.

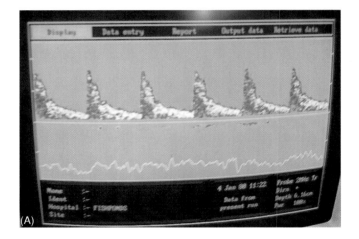

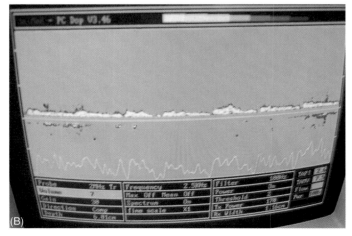

Figure 40.9 Transcranial Doppler tracing (**A**) prior to clamping of carotid arteries and (**B**) following clamping and prior to insertion of shunt.

supply is being assessed and extracranial as well as intracranial vessels are likely to contribute.

EARLY POSTOPERATIVE MANAGEMENT

- Immediate neurological testing.

- A perioperative stroke may first be suspected if there is failure or delay in the patient awakening from a general anaesthetic. In this scenario it is important to exclude thrombosis at the operation site by the use of duplex scanning. If thrombosis is present the vessel should be immediately reexplored.

- High dependency unit – careful monitoring of BP, oxygen saturation and electrocardiogram, wound and neurological status. Avoid hypotension and hypertension.

- Dextran 40 – if significant emboli detected on transcranial Doppler. Also used in some units where transcranial Doppler is not available as a prophylactic measure.

COMPLICATIONS

- Neurological – see Table 40.3 for ECST and NASCET outcome.

- Cranial and cervical nerve injury may occur in 3–27%; most resolve, 7% are permanent. Cutaneous nerves at risk: marginal branch of mandibular nerve, transverse cervical nerve. Deep: vagus, hypoglossal, superior and recurrent laryngeal.

- Neck haematoma – 5.5% in NASCET, note confined space, potential for laryngeal oedema.

- Cardiovascular – myocardial infarction (1%), arrhythmias (1–2%), hypertension.

- Hyperperfusion syndrome – 1–2% headache, seizures, impaired cognitive function mechanism: impaired cerebral autoregulation on background of preoperative vasodilatation.

Less common complications

- Vein patch rupture: 1.5%, increased if ankle vein used.
- False aneurysm formation: 0.7%.
- Prosthetic patch infection: 0.6%.

FURTHER READING

Bamford J, Sandercock P, Dennis M, Burn J, Warlow C. A prospective study of acute cerebrovascular disease in the community: the Oxfordshire Community Stroke Project – 1981–86. *J Neurol Neurosurg Psych* 1990; **53**:16–22

Counsell CE, Salinas R, Naylor R, Warlow CP. A systematic review of the randomised trials of carotid patch angioplasty in carotid endarterectomy. *Eur J Vasc Endovasc Surg* 1997; **13**:345–354

European Carotid Surgery Trialists' Collaborative Group. Randomised trial of endarterectomy for recently symptomatic stenosis: final results of the MRC European Carotid Surgery Trial (ECST). *Lancet* 1998; **351**:1235–1243

European Carotid Surgery Trialists' Group. MRC European carotid surgery trial: interim results for symptomatic patients with severe (70–99%) or with mild (0–29%) carotid stenosis. *Lancet* 1991; **337**:1235–1243

Executive Committee for Asymptomatic Carotid Atherosclerosis Study. Endarterectomy for asymptomatic carotid artery stenosis. *JAMA* 1995; **273**:1421–1428

Gaines PA. Carotid angioplasty. *Vasc Med* 1996; **1**:121–124

Gaunt ME, Naylor AR, Bell PRF. Preventing strokes associated with carotid endarterectomy: detection of embolisation by transcranial Doppler monitoring. *Eur J Vasc Endovasc Surg* 1997; **14**:1–3

Halliday AW. The Asymptomatic Carotid Surgery Trial (ACST) rationale and design. *Eur J Vasc Surg* 1994; **8**:703–710

North American Symptomatic Carotid Endarterectomy Trial Collaborators. Beneficial effect of carotid endarterectomy in symptomatic patients with high-grade stenosis. *N Engl J Med* 1991; **325**:445–453

Rothwell PM, Slattery J, Warlow CP. Clinical and angiographic predictors of stroke and death from carotid endarterectomy: systematic review. *BMJ* 1997; **315**:1571–1577

Tangkanakul C, Counsell CE, Warlow CP. Local versus general anaesthesia in carotid endarterectomy: a systematic review of the evidence. *Eur J Vasc Endovasc Surg* 1997; **13**:491–499

41

Venous and lymphatic diseases and arteriovenous malformations

Douglas R. Harper, K. Simon Cross

VENOUS DISEASE

Chronic venous insufficiency

Chronic venous insufficiency of the lower limb is found when a patient is unable adequately to reduce his pedal superficial venous pressure on walking. Clinically, it takes many forms, the commonest being varicose veins, and more severe venous insufficiency may result in leg ulceration. The various disorders are best understood by first considering the venous physiology of the lower limbs.

Physiology

Venous return from the lower limbs is partly achieved by the 'push' of systemic blood pressure but also by the calf muscle pump. This is the calf muscle surrounded by its tough deep fascia and containing numerous venous spaces or sinusoids. The direction the blood takes through this system is dictated by passive bivalves.

The calf muscle pump is like a peripheral heart. During calf diastole or relaxation, blood passes through the superficial veins to the deep system, i.e. through the perforator veins with their unidirectional valves. The hydrostatic pressure in the veins of the foot or ankle is determined by the height of the heart but the muscular relaxation will allow the pressure in the deep veins and sinusoids to drop further and so open the perforator valves and allow the passive filling of the calf pump. When the calf muscle contracts, these perforator valves shut as the intramuscular pressure rises (calf systole) and this pressure rise also opens the valves of the proximal deep system (the outflow) to return blood towards the heart. The outflow tract of the deep system has a series of valves, the highest of which is usually in the common femoral or external iliac vein. More proximally, other factors drive the venous return, such as abdominal and thoracic pressure.

Epidemiology

The prevalence of varicose veins in the Western world is about 10–25%, depending on population and definition. The female: male ratio is usually about 2.5:1 although recent studies have not found such a major difference. Risk factors include parity, obesity, age and family history. There is a long-held view that heredity plays a part in the predisposition towards varicose veins but the relationship is not clear. For example, native Africans rarely have varicose veins but Americans of African descent enjoy the same incidence as their Caucasian countrymen.

Chronic leg ulcer has a prevalence in Western European peoples of about 1% of whom one in eight will have an open ulcer at any one point in time; 70% of leg ulcers have a venous component and in about 10% an arterial component. In a further 10% arterial and venous factors will co-exist. Diabetes and rheumatoid disease are other important factors in the aetiology (Figure 41.1). In 50%

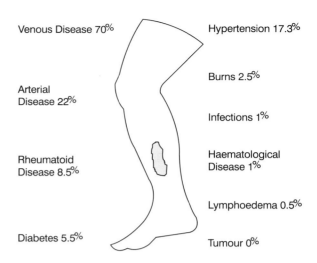

Figure 41.1 Conditions associated with leg ulceration.

there is a family history of a first-degree relative with severe venous disease.

Pathophysiology

The basic pathology of most venous disorders relates to deficiencies in the vein wall which becomes weak and so the bivalves become incompetent. Vein wall weakness is associated with:

- poor elastin/collagen synthesis
- fibrinolytic deficiency
- smooth muscle abnormalities.

These are also some of the factors which relate to increased risk of venous thromboembolism.

The walls of varicose veins have been shown to be deficient in elastin and collagen, resulting in a loss of elasticity. Since collagen is modified during pregnancy it may well be that this explains the higher incidence of varicose veins postpartum, veins which often become less noticeable later. Altered vein wall chemistry might also explain the familial nature of some varicose veins. Failure of the vein wall leads to failure of the bivalves and so flow refluxes. In addition, flow abnormalities might alter the surface of valves and this will encourage platelet deposition and subsequent cusp distortion, especially if fibrinolysis is less than adequate.

Patients with some of the more severe complications of venous disease, such as ulceration, have been noted to have fibrinolytic deficiency and this is thought to result in the failure to clear extravascular fibrin and failure to clear platelet and white cell aggregates from valve cusps. The latter might lead to the development of deep venous thrombosis (Figure 41.2).

Valvular incompetence leads to the development of superficial venous hypertension. Even transient venous hypertension causes changes in white cell function. White cells become marginalised in

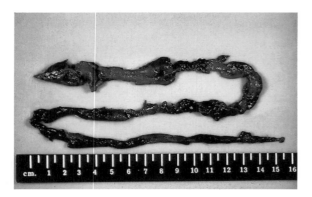

Figure 41.2 Thrombectomy specimen showing foci of white thrombus from within the valve cusps and dark consecutive thrombosis between.

the bloodstream and react with endothelial cells through 'adhesion molecules'. White cells become activated as a result. Such activation in chronic venous hypertension leads to the release of free radicals and other vasoactive substances which damage the endothelium. In addition, white cells aggregate in the dilated and tortuous capillaries and the subsequent focal anoxia again contributes to endothelial damage. Capillary leakage leads to the loss from the circulation of large molecules such as haemosiderin and the subsequent iron stain is pathognomic of venous hypertension. If the lymphatic pathways are overwhelmed, leg swelling results. Another leaked molecule is fibrinogen which promptly coagulates to fibrin in the immediate environs of the capillary, giving rise to the 'fibrin cuff'. The fibrin cuff also contains numerous other substances such as collagen, laminin, fibronectin, tenascin, macrophages and T lymphocytes. It has been suggested that the fibrin cuff might reduce the transfer of oxygen to the tissues but this has not been established. However mediated, the eventual skin damage is thought to be anoxic and reduced skin oxygen tension is the rule. In severe cases of chronic venous insufficiency, this leads to venous ulcer. The final link in the pathological process giving rise to skin anoxia remains to be discovered.

Varicose veins: clinical syndromes

There are several ways of classifying varicose veins and chronic venous insufficiency and a simplified clinical classification might include the following:

- stem varicose veins
- reticular varicose veins
- telangiectasia
- perforator incompetence.

Stem varicose veins

These are sometimes referred to as familial or primary varicose veins and affect the main trunks and their branches. The calf muscle pump is normal in these patients and it is probably working

overtime. Blood is ejected in a proximal direction up the leg through the competent valves until it reaches the saphenofemoral or saphenopopliteal junctions, where a proportion refluxes down the leg to be recycled once again by the pump. This reflux occurs as a result of the weakness of the vein wall, leading to valvular incompetence. There may be a progressive valvular failure down the leg but recent studies have confirmed that this may not always be the case, i.e. valve failure below a competent saphenofemoral valve does occur. It is likely that the deep vein walls will be similarly weak in chronic venous insufficiency but the superficial veins lack the support of surrounding muscle and are easily seen. Superficial venous hypertension over the territory of the stem vein involved is responsible for the leg ache, restlessness, cramps, itch and swelling which complete the syndrome.

Reticular varicose veins

These display no stem and branch pattern and are frequently distributed over the lateral and posterior thigh. Often they are small in calibre and do not respond well to surgery.

Telangiectasia

These are dilated veins in the deep dermis and are very fine. They are also referred to as thread veins, venous stars or spider veins. Commonly they are found in the outer and inner thighs and can be very unsightly. They may or may not be associated with venous hypertension. They often develop in pregnancy and may be precipitated by venous surgery, appearing around the sites of stab avulsions. Other iatrogenic causes include UV radiation and compression sclerotherapy.

Perforator incompetence

Perforating vessels between the deep and the superficial parts of the venous system are widely distributed in the leg but some appear more clinically important than others. In the medial thigh is the Hunterian perforator, there is often one just below the knee anteromedially and usually three lower calf perforators medially. Incompetence of the Hunterian perforator may give rise to thigh recurrence following inadequate surgery as may the upper medial calf one just below the knee. The most clinically important perforators are those on the lower medial calf.

The failure of the calf perforators may be secondary to adjacent primary varicose veins or follow damage from venous thrombosis, or again, isolated perforator failure can occur. Perforator incompetence allows the sudden transmission of the deep venous pressure cycle to the superficial tissues and will be responsible for local or focused superficial venous hypertension. While the development of superficial hypertension may be gradual in stem varicose veins and more precipitate in perforator incompetence, the hypertension must be the same order of magnitude since it is hydrostatic. In both, the ability of the deep system to clear the superficial tissue of venous blood will be impaired and the drop in superficial pressure associated with exercise will be either partially (stem) or substantially (perforator incompetence) reduced (Figure 41.3).

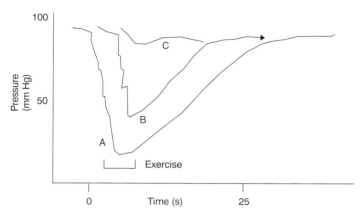

Figure 41.3 Ambulatory venous pressure.

Complications of varicose veins

Varicose veins may be complicated by:

- thrombophlebitis and pulmonary embolism
- haemorrhage
- venous dermatitis
- lipodermatosclerosis
- venous leg ulcer.

Thrombophlebitis

Thrombophlebitis may arise in any part of the venous tree and is more frequently found in varicose veins than in normal veins. The thrombotic component always extends more proximally than the inflammatory one and may allow clot to extend to the ostium of the saphenous and into the external iliac vein beyond. Phlebitis of the thigh saphenous should therefore be treated by saphenous ligation at the groin, care being taken to first remove any clot that may have already progessed that far. Phlebitis below the knee may be treated initially during the acute phase with bedrest, elevation and analgesics and later by ambulation with graduated compression.

Haemorrhage

Haemorrhage from varicose vein rupture is a dangerous condition which can be fatal. Simple pressure and elevation of the limb will always control it before admission and graduated compression bandaging combined with bedrest will allow preparation for definitive surgery.

Venous dermatitis

Venous dermatitis can develop in the skin overlying the varicose veins and may display erythema, weeping, scaling and pigmentation. It may also be associated with venous ulcer when it is often a contact dermatitis related to the treatment of the ulcer.

Lipodermatosclerosis

Lipodermatosclerosis is the syndrome characterised by changes in the subcutaneous tissue of the gaiter area as a result of sustained venous hypertension and associated microcirculatory changes. These manifest themselves as induration, cellulitis, venous flare in the instep and atrophy blanche. Venous ulceration usually follows unless active conservative or surgical steps are taken to control the venous hypertension.

Venous leg ulcer

The most challenging complication of venous disease in the lower limb is chronic venous leg ulcer. The treatment of leg ulcers is a huge drain on community nursing resources, which are responsible for over 80% of the care.

The key to the management of leg ulcers is to understand their aetiology, since not all of them will be venous. For example, ulcers associated with arterial and rheumatoid disease and diabetes may require a different approach from that employed for purely venous ulcers. Unfortunately more than one aetiological factor may be present.

Appearance may be of some value; deep ulcers are associated with rheumatoid disease, etc., but these manifestations may be misleading, especially when more than one factor obtains. Firstly, diabetes must be ruled out by urinalysis (or fasting blood sugar) and secondly, the ankle/brachial systolic pressure index must be determined. The index is not reliable in the diabetic and compression may be contraindicated. Rheumatoid and other connective tissue disorders should be looked for as should haemopoietic and cardiac disease.

Control of oedema is mandatory in the treatment of a leg with an ulcer. Once the leg has been reduced to its normal dimensions, treatment of the ulcer and the leg may commence. A recent randomised controlled trial failed to establish an advantage for hydrophilic dressings in venous ulcers but they appear to be superior to non-adherent dressings in the arterial ulcers. Better evidence exists for the efficacy of graduated compression and specifically of multilayer bandaging as the principal treatment for venous ulceration. Diabetes and other microvascular disorders and arterial insufficiency should be ruled out before starting this therapy. Multilayer systems are certainly superior to monolayer systems. Systems which contain elastic compression are significantly better than those with inelastic compression. The system usually contains four layers but the cost of this is offset by better healing rates, making it a cost-effective treatment.

A healing rate of 75% for venous ulcers in three months should be the target. Those that do not heal in this time should be completely reassessed and this might include biopsy.

Investigation

The precise diagnosis of venous disease cannot presently be made with any single test, although colour flow duplex ultrasound is probably the single most informative investigation. Essentially it is important to quantify the distribution of occlusion (particularly in the deep veins) and reflux (in both deep and superficial systems).

Tests of reflux

The Trendelenberg tourniquet test is perhaps the most basic examination of venous reflux and still the most commonly practised. Unfortunately it suffers from considerable observer error, being very subjective. The patient lies supine and the examiner raises the leg and massages the dilated veins towards the trunk until they are empty. A tourniquet is then applied around the upper third of the thigh and the patient is asked to stand. Filling below the tourniquet indicates an incompetence between the deep and superficial systems (i.e. short saphenous or perforator(s)). Release of the tourniquet will show whether there is reflux from above (i.e. saphenofemoral or a perforator depending on the position of the tourniquet). Repeating this test by applying the tourniquet at different levels will give added information.

The Trendelenberg test may be used in conjunction with probes held over the skin of the ankle as in photoplethysmography (PPG) or light reflex rheology (LRR). These relatively user-friendly devices give more precise information and will usually confirm that an abnormality in venous function exists. They cannot discriminate between deep and superficial disease.

The continuous-wave Doppler may be used in any clinic or domiciliary situation and gives important, albeit limited information. It can detect incompetence at the groin or popliteal fossa but cannot define the vessel in which reflux occurs. The examination is conducted with the patient standing. The vein is insonated and manually compressing and releasing the calf will detect patency, competency or reflux. It may be useful in screening out those patients who require more detailed assessment by duplex.

Colour flow duplex ultrasound is at the moment the most reliable and comprehensive technique for the investigation of venous disease. Reflux can be detected in a specific vessel and its degree semi-quantitatively measured. Debate continues about interpretation of some of the results but confirmation of reflux in the stem vessels, in the calf perforators and in the deep vessels, particularly below the knee can assist the planning of any surgery and inform advice to the patient on prognosis. Occlusion is a much less common feature of venous disease in general, and following DVT in particular, but once again duplex is the most reliable non-invasive way of establishing its distribution below the groin.

Phlebography

Phlebography can be carried out by a number of techniques depending on the clinical situation. The assessment of deep venous patency in the calf or reflux within the calf perforators is performed by ascending phlebography, while assessment of deep venous reflux may be made by descending phlebography from the groin. Varicography, the direct opacification of a varicosity, may be used to define a source of filling, particularly following previous surgery. Finally, iliofemoral phlebography from bilateral groin injection can define pelvic venous disease.

Tests of occlusion

The commonest sequel of deep vein thrombosis is valvular incompetence and non-persistent occlusion, but occlusion will be present in about 10% of symptomatic patients. Phlebography is a helpful investigation. Duplex ultrasound examination needs to be extensive but yields the same information. However, should a collateral circulation develop, say across the pelvis, duplex ultrasound may not identify this as easily as the appropriate phlebogram.

Surgical management of varicose veins

Patients with varicose veins complain of the symptoms of chronic venous insufficiency, namely leg aches, swelling, restlessness, pain over specific veins or skin problems such as phlebitis, venous eczema or ulceration. Many patients are unhappy with the appearance of their leg and are aware of a family predisposition. Surgery may be indicated for any of these complaints depending either on the clinician's perception of the patient's disability or to what extent he believes that surgery can avoid skin or other complications.

The assessment of a patient immediately before surgery is crucial. This involves the painstaking marking of the dilated veins of the leg when the patient stands.

There are three elements to the operative treatment of stem varicose veins:

- high saphenous ligation ± short saphenous ligation
- removal of the long saphenous vein in the thigh or the upper section of the short saphenous vein
- excision of calf varicosities.

High saphenous ligation

The saphenofemoral junction should be exposed by a 3 cm incision in the groin crease immediately medial to the femoral pulse. Care must be taken to identify positively the long saphenous vein before dividing it. Thereafter careful dissection of the various tributaries is straightforward. Nevertheless, this is frequently the site of later recurrences because of technical error resulting from poorly defined anatomy. Included in this is the failure to divide independently the branches of the main tributaries (e.g. Figure 41.4). The tributaries that must be accounted for and divided are the superficial circumflex iliac, the superficial inferior epigastric and the deep external pudendal. More distally are the medial and lateral thigh tributaries.

The saphenous termination is finally positively identified by the close relationship to the superficial external pudendal artery which passes immediately above or, more commonly, immediately below the junction of the long saphenous with the common femoral vein.

Long saphenous stripping

While technical inadequacy in ligating the saphenofemoral junction may be the commonest reason for recurrence in the thigh, there is evidence to suggest that the small branches elsewhere in the femoral triangle may communicate directly with the incompetent saphenous trunk. For this reason there is no longer any question that the saphenous vein in the thigh should be removed if recurrence is to be reduced to acceptable levels. There is probably no need to strip in the lower leg where the risks of damage to the saphenous nerve are high. To further reduce the changes of damage, stripping should always be towards the foot. More recently, techniques of invagination or endo-stripping have been developed in the hope that less tissue and nerve damage results.

Short saphenous surgery

In 10–15% of varicose vein patients the short saphenous vein will be incompetent. The saphenopopliteal junction is at a variable level and may not communicate with the popliteal vein at all. It is therefore strongly recommended that the anatomy be clarified by either duplex mapping or on-table varicography (Figure 41.5). The junction is then best approached through a transverse incision in the popliteal fossa with the patient either prone or in a lateral position with the leg to be operated on uppermost. Variations in the terminal anatomy are common and occasionally the short saphenous vein will have a major connection with the medial thigh vein. After a safe saphenopopliteal ligation, the upper 15 cm of the vein should be excised rather than a longer section stripped. Stripping of the short saphenous vein is not recommended since any damage to the sural nerve will render the heel anaesthetic.

Calf phlebectomy

Calf phlebectomy is necessary to remove the varicose tributaries in the leg and thigh, which will otherwise remain even if the saphenous reflux is dealt with. These veins will continue to be incompetent and since they are still part of the circulation, the hydrostatic pressure will still be transmitted to them throughout the ambulatory cycle. They will continue to place the patient at risk of phlebitis and skin complications. The calf operation may be done under thigh tourniquet (Figure 41.6). There are advantages to carrying out this stage of the operation in a bloodless field but caution should be exercised in patients with a recent history of DVT or pulmonary embolism. Complications of a tourniquet should also be borne in mind, such as damage to diseased femoropopliteal artery or neuropraxia.

Straightforward varicose vein surgery in otherwise fit patients can conveniently be done on a day case basis. The aim should be to return the patient to full activity within two weeks following operation.

Perforator surgery

Incompetence of any leg perforator may be important in the genesis of varicose veins or may follow the development of the varicose veins. On balance there is a good argument for ligating large incompetent perforators at surgery. However, there is some evidence that control of the superficial venous hypertension by superficial venous surgery may reverse perforator incompetence.

Perforator surgery is usually performed through a small incision when the perforator is dissected out from the subcutaneous tissue

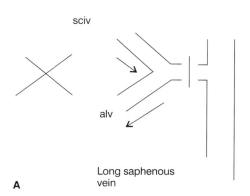
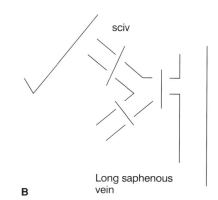

Figure 41.4 Ligating branches of the long saphenous vein. **A** Only the common stem of the superficial circumflex iliac vein (sciv) and the anterolateral thigh vein (alv) are ligated resulting in continued reflux down the thigh and 'recurrent' varicose veins. **B** Correct procedure where all three are ligated.

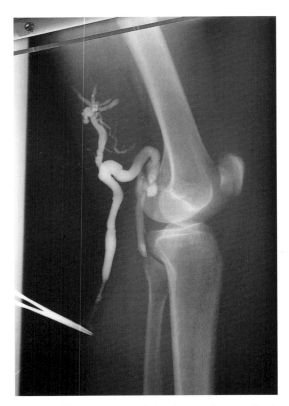

Figure 41.5 On-table varicogram of the short saphenous allowing precise identification of the anatomy before exploration of the popliteal fossa.

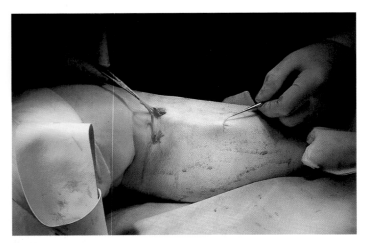

Figure 41.6 Calf phlebectomy by subcutaneous dissection and avulsion, in this case, under tourniquet.

and ligated and divided at the deep fascia – the extrafascial approach. Subfascial ligation may be carried out through a posterior or medial incision from the level of the malleoli to the calf muscle. The incision is carried down directly to the deep fascia which is divided in the line of the incision. Each edge is lifted in turn and a plane developed between the deep surface of the fascia and the muscle. The perforators are seen passing from the muscle to a gap in the fascia and may be ligated and divided at that point (Figure 41.7). More recently, the advantages of the subfascial approach without the

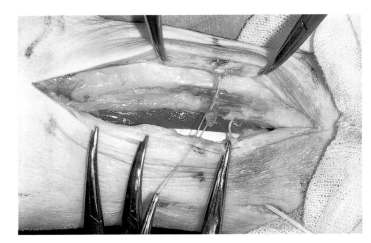

Figure 41.7 Open subfascial approach to a calf perforator. This is now largely superseded by an endoscopic technique (see Fig. 41.8).

difficulties relating to the wound have been overcome by the development of endoscopic techniques through more proximal, smaller incisions (Figure 41.8). The efficacy of this approach, and indeed the benefits of perforator surgery, remain to be established.

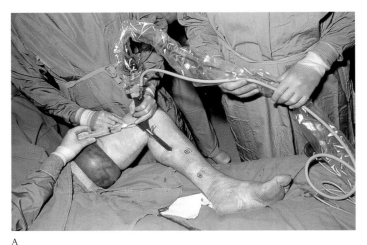

A

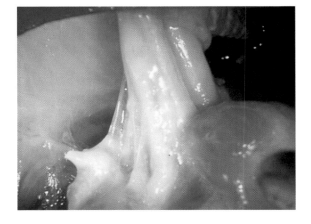

B

Figure 41.8 Subfascial endoscopic perforator surgery (SEPS). **A** the endoscope is inserted and **B** the perforator visualised. Courtesy of C.V. Ruckley.

Open ulceration

It is often best to skin graft larger ulcers, although the long-term results will be no better than with conservative care unless the underlying cause is corrected. For this reason, grafting may be combined with perforator or superficial venous surgery.

Complications

Complications specific to surgery may include:

- damage to the common femoral or popliteal vein
- tie not flush, leaving stump as possible source of pulmonary embolism
- damage to sural, saphenous nerve (particularly at the ankle) and femoral/popliteal nerves
- haematoma, wound infection and wound edge necrosis.

In addition, the application of a tourniquet carries increased risk of neurological damage which must be balanced against the advantages of working in a bloodless field. Graduated compression bandaging must also be applied competently if pressure necrosis is to be avoided.

Non-surgical management of chronic venous insufficiency

Compression sclerotherapy

This may be indicated in reticular veins but is not effective as a treatment of stem varicose veins, when the recurrence rate is unacceptable. Microsclerotherapy can also be used in telangiectasia.

Graduated compression

Graduated compression must not be applied to the swollen limb, so as a preliminary, the patient should be encouraged to elevate the legs. The most effective way of doing this is to place 10cm blocks beneath the foot of the bed.

Graduated compression takes many forms – shaped tubular bandage, multilayer bandaging or compression hosiery – and it forms an essential element in the management of chronic venous insufficiency treated by operative or non-operative methods. The graduation should allow a pressure of 30 mmHg or more at the ankle, reducing to about half that below the knee. It should not be used in the diabetic or in those patients with arterial disease (APBI <0.8) or vasculitic disorders except under the most stringent supervision.

If bandaging is employed, multilayer systems are superior to single bandages. The first layer should be a generous one of wool roll followed by a bandage to compress the wool, such as a white crepe bandage. On this foundation the elastic compression bandage should be applied. Graduated compression should deliver progressively reducing pressure from the foot to the knee. In applying it progressively up the leg from the base of the toes, graduated compression will be assured if:

- the tension applied by the applier is constant as the diameter increases
- the overlap in successive layers is gradually lessened from foot to below the knee
- winding round excess bandage below the knee is avoided.

On top of the elastic compression should be applied a self-adhesive bandage or a large-fitting shaped tubular bandage to ensure all stays in place – the fourth layer.

Graduated compression is an effective treatment of chronic venous insufficiency and, like most effective treatments, it also has complications. Principal among these is tissue necrosis over bony prominences. If the tension on the bandage (stretch) is constant then the pressure on the tissue depends on the radius of the leg surface. (Smaller radii allow higher pressures.) This follows Laplace's law which is illustrated in Figure 41.9. Graduated compression must be applied with great caution, if at all, in patients suffering from peripheral vascular disease and especially diabetes (where the Doppler pressure may be misleading).

In cases of severe chronic venous insufficiency, uncomplicated by peripheral vascular disease or diabetes, graduated compression will need to be indefinite and compression hosiery should be replaced every 4–6 months. Often a second fitting will be required after a few months as the shape of the leg changes. As the patient ages, reassessment of the resting pressure index will be required to ensure that the treatment is still safe.

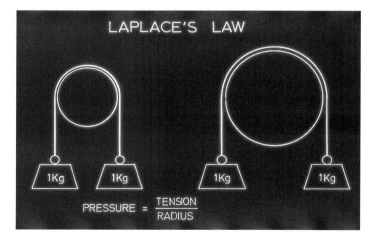

Figure 41.9 High tissue pressure is exerted beneath surfaces of small radii when bandage tension remains unaltered. Laplace's law which is the basis of graduated compression, reminds us of the risks to the tissue overlying bony prominences or tendons. Courtesy of J.J. Dale.

Drugs

Hydroxyethylrutoside may be beneficial in cases of 'restless leg syndrome', night cramps or swelling. These act to reduce capillary leakage and so the interstitial fluid load. They are best used to supplement graduated compression rather than being prescribed on their own. Quinine sulphate has been used for many years for the treatment of leg cramps but its efficacy remains in doubt. Other drugs, such as anabolic steroids, prostaglandins, methylxanthines or aspirin, have not proved to be of benefit.

Prevention of recurrence of venous leg ulcer

The probability of recurrence in an unselected group of leg ulcers is reckoned to be as high as 90% and so while the need to heal is obvious, prevention of recurrence may be the greater challenge. Patients should be fitted and regularly prescribed graduated compression hosiery indefinitely. In a recent study class 3 compression was confirmed to be significantly more effective than class 2 compression, even allowing for slightly poorer patient compliance with a stronger garment. The effect in addition to surgery is as yet unknown but there is renewed interest in the role of superficial varicose veins in the genesis of this disorder.

Venous thromboembolism and methods of prevention

Deep venous thrombosis (DVT) is the process by which thrombus forms in the deep veins of the calf, thigh or pelvis or any combination of these. Pulmonary embolism is another manifestation of the same disease – venous thromboembolism. In this section we will concentrate on the source of emboli and the consequences for the venous function of the lower limb.

Presentation

The thrombosis may be occlusive or non-occlusive and the process may start at any level, usually in the valve sinuses. It may start in the lower leg and progress proximally, but equally may start in the pelvis or synchronously at several levels. Since many of the underlying factors are systemic, DVT is often bilateral.

White thrombus, consisting of activated platelets and white cells with fibrin, usually forms in the valve sinuses and then darker 'consecutive' thrombosis forms much of the bulk of the DVT (see Figure 41.2). Occlusive thrombosis is usually clinically evident since flow is obstructed.

Non-occlusive DVT, however, is usually occult and commonly follows major surgery or serious illness. It is common in patients suffering from cancer and may be the first indication of the illness.

Any DVT may embolise, the larger life-threatening emboli usually coming from the pelvic veins. Commonly, the patient who has sustained a fatal pulmonary embolism has no leg swelling, suggesting that the thrombus was large, pelvic, non-occlusive and so poorly attached to the vein wall ('the silent leg'). About 50% of major, life-threatening pulmonary emboli are preceded by a small herald embolus.

Investigation

If a traumatic cause for leg swelling can be excluded, it is always prudent to heparinise a patient suspected of having a DVT on clinical grounds.

Duplex ultrasound is the best way to look at the deep veins of the leg, the critical areas to scan being the popliteal, femoral and pelvic veins of both legs.

If phlebography is required then it should normally be bilateral and must include good views of the pelvic veins. An exception is the leg which is swollen to the groin. This is most likely to be due to an iliofemoral venous thrombosis and the best way of defining its extent is to carry out a phlebogram via the contralateral groin which will allow access to the upper end by the cross-over technique and provide an opportunity there and then to place a caval filter if indicated (Figure 41.10).

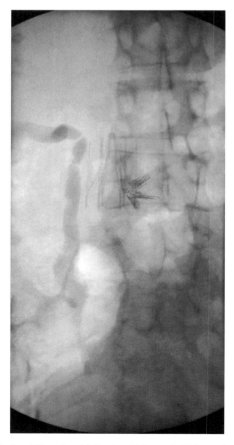

Figure 41.10 Caval filter placed following iliofemoral phlebography. Courtesy of J.E. Barry.

If there is thought to be any risk of pulmonary embolism then this should be confirmed as soon as possible. Usually the procedure of choice is a ventilation: perfusion lung scan. Where this is equivocal or the findings do not support a confident clinical diagnosis then a pulmonary angiogram should be undertaken. Even a small pulmonary embolus may be the first indication of serious venous thromboembolism and its diagnosis provides an opportunity to avoid fatal progression of the disease.

Treatment

Anticoagulation should be started on suspicion of a DVT pending confirmation by investigation. Heparin is prescribed to maintain the APTT at 2.5 times that of the control. Low molecular weight heparin may also be used (150–200 units/kg per 24 hours). This has the advantage of not requiring routine monitoring and so facilitating ambulation, earlier discharge or even outpatient or community management.

Thrombolysis of the pelvic or leg veins may be successful but only with recent thrombosis and since it is usually impossible to age the clot, this is only rarely used. Similarly, the results of thrombectomy are variable and this procedure should be left to the specialist. Both thrombolysis or thrombectomy may have to be considered in phlegmasia cerulea dolens when there is sudden massive swelling and impending venous gangrene, but in less desperate situations the advantage of these treatments is outweighed by the potential complications of bleeding or rethrombosis.

The swollen leg must be elevated well above the level of the heart until the swelling subsides. Elevation, if it is high enough, will always reduce the leg swelling, when graduated compression may be safely applied. Using compression bandages actively to reduce the leg swelling of DVT is dangerous.

Longer term sequelae

In 90% of cases of DVT the occlusion resolves as the clot contracts and recanalises. However, valvular function is lost more often than not and persistent swelling and superficial venous hypertension usually follow. It is mandatory in the early months to ensure that the leg is well supported with properly fitted, good-quality graduated compression, otherwise the patient is likely to develop a venous leg ulcer.

Methods of prevention

Venous thromboembolism is still a common complication of surgery, despite the widespread use of prophylaxis. Fatal pulmonary embolism still occurs in 0.1% of patients. In assessing a patient's requirement for prophylaxis, risk factors should be identified, such as:

- acute trauma
- serious, acute medical illness
- neoplasia
- over 40 years
- a history of venous thromboembolism
- thrombophilia
- for major surgery (especially for cancer)
- immobility
- obesity
- parity (>4).

On the basis of these, high-, moderate- and low-risk patients may be identified. High-risk patients include those with major trauma or facing major surgery, particularly of pelvis, lower abdomen, hip or lower limb; patients with cancer; patients with lower limb paralysis; patients with severe peripheral vascular disease or facing amputation. Moderate-risk patients will be undergoing major surgery and have in addition two other risk factors. Low-risk patients will be those scheduled for minor surgery, without any risk factors being identified.

Methods of prophylaxis

Subcutaneous heparin

This is the most effective method in a dose of 5000 units subcutaneously, twice daily. Dosage, however, has been adjusted in neurosurgical and orthopaedic practice. The injections may give rise to bruising and discomfort at injection sites, particularly if the injection technique is poor. Occasionally thrombocytopenia has been seen.

Low molecular weight heparin

This only requires a once-a-day injection and may have fewer haemorrhagic complications. It is commonly used in orthopaedic patients but is expensive, even when reduced nursing costs are taken into account.

Warfarin

There is good evidence for the efficacy of warfarin prophylaxis in orthopaedics, but it has largely been superseded by low molecular weight heparin. For longer term maintenance of anticoagulation, warfarin is almost universally used.

Compression hosiery/intermittent pneumatic compression

These may be used in conjunction with drug therapy or on their own. They are frequently used in orthopaedics and urology, but the evidence for their effectiveness in other areas is not so strong.

Dextran 70

This is an effective prophylaxis but involves daily IV infusion and is expensive. Rarely, allergic reactions occur.

LYMPHATIC DISEASE

Lymphoedema – congenital and acquired

Lymphoedema describes the accumulation of protein-rich fluid in the interstitial spaces of the skin and subcutaneous tissues as a result of lymphatic system dysfunction. This condition affects women three times as often as men. As in all aspects of clinical practice, in order to understand the pathophysiology of a condition, it is necessary to be familiar with the anatomy and normal physiology of the system concerned.

Anatomy of the lymphatic system

The lymphatics were first recognised as a discrete system in the 17th century and it is now believed that this system arises from endothelial sprouting of the primordial venous system. These endothelial sprouts invade almost all tissues of the body between the third and eighth weeks of gestation and ultimately form the lymphatic channels and regional nodes of each extremity. The lymphatic channels of the lower limbs drain into the cisterna chyli and those of the upper limbs drain directly into the thoracic duct.

The lymphatic system consists of three components:

● initial (terminal) lymphatics

● collecting ducts

● lymph nodes.

The initial lymphatics are quite similar to capillaries although the basement membrane is either absent or poorly defined, allowing the absorption of lymph from the interstitial space. The lymphatic capillaries progress and enlarge to form the collecting lymphatic ducts which have valves and run alongside the primary blood vessels of the extremity.

Lower extremity lymphatics

This consists of both superficial and deep systems. In the superficial lymphatic system, medial and lateral pathways correspond closely to the superficial venous drainage of the leg. The deep lymphatic system runs parallel to the deep veins. Both the superficial and deep lymphatic systems drain into the inguinal lymph nodes. These lymph nodes consist of a superficial group (around the fossa ovalis) and a deep group (within the femoral sheath).

Both these systems drain into the iliac lymph nodes. Lymph from these nodes ultimately drains via the cisterna chyli and the thoracic duct into the venous circulation.

Upper extremity lymphatics

Similar to the lower limb, the superficial lymphatics consist of medial and lateral groups of vessels which parallel the basilic and cephalic veins respectively. The medial group of superficial lymphatics drain into the axillary lymph nodes, whereas the lateral group drain into the supraclavicular lymph nodes. The deep lymphatic system parallels the brachial vessels and drains into the axillary nodes.

Physiology of the lymphatic system

Proteins and fluid that are lost from the capillary system along with any infectious agents are transported by the lymphatics back into the circulation. However, lymphoedema occurs when the formation of protein-rich interstitial fluid exceeds the lymphatic transport capacity. Interstitial fluid is a plasma ultrafiltrate formed by capillary filtration which is determined by the difference in hydrostatic and colloid osmotic pressures between the intravascular capillary space and the interstitial space. The capillaries allow up to 80% of the intravascular protein to enter the interstitial space which is then absorbed by the initial lymphatics and transported back into the circulation.

The propulsion of lymph proximally occurs because of the effects of adjacent muscle contractions and arterial pulsations on the valve-containing lymphatic system. In addition, the alternating negative then positive intraabdominal and intrathoracic pressures associated with respiration act to pump lymph through the abdominal and thoracic cavities.

Pathophysiology of lymphoedema

Lymphoedema is confined to the subcutaneous compartment and the accumulation of protein-rich lymphatic fluid occurs when fluid formation exceeds lymphatic transport capacity. Normal lymphatics have a significant capacity to increase their flow rate by up to a factor of 10. Therefore an increase in the rate of interstitial fluid formation by itself does not produce lymphoedema. The accumulation of protein-rich fluid is a direct result of lymphatic system dysfunction.

Early in the natural history of lymphoedema, the accumulation of protein-rich interstitial fluid results only in a soft pitting oedema. However, with the passage of time, low oxygen tension, decreased macrophage function and the presence of increasing amounts of protein-rich fluid give rise to a chronic inflammatory state and consequent fibrosis. Such an environment is ideal for bacterial proliferation and recurrent episodes of lymphangitis are a common complication in up to 25% of lymphoedema patients.

Recurrent episodes of lymphangitis and cellulitis accelerate the rate of subcutaneous fibrosis and further lymphatic obstruction.

Differential diagnosis of lymphoedema

Since the differential diagnosis of lymphoedema is lengthy, many patients who are assumed to have lymphoedema may in fact have oedema due to other causes. These can be classified in the following manner.

Systemic disorders

- Cardiac failure
- Renal failure
- Hepatic failure (cirrhosis)
- Hypoproteinaemia
- Hereditary angio-oedema
- Allergic disorders
- Idiopathic cyclic oedema

Venous disorders

- Postphlebitic syndrome (reflux)
- Iliac venous disease (obstructive)
- Extrinsic pressure, i.e. pregnancy or tumour
- Klippel–Trenaunay syndrome

Miscellaneous disorders

- Arteriovenous malformations (see later section)
- Lipoedema
- Erythrocyanosis frigida
- Disuse oedema

Cardiac and renal failure are very common and usually present in patients as bilateral pitting oedema. Hepatic failure and hypoproteinaemia will become evident with the results of initial biochemistry. If the hypoproteinaemia appears idiopathic, consideration should be given to the possibility of a protein-losing enteropathy or chylous ascites. Hereditary angio-oedema is inherited as an autosomal dominant condition and is thought to be due to a deficiency of complement regulation. Allergic disorders are usually suggested by the history. Idiopathic cyclical oedema occurs in females and may be assumed to be mild distal lymphoedema. However, lymphoscintigraphy is invariably normal and the patients describe recurrent attacks of facial or extremity swelling that subsequently resolves.

Chronic venous insufficiency remains the most common cause of unilateral oedema. This diagnosis is suspected because of the clinical characteristics of venous eczema and lipodermatosclerosis. Skin ulceration is common in venous disease and extremely rare in lymphoedema. Limb elevation rapidly improves venous oedema whereas lymphoedema resolves more slowly, often requiring days of limb elevation. Venous duplex ultrasound is usually utilised to confirm or establish the diagnosis of chronic venous insufficiency. Venography may be helpful in further characterising the extent of venous disease. It is essential to remember that deep venous thrombosis caused by malignant disease is an important cause of unilateral leg oedema. However, malignant disease can also cause lymphoedema by direct invasion of the lymphatic system.

Lipoedema is due to excess fat deposition in the legs. Often these patients will have generalised gross obesity. Erythrocyanosis frigida occurs in young women. The patients complain of cold peripheries and the skin often has a reddish-blue blotchy appearance. This condition usually affects both lower limbs. Disuse oedema occurs because of immobilisation of a limb and is clearly seen in a patient with long-standing paralysis. However, it can also be seen in patients exhibiting hysterical immobilisation of a limb.

Patients with the Klippel–Trenaunay syndrome (congenital varicose veins, elongation of the limb, capillary naevi ± deep venous system anomalies) may also have lymphoedema due to hypoplasia of their lymphatic system. Patients with arteriovenous malformations may also develop lymphoedema because of hyperplastic lymphatics.

Classification of lymphoedema

Once a preliminary diagnosis of lymphoedema has been made on clinical grounds, it is important to try to identify the cause. Patients with this condition fall into two groups.

- Primary lymphoedema, due to a congenital abnormality intrinsic to the lymphatic system.
- Secondary lymphoedema, due to surgical excision of lymphatic pathways, trauma, malignant disease, infection, inflammation or irradiation.

Primary lymphoedema

This condition can be classified by the age of onset or on the basis of lymphangiographic findings.

CLASSIFICATION BY AGE OF ONSET:
- Congenital lymphoedema, where the oedema is present at birth
- Lymphoedema praecox, which presents during adolescence
- Lymphoedema tarda, which presents after the age of 35

Congenital lymphoedema accounts for 10–15% of cases and may be associated with other diseases of the lymphatic system, i.e. cystic hygroma or lymphangiectasia. Lymphoedema praecox accounts for 80% of cases and probably represents another form of congenital lymphoedema with a later onset of symptoms (Figures 41.11, 41.12). Lymphoedema tarda represents 10–15% of cases. It remains unclear, however, why patients should develop symptoms at this later stage of their lives. It is also interesting to note that we cannot explain why women are affected three times more often than men or why the left leg is more commonly affected or why the upper extremities are seldom involved.

CLASSIFICATION BY LYMPHANGIOGRAPHIC APPEARANCE

Although classification by age is helpful in giving a further understanding about the epidemiology of lymphoedema, classification on the basis of lymphangiographic findings provides an accurate

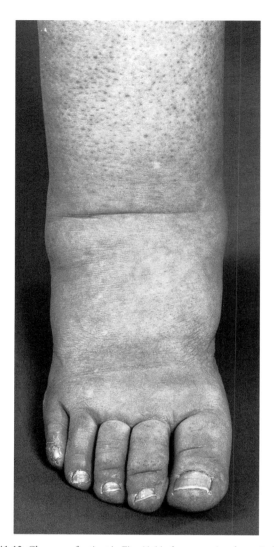

Figure 41.12 Close-up of patient in Fig. 41.11, demonstrating the typical appearance of the oedematous toes and ankles.

description of the anatomical abnormality in terms of obliterative (hypoplastic) or hyperplastic lymphatic disease.

Primary obliterative (hypoplastic) lymphoedema:

- those with distal obliteration
- those with pelvic obliteration
- those with proximal and distal obliteration (a+b).

Primary hyperplastic lymphoedema:

- bilateral hyperplasia
- megalymphatics.

In patients with primary obliterative lymphoedema of the distal variety, lymphangiography will show that the limb lymphatics are few and appear narrow or obliterated. In patients with pelvic obstruction, lymphangiography reveals few lymph vessels or nodes in the groin and pelvic region. However, these patients will

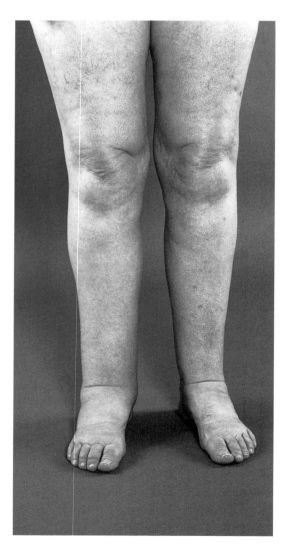

Figure 41.11 Illustration of lymphoedema praecox. The right leg is more significantly affected than the left.

often exhibit numerous and distended lymph vessels distal to the area of hypoplasia. Patients with proximal and distal obliteration will show lymph vessels that are small and few in number.

The importance of the above classification system is that there are significant differences in the clinical features of those patients in the different subgroups. Patients with distal obliterative disease usually suffer from a relatively mild form of lymphoedema. Most of these patients are women, both legs are often affected and this is a common form of the disease. However, those patients with pelvic obstruction often suffer from progressive swelling, usually involving one leg but which may also involve the genitalia. This form of the disease occurs equally in males and females.

About 8% of patients with primary lymphoedema have the hyperplastic form. This may take the form of bilateral hyperplasia or megalymphatics. Patients with hyperplasia are believed to have an obstructive process at the level of the cisterna chyli or the thoracic duct. Valves are present and the lymphatics are not grossly varicose, features which distinguish these patients from those with megalymphatics who have large, valveless, dilated lymphatics.

Secondary lymphoedema

Worldwide, secondary lymphoedema is a much more common condition than primary lymphoedema. It is usually due to infection or inflammation affecting the lymphatics and typically affects patient populations where hygiene levels are poor. In tropical countries the parasite *Wuchereria bancrofti* is often endemic and is recognised as an important cause of lymphoedema. The adult form of this parasite lodges in lymphatics and lymph nodes, causing lymphatic obstruction. There are, however, other non-filarial causes of secondary lymphoedema.

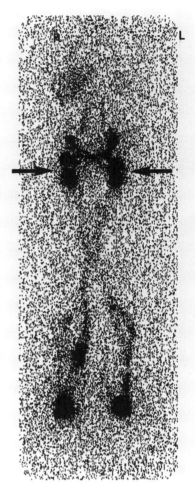

Figure 41.13 Illustration of a normal lymphoscintigram.

Diagnosis of lymphoedema

The diagnosis of lymphoedema can usually be made on the basis of the history and clinical examination. However, if the diagnosis is in doubt then lymphoscintigraphy is indicated. Lymphoscintigraphy is a radionuclide study utilising ^{99}Tc-labelled sulphur colloid and it assesses lymphatic function by quantitating the rate of lymphatic isotope clearance. The major advantage of radionuclide scanning is that it provides functional as well as anatomical information about the patient's lymphatic system and is a relatively simple technique that can be easily repeated (Figures 41.13, 41.14). Lymphoscintigraphy is performed by measuring the amount of radioactivity at the inguinal nodes at 30 minutes and one hour after bipedal subcutaneous isotope injection. The normal range of inguinal node uptake is 0.6–1.6%. Uptake values below 0.3% are considered abnormal and many patients with distal hypoplastic disease demonstrate uptake values of less than 0.1%.

An alternative investigation is lymphangiography. This is performed by injecting a blue dye into the first digital web space bilaterally. Massage promotes dye dispersion and uptake into the subcutaneous lymphatics which are then directly canalised, allowing injection of radio-opaque dye. This provides good anatomical information about the type and extent of the lymphatic vessel disease. It is important to note, however, that lymphangiography may damage remaining lymphatics and exacerbate the patient's symptoms. Other complications of this procedure include skin staining, wound infection, allergic reaction and pulmonary embolisation. For these reasons lymphangiography should not be performed routinely in patients suffering from lymphoedema. However, if a lymph drainage operation is being considered then lymphangiography would be an essential preoperative investigation.

Treatment of lymphoedema

Lymphatic system dysfunction leads to the interstitial accumulation of protein-rich fluid with subsequent inflammation and fibrosis of the subcutaneous tissue. Therefore to effect a cure, lymphatic drainage must be restored to effectively remove the

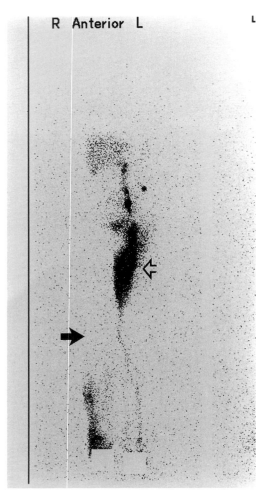

R Anterior L   L

Figure 41.14 Illustration of an abnormal lymphoscintigram demonstrating distal obliteration of the lymphatics in the right leg and the presence of megalymphatics in the left thigh.

protein-rich fluid prior to the development of significant subcutaneous fibrosis. Unfortunately, it is impossible to achieve this for the vast majority of patients and therefore the treatment, whether it be medical or surgical, remains palliative. It has been shown that 60% of patients with primary lymphoedema do not have any significant progression of their oedema following the initial year of symptoms. However, the remaining 40% of patients have an inexorable increase in the girth of the affected limb. Only 16% of these patients underwent limb-reducing surgery.

Medical treatment

Medical treatment which is applicable to the vast majority of patients is aimed at avoiding infection, reducing interstitial fluid volume and treating skin complications.

Cellulitis and lymphangitis episodes can be reduced with good hygiene practice by the patient, including the regular use of mild antiseptic soap. Careful drying between the oedematous toes and the regular use of antifungal agents is very important in reducing the risk of fungal infections. The regular application of hand cream to the skin of a swollen lymphoedematous leg is important to prevent the skin becoming hard and cracked. When infections occur, they must be treated immediately and aggressively. This should include bedrest with elevation of the affected leg and administration of systemic antibiotics.

Reducing interstitial fluid volume is achieved by external compression using elastic support stockings. This is most effectively achieved if the elastic support stocking is fitted after the oedema has been reduced by elevation and/or use of pneumatic sequential compression therapy. Below-knee stockings are often adequate as long as they exert a pressure of 30 mmHg. However, full-length thigh stockings and one-legged tights are also available to control thigh oedema. Elastic support stockings require replacement regularly every 3–6 months. Since the elastic support stockings are removed at night, the foot of the bed should be raised to assist fluid drainage from the legs.

Intermittent sequential compression therapy using a pump (e.g. Centromed®) can be very helpful in controlling daily swelling due to lymphoedema. The pump can be applied up to three times per day. Some patients are able to sleep while undergoing sequential compression therapy at night. Unfortunately, however, compression therapy whether by elastic stocking or pneumatic pump only reduces the water content of the interstitial space. This therapy does not remove protein and therefore fluid reaccumulation is inevitable. Some studies have suggested that the benzopyrones can reduce the concentration of interstitial protein but they have not gained wide acceptance in clinical practice.

Skin complications including hyperkeratosis, vesicles and eczema are quite common in the affected limbs of patients with lymphoedema. These problems usually respond to dressings and bedrest. Eczema may require a course of hydrocortisone cream.

Surgical treatment

The vast majority of patients with lymphoedema can be satisfactorily managed by optimal medical therapy. However, if this is ineffective and the patient is suffering functional impairment caused by the size of their involved extremity, then surgical treatment should be considered. About 15% of patients with lymphoedema may benefit from surgery. The types of operations can be divided into two groups:

● palliative excisional procedures

● lymph drainage operations.

Whatever type of surgery is performed, it is essential that the patient does not have unrealistic expectations about the end results which are palliative rather than curative. To obtain the best surgical result, the skin must not be infected and any cellulitis or lymphangitis should be treated with systemic antibiotics prior to surgery. Similarly, limb oedema should be reduced as much as possible by conservative measures prior to surgery.

PALLIATIVE EXCISIONAL PROCEDURES

In Homan's operation, a medial incision is made in the leg about 2 cm posterior to the tibial border and extended proximally into the thigh. Skin flaps about 1.5 cm in thickness are elevated to reach the mid-line anteriorly and posteriorly. All subcutaneous tissue below the flaps is excised. Incision of the deep fascia allows the development of a good plane of dissection. Redundant skin is excised and the skin flaps are closed over a suction drain. The limb is elevated and the patient kept immobilised for about eight days. Areas of the skin flaps may become ischaemic. Partial-thickness skin loss can be treated conservatively, but areas of full-thickness loss will require excision and subsequent split-thickness skin grafting. A similar procedure can then be performed on the lateral aspect of the leg, 2–3 months later.

In Thompson's operation, skin flaps are developed in a similar fashion to Homan's operation. However, the posterior flap edge is deepithelialised and buried by suturing it down between the gastrocnemius-soleus group of muscles and the deep flexors. Theoretically, this action might permit the formation of lymphatic connections between the subdermal lymphatics of the flap and the deep lymphatics of the muscle compartment. However, postoperative lymphangiography has failed to demonstrate any lymphatic anastomoses. Nevertheless, this operation is associated with satisfactory results in over 50% of cases.

In Charles' operation, the skin is excised along with the oedematous subcutaneous tissue and deep fascia. Split-skin grafts taken from the abdomen and thighs are used for tissue cover. Unfortunately, however, these skin grafts are prone to breakdown and eczema. Therefore the Charles operation is best utilised for patients with severe skin changes.

LYMPH DRAINAGE OPERATIONS

These 'physiological' operations include lymphonodal-venous shunt, lymphovenous shunt and pedicle flaps utilising skin, omentum or small bowel. These sorts of microsurgical reconstruction are most likely to benefit patients with secondary lymphoedema.

Iatrogenic lymph fistula

Lymph fistulas may occur following groin surgery, particularly if there has been previous groin surgery and the dissection required is extensive. Most lymph fistulas will close spontaneously, but this can take 6–8 weeks. However, if large amounts of lymph continue to drain, it may be necessary to explore the fistula tract and ligate the damaged lymphatic.

Arm lymphoedema

This can occur after radical axillary dissection for breast carcinoma. Usually it can be adequately managed by an upper limb compression stocking. Surgery in the form of a modified Homan's operation may be required in severe cases.

Lymphatic system tumours

Lymphangioma

These tumours are benign, the most common example being the cystic hygroma. These lesions appear as a cystic non-tender lesion that transilluminates. They are most commonly found in the head and neck region, but can be found in almost any part of the body. They are usually detected by the end of the first year of life. Surgical excision is the appropriate therapy.

Lymphangiosarcoma

This highly malignant tumour is usually associated with longstanding lymphoedema following mastectomy or filariasis infestation. Treatment has traditionally consisted of radical amputation. Multimodality therapy with radiotherapy and chemotherapy in addition to surgery may offer the prospect of improved prognosis.

CONGENITAL ARTERIOVENOUS MALFORMATIONS

Congenital vascular malformations can involve all elements of the circulation including arteries, capillaries, veins and lymphatics. However, it is only those that have arterial and venous components that may produce significant clinical manifestations. Congenital arteriovenous malformations (AVM) account for about one-third of all congenital vascular malformations.

AVMs become clinically important when they shunt a significant amount of blood directly from artery to vein, bypassing the capillary network. This can result in the following problems:

- tendency to enlarge with time
- development of chronic venous hypertension
- distal extremity ischaemia secondary to steal phenomenon
- cardiac failure due to increased cardiovascular demand.

The vast majority of AVMs occur in the extremities, pelvis, shoulder girdle and body shell of the trunk. However, since AVMs are rare, most surgeons will not have a significant personal experience.

Classification of congenital vascular malformations

There is no universally accepted classification system for the wide spectrum of clinical presentations, from asymptomatic birthmarks to functionally impaired extremities. However, this author finds the classification based on the embryological development of the vascular system as described by Szilagyi helpful.

- Cavernous or simple haemangioma
- Microfistulous AV communications
- Macrofistulous AV communications
- Anomalous development of mature vascular channels

Cavernous or simple haemangioma

These lesions consist of a mass of disorganised capillaries. They are usually identified at birth and grow as the child gets older. Some of these lesions will demonstrate gradual involution. Patients with the Klippel–Trenaunay syndrome have capillary malformations.

Microfistulous AV communications

Histologically, these lesions consist of numerous interconnections between arteries and veins which are too small to be seen at angiography. However, the presence of secondary angiographic findings such as early venous filling and proximal artery dilatation may indicate the presence of significant arteriovenous shunting.

Macrofistulous AV communications

These lesions contain much larger interconnections between arteries and veins and are thus visible on angiography and to the naked eye. If these lesions are superficial in position, they will be palpable and characteristically warm and will have a bruit or thrill because of very high AV shunt flow.

Anomalous development of mature vascular channels

This consists of lesions containing mature but aberrant vessels. An example would be a persistent sciatic artery.

Clinical features

Patients with congenital vascular malformations can present in many different ways. The severity of the lesion is inversely proportional to the age of the patient. Younger patients (i.e. children) tend to present with huge 'birthmarks' or limb enlargements or very obvious vascular lesions. Adults, however, usually present with more subtle signs such as:

- aching/heavy sensation in the involved extremity
- swelling (chronic venous insufficiency) of the involved extremity
- limb length discrepancy
- development of varicose veins.

The most common clinical finding in patients with AVMs is the presence of birthmarks. It should be appreciated that birthmarks are potential indicators of more significant occult AVMs. Venous varicosities are also a common finding. Oedema and asymmetric limb length are much less common. In summary, therefore, patients with birthmarks, early-onset varicose veins and limb asymmetry, either singly or in combination, warrant further clinical follow-up over time.

Methods of diagnosis

With the advent of non-invasive vascular studies along with new non-invasive imaging, much information about the patient's AVM can be obtained, obviating the need for angiography unless intervention is planned. Apart from the potential for morbidity associated with angiography, this investigation does not always provide definitive information about:

- anatomical extent
- microfistulous communications
- characterisation of venous, capillary or lymphatic abnormalities.

Non-invasive vascular tests

Segmental limb pressures

Segmental limb pressures may be helpful in localising arteriovenous fistulas (AVFs). Proximal to a fistula, systolic pressure is often increased. However, distal to a fistula, systolic pressure is usually normal but can be decreased secondary to a 'steal' effect. Therefore segmental limb pressures can help locate AVFs by demonstrating a reduction in systolic pressure from above the fistula to below it.

Pulse volume recordings

This test measures the change in limb volume that occurs with pulsatile arterial blood flow using pneumatic cuffs placed around the extremity at multiple levels. Limb volume changes will be increased proximal to a haemodynamically significant AVF because of reduced vascular resistance.

Doppler velocity waveforms

This investigation measures blood velocity. In a normal extremity, the velocity pattern is triphasic, with major forward flow in early systole, some flow reversal in later systole, minor forward flow in early diastole and negligible forward flow in late diastole. This results in the Doppler waveform lying close to the zero baseline. However, the presence of a significant AVF flow eliminates any end-systolic flow reversal and produces significant flow throughout diastole so that the Doppler waveform proximal to the fistula never drops to near the baseline.

The three forms of non-invasive vascular tests described above are ideal for screening children who have birthmarks, early-onset varicose veins or unilateral limb enlargement. Unfortunately, they are not useful in detecting AVFs proximal to the upper cuff (i.e. the groin or axilla).

Labelled microspheres

This is a radionuclide technique that allows quantification of AV shunting in an extremity. A bolus of technetium-99 labelled human albumin microspheres is injected intra-arterially proximal to an AVF and a gamma camera is used to measure the amount of radioactivity that subsequently arrives at the lungs. Less than 3% of 25–35 micron microspheres will pass through a normal extremity capillary bed. This technique is useful in distinguishing shunting from non-shunting CVMs (i.e. a microfistulous AVM from a purely venous anomaly) and is also of prognostic significance. For example, a value of 8% AV shunting is likely to be associated with only mild future symptomatology. However, a lesion with an AV shunt value of 35% is likely to require significant interventions in the future.

Non-invasive imaging

Successful surgical resection is dependent on the AVM location and its degree of involvement of important surrounding structures. Computed tomography (CT) and magnetic resonance imaging (MRI) both help to define the anatomical relationship of the AVM with the surrounding structures. However, MRI is better than CT for AVM evaluation for several reasons. MRI needs no contrast and it differentiates between muscle, fat, bone and blood and is therefore able to clearly define the tissue involvement (Figure 41.15). This degree of differentiation can be difficult if one is using CT. MRI can distinguish between high- and low-flow lesions which is essential in trying to determine the likelihood of significant haemodynamic or functional impairment in the future. In fact, because MRI accurately assesses both anatomic relationships and flow characteristics, it is more useful

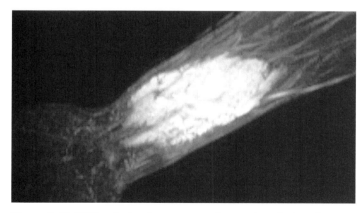

Figure 41.15 MRI study showing a cavernous haemangioma in the volar aspect of the forearm.

than any other single test in the management of AVM. The current development of MR angiography will probably increase the value of this form of imaging in the management of this condition.

Diagnostic and management approach

Having established the existence of a congenital vascular malformations (CVMs) and categorised its nature, it is important to determine its anatomical extent and the degree of involvement of adjacent structures. However, the most important factor to determine is what the local, regional and systemic haemodynamic effects of the lesion are. The answers to this question will allow the vascular surgeon to determine the need for intervention. Intervention is indicated for those lesions which demonstrate significantly increased vascularity and arteriovenous shunting and are causing significant functional impairment. In the absence of significant shunting, most CVMs can be successfully managed conservatively. However, there will be lesions that demonstrate significant high-flow characteristics which because of their anatomical involvement may preclude resection. In these cases, carefully timed palliative interventions may be appropriate. Therefore the absolute indications for intervention are:

- arterial 'steal' producing ischaemia
- non-healing ulceration secondary to venous hypertension
- haemorrhage
- congestive cardiac failure.

The relative indications for intervention are:

- lifestyle-limiting claudication
- persistent severe pain
- functional impairment of an extremity
- major cosmetic deformity.

Limb length discrepancy alone is not an indication for intervention since appropriately timed epiphyseal closure can produce highly satisfactory results.

The most frequently chosen management option is conservative, using support stockings and extremity elevation to control venous hypertension. The alternative interventional options consist of embolisation (Figure 41.16) or surgical resection or a combination of both. Many of these interventions are palliative rather than curative as AVMs have a propensity to recur.

Embolisation is usually performed under general anaesthesia to control pain and improve procedure tolerance, especially amongst children. Multiple embolisation procedures are required for large malformations to reduce contrast volume and excessive tissue necrosis. Agents used for embolisation include Ivalon (polyvinyl alcohol) particles, absolute alcohol and cyanoacrylate adhesive. If a combined embolisation and surgical resection strategy is decided

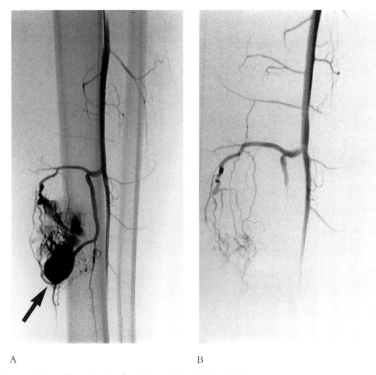

A   B

Figure 41.16 Angiograms demonstrating an AV malformation before (**A**) and after (**B**) embolisation.

upon, there should be no significant delay between the procedures so as to prevent oedema and vasculature recruitment impeding surgical resection. Following embolisation patients typically develop a fever and leucocytosis and complain of significant pain. The major complications of embolisation include extensive tissue necrosis and inadvertent embolisation of normal vasculature. Although the best embolic agent remains a matter for debate, the overall results from published series seem similar with most patients obtaining significant benefit.

Acknowledgements

The authors would like to thank J.E. Barry, J.J. Dale, C.V. Ruckley and colleagues from the Departments of Nuclear Medicine and Interventional Radiology at Aberdeen Royal Infirmary for their help in the preparation of this chapter.

FURTHER READING

Baulieu F, Vaillant L, Baulieu JL et al. The current role of lymphoscintigraphy in the study of lymphedema of the limbs. *J Mal Vasc* 1990; **15**:152–156

Callum MJ. Epidemiology of varicose veins. *Br J Surg* 1994; **81**:167–173

Callam MJ, Harper DR, Dale JJ et al. Lothian and Forth Valley Leg Ulcer Healing Trial, Part 1: Elastic versus non-elastic bandaging in the treatment of chronic leg ulceration. *Phlebology* 1992; **7**:136–141

Ruckley CV, Fowkes FGR, Bradbury AW, eds. *Venous Disease: Epidemiology, Management and Delivery of Care.* London: Springer, 1999

Saharay M, Sheilds DA, Porter JB, Scurr JH, Coleridge Smith PD. Leukocyte activity in the microcirculation of the leg in patients with chronic venous disease. *J Vasc Surg* 1997; **26**:265–23

Szilagyi DE, Smith RF, Elliott JP, Hageman JH. Congenital arteriovenous anomalies of the limbs. *Arch Surg* 1976; **111**:423–429

Wildus DM, Murray RR, White RI et al. Congenital arteriovenous malformations: tailored embolotherapy. *Radiology* 1988; **169**:511–516

42

Vasculitis

Linda Hands

NORMAL VESSEL HISTOLOGY

The standard structure of an artery or vein consists of three layers separated by two membranes (Figure 42.1). The vasa vasorum lie within the adventitia of larger vessels. The relative thickness of each layer depends on whether the vessel is part of the arterial or venous side of the circulation and whether it is a large, medium or small vessel. Large arteries (the aorta, carotids, iliacs and the like) are distinguished not only by vessel size but also by the large amount of elastic tissue in the media. Medium-sized arteries (most of the rest) have a media consisting mainly of smooth muscle.

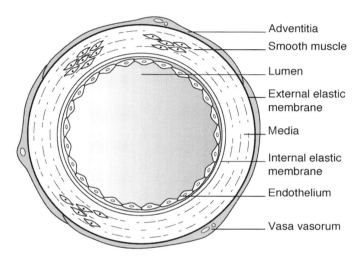

Figure 42.1 Basic structure of arteries and veins.

TYPES OF VASCULITIS

Inflammation of the arterial wall may be found as a secondary feature of a well-described 'systemic' disease such as rheumatoid arthritis, syphilis or malignancy or it may be the predominant feature of a series of much less well-characterised 'vasculitic syndromes'. Attempts have been made to define this latter group on the basis of:

- sites affected
- pattern of inflammation within the vessel wall
- associated immune response.

Vasculitis associated with systemic disease

Rheumatoid arthritis

It is usually confined to small arteries in synovial membranes. In advanced disease there may be widespread involvement of:

- small arteries in the skin (ulceration, gangrenous patches or poor healing)

- peripheral nerves (mononeuritis multiplex), CNS (focal deficits), heart (myocardial infarction) and bowel (perforation/infarction)
- aorta – granulomatous change, rarely symptomatic.

Systemic lupus erythematosus

This affects medium/small arteries in lung, brain, heart and gut (occasionally leading to infarction, perforation or gastrointestinal bleeding).

In the aorta there is granulomatous change and it is rarely symptomatic.

Scleroderma

- Affects small arteries in the skin – fibrosis of intima and media (ulceration of tips of toes and fingers).
- Often associated with Raynaud's phenomenon (see later).
- Intimal fibrosis in pulmonary arteries leading to pulmonary hypertension.
- Rarely fibrosis of other arteries causing peripheral ischaemia.
- Extensive fibrosis in many organs may be linked to vasculitis but this is unproven.

Syphilis

(Any stage but most marked in tertiary stage.)

- Perivascular invasion of inflammatory cells affecting small vessels in the skin, meninges and many other sites.
- Involvement of the vasa vasorum is followed by fibrosis of adventitia and media in large arteries (may lead to aneurysmal dilatation of ascending aorta).

Tuberculosis

Tuberculosis occasionally affects the aorta through haematogenous spread to the vasa vasorum or direct spread from lung or nodes (may cause an aortoduodenal fistula).

Malignancy

Vasculitis occurs in cryoglobulinaemia sometimes associated with multiple myeloma and B cell lymphoma (as well as some non-malignant conditions).

Vasculitic syndromes of surgical interest

Although most of these conditions involve true vasculitis there are three (fibromuscular dysplasia, frostbite, trenchfoot) which fall outside this category but are nevertheless included because they present in a similar fashion and are not described elsewhere.

Polyarteritis nodosa

This affects mainly small arteries, in a multitude of possible sites (Box 42.1). Patients present with vague symptoms of fever, malaise, weight loss, arthralgia and myalgia so that infection, malignancy and connective tissue disorder compete with vasculitis in making the diagnosis. The ESR is usually >20 mm/h, other acute-phase reactants are elevated, albumin is low and renal function may be impaired but unfortunately none of these features is specific to vasculitis. The definitive diagnosis can only be made with a positive biopsy from clinically involved tissue.

Abdominal symptoms usually arise in patients with widespread evidence of the disease elsewhere. Fever, colicky abdominal pain and distension gradually develop over a few days, occasionally longer, and are accompanied by anorexia, nausea and vomiting. Examination reveals diffuse tenderness with rebound in the later stages. Abdominal radiographs may show small bowel distension and fluid levels, occasionally gas in bowel wall, 'thumbprinting' of the mucosa or free gas, as in any case of acute bowel ischaemia. Relatively mild symptoms may respond to increased doses of steroids ± cyclophosphamide but vigilance is essential because symptoms and signs of progressive bowel ischaemia may be masked by steroid treatment. Gas in bowel wall or free in the peritoneal cavity on radiographs or deteriorating clinical status despite aggressive medical treatment are indications for laparotomy. At operation there may be frank perforation or patchy necrosis of large or small bowel. Occasionally peritonitis without bowel involvement is found. The prognosis is poor: surgery improves survival rates slightly but most patients die.

Box 42.1   Polyarteritis nodosa

Incidence	Rare, 2–3/million/year
Course	Remissions and relapses over months/years
m:f	2:1
Age	Mean 45 years (10–80)
Cause	?Response to an infective agent (30% are associated with hepatitis B antigenaemia) ?Response to a drug or toxin
Arteries affected	Small/medium
Sites	Skeletal muscle/kidneys/peripheral nerves/liver/gut/skin/heart
Pattern of inflammation	Acute transmural fibrinoid necrosis associated with microaneurysms (which may be visible on angiography) or thrombosis Healing with fibrosis Lesions are segmental and adjacent lesions may be at different stages
Presentation	Fever, malaise, weight loss, arthralgia, myalgia Skin lesions Renal failure Acute abdomen due to bowel perforation occurs in up to a third of patients
Treatment	Steroids alone in relatively mild cases; cyclophosphamide or azathioprine may be added if the disease is more severe Laparotomy for the deteriorating acute abdomen

---

Giant cell arteritis (temporal arteritis)

Surgeons are often enlisted to help with the diagnosis in an elderly patient who presents with headache, scalp tenderness, jaw claudication or visual disturbance and who requires a temporal artery biopsy to confirm or exclude the diagnosis of giant cell arteritis (GCA) (Box 42.2). The same disease is occasionally encountered in elderly patients with arm ischaemia in whom an angiogram shows a subclavian lesion which is atypical for the presumed diagnosis of atherosclerosis.

Patients presenting with upper limb claudication or digital ischaemia in whom the angiogram reveals localised subclavian disease which lies beyond the origin of the vessel and which is smooth rather than irregular, in contrast to atherosclerosis, should have an ESR checked. A further differential diagnosis is

---

Box 42.2   Giant cell arteritis

Incidence	Highest in those of northern European stock where it reaches 17/100 000/year
Course	Acute onset with maximum symptoms within 1 month
m:f	1:2–3
Age	>50 years
Cause	?Immune response directed at elastin
Arteries affected	Medium-large
Sites	Temporal and other extracranial head arteries Branches of ophthalmic artery (central retinal and ciliary) Occasionally other branches of the internal carotid artery and the vertebral arteries In at least 15% it also involves the subclavian arteries (in particular), aorta/lower limb arteries/coronary arteries/visceral arteries (Figure 42.2)
Pattern of inflammation	Macrophage and lymphocyte invasion – most marked in media in 50% cases – associated giant cells Necrosis and disruption of internal elastic lamina Intimal proliferation leading to thrombosis
Presentation	Headache, fatigue, anorexia, fever Sudden onset of partial or complete visual field loss, initially uniocular but may subsequently affect both eyes and may be permanent Erythema and tenderness over affected arteries (especially temporal) Diplopia, jaw claudication Polymyalgia (proximal myalgia and joint stiffness) Dissecting and fusiform or saccular aneurysms of the aorta (particularly thoracic) Raynaud's phenomenon when limb arteries affected ESR >60 mm/h
Angiographic appearance	Smooth tapering segmental stenosis or tapered occlusion with normal or dilated intervening vessel
Diagnosis	Biopsy of temporal or other affected arteries (need at least 2–3 cm because of skip nature of lesions)
Treatment	Steroids, initially in high dose but tailed off over 2–5 years

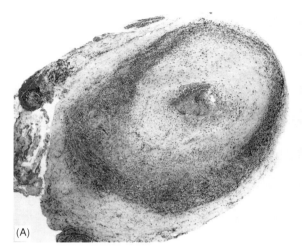

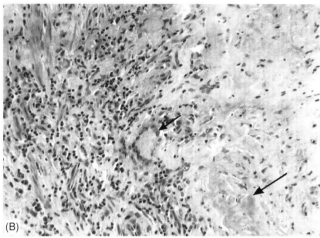

Figure 42.2 A. Histology of temporal artery biopsy in giant cell arteritis (×40) showing large numbers of mononuclear inflammatory cells throughout the wall but mostly in the media, intimal thickening and thrombosis of the lumen. Adjacent small branches are also involved. **B**. Histology of temporal artery biopsy in giant cell arteritis (×200) showing lymphoid cells, histiocytes and giant cells (small arrow) at the internal elastic lamina (large arrow). Courtesy of Dr D. Roskell, Nuffield Dept of Pathology, John Radcliffe Hospital, Oxford.

irradiation arteritis, especially following breast carcinoma, but this should be evident in the history. Where vasculitis seems likely and the ESR is >20 mm/h, a course of steroids may resolve arm claudication. If more severe symptoms are associated with vessel occlusion rather than stenosis, then bypass surgery may be indicated. The discontinuous nature of the vessel changes allows anastomosis to sites not obviously involved but concomitant steroid treatment will slow healing.

Patients with diagnosed and treated giant cell arteritis are 17 times more likely to develop a thoracic aneurysm and 2.4 times more likely to develop an abdominal aortic aneurysm than the general population of the same age. The onset of aneurysmal disease is related to the arteritis rather than steroid treatment. A diagnosis of giant cell arteritis is sometimes made in retrospect after discovery of the aneurysm; in others the aneurysm is noted months or years after diagnosis and treatment. The ascending aorta and aortic arch

are most likely to be affected; aortic incompetence may be the presenting feature. Treatment depends on age and co-morbidity but aortic valve replacement and repair of thoracic and aortic aneurysms in these patients is not associated with a greater mortality than in the general population of a similar age.

Kawasaki's disease

This was first described amongst the Japanese in 1967. It is a systemic vasculitis of children which in most cases resolves with no sequelae (Box 42.3). A few children develop aneurysms, usually during the acute phase, and these are found particularly in the coronary circulation (it is the primary cause of acquired heart disease in childhood in the USA). Ischaemia due to aneurysm thrombosis or spasm associated with the vasculitis can lead to tissue infarction.

Box 42.3	Kawasaki's disease
Incidence	Highest amongst those of Asian origin (Japan 45–195/100 000/year, USA 5–10/100 000/year in children under 5 years)
Course	Acute, self-limiting illness which rarely recurs
m:f	1.5:1
Age	Peak at age 2, 80% cases occur in those aged less than 4 years
Cause	Intense immune response ? to superantigen produced by staphylococci or streptococci (similar to toxic shock syndrome),? to unknown infective agent but increased incidence in Japanese-Americans suggests a genetic predisposition
Arteries affected	Small to medium
Sites	Coronary arteries, aorta and its visceral branches (via the vasa vasorum), subclavian, axillary, brachial and iliac arteries
Pattern of inflammation	Acute inflammation ± aneurysm formation; aneurysms may disappear over time but leave a region of intimal hyperplasia and calcification – a rigid, sometimes narrowed vessel which will not dilate under stress
Presentation	Fever, conjunctival injection, erythema of lips and oropharynx
	Erythema of palms and soles, rash, lymphadenopathy
	Myocarditis, pericardial effusion, myocardial infarction
	Inflammatory changes in lung, brain, kidneys, liver
	Infarction of distal extremities and viscera
	Raised white cell count, anaemia, abnormal lipid profile, raised platelet count in later stages
Treatment	In the acute phase intravenous immunoglobulin and aspirin are the mainstay and surgery plays no part
	Larger aneurysms sometimes fail to regress and are liable to thrombose. A similar risk applies to narrowed, calcified vessels. Long-term anticoagulation may be appropriate
	In the heart, at least, successful revascularisation is possible if necessary, once the acute disease has resolved. Bypass grafting elsewhere is rarely indicated

Behçet's disease

This is a chronic systemic vasculitis which starts in early adulthood and pursues a course of repeated relapses and remissions (Box 42.4). The primary symptoms are of eye inflammation (usually uveitis), oral and genital ulceration but many patients have major arterial or venous involvement. Venous problems arise twice as frequently as arterial problems: recurrent superficial thrombophlebitis occurs in a third, thrombosis of the larger veins, particularly the superior and inferior vena cavae, is not uncommon. Some patients appear to have a defect in thrombolysis which may contribute to the risk of thrombosis. Arterial disease is more likely to be fatal, however. Small arteries are primarily involved and inflammation and thrombosis of vasa vasorum lead to transmural infarction of larger vessels. As a result true saccular aneurysms arise in the weakened wall or the vessel ruptures and a false aneurysm develops. Apparently normal arteries are liable to produce false aneurysms at puncture sites and at anastomosis sites following vascular reconstruction. It is important to avoid arterial puncture in these patients if at all possible: duplex scanning, intravenous digital subtraction angiography, CT or MRI scanning should replace intraarterial angiography whenever feasible.

The diagnosis of Behçet's disease may not have been made prior to presentation with vascular complications. Any apparently spontaneous aneurysm in a patient under the age of 50 years must raise the question of Behçet's disease, the alternative causes being unrecognised trauma or infection.

Box 42.4	Behçet's disease
Incidence	Commonest in those of eastern Mediterranean and Japanese origin (7–8/100 000 in Japan, 2/100 000 in Western Europe) Increasingly diagnosed in USA and UK
Course	Chronic with repeated relapses
m:f	2:1
Age	Peak incidence at 20–30 years, rare under school age
Cause	?Inherited predisposition but otherwise unknown
Vessels affected	Small arteries primarily, large vessel disease via vasa vasorum
Sites	Superficial veins including long saphenous, SVC, IVC, femoral, subclavian, common iliac and hepatic veins, aorta and its major branches, common, superficial and deep femoral arteries (Figure 42.3)
Pattern of inflammation	Vasculitis of vasa vasorum and other small vessels, with mononuclear cell infiltration and fragmentation of elastic fibres in the media
Presentation	Eye inflammation (usually uveitis), oral and genital ulceration 60% have arthritis 30% have GI involvement 15–20% have neurological problems 33% have superficial thrombophlebitis Large vein thrombosis (including Budd–Chiari syndrome from hepatic vein occlusion) 2–3% have true or false aneurysms of larger arteries (Figure 42.4) Occasional myocarditis and pericarditis
Treatment	Steroids ± immunosuppression are the mainstay of treatment with the dose(s) tailored to disease activity measured by clinical and haematological parameters Thrombolysis may be considered for major venous thrombosis but has to be accompanied by increased immunosuppression if it is to have any lasting effect Surgery – most aneurysms develop during an active phase of the disease and can expand rapidly. Those in aorta, whether false or saccular, will need replacement with a synthetic graft. The risks are high: further aneurysms can develop at each anastomosis site and graft infection is a distinct possibility because of immunosuppression. When aneurysms develop at a more peripheral site, non-synthetic material should be used and consideration given to primary ligation of the vessel without reconstruction All patients undergoing reconstruction need regular, frequent follow-up by duplex ± CT or MRI to exclude anastomotic or new aneurysms

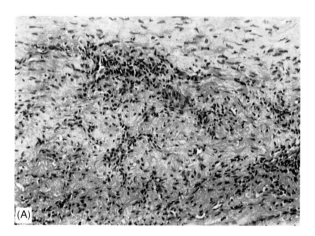

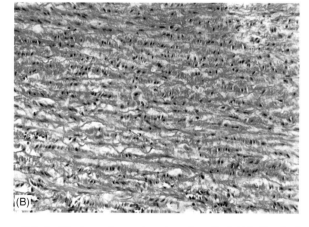

Figure 42.3 A. Histology of normal aortic wall media (×100). **B**. Histology of aortic wall media (×100) in patient with Behçet's disease showing invasion of mononuclear cells. Courtesy of Dr D. Roskell, Nuffield Dept of Pathology, John Radcliffe Hospital, Oxford.

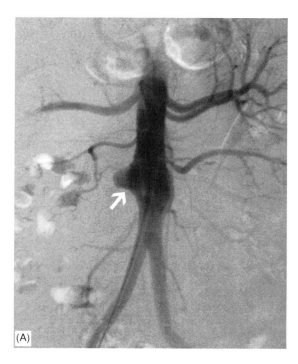

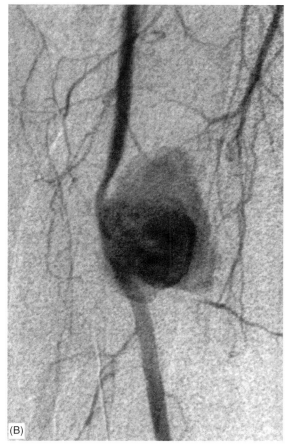

Figure 42.4 A. Angiogram in Behçet's disease showing saccular aneurysm of aorta (arrowed). **B**. Angiogram in Behçet's disease showing aneurysm of superficial femoral artery. Courtesy of Dr J. Phillips-Hughes, Dept of Radiology, John Radcliffe Hospital, Oxford.

Takayasu's disease (Box 42.5)

This is a disease of the aorta, its main branches and the pulmonary arteries. It is found predominantly in young women, often of

Box 42.5	Takayasu's disease
Incidence	2.6/million/year in USA but much higher in Far East
Course	Onset acute or gradual, most cases respond to a course of steroids with sustained remission
m:f	1:>10
Age	Peak onset between 10 and 24 years but may range up to 40 years (American College of Rheumatology criteria)
Cause	Unknown but presumed genetic susceptibility
Arteries affected	Large elastic and some muscular arteries
Sites	Subclavian (approx 90%) (Figure 42.5) Aorta (particularly the arch and the abdominal aorta), carotid, vertebral, coronary, renal and iliac arteries Pulmonary arteries (50%)
Pattern of inflammation	Acute stage – periarteritis spreading to media and intima with granulomata and occasional giant cells (similar to GCA), associated with disruption of elastic fibres Chronic – fibrosis
Presentation	Sometimes acute fever, arthragia, myalgia, malaise, weight loss, raised ESR, anaemia Arm (or leg) claudication or Raynaud's phenomenon Hypertension (>50%) Dizziness, impaired vision due to ischaemic retinopathy CVA due to hypertension or extensive carotid and vertebral disease Aortic regurgitation Aortic aneurysm
Treatment	Steroids in acute phase, cytotoxic agents (e.g. cyclophosphamide) if poor response Balloon dilatation – stenosis due to acute vasculitis may resolve with drug treatment but in the later stage of the disease, when acute inflammation (and inflammatory markers) has settled down, a fibrotic stricture may develop and persist. Balloon dilatation should be considered if there are significant associated symptoms. It can be successful in at least the short to medium term and does not seem to be associated with an increased risk of vessel rupture although occasionally aneurysmal dilatation at the dilatation site has been observed
Treatment	Surgery may be considered when balloon angioplasty fails or is imposssible. Endarterectomy is not an option because the disease affects the full thickness of arterial wall but bypass grafting is possible. Aortic aneurysms due to Takayasu's disease rarely rupture and repair is not usually necessary unless the aortic valve becomes incompetent as a result of a dilatating ascending aorta. Aortic replacement and bypass grafts work well when necessary and there is no evidence of an increased tendency to graft thrombosis or false aneurysms at anastomoses

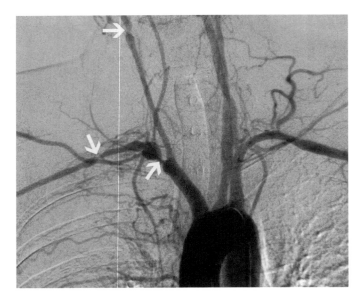

Figure 42.5 Angiogram in Takayasu's disease showing stenoses of R subclavian and carotid arteries (arrowed). Courtesy of Dr J. Phillips-Hughes, Dept of Radiology, John Radcliffe Hospital, Oxford.

Asian origin. Its onset may be marked by an acute febrile illness, with muscle and joint pain and general malaise, or it may be more insidious with symptoms arising due to large vessel complications. Recognition and treatment in the early stages protect against later, possibly life-threatening complications. Fifteen-year survival with treatment is about 80%; death when it does occur is usually due to congestive cardiac failure or stroke. Arterial involvement leads to stenosis and thrombosis and, in about 20%, aneurysmal dilatation of the aorta, usually in the chest.

Buerger's disease (thromboangiitis obliterans)

This is predominantly a disease of young cigarette-smoking men (Box 42.6). It affects the medium-sized muscular arteries of the calf and, less commonly, the palmar and digital vessels of the upper limb but it rarely involves visceral arteries. It does not confine itself to arteries but frequently presents as a migratory superficial thrombophlebitis in the same limb. If the patient continues to smoke he faces amputation of several limbs: if he stops smoking the disease almost always comes to a halt. It should always be considered as a possible diagnosis in a young man presenting with distal arterial disease, especially if there is also upper limb involvement.

Revascularisation of the lower limb is often imposssible because no distal vessel is available for anastomosis. Any proposed graft will need to run into ankle or pedal vessels: graft failure is a distinct possibility and may lead to amputation. Any reconstructive surgery is therefore usually reserved for those patients with advanced disease, i.e. rest pain and tissue necrosis, who are already threatened with limb loss. Bypass grafting performed in a

Box 42.6	Buerger's disease
Prevalence	Higher in the Far East, India, SE Asia, Eastern Europe and Israel than in USA and UK 1 in 5000 male Ashkenazi Jews over 25, 6.8/100 000 white males aged 20–44 in USA
Course	Insidious onset and chronic progression unless patient stops smoking
m:f	30:1
Age	<40 years
Cause	Genetic predisposition and tobacco
Arteries affected	Small to medium
Sites	Upper and lower limbs
Pattern of inflammation	Arteries and veins: *acute* – segmental, thrombosis with associated polymorphonuclear infiltration throughout vessel wall and thrombus, giant cells on surface of thrombus, preservation of elastic fibres and no necrosis *subacute* – lymphocytic infiltration of thrombus *chronic* – recanalisation of thrombus, branches of vasa vasorum infiltrate media and connect to recanalised lumen, perivascular fibrosis
Presentation	Progressive ischaemic symptoms in lower and upper limbs, followed by tissue necrosis in the feet and hands Superficial thrombophlebitis Angiographic appearance (Figure 42.6), smooth tapering segmental occlusions of upper and lower limb arteries 'Corkscrew' collaterals (enlarged vasa vasorum) Corrugated appearance to intervening arteries
Treatment	Stop smoking Limited scope for surgery

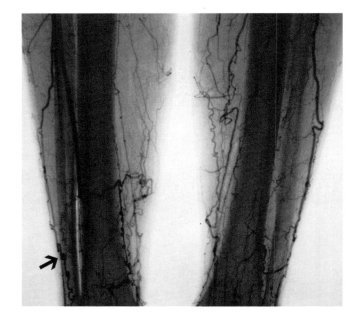

Figure 42.6 Angiogram of calf arteries in Buerger's disease showing occlusion of the main infrapopliteal vessels and corkscrew collaterals (arrowed). Courtesy of Dr E.W. Fletcher, Dept of Radiology, John Radcliffe Hospital, Oxford (retired).

patient who continues to smoke is doomed to early failure. Upper limb ischaemia is caused by relatively more distal disease and reconstruction is rarely feasible. Unfortunately operative intervention in most of these patients takes the form of amputation. It should be recognised, however, that patients with Buerger's disease may also have proximal disease due to atherosclerosis. Treatment of such disease is often worthwhile: it may save the limb or lower the amputation level.

Irradiation arteritis (Box 42.7)

Patients who have had radiotherapy up to 20 years or more previously occasionally present with claudication of arm or leg or acute digital ischaemia. The symptoms are associated with arterial damage within the field of irradiation and occur particularly after treatment of breast cancer but also after irradiation for lymphoma, pelvic malignancy and other tumours. The condition is uncommon and bears no consistent relationship with irradiation dose but appears to depend more on individual susceptibility.

Box 42.7	Irradiation arteritis
Sites	Anywhere in irradiated field
	After breast cancer – subclavian or axillary arteries
	After pelvic irradiation – iliac disease
Pathology	Rarely – full-thickness arterial wall necrosis leading to rupture (within 2 years of DXT)
	Endothelial damage and disruption of the internal elastic membrane, leading to mural thrombus (within 5 years of DXT)
	Intimal thickening in vasa vasorum results in relative ischaemia of media and adventitia and fibrosis within and around the artery (within 10 years of DXT)
	Early-onset atheromatous change (20 years after DXT) more likely in those with hypertension or raised cholesterol levels
Presentation	Either progressive symptoms of upper or lower limb claudication or acute onset of digital ischaemia due to embolisation

Treatment

The natural history of this condition is of gradual progression of stenosis to occlusion. Collateral vessels lie within the irradiated field and cannot be relied upon to take over the supply of distal tissues. Thus if the patient presents with significant ischaemia due to proximal disease, vascular intervention will be required.

Balloon angioplasty has been tried with some success in the short term and has the advantage of relatively easy access to the arterial lesion. There is an immediate risk of distal embolisation and the underlying fibrosis tends to produce recurrent stenosis within a year or so. The place of arterial stenting in this condition has not yet been defined.

Bypass grafting has the advantage of good long-term patency and relief of symptoms but access through the irradiated field is often difficult because of dense fibrosis, loss of tissue planes and lymphoedema and healing is slow. Carotid–subclavian grafts, preferably with vein because of the infection risk, have been used in many cases. When the occlusion is more distal or the tissues particularly hostile, extraanatomical bypass grafting from the opposite subclavian to the axillary or brachial artery or the ipsilateral carotid to brachial artery via a lateral route may be preferable.

When the problem is of distal embolisation with local ischaemia but good limb perfusion otherwise, antiplatelet agents or anticoagulation may control the situation with local amputation of dead tissue if required. The alternative is bypass grafting to exclude the embolic source but this is usually unnecessary.

Experimental use of endovascular or external beam irradiation has been tried in an attempt to reduce intimal hyperplasia associated with intraarterial stents. Promotion or inhibition of hyperplasia is a delicate balance which seems to depend critically on the dose of radiotherapy. Encouraging short-term results have been published but the long-term consequences are unknown and may mirror those seen with irradiation arteritis.

Fibromuscular dysplasia (FMD) (Box 42.8)

This disorder of larger arteries is usually diagnosed in young to middle-aged Caucasian women. Its cause is unknown: the pathological change is fibroblastic transformation of smooth muscle cells but whether this is a primary developmental abnormality or secondary to ischaemia from the associated obliteration of vasa vasorum is unclear. There is a clear association with intracranial aneurysms and, despite their relative youth, 20% patients with FMD have atherosclerosis of the carotid bifurcation. Familial clustering suggests autosomal dominant inheritance with variable penetrance.

Three patterns of disease are described. The commonest (60–85% cases) is medial fibrodysplasia in which fibrous tissue in the media creates alternating ridges and thinned microaneurysms, producing the classic 'string of beads' sign on an angiogram (Figure 42.7). The remainder of cases fall into the category of either intimal or periadventitial dysplasia.

The disease often goes undetected in life. Ischaemia associated with arterial stenosis secondary to the disease is the commonest complication, in particular hypertension associated with renal artery involvement. Occasionally the media dissects (particularly in the carotid artery), aneurysms develop or arteriovenous fistulas occur as a result of FMD.

Treatment

Percutaneous transluminal (balloon) angioplasty for symptomatic disease of the renal, mesenteric or iliac vessels provides effective,

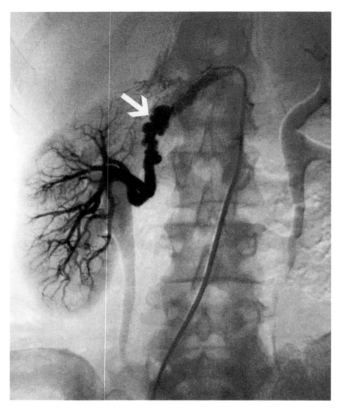

Figure 42.7 Angiogram showing 'string of beads' sign (arrowed) in a renal artery affected by fibromuscular dystrophy. Courtesy of Dr E.W. Fletcher, Dept of Radiology, John Radcliffe Hospital, Oxford (retired).

Box 42.8	Fibromuscular dysplasia
Prevalence	1% Caucasian population
m:f	1:2
Age	Mean 40–50
Cause	Unknown
Sites	Renal (usually in distal 2/3) – most patients
	25–35% – distal internal carotid (or vertebral) arteries
	9% – mesenteric or subclavian arteries
	5% iliac arteries
	Rarely coronary arteries
Presentation	Hypertension (but fewer than 2% hypertensive patients have FMD)
	CVA as a result of hypertension, carotid atheroma or dissection and occasionally carotid stenosis due to FMD

durable and low-risk correction of the stenosis. If renovascular hypertension is suspected in a young patient and renal angiography shows a distal renal artery stricture, consistent with FMD, balloon dilatation will be diagnostic (of renovascular hypertension) and curative (if it is FMD). Success is such that early angiography to look for and treat these lesions is indicated, in contrast to the older patient with renovascular hypertension due to atherosclerosis where balloon dilatation carries a higher risk and

is much less likely to be successful both immediately and in the longer term.

If FMD has progressed to occlusion (uncommon) then bypass grafting may be indicated but only, in the case of renal artery disease, if the kidney is still large enough to justify the procedure (>8 cm in length on ultrasound).

Carotid FMD rarely progresses sufficiently to cause problems and usually requires no treatment.

Cryoglobulinaemia

Circulating proteins which precipitate with cold are found in low concentrations in normal individuals. Elevated levels occur in association with increased activity in the immune system and occasionally with no obvious abnormality. Cryoglobulinaemia is associated with localised areas of vasculitis where the protein has precipitated. Analysis of these proteins shows that most are immunoglobulins, either IgG or IgM, or circulating immune complexes, usually of IgG and IgM (Box 42.9).

Box 42.9	Cryoglobulinaemia
Histology of the skin	Fibrinoid necrosis of the vessels with surrounding acute inflammatory infiltrate of polymorphonucleocytes and intravascular hyaline casts of cryoglobulin
Other manifestations of cryoglobulinaemia	50% have Raynaud's phenomenon
	35% have arthralgia
	20% have renal symptoms (anuria or glomerulonephritis)
	17% have a peripheral neuropathy, usually sensory in the early stages but motor a few years later. Central neurological disturbance and GI symptoms occur occasionally
	Some or all of these symptoms may be related to protein precipitation but, if so, suggest that some of these proteins will precipitate at central core temperature as well as in the cold
Associated disease	15% Waldenstrom's macroglobulinaemia
	10% multiple myeloma
	10% chronic lymphocytic leukaemia or lymphoma
	10% Sjögren's syndrome
	6% systemic lupus erythematosus
Associated disease	6% rheumatoid arthritis
	Acute viral infection (EBV or CMV)
	1° or 2° syphilis, leprosy, protozoal disease such as trypanosomiasis
	30% idiopathic
	Symptoms associated with the cryoglobulins may appear several years before the associated disease is manifest
Treatment	Supportive measures such as avoidance of cold, analgesia and dialysis
	Emergency plasmapheresis if major visceral involvement or skin necrosis
	Immunosuppression
	Treatment of associated disorder

Up to half of subjects with increased levels of cryoglobulins have no cold-associated symptoms but the commonest cold-related phenomenon is reticulate purpura affecting the lower leg or thigh, occasionally spreading to the lower abdomen or buttocks and precipitated not only by cold but also sustained effort or prolonged dependency of the legs. A few cases develop ulceration of the tips of toes, fingers, the nose, ears or lower legs but usually only on exposure to extreme cold. Cold urticaria appears to be a milder manifestation of the disorder. Individuals with the disorder usually suffer repeated attacks of purpura, each lasting 1–2 weeks, repeated once or twice a month and leaving a permanent brown skin discoloration after some years.

Frostbite

Cold exposure leads to alternating cycles of vasoconstriction and vasodilatation in the microcirculation as the body seeks to maintain both core temperature and local tissue viability. Excessive cold exposure during sporting activities, military exercises or inability to take cold avoidance measures (because of poverty, vagrancy, age, psychiatric disorder, etc.) leads to persistent vasoconstriction in an effort to maintain core temperature. As a result local tissue viability may be sacrificed. At temperatures of 2°C or less ice crystals start forming in the extracellular fluid of the extremity. This leads to an increased osmolality of the extracellular fluid which draws out intracellular fluid. Cells can still survive provided that intracellular dehydration is not excessive and that intracellular ice crystals do not form. Capillary endothelial cells tend to lift off the internal elastic membrane and this and other tissue damage may impair subsequent function even if cells survive. Rewarming causes the ice crystals to melt. The disrupted capillary endothelial cells are 'leaky', allowing excessive fluid and protein loss into the interstitial tissue, resulting in generalised oedema in the extremity. Ischaemia/reperfusion leads to free radical release, causing further tissue damage and endothelial malfunction. Patchy thrombosis occurs.

The severity of frostbite can be classified after rewarming as follows.

Superficial

- First degree (partial skin freezing):
  - hyperaemia and swelling
  - no blisters or necrosis
  - stinging ± throbbing
- Second degree (full thickness):
  - as above + blisters or superficial necrosis
  - numbness

Deep (including subcutaneous tissue ± muscle and bone)

- Little or no oedema

- Haemorrhagic blisters
- Dusky, mottled appearance eventually progressing to dry gangrene (Figure 42.8)
- Absent sensation initially, later throbbing/burning/shooting pains

Treatment

If still cold:

- avoid friction (rubbing with hands or snow)
- avoid rewarming then recooling; both will lead to increased tissue damage
- move to secure warm environment then rapid rewarming in water bath at 40–42°C
- analgesia
- tetanus cover
- antibiotics probably best reserved for supervening infection rather than prophylaxis
- treatment of co-existent hypothermia takes precedence over treatment of frostbite.

Once warm:

- prevention/treatment of infection
- physiotherapy
- await demarcation of dead tissue (this may take several months) then escharectomy or amputation if necessary

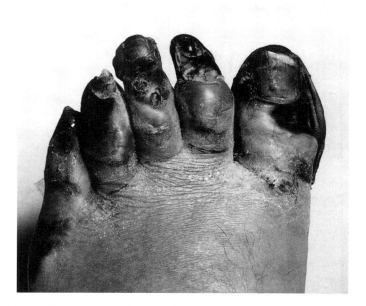

Figure 42.8 Gangrene of the toes in frostbite.

- various systemic treatments (prostaglandins, heparin, strepto-kinase, sympathectomy, low molecular weight dextran) have been tried but with no proven benefit.

Long-term sequelae of frostbite in the extremity include:

- cold or heat sensitivity
- hyperhidrosis
- hyperaesthesia or persistent pain
- arthritis
- skin discoloration
- tissue loss
- increased liability to further cold injury.

Trenchfoot (immersion foot)

Prolonged exposure of the foot to a moist environment results in certain distinct changes which have been variously described under a variety of names depending on the circumstances (trenchfoot, immersion foot, jungle rot, etc.) (Box 42.10). The underlying changes are similar although the speed of onset and severity of tissue damage depend on temperature and salinity of the water (worse with cold salt water immersion). Most descriptions originate in wartime or shipwreck but the condition may be recognised amongst the homeless or psychologically impaired members of a civilian population. Prolonged wearing of footwear soaked by rain or discharging leg ulcers are usually the cause in the latter group.

Box 42.10	Trenchfoot
Pathology	Waterlogging of the stratum corneum, particularly of the sole which is more liable to such changes than the dorsum of the foot. There may be dermal oedema and some absorption into the circulation. Tissue necrosis, nerve damage and thrombosis (usually venous) sometime occur
Presentation	Painful feet with swollen, wrinkled, tender soles Cold (not freezing) immersion produces a white numb and pulseless foot initially because of associated vasoconstriction; this is followed by a hyperaemic phase a few hours later when the foot is hot, red and painful. Blistering, oedema, gangrenous patches and paraesthesiae may then develop Sometimes fever and local lymphadenopathy In the long term the feet may be permanently cold and sweaty
Treatment	Elevation, exposure and air drying of the extremity Antibiotics if evidence of infection Amputation where necessary once demarcation established (may take weeks)
Prognosis	Dependent on extent of tissue necrosis and nerve damage

VASOSPASTIC DISEASE

Control of vessel size

Central cardiovascular control lies in the medulla but this receives important inputs from the hypothalamus, especially relating to temperature and emotion, which are known to affect vascular tone. Descending fibres from the medulla reach the lateral horn cells of the spinal cord from which arise the nerve fibres of the autonomic nervous system. Sympathetic outflow comes from all the thoracic and the first two lumbar segments of the spinal cord (Figure 42.9): parasympathetic outflow arises in various cranial nerve nuclei (III, VII, IX and X) and the third and fourth sacral segments of the cord. Autonomic fibres leave the cord with the spinal nerve serving that segment but most of the sympathetic fibres soon divert to synapse in ganglia of the nearby sympathetic chain. The majority of their postganglionic fibres rejoin the spinal nerves for distribution to the periphery but a few form a plexus around the largest arteries which they supply for several centimetres. Parasympathetic fibres are relayed in peripheral ganglia, much closer to their target organ.

Out in the periphery fingers and toes have a rich blood supply but only a small part of this is nutritional, the remainder playing an important part in temperature control. There are multiple arteriovenous (AV) fistulas in the digits which allow increased

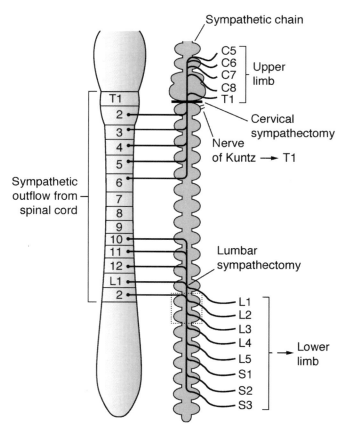

Figure 42.9 Sympathetic outflow to the limbs from the spinal cord.

blood flow to dissipate heat but which bypass the capillary bed. These AV shunts are richly innervated by sympathetic fibres which impose vasoconstriction in response to cold or emotional stimuli. Parasympathetic input, on the other hand, leads to vaso-dilatation. There is a third neural input; small sensory fibres in the skin are capable of efferent control. They release calcitonin gene-related peptide (CGRP) and substance P (SP), both of which cause vasodilatation but by different mechanisms. SP needs an intact endothelium for its effect, presumably via an intermediate messenger, whereas CGRP acts directly on smooth muscle (Figure 42.10).

The picture is even more complicated because of vasoactive agents released within the vessel wall or lumen. Endothelium is capable of generating both a potent vasoconstrictor, endothelin and vasodilators, nitric oxide (EDRF) and prostacyclin. Platelets within the lumen can release thromboxane, serotonin or platelet factor 4, all leading to vasoconstriction. The final outcome depends on a delicate balance which is susceptible to distortion by changes at a number of different points.

Raynaud's syndrome

This describes a clinical syndrome of sharply demarcated colour change in the fingers, sometimes the toes and occasionally the ears and nose in response to cold and sometimes emotion (Box 42.11). The classic description is of one, some or all of the fingers turning white, then blue and finally red as a painful hyperaemia accompanies reperfusion (Figure 42.11). It may occur as an isolated phenomenon, particularly in young women, when it is known as Raynaud's disease. Somewhere between 50% and 70% cases prove secondary to a systemic disease although it may be several

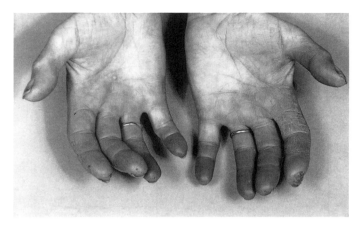

Figure 42.11 Fingers affected by Raynaud's phenomenon.

(even 20) years before the cause becomes manifest. The changes described are due to vasospasm in the distal arteries and are reversible in the majority. A few patients have more severe disease where the changes do not reverse and the arteries occlude, resulting in ulceration or gangrene in distal tissue.

Treatment

Patients are advised to:

● stop smoking (since this contributes to vasoconstriction)

● stop vasconstricting drugs

● keep their hands and feet warm with woollen gloves and socks, if necessary with inbuilt electrical heating.

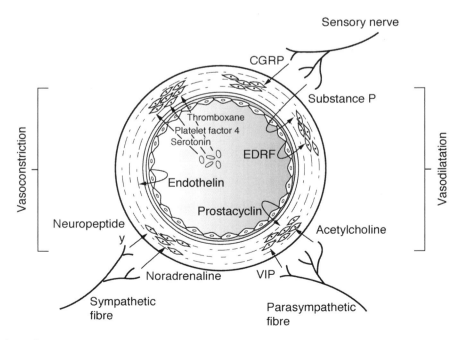

Figure 42.10 Local control of arterial tone.

Box 42.11	Raynaud's syndrome
Prevalence	5–20% females and 4–14% males. Higher prevalence in Northern latitudes
Course	Relapses and remissions, dependent on ambient temperature. Improves during pregnancy but may be worse at particular times of the menstrual cycle
m:f	1:4
Age	Onset occurs predominantly in the second and third decades but there is a further peak after 60 years when the phenomenon is secondary to upstream occlusive disease
Cause	There is much speculation over this. Originally it was thought to be due to increased central sympathetic stimulation but it has gradually become obvious that this plays little if any part. An increase in α2-adrenoceptors and a decrease in CGRP in skin together with increased levels of circulating endothelin and serotonin have been documented and it may be that a subtle adjustment at local level biases the vasculature to vasoconstriction. Increased platelet activity, raised levels of von Willibrand factor, cryoglobulins and increased fibrinogen in circulating blood may also play a part but could be secondary effects. In secondary Raynaud's phenomenon a thickened vessel wall in connective tissue disease or reduced arterial pressure due to upstream stenosis by atherosclerosis, Buerger's disease or a thoracic rib predispose the artery to exaggerated narrowing with normal vasoconstriction. 14% patients with Raynaud's disease have a family history of the disorder
Arteries affected	Digital predominantly
Associated disease	Connective tissue disorders – 24% patients have scleroderma, up to 10% rheumatoid arthritis or SLE
	Thoracic outlet syndrome – due to arterial and possibly nerve compression
	Carpal tunnel syndrome – presumed secondary to nerve damage
	Drugs (vasoconstrictors) beta blocking agents, ergot derivatives for migraine
	Cytotoxic drugs e.g. vinblastine, bleomycin, cisplatin, cyclosporin
	Chemicals – e.g. vinyl chloride
	Malignancy – occasionally associated with haematological malignancy, myeloma, breast, bronchial or visceral tumours
Diagnosis	Clinical presentation
	Digital artery pressure or flow changes with cold immersion and warming (faster fall to lower levels than in controls and slower recovery on rewarming)

In a minority of patients the symptoms may cause significant discomfort or restriction and in these cases the following drugs may be useful:

- Vasodilators, e.g. naftidrofuryl, inositol nicotinate, gylceryl trinitrate paste

- calcium channel blockers – nifedipine appears most effective but has significant side effects

- diltiazem has fewer side effects but also less benefit

- ketanserin – serotonin receptor blocker (on a named patient basis in UK) has been shown more effective than nifedipine in one study

- prostacyclin (currently IV but oral preparations likely in future) – given for about five days but detectable benefit persists for at least a month.

In very severe cases sympathectomy may be considered. However, upper limb sympathectomy provides only short-term benefit in this condition; improvement is unlikely to last longer than six months. Phenol or operative lumbar sympathectomy to treat the feet is much more likely to provide long-term improvement but lower limb Raynaud's phenomenon is rarely a significant problem.

Vibration white finger

This is a vasospastic condition affecting the fingers of those who work with vibrating tools (Box 42.12). Cold-induced colour changes occur in a similar fashion to Raynaud's phenomenon but there is sometimes persistent pain and paraesthesiae even on warming. It is well described in those using pneumatic drills, chain saws and buffs. The disorder is more likely to occur if the equipment has to be held tightly because of its weight, if it is used for long periods at a time without interruption in a cold environment and in the young and female. There was thought to be an association with low-frequency vibration but recently it has become clear that it occurs over a wide range of vibration frequencies. It is worse in those who smoke and in the advanced form there are irreversible colour changes in the fingers and, in 1%, ulceration of the finger tips.

Box 42.12	Vibration white finger
Prevalance	40–90% of those using heavy vibrating equipment
Course	Continued deterioration unless use of vibrating tools stopped and even then may still progress if patient over 45 years
Age, m:f	Linked to local employment pattern
Cause	There is evidence for a central disturbance of autonomic regulation. The phenomenon can be prevented by digital nerve block and there are increased circulating levels of catecholamines. In this it seems to differ from Raynaud's phenomenon but in other ways it is very similar. There are local changes: α-adrenoceptors increase in number and there is a reduction in CGRP detectable in skin, in advanced cases there is medial hypertrophy and subintimal fibrosis in the digital arteries. There is systemic evidence of platelet activation
Treatment	Stop use of vibrating tools
	Stop smoking and and vasoconstrictor medication
	Keep hands warm
	Drug treatment as for Raynaud's phenomenon if necessary

Erythromelalgia

This is an uncommon condition characterised by periodic burning discomfort, usually in the feet and lower leg, sometimes in the hands (Box 42.13). There is an associated subjective feeling of warmth in the extremity. The symptoms are precipitated by warmth, dependency and exercise and relieved by cooling and elevation. Patients may spend several hours a day with their feet in cold water. Most cases are thought to be primary conditions but a third are associated with another 'primary' disorder, most commonly thrombocythaemia or other myeloproliferative disorders, connective tissue disease, diabetes, infection (HIV, occasional epidemics of erythromelalgia associated with pox virus) and previous frostbite. The 'primary' disorder may not be manifest for several years after onset of erythromelalgia symptoms and so the diagnosis of primary erythromelalgia is always provisional. A few cases also have Raynaud's phenomenon. Occasionally there is associated tissue necrosis in the extremity.

Box 42.13	Erythromelalgia
Prevalance	Uncommon
Course	Either acute (maximum symptoms within one month then resolution) or chronic and stable
m:f	1:2
Age	Mean 5th decade, range 1st–9th decades
Cause	Histological studies of skin biopsies in this condition show reduced sympathetic innervation of arterioles and sweat glands together with endothelial swelling, perivascular oedema and a thickened arteriolar basement membrane. The condition was thought to be secondary to increased microvascular blood flow through arteriovenous shunts with relative ischaemia in the nutritive bed but recent studies have demonstrated reduced basal skin temperature in the toes, feet and lower leg, reduced skin basal RBC flux measured by laser Doppler and impaired hyperaemic response to heating. The latter finding suggests that the underlying fault lies in the vessel wall which is unable to dilate normally in response to heat
Treatment	Cooling and elevation of the limb
	Carbamazepine or amitriptyline may relieve discomfort
	Prostacyclin infusion in those few patients with tissue necrosis is sometimes beneficial. Rarely is amputation necessary
	Those cases associated with thrombocythaemia may respond to aspirin
	Beta-blockade has been reported to help but needs careful monitoring as it may make the symptoms worse

Hyperhidrosis

This autonomic disorder affects sweat glands rather than blood vessels (Box 42.14). The commonest presentation is with sweaty hands: under the mildest heat or emotional stress the patient has sweat dripping from their hands, soaking paperwork, making it impossible to grip a pen or other tool and driving them away from social interaction, in particular shaking hands. The axillae can also be affected and the patient has to change shirts several times a day. The feet are sometimes affected: shoes deteriorate quickly and odour may be difficult to control but problems here are easier to hide than in the upper limb.

Box 42.14	Hyperhidrosis
Prevalance	1% population
m:f	Equal
Age	Onset usually in childhood
Cause	Occasionally hyperthyroidism, phaeochromocytoma or neurological disorders but usually idiopathic
Sites affected	Palms, axillae, soles of feet
Presentation	Excessive sweating with minimal stimulation
Treatment	Aluminium chloride sprays or roll-on
	Sympathectomy
	Botulinum toxin intradermal injection

Treatment

Topical antiperspirants are the first-line treatment but if symptoms are incapacitating and still poorly controlled, sympathectomy should be considered. Minimally invasive techniques have made this an attractive treatment option (see below). When excessive sweating is confined to the palms, division of the sympathectic chain above T2 ganglion (Figure 42.9) should suffice and is successful in more than 90% cases. This procedure will reduce or abolish axillary sweating in about 60% cases but if T2 and 3 sympathetic ganglia are removed then more than 80% of patients have relief from axillary sweating.

There are six side effects or complications the patient must be warned about.

1. *Dry hands* – all patients require regular use of moisturising cream to avoid cracking.

2. *Compensatory sweating on the trunk, thighs or face* – occurs in most patients to a minor extent but can be troublesome (and occasionally outweigh any benefit) in those having bilateral sympathectomies. In most cases it improves to some extent in the year following surgery.

3. *Gustatory sweating* – head and neck sweating in response to taste or smell occurs in up to 30% of patients.

4. *Horner's syndrome* – implies damage to the stellate ganglion immediately above T2 ganglion, assumed to be diathermy damage in most cases because the stellate ganglion is out of view on thoracoscopy and unlikely to be removed in error. Most audits report less than 1% incidence but if rhinitis alone is accepted as a manifestation of incomplete Horner's syndrome then the incidence rises to about 8%.

5. *Pneumothorax or haemothorax at the time of surgery* – 1–2% of cases will need an intercostal chest drain at or following surgery.

6. *Intercostal neuralgia* (probably related to trauma at port site) is an occasional and temporary complication.

Mild palmar sweating returns within two years of surgery in 10–20% patients but in only about 5% is it sufficient to require intervention. Repeat sympathectomy is an option for that small percentage where the first operation failed (when incomplete division of the sympathetic chain or a nerve of Kuntz is frequently discovered) or when sweating recurs (when nerve regeneration may be discovered and more extensive sympathectomy, i.e. removal of T2 and 3 ganglia for palmar sweating, can produce a more durable result).

Lumbar sympathectomy for sweaty feet is occasionally undertaken but patients often have sweaty hands as well which take precedence. The prospect of even more compensatory sweating with both upper and lower limb sympathectomy usually precludes lumbar sympathectomy in this situation.

Patients who suffer from isolated axillary hyperhidrosis may benefit from subcutaneous injection of botulinum toxin. This binds irreversibly to block the sympathetic fibres in the area and suppresses local sweating for several months, until sympathetic fibres regenerate.

Causalgia and reflex sympathetic dystrophy

Injury to a limb, sometimes trivial, can result in local changes which appear to be due to autonomic dysfunction. A variety of names have been used for what is probably a hotch-potch of conditions.

Causalgia

The first described and best characterised is causalgia (Box 42.15). This is a burning pain, usually affecting only the hand or the foot, occasionally the forearm or leg, developing within days or weeks of injury to a major nerve.

Box 42.15	Causalgia
Cause	Partial (rather than complete) nerve division appears to cause sympathetic overactivity
	?Denervation hypersensitivity due to increased expression of adrenoceptors in the afferent neurones
Site	Most common in the upper limb
Presentation	The affected extremity is hypersensitive to any stimulation and the patient usually holds the limb flexed and the part protected. There are often associated colour and temperature changes but the extremity may equally well be warm and pink as cold and pale or cyanosed. Increased sweating is found in about one-third. Some patients improve spontaneously but others have persistent symptoms which, with time, are accompanied by non-specific changes of disuse such as atrophy, oedema, joint stiffness and osteoporosis
Treatment	Physiotherapy to encourage passive and active limb movement and compression and elevation if oedema is a major component. If this fails to improve the situation then sympathetic blockade or sympathectomy are frequently used although there is no clear advantage over placebo in randomised trials

Reflex sympathetic dystrophy

Reflex sympathetic dystrophy (RSD) encompasses a multitude of other poorly characterised conditions (e.g. Sudek's atrophy, algodystrophy, shoulder-hand syndrome) which probably vary in pathogenesis and which have an uncertain response to treatment. The changes are similar to those seen in causalgia but are precipitated by injury to the limb, which may be as trivial as a minor knock, in which there is no obvious nerve injury, or by myocardial infarction or stroke (the latter two in shoulder-hand syndrome). There is pain in the extremity but it is not burning in nature. The extremity is hypersensitive and again held in a protective fashion. The hand or foot is usually pale and cold and excess sweating is evident in about one-third. Those patients who have persistent symptoms again go on to develop accompanying changes of disuse. Treatment is again physiotherapy, compression and elevation: the response to sympathetic blockade or sympathectomy is uncertain and, in some cases, such intervention results in deterioration. Systemic steroids may be beneficial.

It has been suggested that the likelihood of RSD should be based on the presence or absence of the following symptoms:

- *definite* – pain + tenderness + swelling + vasomotor instability
- *probable* – pain + tenderness + (swelling or vasomotor instability)
- *possible* – pain ± tenderness only, not attributable to another cause or vasomotor instability and swelling without pain or tenderness

SYMPATHECTOMY

Interruption of the sympathetic supply to a limb may be beneficial in certain cases of autonomic dysfunction (see above). The 2nd to 4th thoracic ganglia of the sympathetic chain supply the upper limb, the 2nd to 4th lumbar ganglia supply the lower limb (see Figure 42.9). Open surgery to divide this supply has been supplanted by either thoracoscopic techniques, via one or two axillary ports, when treating the upper limb (Figure 42.12), or transcutaneous injection of phenol under radiographic control to treat the lower limb. Complications of thoracoscopic sympathectomy are listed above (see hyperhidrosis) although compensatory sweating is not usually a significant problem when hyperhidrosis is not the underlying problem.

Complications of lumbar sympathectomy include postsympathectomy neuralgia – up to 35% of patients develop an anterior thigh ache within a few days of the procedure which resolves after a few months but can be successfully treated with carbamazepine in the interim. The following are rarely encountered:

- ureteric damage
- erectile impotence if both L1 ganglia are ablated
- postsympathectomy hypotension with bilateral procedures.

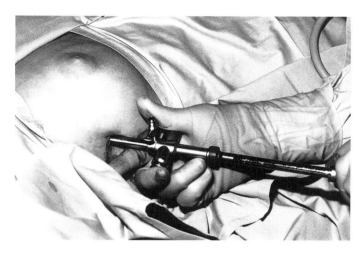

Figure 42.12 Thoracoscopic sympathectomy.

Sympathectomy for atherosclerotic disease

Claudication

The sympathetic supply to muscle is vasodilatory so sympathectomy is unlikely to help in theory. This is borne out in practice: a randomised trial of phenol sympathecomy versus local anaesthetic infiltration of the sympathetic chain demonstrated a better response in the placebo (local anaesthetic arm).

Rest pain

There is some evidence of benefit here. Uncontrolled trials have shown that up to two-thirds of patients have a subjective improvement with sympathectomy. Such an improvement is more likely in the absence of significant gangrenous changes and neuropathy and with an ankle:brachial pressure of at least 0.3. Cross and Cotton performed a randomised study of 41 limbs with rest pain due to large vessel disease, none with more than minimal digital gangrene, peripheral neuropathy or in patients dependent on insulin. Patients were randomised to phenol sympathectomy or local anaesthetic injection of the sympathetic chain. One week after intervention 84% of the phenol group had subjective improvement in pain scores and reduced analgesic use, compared with only 24% in the placebo group. At six months, 67% of the phenol group still had significant pain relief compared with 24% in the placebo group. Many of the latter group had required reconstruction or amputation by this stage. Interestingly there appeared to be no change in ankle:brachial indices or total foot

perfusion associated with pain relief after sympathectomy. The authors suggested an effect on pain pathways but there may have been redistribution of blood flow within the extremity.

So phenol sympathectomy probably does have something to offer the patient with rest pain provided that perfusion has not fallen to a level where there is extensive tissue loss and arterioles already are maximally vasodilated. It may be a temporising move when reconstruction is technically unattractive or the perioperative risk is high and sometimes it removes the need for amputation completely.

FURTHER READING

Barron KS. Kawasaki disease in children. *Curr Opin Rheumatol* 1998; **10**:29–37

Belch JJF, Ho M. Pharmacotherapy of Raynaud's phenomenon. *Drugs* 1996; **52**(5):682–695

Campbell WB. Sympathectomy. *Vasc Med Rev* 1994; **5**:61–71

Cross FW, Cotton LT. Chemical lumbar sympathectomy for ischemic rest pain. *Am J Surg* 1985; **150**:341–345

Evans J, Hunder G. The implications of recognizing large-vessel involvement in elderly patients with giant cell arteritis. *Curr Opin Rheumatol* 1997; **9**:37–40

Fox AD, Hands L, Collin J. The results of thoracoscopic sympathetic trunk transection for palmar hyperhidrosis and sympathetic ganglionectomy for axillary hyperhidrosis. *Eur J Vasc Endovasc Surg* 1999; **17**:343–346

Kahaleh B, Mattucci-Cerinic M. Raynaud's phenomenon and scleroderma. *Arthritis Rheum* 1995; **38**:1–4

Kalgaard OM, Seem E, Kvernebo K. Erythromelalgia: a clinical study of 87 cases. *J Intern Med* 1997; **242**:191–197

Kent PJ, Williams GA, Kester RC. Platelet activation during hand vibration. *Br J Surg* 1994; **81**:815–818

Mills JL. Buerger's disease: current status. *Vasc Med Rev* 1994; **5**:139–150

Palmer RA, Collin J. Vibration white finger. *Br J Surg* 1994; **80**:705–709

Parums DV. The arteritides. *Histopathology* 1994; **25**:1–20

Perl ER. Causalgia, pathological pain and adrenergic receptors. *Proc Natl Acad Sci USA* 1999; **96**:7664–7667

Schott GD. Interrupting the sympathetic outflow in causalgia and reflex sympathetic dystrophy. *BMJ* 1998; **316**:792–793

Swannell AJ. Polymyalgia rheumatica and temporal arteritis: diagnosis and management. *BMJ* 1997; **314**:1329–1332

Tuzun H, Besirli K, Sayin A et al. Management of aneurysms in Behcet's syndrome: an analysis of 24 patients. *Surgery* 1997; **121**:150–156

Weinberger J, Simon AD. Intracoronary irradiation for the prevention of restenosis. *Curr Opin Cardiol* 1997; **12**(5):468–474

Section 7

Transplantation

43

Transplantation immunology

J. Andrew Bradley

An understanding of relevant transplant immunology is an essential requirement for surgeons involved in the care of patients undergoing organ transplantation. Aspects of the subject are also likely to be of general relevance in the wider field of surgery.

It is now over half a century since the pioneering studies of Peter Medawar firmly established that tissue grafts are rejected because of the specific immunological response they provoke and not, as many had previously thought, because of a non-specific inflammatory response. Since this landmark observation, remarkable progress has been made in our understanding of graft rejection and in how best to try and overcome it. To those readers not familiar with the specialty of transplantation, the prospect of transplant immunology can seem somewhat daunting and the apparent complexity of the terminology used may do little to allay this view. The reader should not be deterred. The key concepts in transplant immunology are not very difficult to grasp and the importance of the science in underpinning progress in the clinic cannot be overstated. This chapter, written with the generalist in mind, outlines the immunopathology of graft rejection and the role of the histocompatibility laboratory in transplantation. The different immunosuppressive agents and regimens used to prevent allograft rejection are described along with the complications of non-specific immunosuppression, namely opportunistic infection and malignancy.

TERMS AND DEFINITIONS

To aid the reader, some of the important terms used extensively in transplantation immunology are defined below.

An *allograft* is a graft between two genetically dissimilar individuals of the same species (the old term *homograft* is no longer used). *Allogeneic* cells or tissue are genetically dissimilar but of the same species.

A *syngeneic* graft (or *isograft*) is a graft between two genetically identical individuals, as in the case of identical twins. An *autograft* is a graft originating from and applied to the same individual as in the case of a skin graft.

A *xenograft* is a graft between two different species.

Human leucocyte antigens (HLA or HLA antigens) comprise two classes (class I and class II) of cell surface proteins whose principal function is to display peptide antigens so they can be recognised by T cells. In the context of transplantation they are the principal transplant antigens or *alloantigens*.

The *major histocompatibility complex (MHC)* is a region of the mammalian genome (designated the HLA region in humans) encoding for proteins that have an important role in immunity. These include HLA antigens in the human.

Polymorphism refers to differences in a particular gene (*genetic polymorphism*) or the amino acid sequence of a protein, e.g. *HLA polymorphism* between different individuals.

ALLOGRAFT REJECTION

Organ and tissue allografts provoke a very strong immunological response and, unless potent immununosuppressive therapy is given, rapid and complete graft destruction within one or two weeks is usually inevitable. The immune response to an allograft is directed against so-called transplant antigens (histocompatibility antigens) expressed on the surface of cells within the graft. Graft rejection is an adaptive rather than an innate or non-specific immune response and experiments where grafts are performed between different inbred strains of mice show that it has both antigen specificity and immunological memory – the two cardinal features of an adoptive immune response (Figure 43.1). The antigen specificity of rejection is provided by T and B lymphocytes that recognise transplant antigens by their antigen-specific cell surface receptors.

Transplantation is not a natural phenomenon and no special immunological effector mechanisms exist solely to prevent successful transplantation. Graft rejection is mediated instead by the cellular and humoral effector mechanisms that have evolved naturally to provide protection against invading pathogens. Allograft rejection is a T cell-dependent immune response and cytotoxic T cells, delayed-type hypersensitivity (DTH) responses and T cell-dependent antibody responses may all contribute to the rejection process.

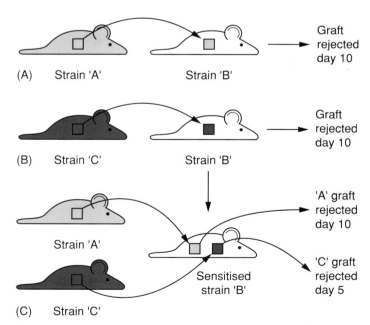

Figure 43.1 Graft rejection is due to an adaptive immune response. **A,B**. Inbred 'B' strain mice reject 'A' strain and 'C' strain skin grafts by 10 days. **C**. When 'B' strain mice that have been sensitised by a previous 'C' strain skin graft are challenged with second grafts they reject 'C' strain but not 'A' strain grafts more rapidly. Graft rejection therefore shows both antigen specificity and memory, the two cardinal features of an adaptive immune response. Adoptive transfer of T lymphocytes alone can transfer accelerated donor specific rejection from a sensitised to a naive recipient.

The ABO blood group barrier

The A, B, O blood group antigens are a crucial consideration in organ transplantation. These antigens result from structural polymorphisms in carbohydrate residues on glycolipids expressed on the surface of red blood cells. Individuals who do not possess a particular blood group antigen develop cross-reactive antibodies against that antigen through exposure of lymphocytes to normal intestinal bacteria bearing similar or cross-reactive antigens. Because blood group antigens are also expressed on the vascular endothelium of organs, it is essential to ensure that allografts are ABO blood group compatible otherwise preformed antibodies are likely to result in hyperacute rejection. Blood group O individuals have naturally occurring antibodies to blood group A and group B antigens and can only be given grafts from blood group O donors (the universal donor). Blood group A recipients can be given grafts from blood group O or A donors. Conversely, blood group B recipients can receive grafts from blood group O and B donors. Recipients who are blood group AB have no ABO antibodies and are universal recipients. Although organ allografts must be ABO compatible there is no need to ensure compatibility for Rhesus blood group and it is not considered when allocating organs for transplantation.

The MHC

Any protein that differs in amino acid composition between donor and recipient may, in principle, act as a transplant antigen. Assuming blood group compatibility, by far the most important transplant antigens are those encoded by genes in two regions (the class I and class II regions) of a segment of the genome designated the major histocompatibility complex (MHC). The major histocompatibility genes that are located collectively in this region of the mammalian genome were first identified in rodents through their influence in controlling acute rejection of skin grafts – hence the designation of the region as the major histocompatibility complex. The MHC did not, of course, evolve as a barrier to transplantation since this is an entirely non-physiological situation created by transplant surgery. The role that products of the MHC play as transplant antigens is instead a byproduct of their fundamental physiological function as immune recognition elements.

Membrane glycoproteins encoded by genes in the class I and class II regions of the MHC act like a scaffold to selectively display foreign antigens as linear peptide fragments at the cell surface for surveillance by T lymphocytes. This, coupled with the fact that

MHC molecules are highly polymorphic and abundantly expressed on the surface of most cell types, explains their unique potency as transplant antigens. The extensive polymorphism of MHC molecules between individuals is unfortunate from the perspective of organ transplantation because it ensures immunological incompatibility unless the prospective recipient and donor are genetically identical. However, it is clearly of great biological advantage for the species as a whole because it maximises the chance that there will always be individuals able to mount an effective immune response to new and potentially dangerous pathogens that might otherwise threaten the entire species.

HLA

In humans the major histocompatibility antigens were first identified using serological techniques to detect their presence on leucocytes. This led to their designation as human leucocyte antigens, abbreviated to HLA, and the same term is used to describe the human MHC. The HLA complex is the most polymorphic region of the human genome and was the first region to be sequenced in detail. It spans around 4000 kilobases of DNA and is located on the short arm of chromosome 6. The genes within the HLA are divided into three regions, known as class I, class II and class III (Figure 43.2). Genes in the class I region encode, in order of discovery, HLA-A, HLA-B and HLA-C (the so-called classic class I MHC antigens) along with other non-classic class I molecules such as HLA-E, HLA-F and HLA-G. Genetic loci in the class II region encode the class II antigens HLA-DR, HLA-DP and HLA-DQ, along with other proteins that are involved in antigen processing but do not act as transplant antigens. The class III region is situated between the class I and class II regions and encodes a number of proteins of importance in immunity although none are major transplant antigens. The most important transplant antigens are all encoded by distinct genes in the class I and class II regions. The class I region gene products of most relevance to organ transplantation are HLA-A and HLA-B (in order of discovery) and the most important class II region product is HLA-DR (for D Related). These three loci or their products are those that are routinely typed to determine the tissue match before organ transplantation.

Inheritance of HLA and HLA type

The HLA genotype or HLA profile of an individual is determined by the particular combination of HLA alleles (different forms of

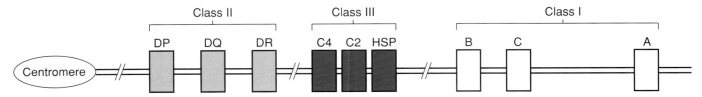

Figure 43.2 Organisation of HLA on the short arm of chromosome 6.

the same gene) that they have inherited from each of their parents. HLA genes are co-dominantly expressed so that, depending on whether an individual inherits the same or a different HLA gene polymorphism from each parent, they will express one or two different isoforms of each HLA molecule. During meiosis the HLA genes of a particular chromosome remain closely linked together so that the HLA haplotype inherited from each parent is generally inherited as a complete unit. HLA haplotypes are inherited according to simple Mendelian genetics. As shown in Figure 43.3, there is a one in four chance that two siblings will share the same parental haplotypes, or that they will share neither HLA haplotype, and a one in two chance they will share one HLA haplotype.

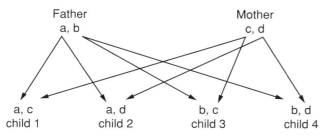

Figure 43.3 Inheritance of HLA. Each child inherits one HLA haplotype (designated a–d) from each parent. In the example shown, child 1 shares one HLA haplotype (i.e. is haploidentical) with child 2 and child 3 but does not share either haplotype with child 4.

As already noted, in clinical organ transplantation the HLA molecules of most importance are HLA-A, HLA-B and HLA-DR. Each chromosome 6 encodes a single HLA-A, -B and -DR antigen. An individual may therefore express between three and six different isoforms of these HLA antigens depending on whether they are homozygous or heterozygous at each of the three loci. The situation for HLA-DR is sometimes rather more complex because chromosome 6 occasionally carries an additional HLA-DR gene so an individual could express up to four different HLA-DR molecules.

Occasionally, a parental HLA haplotype is not inherited intact and crossover and recombination of DNA occur so that part of one haplotype recombines with part of another haplotype, giving rise to a new combination (or allele) of HLA genes. Genetic recombination of HLA is not entirely random in nature and certain combinations of HLA genes are found associated with each other more frequently than would be predicted. This non-random gene association of HLA genes is known as linkage disequilibrium and sometimes extends to an entire HLA haplotype. It probably arises because the resulting combination of genes making up the haplotypes confers a survival advantage by providing better protection against pathogens present in the geographical environment of a particular population or ethnic group.

HLA polymorphism

The MHC is the most polymorphic region of the human genome and there is extensive polymorphism of both HLA class I and class II molecules. Much of the genetic polymorphism observed encodes for amino acids situated in the regions of the HLA molecule that form the peptide binding groove and that bind with the T cell receptor. The number of amino acid differences between different HLA allotypes varies between one and 50 but even very small differences in amino acid sequence are sufficient to create a strong histocompatibility barrier to transplantation.

Before molecular typing techniques became available, HLA typing was performed by serological techniques. As new allelic variants were discovered and their serological specificity defined, they were assigned numerically under the letter designating their allele. In many cases the original antigen was subsequently *split* as further serological analysis revealed further variants and the nomenclature became increasingly complex. Using carefully defined panels of sera from individuals who had been sensitised to HLA molecules, around 20 different alleles at the HLA-A, 40 at the HLA-B and 20 at the HLA-DR locus were identified. DNA analysis has revealed that the true number of functional allelic variants is several times greater than that revealed by serological analysis, with over 100 HLA-A alleles, 200 HLA-B alleles and 200 HLA-DR alleles.

To standardise the designation of HLA genes and their protein products, a new nomenclature was introduced under the auspices of the World Health Organisation (WHO). In this system, all HLA allotypes are classified on the basis of their DNA sequence. Individual HLA alleles are identified first by their gene locus followed by a four-digit number, with the first two digits signifying the HLA specificity and the next two digits denoting the HLA subtype. Under the WHO nomenclature, for example, all alleles of the HLA-A gene are given the prefix A★ followed by the digits 01 for alleles encoding the serologically defined A1 antigen, 02 for alleles encoding A2, etc. The two individual alleles of HLA-A1 are designated A★0101 and A★0102 and the numerous alleles of HLA-A2 are designated A★0201 to A★0226 respectively. Additional digits are used to indicate DNA polymorphisms that do not result in functional allelic variants and the suffix N is used to denote null alleles where a particular polymorphism prevents gene expression.

Structure and function of HLA class I and class II molecules

HLA molecules are of such fundamental importance to graft rejection that a full description of their structure and function is merited. The physiological function of HLA class I and class II molecules is to bind foreign antigen in the form of linear peptide and display it at the cell surface for surveillance by T cells. Antigen displayed in this form is recognised by antigen-specific T lymphocytes and these then trigger a protective cellular immune response. The role of HLA molecules in this regard is crucial since the antigen receptor on T lymphocytes cannot recognise proteins from pathogens in their native form but only after they have been broken down and displayed as peptides bound to HLA class I or class II molecules. Moreover, the specificity of the T cell receptor is such that it cannot recognise peptide *per se* but instead recognises a molecular composite comprising the antigenic peptide along with adjacent parts of the HLA molecule to which it is bound.

The three-dimensional structure of class I and class II molecules is broadly similar in that they both possess a deep peptide-binding groove walled by two parallel alpha helices and floored by a beta-pleated sheet (Figure 43.4). This functional structure is achieved in a different way by the two classes of HLA molecule. Class I HLA molecules are made up of a transmembrane heavy chain (the alpha chain) associated non-covalently with a small non-polymorphic molecule called beta-2 microglobulin that is encoded by chromosome 15. The alpha chain of class I has three extracellular immunoglobulin-like domains and two of these (the alpha-1 and alpha-2 domains) make up the peptide-binding groove. Class II HLA molecules, on the other hand, comprise two membrane bound chains, the alpha and the beta chains, each of which has two extracellular immunoglobulin-like domains. The peptide-binding groove is formed by the alpha-1 domain of the alpha chain and the beta-1 domain of the beta chain.

Peptides can only bind within the groove of a MHC molecule if they contain the relevant amino acids, or *anchor residues*, which collectively constitute a peptide-binding motif for that particular

HLA molecule. The lengths of peptides that can be accommodated in HLA molecules are also constrained by the architecture of the peptide-binding groove and this differs for HLA class I and class II. HLA class I molecules have a binding groove that is closed at each end and bound peptides are usually 8–10 amino acids in length. The peptide-binding groove in class II molecules is open ended, allowing longer peptides, typically 12–25 amino acids in length, to be accommodated.

An important point to appreciate, particularly in the context of transplantation, is that cell surface HLA molecules rarely have 'empty' peptide-binding grooves. When they are not occupied by an antigenic peptide derived from pathogens, they are filled instead by non-antigenic peptides derived from intracellular and cell surface proteins. In fact, even in the presence of an infection, the majority of bound peptides in HLA are still derived from self-proteins rather than from the invading microorganism.

Peptides presented by the two classes of HLA molecule are derived from two different antigen-processing and presentation pathways (Figure 43.5). HLA class I molecules present peptides derived from the intracellular environment. Endogenous proteins synthesised in the cytosol (self-proteins, viral proteins and intracytoplasmic bacteria) are broken down into peptides and transported to the endoplasmic reticulum where they bind to HLA class I molecules and are then transported to the cell surface. HLA class

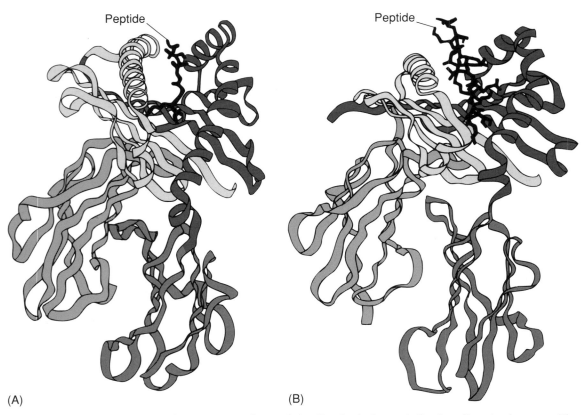

(A)   (B)

Figure 43.4 Structure of HLA class I (**A**) and HLA class II (**B**). HLA class I and class II molecules have a similar three-dimensional structure. The membrane distal domains of the molecules form a cleft in which is bound an antigenic peptide for recognition by a T lymphocyte. Redrawn with permission from Stern and Wiley, *Structure* 1994; **2**:245–252.

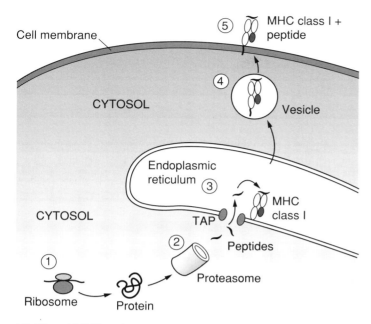

(A) Class I MHC pathway

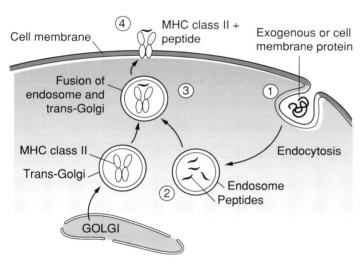

(B) Class II MHC pathway

Figure 43.5 Antigen processing and presentation. **A**. MHC class I molecules present peptides derived from intracellular proteins. The proteins are broken down into peptides by the proteasome and then transported to the endoplasmic reticulum by the ATP-dependent TAP transporter where they are loaded into class I molecules before transfer to the cell surface in a vesicle. **B**. MHC class II molecules present peptides derived from proteins at the cell surface or from the extracellular environment. After endocytosis, the protein is broken down into peptides within the endosome. The endosome then fuses with a trans-Golgi containing class II molecule and the class II MHC/peptide complexes are transported to the cell surface.

II molecules, on the other hand, present peptides derived from the extracellular environment. Cell surface molecules (including HLA molecules themselves) and extracellular proteins (such as bacterial proteins) are taken up within endosomes or lysosomes. There they are degraded by proteases into peptides before fusion

of the endocytic vesicle with the trans-Golgi network results in loading of the peptides into class II molecules and transport back to the cell surface.

There are important differences in the cellular distribution of HLA class I and class II molecules. HLA class I is expressed on the surface of nearly all nucleated cell types. HLA class II, in contrast, has a more restricted cell distribution and is expressed most abundantly on cells of the immune system that have a special role in antigen presentation, notably dendritic cells, macrophages and B lymphocytes, the so-called *professional antigen presenting* cells. Some other cell types, such as the vascular endothelium and parenchymal cells of an organ graft, can also express HLA class II and such expression is upregulated during inflammatory responses, such as allograft rejection, by the proinflammatory cytokine interferon-γ.

Alloantigen recognition by T cells

The initial cellular interaction that triggers graft rejection is the cognate interaction of alloantigen on the surface of an antigen-presenting cell with an antigen-specific T cell through its T cell receptor (TCR) (Figure 43.6). The TCR is a membrane-bound immunoglobulin-like molecule comprising two similar polypeptide chains (designated alpha and beta). Each individual T cell clone expresses a unique TCR with particular antigen specificity and all the TCRs on a given T cell have the same antigen specificity. Although the TCR molecule itself lacks a full cytoplasmic tail and cannot deliver an intracellular signal, it is closely associated at the cell surface with a series of non-polymorphic proteins called the CD3 complex and these are responsible for intracellular signalling following engagement of the TCR with antigen. Together, the TCR and the CD3 complex form a functional unit for antigen recognition called the TCR complex. Mature T cells

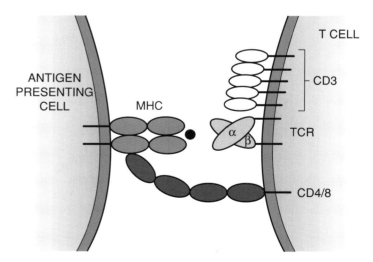

Figure 43.6 Interaction of the T cell receptor complex with MHC/peptide complex. The T cell receptor complex comprises the TCR, the CD3 complex and either CD4 or CD8. The CD3 complex transduces the intracellular signal from the TCR. CD8 and CD4 bind to non-polymorphic regions of the class I and class II MHC respectively.

can be divided into two subclasses according to whether they express CD4 or CD8 cell surface glycoprotein molecules. Whereas CD8 T cells are cytotoxic and able to kill target cells bearing antigen, CD4 T cells have a helper function and are known as helper T cells. The non-polymorphic CD8 and CD4 molecules function as co-receptors during antigen recognition by binding to non-polymorphic regions of HLA molecules on the antigen-presenting cell. Because CD8 binds only to HLA class I and CD4 only to HLA class II, the two functionally distinct T cell subsets recognise peptide antigens derived from different antigen-processing pathways.

The ligation of the TCR complex by HLA-antigen leads to activation of ZAP-70, a cytoplasmic tyrosine kinase molecule. Activation of ZAP-70 initiates a series of complex downstream signalling cascades that culminate in the activation of a set of transcription factors comprising NFκB, NFAT and AP1. These three transcription factors then turn on the genes necessary for T cell activation and differentiation. However, the signals arising from the TCR complex are not by themselves sufficient to cause full T cell activation. Indeed, ligation of the TCR alone (so-called signal 1) may encourage the T cell to become unresponsive or anergic instead of fully activated. To achieve full activation, the T cell also requires the delivery of additional or co-stimulatory signals (collectively comprising signal 2). These are provided when non-polymorphic receptor molecules on the T cell surface bind to their ligands on the surface of the antigen-presenting cell and provide supplementary activation of ZAP-70. Important co-stimulatory molecules expressed on antigen-presenting cells include CD80 and CD86, that both bind to CD28, and CD40 whose ligand is CD154.

Allorecognition pathways

HLA antigens in a transplanted organ can be recognised by two different routes designated the direct and indirect pathways of allorecognition. Until recently, the direct pathway of allorecognition was regarded as the principal route for allorecognition but it has become increasingly clear that indirect allorecognition is also important.

DIRECT ALLORECOGNITION

During direct allorecognition, which is unique to transplantation, the recipient T cell recognises intact donor HLA molecules complexed with endogenously derived peptide expressed on the surface of a donor strain antigen-presenting cell (Figure 43.7). The most effective type of donor strain antigen-presenting cell (APC) is the interstitial dendritic cell, known, in the context of transplantation, as a passenger leucocyte. The interstitial dendritic cell is a bone marrow-derived leucocyte that is widely distributed throughout all of the commonly transplanted organs. These cells are richly endowed with both class I and class II HLA molecules and are armed with the full complement of co-stimulatory molecules needed to cause T cell activation.

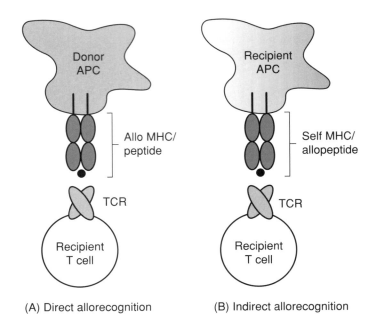

(A) Direct allorecognition   (B) Indirect allorecognition

Figure 43.7 Alloantigen recognition pathways. **A.** In direct allorecognition, the recipient T cell recognises allogeneic MHC (plus bound endogenous peptide) on the surface of a donor APC. **B.** In indirect allorecognition the recipient T cell recognises and responds to shed donor-derived alloantigen after it has been taken up by a recipient APC and presented as peptide bound to self-MHC.

Why should T cells recognise and respond to allogeneic HLA molecules but not self-HLA molecules? To answer this question it is necessary to consider how the normal T cell repertoire is selected as it develops within the thymus gland. As T cells mature they undergo a two-stage selection process. First, they undergo positive selection during which only those T cells that are specific for complexes of self-HLA molecules and peptides derived from breakdown of self-proteins are allowed to survive. All remaining non-reactive T cells are destined to die by apoptosis. Next, the developing T cells undergo a negative selection process during which any T cells whose antigen receptors bind too strongly to self-HLA and self-peptide are deleted. This is an important selection process because if high-affinity autoreactive T cells were not purged in this way autoimmunity would develop. The final T cell repertoire remaining after thymic selection, therefore, comprises T cells with a wide range of antigen specificities, all recognising self-HLA and bound endogenous peptide but with insufficient binding affinity to cause T cell activation. During an immune response to a foreign protein antigen, T cells recognise the complex of antigenic peptide and self-HLA with high affinity and respond accordingly.

When, following organ transplantation, T cells encounter intact allogeneic HLA molecules and their bound endogenous peptides on donor APC, about 5% of them are activated. This is an enormous response considering that only around one in 10 000 T cells recognises a foreign protein antigen during a physiological immune response. Two hypotheses have been advanced to explain why so many T cells respond so strongly to intact allogeneic HLA. The 'multiple binary complex hypothesis' states that the responding T cells comprise multiple T cell clones each responding to a molecular complex of foreign HLA and one of the thousands of different endogenous peptides bound within the groove of the allogeneic HLA molecule. The 'high determinant density hypothesis' states that the specificity of the alloreactive T cells is predominantly directed against the allogeneic HLA molecule and that the identity of the bound peptide is not critical. Accordingly, all of the hundreds or thousands of HLA molecules expressed on an individual APC will be recognised as 'foreign'. This is in marked contrast to a physiological immune response where only a relatively small percentage of self-HLA molecules present a foreign antigenic peptide and the remainder continue to present non-immunogenic self-peptides. The high density of antigenic HLA molecules present during direct allorecognition exceeds the threshold for the number of TCR molecules needed to trigger T cell activation, even when the affinity of the TCR for allogeneic HLA is not very high. These two hypotheses outlined above are not mutually exclusive and a combination of both is the likely explanation for the strength of the direct alloimmune response.

INDIRECT ALLORECOGNITION

During the indirect pathway of allorecognition, recipient T cells recognise allogeneic HLA molecules (or any other polymorphic protein unique to the donor) after they have been processed and presented as antigenic peptides by recipient HLA molecules on the surface of a self-APC (see Figure 43.7). The indirect pathway is therefore analogous to the normal immune response to a foreign protein and the donor interstitial cell plays no role other than acting as a further source of allogeneic HLA molecules for uptake and processing by recipient APCs. Within a few days of transplantation, donor interstitial dendritic cells migrate from the donor organ into the recipient lymphoid tissue. This leaves the graft devoid of 'professional' APCs and considerably reduces the scope for further activation of T cells by the direct allorecognition pathway. It has been postulated that once donor dendritic cells have disappeared, the indirect allorecognition pathway assumes an increasingly important role in graft rejection. The indirect allorecognition pathway may be particularly important during chronic allograft rejection. As noted earlier, extracellular protein antigens are taken up by APCs via the endocytic pathway and the processed antigen is then presented to CD4 T cells by HLA class II molecules. HLA antigen shed from donor cells is treated the same way and therefore generates a predominantly CD4 T helper cell response. In contrast to T cells that recognise HLA directly, CD4 T cells activated by the indirect pathway are not able to directly damage the graft since they do not recognise intact donor HLA on target cells. They are able, however, to provide essential T cell help for CD8 T cells activated via the direct pathway. They can also provide cognate help for alloantibody and can mediate an intragraft DTH response.

Minor histocompatibility antigens

Although HLA antigens are the most important barriers to successful transplantation, peptides derived from other polymorphic proteins expressed in the donor can also act as transplant antigens. These antigens, known collectively as minor histocompatibility antigens, are presented by recipient APCs via the indirect pathway of allorecognition. Multiple minor histocompatibility antigens are likely to be present in all organ transplants and one of the best characterised in experimental mouse studies is the male or HY antigen. Although minor histocompatibility antigens are, as their name implies, weak transplant antigens, multiple minor antigens can exert a cumulative effect and they can cause rejection episodes when kidney transplants are performed between HLA identical sibs.

B cell allorecognition

In contrast to T cells that can only recognise HLA molecules as peptide fragments, B lymphocytes are able to recognise, through cell surface immunoglobulin receptors, conformational antigenic epitopes expressed by the intact allogeneic HLA molecule. Alloantibody production by B lymphocytes is critically dependent on the provision of T cell help. The B cell internalises allogeneic HLA molecules by receptor-mediated endocytosis and then processes and presents HLA-derived peptide in the peptide-binding groove of HLA class II on its cell surface. The processed alloantigen is recognised by T cells activated by the indirect pathway and these then deliver the essential help required for B cell activation and alloantibody production. T cell help for B cells takes the form of cognate receptor ligand interactions such as CD40 with CD154 and cytokines such as IL-4, IL-5 and TGF-β. Cytokines are important for promoting B cell maturation into antibody-producing plasma cells and for promoting the production of different antibody classes (IgM to IgG) and subclasses (IgG1, IgG2a and IgG2b). The antibody isotypes retain their original antigen specificity but display different effector functions. As will be outlined later, alloantibodies make an important contribution to graft rejection. They may cause hyperacute rejection of a kidney allograft in a sensitised recipient and they may contribute to both acute and chronic rejection in all types of organ allograft.

Lymphocyte activation, differentiation and expansion

During the first few days after transplantation, donor-derived dendritic cells migrate from the graft into the secondary lymphoid tissue of the recipient. Here they present intact donor alloantigen to naïve alloreactive T cells and B cells. In addition, intact alloantigen is released or shed from the graft as membrane fragments and circulates to the secondary lymphoid tissue where it is taken up by recipient APCs which then activate alloreactive lymphocytes. After T and B cells are activated they undergo a period of clonal expansion and differentiate into regulatory and effector cells. Circulating naïve T and B cells may also first encounter alloantigen within the graft rather than the peripheral lymphoid tissue and then undergo clonal expansion in situ. Activated T cells acquire the ability to produce a range of regulatory cytokines, upregulate or downregulate the expression of various cell surface molecules and develop the capacity to kill target cells by producing lytic granules. B cells differentiate, with the aid of T cells, into antibody-producing plasma cells. The differentiation and clonal expansion of lymphocytes is dependent on a range of cytokines, including IL-2, IL-4, IL-7, IL-9 and IL-15. These cytokines therefore play a critical role in allograft rejection.

Lymphocyte cell surface receptors for the different T cell growth factors comprise units of two or three polypeptide chains. All of the receptors share a common gamma chain. IL-2 and IL-15 are particularly important T cell growth factors and although their receptors each have a unique alpha chain, they also share the same IL-2β chain. Not surprisingly, therefore, IL-2 and IL-15 have a very similar biological function. There is considerable redundancy and functional overlap among all the T cell growth factor family of cytokines and this may explain why targeting an individual cytokine or its receptor (e.g. IL-2/IL-2 receptor) does not necessarily prevent graft rejection.

After activation, T cells may differentiate into at least three functionally distinct populations. CD8 T cells differentiate into cytotoxic effector cells. CD4 T cells, on the other hand, may differentiate into either Th1 or Th2 cells. These two T helper cell subsets are defined in terms of the pattern of cytokines they produce and have a counter-regulatory effect on each other that may polarise towards either a Th1- or a Th2-dominated response. Th1 cells produce IL-2 and IFN-γ and are responsible for directing cell-mediated immune responses whereas Th2 cells secrete IL-4, IL-5, IL-10 and IL-13 and are mainly responsible for promoting alloantibody responses. Through release of cytokines, CD4 T cells play a pivotal role in orchestrating the different cellular and humoral effector mechanisms that contribute to graft rejection (Figure 43.8).

As the alloimmune response develops there is progressive mononuclear cell infiltration and deposition of alloantibody within the graft. In unmodified animal models of transplantation, there is complete graft destruction by 7–10 days. Infiltration of the graft by mononuclear cells starts very soon after transplantation and is facilitated by tissue injury arising during the transplant procedure. An organ graft inevitably suffers a degree of ischaemic injury during transplantation and this contributes to the early inflammatory response. Activated macrophages that have been resident or recently recruited to the graft produce cytokines such as IL-1, IL-6 and IL-8. These cause upregulation of adhesion molecules such as P- and E-selectins, vascular addressins and intercellular adhesion molecules-1 and -2 (ICAM-1 and ICAM-2) on the endothelial cell surface and facilitate binding of lymphocytes that express complementary adhesion molecules. Over the course of the next few days, increasing numbers of lymphocytes home to the graft where, after binding to endothelial cells, they migrate into the graft tissue under the control of chemokines such as IL-8, macrophage inflammatory protein (MIP), RANTES and macrophage chemoattractant protein-1 (MCP-1).

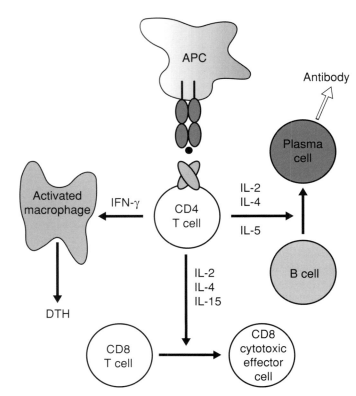

Figure 43.8 Central role of the CD4 T helper cell in orchestrating allograft rejection. After activation the CD4 T cell produces a range of cytokines that promote the development of DTH, CD8 cytotoxic effector cells and antibody.

Intragraft effector mechanisms

Most of the different cellular and humoral effector mechanisms that the immune system has evolved to protect against invading pathogens can play a role in allograft rejection. As already noted, alloantibodies play an important role in tissue destruction, especially in the sensitised recipient. After binding to target antigens within the graft vasculature, antibodies may induce target cell damage by a variety of mechanisms. Bound antibody may activate the complement cascade via the classic pathway, culminating in formation of membrane attack complexes and cell injury or death. Antibody may also cause cell damage indirectly by guiding non-specific effector cells such as macrophages and non-specific cytotoxic cells onto target cells in the graft. Finally, alloantibody may, through cross-linking cell surface molecules on endothelial cells, cause endothelial cell activation leading to release of cytokines and growth factors.

Specific cytotoxic CD8 T cells recognising donor HLA class I antigens are able to kill target cells by release of lytic enzymes such as perforins and granzymes, by triggering the Fas death pathway and through release of the proinflammatory cytokines such as tumour necrosis factor alpha (TNF-α). CD4 and CD8 T cells are able to initiate a DTH response through release of proinflammatory cytokines, such as IFN-γ, leading to recruitment and activation of macrophages. Activated macrophages function as non-specific effector cells by releasing a wide range of noxious agents. These include proinflammatory cytokines such as TNF-α, enzymes such as lysozyme and hydrolase and oxygen derivatives such as hydrogen peroxide and nitric oxide. Activated eosinophils may also contribute to allograft rejection by releasing a range of toxic molecules, enzymes, cytokines and lipid mediators. Finally, natural killer (NK) cells may play a role through release of IFN-γ and through cell-mediated killing. There is considerable redundancy in the effector mechanisms responsible for allograft rejection and attempts to prevent rejection are most likely to be effective if they disrupt the alloimmune response at the level of the T cell rather than at the level of the effector mechanisms themselves.

Patterns of allograft rejection

Three distinct patterns of allograft rejection are recognised. These occur at different times after transplantation and each has a different histopathological appearance.

Hyperacute rejection

This occurs within minutes or hours of transplantation and is due to the presence of preformed antibodies in the recipient. These bind to the vascular endothelium of the graft as soon as it is reperfused with recipient blood. Antibody binding activates complement and also causes type I activation of the vascular endothelium. The net effect is rapid and extensive intravascular thrombosis and irreversible loss of graft function. Hyperacute rejection occurs when an organ is transplanted into a blood group-incompatible recipient and it is essential for all types of organ transplant to ensure ABO compatibility. Hyperacute rejection also occurs when a recipient has preformed cytotoxic alloantibodies directed against HLA class I expressed by the graft. Anti-HLA antibodies may arise following allogeneic blood transfusion, pregnancy or a previous organ transplant. For unknown reasons, kidney allografts are more vulnerable to hyperacute rejection than other types of solid organ transplant whereas liver transplants are relatively resistant. In clinical practice, hyperacute rejection of kidney allografts can be avoided completely by performing a pretransplant cross-match test to make sure that there are no anti-donor HLA alloantibodies present.

Acute rejection

Acute rejection occurs within days or weeks of transplantation and it is not commonly encountered beyond the first six months. It is generally attributed to cellular effector mechanisms although alloantibody may also play an important role. When rejection occurs within the first week it is known as accelerated acute rejection and is a consequence of previous sensitisation to HLA antigens. Acute rejection is usually accompanied by progressive mononuclear cell infiltration of the graft (Figure 43.9). The infiltrate is heterogeneous in nature and includes large numbers of T

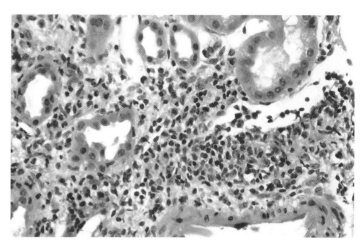

Figure 43.9 Acute renal allograft rejection. There is a heavy interstitial infiltrate of mononuclear cells associated with inflammation of the renal tubules.

cells, B cells, activated macrophages and NK cells. Alloantibody deposition may also occur. Initially the cellular infiltrate is predominantly perivascular in distribution but soon it becomes distributed throughout the interstitium of the graft and is associated with a variable degree of graft cell injury. In around 10–20% of cases, infiltration and damage of the graft vasculature is a dominant feature and this is known as acute vascular rejection. Severe acute rejection is characterised by interstitial haemorrhage, necrosis and eventually thrombosis and irreversible graft destruction. The graft becomes swollen and haemorrhagic and may even rupture.

In the era before cyclosporin, acute rejection used to be accompanied by pyrexia together with swelling and tenderness of the graft and was a common cause of graft loss. Episodes of acute rejection are still common (occurring in 25–40% of transplants). However, they are not usually associated with such florid clinical signs and in most cases are reversible with supplementary immunosuppressive therapy. Few grafts (<10%) are now lost through acute rejection.

Chronic rejection

Chronic rejection usually occurs beyond the first six months and is the major cause of long-term graft failure. The pathophysiology of chronic rejection is less well understood than that of hyperacute and acute rejection. Alloantigen-dependent effector mechanisms undoubtedly play a key role in chronic rejection but alloantigen-independent factors are also important. The characteristic histological feature of chronic rejection is progressive myointimal proliferation within the arteries of the graft leading to ischaemia, fibrosis and deterioration in graft function (Figure 43.10). Both alloantibodies and cellular effector mechanisms have been shown to trigger chronic rejection and the arterial pathology observed likely represents the stereotypical remodelling response of the arterial tree to injury.

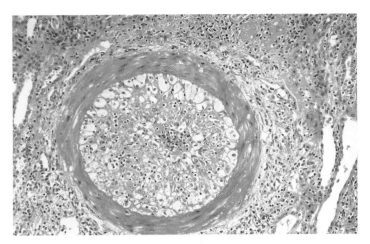

Figure 43.10 Chronic renal allograft rejection. The medium-sized artery shows gross myointimal proliferation causing concentric narrowing and almost complete obliteration of the lumen.

Although chronic rejection occurs months and years after transplantation it is clear that events occurring during the peri-transplant period may have a major influence. In particular, factors that produce early graft injury appear to exacerbate chronic rejection. A number of risk factors for the development of chronic rejection have been identified. Of these, previous episodes of acute rejection that are either multiple or resistant to steroid therapy are the most important. Other risk factors are poor HLA matching, long cold ischaemic time, inadequate levels of immunosuppression and CMV infection. Unlike acute rejection, chronic rejection is largely resistant to treatment with available immunosuppressive therapy.

THE HISTOCOMPATIBILITY LABORATORY

The histocompatibility laboratory has two important roles in clinical transplantation. First, and perhaps most important, the sera of potential transplant recipients are screened for the presence of antibodies which would be detrimental to graft survival. Second, HLA typing of donors and recipients is performed so that matching can be undertaken to reduce the risk of graft loss from rejection. These laboratory investigations are of most relevance to kidney transplantation. In the UK, the histocompatibility laboratory is also responsible for establishing, by means of genetic tests based on DNA variations, the genetic relationship between a proposed living donor and their potential recipient as required by the Human Organ Transplants Regulations 1998.

Antibody screening

Patients awaiting organ transplantation may have developed antibodies to HLA through blood transfusion, pregnancy or a previous organ transplant. In the case of kidney transplantation it is important that a recipient is not given a kidney bearing HLA antigens against which they have developed antibodies. If transplantation were to proceed in the presence of preformed anti-HLA antibodies it would likely result in hyperacute rejection and immediate graft loss. Other types of solid organ transplant are less susceptible to hyperacute rejection but may instead undergo accelerated acute rejection. Liver transplantation can be performed safely in the presence of preformed anti-donor HLA antibodies without hyperacute or accelerated rejection but there may be a detrimental effect on long-term graft survival.

The sera of patients on the waiting list for renal transplantation is routinely screened to determine the presence and specificity of HLA antibodies. Screening of sera should be undertaken before activation on the transplant waiting list and then periodically thereafter. It can be performed in a variety of ways. Commonly, the patients' sera are screened in a microlymphocytotoxicity test using lymphocyte target cells obtained from an HLA-typed panel of donors carefully chosen to represent a wide range of the more commonly encountered HLA antigens. Typically the extent to which a patient is sensitised to HLA is expressed as the percentage of the donor panel against which they have cross-reactive antibodies, so-called 'panel reactivity'. Highly sensitised patients are arbitrarily defined as those who react with more than 85% of the panel cells. A range of commercial assays is now also available for screening sera for the presence of HLA antibodies. These are in widespread use and employ purified HLA class I antigens bound to either microtitre plates or microbeads and rely on ELISA and flow cytometry, respectively, to detect the presence of bound HLA antibody.

When a prospective cadaver or living donor has been identified for a kidney recipient, a lymphocyte cross-match test is routinely performed to ensure the absence of harmful anti-HLA antibodies. In this assay, the most recent recipient serum (along with historical sera) is tested against donor lymphocyte target cells. For many years, all laboratories undertook this analysis using a complement-dependent microlymphocytotoxicity assay in which donor lymphocytes are incubated with recipient sera in the presence of rabbit complement. Antibody binding causes target cell lysis that is detected by microscopy using a dye to distinguish between living and dead target cells. Separated T and B lymphocytes are used as targets in order to detect the presence of class I and class II antibodies respectively. A positive T cell cross-match is a contraindication to renal transplantation. A negative T, positive B cell cross-match is also associated with poor renal allograft outcome if it is due to the presence of anti-HLA IgG antibodies. Often, however, a positive B cell cross-match test arises because of the presence of autoreactive antibodies and these are not detrimental to graft outcome. Since autoantibodies are mostly of the IgM class they can be inactivated by treating the sera with a reducing agent such as dithiothreitol (DTT), thereby allowing a distinction to be made between IgG class anti-HLA antibodies. In sensitised patients, the levels of HLA antibodies may vary over time. So long as a cross-match test using the most recent pretransplant serum sample is negative, renal transplantation can usually be undertaken safely even when a historical serum sample gives a positive cross-match. Retransplantation is, however, not normally advisable under such circumstances.

Although some laboratories still use the lymphocytotoxic cross-match test, many now use the more sensitive flow cytometric cross-match instead. In this test, recipient antibodies that bind to donor lymphocytes are detected by adding a fluorescent anti-human IgG antibody and then identifying labelled cells by passage through a flow cytometer. Additional staining can readily identify T and B cells, thereby avoiding the need to physically separate them in order to distinguish HLA class I from HLA class II antibodies.

HLA typing

HLA typing used to be undertaken exclusively by serological analysis using the complement-dependent microlymphocytotoxicity test and some centres still use this approach. Carefully selected panels of well-characterised antisera from multiparous women who have developed antibodies against paternal HLA antigens together with monoclonal antibodies directed against defined HLA specificities are used to prepare Terasaki microtitre trays. These are then frozen until required. Serological typing is usually performed on lymphocytes prepared from a sample of peripheral blood. Purified lymphocytes are added to thawed microtitre trays and rabbit complement is added. After incubation an intravital dye is added and the trays are examined by an inverted microscope to determine whether cells in a particular well have undergone lysis, indicating that they have bound antisera against a particular HLA specificity.

The majority of histocompatibility laboratories now perform HLA typing by molecular techniques although a minority still rely on serological methods to type HLA class I. Molecular typing has clear advantages over serological typing. It is usually performed on genomic DNA isolated from peripheral blood cells and because viable cells are not required, patient samples are easier to transport and to store. The oligonucleotide primers used for molecular typing are standard from laboratory to laboratory and can be readily synthesised on demand. Finally, molecular typing provides a much greater resolution of HLA polymorphism than serological analysis and allows identification of HLA specificities that cannot otherwise be detected.

The molecular typing procedures commonly used are all based on the amplification of genomic DNA using specific oligonucleotide primers in the polymerase chain reaction (PCR). There are a number of different approaches. In one approach (PCR-SSOP), DNA encoding the HLA locus of interest is amplified by PCR and the particular HLA allele is then identified by probing the PCR product with a series of labelled sequence-specific oligonucleotide probes (SSOP). Sequence-based typing (SBT) is an alternative approach where PCR is first used to produce a product encompassing the particular HLA allele of interest. The nucleotide sequence of the amplified PCR product is then determined using a DNA sequencer and matched to the known HLA

sequences to determine the HLA allotype. A third approach, PCR-SSP, uses a panel of sequence-specific primers (SSP) designed to amplify particular HLA alleles or groups of alleles in the PCR. The PCR products generated are subjected to gel electrophoresis and the resulting pattern reveals the HLA type.

Attempts to reduce the HLA mismatch between organ donor and recipient are made only for kidney and not for other types of solid organ transplant. It is not practicable for heart transplants and in the case of liver transplants appears to offer no immunological advantage.

In the context of kidney transplantation, HLA typing allows detection of HLA antigens in the donor against which a recipient may be sensitised and it allows the opportunity to reduce the mismatch when allocating a cadaveric kidney for transplantation. Mismatches for common HLA antigens should when possible be avoided, especially in young patients, because if the recipient becomes sensitised and graft failure occurs, retransplantation will be made more difficult because of antibodies to a high proportion of potential donors. There is a progressive increase in renal allograft survival as the HLA-A, -B, -DR MM grade decreases from 6 to 0. However, a balance between the practicalities and the benefits of HLA matching is needed. In the USA many centres do not attempt to match cadaveric kidneys for HLA antigens and rely on the use of additional immunosuppression to overcome increased rejection in poorly matched grafts. In the UK an attempt is made to obtain a favourable match, i.e. 0 MM at HLA-DR and no more than 1 MM at HLA-A and/ or -B.

IMMUNOSUPPRESSIVE THERAPY

Historical perspective

The successful development of organ transplantation was to a large extent dictated by developments in immunosuppressive therapy and an understanding of the history of immunosuppression provides a valuable perspective on modern immunosuppressive regimens. Early attempts to prevent rejection of kidney allografts used whole-body irradiation but with few successes and considerable side effects. A breakthrough in the search for chemical agents that could replace irradiation came in 1959 when Schwartz and Damashek found that non-myeloablative doses of 6-mercaptopurine, an anti-cancer drug, were immunosuppressive. Azathioprine, an analogue of 6-mercaptopurine that could be given orally, was then shown by Calne and Murray in Boston to prevent rejection of canine renal allografts. Azathioprine was, when used alone, less effective at preventing renal allograft rejection in humans but it was soon realised that its efficacy improved when it was combined with steroids in the form of prednisone. The combination of azathioprine and steroids gave a one-year renal allograft survival rate of 65–75% and became, for the next 20 years, the standard immunosuppressive regimen for renal transplantation. In 1966, Starzl and colleagues in Denver described the use of polyclonal anti-lymphocyte serum (ALS) as an adjuvant to azathioprine and steroids. ALS was a valuable addition to existing therapy and provided, when necessary, a means for increasing the level of immunosuppression after renal transplantation. ALS also contributed to the early successes in heart and liver transplantation. In the early 1980s the first monoclonal antibody to be used in transplantation was introduced. This was a mouse antibody (OKT3) directed against the human CD3 molecule found on the surface of T cells and it provided a potent alternative to anti-lymphocyte serum for induction therapy and treatment of steroid-resistant rejection.

The introduction of cyclosporin (cyclosporin A) in the early 1980s was the most significant development since the discovery of azathioprine. Cyclosporin was first discovered during routine screening of fungal extracts at the Sandoz laboratories in Basle and was shown there by Jean Borrel to have immunosuppressive properties. Roy Calne, David White and colleagues in Cambridge, UK, first demonstrated the potential of the new compound as an immunosuppressive agent for organ transplantation and cyclosporin quickly became the mainstay of immunosuppressive regimens around the world. In the UK it was most often used alongside azathioprine and steroids (triple therapy) whereas in North America either ALS or OKT3 was often added as well (quadruple therapy). The use of cyclosporin not only led to a significant improvement in graft survival after kidney transplantation but also facilitated the widespread introduction of heart and liver transplantation.

Towards the end of the 1980s Japanese scientists discovered another fungal metabolite with potent immunosuppressive activity. The new agent, designated FK-506 and later named tacrolimus, was, like cyclosporin, a calcineurin inhibitor and was soon shown by Starzl and colleagues in Pittsburgh to be an acceptable alternative to cyclosporin for kidney and liver transplantation. Some centres, particularly those undertaking liver transplantation, chose to use tacrolimus in preference to cyclosporin-based regimens on account of its potency. The availability of tacrolimus also facilitated early success with small bowel transplantation.

During the late 1990s, the immunosuppressive armamentarium was strengthened further by the addition of several new agents. Mycophenolate mofetil (MMF) was introduced as a more effective alternative to azathioprine after it had been shown to reduce the number of acute rejection episodes when used along with cyclosporin and steroids after kidney transplantation. It quickly replaced azathioprine in most North American centres and many European transplant units. Two new anti-CD25 monoclonal antibodies (a chimaeric and a humanised antibody) were also licensed for use as induction agents for kidney transplantation after they had been shown to reduce the incidence of acute rejection and are in widespread use. Finally, sirolimus, another potent immunosuppressive agent with a mode of action distinct from that of cyclosporin and tacrolimus, was recently licensed for use in kidney transplantation after it too had been shown to reduce the incidence of acute rejection. A number of other new chemical and biological agents are currently undergoing clinical evaluation and when licensed will further increase the choice of immunosuppressive agents for use in organ transplantation.

Immunosuppressive agents

Pharmacological agents

Calcineurin antagonists

A calcineurin antagonist, in the form of either cyclosporin (Cyclosporin A, Neoral®) or tacrolimus (FK-506, Prograf®), is the mainstay of most immunosuppressive regimens for organ transplantation. The two calcineurin antagonists share many similarities but there are also important differences.

Although cyclosporin and tacrolimus are structurally distinct they have a similar mode of action and their efficacy in preventing allograft rejection is broadly the same. They both exert their principal immunosuppressive effect by inhibiting the activity of the enzyme calcineurin in T lymphocytes, thereby blocking antigen-specific T cell activation (Figure 43.11). After entry into the cytoplasm of the T cell, the drugs bind to their specific receptors or immunophilins. Cyclosporin binds to cyclophilin whereas tacrolimus binds to FK-binding protein (FKBP). The resulting drug/immunophilin complex then binds to and inhibits calcineurin, a calcium/calmodulin-dependent phosphatase. The normal function of calcineurin is to dephosphorylate the cytoplasmic subunit of nuclear factor of activated T lymphocytes (NFAT) after activation of the T cell receptor. This then allows cytoplasmic NFAT to translocate to the nucleus of the cell where it would normally increase transcription of IL-2 and other cytokine genes. By preventing nuclear translocation of NFAT, cyclosporin and tacrolimus block the transcription of key cytokine genes and prevent T cell activation and proliferation.

Cyclosporin was originally produced as an olive oil-based formulation (Sandimmune®) that was dependent on bile salts for absorption and displayed poor and unpredictable bio-availability. A new microemulsion formulation (Neoral®) with improved oral bioavailability, less dependence on bile for absorption and reduced pharmacokinetic variability was introduced in 1995 and has now largely replaced the original formulation. Tacrolimus is well absorbed and absorption is not dependent on bile salts. The mean oral bio-availability is similar to that for cyclosporin at around 30% and, like cyclosporin, there is considerable variability in bio-availability between and within patients.

Cyclosporin and tacrolimus are both metabolised in the liver and gastrointestinal mucosa by the cytochrome P450 (CYP3A4) enzyme system and the metabolites are excreted in the bile. The half-life of the parent compounds is 8–12 hours. Any drugs that induce, inhibit or compete for metabolism by the CYP3A system will have clinically important interactions with cyclosporin and tacrolimus. Cyclosporin and tacrolimus are given in twice-daily doses 12 hours apart. The immunosuppressive activity of the

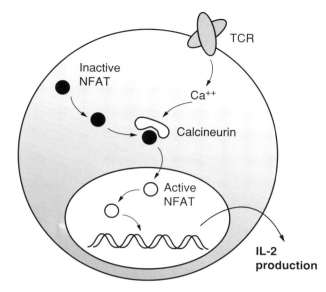

(A) Normal T cell activation

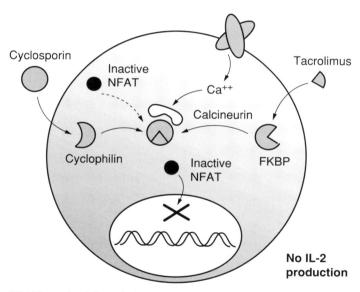

(B) Effect of calcineurin blockade

Figure 43.11 Calcineurin blockade.

agents is related to their blood levels and it is necessary to monitor these on a regular basis after transplantation in order to ensure optimal therapy and avoid potential side effects. In the case of tacrolimus, the trough level (the drug level immediately prior to the next dose) is a good guide to drug exposure. The trough level of cyclosporin is also frequently used as a guide to drug exposure but some units measure the drug level two hours post-dose (C2 level) instead on the grounds that this is a better indicator of cyclosporin exposure.

Cyclosporin and tacrolimus share several agent-specific side effects but there are also differences in their side-effect profiles. Both agents are nephrotoxic, one of their most serious side effects,

and may cause hypertension. Cyclosporin may cause gingival hyperplasia and hirsutism and whilst tacrolimus is largely free from cosmetic side effects, it is more likely to cause post-transplant diabetes and neurotoxicity.

Corticosteroids

Glucocorticoids have a range of anti-inflammatory and immuno-suppressive properties and are used extensively as prophylaxis against rejection as well as to treat acute rejection episodes. Most European units prefer to use prednisolone whereas many North American units prefer the 11-keto analogue prednisone. Both preparations have good oral bio-availability. Glucocorticoids enter the cell and bind to intracytoplasmic glucocorticoid receptors. The resulting complexes translocate to the cell nucleus of T cells and macrophages. Here they interact with various gluco-corticoid response elements – specific DNA sequences - which modulate the transcription of a wide range of genes. In addition, glucocorticoids mediate indirect effects through inhibition of NFκB. Through these pathways, glucocorticoids act at multiple levels of the immune response. They inhibit the production of several proinflammatory cytokines (including IL-1, IL-2, IL-6 and TNF-α and interferon-γ), impair the function of macrophages and monocytes, interfere with T cell activation and influence lymphocyte recirculation. The side effects of steroids are well known and include hypertension, osteoporosis, diabetes mellitus, dyslipidaemia, peptic ulceration and cushingoid features.

Antiproliferative agents

Most immunosuppressive regimens include either azathioprine (Imuran®) or mycophenolate mofetil (MMF, CellCept®) as a maintenance drug. Until recently azathioprine was the only agent in widespread use. It is an inactive prodrug which after ingestion is rapidly absorbed and converted in the liver to 6-mercapto-urine, a purine analogue. Azathioprine interferes with purine synthesis and inhibits the proliferation of both T and B cells. Its principal side effects arise from marrow suppression, resulting in thrombocytopenia and pancytopenia. The blood count should be monitored carefully and the dose of azathioprine adjusted according to the result. Reversible cholestasis and other gastrointestinal symptoms may also occur with azathioprine. Azathioprine is metabolised by xanthine oxidase. Since allopurinol inhibits this enzyme it markedly increases the bio-availability of azathioprine and increases toxicity.

MMF is the ester prodrug of mycophenolic acid (MPA) and in many centres has replaced azathioprine since it is more effective in reducing acute rejection episodes. The mofetil ester of MPA serves to increase stability and improve bioavailability. After ingestion, MMF is rapidly absorbed and converted to its active form. MPA is a non-competitive and reversible inhibitor of the enzyme inosine monophosphate dehydrogenase (IMPDH). This enzyme is a rate-limiting step in the *de novo* synthesis of guanosine nucleotides from inosine. Lymphocytes rely on *de novo* purine synthesis to a greater extent than other cell types because they lack the so-called 'salvage pathway' for purine synthesis. Consequently MPA selectively inhibits the proliferation of both T and B cells. It also inhibits proliferation of arterial smooth muscle cells *in vitro* and this has given rise to hope that it might limit the development of chronic allograft rejection. The side effects of MMF include gastrointestinal symptoms, leucopenia and thrombocytopenia. An enteric-coated form of MMF is in development and may reduce the gastrointestinal side effects sometimes seen with MMF.

Sirolimus

Sirolimus (Rapamycin, Rapamune®) is a macrolide produced by the bacterium *Streptomyces hygroscopis*. It is similar in structure to tacrolimus and binds within lymphocytes to the same cytosolic receptor FKBP-12. Unlike tacrolimus, however, sirolimus is not a calcineurin inhibitor and has little effect on cytokine production. Rapamycin exerts its immunosuppressive effects by inhibiting an enzyme known as mTOR (mammalian target of rapamycin). This intracellular kinase has an important influence on the activity of a number of downstream signalling molecules, including mitogen-activated protein kinase (MAPK). By interfering with signal transduction from the IL-2 receptor and other cytokine receptors, the net effect of tacrolimus is to prevent cytokine-dependent lymphocyte proliferation blocking progression of the cell cycle from the G1 to S phase.

Even though rapamycin and tacrolimus both bind to FKBP-12 the levels are not saturating and hence both sirolimus and tacrolimus can be used together if required. In contrast to the calcineurin inhibitors, sirolimus is not nephrotoxic and does not cause hypertension. Reported side effects include hypercholesterolaemia, hypertriglyceridaemia, thrombocytopenia, impaired wound healing and bone pain. An analogue of sirolimus called SDZ RAD with similar immunosuppressive properties is currently undergoing clinical development.

New pharmacological agents in development

A number of novel small molecule immunosuppressive agents are at various stages of clinical development and some are likely to be licensed for clinical use over the next few years. Promising new agents include FTY720 and the leflunomide analogues. FTY720 is a synthetic analogue of myriocin, a fungal metabolite produced by *Isaria sinclarii*. It is of particular interest because it has a completely different mode of action to existing immunosuppressive agents. FTY720 alters the homing pattern of lymphocytes, diverting them from the peripheral blood into lymph nodes and Peyer's patches. Phase three studies of FTY720 in renal transplantation are currently in progress. Leflunomide, along with other members of the malononitrilamide family, is a potent immunosuppressive agent that affects both T and B cell function. The malononitrilamides block division of activated lymphocytes by inhibiting the enzyme dihydro-orotate dehydrogenase and they also inhibit tyrosine kinase activity. Leflunomide has an excessively long half-life but other family members may prove useful in transplantation.

Biological agents

A number of antibody preparations are available for use as induction agents and to treat rejection episodes. They are only used for limited treatment periods and are unsuitable, therefore, for maintenance immunosuppression.

Polyclonal anti-lymphocyte antibodies

These are produced by immunising animals (horses or rabbits) with human lymphocytes or thymocytes. The gammaglobulin fraction of the serum is purified to yield an antibody preparation directed against a range of lymphocyte cell surface molecules. Polyclonal antibodies are given daily over several days and cause marked depletion of circulating lymphocytes. They commonly cause fever and rigors when first given and occasionally result in anaphylaxis.

OKT3 (Orthoclone®, Muromonab-CD3)

OKT3 is a mouse IgG2a monoclonal antibody directed against the CD3 component of the T cell receptor complex. The antibody binds to T cells, causing rapid depletion of lymphocytes from the peripheral blood. Residual T cells have impaired function because their CD3 complex has either been modulated from the cell surface or is blocked by persistent antibody coating. OKT3 is a potent immunosuppressive agent. When first administered it causes fever, rigors, tachycardia and bronchospasm and in the presence of fluid overload it may cause life-threatening pulmonary oedema. These effects are thought to be due to cytokine release from T cells (cytokine release syndrome) and are lessened by giving an intravenous bolus of methylpredisolone with the first dose. OKT3 may provoke the development of neutralising human anti-mouse antibodies that limit the efficacy of subsequent treatment.

IL-2 receptor antibodies

Two monoclonal antibodies directed against the alpha chain of the high affinity IL-2 receptor (CD25) are now commercially available. They are both mouse anti-human antibodies that have been genetically engineered to make them less immunogenic. Basiliximab (Simulect®) is a 'chimaeric' antibody in which only the variable region of the antibody is of murine origin and the constant region is of human origin. Daclizumab (Zenopax®) is a 'humanised' antibody in which only the antigen-combining site of the immunoglobulin molecule encoded by the six complementarity-determining regions is of murine origin and the remainder is human. Because the alpha chain of the IL-2R is only expressed after antigen-specific T cell activation, anti–CD25 antibody therapy specifically targets activated lymphocytes (Figure 43.12). Anti–CD25 monoclonal antibodies reduce the risk of acute rejection when given as induction therapy at the time of renal transplantation and they appear to be free from unwanted side effects.

Biological agents in development

A variety of engineered antibodies and fusion proteins directed against key cell surface molecules are under development. These include antibodies directed against molecules such as CD4, CD2 and ICAM-1. There is also intense interest in agents that block the delivery of co-stimulatory activity to lymphocytes through the CD40 / CD40L and the CD28 / B7 pathways and these are entering clinical trial.

Immunosuppressive regimens

Immunosuppressive regimens vary between transplant centres but there are a number of important general principles. The aim in all

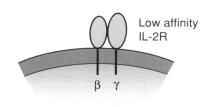

(A) Naive T cell

Low affinity IL-2R

β γ

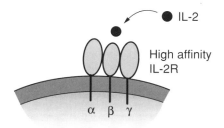

IL-2

High affinity IL-2R

α β γ

(B) Activated T cell

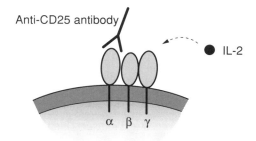

Anti-CD25 antibody

IL-2

α β γ

(C) Blockade by anti-CD25 antibody

Figure 43.12 Anti-CD25 antibody blockade.

cases is to provide a level of immunosuppression that is sufficient to prevent allograft rejection. However, excessive immunosuppression should be avoided so as to minimise the risks of infection and malignancy that result from non-specific depression of the immune system. The levels of immunosuppression required after transplantation are highest during the first few weeks when the risk of acute rejection is greatest. Thereafter the level of immunosuppression can be gradually reduced but immunosuppression cannot be stopped completely even after many years without risking graft loss from rejection. It is likely that occasional patients could tolerate very low levels or even no immunosuppression without rejecting their graft but there is no reliable way to identify such patients at the present time.

Immunosuppressive regimens are broadly similar for kidney, heart, liver, pancreas and lung transplantation although there is a tendency to give more immunosuppression after thoracic organ transplantation since graft rejection is life threatening. Certain groups of recipients are known to be at greater risk of graft loss from rejection, e.g. recipients who are highly sensitised and are receiving a second or third graft. Such patients may also benefit from higher levels of immunosuppression. Now that there is a widening choice of immunosuppressive agents, the concept of tailoring particular immunosuppressive regimens to individual patients is becoming common.

Prophylaxis of rejection

Most regimens are based on cyclosporin or tacrolimus, given along with an anti–proliferative agent (azathioprine or MMF) and steroids. This combination is known as triple therapy. There is not a clear consensus on whether cyclosporin or tacrolimus is superior. Tacrolimus appears to be a more potent agent than cyclosporin although this is not universally accepted. The choice between the two agents is largely dependent on preference of the unit and the need to avoid agent-specific side effects in a particular category of recipient. For recipients of thoracic organ transplants and for renal allograft recipients judged to be at increased risk of rejection it is common to also include induction therapy using either a polyclonal anti-lymphocyte antibody or anti-CD3 monoclonal antibody (quadruple therapy). The anti-CD25 monoclonal antibodies are also being increasingly used as a standard addition to triple therapy. At the other end of the scale some renal transplant units use dual therapy in the form of a calcineurin antagonist and either an anti-proliferative agent or steroids.

Long-term maintenance immunosuppression is variable. Many centres continue with triple therapy but some reduce and attempt to withdraw steroids completely after several months. The occasional centre attempts to maintain selected recipients on monotherapy with a calcineurin antagonist whereas others attempt to withdraw calcineurin antagonists in patients who have stable long-term graft function, leaving them on an anti-proliferative agent and steroids.

The role of rapamycin in immunosuppressive regimens is not yet clear. It is undoubtedly a potent immunosuppressive agent and can be used to replace a calcineurin antagonist or it can be used effectively alongside cyclosporin and possibly tacrolimus.

Treatment of acute rejection

Acute rejection episodes are treated initially with a course of high-dose corticosteroids given either orally or intravenously over a 3–7 day period. In most cases this will reverse rejection but steroid-resistant and recurrent episodes of acute rejection can be treated with either a polyclonal anti-lymphocyte preparation or anti-CD3 monoclonal antibody.

Infection

All of the immunosuppressive agents used in transplantation cause a non-specific reduction in immunity and leave the recipient at increased risk from infection. Recipients are at particular risk from opportunistic infection, especially viral and fungal infections where protection from infection depends on intact cell-mediated immunity. The overall risk of infection is related to the degree of immunosuppression but is also determined by other factors like the type of transplant, whether the recipient has latent infection and their age, general health and immunological memory of previous exposure to infectious agents. All patients should be carefully screened for infection prior to transplantation and, wherever feasible, infections identified should be eradicated before the transplant procedure is undertaken.

Early recognition together with prompt and aggressive treatment of infection are paramount after transplantation. It is important to remember that the symptoms and signs of infection are often masked or atypical and that infection may be at an advanced stage when diagnosed. It is also important to bear in mind that vaccines may be less effective in patients taking immunosuppressive agents. When possible, pretransplant vaccination is recommended. Non-live vaccines rather than live attenuated vaccines should be given to patients taking immunosuppressive therapy.

Bacterial infections

Transplant recipients are at increased risk from the common types of bacterial infections seen after all forms of major surgery. These include wound infection, intra-abdominal or intra-thoracic abscess, postoperative chest infection and urinary tract infections. The organisms responsible are those that commonly cause infection in other types of surgical patient undergoing major surgery. Bacterial infections usually occur during the first few days and weeks after transplantation. They are more common in those patients who are critically ill before their transplant operation, especially if they are in the intensive care unit with multiple invasive lines and catheters *in situ*. Bacterial infections are also more common in recipients who have a long or complicated postoperative course. It is routine

practice to give broad-spectrum antibiotics at the time of organ transplantation to reduce the risk of wound infection and in case there is bacterial contamination of the graft either because of infection in the donor or bacterial contamination during organ procurement and storage prior to transplantation. Acute bacterial infections may be life threatening in the immunosuppressed patient and when identified should be treated aggressively.

Transplant recipients are at increased risk of tuberculosis and chemoprophylaxis should be given to prevent reactivation of disease in those patients who have a past history of tuberculosis or a history of recent exposure. Presentation of tuberculosis may be atypical and for all patients, a high index of suspicion and prompt treatment of suspected tuberculosis are important.

Viral infections

Cytomegalovirus (CMV)

CMV (human herpes virus 5) is one of the most important causes of infection in transplant recipients. Symptomatic CMV disease occurs in up to one-third of recipients of a solid organ and causes considerable morbidity. Before the advent of effective antiviral therapy there was also an appreciable mortality from CMV disease.

CMV is a member of the herpes group of viruses and is widely prevalent in the general population. Around 50% of normal young adults have antibodies to CMV, indicating previous exposure to the virus, and this figure increases progressively with age. The virus is transmitted by direct person-to-person contact through close exposure to body secretions. In a healthy individual with a normal immune system, primary CMV infection is usually subclinical although fever and malaise may sometimes occur. In the presence of immunosuppressive therapy CMV infection can cause a severe and life-threatening disease. CMV disease, as opposed to CMV infection, implies symptomatic or tissue-invasive CMV. Non-specific symptoms including fever, malaise and myalgia are common along with leucopenia, thrombocytopenia and elevated liver enzymes. Depending on the target organ, CMV infection may produce pneumonitis, haemorrhagic gastroenteritis, hepatitis, renal inflammation myocarditis, pancreatitis, retinitis or encephalitis. Infection with CMV may also further reduce cell-mediated immunity and predispose to co-infection with other opportunistic viruses and fungi. The immunological derangement resulting from CMV disease may also be associated with an increased risk of both acute and chronic allograft rejection although this is controversial.

CMV disease after transplantation is most common between one and six months. It may result from a primary infection with the virus in a previously uninfected recipient or it may arise instead from either reactivation of latent virus or reinfection with a different strain of CMV in a previously infected recipient. Recipients who are CMV seronegative at the time of transplantation are most at risk of CMV disease, especially if they receive an organ from a CMV-seropositive donor, since this is an effective vehicle for transmitting CMV. Primary CMV infection usually presents earlier and is more likely to result in severe disease than CMV reactivation or reinfection. Blood transfusion used to be a common means for transmitting CMV but this is no longer a major problem now that filtered or leucodepleted blood is used routinely.

A range of laboratory methods is available for making a diagnosis of CMV infection and CMV disease. Serology is used to determine previous exposure to CMV in the donor and recipient before transplantation but is of only limited value in the diagnosis of acute infection where the antibody response may be slow to develop. Assays for CMV antigen in cultures of blood and tissue samples are commonly used and the level of CMV antigenaemia is a useful marker of disease progression. Identification and quantification of CMV DNA in blood by PCR are also being used increasingly.

Finally, histological examination of tissue biopsy for viral inclusion bodies and CMV antigen may be useful in the diagnosis of invasive CMV infection.

Adopting a CMV matching policy so that high-risk CMV-seronegative recipients only received organs from CMV-seronegative donors would reduce the incidence of CMV infection in this high-risk group but this approach is seldom adopted because of practical constraints. Vaccination of CMV-seronegative patients prior to transplantation is also an attractive concept but available vaccines have limited efficacy. Passive immunoprophylaxis using hyperimmune globulin provides protection from severe CMV disease and is used in some renal transplant centres. However, most centres use anti-viral agents rather than immunoglobulin as prophylaxis against CMV. These include oral aciclovir, valacyclovir (the L-valine ester of aciclovir) and ganciclovir as well as intravenous ganciclovir. The disadvantage of prophylaxis is that it is expensive, causes side effects and is not always completely effective.

There are two approaches to prophylaxis. The first, known as 'conventional prophylaxis', is to give oral prophylaxis to all recipients or to high-risk recipients. The latter would include CMV-seronegative recipients of a CMV-seropositive organ and recipients treated with anti-lymphocyte antibody preparations. Potential disadvantages are that prophylaxis may merely delay onset of CMV disease until completion of prophylaxis and that it may favour the development of resistant strains of CMV. The second approach, known as 'preemptive prophylaxis', is to monitor recipients regularly, for example by measuring CMV antigenaemia, and to treat them with intravenous ganciclovir when it is predicted they will develop CMV disease. There is, however, no clear agreement on the best way to monitor viral activity and the logistics of CMV surveillance can be considerable.

For treatment of established CMV disease intravenous ganciclovir should be used and consideration should be given to reducing the level of immunosuppressive therapy where this is feasible.

Herpes simplex virus (HSV) and varicella zoster virus (VZV) infection

Reactivation of latent HSV is common during the first few weeks after transplantation. It usually causes ulceration of the lips and mouth but sometimes it produces lesions in the cornea or in the anogenital area. Encephalitis and dissemination to visceral organs are occasionally seen and potentially fatal. HSV pneumonia is sometimes seen in recipients of lung transplants.

Herpes zoster is ten times more common in transplant recipients than in the general population. It is usually seen during the first few months after transplantation and results from reactivation of latent VZV in the sensory ganglion with transport of virus along the sensory nerves to give a vesicular skin eruption in the corresponding dermatome (shingles). Primary VZV infection (chickenpox) is potentially very serious in the immunocompromised patient but fortunately it is uncommon because most adults have immunity through previous exposure to the virus during childhood. If a non-immune patient is exposed to a case of chickenpox, it is advisable to give them VZV immunoglobulin. Prophylaxis and treatment of both HSV and VZV are with antiviral agents (aciclovir or ganciclovir).

Human herpes virus (HHV)-6, -7 and -8

HHV-6, -7 and -8 are ubiquitous and infection after transplantation may arise from reactivation of latent virus or from transmission of virus in the transplanted organ. The effects of infection range from a brief viral syndrome to tissue-invasive disease. HHV-6 may cause bone marrow suppression and encephalitis and HHV-8 infection has been associated with the development of Kaposi's sarcoma.

Epstein–Barr virus (EBV)

EBV is a ubiquitous herpesvirus. Over 90% of adults have encountered the virus which is either subclinical or causes a mononucleosis syndrome (glandular fever). EBV-seronegative recipients may develop a primary infection following transmission of EBV in an organ from an EBV-seropositive donor and reactivation of latent EBV may occur in EBV-seropositive recipients. EBV targets B lymphocytes, causing them to proliferate and undergo transformation. In an immunocompetent individual the proliferating B cells are held in check by cytotoxic T cells but in the immunosuppressed transplant recipient they may undergo uncontrolled proliferation, leading to post-transplant lymphoproliferative disease.

Human papoviruses (polyoma virus)

Human papilloma virus (HPV) reactivation is common after transplantation and is associated with cutaneous and sometimes anogenital warts. The papovirus family includes BK virus and JC virus. These are ubiquitous and the majority of healthy adults will have experienced infection during childhood. They remain latent in the kidney and after renal transplantation latent virus in the graft may be reactivated, occasionally causing invasive disease of the graft, bladder and urethra.

Fungal infections

Candida

Oral candidiasis is common after transplantation and candidal oesophagitis is seen occasionally. Topical antifungal agents, e.g. nystatin, are routinely given as prophylaxis. Occasionally candida is responsible for causing deep infections at the site of transplantation and disseminated candidiasis.

Aspergillus

Aspergillus is widespread in the environment and spores are often released in high concentrations during hospital building work. Exposure to aspergillus may lead to the development of aspergillus pneumonia or other forms of tissue-invasive disease. Colonisation is sometimes seen in the absence of invasive disease and chemo-prophylaxis is not routinely used in this situation. The diagnosis of invasive aspergillus can be difficult and is often delayed. Treatment is with amphotericin B. Systemic anti-fungal agents are, however, expensive and commonly cause side effects.

Pneumocystis carinii

Pneumocystis carinii is a ubiquitous fungus that causes pneumonia (PCP) in the immunocompromised host. PCP occurs in the first six months after transplantation and presents with fever, dyspnoea and a non-productive cough. Physical and radiological signs may be minimal and the diagnosis is made by bronchoalveolar lavage and transbronchial biopsy. Prophylaxis against PCP after transplantation is routine, usually in the form of trimethoprim-sulphamethoxazole. Without prophylaxis the incidence of PCP is around 10% and much higher after lung transplantation.

Malignancy following transplantation

Organ transplant recipients are much more likely to develop a malignancy than individuals of comparable age in the general population and this is attributed largely to the immunosuppressive therapy they receive. The risk of malignancy after transplantation increases progressively over time and up to half of transplant patients followed for 20 years or more develop a malignancy. The types of cancer encountered after transplantation are markedly different from those seen in the general population. Much of the increase in malignancy is accounted for by cancers of the skin and by lymphomas although there is also a markedly increased risk of urogenital malignancy. When skin cancers are excluded there is a three- to fourfold increase in the incidence of malignancy. Most of the common solid malignancies show a twofold increase in incidence compared to age-matched controls, although there is no increase in carcinoma of the breast or prostate. Malignancy after transplantation occurs at an earlier age than in the general population and the mean age of patients at the time of diagnosis of malignancy is the mid-40s.

The increased susceptibility of immunosuppressed patients to malignant disease is due to multiple mechanisms. Infection with oncogenic viruses undoubtedly plays an important role and the malignancies with the greatest observed-to-expected ratio are those in which viral infection is known or thought to play an aeti-ological role. Immunosuppression may also enhance the effect of other oncogenic stimuli, for example UV light and carcinogens, and it may impair immunosurveillance and elimination of cells that have undergone malignant transformation. Chronic antigenic stimulation by the allograft may also play a role in the promotion of neoplasia. There is no convincing evidence that any of the commonly used immunosuppressive agents have a significant direct oncogenic effect.

Skin cancer

Cancers of the skin are the most commonly encountered malignancy in transplant recipients and comprise over one-third of all malignancies seen. The majority are squamous cell carcinomas and the normal preponderance of basal cell carcinoma over squamous cell carcinoma in the general population is reversed after transplantation. Exposure to sunlight is a major aetiological factor and squamous cell carcinoma is particularly common in white Caucasian recipients exposed to strong sunlight. Many of the malignancies occur on sun-exposed areas of the body although non-exposed areas including the vulva and vagina are often affected. Squamous cell carcinomas after transplantation are often preceded by premalignant lesions and are commonly multiple. They tend to grow rapidly and are more likely to metastasise and recur than lesions occurring in the general population. Reactivation of HPV has been implicated as an aetiological factor in the development of squamous cell carcinoma.

Transplant recipients should be advised to protect their skin from exposure to strong sunlight and should be assessed regularly for the presence of premalignant and malignant skin lesions. When identified, these should be treated promptly and aggressively. Consideration should be given to reducing the level of immunosuppressive therapy in patients with multiple or rapidly developing skin cancer.

Post-transplant lymphoproliferative disease (PTLD)

After skin cancer, PTLD is the next most common malignancy seen in transplant recipients and affects between 1% and 5% of recipients. The majority (95%) of cases of PTLD are associated with EBV infection and the incidence is highest in recipients who have received a high total burden of immunosuppression. EBV-seronegative recipients of an EBV-seropositive organ allograft are at particularly high risk of developing PTLD and the incidence of PTLD is greatest in paediatric recipients. The disease progresses with varying rapidity through a clinical spectrum ranging from EBV-driven polyclonal B cell activation and hyperplasia to malignant monoclonal B cell lymphoma. PTLD may be confined to secondary lymphoid tissue or it may develop at extranodal sites including the gastrointestinal tract, central nervous system and organ allograft.

The presentation may be varied. Pressure symptoms from an enlarging mass are a common presentation. A high index of suspicion aids early diagnosis. Reducing or, where feasible, even stopping immunosuppression is the most important treatment and may lead to the complete regression of the disease. Localised disease may be amenable to surgical excision or radiotherapy. Anti-viral drugs and IFN-α may also be used. If the disease does not respond promptly to treatment the outlook is usually poor.

Genitourinary cancer

Cancer of the genitourinary tract is common after transplantation, particularly in the female. There is a markedly increased incidence of carcinoma of the uterine cervix and this is associated with HPV infection. Regular screening and early treatment are important.

Kaposi's sarcoma

Kaposi's sarcoma is rarely seen in Western countries except in patients with HIV infection. After organ transplantation there is a 100-fold increase in the incidence of Kaposi's sarcoma, although it still remains uncommon, affecting <0.5% of recipients. It is associated with HHV-8 infection and recipients of Mediterranean origin are particularly susceptible to developing the condition. It usually presents as a cutaneous lesion but may also involve the visceral mucosa. If immunosuppression is reduced or stopped the disease may completely regress but disseminated disease is usually fatal. Anti-viral agents may be beneficial.

FUTURE PROSPECTS IN TRANSPLANTATION

Chronic rejection is the major cause of graft failure and there is a need to better understand the pathophysiology of this condition and to develop effective approaches for preventing it. The shortage of human organs for transplantation means that it is essential to optimise graft survival. For many years a major goal in transplantation has been to develop strategies whereby the recipient is made specifically tolerant to their transplant without the need for non-specific immunosuppressive therapy. A state of transplant tolerance would ensure long-term graft survival and leave the

recipient free from all the complications of immunosuppressive drugs. It has long been known that specific immunological tolerance to organ allografts can be achieved by various methods in experimental animals but achieving transplant tolerance in humans has proved very elusive. One of the more promising approaches for inducing tolerance is the use of monoclonal antibodies directed against molecules that provide essential co-stimulatory signals for T cell activation. Early clinical trials of such antibodies, notably those interfering with CD40–CD40 ligand interaction, are currently in progress but it is too early to assess the efficacy of this approach.

The use of animal organs for transplantation into humans is a potential solution to the shortage of human organs but very considerable problems have to be overcome to make this approach safe and feasible. The use of non-human primates as a source of donor organs is not acceptable by most people because of ethical concerns. Moreover, primates are difficult to breed in captivity and may harbour pathogens that are dangerous for humans. Consequently the pig has emerged as the most suitable potential source of donor organs on the basis of size, physiology and ease of breeding. There are still ethical concerns, however, as well as concern about the potential for transmission of pathogens such as porcine endogenous retrovirus. This virus is embedded within the pig genome and cannot, therefore, be eliminated as a potential hazard.

Until recently hyperacute xenograft rejection was a major barrier to the successful transplantation of pig organs in primates. Most primates, including humans, have naturally occurring IgM and IgG antibodies directed against a carbohydrate antigen, galα(1,3)gal, expressed by pig tissues. This is analogous to a blood group antigen and causes hyperacute rejection and xenograft destruction within minutes of performing xenotransplantation. However, hyperacute xenograft rejection of pig organs in primates can now be overcome using a variety of approaches. Of these, one of the most effective is to use organs from pigs that have been made transgenic for human complement regulatory proteins such as decay accelerating factor. Considerable immunological barriers still remain, however. Accelerated vascular rejection occurs within the first three or four days and if this is overcome acute rejection and probably chronic rejection are major barriers. Conventional immunosuppressive agents are not sufficiently potent to prevent these processes without causing unacceptably high risks from infection because of over-immunosuppression.

FURTHER READING

Arbeit JM, Hirose R. Murine Mentors: transgenic and knockout models of surgical disease. *Ann Surg* 1999; **229**(1):21–40

Goes N, Chandraker A. Human leukocyte antigen matching in renal transplantation: an update. *Curr Opin Nephrol Hypertension* 2000; **9**(6):683–687

Niklason LE, Langer R. Prospects for organ and tissue replacement. *JAMA* 2001; **285**(5):573–576

Pohanka E. New immunosuppressive drugs: an update. *Curr Opin Urol* 2001; **11**(2):143–151

Rose SM, Blustein N, Rotrosen D. Recommendations of the expert panel on ethical issues in clinical trials of transplant tolerance. National Institute of Allergy and Infectious Diseases of the National Institutes of Health. *Transplantation* 1998; **66**:1123

Rydberg L. ABO-incompatibility in solid organ transplantation. *Transfusion Med* 2001; **11**(4):325–342

44

Organ donation

Greg Armstrong, Stephen Lynch

In the early part of the 20th century great advances were made in surgical techniques. Among the pioneers was Alexis Carrel who developed many surgical techniques for vascular anastomosis. His contributions in this area made the transplantation of organs surgically possible. Many attempts at organ transplantation were made in the ensuing years but all were doomed to failure as there was no method of modifying the immune response. The first long-term success in organ transplantation occurred in 1954 in Boston. Murray, Merrill and Harrison performed a live donor renal transplant between identical twins, thus negating the need for immunosuppression. Many advances have been made in the ensuing half-century and so today the process of transplantation is undertaken with great success in numerous centres around the globe.

A number of areas within organ donation have been crucial to this success. The general societal acceptance of organ donation has made the availability of donor organs possible. The recognition of brain death as death has allowed for the retrieval of multiple viable organs from brain-dead, beating-heart cadavers. Advances in organ preservation have expanded the potential donor pool, made possible organ exchange and provided time for better matching. Finally the development of organ retrieval networks or systems has greatly enhanced the overall process.

This process of organ donation and transplantation is no doubt one of the most complex in modern medicine and its success is dependent on the successful coalescence of many factors, some of which can be controlled or influenced by those involved in organ donation and transplantation, some not.

ACCEPTANCE OF BRAIN DEATH AND ORGAN DONATION

Transplantation has achieved an outstanding improvement in both patient and graft survival over the last decade. Better surgical techniques, anaesthesia and perioperative management have allowed more marginal recipients to benefit from this treatment. This has meant a growing acceptance of transplantation as a treatment for end-stage organ failure and opened up transplantation for many more patients than in the past. The consequence of this revolution is ever-expanding transplant waiting lists. Although there is an increasing number of live donor transplants being performed, live donation incurs a risk to the donor and as such must not be undertaken lightly. The number of such donors, suitable both medically and psychosocially, is limited and is confined to kidney, partial liver, partial pancreas and, more recently, lobar lung transplants. Even though the number of live donor transplants is increasing, it continues to fall short of demand. Cadaveric organ donation thus remains the main reservoir of supply of organs for transplantation and as the acceptance of brain death and the donation of organs form the basic foundation for cadaveric organ transplantation, these two concepts remain central to transplantation.

Public acceptance

Public acceptance of organ donation is critical. Without it no cadaveric organ transplantation could occur. Numerous studies of public attitudes to organ donation have been undertaken in the United Kingdom, United States and other Western countries with similar explicit consent laws. In general, approximately 90% of the public believes organ donation is a good thing but only 60–65% would actually donate their organs. Fear appears to be the major reason for this discrepancy between seeing donation as a good thing and actual commitment: fear of inadequate resuscitation, fear of not being 'really' dead and fear of mutilation. In essence the public are mistrusting of the health system. Of those who have stated a commitment to donation, few have actually taken definitive steps to formalise their wishes. The National Organ Donor Registry of UK Transplant has fewer than 10% of the public registered as donors despite easy access to registration forms and five years of public promotion and educational campaigns. The Netherlands' experience has shown similar apathy towards formal registration. The reasons for this failure on the public's part to register their wishes are unknown, but given the decided lack of success of registries most efforts to increase donor numbers are focused on encouraging people to make a decision regarding donation and to inform their family of that decision.

Less is known of the public's acknowledgement of brain death as being definitive death. Little public debate on the issue occurs in most Western countries. One can only assume that at least philosophically, the population has an acceptance of it as being death. However, problems with the acceptance of brain death may arise when a member of the public is confronted with it as a reality, when a family member or close friend is declared brain dead.

The influence of the media is another uncertainty. The most well-known example within the United Kingdom centred on a television programme that questioned brain death. Organ donation rates declined markedly in the ensuing months but rebounded later in that year. In the United States a number of well-publicised transplants occurred in the mid 1990s. The recipients were high-profile citizens who allegedly had inordinately short waiting times prior to transplant. Public outrage and negative publicity towards organ donation occurred at the perception of the favoured treatment of a few. Yet even in this negative environment the organ donation rate remained unaffected. What is known, however, is that most donations occur because of altruism on the part of the donor and the donor's family. That is, most want to donate because it will help other people and most donor families agree to donation for similar reasons. The positive publicity of transplantation successes conveys this message to the public – they know transplantation saves lives. The unanswered question is whether positive publicity has a greater impact than negative publicity. No matter what the answer, public support for donation is crucial to providing transplantation to those in need. Careful attention to accuracy and honesty when publicly representing donation and transplantation is critical to maintaining public faith in the process and therefore the process itself.

Hospital acceptance

Equally important as public acceptance is the acceptance by hospitals of their role in the donation process. This is the second crucial step in the process of successful donation. It is within the hospitals that potential donors need to be identified, that the consent process is carried out in the best possible way and that the donors are maintained in optimal condition.

For this to occur in a consistent manner, hospital staff must be committed to donation. They must recognise it as not just something they do to benefit transplant recipients but as part of their obligation to provide for their patients. As stated earlier, the majority of the population support organ donation and believe it is the right thing to do. There is a public expectation that their wishes will be acted upon. It is incumbent upon hospitals to provide for this expectation and to ensure that should the situation arise, there will be processes in place that ensure that the option of donation is made available. By inaction, institutions are in essence making the decision regarding donation for the deceased and their family. This is not their role, nor is it their right.

The United States and Spain are the two most successful organ donation countries, practising 'explicit consent' donation. Both of these countries have recognised that the major barrier to donation is not within public circles but within the health system itself. Although public promotion of donation and the benefits of transplantation are not ignored, they centre their activities on developing and maintaining defined processes and responsibilities for donation within their hospitals. Differing approaches have been used in both countries but the basic principle of a structured approach to donation with defined roles and responsibilities for those involved is the common theme. They have recognised that for successful donation to occur it must be a part of routine hospital practice. Recently this has been recognised in Belgium where 'presumed consent' is practised. Belgian law does not require hospitals to actively participate in donation, there is no requirement to consult the 'non-donor registry' and thus notify the donor coordinators of potential donors. In a pilot study at one Belgian hospital the introduction of processes to ensure routine notification of deaths saw a doubling of donor numbers.

BRAIN DEATH: CLINICAL AND LEGAL CRITERIA

It was not until techniques of ventilatory support were developed that the issue of brain death arose. Prior to this the common outcome of intracerebral catastrophe was irreversible cardiopulmonary standstill. The development of mechanical ventilation meant that gas exchange could continue and therefore cardiac output was maintained due to oxygenation and the heart's intrinsic rhythm. Despite these conditions, cardiac arrest occurred in some clinical settings. In 1958 Mollaret and Goulon first described what was then termed 'coma dépassé' and defined the diagnostic criteria for this state. The question of when death occurred inevitably arose. Was life dependent on the mechanical support or was an already dead patient being senselessly ventilated? The issue transcended clinical curiosity to become a legal, philosophical and theological phenomenon. The validity of the brain death concept was subject to many debates during the 1960s. In 1968 an ad hoc committee of the Harvard Medical School released recommended criteria for the diagnosis of what was then called irreversible coma. In the same year France released the Jeanneney Circular which defined brain death and authorised the donation of organs from people in such conditions.

Clinical evidence and support for the concept of brain death grew. In 1976 the Conference of Medical Royal Colleges and their Faculties in the United Kingdom published a statement on the diagnosis of brain death. Subsequently the clinical, legal and theological recognition and acceptance of brain death has occurred in most countries.

Clinical criteria: brain death

Aetiology and pathophysiology

Although there are many situations that may lead to brain death, a general classification is possible (Box 44.1). Events may be sudden and unexpected, such as a spontaneous intracranial haemorrhage from an arteriovenous malformation, or may follow a protracted course of treatment and hospitalisation, as with a primary brain tumor. Whilst the aetiology of the cerebral insult is protean, the final common pathway is an inexorable rise in intracranial pressure as a consequence of cerebral injury. Brain oedema leads to compression of cerebral venous outflow, further increasing intracranial pressure and decreasing cerebral perfusion. Unless cerebral oedema is successfully treated cerebellar tonsillar herniation eventually occurs with virtually complete cerebral infarction. Brainstem herniation, commonly described as coning causes a loss of the centres of control for vasomotor function, temperature regulation and respiration.

Box 44.1   Events that may lead to brain death

- Trauma
- Intracranial haemorrhage
- Anoxia
- Space-occupying lesion
- Infection
- Toxins

Assessment

A number of different methods may be employed to determine if brain death has occurred. (Box 44.2). Currently the most

Box 44.2   Methods of assessing brain death

- Clinical examination
- Contrast cerebral angiograph
- Radionucleotide cerebral scan

(± EEG)

common method is by clinical examination of the cranial nerves and the testing for respiratory effort, which has become the method of choice in most instances, as it is non-invasive and harmless. Unless stipulated by law, as is the case in some countries, other forms of testing are usually only undertaken when a clinical examination is not possible due to complications such as facial trauma, C1/C2 fracture or known respiratory disease.

Clinical examination

Prior to clinical examination a number of prerequisites must be met (Box 44.3). There should be a known cause of coma. If a cause cannot be established then a diagnosis of brain death based on clinical examination cannot be supported as unknown extraneous factors may influence the observations. Body temperature must be above 35°C as hypothermia may mimic brain death. There must be no metabolic or endocrine disturbances that may confuse the findings. Pharmacological agents such as neurodepressants or muscle relaxants must also be excluded as these may mask or block responses to attempts at eliciting cranial nerve reflexes and respiratory effort.

Box 44.3   Prequisites for declaration of brain death

- Known cause of coma
- Absence of hypothermia
- No muscle relaxants
- No depressant drugs
- No metabolic or endocrine disruptions

The clinical examination for brain death is based on three principles.

- First, there is deep coma of known cause and sufficient in extent as to be likely to cause brain death.

- Second, the observation of certain responses to the stimulation of the cranial nerves must be possible.

- Finally the confirmation of complete lack of respiratory effort stimulated by hypercapnia following cessation of mechanical ventilation.

A number of professional societies have produced guidelines for the determination of brain death and although there may be minor and insignificant differences between the various guidelines, they are in essence uniform.

Steps in clinical examination for brain death

Initially it is necessary to establish a cause for the deep coma. It is usual that the cause has already been determined during admission and thus prior to any consideration of brain death. However, once the patient has been comatose with a Glasgow Coma Score of 3, has demonstrated non-reacting pupils, absent cough and gag reflexes and no spontaneous respiratory effort most guidelines recommend a further period of observation of 4–6 hours prior to any clinical examination for brain death. If during this period of observation no change in the patient's condition is observed it is usual to carry out the first set of brain death tests. In the setting of hypoxic brain injury and encephalitis it is commonly recommended that a longer period of observation is appropriate.

Following the first set of tests a period of 2–4 hours of further observation is recommended before the second confirmatory set of tests is undertaken. This period of observation and the second set of tests are done in order to demonstrate irreversibility and avoidance of observer error. Each set of tests must be carried out by appropriately trained and experienced clinicians. Both may or may not be present at each examination but each must be responsible for performing one of the two sets of tests. In most jurisdictions two independent examinations are a legal requirement.

The sequence in which the components of the examination are undertaken is also important. It should be remembered that although death may be indicated by general clinical observation, the patient must be considered to be alive and therefore should not be subjected to the apnoea test, which is potentially harmful, until all other tests show no response. The sequence of testing is outlined in Box 44.4. To confirm brain death all reflexes in both sets of tests must be absent.

Box 44.4   Reflexes tested and sequence of testing

- Papillary responses to light
- Corneal reflexes
- Response to painful stimuli within the distribution of the cranial nerves
- Occulovestibular reflexes
- Gag reflex
- Cough reflex
- Respiratory reflex – passive oxygenation, PCO_2 >60 mmHg and arterial pH <7.3)

Other confirmatory investigations

In some jurisdictions four-vessel cerebral angiography is mandated and must be carried out as part of the examination to determine brain death. In other jurisdictions such as the United Kingdom it is not mandated and is used only when it is either not possible to carry out a clinical examination or other factors indicate the necessity for confirmatory testing, such as in the case of a C1/C2 injury. Radiological evidence of the absence of cerebral blood flow is by itself confirmatory evidence of brain death. The legal position regarding the interpretation of the results will be discussed later in this chapter.

Electroencephalography was commonly used in addition to the clinical examination for the determination of brain death but it is now rarely performed as a confirmatory investigation in the UK, USA and Australia. It is, however, still used in some European countries and is a mandated part of brain death testing in Japan. Unlike cerebral angiography, EEG is not used as a sole method of determining brain death but rather as an adjunct to either clinical or radiological examination.

It needs to be stressed that death in all but the most extreme circumstances is a process and not a single event. Regardless of which criteria are used to declare death (cerebral or circulatory), the time of death is an arbitrary time set down by society. It indicates a point where irreversibility of the process has been reached. It should also be recognised that in the setting of brain death, lower motor neurone function is variously preserved and may give rise to spontaneous spinal movements of the limbs, shoulder elevation and abduction and back arching. Sweating, abdominal and deep tendon reflexes may sometimes be elicited. Diabetes insipidus may not be absent.

Legal criteria: brain death

The clinical appreciation of brain death predated that of its legal acceptance. The first laws recognising brain death as legal death were enacted in the 1970s. Since that time the legal acceptance of brain death has slowly spread across the globe. As recently as 1997 brain death was legally recognised in Japan. Other countries have not passed laws defining brain death but have placed the determination of death in the hands of the medical community. The United Kingdom does not have a legal definition of brain death nor does it have a legally prescribed method or standard of qualification for those determining brain death. Full reliance is placed on adherence to the guidelines as outlined by the Royal Colleges statement on the diagnosis of brain death (Box 44.5).

Box 44.5   Legal definition of brain death
Irreversible cessation of all functions of the brain

In countries where formal legal definitions exist legislators have applied a number of approaches in addressing how brain death is to be determined and/or who can make such a declaration. The components of these differing approaches can be divided into a number of general categories (Boxes 44.6, 44.7). In countries such as Australia there are no legally defined criteria by which brain death is determined. It is left to accepted clinical standards. The law does, however, state that two medical practitioners, each of whom has attained specific minimal registration requirements, must determine it. In other countries the law requires specific methods for determining brain death such as cerebral angiography

Box 44.6   Legal approaches to the determination and declaration of brain death
● No defined tests – based on current clinical criteria
● Defined tests
● Defined professional status of testers
● Defined exclusion of certain persons

Box 44.7   Countries and requirements
Australia
● No defined tests – current clinical criteria
● Defined status
● Defined exclusion of certain persons
USA
● No defined tests – current clinical criteria
● Defined status
● Defined exclusion of certain persons
Japan
● Defined tests
● Defined status
● Defined exclusion of certain persons

or EEG. Furthermore, the law in most countries excludes those who may potentially have a conflict of interest from being able to legally declare brain death (Box 44.8).

Regardless of the legal position, it is essential that only well-trained, qualified and experienced medical practitioners declare brain death. Additionally it must always be remembered that brain death is, to most, an abstract concept. The acceptance of brain death by the deceased's family may be difficult. The body is warm and well perfused, the monitor shows a heart rhythm, the chest rises and falls with the help of mechanical ventilation. All of these indicate life to the unaware observer. The difficulty of some families in accepting brain death is real. Often it is best to demonstrate apnoea or complete absence of pupillary reflexes to the family members.

Box 44.8   Excluded from declaring brain death
● Medical practitioners who propose to treat the recipients of the donation
● Medical practitioners who propose to remove tissue
● Medical practitioner who is the designated person who gives the authority

DONOR SUITABILITY

Driven by the increasing demand for donor organs, suitability criteria for organs are in a constant state of flux. Donor age limits have expanded while suitability criteria with respect to infectious diseases have cycled between expansion and contraction as experience, knowledge and technology have grown. Disease or trauma are no longer necessarily contraindications to donation. The urgent need to transplant specific recipients may often dictate using less than optimal organs in some circumstances. Referring centres are encouraged to notify the donor coordinators of all potential donors regardless of age and co-morbidity. Therefore detailed donor suitability criteria are avoided if possible. This approach alleviates the need for continuous updating of detailed donor criteria, removes the real potential for inappropriate exclusion of possible donors and allows decisions regarding donor and organ suitability to be made by those working within the specialty.

Assessment of the potential donor

Donor suitability criteria for referral for organ donation should be set at the bare minimum. The suitability criterion 'brain death with intact circulation' is sufficient and should be used to initiate referral for assessment. In those hospitals with active non-heart-beating donor programmes all deaths should be referred. The initial assessment of potential donors is made by the donor coordinators and then for specific organs by the relevant transplant units at the time of organ allocation. Accurate data collection is essential in determining suitability and therefore protecting the recipients from unnecessary risk. Referral of potential donors for assessment may occur either when death is thought to be imminent or after death has been declared. Referral prior to death should be done in those instances where the donor coordinators are independent of the transplant units and/or the family has volunteered donation based on a hopeless prognosis. Early referral allows the treating doctor to have a clearer indication of the possibilities should death occur and, in the setting of volunteered donation, the ability to provide the family with accurate information. Additionally early referral makes possible an on-site assessment by the donor coordinator and their inclusion in the consent process.

The initial assessment is aimed at three specific areas:

- that death has been or is likely to be declared

- to ascertain the existence of any total exclusion criteria and lastly

- to identify potential organ-specific exclusion criteria

These last two areas are based on exclusion rather than inclusion. Potential organ donor assessment is not a process of finding reasons why someone can be placed in the category 'potential organ donor' but rather of ascertaining if there are valid reasons to remove them from the category.

The final assessment for suitability of organs for donation is made at the time of removal.

Brain death

In circumstances where death is thought to be imminent no further action is taken other than the assessment for suitability and arrangements regarding the discussion of donation with the family

should donation be possible and death is declared. In those circumstances where death has been declared full details regarding the declaration of death should be obtained and recorded (Box 44.9). In countries where legislation applies to the declaration of brain death, full compliance with the legislative requirements must be verified. Written confirmation of the test results usually takes the form of a signed and dated declaration or medical record note. The donor coordinator, prior to discussion of donation with the family, should have sight of these, as should the donor surgeons prior to organ removal.

Box 44.9 Details of brain death testing

- Name and qualifications of medical practitioners who performed first and second sets of tests
- Date and time of tests
- Method of testing

Exclusion criteria

In the United Kingdom the specific criteria for exclusion to donation are very similar to those used elsewhere in the world. UK Transplant includes within its Operating Principles for Transplant Units guidelines on contraindications to donation. These contain not only general contraindications but also organ-specific ones (Box 44.10). The National Health Service Executive circular 'Guidance on the microbiological safety of human tissues and organs used in transplantation' defines four main categories of absolute exclusion from organ donation:

- patients with high-risk factors for transmissible diseases

- patients with a history of malignancy (except proven primary brain tumour)

- patients with diseases of unknown aetiology

- patients with other untreated systemic infections.

The risk categories as defined by the Chief Health Officer as contraindications to donation for organ transplantation apply to all organs except the liver. In this case the only definitive contraindication is human immunodeficiency virus antibody positivity. Therefore even in cases where a risk factor exists, donation is possible. The final decision to proceed to organ

---

Box 44.10 General and organ-specific contraindications to donation

General exclusions
- Patients with high-risk factors for transmissible diseases
- Patients with a history of malignancy (except proven primary brain tumour)
- Patients with diseases of unknown aetiology
- Patients with other untreated systemic infections

Organ specific
- Disease or trauma to the organ

---

retrieval and transplantation remains with the transplanting unit. If there is evidence of the existence of a definitive contraindication to all donation, such as recent intravenous drug use, then no further action regarding donation is taken.

Assessment process

In order to fully assess a donor referral it is essential that full and accurate information is obtained from the treating unit. Initially information is obtained from both the treating doctor and the medical record. Details of the events leading up to admission, the cause of death, course of treatment, results of pathology and radiology investigations and significant haemodynamic, ventilatory and observational events are obtained and recorded. The current haemodynamic and ventilatory parameters, observations and fluid status as well as pharmacological support requirements are noted (Box 44.11). A full detailed medical, surgical and social history is obtained from the medical notes, the caring doctor and if necessary the family and the general practitioner. A physical examination of the body should also be carried out. A record of any tattoos, signs of intravenous drug use, skin lesions or surgical procedures should be made. A note is made of the age, sex, height, weight and build. In the absence of any definitive contraindications to donation, an assessment of individual organs based on the above data is undertaken. The approach to this is aimed at identifying anything within the history that may potentially exclude the donation of any organ or organs. It is not aimed at a definitive exclusion of those organs but at ensuring there is detailed information available.

Box 44.11 Information required – details since admission

- Date and time of admission and ventilation
- Principal cause of admission and additional injuries
- Age, sex, weight, height and build
- Medical, surgical and social history
- Investigation results
- Significant events
- Current observations
- Drugs administered
- Physical examination results

Based on this information, each of the individual transplant units, when offered an organ, will make an informed decision on suitability. The donor coordinator's assessment of the information also provides a guide during discussions with the potential donor's family. It aids in providing realistic information on the likely outcome of a donation and enables an informed discussion to take place. The assessment of individual organs is, as stated, a process of exclusion. Preexisting medical conditions, trauma, localised infection or adverse haemodynamic events may not necessarily contraindicate donation. Once the basic criteria of actual or imminent brain death with intact circulation are met, a referral to the donor coordinators should be made. An assessment of donation potential will then be undertaken.

The process of referral to transplant units varies from country to country. In the United Kingdom all potential kidney, liver, heart and lung donors must be reported to UK Transplant and a core donor data form is completed by the donor coordinators and forwarded to the Duty Office of UK Transplant. Conversely, in Australia the referral of potential donors to transplant units is usually not done until such time as there is consent for donation. Transplant units may, however, be contacted regarding suitability in marginal cases.

Authority to remove and transplant organs: consent

In many countries there are legal provisions for the removal and transplantation of organs from deceased persons. In some countries this legal authority is principally dependent on an expressed agreement or request by the deceased person. In others the legal authority is dependent on a lack of objection to the removal and transplantation of organs upon death. The first approach is known as 'explicit consent' while the latter is termed 'presumed consent'.

Explicit consent

Explicit consent laws require that the deceased prior to death has given consent or has made a request to donate. Based on true autonomy and altruism, advocates argue that the individual has a right to choose to donate, not to donate or to make no decision at all. Although they recognise the benefits to society of donation and the religious support for donation, there is a belief that presumed consent removes the true nature of donation from the act. This form of legislation is currently enacted in the United Kingdom, the United States and numerous other countries. Only the United States has donation rates similar to those of the major presumed consent countries. Through the use of a structured procedural approach to potential donor identification, referral and the consent process organ procurement organisations in the USA achieve high donation rates based not only on a high rate of donor identification but also consistently high consent rates.

Presumed consent

It is thought that the first presumed consent law was enacted by the Austrian Empress Marie-Thérèse. This decree provided blanket consent to autopsy and for the use of autopsy specimens for medical purposes. In 1978 the Council of Europe recommended a presumed consent approach which allowed for the automatic removal of organs for transplantation from citizens but provided a provision for those who object to register that objection to donation. The objection would be given legal weight and donation would not occur. It would be presumed that those who did not register an objection were in agreement with donation. Proponents for presumed consent argue that transplantation is legal, is beneficial to the society as a whole, has been embraced by virtually all religions and is acceptable to the majority of the populace. Personal autonomy is preserved by the provision of the option of registering as a 'non-donor' and donor families are spared the consent process at the time of bereavement.

A number of European countries have since enacted this 'presumed consent' legislation, the most noteworthy of these being Belgium. In 1986 the Belgian Parliament passed presumed consent legislation. The law applies to Belgian citizens and foreign nationals who have resided in the country longer than six months. Less than 0.1% of the Belgian population have registered an objection. An explicit consent law applies in all other cases. Whenever a potential donor is identified the treating unit is expected to contact the donor coordinator who then checks the registry for an objection. Referral of potential donors is not mandated. Should an objection be registered no further action regarding donation is taken. If there is no registered objection then the intent is to proceed to donation. Should the family wish to know what will happen now that their family member is dead they are informed of the intent to proceed to donation. If at this point the family objects to donation then that objection is respected and donation does not occur.

The introduction of this form of legislation saw a dramatic increase in the organ donation rate in Belgium. Although there has been a minor decline in this rate in recent years it still remains well above the European average. Recent evidence, however, indicates that not all potential donors are referred to the donor coordinators and therefore room for further improvement in the system exists. The introduction in the United Kingdom of presumed consent legislation was supported by the British Medical Association at their 1999 conference.

Legal requirements

In the United Kingdom the Human Tissue Act was passed by Parliament in 1961. The original purpose of the Act was to enable the use of parts of bodies of deceased persons for therapeutic purposes and purposes of medical education and research. The Act also refers to postmortem examinations and permits the cremation of bodies removed for anatomical examination. Section (1) of the Act covers the circumstances under which an authority to remove body parts may be given by the person lawfully in possession of the body. Lawful possession of the body rests with the person in control and management of the hospital or any officer or person designated by that person. Such an authority may be given when 'any person either in writing at any time or orally in the presence of two or more witnesses during his last illness, has expressed a request that his body or any specified part of his body be used after his death for therapeutic purposes . . .'. It also states that the person in control of the body cannot issue an authority if he has reason to believe that the request has been withdrawn. In simple terms a written request to donate or a witnessed verbal statement during the last illness is sufficient for an authority to be given (as long as it has not been withdrawn). This is similar to other explicit consent

laws except that most do not stipulate that the verbal request to donate has to be made 'during the last illness'. It can be made at any time during adult life. Additionally most do not require the authorization of the person in lawful possession of the body if there is a written consent by the deceased.

Subsection (2) is similar to a presumed consent law in that the aim is to establish if there is an objection to the removal of body parts. Without prejudicing subsection (1), the person lawfully in possession of the body may authorise the removal of any part from the body 'if after having made such reasonable enquiry as may be practical has no reason to believe –

> that the deceased had expressed an objection to his body being so dealt with after his death, and had not withdrawn it; or

> that the surviving spouse or any surviving relative of the deceased objects to the body being so dealt with.'

As can be seen, the aim is to establish if there is an objection to donation, not to establish a willingness to donate. Although, under this subsection, the establishment of a lack of objection is all that is necessary to proceed to donation the practice is to establish an agreement from the family before proceeding. Other jurisdictions require consent from the next of kin in such circumstances. No matter how the law is framed and therefore what the minimal legal requirements are, the general practice in countries with explicit consent laws is to only proceed to donation and transplantation on a written, signed and witnessed agreement or consent from the next of kin.

Two other sections of the Act are of direct relevance to organ donation. Subsection (4) stipulates that no removal of body parts under an authority given under the Act shall be 'effected except by a fully registered medical practitioner who has satisfied himself by personal examination of the body that life is extinct'. Many other explicit consent laws do not deal with prescribed qualifications for those who effect the removal. The last subsection of concern to those working in donation and transplantation covers deaths that may require an inquest or a coroner's postmortem examination. Subsection (5) states that 'Where a person has reason to believe' that an inquest or coroner's postmortem may be required

> 'he shall not, except with the consent of the coroner, –
> give an authority under this section in respect of the body; or
> act on such an authority given by any other person.'

This is a common provision in laws addressing donation. The body of the deceased is evidence in the investigation of the person's death and therefore comes under the control of those charged with investigating the death. It cannot be tampered with without the consent of those so charged.

Consent process

Within an explicit consent system each and every donation is the culmination of the successful coalescence of many additional factors. The first of these critical factors is the identification and referral of potential donors for assessment. The second is the discussion of donation with the next of kin. The discussion of donation is not just a process whereby the aim is to meet legal requirements and gain agreement to donation but it is also one of ensuring that the option of donation is presented in a sensitive and honest fashion. The principal focus is to determine the wishes of the deceased and then the family's feelings towards those wishes. Although somewhat paradoxical, a successful outcome may actually be a decision not to donate. However, given that the large majority of the population agree with donation it is more likely that there will be an agreement to donate provided that the process is conducted in an appropriate way.

Successful donation programmes have shown a formalised and consistent approach to the consent process to be the most effective. It is inappropriate that the discussion of donation be carried out in an *ad hoc* fashion. There are a number of key aspects to successful donation discussions. The use of these guidelines is more likely to provide a degree of comfort and control for the next of kin, reducing stress for all involved and achieving a greater likelihood of an 'informed consent'.

Timing

The timing of donation discussions should never be governed by staff convenience. Donation should not be discussed until after death has been declared and the family has been informed of this and have understood and accepted it. A decoupling of the discussion of death and the discussion of donation is highly advised. By allowing a number of hours between these discussions the family is given time to be with the deceased, time to talk, time to move towards an acceptance of the situation. This separation is important as it partitions death from donation, treating them as the two separate issues that they are, and allows donation to be seen as something positive arising from the otherwise negative situation. If the family have spontaneously volunteered donation prior to the declaration of death it is acceptable to acknowledge their wishes and provide information but it is best not to enter into a formal discussion of donation at that time.

Setting

The setting in which donation is discussed should be well chosen, private, quiet and comfortable. The bedside or the hallways are inappropriate. A venue should be available which is non-threatening with adequate seating for all involved and free of physical barriers.

Staff participants

Experience has shown that the mix and role of those conducting the discussion have an influence on outcome. Ideally the participants should be the doctor who discussed brain death with the

family, the nurse caring for the deceased and the donor coordinator. Each of these participants has defined roles that have been accepted by the group prior to the discussion with family. The doctor's role is to comment on the course of treatment culminating in death should the family have further questions. The nurse's role is that of comforter and the provider of reassurance and support. The donor coordinator's role is to discuss the option of donation. There should be no mixing of roles if at all possible. This approach gives the family a point of reference for expertise, avoids mixed messages and contradictions and demonstrates cohesiveness on the part of the health professionals towards donation. Prior to the discussion these participants must familiarise themselves with the deceased's admission history, the family dynamics and their perceived level of understanding and acceptance of the situation. If at any time during the discussion of donation it becomes apparent that death has not been accepted then the clinician should intervene and the discussion of donation should cease.

Family participants

It is not uncommon for the immediate family and members of the extended family to be present at the hospital. It is advisable that discussion of donation be limited to members of the immediate family but at times this may not be possible and it may be necessary to negotiate for a family spokesperson when dealing with large groups.

Attitude and approach

The aim of the discussion of donation is to try to determine the wishes of the deceased. The discussion is not aimed at 'getting consent' and therefore should not contain any statements or comments that may be construed as putting pressure on the family to agree to donation. The discussion should present the family with the option of donation in an honest and open fashion.

Information gathering and discussion

The discussion itself should follow a loosely structured format. The discussion is centred on determining the known or perceived wishes of the deceased and not those of the family. Their agreement with donation is explored if it is felt the deceased wanted donation. If the family are ambivalent or do not agree it is worthwhile exploring their reasons for this as it may be based on a lack of knowledge or misunderstanding of donation. Throughout this discussion the staff participants should avoid monologues and should allow time for questions from the family. The word 'dead' should not be avoided and the discussion should be open and honest. If there is an agreement to donate it is necessary to reach a mutually agreed definition of donation in terms of what organs and tissues will be donated.

Recapping

Assuming an agreement to donate has been reached, the donor coordinator should briefly recap the discussion and its conclusions. An agreement that this is an accurate summation should be sought.

Formalities

Often this is the hardest part of all for the family as it is when the events must be acknowledged on paper. The donor coordinator should go through the forms word for word and clarify any points.

ORGAN ALLOCATION

The rules by which cadaveric organs are allocated for transplantation have been and most likely will continue to be subject to much discussion. Issues of justice, equity and utility dominate the debates. Should organs be distributed on the basis of duration of time on the waiting list, greatest need or likelihood of best outcome? Various national and international cadaveric organ allocation systems have evolved. The dominant philosophy of these systems is utility. Given that the supply of cadaveric organs is far less than the demand and that donated organs are deemed to be a societal resource, it is incumbent upon any system to deliver the greatest benefit to the society. Cadaveric organ allocation is therefore principally based on mechanisms to maximise outcomes balanced against equity and justice. Access for patients with acute end stage organ failure where no alternative therapy is possible, but who have good predicted survival, is facilitated through priority listing mechanisms. In this group of patients the time from listing to death may be only a matter of hours or days. In general there are two systems of allocation: patient and centre based.

Patient-based allocation

Patient-based allocation systems allocate organs to specific patients. The organ offer is most commonly derived by a points algorithm whereby the organ is offered to the patient with the most points. This type of system is most commonly applied to renal allocation although countries such as the United States also use it for extrarenal organ allocation. Patient-centred systems work well in renal allocation as ABO blood group compatibility and human leucocyte antigen (HLA) matching between donor and recipient predict outcome and are easily quantified.

Centre-based allocation differs from patient-centred allocation in that the organ offer is made to the transplant centre and not to a specific patient. Patient selection is then the clinical decision of the centre, thereby giving primacy to clinical judgement.

Centre-based allocation is usually applied to the allocation of organs such as hearts, lungs and livers where predictors of outcome are not easily quantified. It should be noted that no matter which method of allocation is used, the basic unit of priority for organ allocation is most usually citizenship or permanent resident status of the country or citizenship of a country with reciprocal arrangements.

Renal allocation

Tissue typing

This is the common term used for the process whereby various immunological parameters of both donors and recipients are determined. In both donors and recipients it involves the determination of ABO blood group and the specification of certain HLA antigens. The HLA locus, located on the short arm of the sixth chromosome, has a key role in defining 'self' as opposed to 'non-self'. Matching donor and recipient HLA therefore is viewed by many as an important determinant of outcome in transplantation. Each known HLA antigen is designated by its locus and a numeral, e.g. A2 or DR3. A patient's or donor's tissue type will therefore encompass the relevant loci and the numeric value of each antigen at these loci, i.e. A2A3, B5B7, DR8DR11. Additionally in recipients the level of any preformed cytotoxic antibodies is determined by direct cytotoxic (antibody/antigen) crossmatch. Recipient serum is tested against a panel of general population antigens. The percentage of positive crossmatches is then calculated. This percentage is designated as the patient's panel reactive antibody level or PRA and is indicative of the percentage of donors with whom the patient is likely to be incompatible. Normally patient serum samples are tested on a monthly basis for PRA levels. The 'current' sample as well as an historical 'peak' PRA sample is stored for future donor/recipient crossmatch.

The degree to which these parameters impact on outcomes depends on the level of incompatibility between donor and recipient. The impact also varies from organ to organ. Recipient tissue typing is most usually carried out at the time of registration on the waiting list and is entered into the waiting list database along with other information such as patient demographics, location, residence status and registration date. Naturally donor tissue typing and recipient donor matching occur at the time of donation.

Renal allocation is most usually a patient-centred system primarily based on:

- ABO compatibility
- the level of HLA mismatching between the donor and potential recipients and
- the presence of a negative donor/recipient cytotoxic crossmatch.

Although there are many variations on the theme, the essential elements of the UK system are paralleled in other national and supranational renal allocation protocols (Box 44.12). Initially patients must be registered on the national renal recipient database. In the UK it is the National Transplant Database maintained by the UKT. The patients are grouped according to their resident status (either Group 1 or Group 2 patients in the UKT system) and as either paediatric (<18 years or an adult <35 kg) or adult patients. At the time of donation the donor's ABO group is determined and the HLA is established from lymphocytes isolated from either peripheral blood or lymph node samples, using either serological or DNA typing methods. These parameters, as well as the donor's identity number, location and age, are entered into the database and a computer match run is undertaken. The patients are sorted and listed according to the allocation algorithm.

Box 44.12   Key elements of renal allocation algorithm – UK

- Patient registered - National Transplant Database – UKT
- Patient group:
  - Group 1: citizenship or permanent resident status or citizenship of a country with reciprocal arrangements (have priority over Group 2 patients)
  - Group 2: other patients
- ABO and HLA compatibility – high level match to low level match, PRA level (high to low)
- Paediatric patients – have priority
- Local patients (same region as donor)
- National patients
- Exchange balance

In some systems such as in the United States and Europe, the kidneys are offered prior to the cytotoxic crossmatch being done. If accepted, the crossmatch is carried out in the local laboratory with donor samples forwarded with the kidney. A positive crossmatch is a strong predictor of hyperacute rejection. In the presence of a positive crossmatch the kidney will be offered on to the next patient on the list. Given the large number of patients on these waiting lists and the numerous tissue typing laboratories involved, it is not possible to maintain current serum samples for all on the waiting lists in all the laboratories. Therefore, although not ideal, pre-crossmatch allocation is necessary.

In the UKT and Australian systems current serum samples are maintained in all tissue typing locations and therefore the cytotoxic crossmatch is performed prior to the kidneys being offered. Those patients with positive crossmatches are removed from the list of potential recipients. The kidneys are then offered according to the results of the allocation algorithm.

Allocation of other organs

The UK extrarenal allocation systems are centre based with organs offered to the transplant centres and internal procedures determining recipient selection.

ABO compatibility and size matching

Matching for ABO compatibility and donor/recipient body size form the basis of recipient selection. Although there is evidence of some beneficial effect from close HLA matching in extrarenal transplantation, particularly with hearts, it is not taken into account in allocation as it is felt that the small advantages gained are far outweighed by the additional complexity the system would require. The comparatively small numbers of patients also means that a close HLA match is less common. Heart and lung transplantation requires a negative cytotoxic crossmatch especially in patients with preformed antibodies.

Age

Organs from children or the very elderly are age matched in some centres.

Organ storage times

Projected organ storage times may influence recipient selection especially when taken into account with other donor or recipient parameters such as the donor age. The allocation of extrarenal organs occurs prior to the organ retrieval being performed. There are a number of reasons why this is so, not the least being the avoidance of unnecessary procedures being performed on the donor. Limited organ storage times dictate that ischaemic time is kept to a minimum. This also avoids the necessity of mobilising and transporting retrieval teams until proven necessary. As with renal allocation, patients must be registered within the system and are grouped according to their residence status.

Priority

Most systems also have a mechanism by which priority patients can be listed. When extrarenal organs are offered the first offers are made to the urgent or priority patients within the same geographical region as the donor. If there are no such patients listed within the region then the organs are usually offered to priority-listed patients from other regions on ABO compatibility and length of time listed. Eurotransplant and the UKT Urgent Heart Allocation Scheme limits the number of urgent patients any one unit can list at any one time and also the total number of urgent cases a unit can list in any one year.

Within centre-based allocation systems if the organ is not used by an urgent patient the offer reverts back to the local unit. If the local unit cannot use the organ it is then usually offered to the other transplant units on a rotational basis. In the UKT liver system the order of offers is based on the balance of organs exchanged between transplant centres. Time since last offer is used as a tiebreak when two or more units have an identical balance of exchange. The UKT heart rota bases changes in the order of offers on the acceptance and transplantation of an organ

(Box 44.13). Although centre-based allocation provides for recipient selection based on clinical judgement, it must be a very open system so as to avoid the perception of favoured patient selection.

Patient-centred extrarenal allocation functions in a similar way to renal allocation, i.e. a patient accrues points based on criteria such as time on the waiting list and clinical status. Organs are offered to the urgent patients first then by point scores with local, regional and national priorities. Patient-centred allocation can, at times, be a cumbersome and time-consuming process but it does ensure openness in allocation.

Box 44.13 Extrarenal allocation mechanisms

- Patient registered – National Transplant Database – UKT
- Patient group:
  - Group 1: citizenship or permanent resident status or citizenship of a country with reciprocal arrangements (have priority over Group 2 patients)
  - Group 2: other patients
- Urgent patients
- Paediatric patients
- Local patients
- National patient according to rota

ORGAN RETRIEVAL

The scheduling of a multiple organ retrieval procedure is in most cases undertaken after the extrarenal organ allocation process is completed and the various teams to be involved are confirmed. The timing of the procedure is based upon a number of interrelated factors. The central focus is the provision of adequate time for the donor's family to say their final farewells. The availability of donor hospital operating theatre time, retrieval team preparation and travel time, organ transportation time, availability of crossmatch and donor serological results and projected recipient preparation times must all be taken into account and balanced to arrive at a donor theatre time that is acceptable to all. Recipient theatre times are usually scheduled based upon the donor theatre time so as to minimise allograft ischaemia. A multiple organ retrieval may include up to four separate surgical teams but is most usually undertaken by two teams, one abdominal and one thoracic. It is common practice in the UK, Europe and Australasia that wherever possible a local or regional retrieval team will perform the retrieval procedure and the organs will be shipped to the transplanting centre. In the United States this is also the common practice for kidneys and at times livers but not for hearts and lungs as the transplanting centre will send a retrieval team to the donor hospital.

The method of transport is dependent on a combination of factors. The safe storage time (cold ischaemic time) varies from organ to organ and therefore is the principal determinant of the type of transport employed. The time of retrieval will dictate whether commercial freight services or specific purpose transport is used. The distance between the donor hospital and the transplant centre will also determine if ground or air transport is utilised.

The retrieval procedure is a full surgical procedure. Anaesthetic support is required for maintenance of donor cardiovascular stability and oxygenation until such time as the organs are preserved. The anaesthetist is also required to administer various pharmacological agents (methylprednisolone 50–1000 mg and chlorpromazine 25–300 mg) aimed at improving organ preservation. Where lung donation is to occur prostacyclin is substituted for chlorpromazine due to its greater vasodilatory effect. This is given either as a slow infusion or as a bolus dose. The methylprednisolone is usually administered at the commencement of the case with the chlorpromazine or prostacyclin given just prior to organ perfusion. Additionally the donor is heparinised (5000–20 000 units) just prior to the placement of the preservation perfusion cannulas. A muscle relaxant is administered to counter the abdominal muscle reflex and facilitate exposure during the surgery.

Upon arrival in the operating theatre it is the retrieving surgeon's responsibility to review the donor's medical notes and discuss the case with the donor coordinator should there be any questions. They must satisfy themselves that no contraindications to donation exist, that the requirements of brain death have been met and that there is a lawful consent for the donation to occur. As in any other medical procedure, the identification band must also be checked against the medical chart.

The organ retrieval procedure encompasses a number of components:

- the assessment of the organs
- the surgical dissection and
- the preservation and removal of the organs.

The principal objectives of the procedure are the exclusion of disease, trauma or malignancy that may preclude transplantation, the rapid cooling of the organs by means of flushing with a cold (4°C) solution and the removal of the organs without damage. The cold flush solutions are used to induce hypothermia, which is the basic principle of organ preservation. Hypothermia decreases the rate at which enzymatic degradation of cellular components occurs. For every 10°C decrease in temperature, enzyme activity is approximately halved. Additionally most preservation solutions contain components that reduce hypothermic cell swelling caused by a reduction in sodium pump activity, prevent interstitial swelling and acidosis. A number of different solutions are in use for each of the different organs.

There are two basic surgical approaches employed by retrieval teams. The major differences between the two approaches are in the amount of dissection that is undertaken prior to the placement of the preservation perfusion cannula. There may be minimal dissection followed by placement of the cannula, organ perfusion and then removal. This is the preferred approach in the setting of a donor with cardiovascular instability as the focus will be on the perfusion and preservation of the organs. Alternatively a detailed dissection of the organs and their vascular attachments followed by cannula placement, perfusion and removal may be preferred in the stable donor. The approach used can vary from surgeon to surgeon, unit to unit, and donor to donor, with the detail depending on individual surgical preference (Box 44.14). When pneumonectomy is contemplated it is common practice for an intraoperative bronchoscopy to be performed.

Box 44.14 General sequence of the surgical procedures

- Incision and inspection for disease, trauma and malignancy
- Dissection and placement of cannulas
- Organ flush and perfusion with preservation solution
- Organ removal and packaging
- Specimen removal – lymph nodes and iliac vessels
- Wound closure

No matter which approach is used, a mid-line incision from the suprasternal notch to the symphysis pubis is made. The abdomen is opened and the sternum is split. An inspection of the abdominal contents is then done. Following either the minimal or detailed dissection in the abdomen and the placement and priming of a portal perfusion cannula in either the splenic or superior mesenteric vein, a slow infusion of cold Hartmann's or normal saline solution is commenced. This is commonly termed precooling. Where the donor is very unstable this manoeuvre is not undertaken and the portal circulation of the liver is flushed on the backtable after removal.

The thoracic team will now open the pericardium and pleural spaces, inspect the organs and commence their dissection. A slow prostacyclin infusion may be commenced around this time. Upon completion of the thoracic dissection the donor is heparinised and cannulas are placed in the ascending aorta and pulmonary artery for heart and lung perfusion. These are then primed by backflushing and connected to infusion sets primed with cold preservation solution.

The abdominal team will now cannulate the distal aorta below the renal arteries and again the primed cannula will be connected to a large-bore infusion set primed with cold Hartmann's or normal saline solution.

Once both teams have rechecked their dissection and cannula placement the chlorpromazine or, where an infusion has not been commenced, the bolus dose prostacyclin is administered. One to two minutes are allowed for the drug to circulate but it is not uncommon for gross hypotension to occur before this time has elapsed.

The aorta is crossclamped in the abdomen immediately inferior to the diaphragm and just distal to the ascending aortic cannulas in the chest. Rapid infusion is commenced on all cannulas. Vascular decompression is achieved by venting the venous system in the chest at the inferior vena cava, by transection of the pulmonary

vein and by either transection or cannulation of the distal abdominal vena cava. All support of the donor is ceased at this time. The perfusion will rapidly flush the blood from the organs and cool them to 4°C. Once the abdominal organs are pale and cool to the touch the Hartmann's or saline solution is replaced with preservation solution. Although a number of solutions are available, Viaspan® has been the standard solution for abdominal organ preservation throughout the 1990s. It is not uncommon for saline or Hartmann's slush to be placed in the chest and abdomen for additional surface cooling. Although various solutions are used for thoracic organ preservation the principle of core cooling and flushing the organ remains the same.

When adequate cooling and flushing have been achieved the organs are excised in order of shortest to longest preservation times. The thoracic organs are removed first followed by the liver, pancreas and lastly the kidneys. If heart and lungs are to be transplanted separately it is common practice to remove them *en bloc* and divide them on a backtable. The heart, lungs and kidneys are most commonly placed in saline or Hartmann's slush while the liver is usually immersed in cold Viaspan®. A final check of the organs is made and a further flush with preservation solution may be undertaken at this point.

The organ is placed into a sterile plastic bag, covered with solution and the bag is tied. This is then placed into a second and possibly a third bag with each being tied and the outer bag labelled. The packaged organ is placed into an insulated box filled with ice and the box is sealed (simple cold storage). Alternatively the kidneys may be placed on a pulsatile perfusion machine (machine perfusion). Machine perfusion is capable of extending renal storage time to 72 hours.

The organs are now transported to the various transplant hospitals. A section of spleen and a number of mesenteric lymph nodes are removed for tissue typing and iliac vessels will be taken if liver donation occurs. The vessels are immersed in preservation solution in a sterile specimen jar and placed with the liver in the insulated box prior to the box being sealed. The wound is now closed and dressed and normal postmortem procedures follow.

In the UK the Cadaveric Donor Assurances and Damage Reporting protocol outlines the responsibilities of the retrieving surgeon. It states that 'the retrieving surgeon(s) will sign the Organ Specific Donation form to confirm the absence of contraindications to donation and to report any relevant damage or physical features'. Further: 'It is the responsibility of the retrieving surgeon(s) to ensure that full information regarding any possible contraindications for the use of any organ(s) reaches the recipient transplant surgeon(s)'.

NON-HEARTBEATING DONORS

The acceptance of brain death saw donation shift from nonheartbeating to heartbeating donation as it allowed for the safe retrieval of extrarenal organs and a more controlled procedure to take place. This shift to heartbeating donors resulted in the number of non-heartbeating donors (NHBD) falling to almost negligible levels. The growing disparity between the number of available organs and the number of people awaiting transplant along with an improvement in preservation solutions and techniques, have seen a renewed interest in non-heartbeating donation. This renewed interest is primarily in the area of renal donation but at some centres it has expanded to include livers.

Initially the organs (principally kidneys) were retrieved in the operating theatre following withdrawal of ventilation and subsequent cardiac arrest. A rapid bilateral nephrectomy was performed and the organs flushed and preserved on a backtable. Today established non-heartbeating programmes commonly employ an *in situ* perfusion technique utilising a double balloon catheter inserted via the femoral artery with venous drainage via a urinary-type catheter placed into the femoral vein. The catheter is placed so that the proximal and distal balloons isolate the renal vessels. The catheter balloons are inflated using a mixture of sterile water and radiological contrast. Perfusion is commenced and a check abdominal radiograph is done to ensure correct catheter placement. Catheter insertion is usually done in the ward or emergency department following cardiac arrest. A period of up to 45 minutes warm ischaemia is acceptable. In some centres the catheters are routinely inserted and perfusion commenced prior to discussion of donation with the family. In other centres the catheters are not inserted until agreement to donate has been gained. If donation is to occur the donor is moved to the operating theatre and bilateral nephrectomy is performed. Non-heartbeating donor kidneys are usually machine perfused as this provides superior outcomes with ischaemically damaged kidneys.

Established NHBD programmes report low primary non-function (7–8%) and long-term graft survival rates similar to those achieved with heartbeating donor kidneys. NHBD programmes require an increased level of support and donor hospital cooperation but do have the potential to increase cadaveric renal transplantation rates by 20–40%.

ORGANISATION OF ORGAN DONATION SERVICES

Of those countries that have developed an organised national approach to organ donation, most have established two-tiered systems. These comprise a national data management, organ allocation and oversight body (Box 44.15) and local or regional organ procurement services. In the UK the UKT, a Special Health Authority of the National Health Service, is the national body for organ donation. The United Network for Organ Sharing (UNOS) in the United States performs very similar functions, as does the supranational Eurotransplant in Europe. These organisations are

---

Box 44.15 Principal functions of UKT and organ procurement organisations

UKT
- Tissue typing
- Organ allocation
- Policy development and enforcement
- NHS Organ Donor Registry
- National Transplant Database
- Organ Donation

OPO
- Donor assessment and provision of advice on donor maintenance
- Coordination of organ retrieval (± organ allocation)
- Development and implementation of policies and procedures to increase donation
- Public promotion of donation

---

extremely important as they maintain openness, consensus, safety and structure in donation.

At the local level the most successful organisational approaches are those of the independent organ procurement organisations (OPO) of the United States and the independent regional services of the Spanish system while those that have remained as transplant hospital-based services are the least successful. Although the principal aim of an OPO is to maximise donation its primary function from an operational perspective is that of coordinating organ and tissue donation.

CONCLUSION

Organ donation and transplantation is no doubt a complex process. It has the potential to benefit a broad spectrum of patients with end-stage organ failure. The ability to provide this treatment is dependent not only upon the public's support for organ donation but also the commitment of those within the health system to ensure the option of donation is made available whenever medically possible.

FURTHER READING

Gridelli B, Remuzzi G, Current concepts: strategies for making more organs available for transplantation. *N Engl J Medi* 2000; **343**(6):404–410

Hauptman PJ, O'Connor KJ. Medical progress: procurement and allocation of solid organs for transplantation. *N Engl J Medi* 1997; **336**(6):422–431

Wijdicks EFM. Current concepts: the diagnosis of brain death. *N Engl J Med* 2001; **344**(16):1215–1221

www.unos.org The website for the United Network for Organ Sharing. It provides information on organ transplantation in the United States.

www.uktransplant.org.uk for information on UK Transplant. The site provides statistics related to organ transplantation in the UK.

45

Renal transplantation

Andrew T. Raftery

Renal transplantation has developed from an experimental procedure of 40 years ago to the preferred therapeutic option for end-stage renal failure. For cadaver renal transplantation a one-year graft survival in excess of 85% may be expected with one-year graft survivals in excess of 95% for well-matched live-related donors.

THE DONOR

The donor may be a:

- cadaver donor
- living related donor
- living unrelated donor.

Cadaver donor

Donors should be between two and 75 years and have normal renal function. The general criteria for cadaver donors are shown in Box 45.1. Cadaveric organ donation remains the most important source of grafts for all forms of transplantation. The majority of kidneys come from brainstem-dead, heart-beating multiorgan donors, although there has been a recent increase in the use of non-heart beating donors which reflects the shortage of organs. Kidneys from non-heart beating donors must be perfused with cold preservation solution within 30 minutes of cardiac arrest.

Box 45.1   General criteria for cadaver donors

Brainstem dead, intact circulation

Age
- 2–75 years

Cause of death
- Cerebral trauma
- Cerebral haemorrhage
- Suicide
- Primary cerebral tumour (proven histologically)
- Cardiac arrest with brainstem death

Exclusions
- Extracranial malignancy
- HIV
- Hepatitis B
- Hepatitis C
- Severe untreated systemic sepsis
- Rare viral disease, e.g. Jakob–Creutzfeldt disease, or high suspicion of transmissible spongiform encephalopathy, e.g. previous recipient of dura mater graft or human pituitary growth hormone

---

Donor management

The following factors need to be addressed:

- haemodynamic instability
- fluid management
- diabetes insipidus
- ventilation
- hypothermia
- hormone levels.

A systolic pressure of around 100 mmHg is required to ensure adequate organ perfusion. Hypotension should be treated by treating hypovolaemia until the CVP is adequate. Catecholamines may be required. Dopamine is the preferred vasopressor because of its potential in maintaining renal blood flow. Destruction of the hypothalamic-pituitary access results in diabetes insipidus. Desmopressin should be given because of its long duration of action and low pressor activity. Ventilation should be maintained at an inspired oxygen level sufficent to maintain normal blood gases with an arterial saturation of 95–100%. Maintenance of a core temperature of greater than 33°C is necessary to ensure an accurate diagnosis of brainstem death. Low levels of tri-iodo-thyronine have been described after brain death. Replacement with intravenous T3 may reduce the requirement for inotropes in unstable braindead donors.

Living donor

Living donation is increasing. Live-related donation is the more common but there has been a recent increase in live-unrelated donation. In fact, the results with live-unrelated donors are better than those with well-matched cadaveric donors. The preparation of the living donor does not differ whether they are related or unrelated except that the latter have to be reported to the Unrelated Live Transplant Regulatory Authority (ULTRA) who will give permission to proceed. Unrelated donors need to be assessed by a third party who will also submit an independent report to the ULTRA.

Living donor evaluation

The following are important in living donor evaluation.

- Full history and examination
- Normal renal function
- ABO compatibility
- Negative cytotoxic crossmatch
- Confirmation of relationships (DNA testing for related donors)
- Urinalysis
- Urine culture
- Hb, FBC, ESR
- Urea and electrolytes
- Creatinine
- Liver function tests

- Blood sugar

- Virology (HBV, HBC, HIV, CMV, EBV)

- Creatinine clearance

- MRI angiography with delayed films to assess lower tract

- IVU (if MRI unavailable)

- Angiography (if MRI unavailable or for delineation of unusual vascular anomalies seen on MRI)

The procedure and the risk should be explained to the donor and their next of kin.

- Risk of general anaesthesia

- Wound infection

- Haemorrhage

- DVT

- Pulmonary embolus

- Pneumothorax

- Long-term hypertension

- Trauma to remaining kidney

- Tumour in remaining kidney

- Time off work and need to inform employer

- Life insurance – check with insurance company

Every effort must be made to ascertain that the consent is freely given and that there is no reward, coercion or threat involved. If there is any concern about the mental state of the donor, a psychiatrist should be asked for an opinion. In the case of the live-unrelated donor, both donor and recipient will be required to sign declarations indicating that the consent is freely given and this will be checked by the independent third party before a report is sent to the ULTRA.

THE RECIPIENT

The following factors need to be taken into account:

- age

- history of malignancy

- infection

- cardiovascular status

- bladder function.

Age

Biological age is more important than chronological age. Depending on fitness for anaesthesia, patients may be transplanted up to the age of 75 years.

Malignancy

Patients may be accepted for transplantation if the cancer is considered to be cured. The decision to transplant is often difficult and the time interval before transplantation varies according to the type of malignancy and the policy of the unit.

Infection

Patients with hydronephrosis, stag horn calculi and polycystic kidneys which are subject to recurrent infection should undergo nephrectomy. Occasionally, polycystic kidneys need to be removed because of sheer size and the inability to find the space below a polycystic kidney for insertion of the transplant. Patients with tuberculosis should have the disease eradicated prior to transplantation. Those with a history of TB should undergo prophylaxis with isoniazid. HIV-positive patients should not be transplanted.

Cardiovascular status

For patients with a history of angina, ECG and echocardiography should be carried out. Coronary angiography with angioplasty or bypass grafting may be required prior to transplantation. Patients with peripheral vascular disease should have pelvic and peripheral vessels checked by MRA or IVDSA.

Bladder function

Patients with urological problems, especially outflow obstruction and neurogenic bladders, should be fully investigated before transplant. Urodynamics should be carried out and ultrasound to assess residual urine should be undertaken. Bladder augmentation or creation of an ileal conduit may be required. Expert urological advice should be sought.

Absolute contraindications to renal transplantation are shown in Box 45.2.

Box 45.2 Absolute contraindications to renal transplantation
Unresolved malignancy
AIDS
Active hepatitis
Active tuberculosis
Active intravenous drug abuse
Severe vascular disease
Metabolic disorders, e.g. primary oxalosis
Life expectancy <5 years
Other untreated end-stage organ failure

Organ preservation

Preservation allows the necessary time after removal of the kidneys to complete the necessary tissue match, selection of recipient, transportation of the organ, crossmatching and the preparation of the recipient for surgery. The basic aim of preservation is to prevent delayed graft function and especially primary non-function. Two techniques are available for kidney preservation – simple hypothermia and continuous hypothermic pulsatile perfusion. With simple hypothermia the organs are flushed with a balanced salt solution, the commonest in use being Collins' solution, Marshall's solution (hyperosmolar citrate) and University of Wisconsin (UW) solution. These solutions contain osmotically active but non-permeable solutes, e.g. mannitol, sucrose, their main effect being to reduce cellular swelling during hypothermic storage. UW solution is superior to others but is also the most expensive and is superior for liver and pancreas preservation and is therefore used for multiorgan donors. It contains lactobionate and raffinose to prevent cells swelling and a colloid, hydroxyethyl starch, to prevent interstitial oedema. It also contains allopurinol and glutathione to limit damage by oxygen free radicals. Marshall's solution has a composition similar to intracellular fluid and is considerably cheaper than UW and is commonly used for renal preservation.

Kidneys can be safely stored for up to 30 hours but after this time the incidence of acute tubular necrosis increases, resulting in delayed graft function, such that it is about 80% in organs preserved for 48 hours.

With continuous hypothermic pulsatile perfusion a machine is used which is expensive. Kidneys may be preserved for up to three days with a low incidence of delayed graft function. However, in the UK, preservation for this time is rarely required and the cheaper technique of simple hypothermia is used.

Preoperative preparation

Any change in the patient's condition since the time of initial assessment in the transplant clinic should be sought on admission. In particular, a history of recent infections or blood transfusions should be sought. A full history and examination must be carried out in addition to the following investigations.

- Hb, FBC
- U&Es, creatinine
- LFTs
- Serum calcium
- Random blood sugar
- Clotting screen
- Crossmatch for four units of blood
- Cytotoxic crossmatch
- Throat swab, perineal swab, urethral swab
- Urine culture

- Chest X-ray
- ECG

Preoperative dialysis may be required, depending on blood results and the timing of the last dialysis session. Informed consent to operation is obtained and prophylaxis against DVT undertaken with graded compression stockings and subcutaneous low molecular weight heparin.

THE OPERATION

The details of the operation are described in the second part of the chapter.

POSTOPERATIVE MANAGEMENT

Immediate function occurs in 70% of cadaver kidney transplants. The following require monitoring in the early postoperative period.

- Pulse, blood pressure, respiration
- CVP
- Urine output
- Hb, FBC
- U&Es, creatinine

Intravenous fluids are administered to maintain a CVP of at least $10\,cmH_2O$ and fluid is replaced as required, the usual regime being 50 cc of intravenous fluid hourly plus the fluid equivalent of the previous hour's urine output. However, bolus doses of fluid may be necessary to maintain an adequate CVP.

A DTPA scan is required on the first postoperative day, especially in the presence of delayed function.

The following factors should be addressed in the postoperative period.

Daily

- Hb, FBC, platelets
- U&Es, creatinine
- LFTs
- Calcium
- Phosphate
- Glucose

Alternate days

- Cyclosporin/tacrolimus levels

As indicated

- DTPA scan

- Hippuran scan

- Ultrasound scan

- Creatinine clearance

Recipient of live donor kidney

The management in the preoperative and postoperative period is basically the same as for a recipient of a cadaver kidney. However, some of the investigations can be carried out in a more leisurely manner and it is our practice to check the cytotoxic crossmatch a few days before transplant to make sure that there has been no change since the initial investigations.

Delayed graft function

Delayed graft function occurs in about 30% of cadaver renal transplants. It is rare in living donor transplantation. Causes of delayed graft function include the following.

IRREVERSIBLE

- Non-viable kidney

- Hyperacute rejection

- Vascular thrombosis

REVERSIBLE

- Hypovolaemia

- Acute tubular necrosis

- Ureteric obstruction (usually technical complication)

- Drug toxicity, e.g. cyclosporin, tacrolimus, aminoglycosides

Irreversible causes can be diagnosed by isotope scan and/or duplex Doppler. Early diagnosis of irreversible causes is required to avoid unnecessary immunosuppression. Ultrasound scan (ureteric obstruction) and biopsy will identify reversible causes of delayed graft function.

Consequences of delayed graft function include:

- need for postoperative dialysis

- prolonged hospitalisation

- difficulty in diagnosis of acute rejection and other graft insults

- poorer long-term graft survival

Immunosuppression

The optimal immunosuppressive regime after renal transplantation has yet to be established. Numerous immunosuppressive drugs, polyclonal and monoclonal antibodies are available and are used in various combinations.

Immunosuppressive agents

Corticosteroids

Corticosteroids have been the mainstay of immunosuppression since the 1950s. They inhibit T cell activation by blocking IL-1, IL-2, IL-6 and IFN-γ. They also exert a local inflammatory effect. They are used as part of most induction and maintenance immunosuppressive regimes and are first-line treatment for acute rejection episodes. They have many long-term side effects and are usually gradually reduced and then discontinued in many patients with stable allograft function. Side effects include Cushingoid appearance (moon face, buffalo hump, striae, obesity), hypertension, weight gain, proximal myopathy, osteoporosis, avascular necrosis of the bone, cataracts, diabetes, stunted growth in children, peptic ulceration, pancreatitis, delayed wound healing, capillary fragility, bruising and psychosis.

Antiproliferative agents

The antiproliferative agents include azathioprine and mycophenolate mofetil (MMF). Azathioprine was one of the first agents used in transplantation and most of the patients who were transplanted more than 20 years ago remain on azathioprine in combination with steroids. The main complication is myelosuppression and careful monitoring of the white cell count is required.

MMF was introduced in the UK in 1996. MMF used in combination with a cyclosoporin (CsA) and steroids significantly reduces the incidence and severity of acute rejection episodes. However, MMF does not improve graft survival at one or three years, suggesting that it does not reduce chronic rejection despite suggestions to the contrary in animal models.

Calcineurin antagonists

These are the mainstay of current immunosuppressive therapy and include CsA and tacrolimus. The short- and long-term results using CsA or tacrolimus as maintenance therapy are similar. The selection of one or the other or the decision to change from one to the other is based on the incidence of side effects. Although nephrotoxicity is similar with both there is a higher incidence of neurotoxicity (tremor), post-transplant diabetes and alopecia with tacrolimus while there is a lower incidence of hirsuitism and gingival hyperplasia with tacrolimus.

Sirolimus

Sirolimus prevents the cytokine-dependent proliferation of T cells but acts at a different stage of the T cell activation compared with CsA and tacrolimus. It is a more potent immunosuppressive agent than CsA and is not nephrotoxic. Used in combination with CsA, it reduces the incidence of acute rejection episodes. There is experimental evidence that it may be beneficial in chronic rejection.

Monoclonal antibodies

ANTI-CD3 MONOCLONAL ANTIBODIES

OKT3 plays an established role in the reversal of steroid-resistant acute rejection episodes. It has been shown that OKT3 will reverse 80% of steroid-resistant episodes. Side effects occur due to the cytokine release syndrome and include fever, headache, rigors, chest pain, wheezing, nausea and vomiting. Severe pulmonary oedema may occur, particularly in the fluid-overloaded patient. There is an increased incidence of lymphoproliferative disease and opportunistic infections.

ANTI IL-2R MONOCLONAL ANTIBODIES

Basiliximab in combination with CsA and steroids decreases the incidence and severity of acute rejection episodes. Basiliximab-treated patients also display better renal function during the first transplant year than placebo-treated controls. Basiliximab is most appropriately used for induction therapy, reserving OKT3 for any subsequent rejection episodes. Side effects have not been reported and cytokine release syndrome does not occur.

Classification of immunosuppression

Immunosuppression for transplantation may be classified as follows.

- Induction therapy
- Prophylaxis against acute rejection
- Maintenance therapy
- Anti-rejection therapy
- Refractory rejection therapy

Induction therapy

Induction therapy attempts to avoid the occurrence or to delay the onset of an acute rejection episode. This is based on the view that early rejection episodes may have a long-term detrimental effect on the kidney. However, using ALG, ATG or OKT3 as induction therapy has not been shown to improve one-year graft survivals. Another reason for using induction therapy is to avoid using high doses of calcineurin inhibitors which cause renal dysfunction. However, there is a tendency to use lower doses of calcineurin inhibitors at the present time and therefore induction therapy with antilymphocyte sera has largely been abandoned due to its toxicity and expense.

The introduction of anti-IL-2R monoclonal antibodies has, however, been beneficial. These agents have been shown to reduce acute rejection rates when used as induction therapy and in combination with CsA. They are less toxic than antilymphocyte sera, almost as potent and cost less.

Prophylaxis against acute rejection

Patients are started on a combination of immunosuppressive agents immediately following transplantation. The main reason for using combinations is to allow reduction in the dose of each agent to attempt to reduce toxicity. Although the agents used are effective in prevention of acute rejection, there is no evidence that they are effective against the occurrence or progression of chronic rejection, with the possible exception of MMF.

Cyclosporin microemulsion remains the backbone of most immunosuppressive regimes. Triple immnosuppression with prednisolone, azathioprine and CsA results in a rejection-free patient in 40% of transplants. There is, however, a move towards other immunosuppressive regimes, e.g. prednisolone, CsA in reduced dose with the addition of MMF or prednisolone, azathioprine and tacrolimus. Results of multicentre trials show that steroids, CsA and MMF, and tacrolimus-based triple therapy have no benefit on graft or patient survival at one year but do show a further reduction in the incidence of acute rejection episodes.

Maintenance therapy

The drugs used as prophylaxis against acute rejection are usually continued as maintenance therapy, the dose being gradually reduced over a period of time. In some cases, one of the drugs may be eliminated with time, e.g. steroids to prevent long-term complications. Reduction in the dose of maintenance therapy is based on the concept of graft 'accommodation', i.e. the gradual acceptance of graft by the host.

Antirejection therapy

Ideally this should not be used without histological evidence of acute rejection. Acute rejection episodes may be mild, moderate or severe. Treatment of rejection depends on the severity of the episode and may be treated with pulsed doses of steroids or anti-lymphocyte antibodies.

Refractory rejection therapy

Refractory rejection is defined as a rejection episode which is resistant to both steroid therapy and antilymphocyte antibodies and is confirmed by biopsy. 'Rescue' therapy may then be attempted. The addition of tacrolimus to a CsA and prednisolone regime, and of sirolimus to a CsA and prednisolone regime, and a tacrolimus and prednisolone regime, have been demonstrated to improve renal function.

COMPLICATIONS

Complications of renal transplants are as follows.

- Related to the operation
- Rejection
- Infection
- Malignancy
- Recurrent disease

Complications related to surgery

Vascular complications

- Renal artery thrombosis
- Renal vein thrombosis
- Renal artery stenosis
- Lymphocoele

Urological complications

- Ureteric leak
- Ureteric obstruction

Vascular complications

Renal artery thrombosis

Renal artery thrombosis occurs with an incidence of about 1% and is usually the result of technical complications. It may be suspected if there was a technically difficult arterial anastomosis.

SYMPTOMS AND SIGNS

- Postoperative anuria
- Sudden cessation of urine flow

INVESTIGATIONS

- Duplex Doppler – no flow in renal artery
- DTPA scan – absence of renal outline

TREATMENT

- Transplant nephrectomy

Renal vein thrombosis

This may follow technical problems with the venous anastomosis and occurs with an incidence of 1–4%. Complete renal vein thrombosis may present in a similar manner to renal artery thrombosis, but occasionally arterial blood continues to pump into the kidney, so that the kidney swells and splits with life-threatening haemorrhage. An urgent graft nephrectomy is required. Partial renal vein thrombosis presents with deteriorating renal function and proteinuria. The following are features.

SYMPTOMS AND SIGNS

- Ipsilateral leg swelling
- Proteinuria
- Ipsilateral deep vein thrombosis

INVESTIGATIONS

- Duplex Doppler
- Angiography with venous phase

TREATMENT

- Complete renal vein thrombosis – transplant nephrectomy
- Thrombectomy (rarely successful)
- Anticoagulation (partial renal vein thrombosis)

Renal artery stenosis

This should be suspected if poorly controlled hypertension occurs in a transplant recipient. It occurs with an incidence of 2–5%. The following are features.

Symptoms and signs

- Refractory hypertension
- Deteriorating renal function
- Bruit over kidney

INVESTIGATIONS

- Duplex Doppler
- Angiography

TREATMENT

- Percutaneous transluminal angioplasty with or without stenting
- Surgery

Lymphocoele

Lymphocoeles, which are lymph collections around the kidney, occur with an incidence of 1–15%. They have been ascribed to inadequate ligation of lymphatics surrounding the iliac vessels. Most lymphocoeles are small and asymptomatic. Rarely is a lymphocoele palpable. The following are features.

SYMPTOMS AND SIGNS

- Ipsilateral leg swelling
- Rarely a palpable mass

INVESTIGATIONS

- Ultrasound/CT scan – Fluid collection ± hydronephrosis

TREATMENT

- Percutaneous drainage under ultrasound control – high incidence of recurrence
- Percutaneous drainage under ultrasound control with indwelling drain and repeated injections of sclerosant agents, e.g. povidone iodine
- Laparoscopic drainage via a window into the peritoneal cavity
- Open surgical drainage via a window into the peritoneal cavity

Recurrence often occurs following percutaneous drainage with or without injection of a sclerosing agent. Laparoscopic drainage into the peritoneal cavity is probably the best approach.

Urological complications

Ureteric leak

This occurs with an incidence of 1–5% and may be due to anastomotic problems at the bladder or to ureteric necrosis consequent on inadequate ureteric blood supply. The latter may be caused by poor technique at the time of donor nephrectomy as a result of stripping periureteric tissue or thrombosis of the ureteric blood supply during a severe rejection episode. If the drain is still *in situ*, urine will leak down the drain. The following are features of ureteric leakage.

SYMPTOMS AND SIGNS

- Pain, swelling, tenderness around the kidney
- Urine leakage from drain or wound
- Decreased urine output
- Fever

INVESTIGATIONS

- Elevated serum creatinine
- Ultrasound scan – fluid collection
- DTPA scan – leakage of contrast into the retroperitoneum
- Cystogram
- Antegrade pyelogram

TREATMENT

- Expectant – if small leak and drain *in situ*
- Surgical reexploration with reimplantation of ureter, uretero-ureterostomy or Boari flap

Ureteric obstruction

This occurs with an incidence of 1–5%. It may be due to faulty anastomotic technique or partial ischaemia of the lower ureter with subsequent fibrosis. The following are features of ureteric obstruction.

SYMPTOMS AND SIGNS

- Decreased urine output
- Urinary tract infection
- Pain over graft

INVESTIGATIONS

- Increasing serum creatinine
- Ultrasound scan – hydronephrosis
- Antegrade pyelogram confirms diagnosis and defines site of obstruction

TREATMENT

- Short distal strictures – percutaneous nephrostomy with balloon dilatation and stenting or resection and reimplantation of ureter

- Long ischaemic strictures or proximal obstruction – pyelo-ureterostomy or ureteroureterostomy if native ureter available. If native ureter not available, psoas hitch or Boari flap

Rejection

Rejection occurs in three main forms:

- hyperacute
- acute
- chronic.

Hyperacute rejection

This is an irreversible antibody-mediated rejection occurring within minutes or hours of transplantation. It is exceedingly rare due to pretransplant crossmatching between recipient serum and donor lymphocytes. It may be due to an error in transplanting across blood group incompatibility. It is irreversible and graft nephrectomy is required.

Acute rejection

This is most common in the early transplant period, especially during the first three months, but may occur at any time. Acute rejection is diagnosed on the following criteria.

- Pyrexia
- Oliguria
- Weight gain
- Graft tenderness
- Rising serum creatinine
- Radioisotope scan (DTPA – reduced perfusion)
- Ultrasound scan
- Core biopsy

Treatment of acute rejection

The three most useful approaches are:

- high-dose intravenous steroids
- ATG
- OKT3.

Most units use pulsed doses of methylprednisolone, usually 500 mg IV over one hour daily for three days. About 75% of acute rejection episodes respond to this regime. ATG is usually reserved for acute rejection episodes that do not respond to high-dose steroids. Treatment is expensive, requires hospitalisation and predisposes the patient to viral infection. OKT3 is significantly more effective than steroids in reversing the first acute rejection episode and can also reverse steroid-resistant rejection episodes. OKT3 has more side effects than ATG. The first treatment causes cytokine release syndrome with fever, rigors, tremor and pulmonary oedema in overhydrated patients. Basic immuno-suppression should be reduced during OKT3 which is usually administered for 7–10 days. There is a high incidence of viral infections in patients treated with OKT3 and ganciclovir should be administered. Steroid-resistant rejection may also respond to rescue treatment with either tacrolimus, MMF or sirolimus.

Chronic rejection

Chronic rejection is the main cause of late failure in renal grafts. About 5% of renal grafts per year are lost from chronic rejection. There is a slowly progressive decline in renal function appearing months or years post transplant, the rate of decline being variable.

Risk factors for chronic rejection include:

- poor HLA matching
- acute rejection
- immunosuppressive drugs, e.g. calcineurin inhibitors
- delayed graft function – ischaemia/reperfusion injury
- hyperlipidaemia
- hypertension
- CMV infection
- non-compliance with treatment
- donor source – lower incidence with live donors than cadaver donors.

There is no effective treatment for established chronic rejection.

Infection

In patients undergoing transplantation, infections can be caused by common bacteria and nosocomial infections but a greater threat is posed by the risk of developing opportunistic infection. Infections occurring in the first month postoperatively are similar to those experienced by general surgical patients. In the period between one and six months, opportunistic infections predominate whereas after six months, the type of infection is similar to that observed in the general population although fungal infections may occur, particularly if further immunosuppressive therapy is required for late rejection episodes.

A timetable of occurrence of infections in renal transplant recipients is shown in Box 45.3.

The methods of investigation and treatment of these conditions are outside the remit of this chapter.

Malignancy

The incidence of neoplasia as a whole is about 3–4 times more frequent among transplant recipients than in age-matched controls. The incidence of some cancers is much greater than others. The risk ratio is highest when a viral aetiology has been implicated, as in lymphomas, Kaposi's sarcoma, skin cancers and cancer of the perineum.

The following gives a comparison between the incidence of cancer in renal transplant recipients and in the general population.

- Kaposi's sarcoma (1000 times)

- Skin cancers (100 times)

- Vulvar and anal cancers (100 times)

- Non-Hodgkin's lymphoma (40 times)

- Hepatic carcinoma (30 times)

- Renal carcinoma (8 times)

Treatment of post-transplant malignancy includes reduction or withdrawal of immunosuppression, antiviral agents and interferon as adjuncts to conventional treatment of malignancy.

Recurrent disease

Recurrence of the original disease following renal transplantation is a relatively frequent event which may lead to allograft dysfunction and occasionally loss of the kidney. All forms of glomerulonephritis may recur after transplantation but focal segmental glomerulosclerosis (FSGS) is associated with the highest rate of graft failure, being reported as between 15% and 50%, and is even higher among children. Membranous nephropathy, membranoproliferative glomerulonephritis and IgA nephropathy may also recur. Anti-GBM glomerulonephritis is the least likely to recur but graft failure does occur in a very small percentage of patients with this condition.

Other diseases that may recur in the graft include Henoch–Schönlein purpura (18%), primary and secondary amyloidosis (10–40%) and haemolytic-uraemic syndrome (10–45%). Recurrence of lupus nephritis and Wegener's granulomatosis is rare. Of the metabolic diseases, oxalosis may show rapid recurrence with deposition of oxalate crystals in the graft, resulting in graft loss. Although histological changes of diabetic nephropathy may recur in diabetic recipients, their progression is slow and the incidence of graft loss is low (around 2%). Cystinosis does not recur in the transplanted kidney.

OPERATIVE SURGERY

Donor nephrectomy (Figure 45.1)

This is usually the last part of multiorgan harvesting. Occasionally, however, only kidneys are removed due to contraindications to removal of other organs but the procedure is basically the same. For multiorgan donation a mid-line incision is made extending from the suprasternal notch to the symphysis pubis. The sternum is split. This section will concentrate only on the preparation of the kidneys for removal.

- Self-retaining retractors are inserted into the abdomen.

- The posterior peritoneum lateral to the ascending colon is mobilised, the incision being carried medially around the caecum and upwards towards the ligament of Treitz. The duodenum is 'Kocherised'.

- The posterior peritoneum lateral to the descending and sigmoid colon is then incised.

- The right colon, small bowel and left colon are reflected superiorly superficial to the gonadal vessels.

- The abdominal aorta and IVC are exposed proximal to the bifurcation and encircled with slings.

- The origin of the inferior mesenteric artery is divided between 0 Vicryl ligatures.

- Care must be taken to avoid injury to polar arteries crossing anterior to the IVC to the lower pole of the right kidney or from the aorta to the left kidney.

- The left renal vein is identified crossing anteriorly to the aorta. The superior mesenteric artery (SMA) is immediately above.

- The SMA is doubly ligated with 1 Vicryl and divided.

- The lesser sac is entered and the aorta above the SMA isolated following division of the crura of the diaphragm.

- The aorta is encircled with a sling.

- A sling is placed around the IVC just below the liver.

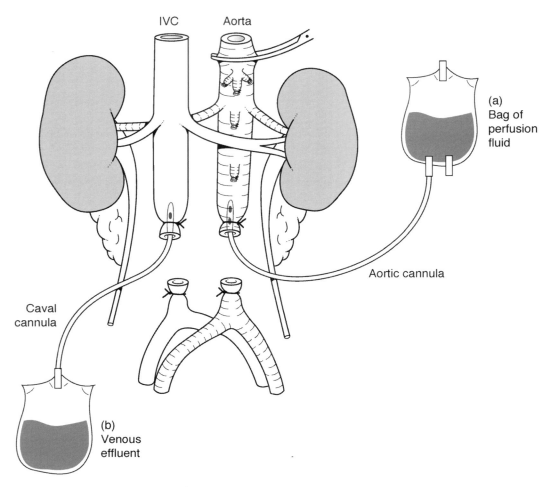

Figure 45.1 Cadaver donor nephrectomy. *En bloc* dissection of kidneys in cadaver donor. (a) Perfusion fluid is delivered by a cannula into the aorta which is clamped at the level of the crura of the diaphragm. (b) The venous effluent drains from the inferior vena cava into a bag.

- 5000 units of heparin are administered intravenously.

- A cannula is placed in the distal aorta so that its tip lies adjacent to the origins of the renal arteries. It is then tied in place.

- A large-bore cannula is placed in the distal IVC and tied in place so that blood can drain out through it.

- The proximal aorta is clamped at the level of the diaphragm and the abdominal aorta perfused with cold preservation fluid, e.g. UW or Marshall's. The drainage cannula in the lower IVC is allowed to drain via gravity.

- Iced slush of sterile saline may be directly applied to the kidneys to provide surface cooling.

- The kidneys usually become pale and cool after rapid infusion of 500 ml of preservation fluid but perfusion is continued throughout the procedure.

- The ureters are mobilised as far down into the pelvis as possible and divided. Plenty of extraneous tissues must be left on the ureter.

- The final mobilisation of the kidneys takes place within the plane of Gerota's fascia.

- The distal aorta and IVC are divided and the entire block lifted anteriorly to expose the lumbar vessels posteriorly. These are divided after being clamped with Liga clips.

- The proximal aorta and IVC are then divided above the level of the coeliac axis and the kidneys, ureters and IVC removed *en bloc* and placed in a bowel of cold perfusion fluid. Excess perinephric fat is removed and the kidneys separated by division of the aorta and IVC in the mid-line. (Figure 45.2).

- If perfusion appears poor each kidney may then be individually perfused via a cannula in the renal artery.

- The kidneys are then packed individually in sterile bags surrounded by cold perfusion fluid, each bag being placed in an outer bag containing cold perfusion fluid. They are then stored in boxes surrounded by crushed ice until transplantation.

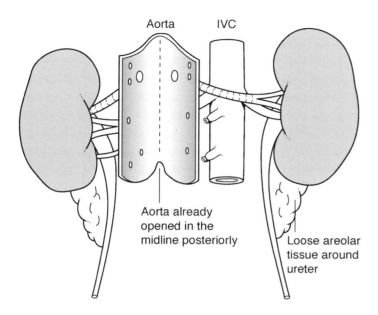

Figure 45.2 Dissection of the *en bloc* specimen (posterior view). The aorta has already been divided longitudinally in the mid-line posteriorly. The anterior wall of the aorta is then carefully divided along the dotted line. This leaves the renal arteries on patches of aorta. The inferior vena cava is then dealt with similarly. It is important at this stage to make sure that when the fat has been dissected from around the kidney, enough loose areolar tissue is left between the lower pole of the kidney and the ureter to ensure adequate blood supply to the ureter.

- Donor mesenteric lymph nodes and spleen are taken for tissue typing and crossmatching.
- The incision is closed and dressed in the normal way.

Living donor nephrectomy

This may be carried out via the following approaches:

- loin approach through bed of 12th rib (extraperitoneal)
- subcostal anterior transperitoneal approach
- laparoscopically.

Careful dissection of the renal vasculature and ureter is required. The advantage of living donor nephrectomy is that preoperative renal angiography has been obtained and this facilitates identification of the vessels. The left kidney is usually chosen if it has a single renal artery as there is a good length of vein. Perfusion of the kidney is carried out using 1 litre of cold perfusion solution and the kidney delivered in sterile bags surrounded by cold preservation fluid to the recipient surgeon.

Laparoscopic living donor nephrectomy is becoming more popular although there may be problems with the procedure. These involve:

- injuries to other structures
- longer operating time

- increased incidence of ureteric complications
- prolonged warm ischaemic time during extraction phase
- need for extensive experience at laparoscopic surgery.

Preparation of the kidney

If the kidney is removed by the transplant team who are to transplant it, preparation of the kidney may be carried out at the same time as the donor nephrectomy. However, if the kidney comes from another source then it will need to be examined and prepared prior to taking the recipient to theatre. Inspection of the kidney takes place in theatre under full aseptic conditions. The kidney is removed from the bags and immersed in fresh perfusion fluid. The following factors are important in inspection of the kidney.

- Assess that the kidney is well perfused.
- The perinephric fat may need removing to expose the kidney to make sure that perfusion is adequate.
- The renal vein should then be inspected and dissected to make sure that all branches have been tied. If they have not they must be tied at this point. The vein should not be dissected too far back into the pelvis for fear of damaging the vascular supply. At this point the vein should be back-perfused with perfusion fluid to make sure there are no leaks from it.
- The renal artery should now be inspected. Check the patch to make sure there is no gross atheroma or narrowing of the ostium of the renal artery. Check that there are no additional arteries that are not attached to the patch. Having ascertained this, clean up the renal artery but not too deep into the renal hilum.
- The ureter should now be inspected. Make sure that there is an adequate length of ureter and that there is plenty of tissue around the ureter to protect its blood supply. Once the surgeon is happy that this is a technically sound kidney, it should be repacked in sterile bags surrounded by crushed ice until it is required for transplantation.

Recipient operation

Regardless of the source of the donor kidney the preferred site of implantation is onto the iliac vessels in the pelvis. Many surgeons prefer to place a right kidney into the left iliac fossa and vice versa, the rationale being to keep the renal pelvis and ureter anterior to the renal vessels in case access is required to these, e.g. following ureteric necrosis.

The patient is positioned supine on the operating table. The anaesthetist inserts a peripheral line and a central line to measure CVP. A urethral catheter is inserted and connected to a 500 ml bag of normal saline such that the bladder may be distended prior to ureteric anastomosis. Intravenous antibiotics are administered at the time of induction of the anaesthesia, the author's preference being for cefuroxime.

The following steps are then carried out.

- Rutherford Morrison incision with extraperitoneal approach to the iliac vessels.

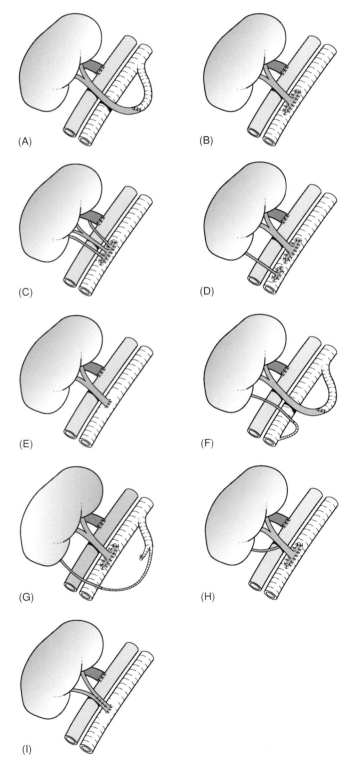

(A)

(B)

(C)

(D)

(E)

(F)

(G)

(H)

(I)

- The peritoneum is reflected medially and the common, external and internal iliac arteries and veins exposed. If the renal artery is on a Carrel patch only the external iliac artery is exposed. If the renal artery is not on a Carrel patch (as in a live donor) the three iliac arteries need to be exposed and slinged.

- With a short right renal vein the internal iliac vein(s) may need to be divided to free the common and external iliac veins. With a long left renal vein only the external iliac vein may require mobilising.

- The donor renal vein is anastomosed end to side to either the external iliac vein or common iliac vein using a continuous 5/0 Prolene suture.

- If the donor renal artery is on a Carrel patch it is anastomosed to the side of the external iliac artery using a continuous 5/0 Prolene suture. If there is no patch the donor renal artery is anastomosed end to end to the divided and mobilised internal iliac artery. It may be necessary on occasions to carry out endarterectomy on an arteriosclerotic internal iliac artery. Alternatively, the renal artery may be spatulated and anastomosed to the side of the external iliac artery if the internal iliac artery is unsuitable.

- Depending on the vascular anatomy, there are many variations in the types of anastomosis carried out. Some of these are shown in Figure 45.3.

- Prior to release of the clamps it is the author's practice to administer 500 mg of methylprednisolone and 80 mg frusemide IV.

- Following release of the clamps additional sutures may be required in the anastomosis. It is usual for some bleeding points to occur in the fat around the hilum of the kidney and these should be carefully dealt with at this point.

- The ureter is then implanted into the bladder (Figure 45.4). The bladder should be distended with normal saline via the urethral catheter. The author's preference is to anastomose the ureter to the dome of the bladder. In the male, the ureter is lead under the spermatic cord.

Figure 45.3 Variations in arterial anastomosis. In each case the venous anastomosis is shown as a single renal vein anastomosed end to side to the external iliac vein. **A**. The donor renal artery is anastomosed end to end to the recipient internal iliac artery. **B**. A single donor renal artery on a Carrel patch is anastomosed to the side of the recipient external iliac artery. **C**. Multiple (three) donor renal arteries on a Carrel patch are anastomosed to the side of the recipient external iliac artery. **D**. Two separate arteries, a main renal artery on a Carrel patch and a lower polar artery on a Carrel patch, are anastomosed to the side of the recipient external iliac artery. **E**. The donor renal artery, without a patch, is anastomosed end to side to the external iliac artery. **F**. The main renal artery is anastomosed end to end to the recipient's internal iliac artery. The lower polar artery is anastomosed end to end to the recipient inferior epigastric artery. **G**. The main renal artery on a Carrel patch is anastomosed end to side to the external iliac artery. The lower polar artery is anastomosed end to end to a branch of the recipient internal iliac artery. **H**. The lower polar artery is anastomosed to the side of the main donor renal artery. **I**. Two equal-sized renal arteries are joined in a 'double barrel' anastomosis and subsequently anastomosed end to side to the recipient external iliac artery. Reprinted from Coen LD, Raftery AT 1992 with permission of the publishers of *Clinical Anatomy*.

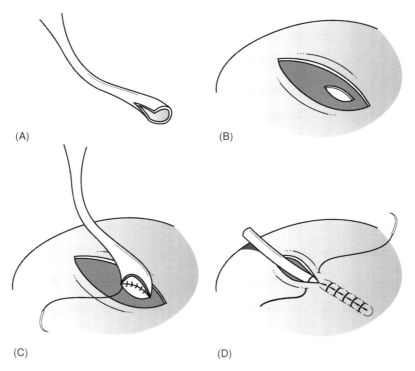

(A) (B) (C) (D)

Figure 45.4 Procedure for ureteroneocystostomy. **A**. The end of the ureter is spatulated. **B**. An incision is made through the muscular wall of the bladder down to the bladder mucosa. An opening is then made in the bladder mucosa. **C**. The ureterovesical anastomosis is then carried out using interrupted 4/0 absorbable sutures. **D**. Creation of a submucosal tunnel by approximation of the muscular layers over the ureter.

- The dome of the bladder is cleared of extraperitoneal fat and the muscle exposed.

- The muscle is opened with a curved haemostat until the mucosa is exposed. This is done over a length of approximately 4 cm. The mucosa is then opened over the distal end of the incision and the bladder emptied via suction. The tip of the ureter is spatulated over about 2 cm and anastomosed to the bladder mucosa using interrupted 4/0 absorbable sutures. The muscle layer is then closed over the ureter using interrupted 2/0 Vicryl sutures so that the ureter runs in a muscular tunnel before entering the bladder. The ureteric anastomosis is usually carried out over a double J stent which is subsequently removed at flexible cystoscopy 4–6 weeks postoperatively. Care must be taken that the ureter is not too long so that it kinks or not too short such that it is under tension.

- Check carefully for haemostasis, especially at the hilum of the kidney.

- Check the position of the kidneys such that there is no kinking of the vessels.

- Insert a closed low-pressure suction drain into the retroperitoneal space.

- Close the wound in layers using 0 or 1 Vicryl sutures.

- Connect the catheter to the urinometer so that hourly urine output can be accurately measured.

Reoperation for ureteric complications

Investigations of urinary leak/obstruction are described earlier in the chapter.

Ureteric obstruction

Depending on the cause and site this may be managed by:

- nephrostomy:
  - relief of dilatation
  - recovery of renal function
  - temporary while clots lyse and oedema settles

- nephrostomy with percutaneous dilatation of the site of obstruction with insertion of stent

- surgery:
  - short segment distal obstruction: resection and reimplantation of ureter
  - long segment obstruction or limited length of donor ureter: uretero-pyelostomy (to native ureter), psoas hitch and pyelovesicostomy, Boari flap.

Ureteric leak

Minor leaks may be treated expectantly provided there is still a drain *in situ* and the ureteric stent remains. Most leaks, however, usually occur after the drain has been removed.

723

Re-exploration for ureteric problems

The procedure is carried out under general anaesthesia and anti-biotics are administered intravenously at the time of anaesthesia induction. If the urine is infected the antibiotic appropriate to prior cultures and sensitivities is used. A urethral catheter is inserted (if not already present) and connected to a bag of normal saline.

The transplant incision is opened and the diagnosis confirmed.

For distal obstruction or distal ureteric necrosis with an adequate length of ureter:

- the area of obstruction/necrosis is excised back to fresh bleed-ing ureter

- the ureter is spatulated and reanastomosed to the same site in the bladder using interrupted 4/0 absorbable sutures between ureter and bladder mucosa and interrupted 2/0 absorbable sutures to form a muscle tunnel. A double J stent is used

- the bladder is tested for leaks by distending with normal saline.

For proximal obstruction, long-length stenoses, limited length of donor ureter and total ureteric necrosis:

- mobilise the recipient native ureter leaving as much extraneous tissue on it as possible

- ligate the proximal ureter with 2/0 Vicryl. This can usually be done with impunity, although occasionally in the presence of pyelonephritis the native kidney may form a pyonephrosis and have to be removed at a later stage

- carry out uretero-pyelostomy across a double J stent using interrupted absorbable 4/0 sutures

- insert a soft latex tube drain to the area of the anastomosis. This will create an excellent track if any urine leakage occurs.

If the recipient's native ureter has been previously removed:

- carry out a pyelovesicostomy following mobilisation of the bladder and a 'psoas hitch'

- alternatively, create a Boari flap and anastomose it to the trans-plant renal pelvis.

The assistance of a urologist will usually be required with the above two approaches.

- The wound is closed in layers as for the initial transplant.

If a percutaneous nephrostomy has been inserted preoperatively, this may be left *in situ* and an antegrade pyelogram carried out at five days postoperatively. If there is no leakage/obstruction then the nephrostomy tube is clamped and, in the absence of problems, may be removed two days later. The drain is usually removed at five days and the stent at about 30 days. If the renal pelvis is friable, leakage of urine may occur around the drain. Latex tube drains form a good track and if urine leakage continues the drain may be safely removed at 10 days and a bag applied over the drain

site. In the absence of distal obstruction, the urine leakage usually settles spontaneously.

Transplant nephrectomy

Most transplant units have a policy to remove grafts that fail within 90 days of transplantation. After this time, only those that cause problems, e.g pain or haematuria, are removed. The indi-cations for transplant nephrectomy are shown in Box 45.4.

The technique of donor nephrectomy depends upon the time post transplant when it is performed. An extracapsular approach is performed in the first four weeks post transplant together with complete removal of the donor artery, vein and ureter. After this time, because of adhesions between the capsule and surrounding tissues, a subcapsular approach is used and part of the vein, artery and ureter remains.

Box 45.4   Indicators for transplant nephrectomy

Hyperacute rejection
Graft thrombosis
Recurrent pain/infection in failed graft
Persistent haematuria in failed graft
Recurrent renal disease with severe proteinuria

Technique

The procedure is carried out under general anaesthesia. Antibiotics, usually cefuroxime, are given IV following induction of anaesthesia. The bladder is catheterised and the catheter attached to a bag of normal saline.

The transplant incision is opened, being careful not to enter the peritoneum which is often adherent to the kidney and must be carefully dissected off.

Extracapsular approach (within four weeks of transplantation)

- The vascular anastomoses are exposed and clamps applied above and below.

- The Carrel patch is removed from the external iliac artery and heparinised saline is injected distally.

- The renal vein is removed from the external iliac vein.

- The ureter is then clamped and divided and the kidney removed and sent for pathological examination.

- The arteriotomy in the external iliac artery is closed with a continuous 5/0 Prolene suture. If this narrows the artery the defect should be repaired with a vein patch.

- The external iliac vein is closed with continuous 5/0 Prolene sutures.

- If the arterial anastomosis is end to end with the internal iliac artery, the internal iliac artery is ligated with 1 Vicryl proximal to the anastomosis.

- The clamps are removed and the suture lines examined for haemostasis.

- The clamped ureter is then traced to the bladder and excised *in toto*. The bladder mucosa is closed with a 4/0 absorbable suture and the muscle is closed with an absorbable 2/0 suture.

The subcapsular approach (more than four weeks post-transplantation)

- The renal capsule is incised and a plane developed towards the hilum.

- The ureter is exposed and ligated with 0 Vicryl as near the bladder as possible but not totally excised.

- The hilum is exposed and a Satinsky clamp applied close to the hilum encompassing both renal artery and renal vein.

- The kidney is then excised following division of the vessels close to the hilum.

- The renal artery (or arteries) is then doubly ligated with 0 Vicryl and the renal vein(s) closed with a continuous 5/0 Prolene suture and the Satinsky clamp removed.

- The bladder is then distended with normal saline to check that there is no leak.

- The wound is closed in layers as for the transplant operation following insertion of a low-pressure suction drain to the transplant bed.

Antibiotics are continued until the urethral catheter is removed, the suction drain being removed if drainage is minimal around 48 hours. The urethral catheter is removed on the fifth postoperative day.

Complications of transplant nephrectomy

- Haematoma
- Wound infection
- Abscess formation
- Major haemorrhage from infected suture line

FURTHER READING

Barry JM. Renal transplantation. *Curr Opin Urol* 1999; **9**(2):121–127

Fabrizii V, Horl WH. Renal transplantation in the elderly. *Curr Opin Urol* 2001; **11**(2):159–163

Waller JR, Nicholson ML. Molecular mechanisms of renal allograft fibrosis. *Br J Surg* 2001; **88**(11):1429–1441

Wilkinson A. Progress in the clinical application of immunosuppressive drugs in renal transplantation. *Curr Opin Nephrol Hypertension* 2001; **10**(6):763–770

Wuthrich RP. Factor V Leiden mutation: potential thrombogenic role in renal vein, dialysis graft and transplant vascular thrombosis. *Curr Opin Nephrol Hypertension* 2001; **10**(3):409–414

46

Liver transplantation

Daniel M. Jaeck, Elie Oussoultzoglou

INTRODUCTION

The first human orthotopic liver transplantation was performed by Thomas Starzl in 1963 in Denver at the University of Colorado, USA. Even if the survival of this patient and of several subsequently transplanted patients was poor, this pioneering effort has since come a long way. Improved results and survival were obtained in the following decades (30% one-year survival in 1970, 80% in 1990, around 90% currently, in elective cases). These excellent results were achieved following improvements not only in surgical techniques but also in organ preservation and in the use of new and powerful immunosuppressive treatments. Cyclosporin was introduced around 1980 in kidney and liver transplantation, followed by FK-506 in 1989.

Although it was initially considered a procedure reserved for patients with end-stage chronic liver disease or unresectable primary liver malignancy, the indications for liver transplantation evolved rapidly in the 1980s. The National Institutes of Health Consensus Conference held in June 1983 in Washington recognised liver transplantation as an accepted therapeutic procedure which 'should be performed in a late enough phase of the disease to offer the patient all opportunity for spontaneous stabilization and recovery but in an early enough phase to give the surgical procedure a fair chance of success'. Ten years later a Consensus Conference held in Paris (June 1993) clarified the indications as well as the contraindications of liver transplantation.

During this period the number of liver transplants performed each year increased dramatically, rising in Europe, for instance, from less than 30 in 1980 to 3500 in 1998. The shortage of donor organs has now become a major problem, restricting the development of liver transplantation. New ways have been devised to increase the pool of grafts:

- the split-liver technique (first *ex vivo*, then *in situ*)
- the use of 'marginal quality' donor liver
- the living related donor (first adult to child and now even adult to adult).

In addition to the above, other approaches such as xenotransplantation or hepatocyte transplantation are also currently being explored.

This spectacular evolution and the fabulous success of liver transplantation 'fostered such changes in practically every aspect of hepatology and liver surgery that it was no longer possible, since 1985, to have a liver disease centre without hepatic transplant capability'.

INDICATIONS FOR LIVER TRANSPLANTATION

Liver transplantation is no longer restricted to patients with a life-threatening illness such as end-stage chronic liver disease or fulminant hepatic failure. The remarkable improvements in the results of this technique have led patients who are not in immediate danger of death to be considered as candidates – patients who experience a poor quality of life due to severe lassitude or pruritus, intractable ascites or recurrent cholangitis. The current indications may be classified into two groups:

- indications unanimously accepted and validated
- other indications still being debated.

Indications unanimously accepted and validated

For these patients, all the criteria represented in Box 46.1 are present. These indications can be classified into three groups:

- cholestatic liver diseases
- fulminant hepatic failure
- other miscellanous rare diseases (mainly metabolic diseases).

Box 46.1 Criteria present in patients with unanimously accepted indications for liver transplantation

- Liver transplantation offers a higher five-year survival rate than any other therapeutic procedure
- Liver transplantation offers a better quality of life than any other therapeutic procedure
- There is no (or very little) risk of recurrence of the primary disease on the graft

---

Cholestatic liver diseases

Three diseases are clear indications for liver transplantation as soon as they induce a poor quality of life or become life-threatening.

- *Primary biliary cirrhosis* (PBC), an autoimmune disease which affects mainly middle-aged and elderly women, is considered as the best indication for liver transplantation. The use of ursodeoxycholic acid seems able to delay the timing for transplantation; however, as soon as bilirubinaemia is higher than $100 \mu mol/l$ (together with some other prognostic factors) the decision for liver replacement should be taken.

- *Primary sclerosing cholangitis* (PSC) is a rare condition often associated with inflammatory bowel disease, mainly in young male patients. Progression of PSC is difficult to predict; however, up to 30% of the patients will develop cholangiocarcinoma within 10 years after diagnosis. If liver transplantation is undertaken after occurrence of a symptomatic cholangiocarcinoma, the two-year survival rate will be very low (around 20%). Therefore, earlier timing for grafting seems justified for these patients.

- *Biliary atresia* is the most common cause of chronic liver failure in children. This disease leads rapidly to biliary cirrhosis and lethal complications within the first two years of life. Therefore, as soon as the diagnosis is established, a porto-enterostomy (Kasai operation) should be performed in order to delay the progression of liver disease. Some patients will not need liver transplantation; others will require a liver graft but may be able to wait. This is important because survival rate is significantly better when children are older than one year (weight over 10 kg). Some other diseases share the same valid indication for liver transplantation in children, such as alpha-1 antitrypsin deficiency, familial intrahepatic cholestatic syndrome (Byler's disease) or ductular hypoplasia syndromes (Alagille's syndrome or arteriohepatic dysplasia).

Fulminant hepatic failure (FHF)

Liver transplantation has completely changed the prognosis of FHF. This disease is frequently lethal due to the development of cerebral oedema, severe encephalopathy and coagulopathy. Specific prognostic factors have been reported for spontaneous recovery; they are also helpful in decision making about transplantation. In almost all countries, a high priority policy has been developed ('super-urgent' procedure) in order to allocate a graft for these patients. FHF has been accepted as an emergency indication for liver transplantation in order to avoid severe encephalopathy. Acute (within eight weeks of onset of symptoms) or subacute (between eight weeks and six months) liver failure is characterised by the sudden onset of liver failure associated with encephalopathy and coagulopathy in a previously healthy person. The aetiologies are numerous (Box 46.2). The decision to undertake transplantation in a patient with FHF is taken when the patient meets well-defined criteria. Criteria for liver transplantation are different according to the cause of FHF and largely related to whether the disease is paracetamol induced (Box 46.3).

Controversy still persists with regard to the timing of the operation because of the difficulty in predicting the natural history of the disease. If the decision is taken too late clinical deterioration may occur

---

Box 46.2 Cause of fulminant hepatic failure (FHF)

Paracetamol overdose

Viral (mainly hepatitis A, B, E)

Drugs
- Antidepressants (e.g. imipramine)
- Antimicrobials (e.g. rifampicin)
- Anticonvulsants (e.g. valproate)
- Anaesthetic (e.g. halothane)
- Cardiovascular (e.g. amiodarone)
- Others (e.g. ecstasy)

Poisons
- Mushrooms (e.g. *Amanita phalloides*)

Others
- Wilson's disease
- Acute fatty liver failure (pregnancy)
- Acute Budd–Chiari syndrome

Box 46.3 Criteria for emergency liver transplantation in case of fulminant hepatic failure (FHF)

Non-paracetamol induced FHF
  Age <30 years and factor V <20%
  or
  Age >30 years and factor V <30%

(A) Non-paracetamol induced FHF
  Presence of three of the following:
  - Age <10 years or >40 years
  - Non-A, non-B or drug/halothane-induced FHF
  - Bilirubin >300 µmol/l
  - Prothrombin time >50 seconds

(B) Paracetamol-induced FHF
Arterial pH <7.3 or presence of the following together:
- prothrombin time >100 seconds
- grade III–IV encephalopathy
- creatinine >300 µmol/l

---

and brain death may occur rapidly. By contrast, to transplant too early has many drawbacks and at the very least, the acute patient might become a chronic patient exposed to the risks related to long-term immunosuppression. Auxiliary liver transplantation (ALT) has been developed in an attempt to overcome these problems. An additional liver or lobe is implanted in the abdominal cavity, better orthotopically after recipient partial hepatectomy, using a reduced or split-liver graft (see below). This procedure restores liver function, reverses encephalopathy and allows regeneration of the native liver, offering to these patients a life free of immunosuppression.

Other miscellaneous rare diseases

Metabolic liver diseases

INBORN ERRORS OF METABOLISM WITH STRUCTURAL LIVER DAMAGE

This group includes alpha-1 antitrypsin deficiency, Wilson's disease with advanced encephalopathy or FHF, some glycogen storage diseases (type IV), galactosaemia in which cirrhosis and even hepatocellular carcinoma (HCC) may occur.

INBORN ERRORS OF METABOLISM WITHOUT STRUCTURAL LIVER DAMAGE

When the liver is exclusively involved and is the only site of the metabolic defect, the decision to replace the liver is easy to make. This situation occurs in several diseases such as familial hyper-cholesterolaemia (type IIA), Crigler–Najjar syndrome type I (severe non-haemolytic unconjugated hyperbilirubinaemia) or hyperoxalaemia type I which needs combined liver and kidney transplantation when kidney failure has occurred as a consequence of oxalate overproduction.

In the near future either partial liver replacement (ALT) or a graft of allogeneic hepatocytes may be able to provide the enzyme activity which is necessary to correct the metabolic disorder. Both strategies have already been successfully used in the treatment of Crigler–Najjar syndrome type I.

In cases of inborn errors of metabolism without structural liver damage, the patient's liver may be used for another patient who is on the waiting list to receive a liver and for whom life expectancy without a graft is short. This procedure, called 'domino grafting', has already been used with the liver of a patient suffering from amyloid polyneuropathy (Portuguese amyloidosis).

Autoimmune chronic active hepatitis

This is a progressive inflammatory liver disease of unknown cause and most commonly seen in young women. The diagnosis is based on the detection of circulating autoantibodies and polyclonal hyperglobulinaemia. Liver transplantation may be indicated either in case of acute liver failure or as a treatment for severe cirrhosis with life-threatening complications. There is a possible but uncommon risk of recurrence of the disease after liver transplantation.

Other indications still being debated

Liver transplantation for these conditions remains controversial because of the risk of recurrence of the disease on the graft. For some diseases, the risk can be reduced with new efficient drugs (i.e. hepatitis B, C) and in other cases by a better selection of the candidates (i.e. alcoholic cirrhosis).

Chronic viral hepatitis

An increasing number of patients develop chronic viral hepatitis and subsequent cirrhosis. Moreover, these patients are at risk of developing hepatocellular carcinoma (HCC).

Hepatitis B

The hepatitis B virus (HBV) is a a major world health problem with an estimated 300 million carriers. In Western Europe and North America, however, the HBV carrier rate is low (0.5 %) and is mainly confined to high-risk groups. The Paris Consensus Conference recommended the avoidance of liver transplantation in viraemic patients due to the high risk of early recurrence after grafting. Patients who show serological indicators of viraemia such as presence of hepatitis Be antigen (HBe Ag) or HBV-DNA have a reinfection rate of the graft of 60–90%. Several prophylaxis programmes have used high doses of hepatitis B hyperimmune globulins as well as antiviral drugs such as lamivudine. This drug is already given prior to transplantation to reduce viraemia. Using these therapeutic protocols, the frequency of recurrence in non-viraemic patients has been lowered from approximatively 80% to 30%. However, in the case of recurrent hepatitis B after liver transplantation, the disease appears to be much more aggressive than in the non-transplant setting, due to the role of immunosuppressive therapy. Under these circumstances, it appears justified to transplant only the non-viraemic patients, suffering from severe complications of cirrhosis (hepatorenal syndrome, intractable ascites, recurrent bleeding from oesophageal varices). Recurrent spontaneous bacterial peritonitis or recurrent episodes of septicaemia are not contraindications to grafting. Hopefully, the incidence of HBV is expected to be lowered in the near future as a result of vaccination programmes.

Hepatitis B-D

This co-infection, mainly described in Italy and the southern part of Europe, tends to be more aggressive than standard chronic hepatitis B and may progress to cirrhosis and to end-stage liver disease more rapidly (over periods as short as 3–5 years). The indications for transplantation are similar to those for chronic hepatitis B. The rate of hepatitis B recurrence after grafting is lower in patients with HBV and HDV co-infection (around 10%). However, there is a need for immunoprophylaxis similar to that after transplantation for HBV alone.

Hepatitis C

Hepatitis C virus (HCV) is now recognised as a major cause of viral hepatitis leading to chronic liver disease, liver failure and HCC. Recent data suggest that in the United States an estimated 3.9 million persons are currently infected with HCV and 8000–10 000 deaths each year are attributed to HCV-associated chronic liver disease. Improvement in the treatment of HCV infection has been achieved during the last few years with a combination of interferon and ribavirin: the overall sustained virological response rate is around 40%. However, patients infected with HCV genotype 1, the most common genotype, remain less responsive to this combination therapy.

Cirrhosis resulting from HCV infection, alone or in combination with alcohol abuse, has become the leading indication for liver transplantation among adults in the United States and Western Europe, accounting for approximately 30–50% of the number of transplantations in many centres. However, recurrence of hepatitis C after liver transplantation is an increasing problem because it is nearly universal; fortunately, in the short term, severe graft dysfunction is rare. The risk of developing recurrent liver cirrhosis is estimated at around 20% after seven years and may lead to a need for a second liver transplant. Factors influencing the rate of progression are largely unknown, but can be related to the intrinsic characteristics of the infecting viral strains, the genetic characteristics of the infected individual and also some iatrogenic influences such as immunosuppression or alcohol consumption. For instance, among variables associated with higher risk of recurrence are viral factors (genotype 1b, high HCV RNA levels before and especially after transplantation), iatrogenic factors (high amount of immunosuppression and particularly frequent methyl-prednisolone boluses, cumulative steroids therapy or OKT3) or host factors (race, more recent year of transplantation).

The major goal of the treatment strategies is to prevent the development of HCV-related graft failure in using pretransplant antiviral therapy as well as early posttransplant preventive therapy with interferon either alone or in combination with ribavirin. However, the inability of currently available antiviral therapy to eliminate HCV in the setting of liver transplantation suggests that indefinitive treatment will be necessary unless new drugs become available. As yet, no vaccine is available to prevent HCV infection but the main cause of contamination, i.e. blood transfusion, is currently under control and the transmission of HCV has declined substantially.

Alcoholic cirrhosis

Alcoholic liver disease is the most common cause of end-stage liver disease in the Western world. Whether to consider patients suffering from this self-inflicted disease as candidates for liver transplantation is still being debated. Many transplant centres were initially reluctant to consider liver grafts in these patients because of the risk of recurrent drinking and also of diseases associated with alcoholism (cardiomyopathy, pancreatitis, malnutrition, oesophageal and/or throat cancer, psychiatric disorders). The objective is to ensure at least six months abstinence before transplantation in order to evaluate the patients properly and to select the good candidates. It has been shown that, following this policy, the results are equivalent to other indications and that recidivism is uncommon. As a result, an increasing number of such individuals are now being grafted with a high five-year survival rate. In our experience, liver transplantation is considered to be a valid therapeutic option for less than 10% of patients with alcoholic cirrhosis.

Hepatocellular carcinoma (HCC)

HCC is one of the most common fatal tumours worldwide with an estimated annual incidence of 1 million cases. Chronic hepatitis B infection appears to be the major cause of HCC; however, in Japan and the Western world, hepatitis C appears more and more to be an independent risk factor. Some patients have surgically resectable HCC but most cases occur in a cirrhotic liver and, after resection, there is a high morbidity and even mortality rate and also a high rate of recurrence. Liver replacement seemed to be a very satisfactory option because it could treat both HCC and cirrhosis. Unfortunately, recurrence rates on the graft are high once the tumour is large. It is now generally accepted that transplantation should be performed only in selected patients with less than three tumours of less than 3 cm in diameter. In this group, the three-year survival rate is excellent (over 80%). Portal vein thrombosis and extrahepatic disease (positive lymph nodes) are contraindications to transplantation.

Other rare primary hepatic tumours that are unresectable might be considered for transplantation; they include epithelioid haemangioendothelioma, fibrolamellar carcinoma or some sarcomas. Hilar cholangiocarcinomas as well as intrahepatic cholangiocarcinomas with a few exceptions are no longer considered appropriate candidates due to high recurrence rates, despite posttransplant adjuvant therapy. It is really a tragedy to consider that liver transplantation is currently not a therapeutic option for unresectable liver malignancies.

Liver metastatic disease

Liver transplantation for metastatic disease has been performed with very poor results, except in rare cases of neuroendocrine tumours, which are slow-growing, in which pharmacological control of hormonal syndromes was not efficient or in patients with symptomatic bulky disease. Under such circumstances, recurrence appears usually only many years later. For instance, in the case of metastatic carcinoid tumours the five-year survival rate is nearly 70%.

Other rare indications

There is a long list of rare indications including:

- the Budd–Chiari syndrome provided it is not associated with a malignant untreatable aetiological factor (myeloproliferative disorder, malignant liver tumour)
- congenital haemochromatosis when associated with small HCC
- tyrosinaemia
- rare giant benign tumours which become life-threatening due to complications, such as giant haemangioma or polycystic liver disease
- diffuse Caroli disease
- secondary biliary cirrhosis
- congenital hepatic fibrosis
- cryptogenic cirrhosis and some other rare diseases.

CONTRAINDICATIONS TO LIVER TRANSPLANTATION

The established contraindications to liver transplantation are constantly being challenged. Some conditions that were previously considered to be absolute contraindications, such as portal vein thrombosis, or age over 65 years, have now become relative contraindications. Some of the main absolute and relative contraindications are outlined in Box 46.4.

Box 46.4 Absolute and relative contraindications to liver transplantation

Absolute contraindications	Relative contraindications
HIV disease	Portal vein thrombosis
Extrahepatic malignancy	Hepatitis Be antigen, DNA positive
Uncontrolled infection	Age >65 years
Failure of another major organ	UNOS status 4
(except the case for multiple	HIV positive serological status
transplantation: heart, lung,	
kidney)	
Severe pulmonary hypertension	

TIMING OF LIVER TRANSPLANTATION

The dilemma is to choose the optimal timing: not too early, not too late. Several studies have addressed the impact of timing and outcome after liver transplantation. For instance, higher survival rate with decrease in overall morbidity could be reached in patients who undergo transplantation relatively early in the course of the primary biliary cirrhosis. Many patients with chronic liver disease remain stable for long periods and then, suddenly, decompensate. This is often due to a complication such as portal vein thrombosis, development of hepatic malignancy or spontaneous bacterial peritonitis. Variceal haemorrhage is one of the most dangerous complications of cirrhosis; transjugular intrahepatic portosystemic shunt (TIPSS) has proved to be useful in prevention of such bleeding and allows the patient to wait more safely on the waiting list. In cases of acute or subacute liver failure the use of prognostic factors has demonstrated its efficiency in selecting the candidates for transplantation. It is clear that one major argument for developing living-related donor liver transplantation procedures is the ability to choose electively the most appropriate timing for grafting.

PATIENT ASSESSMENT

Psychological as well as complete medical assessment is needed before the patient is placed on the transplant waiting list. This procedure is best performed by a joint team of hepatologists, anaesthesiologists and transplant surgeons with the help of consultants in cardiology, respiratory physicians, nephrology, immunology, infectious diseases, neuropsychiatry or any other necessary advice. The important message to deliver is that the referral should not be too late in order to allow time to assess completely and very carefully not only the liver disease but also the medical and psychosocial aspects.

Detailed evaluation of cardiorespiratory system is mandatory: this may require several investigations, from simple exercise ECG tests to Swan–Ganz catheterisation for patients with raised right cardiac pressures or major pulmonary shunts (such as seen in hepato-pulmonary syndrome).

It is crucial to determine the functional reserve (of the heart, lung, kidney), as it greatly influences the postoperative outcome.

A careful medical history needs to be documented regarding alcohol consumption and medications. Furthermore, psychosocial evaluation is important to consider as well as the estimated compliance with transplant procedure and daily intake of immunosuppressive treatment.

Of surgical importance is a history of previous extensive biliary surgery or portocaval shunting. Portal vein patency has to be documented (with Doppler ultrasound, CT scan, angio-MRI or angiography). Patients with HCC require detailed investigation to exclude any detectable extrahepatic involvement. They may also receive preoperative treatment, such as chemoembolisation, while on the waiting list.

Patients with unexplained cirrhosis should be thoroughly investigated in order that rare diseases such as Wilson's disease, alpha-1 antitrypsin deficiency and autoimmune chronic active hepatitis are diagnosed; this will decrease the number of cases labelled as 'cryptogenic cirrhosis'.

Infectious disease screening for viruses, bacteria, parasites and fungi is also mandatory before transplantation, as immunosuppressive treatment leads to a form of acquired immunodeficiency state.

Nutritional aspects are also a central issue throughout the transplantation process. Patients with advanced muscle wasting pose major problems for recovery after grafting. Enteral feeding, particularly in children, may help to prevent posttransplantation complications related to malnutrition.

Renal failure due to the hepatorenal syndrome is often present in patients with end-stage liver disease. Usually, liver transplantation will reverse this condition.

Finally during the pretransplant period the patient will be in close communication with the clinical nurse coordinator whose role is essential as a patient advocate and an administrative facilitator.

Pretransplant assessment of children

The basic pretransplantation evaluation of children is similar to adult patients with regard to the diagnosis, severity of liver failure and the need for transplantation. Children must also be carefully evaluated to judge the patency of the portal vein, the type of portoenterostomy (if required) and the degree of discrepancy between recipient hepatic fossa and graft. All this information is important in order to select the adequate approach, size of graft and type of reconstruction technique.

The potential risk of infection after liver transplantation should also be evaluated, particularly for cytomegalovirus (CMV). Small children with negative CMV serological status should receive seronegative graft and blood products which greatly reduces the risk of infection. For seropositive children this rule is not justified.

Epstein–Barr virus (EBV) is also important because of its association with lymphoproliferative disorders which occur in 4% of immunocompromised paediatric recipients.

All children should receive routine immunisation against the usual infectious diseases. Because splenic dysfunction may occur, vaccination against *Streptococcus pneumoniae* and *Haemophilus influenzae* should also be considered.

The patient is then placed on the transplant waiting list early enough to avoid risk of death during the waiting period. In our experience, this period varies with the severity of the disease but also the limited donor pool, particularly in some blood groups such as the B blood group. Patients are sometimes excluded from the waiting list because of significant worsening of their condition (such that a poor outcome of the transplant procedure is predicted) or due to improvement in their condition (for instance, in some cases of alcoholic cirrhosis, strict abstinence may result in an improvement of liver function; in cases of FHF, regeneration of the liver may reverse encephalopathy). In such circumstances, it is important that the medical staff together with the transplant surgeons remain responsible for the allocation of the liver grafts. The waiting list thus needs to be regularly reviewed.

LIVER DONORS AND ORGAN PRESERVATION

There are currently two ways to obtain a liver, or part of a liver, to be grafted: either by harvesting a whole liver from a cadaveric donor or by taking part of the liver of a living healthy donor related to the recipient.

Cadaveric donors

The best donor profile is represented by young brain-dead patients without previous history of disease and who are in a stable haemodynamic condition. However, successful outcome is possible even in haemodynamically unstable donors and those with abnormal liver function tests.

The quality of the liver is best assessed by an experienced transplant surgeon at the time of retrieval by examining liver colour, size, consistency and fatty change. In case of doubt, a frozen section for histological assessment can be helpful. Usually, less than 30% steatosis is recommended; however, shortage of organs has led to the successful use of marginal donor livers with higher fatty infiltration. These marginal grafts are better used in a relatively fit recipient; a poor-risk recipient, conversely, will need a graft which functions without delay.

With regard to the donor's age, there is a trend to routinely accept older donors if they are free of hepatobiliary disease; clear upper age limits no longer exist. At present, the only absolute contraindications to organ donation are positive serology for HIV, positivity of hepatitis B surface antigen and extracerebral malignancy. Size-matching of donor and recipient is only attempted in the case of a small recipient because grafting too large a liver in such patients may cause major technical problems with subsequent severe complications. Graft splitting, either *ex vivo* or better *in situ*, is a good way to increase the pool of organs. However, this procedure should be performed only by experienced liver surgeons and both grafts implanted simultaneously by two transplant teams in order to reduce the cold ischaemia time.

Good organ preservation is important for the success of organ transplantation. The aim is to preserve the viability of the cells, thus allowing immediate function after transplantation. Transplanted organs are exposed to different periods of ischaemia and injuries and the liver parenchyma is highly sensitive to ischaemia. Simple hypothermia slows the process of ischaemic damage.

Three periods of ischaemia can be distinguished.

- *Warm ischaemia*: while the liver is no longer perfused by the donor blood but not yet perfused by a cold storage solution. This period should not exceed a few minutes.

- *Cold ischaemia*: starts after vascular flushing and cooling until the graft is refrigerated in a cold (0–4°C) storage solution and packed in an isotherm container.

- *Relative cold ischaemia*: starts when the liver is brought into the recipient for vascular reconstruction until graft reperfusion. During this period vascular anastomoses are performed and the graft is washed by a cold albumin-containing solution to eliminate accumulated potassium and oxygen free radicals.

The University of Wisconsin (UW) cold storage solution, which has found widespread clinical use, allows effective preservation of most organs for at least 24 hours. This solution (Table 46.1) improved quality of preservation for the liver and the percentage of primary non-function (PNF) in liver transplantation could be significantly reduced. Currently, our policy is that if no risk factors are present and if the patient does not suffer from acute liver failure, extended preservation is accepted (10–15 hours) so that elective surgery can be accepted with the same quality of outcome. However, when risk factors are present related to the donor and/or recipient conditions, preservation times are kept as short as possible.

Table 46.1 Main components of the University of Wisconsin solution (UW)

Main components	Expected role
Lactobionate	Impermeant; calcium and iron chelator
Raffinose	Impermeant saccharide
Hydroxyethyl starch	Colloid
Adenosine	Precursor of adenine nucleotide synthesis
Glutathione	Oxygen free radical scavenger
Allopurinol	Inhibitor of xanthine oxidase

Living related donors

The procedure of living related donor liver transplantation, first reported by Raia in Brazil, has developed rapidly over the past decade. Strong was the first to report successful transplantation in a child using the left lobe of the mother's liver. The first programme in living related donor liver transplantation was established at the University of Chicago. This technique was rapidly adopted in Japan with the development of a programme at Kyoto University, which is currently the largest in this field. The results are impressive, with an overall survival near 90%. More recently, this procedure has been used successfully in adults with adult-to-adult living related donors.

After completion of the donor hepatectomy, the graft is immediately flushed with heparinised preservation solution on the back-table and then implanted into the recipient. The main advantages of this procedure are: elective procedure with no time limit in evaluation of the quality of the donor, short preservation time and excellent results.

However, the risk of morbidity and even mortality of the donor is the subject of controversy and in Western Europe there has been some resistance to the development of the concept. By contrast, in Japan, where the cultural barrier to cadaver donation has left no alternative for Japanese patients, this approach has become well established.

In cases of adult-to-adult transplantation, controversy remains in Japan regarding whether the right liver from the donor (segments 5, 6, 7 and 8) or the left liver (segments 1, 2, 3 and 4) should be used. The right liver provides more parenchyma for the donation, whereas the left liver is less risky for the donor as far as risk of postoperative liver insufficiency is concerned.

POSTOPERATIVE MANAGEMENT

Immunosuppression

It is well known from early experimental work that the liver is less vulnerable to rejection than other organs such as heart, lung and kidney. In addition, late rejection of liver grafts is uncommon. It has also been shown that combined liver–kidney transplantation protects the kidney graft against rejection. Most patients with a liver graft can be maintained on relatively low doses of immunosuppressive drugs and some are even able to stop their immunosuppression after several years without incurring much risk of acute rejection and graft loss. Kupffer cells in the grafted liver change from donor to recipient within a few months. Donor leucocytes (principally dendritic cells) can also be demonstrated in the skin, nodes, heart and other tissues of the long-surviving host. These chimeric cells that had emigrated from the graft and then perpetuated themselves for many years are present in larger number in liver recipients than in patients carrying other grafts. This subject is currently under intensive study in order to understand graft tolerance and also to be able to identify those patients who will manage without immunosuppression.

Currently transplant centres are using either the cyclosporin–steroid or the tacrolimus (FK-506)–steroid combination (Box 46.5). Cyclosporin is now available as a microemulsion (Neoral®) which has a better intestinal absorption and is bile independent. The aim of immunosuppressive therapeutic regimens is to suppress the patient's immune response to the transplanted allograft while preserving an adequate functional immunity to prevent the development of opportunistic infection and malignancy. There has been a trend to rapidly decrease oral steroids (in order to avoid some of their disadvantages) and this practice has not been accompanied by a deleterious effect on graft survival. For some teams, steroids can be withdrawn in order to improve quality of life and avoid steroids side-effects.

Several new immunosuppressive medications have been developed recently (mycophenolate mofetil sirolimus, anti-IL-2 receptors). They seem to be useful in reducing the incidence and severity of rejection, reducing the concomitant use of steroids and decreasing the dose of cyclosporin or tacrolimus in order to minimise their toxicity.

Postoperative course

Successful liver replacement results, within 48–72 hours, in evident postoperative changes in the recipient. Correction of pre-

---

Box 46.5 Immunosuppressive protocols currently used after liver transplantation

Protocol A (cyclosporine (Neoral) + steroids)			Protocol B (tacrolimus (FK-506) + steroids)		
Neoral	Steroids		FK-506	Steroids	
Day 0: 5 mg/kg (through the gastric tube) 6h after surgery	Day 0	1 g IV hydrocortisone	Day 0: 0.075 mg/kg (through the gastric tube) 6h after surgery	Day 0	1 g IV hydrocortisone
D1, etc.: 8–10 mg/kg/day	D1 + 2	1.5 mg/kg/day prednisolone		D1 + 2	1.5 mg/kg/day prednisolone
Aim: maintain blood level of 300–400 ng/ml	D3 → 8	1 ,,	Aim: maintain blood level of D1–30: 10–20 ng/ml > D30: 5–15 ng/ml	D3 → 8	1 ,,
	D9 → 13	0.5 ,,		D9 → 13	0.5 ,,
	D14 → 30	0.3 ,,		D14 → 30	0.3 ,,
	D31 → 60	0.2 ,,		D31 → 60	0.2 ,,
	>D60	0.1 ,,		>D60	0.1 ,,

existing liver function abnormalities, bile production, rapid recovery of normal consciousness allowing early removal from mechanical ventilation occur together with recovery of a good renal function. Monitoring graft function includes close clinical, biological and radiological controls. Normalisation of hepatic function is assessed by daily liver function tests (bilirubin, transaminases, prothrombin time). The Doppler ultrasound examination provides accurate images of the blood flow throughout all major vessels of the liver, assessing patency of the vascular anastomosis (mainly arterial and portal anastomosis). When a bile duct catheter is present (T-tube usually), the bile production can be monitored which is a reliable index of liver function.

Complications

Several complications may occur after liver transplantation. It is convenient to consider them chronologically as immediate (during the two first postoperative days), early (during the first three months) or late (after three months).

Immediate complications

Among them, primary non-function (PNF) of the liver is so severe that it often requires prompt retransplantation. Most centres experience an incidence of primary poor function ranging from 5% to 10%. Fortunately real PNF is rare. As soon as the diagnosis of PNF is established, urgent retransplantation is undertaken. Most organ allocation organisations consider PNF a priority for emergency retransplantation. The PNF syndrome may be due to preservation injury or may be related to poor quality of the donor liver; sometimes it may be secondary to pre-existing occult recipient disease (such as endotoxin or hepatotoxic drug exposure).

The diagnosis of PNF is recognised in the following circumstances: rapid development of coagulopathy, persistent acidosis, poor bile production, very high levels of transaminases or continued hepatorenal failure. These patients present often with continued ventilatory dependency and deteriorating encephalopathy. Haemodynamic instability and death rapidly follow unless urgent retransplantation is undertaken.

Besides the real PNF syndrome, primary poor function is more often observed. In such cases, some features of liver failure (such as coagulopathy, high transaminase levels, persistent hyperbilirubinaemia) are seen but early supportive treatment is usually successful and improvement observed within two weeks while the liver recovers. However, these patients often remain asthenic and cholestatic for several weeks and recovery is slow.

Haemorrhage

Elective routine cases without previous abdominal surgery often require minimal or no blood transfusion. Conversely, patients with portal hypertension and previous major upper abdominal surgery can develop extensive bleeding. Better preoperative management of the recipient, meticulous intraoperative haemostasis, use of warmed blood and blood products will be of great help in avoiding unnecessary bleeding.

Renal failure

Renal failure often complicates the postoperative course of liver transplant recipients. Many patients present with preoperative hepatorenal syndrome. Furthermore, some intraoperative factors may produce renal dysfunction such as haemorrhage or vena caval clamping. Optimal hydration and use of dopamine are helpful in treating these factors.

Renal function may be affected by drugs such as the immunosuppressive drugs (cyclosporin, tacrolimus), sepsis or other nephrotoxic drugs (antibiotics). Patients with hepatorenal syndrome can be successfully treated with liver transplantation, even if initial haemodialysis may be necessary. Combined liver–kidney transplantation is highly successful in some cases with preoperative chronic irreversible kidney failure. In liver transplant recipients, reduction of dosage of immunosuppressive therapy is sometimes required to avoid nephrotoxicity.

Early complications after surgery

Technical failures

Technical failures include:

- hepatic artery thrombosis
- portal thrombosis
- biliary leakage or obstruction.

Hepatic artery thrombosis (HAT) can be a devasting complication. It occurs most frequently during the first postoperative month, leading to graft ischaemia. The incidence of this complication is less than 5% but can be higher in paediatric recipients due to the very small diameter of hepatic artery in very young children. Clinical presentation varies from acute hepatic failure with necrosis of the graft to sepsis with hepatic abscesses or biliary necrosis with cholangitis, bile leaks or bile duct strictures. The onset of HAT is usually detected by a massive rise in transaminases and altered coagulation profile; the diagnosis is assessed by Doppler ultrasound and confirmed by angiography. For patients in whom HAT develops in the immediate postoperative period, an attempt to perform urgent rearterialisation has to be undertaken. Reconstruction of the hepatic artery may be successful in some cases but in most patients regrafting will be necessary. Conversely, late arterial thrombosis (several months after transplantation) may be asymptomatic with normal liver function and can sometimes be ignored if no further biliary complications occur.

Portal vein thrombosis is rare but can be seen mainly in children. Early detection is assessed by routine Doppler ultrasound leading to emergency desobstruction.

Biliary complications remain a significant source of morbidity after liver transplantation. They include mainly bile leaks and anastomotic strictures. The overall incidence is around 10% despite a variety of procedures and techniques used in order to reduce the risk of these complications. The use of a T-tube was advocated in order to decompress the biliary anastomosis, to be able to control bile production in the early phase and finally to check, by performing a cholangiogram, the biliary anatomy as well as the healing of the biliary anastomosis. However, the risk of bile leak and of subsequent biloma, following T-tube removal, resulted in loss of favour for this procedure. Moreover, MRI-cholangiography has been shown to produce excellent imaging of the biliary tree. Biliary complications have been reported to occur more frequently with several associated conditions and particularly in cases of hepatic artery thrombosis which should always be looked for. Simple bile leaks may be treated by temporary internal stenting through endoscopic retrograde cholangiography (ERCP). Conversely, the presence of a major biliary disruption is an indication for an urgent reconstruction using a Roux-en-Y jejunal loop. Biliary obstruction can be treated by balloon dilatation if it does not occur within the first postoperative weeks. Failure of this endoscopic treatment, or early stenosis, will require biliary reconstruction using a jejunal loop.

Medical complications

Medical complications include primary poor function and acute renal failure that have already been described, but also rejection (acute and/or chronic) and infections (bacterial, fungal and viral).

REJECTION

Rejection is not usually a major clinical problem following liver transplantation. However, on light microscopy, features of acute rejection can be found in around 70% of cases on liver biopsy performed one week after grafting. If other parameters (liver function tests) are satisfactory, there is a trend towards avoiding additional immunosuppression. Nevertheless, patients experiencing severe cellular rejection or milder rejections together with significant biochemical abnormalities will require specific treatment, either a tapering of high-dose steroids or a series of intravenous steroid boluses (two or three). Steroid-resistant rejection will usually respond to other agents such as monoclonal (OKT3) or polyclonal antibodies (ATG) currently, more often, immunosuppression regimen will be changed, switching from cyclosporin to tacrolimus or other new drugs. After transplantation of a liver graft in the presence of a positive crossmatch, early inferior graft function or even, rarely, hyperacute rejection has been reported. Finally, when liver from ABO blood group-compatible, but not identical, donors is used, graft-versus-host (GVH) disease may be rarely observed.

Chronic or irreversible rejection in the liver is mainly an epithelial rather than a vascular phenomenon, in contrast to other transplanted organs. It is an insidious process with few symptoms and is microscopically characterised by ductopenia and portal fibrosis. If this process cannot be stopped it may lead to the so-called vanishing bile duct syndrome which is usually irreversible. High-dose steroid therapy may, at best, postpone a retransplantation.

INFECTIONS

Infections can be a major problem and may even lead to life-threatening complications. About 55% of all infections are bacterial, 25% viral, 15% fungal and about 5% due to *Pneumocystis carinii* or toxoplasma. Most infections occur in the first two months after transplantation. The main potential septic problems relate to the biliary tract, the peritoneal cavity and the lungs.

Over half of the bacterial infections are observed within the first two postoperative weeks. This is also the time period in which the highest levels of immunosuppressive therapy are encountered. In many cases, biliary and peritoneal infections are related to technical difficulties (biliary obstruction, hepatic artery stenosis or thrombosis). The pathogens most frequently encountered are aerobic Gram-positive organisms and Gram-negative bacilli. Most pulmonary infections are nosocomial and caused by Gram-negative bacilli, although legionella should always be kept in mind.

The highest incidence of fungal infections occurs during the first eight weeks after transplantation. Candida is the most frequent isolated fungal infection. Prophylaxis treatment is effective in reducing the risk of invasive disease. Aspergillus-related disease is associated with a high mortality rate.

Amongst the viral infections, CMV is the most common viral pathogen found after liver transplantation. Primary CMV infections (transmitted by the donor liver) should be avoided by using CMV-matched donors. Most CMV infections are seen between three and eight weeks after liver transplantation. They provoke fever and leucopenia and may involve lungs or liver. Usually, they respond well to a combination of ganciclovir therapy and reduction in doses of immunosuppressive therapy. Herpes simplex virus (HSV) may be reactivated during the first postoperative weeks. Epstein–Barr virus (EBV) is not usually seen until after the first six months. It presents a spectrum of illness from mononucleosis syndromes to posttransplant lymphoproliferative disease.

Late complications

More than 80% of liver transplant recipients survive the first year and most of them experience an excellent quality of life. However, it is important to be aware of late complications (i.e. those occurring more than three months after the operative procedure and usually much later).

737

Chronic rejection

Chronic rejection remains a significant clinical problem after liver transplantation. It is usually seen within the first 12 months. The differentiation from other causes of late graft damage, particularly chronic hepatitis, is sometimes difficult. Resolution can occur in mild cases but slow progression to graft failure is usually the rule and will often lead to the need for a second liver transplantation. However, in contrast with other grafts, chronic liver rejection affects only a minority of patients.

Recurrent non-malignant disease

The recurrence of HCV infection is universal after liver transplantation. However, the five-year survival rate is high. Trials with combination interferon-ribavirin are under way; their aim is to reduce the risk of HCV-related allograft failure. This has been achieved rather successfully in case of HBV infection using lamivudine together with long-term HBV immunoglobulin treatment after liver transplantation. Histological examination of the transplanted liver, even in stable long-term patients, shows frequent abnormalities. They have to be considered in conjunction with both the clinical state and the liver function tests. Recurrence of the primary disease, chronic rejection or viral infections are the main causes to discuss.

Malignancy

Malignancy can be recognised in patients grafted for primary liver malignancy and who develop recurrence. It may also be observed as a complication of long-term immunosuppression and include lymphomas, sarcomas or skin cancers.

Hypertension

This is seen in patients receiving either cyclosporin or tacrolimus and needs appropriate treatment.

In conclusion, the importance of careful and detailed follow-up of liver transplant recipients has to be emphasised. Such attention will help to detect early and to treat efficiently the late complications which may occur.

OPERATIVE SURGERY

The donor operation

The cadaveric donor

Standard operation

Liver retrieval is usually carried out as part of a multiorgan procurement. Key features include recognition of arterial anatomical variants, maintenance of the organ anatomical integrity and avoidance of warm ischaemia.

INCISION

A long mid-line incision, from sternal notch to pubic symphysis, provides adequate exposure for all procurement teams.

TECHNIQUE

- The basic technique for liver procurement consists of mobilisation of the liver with division of its ligaments, dissection of the bile duct, the portal vein trunk, the hepatic artery as far as the coeliac axis and the inferior vena cava, above and below the liver. The main difficulty is due to the anatomical variations of the hepatic artery. Instead of arising from the coeliac axis (60–70% of cases), there can be some anatomical variations: a left hepatic artery arising from the left gastric artery and a right hepatic artery from the superior mesenteric artery. Sometimes a common hepatic artery arises from the superior mesenteric artery. It is essential to recognise these variations and to preserve these vessels.

- The right colon and duodenum are mobilised to expose the retroperitoneum.

- The aorta is encircled with a tape as well as the vena cava, just above the iliac vessels.

- The hepatic pedicle is then dissected. The common bile duct is divided above the head of the pancreas and the bile tract is washed out after opening the fundus of the gallbladder.

- The aorta is isolated and cannulated as far as the inferior mesenteric artery which is ligated so that unnecessary organs are not perfused with the preservation solution. When the heart is perfused with cardioplegic solution, the abdominal organs are washed with a hypothermic preservation solution (UW solution).

- The left gastric and the splenic arteries are also ligated and divided.

- The portal vein is cannulated through the inferior mesenteric vein. Aortic and portal perfusion are achieved *in situ* with cold UW preservation solution.

- When the liver is cool and blanched the cold-phase dissection is undertaken. After performing a Kocher's manoeuvre, the superior mesenteric vein can be palpated. Careful dissection of the right edge of the superior mesenteric artery will preserve any abnormal right hepatic artery.

- The aorta is divided at the supracoeliac and infracoeliac levels. If the right hepatic artery arises from the superior mesenteric artery the aorta patch includes both coeliac axis and superior mesenteric artery.

- The superior mesenteric vein and the splenic vein are divided after removal of the cannula.

- The subhepatic suprarenal vena cava is dissected and divided above the right renal vein.

- The diaphragm is cut, leaving a wide cuff containing the suprahepatic vena cava.

- The donor liver is taken to the back-table, placed in a bowl and given a second flush with cold UW preservation solution into the hepatic artery, the portal vein and the common bile duct. The liver is placed in fresh UW solution and the bowl is placed in two sterile plastic bags which are then stored in an ice box for transport.

The donor operation can be modified to a rapid technique if the donor becomes unstable. In such cases, the dissection of the hepatic pedicle is undertaken after the cooling with the preservation solution.

Reduced grafts and split-liver transplants

Reduction in size, carried out on the back-table, was initially described by Bismuth. Three different types of reduced livers can be obtained.

- The whole right liver (Couinaud's segments 5, 6, 7 and 8)

- The whole left liver (segments 2, 3 and 4)

- The left lateral lobe (segments 2 and 3)

The further development of the concept of size reduction has led to the possibility of using the same liver for two different recipients, usually an adult for the right liver (segments 5, 6, 7, 8) and a child for the left liver (segment 2, 3, 4) or the left lobe (segments 2, 3) according to the size of the recipient. In such cases all the liver parenchyma is used, contrary to the reduced-size technique in which part of the liver is lost. This explains why reduced-liver grafts are currently less and less used.

The split-liver technique has been developed in several centres with satisfactory results. The ultimate development of this technique is to perform this procedure *in vivo*: the so-called *in situ* splitting procedure was advocated in order to decrease the ischaemia time and to perform better haemostasis of the liver. However, this technique requires an experienced donor surgery team.

The living-related donor

The donor operation may be either a left-sided or a right-sided hepatectomy. Initially, the left lobe only was considered to be removed and used as a graft for a child. Further development of living related liver transplantation allowed this procedure to be considered for adult recipients. Both techniques have been used:

- either removing the left liver (segments 2, 3 and 4) and recently the left liver together with the Spiegel lobe (segments 2, 3, 4 and 1)

- or removing the right liver (segments 5, 6, 7 and 8).

Informed consent and permission from the ethical committee have to be obtained before performing this hepatectomy in a living related and healthy donor. In the donor particularly, morbidity has to be very low and mortality should be nil.

For the left-sided hepatectomy three types of resection have been described according to the amount of parenchyma which is taken out :

- lateral segmentectomy (segments 2 and 3)

- extended lateral segmentectomy (segments 2, 3 and partially 4)

- whole left hemihepatectomy together with the middle hepatic vein (segments 2, 3, 4).

The left lateral segmentectomy is the most widely used procedure. The left hepatic artery and portal vein are carefully dissected. If possible, a branch from the artery or the portal vein to segment 4 is saved. Small portal branches to the caudate lobe are suture-ligated and divided. Dissection is carried out to the right side of the round ligament. Liver transection is usually carried out without hepatic pedicle clamping in order to avoid any ischaemic injury. Portal branches to segment 4 are suture-ligated and cut so that the ligament is progressively rolled to the left. A free view of the hilar plate and the portal bifurcation is finally obtained. At the end of this dissection, some blue discolouration of the tip of segment 4 may be apparent. The hilar plate containing the bile duct to segments 2 and 3 can now be divided.

For the right lobe living donor operation, the left lobe should not be mobilised. The cystic duct is first identified and an intraoperative cholangiogram is performed, followed by a cholecystectomy. Intraoperative ultrasound is used to define the course and relationship of the middle hepatic vein. The presence of accessory hepatic veins draining the right lobe is assessed. The right hepatic artery is identified, as well as the right portal vein. The right bile duct is then visualised. All vascular branches and bile duct going to segment 4 have to be identified and protected from any injury. Transection of the parenchyma is then performed. Doppler assessment of the left lobe vessels is performed several times during the liver resection in order to control the integrity of its vascular supply. Transection of the hepatic parenchyma is usually carried out without vascular occlusion to avoid any ischaemic injury. Finally, the partial liver graft is removed and preservation UW solution is infused through the portal pedicle and hepatic artery. In the living related liver transplantation procedure the total ischaemia time is significantly less than in the cadaveric procedure.

The procedure has earned an important place in the treatment of children with end-stage liver disease. To date there have been six donor deaths reported after living related liver donation (particularly due to massive pulmonary embolism). Complications have been very limited and similar to those of elective minor liver resection. The procured organ has generally been of excellent quality and long-term results are even better than those obtained with cadaveric donor.

The recipient operation

Anaesthetic management

Anaesthesia for liver transplantation is complex and challenging. The patient with end-stage liver disease frequently presents with associated disease of other major organs and metabolic disturbances. High cardiac output and low peripheral vascular resistance, secondary hyperaldosteronism with consequent sodium retention and decreased total exchangeable potassium are often present. Other preoperative electrolyte abnormalities frequently seen include hypocalcaemia, hyperphosphataemia and hypomagnesaemia. Moreover, the coagulation parameters may be grossly abnormal (elevated prothrombin time, decreased platelets and fibrinogen). There may also be some degree of renal failure as well as hypoalbuminaemia. Continuous monitoring of many different parameters requires several intravascular cannulas including:

- two radial arterial lines (one for pressure monitoring and the other for blood sampling)

- one large peripheral intravenous catheter in the arm opposite to the side of the venous bypass

- one large external jugular catheter (to serve as access for the rapid infusion system) and

- a Swan–Ganz catheter inserted usually through the right internal jugular vein in order to monitor central venous and pulmonary arterial pressures.

A rapid infusion system, blood pump with warmer, warming blanket and cardiac defibrillator (with external and internal pads) are needed. Most patients undergoing liver transplantation today require less than 10 units of blood. However, in some difficult cases, when rapid blood transfusion is needed, the rapid infusion system with a blood warmer may be life saving. The blood bank must be able to provide large amounts of blood or blood products in a very short period of time. The laboratory must be in a position to provide immediate results at any time, day or night.

During the liver transplantation procedure there are three phases:

- hepatectomy

- anhepatic phase

- reperfusion of the transplanted liver.

During hepatectomy clotting is poor, fluid and electrolytes are often lost in large amounts and there may be considerable shifts in the acid–base status.

The anhepatic phase, if no venous bypass is used, is characterised by low venous return and low renal function. Replacement of fluids and electrolytes is necessary but the potassium level must be kept relatively low to prevent reperfusion hyperkalaemia. The body temperature decreases and thus warmed blood should be used.

During reperfusion, cardiovascular changes frequently occur with hypotension, bradycardia due to release of high potassium and

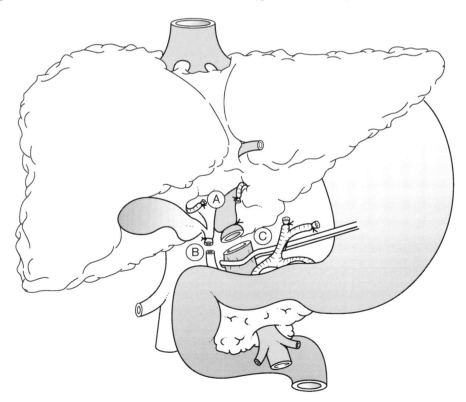

Figure 46.1 The recipient hepatectomy. **A.** The right and left branches of the hepatic artery are ligated and divided. **B.** The common bile duct is divided below the cystic duct. **C.** The portal vein is divided at its bifurcation with ligation of left and right portal branches and clamping of the portal trunk.

catabolic products from the liver and bowel. Treatment consists of volume replacement, Ca Cl$_2$ and atropine.

Early treatment of electrolyte changes is necessary, especially regarding hyperkalaemia and acidosis. Fibrinolysis may occur and coagulation products as well as ε-aminocaproic acid may be necessary. Hypothermia is very common and should be treated. In most cases, the patient's condition improves rapidly and stabilises. The lactate level decreases; the coagulation parameters and urine output improve. The pulmonary function, pulmonary artery pressures and other parameters normalise.

Conventional technique with use of a venovenous bypass

Before beginning the abdominal incision, the access routes for the venovenous bypass are prepared: the upper part of right (on left) saphenous vein is isolated as well as the left axillary vein. The abdominal incision most commonly used is a bilateral subcostal incision with upper mid-line extension ('Mercedes incision'). However, a J-shape right subcostal incision may be used with less morbidity (fewer pulmonary complications and abdominal eventration). The use of an adequate abdominal wall retractor allows an unrestricted view of the operative field.

Recipient hepatectomy (Figure 46.1)

The liver is mobilised after division of the falciform ligament and the umbilical ligament, and then of the left triangular ligament and the lesser omentum. Hilar dissection starts after incision of the anterior peritoneal layer of the hepatoduodenal ligament. The right and left branches of the hepatic artery are ligated, as well as the common bile duct immediately below the cystic duct. The portal trunk is completely isolated from the lymphatic tissue and the vein is followed as far as the bifurcation where the portal vein will be divided and the cannula inserted for the bypass. The right triangular ligament is divided and the right adrenal vein is ligated. The vena cava is controlled and encircled with a tape above and under the liver. The venovenous bypass is filled with saline solution and connected to the Bio-Pump after cannulation of the axillary, the iliac and the portal vein (Figure 46.2). The Bio-Pump is then activated. The vena cava is clamped below the liver and then above the liver with a large, curved, safe clamp. The upper vena cava is divided a few centimetres inside the liver parenchyma in order to keep a longer segment of vena cava. The lower section of the vena cava is performed above the lower clamp and the recipient liver is removed.

Anhepatic phase

Haemostasis of the retrohepatic space is ensured by coagulation and sutures. This stage is very important to avoid further bleeding behind the graft which could be difficult to control. The upper

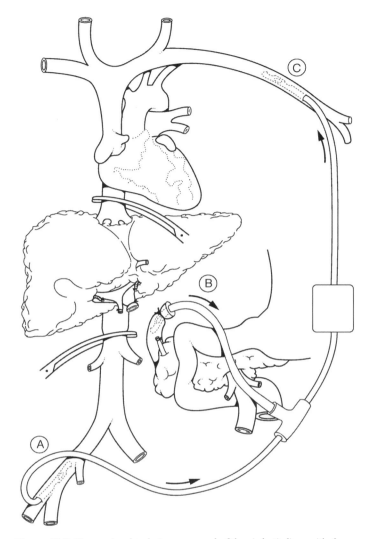

Figure 46.2 Conventional technique: removal of the cirrhotic liver with the use of a venovenous bypass. **A**. One cannula is inserted in the (left or right) iliac vein. **B**. One cannula is inserted in the portal vein. **C**. One cannula is inserted in the left axillary vein. The inferior vena cava is crossclamped above and below the liver.

vena cava is prepared to obtain a wide venous cuff by opening the right and left hepatic veins into a common cavity.

Implantation of the liver graft. Vascular and biliary reconstruction (Figures 46.3 and 46.4)

The upper caval anastomosis is constructed first with a 3/0 Prolene suture. Then the lower caval anastomosis is performed with a 4/0 Prolene suture while washing out the liver through a cannula placed in the portal vein, using a cold albumin solution to remove the preservation UW solution, rich in potassium. After removal of the portal cannula of the venovenous bypass, the portal anastomosis is performed using a 5/0 Prolene. This suture is not tied immediately to allow complete distension of the anastomosis to avoid any stricture. The suprahepatic vena cava is unclamped, then the lower vena cava and finally the portal vein.

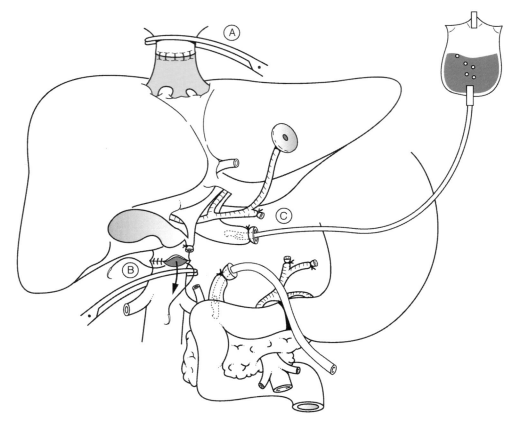

Figure 46.3 Conventional technique: implantation of the liver graft. **A.** The suprahepatic cavocaval anastomosis and the **B.** infrahepatic cavocaval anastomosis are successively performed. The liver graft is washed out (**C**) with albumin solution infused through a cannula inserted in the portal vein.

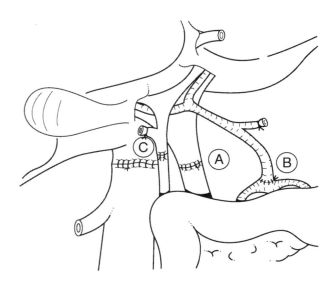

Figure 46.4 Implantation of the graft: arterial and biliary reconstruction. **A.** Portoportal end to end anastomosis is already performed. **B.** Arterial reconstruction is performed by an end-to-side anastomosis between the patch of the coeliac axis of the graft and the common hepatic artery of the recipient near the origin of the gastroduodenal artery. **C.** Biliary reconstruction is made by an end to end duct-to-duct anastomosis.

The liver recovers and rapidly returns to a normal colour. At the same time, the venovenous bypass is interrupted.

Successful hepatic artery reconstruction is crucial for the graft to function. A variety of methods can be used. In the routine, a Carrel patch of donor aorta or coeliac trunk is anastomosed to the recipient common hepatic artery, at the level of the gastro-duodenal artery outlet.

Finally, biliary reconstruction is performed with an end to end common bile duct anastomosis, using 6/0 absorbable mono-filament and interrupted sutures. T-tubes are no longer routinely used, as has been discussed previously. In cases of inadequate common bile duct in the recipient due to previous surgery, sclerosing cholangitis or transplantation in children, biliary reconstruction is performed with a Roux-en-Y loop.

The 'piggy-back' technique

This technique maintains the recipient's vena cava and also the vena caval flow during the anhepatic phase, avoiding the need for venous bypass. The original technique was described in children;

then a temporary portocaval anastomosis was proposed to avoid splanchnic stasis during the anhepatic phase. The 'piggy-back' technique has become increasingly popular in many transplant teams.

During the hepatectomy, the liver is raised and the accessory hepatic veins are ligated, proceeding in a caudocranial direction. The whole anterior wall of the vena cava is progressively freed and separated from the liver as far as the outlet of the right hepatic vein. Then, the left edge of the caudate lobe is detached from the vena cava. If clamping of the portal trunk is not well tolerated temporary portocaval shunt is performed (Figure 46.5).

After removing the liver, the orifice of two (middle and left) or three main hepatic veins is modelled by dividing the septa and sometimes widening the incision on the vena cava by around 1 cm. Caval anastomosis may be carried out either at the outlet of the three main hepatic veins or laterally on the vena cava or on the outlet of the middle and left hepatic veins (Figure 46.6). Liver flushing is started during caval anastomosis. When the graft has been irrigated with about 700 cc of albumin solution, the infra-hepatic stump of the vena cava is closed (with a vascular stapler or by suture). The procedure then follows the conventional steps

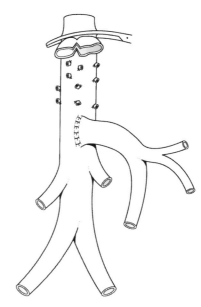

Figure 46.5 The 'piggy-back ' technique. During the hepatectomy and the anhepatic phase, a temporary portocaval shunt is performed.

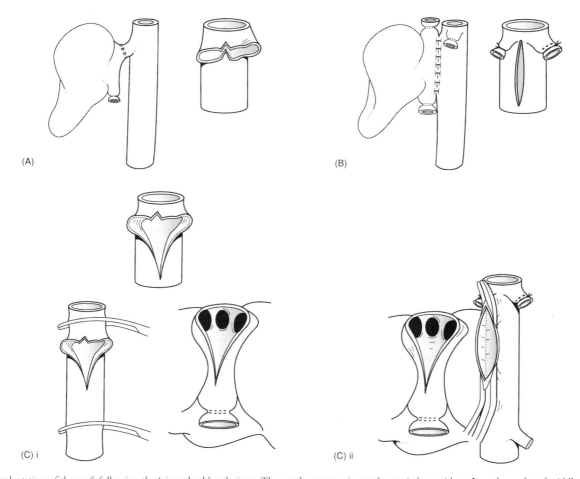

(A)

(B)

(C) i

(C) ii

Figure 46.6 Implantation of the graft following the 'piggy-back' technique. The caval anastomosis may be carried out either: **A**. at the outlet of middle and left hepatic veins or **B** laterally on the inferior vena cava (IVC) or **C** on the outlet of the three main hepatic veins (sometimes widening the incision on the vena cava) (**Ci** with complete clamping of the IVC or **Cii** with lateral clamping of the IVC (the most commonly used)).

with portal anastomosis and revascularisation of the graft followed by arterial and biliary reconstruction.

The living donor recipient operation

The diseased liver is removed as in the 'piggy-back' technique. In patients without portal hypertension, a temporary portocaval shunt is placed to avoid splanchnic congestion and bleeding. In the case of a left liver graft, the temporary portocaval shunt is placed using the right portal venous branch. An outflow tract is reconstructed by anastomosing the left hepatic vein of the graft end to side to the recipient's vena cava. In the case of a right lobe graft, the right lobe is piggy-backed to the native right hepatic vein. Arterial reconstruction is particularly critical in children and an operating microscope should be used.

Auxiliary liver transplantation

Over the past decade there has been a renewed interest in the use of auxiliary liver transplantation (ALT) either in patients with fulminant or subfulminant liver failure or for some metabolic diseases. In patients with acute liver failure the rationale for ALT

is to allow the native liver to recover from the acute injury so as to be able, in the long term, to discontinue immunosuppression and to avoid lifelong treatment. The lessons learned from previous heterotopic auxiliary liver grafting clearly showed that the portal blood inflow is crucial for the outcome of the procedure and that the hepatic vein outflow should be as near as possible to the heart.

The concept of auxiliary partial orthotopic liver transplantation (APOLT) was then developed and proved to be efficient. APOLT requires that both the graft and the recipient's liver are reduced. A frozen section of the recipient liver is sampled in order to assess the absence of fibrosis and the presence of viable hepatocytes. In children we use a left liver graft (segments 2 and 3 or 2, 3 and 4); in adults it is necessary to use a right liver graft (segments 5, 6, 7, 8) in order to provide more liver parenchyma according to the weight of the recipient. The hepatic vein of the graft is anastomosed to the hepatic vein of the recipient or end to side to the inferior vena cava (Figure 46.7). The portal vein of the graft is anastomosed to the portal trunk of the recipient. The graft's artery is anastomosed to the infrarenal aorta. Bile flow is restored through a Roux-en-Y hepaticojejunostomy.

Postoperative assessment focuses on the evaluation of the native liver function (bile production, liver scintigraphy, MRI-

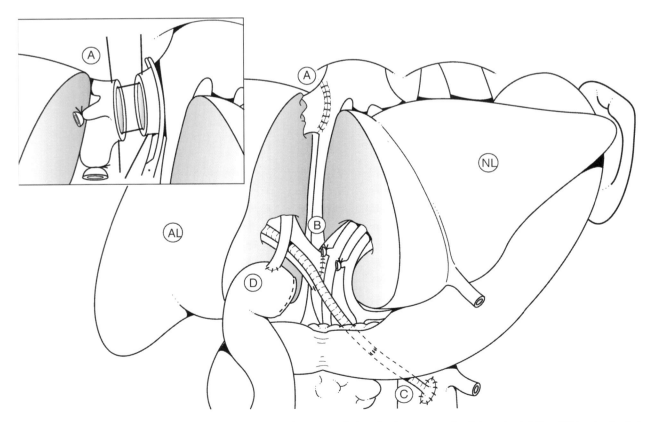

Figure 46.7 Auxiliary partial orthotopic liver transplantation (APOLT). The native right liver has been removed and the native left liver (NL) maintained. An auxiliary right liver (AL) is implanted orthotopically with: **A** the right hepatic vein of the graft anastomosed to the right hepatic vein of the recipient, **B** the right portal vein of the graft anastomosed to the portal trunk of the recipient, **C** the hepatic artery of the graft anastomosed to the recipient's aorta and **D** the bile duct of the graft implanted in a Roux-en-Y loop.

cholangiography, CT scan) in order to decide when immuno-suppression can be tapered or even, in some cases, the auxiliary graft removed.

Acknowledgement

The authors thank Mrs Veronique Rohfritsch for her help with preparation of the manuscript.

FURTHER READING

Allen KJ, Soriano HE. Liver cell transplantation: the road to clinical application. *J Lab Clin Med* 2001; **138**(5):298–312

Boudjema K, Jaeck D, Simeoni U et al. Temporary auxiliary liver transplantation for subacute liver failure in a child. *Lancet* 1993; **342**:778–779

Broelsch CE, Emond JC, Whitington PF et al. Application of reduced-size liver transplants as split grafts, auxiliary orthotopic grafts and living related segmental transplants. *Ann Surg* 1990; **212**:368–373

Busuttil RW, Klintmalm GB. *Transplantation of the Liver*. WB Saunders, Philadephia, 1996

Calne RY, Rolles K, White DJG et al. Cyclosporine A initially as the only immunosuppressant in 34 recipients of cadaveric organs: 32 kidneys, 2 pancreas, and 2 livers. *Lancet* 1979; **2**:1033–1036

Consensus Conference on indications of liver transplantation. Paris, June 22–23, 1993. *Hepatology* 1994; **20** (suppl):15–68S

Lacaille F, Sokal E. Living-related liver transplantation. *J Pediatr Gastroenterol Nutrition* 2001; **33**(4):431–438

Le Treut YP, Delpero JR, Dousset B et al. Results of liver transplantation in the treatment of metastatic neuroendocrine tumours. A 31 case French multicentric report. *Ann Surg* 1997; **225**:355–364

Mazziotti A, Cavallari A. *Techniques in Liver Surgery*. Greenwich Medical Media, London, 1997

Merritt WT. Bridge therapy to liver transplantation in fulminant hepatic failure. *Curr Opin Anaesthesiol* 2001; **14**(6):713–719

Mirza D, Gunsen BK, Da Silva RF et al. Policies in Europe on 'marginal quality' donor liver. *Lancet* 1994; **344**:1480–1483

National Institutes of Health. Consensus Development Conference statement: liver transplantation. Washington, June 20–23, 1983. *Hepatology* 1984: **4** (suppl 1): 107S–110S

Prasad KR, Lodge JPA. Transplantation of the liver and pancreas. *BMJ* 2001; **322**(7290):845–847

Rogiers X, Malago M, Gawad K et al. In situ splitting of cadaveric livers. The ultimate expansion of a limited donor pool. *Ann Surg* 1996; **224**:331–341

Starzl TE, Marchioro TL, Von Kanlla KN et al. Homotransplantation of the liver in humans. *Surg Gynecol Obstet* 1963; **117**:659–676

Starzl TE, Todo S, Fung J et al. FK-506 for human liver, kidney and pancreas transplantation. *Lancet* 1989; **2**:1000–1004

Strong RW, Lynch SV, Ong TN et al. Successful liver transplantation from a living donor to her son. *N Engl J Med* 1990; **332**:1505–1507

Section 8

Paediatric surgery

47

Paediatric surgery of the upper gastrointestinal tract

Edward R. Howard, Mark Davenport

OESOPHAGEAL ATRESIA AND TRACHEO-OESOPHAGEAL FISTULA

Incidence and presentation

Tracheo-oesophageal fistulas (TOF) (Figure 47.1) and oesophageal atresia occur with an incidence of approximately 1 in 3000 live births. The most frequent type of atresia is associated with a fistula between the distal oesophagus and the right main bronchus or tracheal carina but other variants occur (Figure 47.2). Difficulty with swallowing causes an excess of frothy saliva and any attempt at feeding provokes a cyanotic attack from bronchial aspiration.

Fistulas without atresia are seen in approximately 5% of cases when the communication is situated in the lower cervical region of the oesophagus. These are known as 'N' or 'H' type fistulas (Figure 47.1) and present with episodes of recurrent chest infection but no difficulty in swallowing. The infections are precipitated by contamination of the upper respiratory tract during feeds.

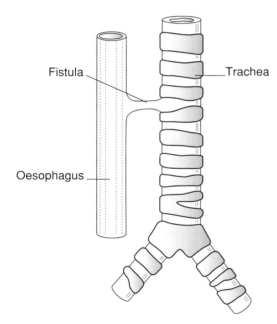

Figure 47.1 Diagrammatic illustration of isolated tracheo-oesophageal fistula.

Diagnosis

There is a history of polyhydramnios in 25–30% of cases due to oesophageal obstruction from atresia and excessive salivation in the newborn infant. The introduction of a firm, blunt-ended catheter through the mouth in suspected cases will demonstrate the atretic obstruction. Associated conditions should be sought as approximately 40% of cases have other anatomical abnormalities such as congenital cardiac disease, vertebral abnormalities and imperforate anus.

In the case of a fistula without atresia the fistula may be visualised using contrast injected via a nasogastric tube lying in the upper oesophagus and cineradiography of the study is particularly useful for the identification of very small fistulous tracks (Figure 47.2).

Treatment

The common type of TOF with atresia is corrected completely through a right thoracotomy using an extrapleural approach. The fistula at the apex of the lower segment of the oesophagus is ligated and divided. An end-to-end anastomosis is then constructed between the upper and lower oesophageal segments using interrupted sutures.

Closure of an isolated H-type fistula in the cervical oesophagus is performed through a transverse incision placed above the clavicle.

Complications of treatment

Primary surgical correction may be followed by anastomotic leakage and this may occasionally cause recurrent fistulation into the trachea. Excessive mobility of the posterior wall of the trachea (tracheomalacia), diagnosed on bronchoscopy, may give symptoms of respiratory obstruction. Severe symptoms of

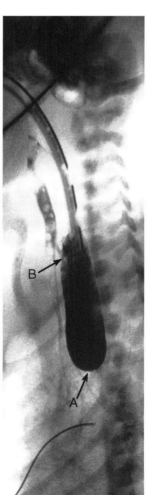

Figure 47.2 Contrast study of oesophagus in a four-week-old girl with 'long-gap' oesophageal atresia (A) awaiting delayed primary surgery. The contrast has spilled into the trachea via an additional 'H' type fistula from the upper pouch (B).

tracheomalacia respond well to aortopexy in which the aortic arch is fixed to the back of the sternum to hold the anterior tracheal wall firmly forwards. This manoeuvre ensures a good tracheal lumen. Late complications include oesophageal motility disorders, which are not uncommon after repair of TOF, and stricture formation at the site of the primary anastomosis. The latter may follow an episode of anastomotic leakage.

DIAPHRAGMATIC PROBLEMS

Anatomy and phrenic nerve injury

The diaphragm is composed of a central fibrous sheet derived from the septum transversum and a rim of striated muscle derived from the body wall. The phrenic nerve (C3, C4, C5), arising from the cervical plexus, supplies the muscle. It descends through the cervical inlet, entering the chest cavity to pass in front of the lung root to supply the diaphragm from the thoracic aspect. Because of its long pathway the nerve is at risk of damage from a variety of causes.

The typical phrenic nerve injury in infants occurs after a history of a prolonged and difficult birth and may be associated with damage to the upper roots of the brachial plexus. It may, for example, be seen in association with Erb's palsy (fifth cervical root damage) in which there is loss of the ability to externally rotate or to elevate the arm. The phrenic nerve may also be damaged during intrathoracic surgical procedures such as ligation of a patent ductus arteriosus.

Loss of hemidiaphragmatic function may be asymptomatic but it frequently causes symptoms of respiratory distress. A chest radiograph shows a high hemidiaphragm which is inert on fluoroscopy. Paradoxical movement, with elevation of the diaphragm during inspiration, may also be observed.

Surgical plication of the diaphragm is an effective method of reducing symptoms in the absence of spontaneous recovery of function. The operation is performed via a thoracotomy and converts a flaccid, stretched diaphragm into a thickened, flattened muscle which maximises intrathoracic volume and improves the efficacy of the accessory muscles of respiration.

Diaphragmatic hernia

Congenital

The incidence of diaphragmatic hernia in the newborn is approximately 1 in 3500 live births and 80% are on the left side. The commonest type is posterolateral in position (Bochdalek hernia) and results from a failure of closure of the pleuroperitoneal canal in the embryo. Gut passes into the chest and interferes with lung development. Respiratory distress is apparent soon after birth and survival depends on residual lung volume and function rather than on the timing of surgery. The classic signs at birth are of cyanosis,

mediastinal shift and a scaphoid abdomen. However, the diagnosis is now frequently made earlier during a routine antenatal ultrasound examination.

A chest radiograph after birth confirms the diagnosis and the early placement of a nasogastric tube will help to prevent intestinal distension in the chest. Ventilation and correction of acid–base abnormalities may be necessary before referral to a specialist centre for surgical correction.

Repair of the hernia is performed through a subcostal abdominal incision and commonly there is a residual rim of diaphragm which can be sutured to close off the thoracic cavity. Prosthetic material is used if there is no available diaphragmatic tissue.

The mortality rate in all cases of congenital diaphragmatic hernia is 40–50%.

Presentation in older children

Occasionally herniation through the diaphragm occurs after closure of the pleuroperitoneal canal and in these cases there is a hernial sac made up of peritoneum and pleura. Usually there is only a minimal effect on lung growth and development although mild, unrecognised, respiratory symptoms may be accentuated by a chest infection. A rare presentation with intestinal obstruction can result from intestinal kinking within the hernial sac. Bowel sounds within the chest are diagnostic and confirmation of the diagnosis is provided by a chest radiograph.

Traumatic diaphragmatic hernia

Traumatic diaphragmatic rupture is rare in children because of the inherent elasticity of the thoracic cage. It should, however, always be considered in patients with injuries to the upper abdomen or lower thorax. The diaphragm may be injured by either penetrating or blunt injuries and a diaphragmatic disruption is frequently accompanied by injuries to adjacent organs such as the spleen or liver. The right diaphragm is protected to some extent by the liver and the left is therefore injured more frequently. Acute symptoms include respiratory distress and chest or abdominal pain. The initial chest radiograph is diagnostic in 25–50% of cases but small lacerations may not be diagnosed in the posttraumatic period and may take months or years to manifest as a true hernia. It is not uncommon for this type of injury to be eventually recognised by chance, perhaps on a chest radiograph performed either for indeterminate symptoms of respiratory or gastrointestinal dysfunction, or for an unrelated condition.

Hiatus hernia and gastro-oesophageal reflux

A hiatus hernia is a structural abnormality of the oesophageal hiatus and, as in adults, may be classified into two types (Figure 47.3). In the more common 'sliding' type the gastro-oesophageal junction lies above the diaphragm and the acute gastro-oesophageal

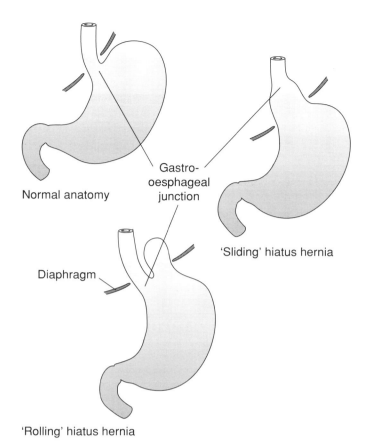

Figure 47.3 Diagrammatic illustration of hiatus hernia.

Normal anatomy

Gastro-oesphageal junction

'Sliding' hiatus hernia

Diaphragm

'Rolling' hiatus hernia

junction is lost. In the less common 'rolling' type the fundus of the stomach migrates through the hiatus into the mediastinum but the gastro-oesophageal junction lies below the diaphragm. Gastro-oesophageal reflux, which is associated particularly with the 'sliding' type of hernia, is a functional problem which may cause mucosal irritation and inflammation in even the youngest infant and which may eventually induce submucosal fibrosis and stricture formation. Reflux in children is recognised as a late complication of oesophageal atresia, diaphragmatic hernia and neurological abnormalities such as cerebral palsy.

Immaturity of the gastro-oesophageal sphincter (chalasia) is not uncommon in normal children during the first few months of life. It is recognised by effortless, non-bile stained vomiting after milk feeds. In the presence of normal weight gain the condition gradually resolves. However, failure to thrive and signs of oesophagitis such as haematemesis or difficulty with feeding are indications for investigation. The diagnosis will be confirmed with a barium study (Figure 47.4) and the severity of reflux gauged from an extended period of intra-oesophageal pH monitoring.

Treatment of reflux

The maintenance of an upright sitting posture after feeds is useful together with feed thickening and medication with Gaviscon to produce a floating liquid gel in the fundus of the stomach. H_2 receptor antagonists are also useful in children.

Fundoplication (Nissen operation) is the operation of choice in children who fail to respond to conservative measures and is particularly useful when reflux is associated with neurological abnormality. Results are good but there is a surgical mortality and reoperation is sometimes necessary.

PYLORIC STENOSIS

Infantile pyloric stenosis is the most common surgical cause of vomiting in young infants with an incidence of approximately 1 in 250 live births. The male to female ratio is 5:1 and the infants commonly present at between four and six weeks of age. The role of breastfeeding is controversial and an increased incidence in breastfed infants has been reported.

Genetic factors are well recognised although as yet candidate genes have not been isolated. Mothers who have been treated for pyloric stenosis are more likely to have affected children than fathers with the condition.

Clinical features

The vomiting is forceful or projectile and does not contain bile. It tends to occur after a feed and the infant appears hungry between feeds. The stools become hard and infrequent (starvation stools) and without treatment there will be weight loss and dehydration. The vomitus is mostly gastric acid which results in loss of electrolytes and water. The metabolic result is a hypochloraemic, hypokalaemic, metabolic alkalosis (Figure 47.5), with renal compensation for the loss of sodium ions by an exchange for potassium.

The diagnosis of pyloric stenosis is made by palpation of an olive-shaped mass in the upper abdomen, just to the right of the mid-line. The 'tumour' may be felt more easily if the stomach is emptied through a nasogastric tube and the infant relaxed with feeding. Gastric peristalsis may be observed in the epigastrium. Other methods of diagnosis include ultrasound which reveals the hypertrophied muscle as a broad ring with a low echo density whilst the mucosa of the pyloric canal is recognised as an inner layer of high echo density. In doubtful cases a barium contrast study will confirm gastric outlet obstruction and a narrowed pyloric canal.

Surgery (see below)

Pyloromyotomy, first described by Conrad Ramstedt in 1912, is the definitive treatment of pyloric stenosis. The abdominal incision is either a transverse muscle split in the right hypochondrium or a periumbilical incision which heals with an almost invisible scar.

A longitudinal incision is made through the thickened pyloric muscle which is then split, or spread, with a blunt spreading

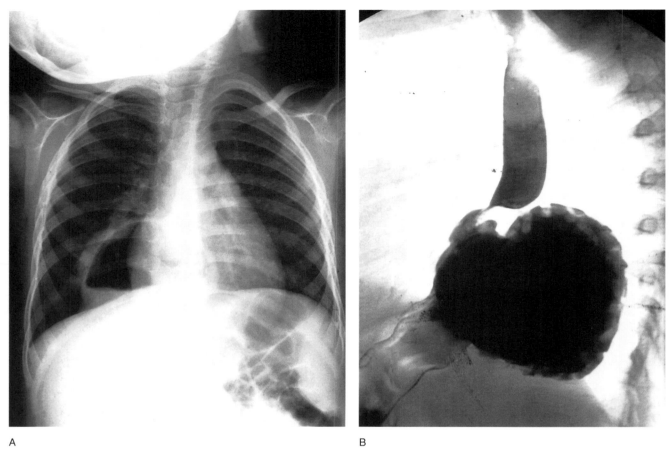

A   B

Figure 47.4 Plain radiograph of chest (**A**) and contrast study of stomach. (**B**) There is a large fluid level behind the heart shadow, which is shown by the contrast study to be a large 'sliding' hiatus hernia. A six-year-old child who presented with failure to thrive.

forceps down to the mucosa of the pyloric canal. The duodenal fornix marks the distal limit of the myotomy. The integrity of the mucosa must be checked by milking some air from the stomach into the duodenum. Laparoscopic pyloromyotomy is also practised by some surgeons using exactly the same principle of splitting the pyloric muscle.

Postoperatively normal feeds are reestablished within 48 hours and the infant is usually discharged on the fourth or fifth postoperative day. Complications of surgery include wound infection (*Staph. aureus*) in 5–10% of cases. There may also be some abnormalities of gastric emptying and gastric acid output in older children and adults.

$$H^+ + HCO_3^- \rightleftharpoons H_2CO_3 \rightleftharpoons H_2O + CO_2$$

loss of $[H^+]$ causes further dissociation of $[H_2CO_2]$ and increase in $[HCO_3^-]$

Figure 47.5 Equation for bicarbonate dissociation in alkalosis associated with pyloric stenosis.

OTHER SURGICAL CAUSES OF INTERMITTENT VOMITING

Structural abnormalities of the upper gastrointestinal tract, although rare in childhood, may be responsible for intermittent attacks of vomiting and a key diagnostic sign in these cases is whether the vomitus contains bile or not; that is, whether the site of obstruction lies above or below the ampulla of Vater. The least rare anatomical abnormalities are annular pancreas, duodenal stenosis, duodenal web and mid-gut malrotation.

Annular pancreas

Encirclement of the second part of the duodenum by pancreatic tissue is termed annular pancreas and is the result of abnormal migration of the ventral and dorsal primordial glands (see below). It may be associated with duodenal atresia in the neonatal period when it presents as complete upper intestinal obstruction. Partial duodenal compression by the annular pancreas may not, however, present until later in childhood. Barium studies are diagnostic and treatment is with either duodenoduodenostomy or duodenojejunostomy. The ring of pancreatic tissue must not be divided as it contains branches of the pancreatic ducts.

Duodenal stenosis or web

Isolated duodenal abnormalities may occur without pancreatic malformations and may present with intermittent vomiting of bile-stained material. The abnormalities occur within the second part of the duodenum and, as with duodenal atresia, may be associated with trisomy 21 (Down's syndrome). Duodenal webs can be excised whilst duodenal stenosis is best treated with a duodenoduodenostomy.

Malrotation

The commonest type of malrotation is an incomplete, anticlockwise rotation of the mid-gut loop which leaves the caecum in the right upper quadrant in close proximity to the duodenum (Figure 47.6). Peritoneal bands lying across the duodenum may cause intermittent bile-stained vomiting. The diagnosis is confirmed with barium contrast studies which will also show a right-sided duodenojejunal flexure and predominantly right-sided jejunal loops of bowel.

The malformation includes an abnormally short mesenteric attachment and a very mobile mid-gut which can twist on the mesentery containing the superior mesenteric vessels. A complete volvulus (twist) of the mid-gut may therefore occlude the mesenteric blood supply and cause an infarction of the whole of the mid-gut from the duodenum to the transverse colon. The clinical features include abdominal pain, bile-stained vomiting and circulatory collapse. Emergency surgery is mandatory.

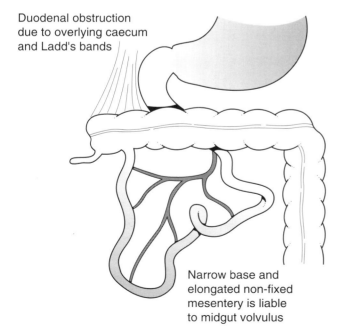

Figure 47.6 Diagrammatic representation of intestinal malrotation.

FOREIGN BODIES AND BEZOARS

Foreign bodies

Most children swallow small foreign bodies without ill effect and these usually pass rapidly through the gastrointestinal tract. A few will cause problems and present as an emergency. Occasionally small items, such as peanuts, will be inhaled through the larynx during swallowing and will lodge in the bronchial tree where they may cause an inflammatory reaction, bronchial obstruction, pneumonitis and lobar collapse.

Foreign bodies may also impact in the oesophagus at sites of relative narrowing, which include the region crossed by the right main bronchus and the gastro-oesophageal junction. Children with a history of oesophageal surgery are particularly at risk from impaction of even small objects at the site of a previous anastomosis. Objects which do not pass through the oesophagus within a few hours should be retrieved endoscopically with grasping forceps.

A minority of oesophageal foreign bodies may not be identified for weeks or even years and may cause symptoms of excessive salivation, recent onset 'asthma' and recurrent respiratory infection. These late presentations may be complicated by erosion of the oesophageal wall and by a vigorous inflammatory response. The safe removal of such an object may require thoracotomy.

In most cases, those objects that pass into the stomach will pass through the whole of the gastrointestinal tract.

Bezoars

A bezoar is a cast of the body of the stomach formed by the chronic ingestion of foreign material. The cast reduces intragastric volume and causes symptoms of gastric outlet obstruction. A mass of undigested vegetable matter is known as a phytobezoar and undigested hair as a trichobezoar (Figure 47.7). The latter is most commonly diagnosed in young girls with long hair with which they play and swallow loosened strands (Rapunzel syndrome).

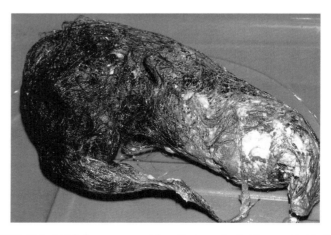

Figure 47.7 A trichobezoar removed from the stomach of a 12-year-old girl who presented with intermittent vomiting.

The clinical presentation includes depression of appetite, feelings of gastric fullness and intermittent vomiting. The bezoar may be palpated as an epigastric mass.

The diagnosis is confirmed on barium contrast studies or endoscopy and the material removed from the stomach by laparotomy and gastrotomy.

GASTRIC VOLVULUS

Gastric volvulus, well recognised in adult surgical practice, is a rare condition in childhood (<12 years). About half of these patients are less than one year at presentation with about a quarter of them under one month of age.

Pathology

Gastric volvulus is a rotation of one part of the stomach around another and is described as either an organoaxial type (the commoner variant), when the stomach rotates around an imaginary line joining the oesophageal hiatus and the pylorus, or a mesentericoaxial type which rotates around a line joining the mid-points of the greater and lesser curves (Figure 47.8).

In organoaxial rotation the greater curve rotates upwards above the lesser curve, resulting in a variable degree of compression of the intraabdominal oesophagus and the pylorus (Figure 47.9).

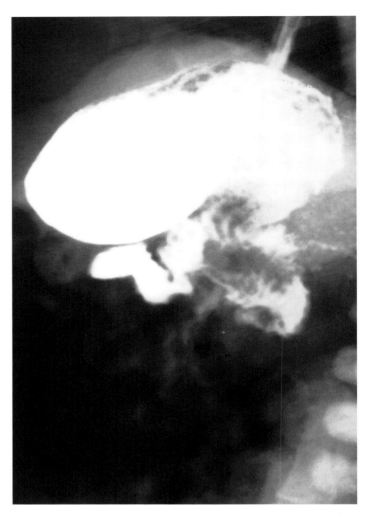

Figure 47.9 Barium radiograph of an organoaxial rotation of the stomach in an infant of seven days who presented with intermittent vomiting.

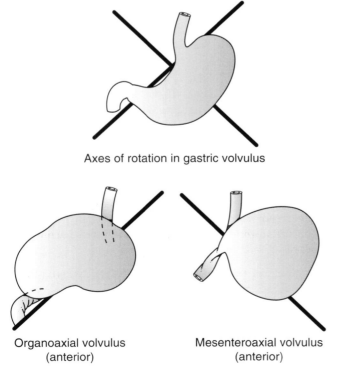

Axes of rotation in gastric volvulus

Organoaxial volvulus
(anterior)

Mesenteroaxial volvulus
(anterior)

Figure 47.8 Diagrammatic illustration of the two types of gastric volvulus, organoaxial and mesenteroaxial.

This process tends to be chronic in the adult but acute and complete volvulus may occur rapidly in the young infant.

Gastric volvulus is possible when the normal ligamentous attachments of the stomach, which comprise the gastrophrenic, gastrosplenic, gastrocolic and gastrohepatic ligaments, are either absent or abnormally lax. Not surprisingly, many of the reported cases in young children are associated with diaphragmatic defects when the displacement of the stomach into the chest results in lengthening of the surrounding ligaments. This association is present in most cases under one year of age. The role of ligamentous laxity in gastric volvulus has been demonstrated in the cadaver by division of the gastrocolic and gastrosplenic ligaments, a manoeuvre which allows the stomach to rotate through 180°.

Other reported associations with gastric volvulus in children have included pyloric stenosis, aerophagy, congenital bands or adhesions, distension of the transverse colon, absence or resection of the left lobe of the liver, intestinal malrotation and congenital absence of the spleen.

Clinical presentation

Acute gastric volvulus

Borchardt's triad (1904) is typical of the presentation of acute gastric volvulus in adults. The triad comprises:

- unproductive retching
- epigastric distension
- inability to pass a nasogastric tube.

This triad is, however, rarely diagnosed in children because the signs are less well defined than in adults. Furthermore, the regurgitation and vomiting which are typical features in adults can occur in many different types of gastrointestinal dysfunction in young children. Forceful vomiting and an absence of bile because of pyloric obstruction may be misdiagnosed as hypertrophic pyloric stenosis.

It should also be noted that respiratory distress and tachypnoea may be the dominant presenting features when the volvulus occupies an intrathoracic position in a child.

Chronic volvulus

Lesser degrees of volvulus, presenting as intermittent, recurrent vomiting, have been described in children.

Investigation

Plain abdominal radiographs show a dilated stomach, often with a fluid level on an erect film. Contrast studies will confirm the abnormal anatomy and the site of obstruction at the pylorus. An associated diaphragmatic defect may allow the antrum of the stomach to rotate into the chest and a fluid level may be seen behind the heart.

Treatment and results

Acute volvulus

Nasogastric decompression is performed urgently whenever possible, as acute volvulus in the small infant may progress to gastric perforation. Inability to pass a nasogastric tube into a severely dilated stomach may occasionally be an indication for percutaneous needle aspiration. Decompression by this technique will relieve respiratory embarrassment and may allow the subsequent passage of a nasogastric tube.

The surgical treatment in both children and adults is relatively straightforward and is always performed through an abdominal incision. Recurrence of a volvulus in small infants can be prevented with a simple gastrostomy using, for example, a Malecot or Foley catheter brought through the abdominal wall. In older children the gastric rotation is corrected and the stomach sutured to the anterior abdominal wall and to the diaphragm, a procedure known as anterior gastropexy. Any associated diaphragmatic defect is repaired. More complex procedures such as gastrectomy or gastroenterostomy are not necessary in these patients.

Mortality (about 10%) results from missed diagnoses or from failure to fix the stomach effectively at laparotomy.

Chronic volvulus

This can be managed conservatively by maintaining the babies in the prone position. Improvements can be expected within six months although radiological signs may be visible for up to 12 months.

SURGICAL JAUNDICE

General introduction (Box 47.1)

The presentation, investigation and diagnosis of obstructive jaundice (conjugated hyperbilirubinaemia) in the older child are similar to those described in adult patients but the separation of conjugated from unconjugated hyperbilirubinaemia in neonates and young infants is more difficult.

Box 47.1 Surgical causes of obstructive jaundice in infants and children

- Biliary atresia
- Choledochal cyst
- Inspissated bile syndrome
- Gallstones
- Perforation of the bile duct
- Segmental inflammatory stricture
- Peritoneal band compression (in gut malrotation)
- Rhabdomyosarcoma of the bile duct

A majority of newborn infants have a physiological unconjugated hyperbilirubinaemia during the first week of life secondary to low glucuronosyl transferase activity and approximately 50% of babies are noticeably jaundiced. The jaundice disappears within a few days but may be aggravated by other factors such as prematurity, breastfeeding and maternal diabetes mellitus. Raised levels of bilirubin in the newborn may also be associated with haemolysis, sepsis, pyloric stenosis and hypothyroidism.

It is imperative that any newborn infant who remains jaundiced for more than two weeks should be thoroughly investigated to determine whether the raised bilirubin is either conjugated or unconjugated because surgical conditions causing bile duct obstruction in young infants, such as biliary atresia, need urgent correction to prevent ongoing liver damage.

The differential diagnosis of prolonged conjugated hyperbilirubinaemia in young infants includes hepatic inflammation, known as the neonatal hepatitis syndrome, as well as structural abnormalities which require surgical correction. Unfortunately routine liver function tests are unhelpful in diagnosis as they show similar abnormalities in the two groups of infants.

There are many causes of neonatal hepatitis syndrome which include infection (e.g. toxoplasmosis, hepatitis B and C), endocrine abnormalities (e.g. hypothyroidism), genetic problems (e.g. trisomy 18 and 21) and metabolic abnormalities (e.g. cystic fibrosis, tyrosinaemia, glycogen storage disease). To exclude the many causes of neonatal hepatitis syndrome, the investigation of these young patients is therefore necessarily wide ranging.

The diagnosis of neonatal surgical causes of hyperbilirubinaemia is aided by ultrasound imaging of the bile ducts, which will detect choledochal cysts or obstruction with inspissated bile, and by liver biopsy which may reveal typical features of biliary atresia. In a small number of cases the histological appearances may be equivocal and not allow a definitive diagnosis of neonatal hepatitis syndrome or biliary atresia. ERCP, which is now possible in small infants, is recommended for this difficult minority of cases.

The most common causes of bile duct obstruction in the young infant are biliary atresia and a variety of cystic lesions of the bile ducts known as choledochal cysts and these will be described in detail. Other surgical conditions, outside the scope of this chapter, are included in Box 47.1.

Biliary atresia

Presentation and investigation

Jaundice is present from birth although it may be confused with physiological jaundice in the first few days. The important clinical signs are dark urine and pale stools. (In normal infants the urine is almost colourless and the stools are yellow.) The liver is enlarged from an early stage but splenomegaly is a relatively late sign. Failure to thrive becomes noticeable within a short time and the absence of bile results in vitamin K deficiency and a coagulopathy which may present in a variety of ways, for example as abnormal bruising or intracranial haemorrhage. Initial investigations will confirm the presence of conjugated hyperbilirubinaemia and subsequent tests with hepatobiliary nuclide scanning and percutaneous liver biopsy will demonstrate an absence of bile in the gut and the histological features of bile duct obstruction. Further confirmation of the diagnosis may be gained by an endoscopic retrograde cholangiogram (ERC) to demonstrate that the bile duct is obstructed. However, ERC in a small infant requires considerable skill and this investigation is not available in all centres.

Pathology

The term 'biliary atresia' refers to an inflammatory obliteration of the bile ducts which occurs in the newborn with a frequency of approximately 1:14 000 live births. The extent of the bile duct

destruction varies from case to case but a simple classification describes three main types (Figure 47.10).

- *Type 1* – occlusion of the common bile duct. Preservation of a proximal segment of hepatic duct containing bile.

- *Type 2* – occlusion of both the common bile duct and the common hepatic duct. Residual patency of the right and left hepatic ducts.

- *Type 3* – occlusion of the bile ducts up to the liver capsule. The hepatic ducts are replaced by an inflammatory mass which varies in size from case to case and which tends to diminish with age. The mass contains residual bile ductules which communicate with intrahepatic ducts in the neonatal period. The intrahepatic ducts will tend to disappear as the child grows if successful surgery is not achieved.

Before the development of this classification the cases with residual, bile-containing segments of bile duct (types 1 and 2) were described as 'correctable' atresias whilst the cases with total obliteration (type 3) were known as 'non-correctable'. However, the demonstration of residual biliary remnants in the porta hepatis of type 3 cases and the introduction of the operation of portoenterostomy have made these terms obsolete. The majority of cases (88%) are type 3 atresias.

The pathological changes in the extrahepatic ducts are also associated with intrahepatic changes which have some similarities in common with sclerosing cholangitis. The portal tracts are

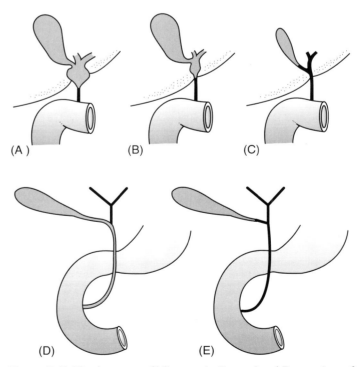

Figure 47.10 The three types of biliary atresia. Figures **A** and **B** are variants of type 1, **C** represents type 2 and **D** and **E** are variants of type 3 disease. Reproduced with permission from *Maingot's Abdominal Operations*, 9th edn; Appleton and Lange.

expanded with oedema and fibrosis and there is proliferation of bile ductules with obvious cholestasis.

The aetiology of biliary atresia remains obscure but there are a few possible clues. Embryological studies of the developing bile ducts, for example, have shown similarities between the appearances of the bile ducts in the porta hepatis in the foetus at the 11th to 13th weeks of gestation and the histology of the tissue resected from the porta hepatis soon after birth from cases of atresia. It has therefore been suggested that atresia may be the end result of arrested bile duct development and that the inflammatory reaction may be caused by bile leakage from malformed bile ducts.

An early embryological insult in aetiology is also suggested by the association of biliary atresia with other extrahepatic abnormalities such as polysplenia, situs inversus and malformation of the portal vein. These associations are present in over 20% of cases. Experimental liver lesions reminiscent of atresia have been produced in animals by the injection of viruses such as reovirus and rotavirus. However, studies in patients have not confirmed any consistent association with this type of infection.

Treatment

The operation known as portoenterostomy or the 'Kasai' procedure is now the accepted first line of treatment for infants with biliary atresia. It was first described by Morio Kasai in a Japanese journal in 1959 and was gradually accepted as an effective treatment in the UK and North America. The procedure is performed through a transverse abdominal incision and commences with a full mobilisation of the liver which is rotated to expose the undersurface and the porta hepatis. The typical appearances of atresia include inflammatory thickening of the gallbladder wall and the periductal tissues in the porta hepatis. The occluded bile duct is dissected free of both the portal vein and the hepatic artery and is excised completely from the supraduodenal border to the capsule of the liver above the junction of the right and left hepatic ducts.

Histological studies of the excised tissue from the porta hepatis show that in a majority of cases there are residual biliary ductules which communicate with intrahepatic biliary channels from which bile will drain. Surgical exposure of these biliary channels is therefore followed by the anastomosis of a Roux-en-Y loop of jejunum to the edges of the transected tissue. The most important part of the operation is an accurate and wide excision of all the inflamed residual ductal tissue in the porta hepatis.

The achievement of good bile flow after a portoenterostomy operation is related to the age of the infant at surgery, as well as to the size of the bile duct remnants in the porta hepatis.

Complications

The most frequent early complication of surgery is ascending bacterial cholangitis which is recognised by the sudden onset of pyrexia and increasing jaundice. Repeated attacks of cholangitis may cause increasing damage to the liver parenchyma and it is therefore important to begin treatment of the infection with broad-spectrum antibiotics as promptly as possible. The diagnosis of infection may be confirmed with blood cultures and with percutaneous liver biopsy.

Portal hypertension and splenomegaly are common sequelae of biliary atresia and approximately 60% of the children who survive for more than two years show endoscopic evidence of oesophageal varices. Approximately half of these will bleed and require obliteration with endoscopic sclerotherapy or variceal banding.

Other reported long-term complications include malabsorption, particularly in the presence of persistent cholestasis, fat-soluble vitamin deficiency (vitamins A,D,E and K) and evidence of osteomalacia and rickets. Prolonged postoperative surveillance of these children is essential.

In common with other causes of severe hepatic fibrosis or cirrhosis, biliary atresia may be complicated by hypoxia secondary to intrapulmonary shunting. The underlying metabolic cause of the pulmonary changes is not yet known although the severity of the condition may be quantified using radionuclide ventilation: perfusion lung scans. Severe symptoms are an indication for liver transplantation.

Surgical results

Approximately 70–80% of infants will have evidence of bile flow after portoenterostomy surgery. However, long-term survival is dependent on complete clearance of jaundice and the overall 5–10 year survival rate was reduced to approximately 39% in a large collected series of cases. Liver transplantation is available for young children who do not achieve successful bile drainage after portoenterostomy and for those who develop severe complications at a later age. The early results of transplantation have been very encouraging and one, two- and five-year actuarial survival rates of 83%, 80% and 78% respectively have been reported.

In summary, there have been major advances in the management of biliary atresia in recent years. Thirty years ago long-term survivors were rare except for an occasional type 1 case in whom there was a residual segment of proximal bile duct. Now, however, the development of portoenterostomy and transplantation has resulted in the survival of approximately 90% of cases, many of whom are now reaching adult life.

Choledochal cyst

Presentation and investigation

Congenital cystic malformations of the biliary tract are rare abnormalities which vary in morphology from case to case. The true incidence in the UK is not known although in our own practice one case has been referred for every three of biliary atresia,

759

giving an incidence of perhaps 1 in 42 000 live births. In all large series there is a female:male ratio of 4:1 and more than 60% of cysts are diagnosed in children below the age of 10 years.

Choledochal cysts may be complicated by jaundice (which may be persistent or intermittent), infection, gallstones and carcinoma.

The classic presentation, with the three signs of jaundice, pain and a mass in the right hypochondrium, is rare. The more common presentations are of jaundice (69%) and pain (18%). Pain is associated with pancreatitis secondary to an abnormality at the junction of the bile duct and the pancreatic duct which results in a relatively long and common pancreatico-biliary channel. This abnormal ductal arrangement, which allows the free reflux of pancreatic enzymes into the biliary tract, was present in most symptomatic cysts (Figure 47.11). Liver function tests may indicate biliary tract obstruction, although this may be episodic, and a rise in serum amylase may be detected particularly if there has been a recent attack of abdominal pain. Ultrasonography provides an accurate method of diagnosis and this investigation is frequently supplemented by endoscopic cholangiography (ERCP).

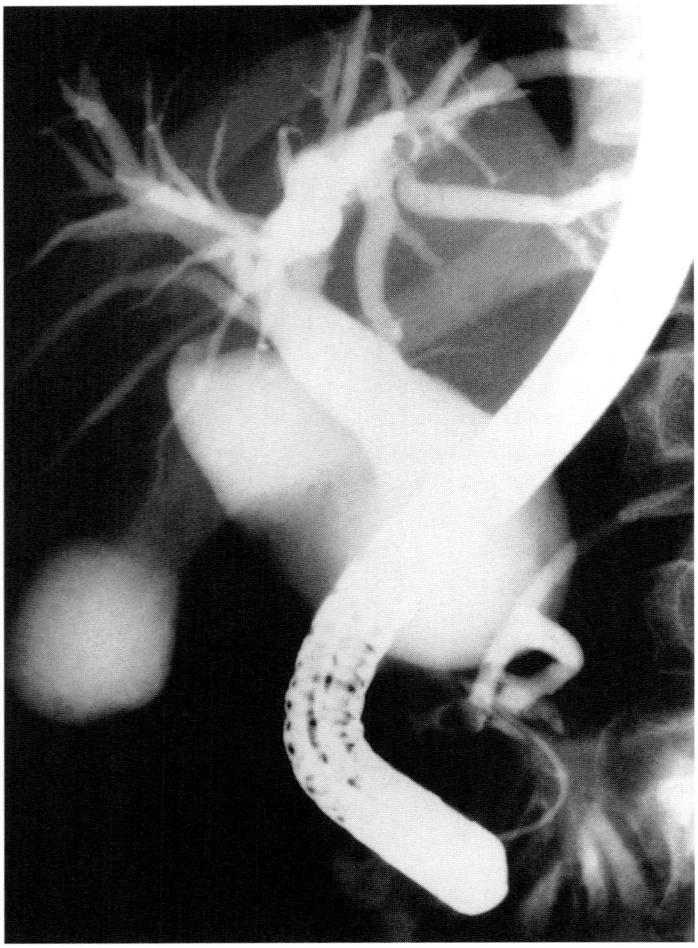

ERCP provides accurate information on the presence or absence of a common pancreatico-biliary channel but should not be performed on patients who have had a recent episode of pancreatitis as the investigation itself may precipitate a severe attack. Magnetic resonance cholangiography (MRC) is now providing accurate images of the biliary tract and pancreatic duct and avoids the possible complications of ERCP.

Pathology

Choledochal cysts are classified into six main types (Figure 47.12).

- *Type Ic* – cystic dilatation of the extrahepatic bile duct.
- *Type If* – fusiform dilatation of the extrahepatic bile duct.
- *Type II* – diverticulum of the common bile duct.
- *Type III* – choledochocoele.

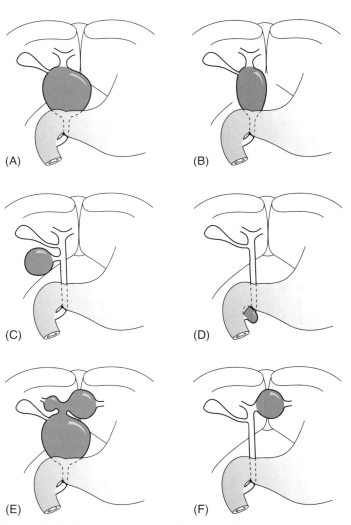

Figure 47.11 A large choledochal cyst in a 12-year-old girl at ERCP. Note that the cyst communicates directly with the pancreatic duct, forming a 'common channel'. Reproduced with permission from *Maingot's Abdominal Operations*, 9th edn; Appleton and Lange.

Figure 47.12 The six types of choledochal cyst. **A** Type Ic – cystic lesions. **B** Type If – fusiform lesions. **C** Type II. **D** Type III. **E** Type IV. **F** Type V. Reproduced with permission from *Maingot's Abdominal Operations*, 9th edn; Appleton and Lange.

- *Type IV* – combined intra- and extrahepatic cysts.
- *Type V* – intrahepatic cysts without an extrahepatic component.

Cystic type 1 cysts are the most common followed by the fusiform type 1 cysts and together account for about 90% of choledochal cysts. Type 4 and 5 cysts account for about 10% whilst type 2 and 3 cysts are rare. Choledochal cysts have now been identified during antenatal foetal scanning with ultrasound, thus providing evidence for their congenital origin. Congenital abnormalities of the pancreatico-biliary junction are also demonstrated in approximately 75% of cases and it has been suggested that the patterns of ductal union are classified into two main types depending on whether the bile duct appears to join the pancreatic duct or vice versa.

Partial loss of epithelium and chronic inflammatory cell infiltration characterise the histological examination of cysts after surgical excision. These features appear to be age related and are more severe in older patients. Similarly, most reports of malignant change in cysts concern adults although the youngest recorded case was in a 12-year-old girl.

Treatment and results

Total excision of extrahepatic cysts is now accepted as the treatment of choice. The proximal line of resection is at the level of the bifurcation of the common hepatic duct and the distal level is just above the junction of the bile duct with the pancreatic duct. The biliary tract is reconstructed with a Roux-en-Y loop of jejunum at least 40 cm in length.

Less extensive operations such as cyst-enterostomy or cyst-duodenostomy have a high risk of late complications such as cholangitis, stone formation and stenosis of the anastomosis.

The removal of isolated intrahepatic cysts may require partial hepatectomy whilst the drainage from bilateral cysts can be improved with a wide anastomosis which incorporates the right and left hepatic ducts above the bifurcation of the common hepatic duct.

Gallstones

Aetiology

Autopsy reports confirm that gallstones are rare in children with a prevalence of less than 0.1%. However, they are well recognised as a complication of certain diseases and it is well known that gallstones are associated with haemolytic disorders such as sickle cell disease, hereditary spherocytosis and thalassaemia. The incidence of gallstones in sickle cell disease, for example, is approximately 25%.

Recent reports have confirmed the relationship between total parenteral nutrition (TPN) and gallstone formation in the young infant and this appears to be related, at least in part, to a lack of gallbladder stimulation by cholecystokinin in the fasting state. However, many other factors have been implicated including the parenteral administration of amino acids and fat, small bowel resection and the duration of TPN administration. Most stones which form during TPN administration remain asymptomatic and few develop complications. A majority resolve with resumption of enteral feeding.

The incidence of idiopathic gallstones, without associated disease, is the same for males and females until puberty. The incidence in females rises rapidly thereafter and as in adults there is an association with pregnancy and with obesity.

Symptoms and diagnosis

Symptoms of gallstone colic in older children may be similar to the well-described features in adults, with intermittent right hypochondrial pain which may radiate to the right shoulder. Diagnosis may be more difficult in younger children who may not localise abdominal pain to the right hypochondrium. Many stones remain asymptomatic in childhood and may only be detected during an investigation for an unrelated illness.

Bile duct stones may be diagnosed after the onset of an episode of jaundice but diagnosis can be difficult in the child with sickle cell disease who may suffer with a persistent hyperbilirubinaemia secondary to the haemolytic disease itself.

The majority of stones are radiolucent and the diagnosis is usually made with ultrasound scanning. A dilated common bile duct identified with ultrasound or abnormally raised liver enzymes suggesting bile duct stones are indications for ERCP which can now be performed in children of all ages.

It should be emphasised that an underlying haemolytic disorder must be ruled out in any child who presents with gallstones.

Treatment

Gallstones identified in infants, particularly those associated with TPN, may resolve spontaneously and conservative management with serial ultrasound is therefore recommended for this age group.

Cholecystectomy is recommended in older children with gallstones secondary to spherocytosis and this can be performed at the same time as they are undergoing splenectomy, either laparoscopically or by open operation. Cholecystectomy is also recommended for sickle cell children in whom gallstones are identified as the symptoms of gallstone colic are difficult to separate from the abdominal pain of sickle crises. Furthermore, complications from gallstones passing from the gallbladder into the bile duct frequently develop in these patients with increasing age.

Symptomatic gallstones in all children should be managed with the same guidelines employed in adults and cholecystectomy should not be withheld simply on age alone. Medical treatment of gallstones has been disappointing.

Laparoscopic cholecystectomy is the surgical treatment of choice in children of all ages and results in a significantly shorter period of hospitalisation compared to open cholecystectomy.

PANCREATITIS AND CONGENITAL PANCREATIC ABNORMALITIES

Acute pancreatitis

The clinical features and complications of acute pancreatitis, which is a rare condition in children, are similar to the well-recognised disease in adults. There are, however, aetiological factors in childhood which are unusual in adults and which include congenital anatomical abnormalities and specific types of abdominal trauma, such as child abuse and car seatbelt injury, (Box 47.2). Pancreatitis may occur in generalised disorders such as cystic fibrosis and haemolytic uraemic syndrome and is also recognised as a complication of mumps and of gallstones.

Box 47.2   Causes of pancreatitis in children

Anatomical:
- annular pancreas
- pancreas divisum
- common pancreatico-biliary channel
- congenital pancreatic cysts

Gallstones
Trauma
Parasites, e.g. ascariasis
Infections, e.g. mumps
Hereditary autosomal dominant disease
Metabolic, e.g. hypercalcaemia, hyperlipidaemia

Acute obstruction of the pancreatic duct has some unusual causes in childhood, which include helminthic infestation with *Ascaris lumbricoides*. These roundworms infect the gastrointestinal tract and may migrate through the duodenal papilla to block the bile ducts or the pancreatic duct, causing jaundice, cholangitis or pancreatitis. Treatment consists of the antihelminthic drug mebendazole and endoscopic removal of the paralysed worms.

Pancreatitis may be precipitated by ERCP examinations and this is a particular risk in the child with a choledochal cyst and 'common channel' malformation.

The principles in the management of acute pancreatitis in children are identical to those described in adults. Complications, such as pseudocyst formation, are similar and there are reported mortality rates of 15–20%.

In the management of postpancreatitic pseudocysts in children about a third resolve spontaneously and the remainder will require some form of drainage procedure, either cystogastrostomy or cysto-jejunostomy.

Chronic pancreatitis

The signs of chronic pancreatitis in childhood include failure to thrive, growth retardation and developmental delay. The condition may result from repeated episodes of acute pancreatitis discussed above although in some cases there is no identifiable aetiology.

Hereditary pancreatitis is a well-defined entity in childhood with an autosomal dominant type of transmission. Most cases become manifest before 10 years of age with attacks of acute pancreatitis which frequently progress to chronic disease identified by pancreatic calcification and dilated pancreatic ducts with or without strictures. The clinical course is variable.

A mutant cationic trypsinogen gene has recently been demonstrated in several families with hereditary pancreatitis. This suggests that during trypsin activation in the normal pancreas, excess trypsinogen and trypsin are hydrolysed and inactivated by trypsin-like enzymes so that the pancreas is protected from autodigestion. The mutation of the cationic trypsinogen gene, which is believed to abolish this protective mechanism, was identified on the 7q35 chromosome and appears to eliminate a trypsin-sensitive hydrolysis site.

Hereditary pancreatitis is also associated with ampullary stenosis and hypertrophy of the sphincter of Oddi causing pancreatic duct dilatation and satisfactory relief from symptoms has been obtained in affected children after surgical sphincterotomy.

Distal pancreatic resection and longitudinal pancreatico-jejunostomy (Puestow procedure) have also been used successfully to improve duct drainage in children with chronic pancreatitis.

Congenital malformations

Embryology (Figure 47.13)

Pancreatitis in children may be associated with malformations of the pancreas or the bile ducts. To understand the origin of these abnormalities it is necessary to understand the embryology of the pancreatico-biliary system.

The pancreas develops from two structures which grow out from the dorsal and ventral aspects of the junction of the foregut and the mid-gut. The ventral outgrowth rotates around the duodenum to reach the dorsal outgrowth with which it fuses.

The common bile duct arises from the pancreatic duct within the ventral portion of the gland and initially the pancreatic–bile duct junction lies outside the duodenal wall. As the foetus develops the junction migrates towards the duodenal wall and at birth it lies within the muscle complex of the sphincter of Oddi.

Pancreatic abnormalities which result from deranged embryology include annular pancreas, pancreas divisum, long common pancreatico-biliary channels, pancreatic cysts and duodenal malformations such as duodenal web. All of these may be complicated by attacks of pancreatitis.

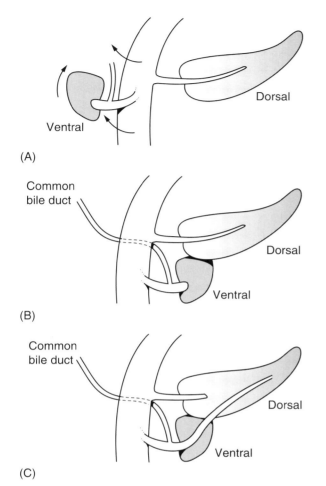

(A)

(B)

Common bile duct

Dorsal

Ventral

(C)

Common bile duct

Dorsal

Ventral

Figure 47.13 Diagrammatic representation of the embryology of the pancreas. Rotation of the ventral segment of the gland around the duodenum (A) is followed by fusion with the dorsal segment (B). The original ventral duct now takes over drainage from the majority of the gland (C).

Annular pancreas

During rotation of the ventral portion of the gland around the duodenum, a portion of the gland is believed to remain fixed to the right side of the duodenum. This persistent fixation disturbs the development of the duodenum, the lumen of which is either narrowed (stenosed) or obliterated (atretic), resulting in high intestinal obstruction at birth (see above). This abnormality is frequently associated with chromosomal abnormalities, particularly trisomy 21 or Down's syndrome, although the reason for this is not understood.

Although pancreatitis in association with annular pancreas has not been reported in children, about one-quarter of adults with annular pancreas suffer attacks of pancreatitis.

Pancreas divisum

During the phase of fusion of the embryonic ventral and dorsal portions of the pancreas the main ducts in each portion join to

form the main duct of Wirsung which drains through the ampulla of Vater. A portion of the dorsal duct remains as the accessory duct of Santorini which drains through an accessory or 'minor' papilla.

A failure of ductal fusion results in two separate and independently draining segments of pancreas (pancreas divisum) with the larger dorsal duct draining through the minor papilla and the smaller ventral duct, from the uncinate process, draining through the ampulla of Vater. The condition is also known as the 'dominant dorsal duct syndrome' and it has been observed in 6–10% of the population. There is a 12% incidence of divisum in patients with a history of pancreatitis which is believed to be a consequence of ductal obstruction caused by stenosis of the minor papilla.

Transduodenal sphincteroplasty in adult patients has been shown to be beneficial. A well-documented case of divisum in an eight-year-old girl who presented with recurrent attacks of acute pancreatitis described stenosis of both the major and minor papilla. She was treated with surgical sphincteroplasty of both papillae and had suffered no further attacks of pancreatitis during the following 22 months.

In summary, pancreas divisum is a relatively common anatomical variation which is associated with recurrent pancreatitis in a proportion of cases who appear to have stenosis of the minor papilla. Currently the recommended treatment is surgical sphincteroplasty to relieve the stenosis.

Common pancreatico-biliary channels

Congenital cystic malformations of the bile duct (choledochal cyst) are associated with an abnormal anatomical arrangement of the junction of the common bile duct with the pancreatic duct. Normally these two ducts either open separately into the ampulla of Vater or join to form a short channel less than 5 mm in length. This channel lies within the muscle complex of the sphincter of Oddi and the arrangement effectively prevents admixture of bile and pancreatic juice.

Longer pancreatico-biliary channels result in the duct junction lying outside the duodenal wall. The resultant free reflux of bile and pancreatic juice is believed to be the cause of recurrent pancreatitis and has been termed the 'common channel syndrome'.

Although abnormally long common channels are found in association with approximately 70% of choledochal cysts, they may also occur in children without significant bile duct dilatation (Figure 47.14). Biliary-pancreatic reflux should be prevented with bile duct excision and Roux-en-Y reconstruction of the biliary tract. This has proved to be an effective treatment for preventing pancreatitis and histological examination of excised bile ducts in these cases shows evidence of inflammatory damage with loss of epithelium and fibrosis in the duct wall.

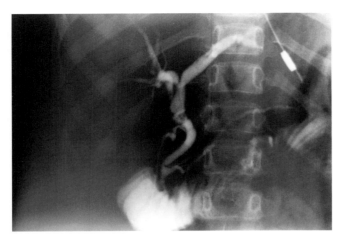

Figure 47.14 A common pancreatico-biliary channel demonstrated at ERCP in an eight-year-old girl who presented with a history of recurrent pancreatitis.

Congenital pancreatic cysts

A range of rare congenital cystic lesions may arise within and in close proximity to the head of the pancreas and may precipitate recurrent attacks of pancreatitis. They include:

- very rare true pancreatic cysts arising within the parenchyma of the gland

- enteric duplications (gastric or duodenal) within the pancreas or adjacent to the duodenum

- duodenal diverticula which do not usually cause symptoms in childhood.

Enteric duplications represent the most common congenital cystic abnormality of the pancreatic head and approximately 18 cases have been reported. They are composed of smooth muscle surrounding gastrointestinal-type mucosa and may share muscle layers with the adjacent duodenum. Duplications may be distinguished on ultrasound from postinflammatory pseudocysts by the demonstration of a hyperechoic inner layer representing the mucosal lining of the cyst. CT scans may also help to identify the exact site of the cyst whilst ERCP is a useful method of identifying any communication with the pancreatic ducts. Surgical treatment depends on the site and size of the lesion but local resection rather than pancreatico-duodenectomy has been successful in a number of cases. Intraoperative ultrasonography is valuable in delineating cysts which are not palpable.

Duodenal web

Duodenal webs are usually situated near to the duodenal papilla and the bile and pancreatic ducts may enter the duodenum on the medial margin. The webs may or may not have a central lumen and although they present most commonly in the neonatal period with signs of high intestinal obstruction, diagnosis may not be made until several years later. Symptoms at late presentation

include epigastric distension, gastro-oesophageal reflux and poor weight gain. Pancreatitis in association with a web has now been described in an adult and a child and excision of the web was reported as curative.

PRIMARY LIVER TUMOURS – BENIGN AND MALIGNANT

A wide range of primary liver tumours occur in children but most present before two years of age. They may be epithelial or mesenchymal in origin and benign or malignant. Although rare, they account for 15% of all abdominal masses in this age group. A particular feature is their occasional association with other congenital disorders such as hemihypertrophy and polyposis coli.

Secondary tumours, particularly from neuroblastomata, also occur and are considered elsewhere in this book.

Box 47.3 lists the more frequent tumours encountered in children and all require surgical resection for cure.

Box 47.3	Primary liver tumours in children
Benign	*Malignant*
Haemangio-endothelioma	Hepatoblastoma
Mesenchymal hamartoma	Hepatocellular carcinoma
Adenoma	Mesenchymoma
Focal nodular hyperplasia	Yolk sac tumour
Non-parasitic cysts	Angiosarcoma

Presentation and investigation

An asymptomatic abdominal mass is the most frequent sign. Pain, fever and weight loss suggest advanced disease and metastases are present in 25% of cases at diagnosis. Alpha-fetoprotein is secreted by hepatoblastomas and other malignant tumours and provides a sensitive tumour marker, both for diagnosis and treatment. Imaging with ultrasound, CT and angiography often differentiates benign from malignant tumours and percutaneous biopsy is only required in cases with a doubtful diagnosis or as a preliminary to chemotherapy. CT scans of the chest are essential to exclude secondary malignant disease.

Treatment

Up to 85% of the liver may be resected in non-cirrhotic children without precipitating liver failure. Surgery is performed through a bilateral subcostal incision and it is never necessary to enter the thoracic cavity. Shrinkage of malignant tumours, particularly hepatoblastomata, is achieved with preoperative chemotherapy and this combination therapy is now mandatory. Transplantation is now available for inoperable hepatoblastomata with a survival rate of over 50%.

Haemangio-endothelioma, mesenchymal hamartoma and hepatoblastoma are the most common lesions in this group of tumours and the following is a synopsis of their main features.

Haemangio-endothelioma

This particular type of infantile haemangioma is often associated with vascular cutaneous lesions. As with the cutaneous haemangiomata, growth is rapid in the first few weeks of life and arteriovenous shunting may result in severe heart failure. Untreated cases have a mortality rate of approximately 75%.

Treatment depends on the severity of symptoms and the anatomical extent of the lesion. Asymptomatic lesions may diminish in size with age and can be monitored with ultrasound. Segmental resection is possible for symptomatic lesions located in one lobe of the liver whilst heart failure secondary to a diffuse haemangioma responds to hepatic artery ligation (HAL).

Mesenchymal hamartoma

Most of these benign cystic lesions, made up of a mixture of mesodermal and endodermal tissues, present before five years of age as an asymptomatic mass. They account for 6% of benign tumours and can grow to over 2 kg in weight. Very large lesions may cause respiratory embarrassment but resection is curative.

Hepatoblastoma

These lesions account for approximately 0.8% of childhood malignancies. A relationship with hemihypertrophy and familial polyposis coli is well documented and an abnormality of chromosome 5 has been suggested as the linking factor with the latter.

Increased survival followed both the introduction of effective chemotherapy and the refinement of resectional techniques. In the 1960s, the resection rate was 50% and the survival rate around 17% whereas in the 1990s resection rates of about 80% and survival rates of over 66% were reported.

OPERATIVE SURGERY

Pyloromyotomy (Figure 47.15)

Patient preparation

- Correction of electrolyte abnormalities (metabolic alkalosis, hyponatraemia, hypokalaemia)

- Nasogastric tube insertion and gastric lavage with physiological saline solution

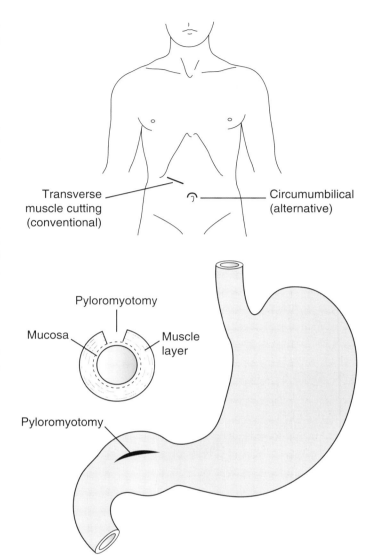

Figure 47.15 Diagrammatic illustration of incisions and technique of pyloromyotomy.

Anaesthesia and patient position

- General anaesthesia with muscle relaxation

- Supine position

- Single dose prophylactic antibiotic (effective against staphylococcal organisms)

Incision

Choice of:

- right upper quadrant transverse muscle cutting, or

- superior circumumbilical skin incision with vertical division of linea alba (cosmetically superior).

Procedure

- Deliver the pyloric 'tumour' into the wound (Figure 47.16A).

- Incise the serosa overlying the pyloric 'tumour', avoiding any prominent vessels.

- Use the convex side of blunt mosquito forceps to open the pyloric incision and split the hypertrophic muscle layer. (Do not use 'points' of forceps which may perforate the mucosa.)

- Extend the muscle split proximally onto the antrum and distally onto the proximal portion of the duodenum.

- The pyloric canal mucosa should 'bulge' into incision (Figure 47.16B).

- Caution must be exercised over the duodenal fornix where the muscle is at its thinnest.

- Confirm that all muscle fibres of the pyloric ring have been split.

- Confirm integrity of the pyloric mucosa by 'milking' air from the stomach into the duodenum and checking for air leaks.

- Any mucosal perforation should be repaired with 5/0 or 6/0 sutures and an omental patch.

- The wound is closed in layers with absorbable sutures.

- A subcuticular absorbable suture is used to close the skin.

Complications

- Incomplete division of the pyloric ring which may lead to persistent postoperative symptoms.

- Accidental perforation of the pyloric canal mucosa which, if overlooked, may lead to leakage of gastric fluid and peritonitis.

Postoperative management

- Continue with intravenous fluids, nasogastric drainage and nil by mouth for 24 hours.

- Commence oral feeding with dextrose solution followed by feeds of increasing strength.

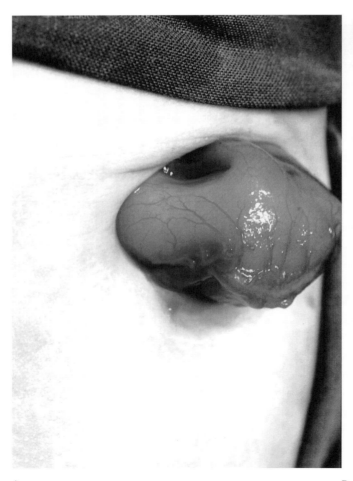 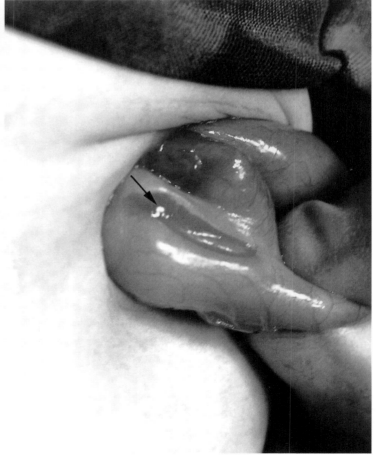

A   B

Figure 47.16 Operative appearances of hypertrophic pyloric stenosis before (**A**) and after (**B**) pyloromyotomy. The bulging mucosa is indicated with an arrow.

FURTHER READING

Al Salem AH, Qaisaruddin S, Al-Abkari H et al. Laparoscopic versus open chole-cystectomy in children. *Pediatr Surg Int* 1997; **12**:587–590

Crombleholme TM, DeLorimier AA, Way LW et al. The modified Puestow procedure for chronic relapsing pancreatitis in children. *J Pediatr Surg* 1990; **25**:749–754

Davenport M, Hansen L, Heaton ND et al. Haemangioendothelioma of the liver in infants. *J Pediatr Surg* 1995; **30**:44–48

Davenport M, Savage M, Mowat AP et al. The biliary atresia-splenic malformation syndrome: an aetiological and prognostic subgroup. *Surgery* 1993; **113**:662–668

Davenport M, Stringer MD, Howard ER. Biliary amylase and congenital chole-dochal dilatation. *J Pediatr Surg* 1995; **30**:474–477

Gilchrist BF, Valerie EP, Nguyen M et al. Pearls and perils in the management of prolonged, peculiar, penetrating esophageal foreign bodies in children. *J Pediatr Surg* 1997; **32**:1429–1431

Goss JA, Shackleton CR, Swenson K et al. Orthotopic liver transplantation for congenital biliary atresia: an 11 year single-center experience. *Ann Surg* 1996; **224**:276–284

Honna T, Kamii Y, Tsuchida Y. Idiopathic gastric volvulus in infancy and child-hood. *J Pediatr Surg* 1990; **25**:707–710

Howard ER. Biliary atresia. In: Stringer MD, Oldham KT, Moriquand PDE, Howard ER, eds. *Pediatric Surgery and Urology: Long Term Outcomes*. London: WB Saunders, 1998; 402–416

Howard ER, Stringer MD. Gastric volvulus in the neonate and infant. In: Puri P, ed. *Neonatal Surgery*. Oxford: Butterworth Heinemann, 1996; 272–276

Okada A, Oguchi Y, Kamata S et al. Common channel syndrome: diagnosis with ERCP and surgical management. *Surgery* 1983; **93**:634–642

Redkar R, Davenport M, Howard ER. Antenatal diagnosis of congenital anom-alies of the biliary tract. *J Pediatr Surg* 1998; **33**:700–704

Siddiqui AM, Shamberger RC, Filler RM et al. Enteric duplications of the pancreatic head: definitive management by local resection. *J Pediatr Surg* 1998; **33**:1117–1121

Spitz L, Kirtane J. Results and complications of surgery for gastro-oesophageal reflux. *Arch Dis Child* 1985; **60**:743–747

Stringer MD, Dhawan A, Davenport M et al. Choledochal cysts: lessons from a 20 year experience. *Arch Dis Child* 1995; **73**:528–531

Tam PKH, Saing H, Koo J et al. Pyloric function five to eleven years after Ramstedt's pyloromyotomy. *J Pediatr Surg* 1985; **20**:236–239

Valayer J. Conventional treatment of biliary atresia. *J Pediatr Surg* 1996; **31**:1546–1551

Warshaw AL, Simeone JF, Schapiro RH et al. Evaluation and treatment of the dominant dorsal duct syndrome (pancreas divisum redefined). *Am J Surg* 1990; **159**:59–64

Whitcomb DC, Gorry MC, Preston RA et al. Hereditary pancreatitis is caused by a mutation in the cationic trypsinogen gene. *Nat Genet* 1996; **14**:141–145

48

Paediatric surgery of the small and large bowel

Paul D. Losty, David A. Lloyd

INTRODUCTION

Paediatric surgeons encounter a complex range of gastro-intestinal pathology in the newborn, usually as a result of disturbances in embryological development, and in the older patient through acquired disease in childhood. This review focuses principally on conditions affecting the small and large bowel that are of interest to the general surgeon.

CONGENITAL SMALL BOWEL OBSTRUCTION

Congenital disorders involving the small bowel frequently present as intestinal obstruction. Clinical features indicating obstruction are bile-stained vomiting, abdominal distension of a varying degree depending on the anatomical level of obstruction (high or low small bowel) and pain. Constipation and failure to pass meconium stool in the newborn are recognised associations. Congenital causes of small bowel obstruction are listed in Box 48.1.

Box 48.1 Common causes of congenital small bowel obstruction

Duodenal atresia
Intestinal malrotation
Jejunoileal atresia
Meconium ileus
Incarcerated inguinal hernia

General principles of management

Clinical management of the newborn surgical patient should involve passage of a wide-bore nasogastric tube (10 F) to decompress the stomach, thereby preventing aspiration and respiratory embarrassment, together with resuscitation using intravenous crystalloid fluids. A suitable fluid regimen is 0.18% saline/10% dextrose with added potassium (2–4 mmol/kg/day). Fluid requirements are calculated individually on a body weight basis. Newborns are given maintenance volumes ranging from 60 ml/kg/day on day 1 of life progressing to 120–150 ml/kg/day by day 4. Factors such as prematurity, presence of obstructed gut, nasogastric fluid aspirate, serum biochemistry and urine output must also be taken into account to refine the ideal volume of fluid needed. Losses from nasogastric tubes are replaced on a volume-for-volume basis with 0.9% saline. Urine output should be ideally 2 ml/kg/h. A plain abdominal radiograph may help to establish the diagnosis in certain cases – the 'double bubble' sign in congenital duodenal obstruction – although it must be generally acknowledged that distinguishing small from large bowel obstruction can be difficult due to the poorly developed colonic haustra in the newborn.

CONGENITAL DUODENAL OBSTRUCTION

This condition is encountered in approximately 1:10 000 births. Diagnosis may have been suspected in the antenatal period from as early as 16–20 weeks because of the known associations with polyhydramnios and the findings of a dilated stomach on foetal ultrasound examination. A careful search for other anomalies (oesophageal atresia and congenital heart disease) should follow because of the recognisable associations with Down's syndrome (trisomy 21) seen in almost one-third of patients. This requires confirmation by karyotyping aided by amniocentesis and may have significant implications for the family in terms of continuation of pregnancy.

Within hours of birth, 90% of patients present with bile-stained vomiting. The abdomen is often flattened or scaphoid in appearance due to the level of obstruction being 'high' in the gastrointestinal tract. An abdominal radiograph may show the typical features of a 'double bubble' appearance formed by the gastric air bubble and an additional air–fluid level in the dilated proximal duodenum (Figure 48.1). The obstruction may be complete (atresia) or incomplete due to a stenosis or mucosal

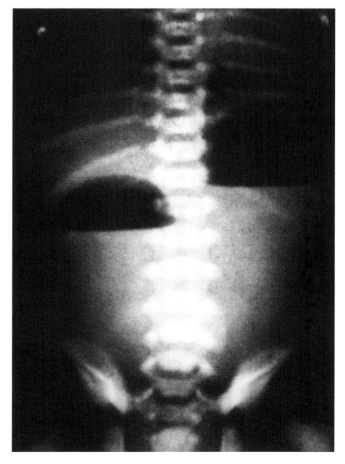

Figure 48.1 'Double bubble' plain radiograph appearance of congenital duodenal obstruction.

diaphragm or 'windsock' web encountered in the second part of the duodenum at the level of the ampulla of Vater. Air seen filling loops of bowel beyond the duodenum on plain radiograph suggests an incomplete or partial obstruction. In 10% of patients the ampulla opens directly into a distal segment of bowel beyond the atresia and bile-stained vomiting can be absent. The distal bowel is frequently normal, although annular pancreas and malrotation have been reported.

Following adequate resuscitation, surgical management entails restoration of gastrointestinal continuity by performing a duodenoduodenostomy between the dilated proximal obstructed segment and the narrowed distal duodenum, taking care to avoid injury to the ampulla. Intestinal abnormalities such as malrotation are dealt with (see below). Postoperatively oral feeding may be somewhat delayed for days or weeks because of associated bowel dysmotility. Intravenous nutrition is frequently required until adequate oral feeds can be established. Outcomes following surgery are generally good for the majority of infants.

INTESTINAL MALROTATION

Malrotation is a term used to define a condition in which the mid-gut loop lies suspended on a narrow-based vascular mesentery nourished by the superior mesenteric vessels. It is an important condition to recognise because of the inherent risks of mid-gut volvulus, a catastrophic event that can threaten major gut loss. The true incidence is difficult to estimate in the population although it is reported at 1 in 500 postmortem examinations.

Embryologically, malrotation is thought to arise as a result of failure of fixation and rotation of the primitive mid-gut loop on its return to the abdominal cavity from the physiological umbilical hernia at around 12 weeks of development. Normally, the mid-gut should undergo a 270° counterclockwise rotation resulting in the duodenojejunal flexure loop, assuming a position to the left of the superior mesenteric vessels on the posterior abdominal wall and the caecocolic loop residing in the right iliac fossa. Fixation in this manner thereby establishes a widened root to the mesentery.

Malrotation usually presents within the first month of life. Thereafter, sporadic cases may be detected throughout childhood and in adults. The most common presenting symptom is bile-stained vomiting, frequently after initiation of feeds. If volvulus co-exists, the infant may be in a state of shock with abdominal distension, accompanied by a profound metabolic acidosis and passing blood per rectum. Occasionally symptoms can be intermittent and milder, suggesting twisting and untwisting episodes.

Diagnosis is based on the clinical history aided by plain film radiology and upper gastrointestinal contrast studies. The plain abdominal film typically shows a gasless abdomen with air in the stomach and duodenum and little elsewhere in the gut. Upper GI contrast studies outline an abnormal configuration of the duodenum with the duodenojejunal flexure lying to the right of the mid-line and vertebral column (Figure 48.2). Ultrasound may

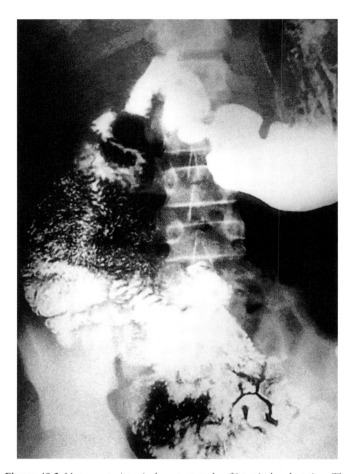

Figure 48.2 Upper gastrointestinal contrast study of intestinal malrotation. The duodenojejunal flexure is lying to the right of the vertebral column and the small bowel loops occupy the right side of the abdominal cavity. The mid-gut lies suspended on a narrrow-based vascular pedicle.

be helpful in showing an abnormal relationship of the superior mesenteric vessels.

Malrotation requires surgical correction. At operation any abnormal peritoneal folds (Ladd's bands) extending from the caecum and ascending colon across the second part of the duodenum are divided. This mobilises the right colon, permitting its displacement to the left side of the abdomen. Attention is then focused on straightening the duodenum and widening the root of the mesentery. The appendix is removed prior to replacing the viscera in the abdomen as the small bowel will now lie on the right side and the caecum in the left upper quadrant of the peritoneal cavity. Future dilemmas with appendicitis should therefore not arise. Patients undergoing surgery for uncomplicated malrotation have an excellent outcome.

Those presenting with mid-gut volvulus require vigorous resuscitation and derotation of the twisted gut without delay. Volvulus occurs around the base of the narrow mesentery. At operation, the bowel is inspected and untwisted by a number of counterclockwise rotations and areas of questionable viability covered with warm moist packs before determining the full extent of ischaemic damage. Gangrenous bowel should be resected. If extensive, limited resection of frankly necrotic bowel and exteriorisation with stomas may be warranted with the intention of performing a second-look procedure at 24–48 hours, providing ventilatory parameters and haemodynamic stability are maintained. Abnormal adhesive bands are divided and the mesentery widened as above. Patients who have undergone massive resection are at risk of short bowel syndrome. Parenteral nutrition may be required for a variable period of time although intestinal adaptation may allow recovery of full enteral intake.

Small bowel transplantation is a recent advance available for those who develop intestinal failure and complications related to long-term parenteral nutrition. This is restricted to highly specialised units.

JEJUNOILEAL ATRESIA

Jejunal and ileal atresias are thought to represent the end result of an intrauterine vascular accident. The classic work of Louw and Barnard in the 1950s established the pathogenic basis of these lesions. Experimentally it was shown that interruption of the vascular supply to the intestine of puppies *in utero* created similar abnormalities to the atresias encountered in humans. Single or multiple, atresias may occur anywhere from the duodenojejunal flexure to the terminal ileum. A classification has been described:

- a simple stenosis to a membrane or web obstruction (type I)

- blind-ending bowel joined by a fibrous cord (type II)

- bowel disconnected and separated by a wide mesenteric defect (type IIIa)

- an 'apple peel' deformity of bowel (type IIIb) and

- multiple atresia (type IV) which can have familial associations (Figure 48.3).

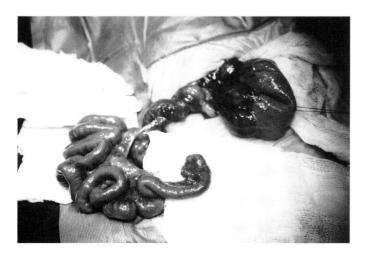

Figure 48.3 Operative findings in a case of jejunoileal atresia (type IIIb). Note the dilated blind-ending proximal small intestine, the wide mesenteric defect and the 'apple peel' appearance of the distal intestinal segment.

Cystic fibrosis is an important co-morbid state that should be excluded promptly in all patients by genotyping.

The diagnosis may be suspected in the antenatal period because of foetal bowel dilatation. Newborns present with bile-stained vomiting and a variable degree of abdominal distension depending on the level of the atresia. Failure or delay in passing meconium is frequently noted. Abdominal X-ray reveals widespread bowel dilatation with air–fluid levels. Contrast enema studies are helpful in demonstrating a 'disused' or small colon as a result of failure of meconium to reach the distal bowel. Operative management involves generous resection of the proximal dilated atretic segment and primary anastomosis. Additional atresias should be excluded by the installation of saline into the segment of bowel beyond the anastomosis to confirm distal patency. Parenteral nutrition may be required in the postoperative period as gut dysmotility is not uncommon. Resumption of normal bowel function allows graded enteral intake. Outcomes for the majority of patients in the absence of multiple atresias or short gut syndrome are usually excellent.

MECONIUM ILEUS

Meconium ileus is a common form of intestinal obstruction in newborns and is invariably associated with cystic fibrosis. Cystic fibrosis (mucoviscidosis) is inherited as an autosomal recessive condition and affects 1:2000 Caucasians with a carrier status of 1:20. Diagnosis in the newborn period is now frequently confirmed by genotyping; ΔF508 is the most common genetic mutation. The sweat test can provide further confirmation but is not usually performed until after six weeks of age. Affected newborns characteristically produce an abnormally viscid meconium deficient of pancreatic exocrine secretions that results in intraluminal obstruction of the terminal ileum. The large bowel distal to the obstructed small intestine is small, narrow and disused, giving rise to a 'microcolon' appearance. The terminal ileum is laden with pellets of meconium and proximally there is widespread dilatation of the small bowel that is prone to volvulus and perforation.

Diagnosis may be suspected in the antenatal period because of foetal bowel dilatation. Following delivery some 50% of newborns are noted to have intestinal obstruction with bile-stained vomiting, abdominal distension and failure to pass meconium stool. Other cases are complicated by volvulus, perforation or harbour intestinal atresias consequent on an *in utero* ischaemic event.

Abdominal radiography reveals a granular 'soap bubble ' appearance of dilated small bowel loops. Those complicated by intrauterine perforation may show intraabdominal calcification.

Management strategies in uncomplicated cases of meconium ileus now frequently employ the use of dilute Gastrograffin as a radiographic therapeutic enema to decompress the obstructed intestine. Gastrograffin is a hyperosmolar wetting agent that disimpacts inspissated meconium. Careful attention to fluid balance before, during and following the procedure is essential in the newborn as the osmolarity of Gastrograffin (1800 mOsm/l) can provoke hypovolaemic crisis. Intravenous fluids are administered judiciously in all patients to ensure an adequate urinary output. The Gastrograffin enema procedure is successful in some 50% of cases.

Patients that fail to respond to a therapeutic enema or those for whom an enema would be contraindicated (volvulus, perforation) undergo operation.

A number of operative procedures have been described, ranging from enterotomy with irrigation of the bowel using saline for simple cases followed by primary closure to intestinal resection with temporary stomas in those with necrotic bowel. Formation of temporising stomas permits postoperative irrigation to disimpact residual meconium. Pancreatic enzyme supplementation is essential to establish adequate feeding schedules, growth and stool patterns in patients. Stoma closure is performed at a later date when these are optimised. The development of specialist cystic fibrosis teams is dedicated to ensuring that families receive state-of-the-art care for affected individuals.

INTUSSUSCEPTION

Intussusception describes an invagination of one portion of the intestine (intussusceptum) into the distal aspect of the other (intussuscipiens). It remains an important cause of intestinal obstruction in the infant and younger child. The typical age for presentation is around 4–8 months and the majority of cases are encountered in the under-2s. Although mostly idiopathic in nature in the younger child, a peak incidence is recorded in spring and autumn months. This suggests a viral aetiology and an association with adenovirus and rotavirus is postulated. A weaning diet and reaction to food allergens are also implicated. The typical site for involvement is the terminal ileum rich in lymphoid tissue (Peyer's patches) which acts as a lead point for an ileocaecal intussusception (Figure 48.4). Ileoileal, jejunoileal and colocolic intussusceptions are encountered less often. As the intussusception evolves, strangulating intestinal obstruction develops, leading to gangrene and perforation. Delay in presentation, diagnosis and treatment can account for appreciable morbidity and mortality. Beyond the typical idiopathic age groups (>2 years) a pathologic lead point should always be suspected. This may be a Meckel's diverticulum, a polyp, duplication cyst of the bowel, neoplasms such as lymphoma or a mucosal haematoma as seen in Henoch–Schönlein purpura. Rarely, intussusception is encountered post-operatively in patients who have undergone abdominal surgery, such as resection of Wilms' tumour or Nissen fundoplication.

Clinical presentation is typically seen in an otherwise healthy infant who presents with colicky abdominal pain, associated with episodic vomiting and rectal bleeding. During attacks of abdominal pain the child goes pale, screams and draws its legs up.

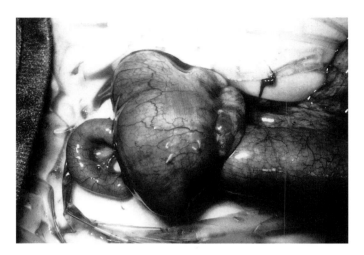

Figure 48.4 Ileocolic intussusception seen at operation.

At other times the child will appear well. As the condition evolves the infant becomes progressively ill, hypovolaemic and shocked. Passage of blood and mucus in the form of a 'redcurrant' jelly stool is often a late and ominous sign. Abdominal examination at a time when the child is free from colic may reveal a sausage-shaped mass palpable in the right upper quadrant. Failure to palpate a mass in the usual location in an infant with a typical history suggests that the intussusception may be hidden under the confines of the liver or it may have progressed along the left side of the colon. In extreme cases an intussusception may protrude from the anus. Peritonitis indicates intestinal perforation or necrotic bowel. Occasionally an infant may present atypically with lethargy and few other symptoms. Abdominal tenderness may provide a clue to the diagnosis which is easily overlooked. A plain abdominal radiograph may reveal the impression of a soft tissue mass in the right iliac fossa. Ultrasound is the investigation of choice. In typical cases the intussusception is seen as a 'pseudo-kidney' shaped mass. A contrast enema is useful when ultrasonography is not diagnostic (Figure 48.5).

Immediate clinical management includes vigorous resuscitation with crystalloid and colloid to correct hypovolaemia. Antibiotics and nasogastric drainage are required in advanced cases with signs of intestinal obstruction and peritonism.

In patients who are otherwise well, reduction of the intussusception may be attempted non-operatively by an experienced paediatric radiologist. Preparation of the patient involves the same attention to detail as for those cases who will require immediate operation (see later). This ensures that the patient experiences no delay in transfer to the operating theatre should radiological reduction fail or the bowel perforate from the enema procedure. The surgeon should accompany the patient to the radiology department. Reduction of the intussusception may be carried out by a paediatric radiologist using air or contrast enema. Most modern units now employ air reduction as the method of choice. The infant is sedated using carefully titrated doses of morphine as the procedure is painful and unpleasant. A catheter is passed per

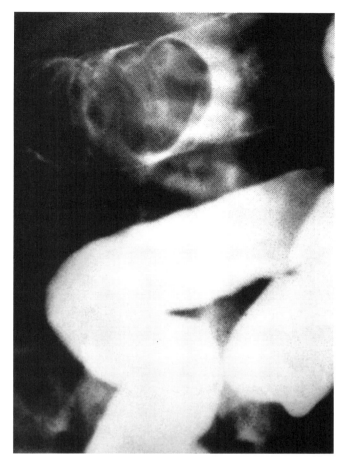

Figure 48.5 Contrast enema diagnostic of ileocolic intussusception.

rectum, gas insufflated into the bowel and the reduction monitored using fluoroscopy. Air or oxygen pressures, controlled manometrically, should not exceed 80–150 mmHg. Initial reduction of the intussusception can be rapid, success being defined when air is seen to enter loops of ileum. Recovery is usually uneventful in these circumstances, feeds are introduced and most patients discharged home in 24–48 hours.

Occasionally a filling defect is seen in the caecum; this may simply represent an oedematous ileocaecal valve. In this situation the patient is returned to the ward and clinical progress monitored.

Recurrence of symptoms whilst in hospital requires reappraisal to consider the need to attempt a second enema or to progress to operation.

Perforation occurring during air reduction warrants decompression of the abdomen by needle paracentesis and immediate laparotomy. A failed reduction and peritonitis are indications for surgery. Intussusception in the older child (>3 years) is likely to be due to a pathological lead point (e.g. Meckel's diverticulum) and a lower threshold for operation should be considered in these cases. Operative management of intussusception is discussed at the end of this chapter.

Mortality for intussusception should be <1%. A recurrence of intussusception days, weeks or months later can occur in some 5–10% of cases after radiological reduction and in <5% of patients following operation. Fortunately for infants who have had an idiopathic intussusception, the risk of recurrence becomes less after two years. Management should be individualised in these circumstances. It is reasonable to consider radiological reduction for first-time recurrences. Second recurrences in the older child suggest the possibility of a pathological lead point and dictate that operation would be the preferred option.

MECONIUM PLUG SYNDROME

Newborns with meconium plug syndrome typically present with abdominal distension, bile-stained vomiting and failure to pass meconium stool. The condition was first described in 1956.

Abdominal radiography reveals widespread bowel dilatation. Contrast enema studies frequently reveal a colon heavily laden with viscid meconium. It is not uncommon for the meconium plug to be expelled by the patient prior to the enema procedure. The enema study nonetheless hastens patient recovery and permits establishment of feeds (Figure 48.6). Cystic fibrosis and Hirschsprung's disease are recognised associations that should be excluded in all patients by genotyping and suction rectal biopsy respectively.

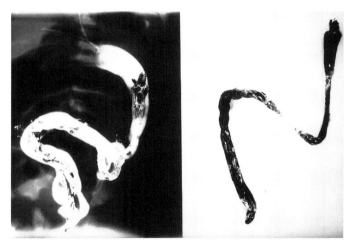

Figure 48.6 Contrast enema typical of meconium plug syndrome. Expelled meconium cast is shown.

HIRSCHSPRUNG'S DISEASE

Hirschsprung's disease is the most common cause of intestinal obstruction in newborns, occurring in 1:5000 live births. The condition is characterised by the absence of ganglion cells in the distal large bowel commencing at the level of the internal sphincter and extending proximally to involve variable lengths of colon. In the majority of patients the aganglionosis is confined to the rectosigmoid region (75%), so-called short segment disease. In others (15–20%) extensive areas of colon (long segment disease) can be affected. Total colonic aganglionosis is a rare condition seen in fewer than 10% of patients. In pathological terms, a functional form of intestinal obstruction develops. The distal bowel fails to relax and propagate normal intestinal peristalsis. Proximal normally innervated bowel becomes grossly distended and hypertrophied in response to the functional obstruction, hence the term congenital megacolon (Figure 48.7).

Embryologically, during development neural crest cells migrate in a craniocaudal direction via the vagal nerves into the alimentary tract. Defects in migration, proliferation, differentiation and survival of the primitive enteric neuroblast may underlie the pathogenesis of Hirschsprung's disease. Genetic and molecular events governing this process are being rapidly elucidated. Abnormalities in the Ret proto-oncogene and the endothelin B receptor genes have been described. Although Hirschsprung's disease is largely a sporadic condition, familial associations are seen in 5–10% of cases. Chromosome anomalies such as trisomy 21 (Down's) and malformation syndromes such as Waardenberg, Ondine's curse (central hypoventilation disorder), von Recklinghausen's disease and Smith–Lemli–Opitz syndrome are recognised associations.

Clinical presentation is frequently seen in the newborn period (80–90%). It is now uncommon to encounter an older child with chronic constipation and megacolon. Infants have delayed passage of meconium stool, gross abdominal distension and bile-stained vomiting. In the healthy full-term newborn, meconium should normally be passed within 24–36 hours of delivery. Diarrhoea may be a feature in one-third of babies due to enterocolitis. This is a life-threatening condition leading to toxic megacolon and bowel perforation. Rectal examination may classically provoke the expulsion of copious amounts of flatus and foul-smelling stool with relief of abdominal distension. In the older child presenting with failure to thrive, recurrent bouts of abdominal distension and irregular stooling, a thorough clinical history will often trace a disturbance in bowel symptoms to the early neonatal period.

Diagnosis is firmly established following the histologic confirmation of an absence of ganglion cells in a rectal biopsy specimen. This can be obtained using a suction biopsy instrument at the bedside in the neonate or by a formal open rectal biopsy in the older child. An experienced pathologist is essential to adequately interpret the biopsy specimen. Histochemistry can aid diagnosis by demonstrating elevated acetylcholinesterase activity in the aganglionic bowel specimens. Contrast enema studies reveal a typical transitional zone (ganglion cells are few in number at this location), a contracted rectoanal canal and dilated proximal ganglionic bowel. Anorectal manometry classically demonstrates failure of relaxation of the internal anal sphincter in response to rectal balloon distension; the 'anorectal inhibitory reflex' is thus absent in Hirschsprung's disease.

Newborns presenting with a diagnosis of Hirschsprung's disease were frequently managed in the past with a temporary 'levelling' colostomy performed in an area of ganglionic bowel confirmed at open operation by frozen section pathologic analysis. This permitted establishment of feeding, reduced the risks of enterocolitis and allowed the infant to go home. At around 3–6 months, infants were readmitted to hospital for a reconstructive pull-through procedure in which the aganglionic bowel was resected, frequently with closure of the stoma at a later date. There are a number of operations described for the definitive treatment of Hirschsprung's disease; the most commonly performed are the Duhamel, Soave and Swenson procedures. Paediatric surgeons are now moving towards performing the pull-through procedure (Soave or Swenson) as a 'one-stage' operation in the neonatal period without the need for a covering colostomy. This has the advantage of a single operation and may further enhance development of rectoanal function.

Patients presenting with total colonic Hirschsprung's disease are a challenging group. An ileostomy is required in the newborn period followed by an ileoanal pull-through (straight or J pouch) at a later date. Laparoscopy has permitted further advances and a number of centres have perfected a minimally invasive pull-through operation.

Long-term outcome and stooling patterns in children with Hirschsprung's disease are generally good. Some patients continue to experience troublesome constipation and soiling. These children are usually managed with the use of laxatives or enemas. The antegrade continence enema (ACE) procedure, in which the appendix is used as a catheterisable stoma for administration of a cleansing enema, is reserved for those cases resistant to conventional laxative therapy.

ANORECTAL MALFORMATIONS

Anorectal malformations occur in 1:4000 live births. The absence of an anal orifice is readily apparent during the routine exami-

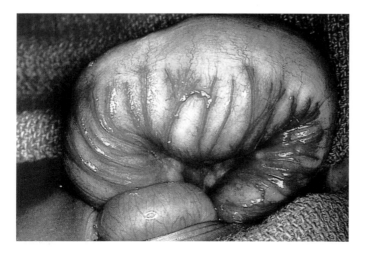

Figure 48.7 Hirschsprung's disease seen at operation. Note the dilated bowel proximal to the zone of transition and the narrowed aganglionic distal bowel.

nation of the newborn. These malformations are generally more common in boys.

A wide spectrum exists and a number of anatomical and morphological classifications (e.g. Wingspread) have been proposed in the past. The system recently described by Peña has proved more practical, is therapeutically orientated and favoured by most paediatric surgeons (Table 48.1). Anatomically, anomalies can be broadly grouped into low, intermediate or high depending on the level at which the bowel terminates above or below the puborectalis complex. Most low anomalies in the male and female, with a visible cutaneous fistula discharging meconium in the perineum, are suitable for an anoplasty procedure and do not require colostomy (Figure 48.8). Intermediate and high lesions require colostomy as the intial operation followed by definitive anorectal reconstruction in the first year of life. A fistulous communication with the genitourinary tract is invariably present with these malformations and requires careful preoperative imaging with the use of contrast studies via the defunctioning colostomy combined with micturating cystourethrography. Posterior sagittal anorectoplasty (PSARP) is the preferred operation to correct the intermediate and high malformations. Using this approach, the aim of surgery is to isolate and divide the genitourinary fistula, mobilise the rectum to the perineum, reconstruct the sphincter complex and fashion a neo-anus.

Outcomes in terms of continence are significantly different for low, intermediate and high lesions. Patients with low anomalies should have continence rates approaching 100%. Those with higher and intermediate lesions have a less favourable outcome – some 50% of children will continue to have troublesome soiling.

It is important to recognise that associated abnormalities are common in patients with anorectal malformations, especially those with intermediate/high lesions. The VACTERL sequence

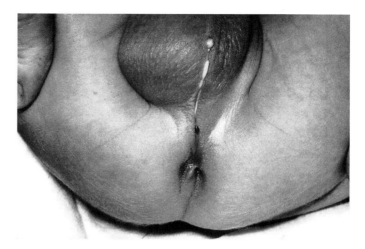

Figure 48.8 Imperforate anus in a newborn male. The meconium-stained perineal cutaneous fistula is clearly seen.

(vertebral, anorectal, cardiac tracheo-oesophageal, renal, radial and limb defects) summarises anomalies that should be screened for in these patients. These may also directly influence functional outcome. Skeletal abnormalities such as sacral agenesis (>2 vertebral segments missing) generally equate with poor bladder and bowel control.

INGUINAL HERNIA

Inguinal hernias are a common condition in infancy and childhood with a peak incidence seen during the first three months of life (Figure 48.9). The premature infant is at increased risk (10%) compared to the term baby (1–5%) of developing an inguinal hernia. Males are affected more often than females (5:1). In 60% of cases the hernia is located on the right side and bilaterality is seen in some 10% of cases. Invariably the hernia is indirect,

Table 48.1 Classification of anorectal anomalies (modified after Peña)	
	Treatment
Males	
Perineal (cutaneous) fistula	No colostomy required Anoplasty or mini-PSARP
Rectourethral fistula Bulbar	
Prostatic	Colostomy required in all cases followed by PSARP
Rectovesical fistula Imperforate anus without fistula Rectal atresia	
Females	
Perineal (cutaneous) fistula	No colostomy required Anoplasty or mini-PSARP
Vestibular fistula	
Persistent cloaca	Colostomy required in all cases followed by PSARP or PSARVUP
Imperforate anus without fistula Rectal atresia	

PSARP = posterior sagittal anorectoplasty, PSARVUP = posterior sagittal anorecto-vagino-urethroplasty (surgical correction for cloaca anomaly in female only)

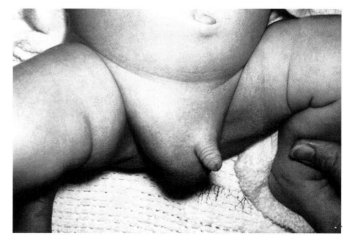

Figure 48.9 Indirect inguinal hernia in a male infant.

transcending the inguinal canal and presenting as an inguinoscrotal or labial swelling. A direct inguinal hernia is rare in childhood. Indirect inguinal hernias invariably arise due to persistence of a widely patent processus vaginalis that permits bowel or other abdominal organs to enter a congenital hernial sac. In the male child undescended testes can co-exist. Parents often notice a bulge in the groin when the infant or child strains, cries or coughs. Reducibility may be reported when the infant is quiet. Examination usually reveals a swelling that gives a characteristic gurgle on reduction indicative of bowel content. In the absence of a demonstrable swelling the cord structures may feel thickened – the 'silk glove sign'. The highest rate of complications is encountered in the first six months of life. These include incarceration of the bowel and gonadal ischaemia with loss of a testis or ovary. In the male entrapment of prolapsed intestine in the inguinal canal results in compression of the delicate testicular vessels with infarction. In the female the ovary and fallopian tube can twist and infarct in a hernial sac.

Early elective surgery is always scheduled following the diagnosis of inguinal hernia to avert such complications. In paediatric practice ligation and division of the hernial sac (herniotomy) is all that is required. A groin crease incision is performed in a natural skinfold and the spermatic cord identified in the male. The inguinal canal in infants is short and need not be opened except in the older child (> 2 years). The cord structures are skeletonised by careful blunt dissection using a pair of fine forceps to identify the hernia sac and the vas and testicular vessels separated using a moistened swab. No attempt should be made to grasp these structures. After identification and isolation of the sac it is opened to check its contents and transfixed at the level of the internal ring with an absorbable suture. In the female, care should be taken when opening the hernial sac to inspect the ovary and ensure that the fallopian tube is adequately free proximal to the transfixing suture. In the male efforts should be made to see that the testis resides in the scrotum at the end of the procedure, to avoid iatrogenic ' high testis'.

Patients presenting with incarceration require prompt reduction. Frequently these are young infants (<6 months). Paediatric practice involves an initial attempt at reduction following administration of sedation. Using gentle taxis efforts are made to manually reduce the contents of the hernia back into the abdomen. If successful, semielective repair is delayed for 24–48 hours later to permit oedema of the cord structures to settle. A hernia that is irreducible requires urgent exploration after adequate resuscitation of the patient with intravenous fluids, nasogastric drainage and antibiotics. No attempt should be made to reduce the hernia under general anaesthesia. An emergency herniotomy procedure, particularly in the preterm or young infant, can be technically challenging. The principles are essentially the same but in these circumstances it is often necessary to formally open the inguinal canal as the external ring may be hindering reduction and then deal with the hernia as previously described. If bowel or ovary is non-viable it may require resection. Bowel resection is most safely accomplished through a

separate higher abdominal incision. Alternatively a preperitoneal approach may be employed from the outset to deal with an incarcerated inguinal hernia. Unless frankly necrotic, the testis is replaced in the scrotum.

Controversy exists as to whether a policy of routine bilateral groin exploration should be adopted in children presenting with an unilateral inguinal hernia given the attendant risks of hernia complications as well as the potential for operative injury to the vas and vessels. It would appear from the literature that fewer than 10% of children go on to develop a contralateral clinical hernia. It is therefore not our current practice to pursue a policy of routine bilateral groin exploration.

OPERATIVE SURGERY

Operative management of intussusception

Preoperative preparation

Patients with acute intussusception frequently are hypovolaemic as a result of fluid lost into the obstructed bowel and preoperative fluid replacement is essential. In most cases isotonic crystalloids are adequate but for severe hypovolaemia a colloid infusion may be required. A nasogastric tube is inserted and allowed to drain freely with regular aspirations.

Broad-spectrum antibiotics are given. Cefotaxime and metronidazole are suitable and provide adequate cover against bowel pathogens. Blood should be crossmatched.

Anaesthesia and assessment

Under general anaesthesia the surgeon palpates the abdomen of the infant. A sausage-shaped mass may be felt in the right or left side of the abdomen. Even if the intussusception is palpated on the left side the surgeon always sites the incision on the right. The abdomen is cleaned with an aqueous solution of chlorhexidine and towelled to expose the abdomen. A large sterile adhesive dressing (Op-site) is applied. This prevents the operating drapes from becoming wet which could lead to the infant becoming hypothermic.

Incision and procedure

A transverse incision is made on the right side of the abdomen, 7–10 cm in length (Figure 48.10). The incision is sited slightly above the level of the umbilicus so that it can be easily extended towards the left should the need arise. Having incised the skin, the lateral abdominal muscles are divided using diathermy to minimise blood loss. The peritoneum is lifted between two pairs of artery forceps and opened carefully with scissors.

On opening the abdomen, yellowish plasma-rich peritoneal fluid is often encountered. The fingers of the right hand are inserted

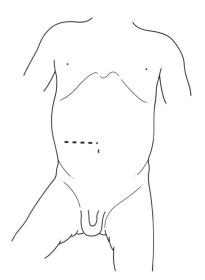

Figure 48.10 Operative incision for intussusception.

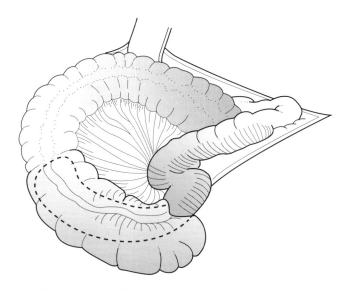

Figure 48.12 Reduction of intussusception.

into the abdominal cavity and the colon palpated to locate the intussusception. If it is lying in the transverse or descending colon, it is gently squeezed back towards the ascending colon by compressing the colon immediately distal to the intussusception (Figure 48.11). Under no circumstances should any attempt be made to reduce the intussuception by pulling from the proximal end.

When the intussusception has been manipulated back to the caecum, it is usually possible to lift the mass out of the abdominal cavity (Figure 48.12). The bowel is carefully inspected for evidence of ischaemia. Further manual reduction is contra-indicated if there is evidence of advanced ischaemia with possible bowel wall necrosis. Provided the bowel appears to be viable, further reduction is attempted under direct vision. If resistance is met, usually at the ileocaecal region, gentle pressure is applied distal to the intussusception, taking care not to allow the wall of the caecum to split. If full reduction is achieved, the bowel is palpated for pathology which may predispose to intussusception,

such as a polyp. This is rare in infants but in children over the age of two years it is important to search for pathology. It is not unusual to find large reactive mesenteric lymph nodes in the ileo-caecal region. In the older child these should be biopsied to exclude a lymphoma which may present in this way. A Meckel's diverticulum may also be encountered as a pathological lead point and, if present, should be removed, preferably by resecting an adjacent short segment of ileum followed by bowel anastomosis using absorbable sutures. An oedematous ileocaecal valve is frequently palpable and may be confused with a polyp; it is not necessary to open the bowel to confirm this. Appendectomy can be performed if the caecum is healthy.

If manual reduction is unsuccessful the involved segment of non-viable intestine should be resected. This usually entails a distal ileal resection or occasionally a limited right hemicolectomy (Figure 48.13). In all cases the resection should be kept to a minimum. Following resection, bowel continuity is restored by end-to-end anastomosis using a single layer of interrupted seromuscular sutures. Any mesenteric defect must be closed.

The abdomen is closed in layers with 3/0 or 2/0 absorbable sutures, The skin is approximated with a 5/0 running subcuticular suture or Steristrips.

Postoperative management

Postoperatively attention to fluid balance is essential, monitoring fluid intake, urine output and nasogastric losses. Nasogastric drainage is maintained until aspirates become minimal. A high temperature and endotoxaemia are not uncommon following surgery. Antibiotics are given for periods up to 48 hours after operation.

Following right hemicolectomy or extensive ileal resection for intussusception, loose stools may be a troublesome feature for

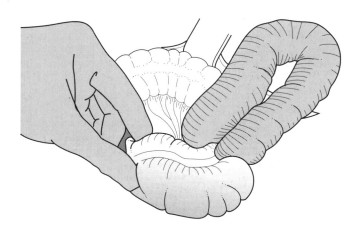

Figure 48.11 Reduction of intussusception.

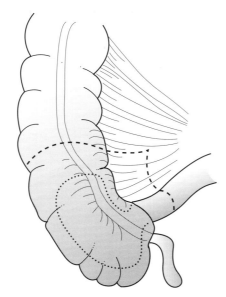

Figure 48.13 Resection of intussusception.

several months. Growth and nutritional parameters should be carefully monitored in these patients.

FURTHER READING

Akhtar J, Guiney EJ. Congenital duodenal obstruction. *Br J Surg* 1992; **79**:133–139

Beasley SW, Myers NA. Intussusception: current views. *Pediatr Surg Int* 1998; **14**:157

Clatworthy HW, Howard WHR, Lloyd J. The meconium plug syndrome. *Surgery* 1956; **39**:131–142

Dalla-Vecchia LK, Grosfeld JL, West KW, Rescorla FJ, Scherer LR, Engum SA. Intestinal atresia and stenosis; a 25 year experience with 277 cases. *Arch Surg* 1998; **133**:490–496

Georgeson KE. Minimally invasive pediatric surgery: current status. *Semin Pediatr Surg* 1998; **7**:193–239

Huddart SN. Hirschsprung's disease: present UK practice. *Ann Roy Coll Surg Engl* 1998; **80**:46–48

Kealey WD, McCallion WA, Brown S, Potts SR, Boston VE. Midgut volvulus in children. *Br J Surg* 1996; **83**:105–106

Louw JH, Barnard CN. Congenital intestinal atresia: observations on its origin. *Lancet* 1955; **2**:1065–1067

Peña A. Advances in anorectal malformations. *Semin Pediatr Surg* 1997; **6**:165–169

Peña A. Posterior sagittal anorectoplasty: results in the management of 332 cases of anorectal malformations. *Pediatr Surg Int* 1988; **3**:94–104

Puri P. Hirschsprung's disease: clinical and experimental observations. *World J Surg* 1993; **17**:374–384

Rao KM, Kiran PR. Midgut malrotation presenting in adult life. 1994; *Br J Surg* **81**:1173–1174

Rescorla FJ, Grosfeld JL. Contemporary management of meconium ileus. *World J Surg* 1993; **17**:318–325

Shankar KR, Losty PD, Kenny SE et al Functional results following the antegrade continence enema procedure. *Br J Surg* 1998; **85**:980–982

Teitlebaum DH, Coran AG. Primary pull through in the newborn. *Semin Pediatr Surg* 1998; **7**:103–107

Torres AM, Ziegler MM. Malrotation of the intestine. *World J Surg* 1993; **17**:326–331

Turnock RR, Jones MO, Lloyd DA. Preperitoneal approach to irreducible inguinal hernia in infants. *Br J Surg* 1994; **81**:251

49

General paediatric urology

John Orr

INTRODUCTION

Patients with paediatric urological problems provide a significant case load which contributes to the subspecialty of general paediatric surgery as encountered by general surgeons. This chapter deals with a number of common conditions of which trainees taking this option will require knowledge in their examination.

The surgically correctable conditions of the male genitalia and inguinal region form the core workload of the general surgeon with an interest in paediatric urology. It is thus important that any surgeon operating in this area has a fundamental knowledge of the common conditions, their natural history, alternative methods of treatment and surgery. The most common abnormalities include those of the foreskin, with circumcision being one of the commonest operations performed worldwide. Hypospadias is becoming an increasingly common condition and undescended testis, inguinal hernias, hydrocoeles and varicocoeles fall within the surgery of this area. The general surgeon has to be prepared to deal with both elective and emergency surgery of the external genitalia and the inguinal canal.

CIRCUMCISION AND PENILE SURGERY

Circumcision

While circumcision is a commonly performed procedure, the medical indications remain controversial. It is gradually being recognised that phimosis, prepucial adhesions, ballooning of the foreskin and balanitis are no longer absolute indications for circumcision. One indication is clear, that of true phimosis with scarring which is typically found in the patient with balanitis xerotica obliterans (BXO). In most newborns the prepuce is adherent to the glans. However, separation takes place and by one year almost half of the male population will have separation of the prepuce from the glans. This process continues and at the age of seven, 90% of boys will have retractable prepuces and at 17 years of age only 1% of foreskins will remain non-retractable. Therefore the question should be asked why, if only 1% of adolescent boys have a non-retractable foreskin, in some regions 7% or more have undergone circumcision by that age. The commonest reason for referral is balanitis where infection occurs beneath the foreskin. It must be recognised that in many of these boys the foreskin is in fact retractable. While the foreskin may be described as phimotic in the absence of symptoms, this is most likely to resolve spontaneously with growth.

Ballooning of the foreskin is another common reason for referral but usually disappears as the foreskin becomes more easily retractable. Prepucial adhesions also give rise to concern. These also will resolve spontaneously in the majority of boys. If they are causing discomfort they may benefit from division. A better understanding of the normal development of the prepuce could result in a significant reduction in the increasing number of circumcisions being carried out worldwide.

Circumcision is performed in a number of different ways, in young infants with either a clamp or plastibel, with excision of the prepuce. In the older child circumcision can be carried out utilising a number of different techniques including excision of the prepuce distal to a pair of forceps based beyond the glans with trimming of the inner part of the prepucial tube or a resection of a sleeve of prepucial tissue. The technique of circumcision is described in detail in a number of major texts. While circumcision is considered a minor surgical procedure, it is not without its complications which include haemorrhage, infection, meatal stenosis and, rarely, urethral fistula. The excision of too much or too little skin will require further surgery. Postoperatively adequate analgesia should be provided by the use of nerve blocks.

Alternatives to circumcision include division of the prepucial adhesions under local anaesthetic, prepucioplasty or conservative management of the phimosis with a steroid cream (triamcinolone acetonide 0.1%) applied topically for six weeks with regular retraction. This conservative approach results in retraction of the foreskin in a significant number of boys with symptoms and thus avoids circumcision. Despite the vogue for conservatism, however, circumcision still has an important part to play in the management of boys with troublesome problems with their foreskin.

Paraphimosis

Paraphimosis occurs when the phimotic foreskin is trapped proximal to the corona and can be seen at all ages in childhood.

It should be reduced by manual pressure carried out under sedation or general anaesthetic. If it proves difficult, a dorsal slit can be utilised to divide the fibrous ring of the prepuce. If reduction is successful, at follow-up it is often noted that the foreskin can be easily retracted and circumcision is thus not always required.

Hypospadias

Hypospadias is a congenital abnormality of the penis which results from the incomplete fusion of the urethra between the 10th and 14th weeks of gestational life. The abnormality is characterised by a urethral meatus which opens in an abnormal position on the ventral aspect of the shaft of the penis or, in the more major forms, proximally on the scrotum or perineum. It is usually associated with a ventral deficiency of the foreskin (hooded foreskin) and in up to 35% of cases chordee – the abnormal ventriflexion of the penis. A number of different classifications for hypospadias have been described but the most useful relates to the anatomical position of the urethral meatus (Box 49.1).

Box 49.1 Anatomical classification of hypospadias

1 Anterior – glanular, coronal or anterior penile
2 Mid shaft
3 Posterior penile, penoscrotal, scrotal and perineal

The more proximal the meatus, the more complex the surgical repair which has to be undertaken. The concept of the urethral plate, which is the strip of urethral mucosa extending from the ectopic meatus towards the glans, has in recent years been recognised as simplifying the surgical approach to hypospadias repair.

Hypospadias is associated with a high incidence of other urogenital abnormalities including testicular maldescent, inguinal hernia and a variety of disorders of the upper urinary tract. Investigation to identify these abnormalities, however, is probably not justified except in those patients with major posterior hypospadias and any patient who has proven urinary tract infections. The surgical treatment of hypospadias has fascinated surgeons for over 150 years with currently in excess of 300 different types of repair recorded.

The ideals of surgical treatment are the formation of a straight penis with a normal-looking ventral meatus at the tip of the glans which allows for a normal, straight urinary stream and normal sexual function. During the last quarter of the 20th century the trend was established towards earlier surgery (between the ages of six and 18 months), single-stage procedures, short stay or day case surgery.

The key principles of hypospadias surgery are:

● the correction of chordee

● the reconstruction of the urethra (urethroplasty)

● re-covering of the denuded penis with suitable skin and the fashioning of a satisfactory urethral meatus.

The modern well-established techniques of hyposapadias surgery include the MAGPI procedure where the meatus is advanced and the glans refashioned with a resultant terminal meatus. When used in carefully selected patients, those with a broad flat glans being ideal, the technique gives excellent cosmetic and functional results.

With anterior hypospadias but no chordee the Mathieu procedure has proved effective, in which parallel incisions are made on either side of the urethral plate through the glans tissue and joined proximally above the meatus. This allows a tubularisation of the urethral plate which is subsequently covered with glans wings.

More proximally the use of adjacent skin flaps or vascularised flaps of prepuce has proved advantageous. The use of the transverse prepucial island flap either as a tube or onlay is well established. More recent developments include the use of the tubularised incised plate (TIP) urethroplasty for distal and mid-shaft hypospadias.

Some authors have challenged the current fashion for single-stage repairs and demonstrate that the two-stage technique can be used for almost any hypospadias deformity whether it be the primary repair in a child or salvage surgery in an adolescent, demonstrating excellent results. Other techniques include the use of free skin grafts and bladder and mucosal grafts. It is outwith the scope of this chapter to describe the many repairs currently in use for hypospadias but the reader is referred to both the major texts and original articles quoted in the Further Reading section.

Modern techniques include the use of optical magnification and fine suture materials, with catgut and polyglactin (Vicryl) in 5/0–7/0 being preferred by many. There is also extensive use of delicate instrumentation, particularly microsurgical instruments. In order to obtain a bloodless or relatively blood-free operating field, a tourniquet at the base of the penis can be used or the soft tissues infiltrated with a solution of adrenaline 1:200 000 in marcaine. Bipolar diathermy can be used safely during hypospadias surgery but usually any bleeding will cease at the end of the operation when the dressings are in place.

The differing methods of urinary diversion remain contentious with individual surgical preference once again being paramount. Techniques include suprapubic penile diversion, urethral Foley catheters or per urethral drip stents which allow urine to drain into the nappy and facilitate early discharge from hospital. It must be recognised, however, that the type and period of urinary diversion, the type of dressing used and the different catheters available do not significantly affect outcome which appears to relate more to patient factors.

Postoperative care must be meticulous with regular follow-up and an awareness of the potential complications which include meatal stenosis, loss of ventral skin, urethrocutaneous fistulas, etc.

Hypospadias cripples are that unfortunate group of patients who have undergone multiple surgical procedures and in order to treat these patients successfully it should be recognised that a radical approach must be adopted. This may require a complete revision of the earlier surgery. For this group of patients and those with severe penile curvature and small hypospadiac penis, the radical procedure of penile disassembly has been described. Its principles include the separation of the penis into its component parts followed by correction of chordee, urethroplasty and reassembly of the penis with full skin cover. This radical technique, developed from principles of epispadias surgery, may prove useful for a small subgroup of patients. In the longer term, uroflowmetry can provide an objective assessment of the functional result.

Hypospadias surgery therefore remains contentious and fascinating. Differing views exist regarding one-stage versus two-stage repairs, the importance of mobilisation of the urethral plate and the extent to which correction of chordee should be undertaken. It is therefore suggested that hypospadias surgery should be undertaken by those who have a particular interest in this condition.

INGUINOSCROTAL SURGERY

Undescended testes

Undescended testes are one of the commonest problems facing the paediatric surgeon. There is a recognised association with an increased risk of infertility and malignancy unless surgical intervention is undertaken at an early stage.

In a full-term male infant, at birth, the incidence of undescended testis is approximately 3% and there is an increasing incidence in premature boys, dependent on their age. During the first year of life spontaneous descent takes place with, at one year, the incidence being recognised as approximately 0.8%.

Testes can be arrested in the normal line of descent, to lie within the abdomen, the inguinal canal or in the neck or upper part of the scrotum. They can be ectopic where they have emerged to lie within the superficial inguinal pouch or, very uncommonly, in an unusual position in the perineum, contralateral scrotal sac or at the base of the penis. The retractable testis accounts for approximately half of the patients seen in the clinic and is due to increased activity of the cremaster muscle. It is defined clinically as a testis which can be brought into the fundus of the scrotum without tension which then retracts.

While parents can be reassured that the great majority of these testes will ultimately descend, it is recognised that the testis can also ascend. This is demonstrated in patients who have been seen for prior examination with either retractable testes or testes in the scrotum and at a later date the testes are noted to be high. The ascending testis is thought to be due to a processus vaginalis which becomes fibrotic and, associated with normal linear growth of the boy, results in testicular ascent.

Undescended testis can also be classified as either being palpable or impalpable. Impalpable testis will either be intraabdominal, in the canal or absent. There is no single identifiable cause for undescended testis but cryptorchidism is usually thought to be due to either a mechanical blockage to descent, endocrine causes or, more rarely, genetic abnormalities.

It is recognised that in the undescended testis, germ cell development is adversely affected and the current recommendations are that if possible, boys should undergo surgery before their second birthday. If surgery is carried out in infancy, however, the surgeon should have considerable experience of operating on the delicate tissues encountered in the spermatic cord at this age in order to avoid iatrogenic damage. The major indication for surgical intervention is to preserve, if not enhance fertility. Failure to intervene will result in lower fertility in a unilateral cryptorchid boy and a significant chance of infertility in the untreated bilateral cryptorchid patient. Thus infertility in the bilateral cryptorchid patient is significantly greater than in the general population and in the unilateral group infertility is approximately twice as great as in the general population. It is simplistic but true that early surgery is better than late surgery.

The same can be said about the potential for malignancy in a patient with an undescended testis where the increased risk is directly related to delay in surgery. There are few, if any, reports of malignancy occurring in patients who have undergone orchidopexy before the age of six years, so treatment before this age will significantly reduce the incident of testicular tumours occur-

ring amongst men with a history of undescended testis. The cryptorchid patient is recognised as having up to a 40-fold increased risk of developing a malignancy with the contralateral also being exposed to increased risk of tumour development if treatment is not offered at the appropriate time. Once again, early surgery is preferable. Recently there have been concerns about a possible increased risk of testicular cancer associated with cryptorchidism and testicular biopsy.

While standard orchidopexy is described in this chapter, the technique used should always be tailored to the individual patient's requirements.

Patients with a palpable testis which can be brought into the upper scrotum will benefit from a scrotal approach for their orchidopexy.

Patients with an impalpable intraabdominal testis present a serious challenge in management. Laparoscopy has been used extensively for the diagnosis of the impalpable testis, identifying the testis in some and obviating the need for groin exploration in others. The technique has also been extended to intervention where a first-stage Fowler–Stephens procedure (division of the testicular artery) can be performed laparoscopically. The second-stage procedure can also be carried out laparoscopically or so assisted. One alternative technique for the intraabdominal testicle is to use a traditional approach with low spermatic vessel ligation which obviates the need for laparoscopy. Another alternative approach for the non-palpable intraabdominal testis is to utilise an inguinal approach with transperitoneal mobilisation of the vas and vessel, which remains the preferred technique for many.

It is now suggested that patients should be treated before the age of two or three to permit optimum tubular development and sperm function. Hypoplastic cryptorchid testes should be removed rather than attempts made at preservation.

Microvascular autotransplantation techniques are an alternative for the treatment of the high intraabdominal testis.

Thus, to successfully manage these patients, they should be referred early and surgery should be undertaken in the hope of increased preservation of fertility and in order to reduce the future risk of carcinoma of the testis.

Testicular torsion

Testicular torsion is an emergency which requires rapid intervention if the testis is to be saved. Unfortunately late presentation to hospital is the major cause of delay leading to orchidectomy in patients with testicular torsion. There are two types of torsion.

- In the neonate the torsion is extravaginal where the spermatic cord rotates proximal to the attachment of the tunica vaginalis. It occurs most commonly in the intrauterine or neonatal period. In the great majority of neonates with torsion, the testis cannot be salvaged and emergency orchidectomy is required. More recently it has been proposed that if an antenatal torsion has occurred, colour Doppler ultrasound will demonstrate the abnormal testicular blood flow and the architecture of the testis, allowing exploration to be deferred. Emergency exploration of neonatal torsion, however, may result in a testicular preservation rate of 20%. Fixation of the contralateral testis should, however, be considered as mandatory in those patients to prevent torsion of the remaining testis.

- In older children torsion of the testis occurs intravaginally and it is recognised that testicular maldescent can be a precipitating factor. Any boy with testicular pain and vomiting should be considered as having a torsion until proven otherwise.

There is no place for conservative management of a child with suspected torsion. Both colour Doppler and radio-isotope scanning have their proponents as diagnostic modalities for torsion but if there is any suspicion that a testicular torsion has taken place, particularly within six hours of the onset of symptoms, exploration, derotation and fixation of the testicle are mandatory. Beyond six hours, it is more likely that the testis will be ischaemic and orchidectomy will be required. Once again the contralateral testis should be fixed.

Operative procedure for torsion of the testicle

A scrotal approach is utilised, either through a vertical incision over the mid-line raphae to allow access to each testicle or through transverse incisions. The tunica vaginalis is incised and the cord delivered and untwisted. The testis is then wrapped in warm swabs and its circulation assessed. There is some benefit in incising the tunica albuginea in order to assess the viability of the underlying structures. If the testis is deemed to be viable, then the tunica is plicated posteriorly and the testis is fixed with three fine, non-absorbable sutures between the mid-line raphae and the tunica albuginea as it is reflected between the epididymis and testis. If the testis is non-viable, then the spermatic cord should be ligated with Vicryl and the testis excised. It is important that the contralateral testis is likewise fixed to the mid-line raphae to prevent it encountering a similar fate.

Inguinal hernia

Inguinal hernia in childhood results from a failure of obliteration of the processus vaginalis.

In childhood, the great majority of inguinal hernias are in infants and young children. They are more common in boys, on the right side and are indirect. The diagnosis requires the identification of the hernia or a reliable history of a recurrent inguinal swelling from the parents. The major risk is that of irreducibility of the hernia leading to incarceration which in turn may lead to strangulation of the bowel. A secondary effect in this event is that testicular atrophy may occur due to the compression of the cord blood supply against the internal ring.

It is also recognised that the incidence of inguinal hernias is higher in premature infants, particularly those with a low birth weight who are subject to an increased risk of postoperative respiratory complications. In this group there may be some merit in the repair being undertaken under some form of spinal/caudal anaesthesia. It should be emphasised, however, that inguinal herniotomy in this at-risk group is extremely safe with under 10% of patients requiring reintubation or ventilation. However, the morbidity is greater in the neonate than the paediatric population as a whole.

Inguinal herniotomy is a very common procedure in childhood and should be undertaken as a matter of urgency once the diagnosis has been made in order to minimise the risk of complications. The recognised risk factors which can be used to predict the serious complications of strangulation and obstruction are early infancy, male sex, a hernia on the right side and a short history. While complications are unusual following inguinal herniotomy, they occur in approximately 4% of cases and include wound infection, recurrence of the hernia, tethering of the testis with the adoption of a high intracanalicular position and, less commonly, injury to the bladder or vas deferens and testicular atrophy.

Those complications are particularly seen in patients who have undergone emergency surgery. The complication of recurrence of an inguinal hernia is associated with incarceration, postoperative complications and concomitant disease, particularly in premature babies who require continued ventilation. Many centres will elect to deal with the hernias of premature babies once ventilation has been withdrawn and they are at less risk.

The operation of inguinal herniotomy is described later in this chapter and while the standard procedure is utilised for elective and emergency cases, some proponents support a transperitoneal closure of the internal ring in those patients with incarcerated inguinal hernia. There has been considerable debate regarding the benefits of routine contralateral groin exploration in patients with occult unilateral inguinal hernias. While this approach is routine in many centres in North America, it is less common in the United Kingdom. Laparoscopy has been proposed as one method of identifying a contralateral patent sac, thus potentially avoiding unnecessary intervention. Irreducible hernias can initially be managed conservatively with elevation of the lower half of the body and sedation with morphine in the correct dose and, if necessary, gentle manual pressure. Failure to reduce the hernia or difficulty in reduction should be an indication for emergency herniotomy. If, however, the hernia is successfully reduced, it is mandatory that elective early repair is carried out within the next 48 hours.

Hydrocoele

Hydrocoeles are due to the fluid which occurs within the tunica vaginalis following persistence of the patent processus vaginalis (PPV). The great majority of hydrocoeles which present in the neonatal period and infancy will resolve and it is only after the child's first birthday, in the absence of any reduction in the size of the hydrocoele, that surgical intervention should be considered. It is usually easy to differentiate between a hydrocoele and hernia both on palpation and with transillumination. An encysted hydrocoele of the cord, however, can cause some confusion but the same principles regarding treatment still apply. Occasionally, hydrocoeles are secondary to epididymitis or torsion of an appendix testis. The operative treatment of a hydrocoele in childhood is virtually identical to that for an inguinal hernia except that it is the PPV which is transfixed and divided and not the hernial sac. The surgeon should always be aware that if a child presents with an acute hydrocoele and the testis is impalpable, a testicular tumour should be excluded with ultrasound.

Varicocoele

Varicocoele describes the dilatation of the veins of the pampiniform plexus of the internal spermatic vein. It is estimated that they occur in 2–10% of adolescent boys and are predominantly found on the left side, this predisposition to the left being related to the differing anatomy of the testicular veins. The varicocoele typically presents as a 'bag of worms' with the symptoms of aching or a dragging sensation in the scrotum. Clinical interest is because of the potential for growth retardation, abnormalities of spermatogenesis and ultimately reduced fertility.

Investigation is usually with ultrasound, measuring the testicular volume and including a scan of the kidneys. In young boys who are asymptomatic, there is no clear indication for surgery. However, in patients who have symptoms or where there is a significant disparity in testicular volume, treatment should be offered.

Treatment of a varicocoele is traditionally:

- by high retroperitoneal approach to the veins (as described by Palomo)
- through an inguinal approach (as described by Ivanissevich).

Both procedures have been described with or without sparing of the testicular artery. More recently, there has been the development of laparoscopic varicocoelectomy and the use of embolectomy and both antegrade and retrograde sclerosing techniques carried out under radiological imaging. There is good evidence that testicular growth will recover following surgery, particularly in those patients with large varicocoeles where the operation improves the patient's fertility potential.

Complications of surgery include haematoma formation, infection and the postoperative development of a hydrocoele or recurrence of the varicocoele and, perhaps more significantly, testicular atrophy in a small number of cases.

VESICOURETERIC REFLUX

Vesicoureteric reflux occurs when there is flow of urine from the bladder in a retrograde manner into the upper urinary tract. There is a well-established relationship between pyelonephritis and reflux which occurs because of incompetence of the valve mechanism at the vesicoureteric junction. Primary reflux is thus due to this inadequate valve mechanism secondary to a deficiency in the length of the intravesical ureteric tunnel compared to the ureteric diameter. Secondary vesicoureteric reflux, while occurring through the same mechanism, is related to bladder dysfunction which may be neurogenic in origin or related to outflow obstruction such as in urethral valves or detrusor sphincter dyssynergia.

The most common presentation of reflux is in young children with pyrexia of unknown origin (PUO) secondary to urinary tract infections. The importance of the febrile urinary tract infection is that it is commonly associated with pyelonephritis whereas a non-febrile urinary tract infection is more commonly associated with cystitis. With the routine use of antenatal ultrasound investigation, abnormalities such as hydronephrosis are detected at an early stage with 15–20% of such cases of hydronephrosis being due to vesicoureteric reflux (VUR). It is those cases which are detected in infancy which are often found to have high grades of reflux. Reflux is also detected in older children who present with abdominal pain secondary to pyelonephritis. Patients with reflux also have a high incidence of bladder instability and dysfunctional voiding. It is recognised that there is a high familial incidence of reflux with a third of the siblings of patients with VUR being likewise affected.

Several grading systems have been used to describe VUR but the most frequently used is the International Study Classification of the International Reflux Study Group. Here grade 1 indicates reflux into the ureter and progresses through to grade 5 where there is massive reflux into grossly dilated ureters and pelvis.

The evaluation of the child with reflux is dependent on the age at presentation and the symptomatology. In the infant with an antenatal diagnosis the ultrasound is repeated at between 24 and 48 hours from birth with an MCU at 2–4 weeks and a DMSA (technetium 99m dimercaptosuccinic acid) scan at 3–6 months to evaluate the presence or absence of renal scarring. In the older patient presenting with febrile urinary tract infection, investigations would be similar. Urodynamic investigation is useful for identifying those patients with severe reflux who may prove resistant to conventional and surgical treatment. The clinical importance of reflux is its well-recognised relationship with infected urine resulting in pyelonephritis with renal scarring. Many patients will have established scarring at the time of diagnosis, thus early investigation of patients with proven urinary tract infections is mandatory.

The management of reflux is governed by the recognition that there is a tendency for VUR to improve spontaneously over a period of time. The higher the grade of reflux, however, the less likely it is that this spontaneous resolution will occur. Whereas in patients with grades 1 and 2 VUR it is recognised that there is a spontaneous resolution rate of 80%, grades 4 and 5 reflux is unlikely to resolve and those patients will benefit from surgical intervention. Initial medical treatment is therefore directed towards maintaining sterile urine with the use of long-term, low-dose antibiotic prophylaxis with the appropriate antibiotics.

The chances of resolution are adversely affected by such factors as duplex ureters, bladder diverticulum and dysfunctional voiding. Treatment with intravenous antibiotics of patients with febrile urinary tract infections may significantly reduce the chance of renal scarring. Prophylactic therapy, however, is the cornerstone of medical management. Factors such as frequent breakthrough infections and poor compliance, side effects of low-dose antibiotics and patients with dysfunctional voiding may weigh in favour of surgical intervention. Follow-up imaging is essential to identify patients who have developed further scars and either MCU or the more recently developed direct puncture nuclear cystogram will allow early identification of resolution of the reflux. It should be recognised, however, that imaging studies carried out on the same patient within a short timescale may differ in up to 30% of patients. After the reflux has ceased, renal growth should be monitored by ultrasound for a further two years or longer if there is scarring with a DMSA scan also at two years post resolution.

The criteria for surgical management are shown below:

- high-grade reflux
- breakthrough urinary tract infections
- new renal scarring
- poor renal growth
- non-compliance with medical therapy
- failure of medical therapy.

Resolution should be expected on medical treatment within five years and if this has not occurred and the grade of reflux remains constant, surgical intervention should be considered.

While the natural history is towards resolution, female patients in late school age should remain under close surveillance since, if their reflux persists, during later pregnancies they are more likely to have episodes of pyelonephritis.

Up until 15 years ago ureteric reimplantation was the treatment of choice for patients with high-grade reflux, with most series showing very high cure rates. The well-established surgical methods of reimplantation include the Politano–Leadbetter procedure, the Cohen and Glenn-Anderson techniques.

During the past 15 years, particularly in Europe, the use of endoscopic submucosal injection techniques has become predominant. The original technique of injection of Teflon paste has proved extremely successful with long-term results now being available in over 6000 injected ureters, showing a cessation of reflux in over 80% of patients treated and a significant downgrading of reflux in a further 10% of patients. It can thus be concluded that the treatment is simple, safe and effective. There have been concerns, particularly in North America, regarding the possible dangers of local granuloma development and distant migration of Teflon paste and thus it is not approved for urological use in the USA. These concerns, however, have not been supported by clinical experience. The simplicity and ease of the STING technique are attractive so other injectable materials have been produced, including collagen, which is approved for use in the USA, Macroplastique and Deflux. The endoscopic injection treatment therefore remains the mainstay of surgical treatment of VUR in many parts of the world.

The management of reflux remains contentious and it is known that renal damage, once it occurs, is non-reversible. Studies have shown that there is no difference in the infection rate between those treated medically or surgically except that there are fewer episodes of pyelonephritis in surgical patients. There is no difference in new scar formation, in the glomerular filtration rate, in the measured renal length or in scar progression. Children under two with severe VUR and associated urinary tract infections remain the target group for early therapy since they are at greatest risk of developing scars.

In order to identify those patients at risk, the Royal College of Physicians guidelines recommend that all patients with a urinary tract infection should undergo investigation with ultrasound to diagnose obstruction, reflux or renal scars. Those under the age of one year should also have a DMSA and MCU. Those under the age of seven years should have an ultrasound and DMSA some three months after any detectable infection. Only by aggressively pursuing the investigation of patients with urinary tract infections and possible VUR will the complications of renal scarring, renal growth retardation, hypertension and renal failure in childhood be reduced.

UROLOGICAL TRAUMA IN CHILDHOOD

Urological trauma remains a significant cause of death in children. Trauma remains a major cause of hospital admission and children suffer most commonly from limb fractures and head injuries, but it is those patients admitted with multiple trauma who have a significant risk of trauma to the genitourinary tract. The great majority of renal injuries are due to blunt trauma but there are a significant number of patients who suffer penetrating injuries and gunshot wounds. There tends to be an increased number of boys sustaining major injuries who require vigorous resuscitation. The great majority of the injuries are, however, minor in nature and can be managed conservatively.

The assessment of the patient requires an accurate history from all available sources followed by a thorough physical examination looking in particular for bruising of the abdomen, pelvic region, perineum or scrotum. Blood at the urethral meatus or significant haematuria must alert the clinician to the possibility of injury to the genitourinary tract. Attempts to relate the significance of haematuria, i.e. greater than 50 RBCs per HPF, to an increasingly severe injury should be balanced by the knowledge that serious injury can occur in the absence of haematuria, but that blood seen at the urethral meatus is a certain indication for further investigation.

While investigation by ultrasound may suffice in those patients with simple injuries, computed tomography (CT scan) is mandatory in those patients with major renal injuries, particularly since these are often associated with other intraabdominal trauma. CT scanning is less effective if the injury is to the bladder or urethra in the pelvis and MRI may have a role in this regard. If there is suspicion of damage to these organs, investigation is best initiated from below, i.e. by ascending urethrography. If this demonstrates that the urethra is intact, it is considered safe to proceed to an MCU and thorough investigation of the bladder. IVP has, to a large extent, been superseded by more modern investigations. However, if nephrectomy is being considered in the emergency situation then the function of the contralateral kidney must be established with either an IVP or an isotope scan.

Renal injuries in children

Children are more likely to suffer from blunt renal trauma since the kidney is relatively exposed. Congenital abnormalities such as a hydronephrosis secondary to PUJ obstruction place the kidney at increased risk. Classification systems have been described which, while becoming increasingly sophisticated, facilitate the clinical decision-making process. A simpler classification is shown in Box 49.2.

Box 49.2 Classification of renal injuries

1 Renal contusion
2 Minor lacerations
3 Major lacerations
4 Vascular injuries

There is still considerable debate regarding the management of children with major renal injuries. However, the current view tends to be that a conservative approach is best, particularly in those patients who are cardiovascularly stable. Those patients with renal vascular injuries who are unstable and are responding poorly to resuscitation will require surgical exploration.

This is best carried out through a long, transverse upper abdominal or mid-line incision. Control of the vessels is key to both attempted repair and nephrectomy and while the kidney can be approached by reflecting the peritoneum lateral to the colon, control of the renal vessels must first be obtained by an incision inferomedial to the inferior mesenteric vein over the aorta. Operative detail is further outlined in major texts.

The complications of surgery for renal trauma are well recognised. They include secondary haemorrhage, urinoma and the leak of urinary collections, infection and abscess formation and at a later stage the development of hypertension. Arteriovenous fistula is also recognised, particularly following penetrating stab wounds. Hydronephrosis can occur secondarily to fibrosis and the development of obstruction to drainage. The development of percutaneous drains and stents has allowed obstructive complica-

tions to be managed without initial recourse to reexploration. In the follow-up of patients with renal trauma the blood pressure should be measured and ultrasound carried out at an early stage followed some three months later by a DMSA scan to assess the renal cortical pattern.

Ureteric injuries

Injuries to the ureter are extremely rare and are probably best managed in a specialised unit. If, however, they are discovered during a laparotomy an attempt should be made at reanastomosis with placement of a urethral stent and external local drainage. The surgical techniques used will relate to the region of the ureter that is damaged and where significant loss of the ureter has occurred, major reconstructive surgery will be required. Temporary ureterostomy can be utilised before complex reconstruction is planned.

Bladder trauma

In young children the bladder is potentially exposed as it is more of an abdominal structure. Bladder trauma can give rise to significant complications unless the initial injury is treated effectively. Extraperitoneal bladder injury is typically associated with fractures of the pelvic ring while intraperitoneal rupture with abdominal signs is less frequent. Clinical suspicion of bladder injury should be raised in patients with pelvic fractures, lower abdominal tenderness following trauma, blood at the urethral meatus and gross haematuria.

The diagnosis of bladder or urethral injury should be considered in all patients who have difficulty in voiding following injury. Diagnosis is best made with a cystogram, ensuring that the bladder is well distended. CT scans are less reliable in this regard and there may be a place for MRI scanning in the pelvis.

Extraperitoneal rupture of the bladder is most commonly managed by Foley catheter drainage for a period of 7–10 days. If, however, there is an extensive injury, exploration may be required. Complications similar to those mentioned in relation to renal surgery should be looked for. Intraperitoneal bladder rupture requires surgical exploration and repair, drainage being with a suprapubic catheter for a period of up to 10 days, with a contrast study being carried out prior to catheter removal.

Urethral injuries

The urethra, particularly in the male, is at risk in pelvic fractures and in straddle injuries. Disruption of the urethra can be either partial or complete and most commonly occurs in the posterior urethra. This leads to extravasation of urine and significant haematoma formation in the pelvis. Suspicion of a urethral injury should be raised when the patient has posttraumatic difficulty in voiding, there is blood at the urethral meatus and perineal bruising and soft tissue swelling are identified. Rectal examination may reveal a high bladder with a boggy swelling in the pelvis.

Ascending urethrogram can be carried out to identify the site of the lesion and any extravasation. If there is no evidence of complete disruption, the catheter can be advanced into the bladder to allow for drainage and a cystogram obtained if there is suspicion of concomitant bladder injury. If there is suspicion of partial disruption the catheter should be left in place for a period of time.

The treatment of posterior urethral injuries has been contentious for some years, but for a surgeon who is not commonly dealing with these injuries it would be advisable to place a suprapubic drain and consider delayed urethral repair in a specialist centre. Primary urethral repair can also be carried out in these centres that have access to the endourological techniques necessary to negotiate the damaged urethra prior to repair. Anterior or bulbous urethral injury usually occurs secondary to a straddle injury. There can be considerable crushing of the urethra and surrounding tissues. The urethra, however, is usually maintained in continuity and extravasation is limited. These patients can be managed with a catheter in situ but the risk of later stricture formation remains high.

Scrotal, testicular and penile trauma

Testicular injuries are less common and are usually as a result of a direct blow. Injury to the scrotum will produce a significant haematoma and while clinical examination is difficult, ultrasound should clearly identify the extent of injury to the testis. Rupture of the tunica albuginea will require exploration with debridement and reapposition of the tunica with postoperative drainage of the scrotum. Zipper injuries to the foreskin are seen in young boys and can be repaired primarily, but occasionally circumcision will be required. Penile fractures result in severe injury and may require catheterisation to relieve retention of urine. Treatment is usually a specialist procedure.

GENITOURINARY TUMOURS IN CHILDHOOD

While most genitourinary tumours are rare in childhood, the general surgeon must always maintain a high index of suspicion when considering the differential diagnosis in a child presenting with a mass in the abdomen or pelvis or with a testicular swelling. The most common solid tumours in childhood, in descending order, are tumours of the central nervous system, lymphomas, neuroblastoma and renal tumours, including Wilms' tumour, followed by bladder and prostate rhabdomyosarcoma. The common groups of genitourinary tumours in childhood are listed below.

● Renal tumours – Wilms'

● Bladder and prostate rhabdomyosarcoma

● Testicular tumours

If tumours of the adrenal gland, sympathetic chain and retroperitoneum are included, there is a wide range of pathologies to be considered when the general surgeon is presented with a child with a possible tumour. While these patients are best managed in specialist centres, their early investigation and treatment are critical.

Wilms' tumour – nephroblastoma

Wilms' tumour is the commonest renal tumour in childhood, other renal tumours being rare in this age group. The management of these patients has improved significantly in recent years with a resultant increase in survival rates, with the four-year survival of patients with favourable histology now approaching 90%. The National Wilms' Tumour Studies (NWTS) in North America and the International Society of Paediatric Oncology (SIOP) studies have added significantly to our increased knowledge in this field.

A child with a Wilms' tumour typically presents with an incidental abdominal mass. Haematuria, acute abdominal pain and acute presentation with a varicocoele in a younger child are less common methods of presentation.

Historically all such patients were originally investigated with an IVP but the dramatic evolution of imaging techniques has meant that ultrasound is now the initial imaging modality of choice in the great majority of children. This allows differentiation between solid and cystic lesions and also identifies whether there is any intracaval extension of a renal tumour.

Use of CT or MRI will provide other information regarding staging. It should be noted, however, that the NWTS Group emphasises the importance of surgical findings and the histological examination of tumour material. Staging, however, demands an accurate assessment of local extension and distant metastases. While imaging may identify bilateral disease, exploration of the contralateral kidney at the time of laparotomy is indicated. Metastatic disease can be found in the chest, liver and, more rarely, dependent on tumour type, in the bony skeleton and brain.

While many patients will benefit from 'downstaging' with chemotherapy, the treatment of Wilms' tumour is essentially with surgery. Radical nephrectomy is performed through a transperitoneal approach, lymph node biopsies are performed in a systematic manner and venous extension excluded. High-risk patients with poor prognosis have been recognised as a subgroup with 'unfavourable' histological features – anaplasia, clear cell sarcoma of the kidney, rhabdoid tumour of the kidney. Effective diagnosis, staging and multimodality therapies dramatically decrease the morbidity and mortality of children with Wilms' tumour. Recently increasing awareness of biology, genetics and epidemiology has led to improved treatment. Primary chemotherapy with delayed resection is evolving as the preferred approach for large inoperable tumours, bilateral disease and those tumours with extensive intravascular involvement. Younger patients with small localised favourable tumours may be treated with surgery alone.

Treatment of all these patients involves a multidisciplinary team with oncologists, surgeons, pathologists, radiotherapists and other therapy staff working closely together. Ideally all such patients should be entered into one of the international trials or treated with a recognised national protocol. It is only with adherence to such that we will see continued improvement in the outcome of treatment for these patients. It should be noted that as the Wilms' tumour is highly chemosensitive, radiotherapy is now used less than in the past.

Bladder and prostate rhabdomyosarcoma

Genitourinary rhabdomyosarcoma commonly presents as a pelvic abdominal mass in a young boy. Symptoms are dependent on the extent of spread at the time of presentation. The tumour is also seen in girls, often at a younger age. Diagnosis can usually be made with biopsy needle specimen or by biopsy at endoscopy. Staging is with the accepted imaging modalities of CT and MRI with the use of isotope scanning to identify the bony metastases. Current therapeutic regimes are based on the use of intensive chemotherapy with surgery and radiotherapy, urinary diversion being required in those patients where radical extirpative surgery is necessary.

Testicular tumours

Testicular tumours are rare in childhood. However, any child presenting with a swelling of the testis or in the scrotum should be considered as having a tumour unless proven otherwise. This is particularly relevant in the case of a boy with a hydrocoele where the testis is not palpable. Delayed surgery for the hydrocoele may delay diagnosis of the testicular tumour. If the testis cannot therefore be palpated, ultrasound should be carried out. Diagnosis in the newborn is particularly difficult, particularly when it is recognised that this group may present with testicular torsion but the possibility of testicular tumour must be considered. The ultrasonographer in this instance may not be able to make a confident diagnosis and the tumour marker alpha-fetoprotein (AFP) is normally markedly elevated in this age group. Tumour markers AFP and beta human chorionic gonadotrophin (β hCG) should be obtained in patients where there is a suspicion of a tumour.

Surgical treatment is by orchidectomy through an inguinal approach with primary ligation of the spermatic cord.

OPERATIVE SURGERY

Orchidopexy

Introduction

Undescended testes are a common condition in childhood, affecting approximately 1% of boys at one year of age. At birth the incidence is 3% with a much higher incidence in preterm boys. It is thus important to recognise that testicular descent can still continue during infancy.

Age for surgery

This has been a matter for considerable debate but it is recognised that ideally surgery should be carried out in the second year of life or later at the time when the patient presents to the surgery. In infancy the cord structures are extremely delicate and at this age the surgery should be carried out by a surgeon experienced in this field.

Preoperative preparation

Antibiotic prophylaxis is not normally required. The operation is usually carried out on a day case basis and premedication is not routinely used. Local anaesthetic (EMLA) cream should be applied during the preoperative period to allow pain-free access to a suitable vein.

Anaesthesia and position

Following the induction of a general anaesthetic and the use of caudal anaesthesia or an ileo-inguinal nerve block, the patient is placed in a supine position on the operating table. The surgeon stands on the appropriate side of the table and the skin is prepared with an iodine-based or other suitable antiseptic solution.

Incision

A transverse incision is made just above and lateral to the palpable pubic tubercle, a few centimetres in length and ideally sited in a skin crease. If an impalpable testis is present a higher incision will facilitate exploration. The skin incision is then deepened through the subcutaneous fat and Scarpa's fascia; superficial veins can be either retracted or divided with bipolar diathermy.

Procedure

- The external ring is identified and the external oblique opened laterally, taking care to avoid damaging the ilio-inguinal nerve.

- The testis and spermatic cord are then delivered through the wound and the gubernaculum divided as required. Bipolar diathermy can be used throughout this procedure.

- The cremaster muscle which surrounds the cord is then incised and reflected, often revealing a hernial sac or processus vaginalis anterosuperior to the cord. Separation of the vas and vessels from the hernial sac is a delicate procedure, particularly in the infant. If the sac is opened it may be easier to complete the dissection under direct vision through the posterior wall of the sac with the scissors between the vas and vessels, and the sac. Otherwise the sac or processus should be dissected intact.

- These structures are then followed proximally to the internal ring where the sac is ligated with 4/0 Vicryl. Just above the internal ring the vas curves medially behind the inferior epigastric vessels and care should be taken with haemostasis to avoid damaging adjacent vessels. The testicular vessels pass proximally and retroperitoneally.

- Mobilisation should allow the testicle to be placed in the scrotum without tension. However, if this is not achieved the testis must be placed under tension and distracted distally and medially to reveal the lateral fibrous bands which are closely adherent to the testicular vessels, which are preserved throughout.

- The bands are then divided, which allows adequate length for the testis to be placed in a dartos pouch. The pouch is fashioned with the insertion of the index or middle finger through the inguinal incision into the scrotum. A transverse incision is then made through the scrotal skin on to the finger. With the finger still in place and using curved scissors, a subcutaneous pouch is fashioned just below the dartos muscle. Care must be taken to obtain haemostasis with the bipolar diathermy.

- The tip of an artery forceps is then placed on the finger through the scrotal incision and the finger then withdrawn, guiding the forceps into the inguinal incision. The artery forceps then grasps the paratesticular tissue, allowing the testis to be pulled into the scrotum, taking care not to twist the vessels.

- The tunica vaginalis should then be opened to allow inspection of the testis and epididymis, with removal of testicular appendages if present.

- The testis can then be placed in the sub-dartos pouch and if there is any concern regarding undue tension, the tunica albuginea of the testis can be fixed to the mid-line raphae of the scrotum with fine non-absorbable sutures.

- The scrotal incision is then closed with fine absorbable sutures using either a subcuticular technique or interrupted sutures with the knots on the inside.

- The inguinal incision is then closed in layers with absorbable sutures and a subcuticular suture to the skin. No dressing is required in these patients but both incisions can be protected with a spray of plastic skin.

Postoperative management

Immediate postoperative analgesia is provided with the continued effects of the caudal epidural or ilio-inguinal nerve blocks. The anaesthesia is usually supplemented with a Voltarol suppository

and paracetamol may be required during the first 24 hours postoperatively. Most boys make a rapid recovery, returning to their normal activities within a few days. Postoperative complications occur in a small number of patients and include wound infection and haematoma which, if it occurs in the scrotal wound, usually results in a breakdown of the wound. This will usually heal with conservative treatment. Other complications include testicular atrophy and retraction of the testis, making follow-up at six months mandatory in order to identify these occasional complications.

The above description is that of a standard orchidopexy for a palpable testis. Many palpable testes can be successfully operated on through a single high scrotal incision which gives excellent anatomical and cosmetic results. In approximately 10–20% of patients the testis is impalpable and there is continuing debate as to the best method of treating this group. The options range from a standard approach with retroperitoneal mobilisation of the spermatic vessels and vas, the Fowler–Stephens procedure with division of the testicular vessel to obtain additional length, laparoscopic techniques which allow identification of the testicular anatomy as a prelude to conventional surgery, laparoscopic or laparoscopic-assisted orchidopexy or free microvascular autotransplantation of the testis. The latter techniques are best performed in centres which specialise in this area of surgery.

Results

Functional results are difficult to assess. However, there is evidence of maintenance of testicular function particularly with earlier operation.

Inguinal herniotomy

Introduction

Congenital inguinal hernias occur when the processus vaginalis fails to fuse following the descent of the testis from an intra-abdominal retroperitoneal position into the scrotum. Inguinal hernias in infancy most commonly occur in boys, with an increased number seen on the right side. The diagnosis is made when the child cries and demonstrates the hernia, but in elective cases a decision to operate can be made when there is a consistent, reliable history of an inguinal swelling given by the parents. The most dangerous complication of an inguinal hernia in infancy is that of incarceration and potential strangulation of the bowel. Thus, when a diagnosis of an inguinal hernia is made in a male infant, every attempt should be made to expedite surgery in order to prevent this complication.

Preparation

Routine antibiotic prophylaxis is not used unless there are concerns regarding incarceration.

Anaesthesia

The procedure is performed under a general anaesthetic but in premature infants with pulmonary complications, a caudal anaesthesia may be preferred. The lower abdomen and inguinoscrotal area are prepared with an iodine-based or other suitable antiseptic solution.

Position

The infant is placed on the operating table in a supine position, taking care to preserve the body temperature with the use of a warming blanket in the preterm baby and infant. The surgeon stands on the side of the hernia.

Incision

A transverse incision is made above the pubic tubercle, in a skin crease extending laterally for a few centimetres.

Procedure

- The incision is deepened through the subcutaneous fat and Scarpa's fascia down to the external ring where the spermatic cord is identified.

- Due to the superimposition of the external and internal rings in infancy, it is usually not necessary to open the external ring. However, if this facilitates surgery, the external oblique should be opened laterally from the external ring, taking care to avoid damaging the ilio-inguinal nerve.

- The spermatic cord is then delivered, if possible without dislocating the testis. However, if this is necessary in order to facilitate surgery, the testis and cord can be delivered complete, but the testis must be relocated in the scrotum at the end of the operation.

- The cremasteric muscle and fascia are then incised along the line of the cord, allowing the cremasteric muscle to be reflected with either blunt or sharp dissection. The hernial sac, which in infancy is usually complete, is then identified lying anteriorly.

- The sac is then grasped with a pair of fine non-toothed dissecting forceps and dissected free from the vas and vessels.

- Once the sac is cleared from these structures it can then be divided between forceps and the proximal portion followed to the level of the internal ring. The distal portion of the sac can be left *in situ*. The hernial sac should be dissected until retroperitoneal fat is identified. Any contents should be reduced and the cord twisted and the neck of the sac suture ligated with 4/0 Vicryl. Care must be taken to preserve the spermatic vessels and vas throughout.

- The wound is then closed in layers with absorbable sutures of the surgeon's choice; a formal dressing is unnecessary and the wound can be sprayed with a plastic occlusive dressing. Postoperative analgesia is usually maintained from the pre- and peroperative analgesia. Most patients make a rapid recovery with little restriction to their normal activities.

Incarcerated inguinal hernia

The most dangerous complication of inguinal hernias in childhood is that of incarceration. This usually occurs in very young male infants who present with a short history and more commonly occurs on the right side. An incarcerated inguinal hernia in the great majority of patients can be successfully managed with the child in a slightly head-down position, sedation and if necessary gentle manual retraction. If the hernia is successfully reduced, the patient should then undergo herniotomy within 24–48 hours. Any further delay is likely to lead to an increased risk of reincarceration. If the hernia does not reduce within a few hours of conservative treatment or if there is concern regarding the viability of the bowel, then urgent exploration should be undertaken although this is rarely required. If the hernial sac contains bowel its viability should be assessed and if viable, it can be returned to the abdominal cavity. If not, ischaemic bowel should be resected and the bowel restored in continuity with an end-to-end anastomosis using a single layer of sero-submucosal 5/0 Vicryl sutures. If the hernia cannot be reduced, the internal ring can be enlarged with a lateral incision. This must be repaired prior to wound closure.

Postoperative management

Postoperative complications include wound infection, recurrence, tethered testis, bladder injury and injury to the vas. There is a higher complication rate in patients with incarceration including atrophy of the testis secondary to compression of the spermatic vessel by the contents of the hernial sac. Recurrence of the inguinal hernia occurs particularly in the group of preterm babies undergoing assisted ventilation. Routine bilateral inguinal exploration has its proponents particularly in North America but more recently this approach has been subject to review. There is an increasing vogue for the use of magnification with binocular loops which may have advantages particularly in the small preterm infant.

Inguinal herniotomy in childhood is a technically demanding operation, particularly in the infant with an incarcerated hernia. These patients are probably best treated in centres which have considerable experience of the condition.

FURTHER READING

Akhtar J, Orr JD. Minimally invasive orchidopexy: the trans-scrotal approach. *Min Inv Ther* 1993; **2**:3

Birmingham Reflux Study Group. Prospective trial of operative versus non operative treatment of severe vesico-ureteric reflux in children: 5 years' observation. *Br Med Clin Res Ed* 1987; **295**:237–241

Bracka I. A versatile two stage hypospadias repair. *Br J Plast Surg* 1995; **48**:345–352

Clarnette TD, Hutson JM. Is the ascending testis actually stationary? Normal elongation of the spermatic cord is prevented by a fibrous remnant of the processus vaginalis. *Paed Surg Int* 1997; **12**:155–157

Duckett JW. MAGPI (meatal advancement and glanduloplasty): a procedure for subcoronal hypospadias. *Urol Clin North Am* 1981; **8**:513–520

Fonkalsrud EW. Current management of the undescended testis. *Semin Paed Surg* 1996; **5**:2–7

Haase GM. Current surgical management of Wilms' tumour. *Curr Opin Paed* 1996; **8**:268–275

Haase GM, Ritchey ML. Neuroblastoma. *Semin Paed Surg* 1997; **6**:11–16

International Reflux Study in Children. Results of a randomised clinical trial of medical versus surgical management of infants and children with grades III and IV primary vesico-ureteral reflux (United States). *J Urol* 1992; **148**:1667–1673

Ivanissevich O. Left varicocoele due to reflux: experience with 4,470 operative cases in forty-two years. *J Int Col Surg* 1960; **34**:742

La Quaglia MP. Genitourinary tract cancer in childhood. *Semin Paed Surg* 1996; **5**:49–65

Lent V. What classification is appropriate in renal trauma? *Eur Urol* 1996; **30**:327–334

Lindgren BW, Darby EC, Faiella L et al. Laparoscopic orchidopexy: procedure of choice for the nonpalpable testis? *J Urol* 1998; **159**:2132–2135

Mee SL, MacAninch JW, Robinson AL et al. Radiographic assessment of renal trauma: a ten year prospective study of patient selection. *J Urol* 1989; **141**:1095

Palomo A Radical cure of varicocoele by a new technique: preliminary report. *J Urol* 1949; 61:604

Pinto KJ, Noe HN, Jerkins GR. Management of neonatal testicular torsion. *J Urol* 1997; **158**:1196–1197

Puri P, Ninan GK, Surana R. Subureteric Teflon injection (STING). Results of a European survey. *Eur Urol* 1995; **27**:71–75

Report of the International Reflux Study Committee. Medical versus surgical treatment of primary vesico-ureteric reflux A perspective. International Reflux Study in Children. *J Urol* 1981; **125**:277–283

Report of a Working Group of the Research Unit, RCP. Guidelines for the management of acute urinary tract infections in childhood. *J Roy Coll Phys Lond* 1991; **25**:36–42

Rescorla FJ, West KW, Engum SA et al. The 'other side' of paediatric hernias: the role of laparoscopy. *Am Surg* 1997; **63**:690–693

Snodgrass W. Tubularised, incised urethroplasty for distal hypospadias. *J Urol* 1994; **151**:464–465

Wacksman J. Modification of the one stage flip flap procedure to repair distal penile hypospadias. *Urol Clin North Am* 1981; **8**:527

50

Paediatric trauma

Paul K.H. Tam, Steve C.L. Lin

INTRODUCTION

Trauma is the most significant threat to the health of children and is the leading cause of death after the first year of life. Most injuries to children and adolescents result from blunt injuries caused by falls, motor vehicle injuries, pedestrian injuries, bicycle injuries and submersion. Penetrating injuries are less common but in some countries such as the United States, firearms are a significant cause of death in older children and adolescents.

Paediatric injuries are not always random events but occur in predictable patterns that are related to age, gender, time of day and yearly season. The main traumatic events during the neonatal period are usually related to birth injury, while injuries during infancy are mostly caused by burns, falling and aspiration or swallowing of foreign bodies. Injuries in school-aged children are often caused by sharp objects, burns, drowning and sports or traffic accidents. Trauma related to child abuse continues to be a worldwide problem and can be found in all levels of society.

The basic principles of management of paediatric trauma are similar to those for adult trauma. Regardless of the type or aetiology of the trauma, early recognition and proper initial management are vital. A significant number of injured children are left with permanent sequelae or disability, which will require long-term rehabilitation. The expenditure of resources and personnel for long-term rehabilitation of children is relatively greater compared to similar traumatic events in adults. In addition, the psychological impact of trauma on a child cannot be estimated. However, properly managed, children have significant potential for full recovery from injury.

EVALUATION AND INITIAL MANAGEMENT

The emergent care of traumatised children calls for a systematic approach and careful planning, including understanding of airway management, control of haemorrhage and the principles of resuscitation. The principles and practice of the Advanced Trauma Life Support (ATLS) introduced by the American College of Surgeons are widely adopted in the Western world. Management of trauma victims begins at the prehospital setting. Good communication ensures that a team (with an assigned leader), comprising a paediatric surgeon, a paediatric anaesthetist and other medical and nursing staff, is prepared to receive the patient at the accident and emergency department. Once the general condition of the child stabilises, the extent of injury should be assessed, followed by establishment of the priorities in further management.

Because of their small size, children are susceptible to multisystem injuries. Children with multisystemic or complex injuries can deteriorate rapidly and develop major complications. Therefore, they should be transferred to paediatric trauma centres that have appropriate expertise and facilities. Initial treatment should take the special characteristics of paediatric anatomy and physiology into consideration.

Blood volume

Actual intravascular volume of children is age and body weight dependent. Therefore, the consequences of blood loss should be interpreted accordingly.

Temperature control

The younger a child, the greater the ratio of total body surface to body weight and the thinner the subcutaneous layer. Consequently, young children are less capable of preventing heat loss. Therefore, posttraumatic hypothermia and metabolic acidosis in young children who have suffered hypovolaemic shock will be more profound and more resistant to resuscitation.

Gastrointestinal function

Posttraumatic intestinal ileus and gastric dilatation due to hypovolaemia are more severe in children than in adults. These may result in vomiting or aspiration pneumonia, further aggravating cardiopulmonary dysfunction.

Pulmonary function

Pulmonary function is not mature until several months after birth. However, requirement of oxygen for neonates and infants with increased metabolic needs is greater than that for older children. Any compromise in pulmonary function due to atelectasis and pneumonia will result in further deterioration of the general condition.

Renal function

Renal function is not fully mature until a child is six years of age. Fluid balance needs to be closely monitored, especially for children younger than two, in order to avoid dehydration or overhydration.

Nutrition

Children at or above the age of eight years have similar nutritional requirements to adults. The metabolic and nutritional needs of normal infants are three- to fourfold greater than those for adults. In addition, these needs are further increased after suffering a major injury.

Airway

The first requirement for life is a patent airway. In an unconscious patient, the tongue may fall back to obstruct the airway. Blood, vomitus, loose teeth or foreign bodies need to be removed from the oropharynx. When emergent intubation is indicated, the child should be oxygenated and orotracheal intubation is undertaken with full protection of the cervical spine. The size of the tube can be judged from the fact that the child's nostril is about the same size as the narrowest part of the airway. Guidelines for the size of the endotracheal tube are listed in Table 50.1.

Table 50.1 Size and the depth of insertion of the endotracheal tube in children

Age	Size of the tube (Fr)	Depth of insertion (cm)
Preterm	2.5–3.0, uncuffed	7.5–8
Term	3.0–3.5, uncuffed	9–10
6 m	3.5–4, uncuffed	10
>1 yr	4+(age/4)#, uncuffed	11
>8 yr	4+(age/4)#, cuffed	12+ (age/2)★

\# age in months ÷ 4
★ age in months ÷ 2

Breathing

Mechanical ventilation with a volume-controlled ventilator should be established once the endotracheal tube is secured in proper position. The rate of ventilation is about 20 inspirations per minute for children of school age; 30 per minute for younger children and 40–60 per minute for infants. The tidal volume of 10–15 ml per kg for a child weighing more than 5 kg should be delivered, with 3–5 cm H_2O positive end-expiratory pressure (PEEP). However, PEEP may have deleterious effects on the hypovolaemic child with a pulmonary contusion. In addition, the application of high PEEP with focal lung injury may further aggravate ventilation:perfusion mismatch and exacerbate hypoxia by increasing capillary resistance in the healthy alveoli. There is no evidence that the prophylactic use of PEEP is efficacious in preventing or reducing the severity of posttraumatic respiratory distress syndrome (RDS).

Frequent arterial blood gas monitoring is mandatory. The aim is to maintain PaO_2 at 80–100 mmHg by adjusting the inspiratory quotient, inspiratory pressure and respiratory rate. In the presence of acidosis (arterial pH less than 7.35) with an increased negative base excess, hyperventilation and sodium bicarbonate infusion are required to correct the metabolic derangement. The required dose of $NaHCO_3$ is calculated by the equation:

$$\text{body weight (kg)} \times \text{base excess} \times 0.3.$$

Half of such a dose can be given first, followed by hyperventilation to reduce $PaCO_2$ to 20–25 torr. The remaining half of $NaHCO_3$ can be given later, depending on the blood gas analysis results.

Symptomatic pneumothorax is treated by tube thoracostomy. To avoid possible intraperitoneal penetration through the elevated diaphragm, the tube should be placed in the mid-axillary line above nipple (fourth or fifth intercostal space) and connected to water seal drainage.

Circulation

Adequate circulation is maintained by control of haemorrhage and treatment for shock. Shock following injury should be presumed to be due to blood loss unless proved otherwise. Trauma to the central nervous system rarely, if ever, causes shock. Circulatory collapse due to autonomic response to fear or pain is usually of brief duration and absent by the time the child arrives at the hospital. Shock resulting from infection or sepsis is usually a late complication.

Healthy children possess a remarkable cardiovascular reserve that allows them to compensate for the early effects of haemorrhage, delaying haemodynamic signs of hypovolaemia until relatively late in their physiological decline. When cardiovascular decompensation occurs in children, it is frequently marked by progressive bradycardia. Changes in heart rate, systolic blood pressure and other indices of peripheral circulation, e.g. urine output, need to be monitored frequently. A child's blood volume relates directly to body weight and is estimated to be 80 ml/kg. The upper limits of normal pulse rate are: 160/min for infants; 140/min for children younger than five years; and 120/min for older ones. Normal systolic blood pressure for children aged 1–10 years is [80 + 2 × age (in years)] mmHg. The normal diastolic pressure is usually two-thirds of the systolic pressure (Table 50.2). Hypotension indicates severe blood loss (>45% circulating volume) and is often accompanied by a change of tachycardia to bradycardia.

Table 50.2 Normal blood pressure in children

Age	Systolic pressure (mmHg)	Diastolic pressure (mmHg)
Term (3 kg)	50–70	25–45
Neonate	60–90	20–60
Infant	85–105	50–65
2 yr	95–105★	50–65
7 yr	95–112	55–72
15 yr	112–128	66–80

★ The lower limit of systolic pressure in children > 1 yr is around [70 (2 × age in years)] mmHg

The goals of effective circulatory support are to restore sufficient intravascular volume and prevent further blood loss. Direct pressure over the bleeding sites and elevation of the bleeding part of the body, if possible, may greatly reduce the loss of blood. Bleeding from extremities may be controlled temporarily by the application of a tourniquet or blood pressure cuff using a pressure that exceeds the systolic blood pressure. Once venous access has been established by percutaneous insertion or cutdown of saphenous or antecubital vein, a bolus of warmed crystalloid fluid, preferably Ringer's lactate, should be given at a volume of three times blood loss (i.e. 3 ml Ringer's lactate for every 1 ml of blood loss). Another method of fluid replacement is 'fluid challenge' by rapid infusion of bolus of Ringer's lactate 20 ml/kg, until pulse rate and blood pressure are normalised. After successful resuscitation, a maintenance rate of 1500 ml/m²/24 hours of crystalloid fluid should be given. Fresh whole blood or packed red blood cells should be transfused for children with unstable vital signs despite having been given an amount of Ringer's lactate infusion equal to one-half of the estimated blood loss. Warmed blood components should preferably be given in boluses, the first bolus being 20 ml/kg. Subsequent transfusion is guided by the estimation of blood loss. Transfusion of 10 ml/kg of red blood cells or 20 mg/kg of whole blood for infants over a 2–3 hour period should raise the haemoglobin concentration by 3 g/dl. Urine output and specific gravity measurement are useful indicators of the adequacy of fluid replacement: urine output should be kept above 1–2 ml/kg and specific gravity of urine should be maintained at between 1.010 and 1.015.

NEONATAL INJURY

Birth injuries rarely cause neonatal death or stillbirths. However, some birth injuries may lead to irreversible loss of physiological function that result in the need for prolonged rehabilitation. Birth injuries affect mostly large babies and occur during difficult labours, such as breech delivery and a protracted course of labour. Advances in prenatal imaging studies allow early detection of risk factors for birth trauma, including foetal size, presentation and abnormal masses that may cause obstruction of delivery.

Birth trauma

Two mechanisms lead to birth trauma during labour or the course of delivery: mechanical damage and asphyxia. Larger babies are prone to mechanical damage but premature or malpresented babies may also be susceptible to mechanical injury.

Three types of birth trauma are frequently encountered:

- nerve injury
- bony fracture
- injuries of visceral organs.

Nerve injury

Brachial nerve injury

The most frequently seen neonatal nerve injury is brachial plexus injury resulting in upper limb paralysis or palsy, which can be further classified into three types.

- *Erb–Duchenne palsy*: Erb's palsy involves injury of C5 to C6 and presents with immobilised shoulder, adducted, prone and internally rotated upper limb, with intact hand function and sensation.
- *Klumpke–Dejerine palsy*: Klumpke's palsy involves injury of C6 to T1 and presents with lack of wrist movement and loss of hand grasp. Horner's syndrome may sometimes accompany Klumpke's palsy.

- *Combined Erb–Klumpke palsy*: This is the most severe form of brachial plexus injury, in which both motor and sensory functions of the upper limb are impaired, and is usually accompanied by fractures of the clavicle and humerus, as well as phrenic nerve palsy.

Treatment is supportive and consists primarily of exercise and, in some cases, splinting. The prognosis for either Erb's or Klumpke's palsy is fair for infants who demonstrate an initial improvement within the first two weeks. Most will have full recovery by one month and no later than 5–6 months. If no signs of recovery are noted for those with severe injuries, microsurgical repair of nerves may be considered after six months of age.

Phrenic nerve palsy

Phrenic nerve palsy is almost always caused by overstretching of the anterior roots of C3, C4 and C5, by lateral hyperextension of the neck during breech or forceps delivery. Most cases of phrenic nerve injury are accompanied by ipsilateral Erb's palsy.

Symptoms of phrenic nerve palsy, which include respiratory distress, tachypnoea and episodes of apnoea and cyanosis, may begin on the first day of life, but sometimes may not be evident till one month old. Phrenic nerve injury should be considered in any newborn baby with respiratory distress, especially when there is history of breech or complicated delivery, or association of Erb's palsy.

Diagnosis is mainly made on clinical suspicion and is confirmed by fluoroscopic examination that reveals paradoxical movement of the diaphragm. There is a mediastinal shift to the uninvolved side during inspiration. In addition to respiratory distress, feeding difficulties due to regurgitation may cause failure to thrive. Infants with mild symptoms are observed.

Surgery is indicated for infants with severe pulmonary dysfunction (i.e. atelectasis, recurrent pneumonia or dependence on assisted ventilation), recurrent aspiration due to regurgitation and failed conservative treatment. Occasionally, it is difficult to differentiate congenital diaphragmatic eventration from phrenic nerve palsy. Operative treatment of both conditions consists of plication with or without partial excision of the diaphragm.

Bony fracture

Clavicle

The most frequent site of fracture during labour is the clavicle. Fracture of the clavicle is most commonly associated with shoulder dystocia, breech presentation or large infants. The severity of the condition ranges from an asymptomatic greenstick fracture to a complete fracture that gives rise to local swelling, irritability, decreased motion of the ipsilateral arm and asymmetric Moro reflex. The fracture site is usually at the mid-point or junction of the middle and outer one-third of the clavicle. A greenstick fracture does not require specific treatment. A complete fracture is treated by immobilisation of the arm and shoulder, with the elbow flexed at 90° or more and the arm adducted. Alternatively, a figure-of-eight dressing can be applied for 10–14 days when callus formation is adequate. Return to normal bony contour takes 2–3 months. Prognosis is good.

Humerus and femur

Fracture of the humerus occurs less frequently and fracture of the femur is even rarer. Both types of fractures are usually associated with prolonged labour, breech presentation or rapid extraction of the baby due to foetal distress. After radiological confirmation, the fractured humerus should be immobilised by strapping and wrapping the arm to the side with the elbow flexed at 90°. The fractured femur is immobilised by a posterior splint extending from the buttock to below the knee or alternatively, traction suspension of both the lower limbs with the legs immobilised in a spica cast. The immobilisation period is usually 2–4 weeks. Long-term prognosis in both cases is excellent.

Visceral injury

Injuries of visceral organs from birth trauma are relatively more severe than other birth injuries and can be life-threatening. The liver is most commonly damaged, followed by adrenal glands, spleen and kidney. Visceral injuries are often associated with difficult delivery, large babies or pathologic enlargement of the involved organs. Derangements of the platelet functions and clotting factors are also contributory factors, especially in premature babies. Spontaneous oesophageal or gastric perforation due to increased intraluminal pressure during delivery occurs rarely. Early detection and prompt treatment for visceral organ injuries are important in reversing the adverse outcome. Shock is usually a late sign and is often irreversible. Haemoperitoneum from visceral injuries should be suspected in neonates with abdominal distension, anaemia, a falling haematocrit or the presence of intraperitoneal fluid.

Liver injury

The liver is the most commonly injured abdominal organ from birth trauma with the incidence ranging from 1% to 9% in autopsies of newborn infants. Liver injuries are usually of two types: subcapsular haematoma and, less frequently, liver laceration.

The onset of subcapsular haematoma is often insidious and asymptomatic for several days until the haematoma ruptures. Occasionally, a large subcapsular haematoma presents with abdominal distension, poor feeding, jaundice, tachypnoea, tachycardia, anaemia and a palpable mass at the right upper quadrant.

Manifestation of liver laceration is more acute; profuse haemoperitoneum and shock may develop immediately after birth and the survival of the neonate depends on the alertness of the medical professionals. Management is similar to that for liver injury caused by blunt trauma. If surgery is needed in the newborn patient, associated coagulation defect must be corrected before operation.

Splenic injury

Most splenic injuries due to birth trauma manifest with symptoms and signs that are similar to those of liver injuries. Splenic injuries are usually seen in large babies after a difficult delivery. Nevertheless, a normal labour history does not preclude the presence of splenic injury. Management is similar to that for splenic injury caused by blunt trauma.

Adrenal injury

The adrenal gland is another visceral organ that is vulnerable to birth trauma. Developmentally, the inner part of the cortex, also known as the foetal cortex, undergoes rapid growth toward the termination of pregnancy. Its sinusoidal vasculature is easily distended by blood in the presence of asphyxia or other causes of visceral congestion. The right adrenal gland sits between the liver and vertebrae with its veins draining directly into the inferior vena cava. These unique anatomical characteristics cause increased susceptibility of the adrenal gland, especially the right one, to haemorrhage as a result of asphyxia or increased abdominal pressure from a difficult delivery. Adrenal haemorrhage can present clinically in two forms: subcapsular haemorrhage and adrenal insufficiency (when both glands are involved).

Symptoms of subcapsular haemorrhage usually arise 2–7 days after birth and include poor feeding, irritability, fever, lethargy, abdominal distension, vomiting or diarrhoea. Some of the mild cases will be asymptomatic in the neonatal period and not be noticed until an abdominal radiograph reveals subcapsular calcification. If the blood loss is severe, signs of hypovolaemia and shock may develop. When both glands are involved, signs of adrenal insufficiency such as pyrexia, purpura, convulsion or even coma, hypoglycaemia or hyponatraemia may occur. Abdominal ultrasound (Figure 50.1) and CT scan are diagnostic tools. Treatment depends on the degree of blood loss. Conservative management is adequate for most patients. For severe cases with massive, continuous bleeding retroperitoneally or intraperitoneally, laparotomy for haemostasis and sometimes adrenalectomy are required.

Postpartum iatrogenic trauma

Apart from the aforementioned birth injuries as a result of difficult deliveries, neonatal trauma may also be iatrogenically induced during the postpartum period. The most frequently seen injuries are pneumothorax and tracheobronchial injury caused by respiratory care manoeuvres, such as endotracheal intubation and inappropriate mechanical ventilation. Oesophageal or gastric perforation

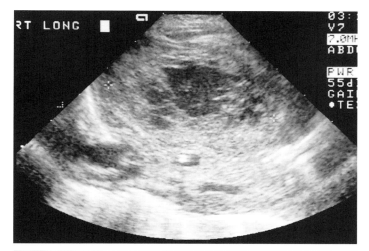

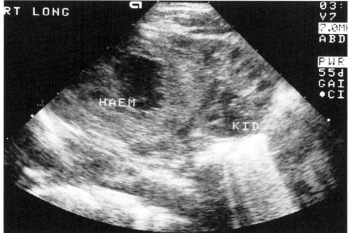

Figure 50.1 Ultrasonography taken in longitudinal plane shows a mixed echogenicity mass with cystic components in the right suprarenal region (*top*) in a neonate with adrenal haemorrhage. Follow-up scan one week later (*bottom*) shows evolution of the mass with increasing cystic change, a feature compatible with liquefaction of an adrenal haematoma (HAEM, haematoma; KID, kidney).

caused by the insertion of a nasogastric tube may also be encountered. The incidence of thrombotic complications after umbilical artery catheterisation has been estimated to be 10–20%. Thrombosis and thrombophlebitis of the umbilical artery can sometimes lead to renal artery occlusion, which may require nephrectomy if medical treatment fails. Other complications from umbilical artery catheterisation include infarction of intraabdominal viscera; pseudoaneurysm of the abdominal aorta; air embolism; haemorrhage; and paraplegia due to lower limb ischaemia. Such complications are also seen in umbilical vein catheterisation.

SPECIFIC INJURIES

Chest injury

The majority of paediatric chest traumatic injuries are blunt injuries, often from falls or traffic accidents. Penetrating thoracic

injury is relatively rare in young children. However, as the chest wall of young children is pliable, severe intrathoracic injuries may occur without detectable external damage or overlying rib fracture. When rib fractures are identified in a child, a high-energy impact can be assumed to have occurred and serious organ injuries should be suspected.

Tension pneumothorax

Tension pneumothorax is the most frequently encountered complication of chest injury and is life-threatening unless treated expeditiously. It can be caused by rib fractures or penetrating injuries, especially stab wounds, resulting in a hyperresonant hemithorax with distant breathing sounds and shifting of the trachea and mediastinum towards the opposite side (Figure 50.2). The shifted mediastinal organs may compress the venous return on the contralateral side, resulting in cardiocirculatory collapse. Physical examination reveals severe respiratory distress, distended neck veins, contralateral trachea deviation, ipsilateral hyperresonance to percussion, decreased breathing sounds and ultimately circulatory collapse. If tension pneumothorax is suspected, a wide-bore needle should be immediately inserted at the mid-axillary line to relieve the pressure. A chest tube should then be inserted and connected to an underwater seal for definite treatment. Gentle suction may be applied if reexpansion of the lung is not satisfactory. If the air leak is rapid and the collapsed lung fails to expand, a tear in the main bronchus or trachea should be suspected. Bronchoscopic evaluation and thoracotomy are therefore indicated.

Haemothorax

Haemothorax may result from pulmonary parenchymal injury due to blunt trauma or penetrating trauma. Fractured ribs may

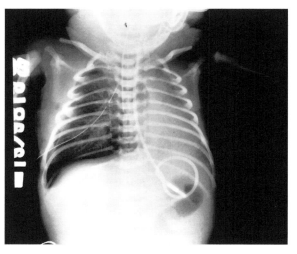

Figure 50.2 Tension pneumothorax. Supine chest radiograph of a neonate shows a right pneumothorax causing shift of the mediastinum to the left. A right chest drain is *in situ* and the right lung is partially expanded.

cause laceration of the lungs, intercostal vessels or internal mammary vessels. Haemothorax may be accompanied by a varying amount of pneumothorax, resulting in a 'haemo-pneumothorax'. Accumulation of a large amount of intrapleural blood may cause compression of the contralateral lung and produce mediastinal shift. As in tension pneumothorax, the immediate goal of management for haemothorax is prompt and complete expansion of the lung. Insertion of a chest tube that is connected to an underwater seal system is the safest way to achieve this. However, if the blood loss from the chest tube exceeds 20 ml/kg, thoracotomy for haemostasis is usually indicated.

Pulmonary contusion

Pulmonary contusion refers to a blunt parenchymal injury that leads to oedema, haemorrhage and desquamative alveolitis; it results from direct transmission of the kinetic energy associated with a severe blunt impact from the overlying chest wall to the underlying lung tissue in the form of a shock wave.

Clinical, radiological and pathological changes similar to those found in the pulmonary contusion may be produced by a variety of causes, resulting in what has been described as 'wet lung', 'traumatic wet lung', 'shock lung' or 'adult respiratory distress syndrome (ARDS)'. The pathophysiology of all these conditions is similar except for the aetiology. Typically, with a resilient chest wall, rib fracture may be absent and the initial chest radiograph may appear normal. Subsequently, severe pulmonary contusion develops over the ensuing 2–3 days and some patients may die of hypoxia. The microscopic characteristics of pulmonary contusion are swelling of endothelial cells of the pulmonary capillaries, followed by leakage of plasma through the endothelial junctions and into the basement membrane and eventually the alveolar spaces. Thus changes in the arterial blood gas analysis may precede clinical and radiographic signs of pulmonary contusion. Initial and serial blood gas determinations are, therefore, recommended for all patients with pulmonary injury. For the same reason, an increased $PAO_2–PaO_2$ (difference in the O_2 pressure between alveoli (A) and arteries (a)) is regarded as a poor early indicator of pulmonary contusion.

The best treatment for pulmonary contusion starts with early recognition. The goals are to:

● prevent clinically significant arterial hypoxaemia with minimal mechanical ventilatory support

● restore lost functional residual capacity and prevent oxygen toxicity

● prevent the progression to ARDS.

PEEP should be used whenever the fraction of inhaled oxygen (FiO_2) required to maintain a PaO_2 of between 70–80 mmHg exceeds 40%. In addition, excessive administration of crystalloid fluid should be avoided. Furthermore, as superimposed lung infection may be life-threatening, administration of broad-spectrum antibiotics is required. The role of corticosteroids in initial therapy remains controversial.

With early recognition and appropriate pulmonary toilet, pulmonary consolidation in patients with minimal pulmonary contusion usually clears within 48–72 hours. If the clinical condition deteriorates, intubation and mechanical ventilatory support are required for at least 48 hours. If a long period of intubation is required, elective tracheostomy should be considered.

Abdominal and pelvic injuries

Splenic injury

The spleen is the solid organ that is most vulnerable to serious trauma in children. Bruises or ecchymoses at the left lower chest wall or left upper quadrant suggest possible splenic injury. Splenic injury in children can occur without rib fracture. Nearly half of all children with a splenic injury have at least one other major injury such as head, chest or musculoskeletal injury.

The typical clinical picture of splenic injury consists of left upper quadrant tenderness and pain that may radiate to the left shoulder. Haemoperitoneum may manifest as abdominal distension, umbilical bruising and, rarely, scrotal bruising as a result of the passage of blood through a patent processus vaginalis. Plain abdominal films are rarely diagnostic. CT scan (Figure 50.3) remains the most reliable and available examination to confirm suspected isolated splenic injury. Typical patterns of splenic injury following blunt abdominal trauma include hilar laceration (the most common type), subcapsular haematoma, splenic fragmentation, and splenic pseudocyst which is likely to be a late sequela of subcapsular haematoma. A varying amount of blood in the peritoneal cavity may be detectable, depending on the type of splenic injuries. Ultrasonography and technetium (Tc9⁹m)

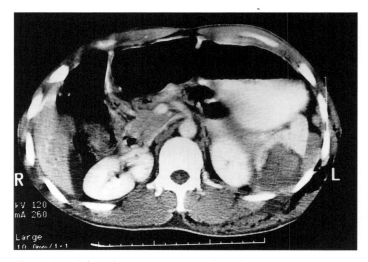

Figure 50.3 Splenic laceration. Contrast-enhanced CT scan in a traumatic patient reveals haemorrhage at the lower pole of the spleen and fluid accumulation at the Morrison pouch.

sulphur colloid scan are alternative imaging modalities. Diagnostic peritoneal lavage can be used to detect haemoperitoneum but is less often practised in children.

Non-operative management of blunt splenic injury in children with blood loss less than 40 ml/kg in the first 24 hours after injury has become the 'gold standard'. Operative management is rarely necessary. The majority of splenic injuries heal spontaneously but require close monitoring and strict bedrest for 3–7 days, followed by three weeks of light activities and three months of non-contact activities. However, splenic lacerations which have ceased bleeding and self-contained subcapsular haematomas may rupture again, usually on the third to fifth day following injury. If bleeding cannot be controlled by conservative treatment, a splenic salvage procedure instead of splenectomy should be attempted, in order to reduce the risks of life-threatening postsplenectomy infection caused by encapsulated bacteria, such as *Streptococcus pneumoniae*, *Haemophilus influenzae*, *Neisseria meningitides*, *Staphylococcus aureus* and *Escherichia coli*. Available options for splenic preservation are segmental resection, splenorrhaphy (suturing with or without omental overlay, application of Vicryl mesh, omental wrap, fibrin sealant or other biological glues) and splenectomy with autotransplantation. Care must be taken to ensure sufficient splenic mass is left behind (at least 50%) to maintain adequate functions. If splenectomy cannot be avoided, omental implantation of splenic remnants fashioned into thin wafers should be performed. Patients who have a splenectomy should be given polyvalent pneumococcal vaccine and maintained prophylactically on long-term oral antibiotic (penicillin).

Liver injury

The liver is the second most commonly injured intraperitoneal organ in paediatric patients and hepatic injury should be considered in all patients with abdominal trauma. The majority of liver injuries in younger children are caused by blunt trauma. Over two-thirds of these children have additional associated injuries, such as head, chest, spleen, renal or long bone fractures. Clinical presentation of liver injuries depends upon the extent of damage and ranges from non-specific abdominal pain to posttraumatic hypovolaemic shock or even cardiac arrest. However, most of the liver injuries encountered in children are minor and may remain undetected unless liver enzymes determinations or imaging studies such as CT scan (Figure 50.4) or ultrasonography are obtained. These children are haemodynamically stable and usually have small capsular lacerations without active bleeding, or self-contained subcapsular haematomas. Non-operative management with close monitoring and bedrest is usually successful.

Generally, children with liver injuries who have no hypovolaemic shock or respond promptly to volume resuscitation will not require laparotomy unless the ongoing blood transfusion requirement exceeds 50% of the estimated intravascular blood volumes (i.e. blood loss greater than 40 ml/kg in the first 24 hours after injury). Most non-operative treatment failures occur in the first

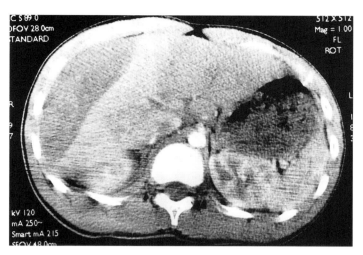

Figure 50.4 Contrast-enhanced CT scan of the liver shows a large subcapsular haematoma. Central hyperdensities are due to more acute haemorrhage.

24–48 hours after the liver injury. For large stellate lacerations and subcapsular haematomas which have eroded through the Glisson's capsule, bleeding usually cannot be stopped without surgical intervention. Lacerations requiring laparotomy can usually be managed by suture repair and drainage. Resection of the liver is rarely required. Uncontrolled bleeding may require initial packing for liver laceration to restore haemodynamic stability. The child should then be transferred to a specialist centre for a second laparotomy. Approximately 2–5% of children with liver injuries have associated injury to the retrohepatic vena cava or hepatic vein. Management of retrohepatic venous injuries is difficult and is associated with a mortality rate of more than 50%. Late haemorrhage occasionally complicates non-operated management of blunt hepatic trauma and should be suspected when right abdominal and shoulder pain persists in children with severe hepatic trauma and high injury severity scores. Children who have non-operative treatment for liver injuries are usually advised to avoid contact sports for at least 3–6 weeks.

Another recognised late complication of hepatic injury is haemobilia, which results from rupture of a traumatic pseudoaneurysm of the hepatic arterial branch into the biliary trees. Bleeding may occur days or even months after liver injury without any warning signs. Mortality is reported as high as 25%. Surgery (hepatic artery ligation, lobectomy, direct ligation of the bleeding vessel) provides good results. Recent results of angiography to embolise the bleeding vessels are encouraging.

Kidney injury

The kidney is the third most common solid organ to be injured by blunt trauma in childhood, after the spleen and liver. Over 75% of the blunt renal injuries result from traffic accidents. Other causes include falls from a height and sports-related injuries. Up to 10% of children with a renal injury were found to have pre-existing congenital anomalies, including pelviureteric junction obstruction, horseshoe kidney, floating kidney, pelvic kidney and an unsuspected Wilms' tumour.

Renal injury can be classified into five categories:

- renal parenchymal contusion
- laceration
- transection
- fragmentation
- renal pedicle injury.

Over 80% of all renal injuries are contusions or lacerations. Flank pain, tenderness and a mass are classic findings of renal injuries, but sometimes they are difficult to elicit in children. The diagnosis of renal injury is therefore usually heralded by the presence of substantial haematuria. The degree of haematuria has no direct correlation with the severity of renal injury.

Ultrasonography is a useful initial screening procedure and provides rapid assessment, but abdominal CT with intravenous contrast is the choice of imaging study for major abdominal injuries, including renal injury. Intravenous pyelography (IVP) remains a useful tool in the evaluation of asymptomatic haematuria in the setting of minimal trauma but findings such as delayed function or poor visualisation are sometimes non-specific. A normal functioning contralateral kidney is an important consideration if surgery to the injured kidney becomes necessary.

CT findings of renal trauma are graded as follows.

- Grade 1: small parenchymal injury without subcapsular or perirenal fluid collection
- Grade 2: incomplete renal laceration with subcapsular or small perinephric collection (Figure 50.5)
- Grade 3: extensive laceration or fracture with large perinephric fluid accumulation
- Grade 4: multiple fragments
- Grade 5: vascular injury

Most blunt renal injuries are grade 1 or 2 and can be managed conservatively: close observation and bedrest until the gross haematuria clears and limited activity until microscopic haematuria disappears.

The management of grade 3 and 4 renal injuries remains controversial and may take the form of either conservative measures or immediate surgical repair, in which the principal guide to management is optimal preservation of renal tissue and function without endangering the health of the child.

Surgery is indicated for grade 5 injury, especially when accompanied by hypotension or shock. If the renal ischaemic time is less than two hours, repair of the injured renal vessels should be considered in order to preserve the kidney. If the kidney has been ischaemic for more than two hours, nephrectomy may be necessary.

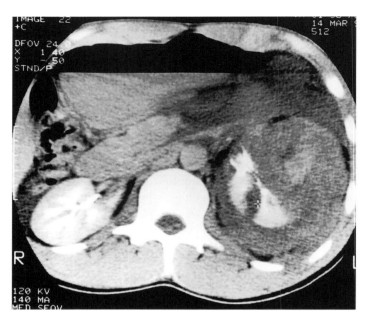

Figure 50.5 Contrast-enhanced CT scan taken at the level of the renal hilum shows a large haematoma from a grade 2 fracture at the mid-pole of the left kidney.

Ureter and bladder injury

Ureteric injury in childhood after blunt injury is relatively rare. It may occur as disruption of the pelviureteric junction in blunt abdominal injury or disruption of the vesicoureteric junction in pelvic fracture. Ureteric leakage may result in massive retroperitoneal accumulation of urine and peritonitis may ensue. Early retroperitoneal repair of the disrupted ureter should be performed after confirmation of the diagnosis by CT scan or IVP.

Bladder injury in childhood may be caused by two mechanisms:

- burst-out rupture, most often at the dome of the distended bladder after blunt trauma
- bladder laceration after pelvic fracture, which is usually associated with urethral injury.

Diagnosis of bladder injury depends on visualisation of contrast extravasation in retrograde cystography (RC). If an associated urethral injury makes RC difficult, suprapubic cystography or IVP are the alternatives. Rupture of the bladder due to blunt injury can be treated with Foley catheterisation for urinary drainage because urinary extravasation is mainly extraperitoneal. In the case of intraperitoneal urinary leakage and penetration-induced bladder perforation, surgical exploration for repair is indicated.

Urethral injury

Urethral injuries in the paediatric population are mainly due to blunt trauma from a pelvic fracture or a straddle injury. Some are caused iatrogenically, such as during insertion of endoscopes or placement of catheters. Most of these injuries are at the membranous urethra in males.

Typical presentation of urethral injuries includes blood at the meatus or a perineal haematoma. In males, if the haematoma ruptures through the penile fascia (Buck's fascia), the haematoma will spread over the perineum, scrotum and lower abdominal wall. Diagnosis of urethral injury depends on imaging studies such as retrograde urethrography (Figure 50.6) or voiding cysto-urethrography (VCUG). Depending on the findings, a urinary catheter can be inserted for stenting and relieving the difficulties in urination. If there is resistance, suprapubic cystostomy or antegrade insertion of a urinary catheter through bladder to the urethra should be considered. Most incomplete urethral disruption injuries can be managed by urethral splinting by the urinary catheters for 2–3 weeks. Complete urethral disruption is indicated by extravasation of contrast material and inability to pass the catheter through the urethra in acute stage. Management involves suprapubic urinary diversion followed 3–6 months later by surgical repair.

Urethral injuries caused by pelvic fracture may be complicated by injuries at the bladder neck and laceration of the anterior rectal wall. Laceration may cause rectourethral fistulas in males and rectovaginal fistulas in females.

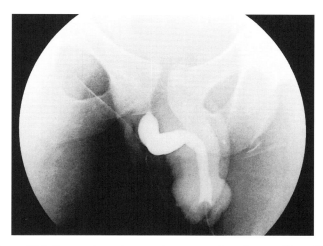

Figure 50.6 Retrograde urethrogram in a teenage boy after a traffic accident shows disruption of the contrast flow at the bulbar urethra, indicating urethral injury and transection.

Gastrointestinal tract injury

Perforation or haemorrhage of the GI tract resulting from penetrating trauma is not difficult to recognise clinically and should be managed by prompt laparotomy. Blunt trauma resulting in GI tract injury, on the other hand, may be difficult to diagnose and repeated examinations are often necessary. Diagnosis is made by a combination of clinical suspicion and radiographic/CT findings of pneumoperitoneum, bowel wall oedema or unexplained free fluid. The majority of GI tract injuries are caused by energy transfer at a discrete point. These include injury from a seat belt or

bicycle handle bar (typically causing duodenal and pancreatic injuries as well) or a blow (non-accidental injury). The types of injuries include perforation, avulsion (GI tract/mesenteric vessels), intramural haematomas and contusions. The most common site of injury is the small bowel, followed by the duodenum, colon and stomach in that order. Intestinal perforation and avulsion are treated by laparotomy, repair or resection. Duodenal haematoma usually responds to conservative treatment and a short course of total parenteral nutrition.

Pancreatic injury

Pancreatic injury is uncommon in children and results from blunt epigastric trauma, e.g. a fall onto a bicycle handle bar. Epigastric bruising and tenderness are typical findings, with an elevated serum amylase level. The initial serum amylase level, however, does not always correlate with the severity of pancreatic injury and in some cases may even be normal. Serial biochemistry and imaging studies (ultrasonography, CT scan, magnetic resonance cholangiopancreatography (MRCP) and/or endoscopic retrograde cholangiopancreatography (ERCP)) are helpful in the management of pancreatic injuries. The majority of pancreatic injuries are low grade and can be managed non-operatively by bowel rest and total parenteral nutrition with or without somatostatin analogue. Pseudocysts need to be drained internally. Penetrating or main ductal injuries require surgical intervention. Distal duct injuries are managed by spleen-sparing distal pancreatectomy whereas proximal duct injuries are managed non-operatively initially with drainage of the pseudocyst subsequently.

Head injury

A newborn infant may suffer from a skull fracture or cephalhaematoma (either subgaleal or subperiosteal) secondary to natural birth trauma or instrument delivery. Blood loss may be significant in relation to body size and may result in shock. Before the age of two, minor trauma rarely results in brain injury. However, a high-speed impact or child abuse may cause intracranial haemorrhage which, in turn, is often associated with bilateral chronic haematoma and retinal haemorrhage. These traumas are often the result of angular acceleration–deceleration of the relatively large head, i.e. shaken baby syndrome.

Older children are more prone to minor head injuries and early posttraumatic seizures which do not require long-term medical treatment are common. In some instances, skull fractures may fail to heal because of the rapidly growing brain (so-called 'growing skull fracture'). This may present as an expanding scalp mass with herniating leptomeningeal cyst.

The response to head injury in young adolescents is similar to adults although fatal brain swelling may sometimes develop due to acute hyperaemia. As a group, children fare better than adults with head injury. The outcome is closely related to the initial neurological state and is worse below the age of three and when associated with shock. In the management of head trauma, the need to be aware of other associated injuries, e.g. cervical spine injury, chest injuries and abdominal injuries, cannot be overemphasised.

OTHER INJURIES

Injuries of extremities

Fractures in children are different from fractures in adults. In children the bones are incompletely ossified and are more elastic, requiring a much stronger impact to result in fractures. Furthermore, because children are growing, treatment of fractures involving growth centres can be difficult.

Fractures of the wrist are the commonest fractures in childhood. Usually these are greenstick fractures which often do not need repositioning. Growth will often correct any large deformity arising from this kind of fracture. Supracondylar humeral fractures are also relatively common in children. Operative reduction of the fracture and K-wire stabilisation are often needed, though Volkmann's contracture is a well-known complication due to ischaemia of the forearm muscles. Femoral fractures and forearm fractures are seen in every age group. Modern treatment includes intramedullary nailing.

Non-accidental injury

Non-accidental injury (the battered/abused child syndrome) is intentional injury of the child by parents, guardians or acquaintances and often occurs in the first year of life. As the pattern of offence is often repetitive, failure to recognise non-accidental injury may result in preventable death. The history may be suspicious: discordance between history and severity of injury, inexplicable delay in seeking medical treatment, history of repeated trauma, inappropriate parenteral response and discrepancies in history given by different child carers. The findings may include multiple subdural haematomas, retinal haemorrhage, perineal/perioral injuries, major internal organ injuries without explicable trauma, cigarette burns, old scars and healed fractures, indicating previous frequent injuries. All suspected cases of non-accidental injury should be reported to the appropriate authorities, including social services and the police.

FURTHER READING

Allen GS, Cox CS Jr, Moore FA, Duk JH. Pulmonary contusion: are children different? *J Am Coll Surg* 1997; **185**:229–233

American College of Surgeons. *Advanced Trauma Life-Support Program Manual.* Washington DC: ACS, 1993; 261–281

Bond SJ, Eichelberger MR, Gotschall CS, Sivit CJ, Randolph JG. Nonoperative management of blunt hepatic and splenic injury in children. *Ann Surg* 1996; **223**:286–289

Firstenberg MS, Volsko TA, Sivit C, Stallion A, Dudgeon DL, Grisoni ER. Selective management of pediatric pancreatic injuries. *J Pediatr Surg* 1999; **34**:1142–1147

Hidalgo F, Narvaez JA, Rene M, Dominguez J, Sancho C, Montanya X. Treatment of hemobilia with selective hepatic artery embolization. *J Vasc Interv Radiol* 1995; **6**:793–798

Li-Ling J, Irving M. Somatostatin and octreotide in the prevention of postoperative pancreatic complications and the treatment of enterocutaneous pancreatic fistulas: a systematic review of randomized controlled trials. *Br J Surg* 2001; **88**:190–199

Shilyansky J, Pearl RH, Kreller M, Sena LM, Babyn PS. Diagnosis and management of duodenal injuries in children. *J Pediatr Surg* 1997; **32**:880–886

51

Paediatric tumours

Paul K.H. Tam, Steve C.L. Lin

INTRODUCTION

Cancer is the leading cause disease of death in children between the ages of one and 15 years. Whereas leukaemia and brain tumours are the most common paediatric cancers, neuroblastoma is the most commonly encountered solid tumour in infants, followed by Wilms' tumour, rhabdomyosarcoma and hepatoblastoma. In recent years, it has been noted that the incidence of cancer in infants has increased. However, because of the refinement in combined treatment modalities, including surgery, chemotherapy and radiotherapy, nowadays the overall survival rate for infants and children with cancers at all sites has been improved to 75%, in comparison with less than 50% in the 1960s. The current five-year survival rate for Wilms' tumour is 88–90%, neuroblastoma 45%, rhabdomyosarcoma 73%, hepatoblastoma 62%, hepatocellular carcinoma 21% and germ cell tumour 65%.

Both environmental and host factors contribute to the development of paediatric cancers. In recent years, genetic mechanisms have attracted the attention of paediatric oncologists because accumulating evidence suggests that genetic changes are intimately involved in the pathogenesis of cancers. Identification of oncogenes, antioncogenes, tumour markers and other biological factors has helped risk classification of specific tumours and provide predictors of outcome.

WILMS' TUMOUR

Pathology

Wilms' tumour, or nephroblastoma, is an embryonal renal tumour that usually presents as a large, solitary, asymptomatic mass in the flank or upper abdomen. It is usually sharply demarcated and variably encapsulated but can invade neighbouring tissues, especially the renal vein, resulting in distortion of the renal outline and compression of the normal renal tissue to a thin rim. Microscopically it contains a mixture of primitive renal parenchymal cells, stromal cells, tubules and glomeruloid features (Figure 51.1). Wilms' tumour with favourable histology generally has a microscopic picture of both stromal and epithelial elements. Three unfavourable histologic patterns associated with aggressive biological behaviour are found in 10% of patients: anaplastic, rhabdoid and clear cell type. The rhabdoid sarcomatous type frequently metastasises to the brain and the clear cell type usually spreads to the bone.

Incidence

The incidence of Wilms' tumour is estimated as 7.8/million under the age of 15 years. It is the most common renal neoplasm in childhood and affects both sexes equally. Eighty percent of patients present before the age of five years with the peak age of incidence at three years. The left kidney is more often involved

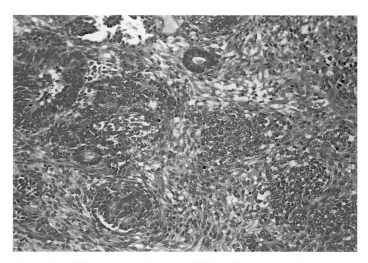

Figure 51.1 Wilms' tumour. This is a 'small blue cell' tumour which has a hyperchromatic blastemal stroma, primitive tubules and glomeruloid features.

than the right. Synchronous bilateral Wilms' tumour occurs in 5–6% of patients, with metachronous lesions in only 1%. Intraoperative examination of the contralateral kidney, therefore, should be regarded as a routine necessity during surgical exploration.

Associated anomalies

An important feature of Wilms' tumour is its frequent association with other anomalies, including congenital aniridia (aniridia-Wilms' syndrome; about 1.1 % of all Wilms' tumour patients), hemihypertrophy (3% of patients with Wilms' tumour) and genitourinary anomalies (4.5% of patients with Wilms' tumour) such as hypospadias, undescended testes, gonadal dysgenesis, duplex kidney, etc. Beckwith–Wiedemann syndrome (BWS), i.e. exomphalos-macroglossia-gigantism, is a renal disorder characterised by abnormal growth of renal, pancreatic, hepatic or other somatic tissues (hemihypertrophy). The incidence of tumour development in BWS is around 10–20%, including Wilms' tumour, hepatoblastoma and adrenocortical tumours. Patients with bilateral or familial diseases have a higher incidence of association with other congenital anomalies.

Loss of heterozygosity of the WT (Wilms' tumour) 1 gene on chromosome 11p13 is found in half of patients with Wilms' tumour. The WT2 gene is located on chromosome 11p15 and is associated with BWS. Chromosomes 16q and 1p are also associated with Wilms' tumour. Resistance to chemotherapy may be linked to the multidrug-resistant gene MDRG-1.

Clinical picture

The most common presentation for children with Wilms' tumour is an asymptomatic abdominal mass, often detected incidentally by a family member or physician. The mass is usually large and crosses the mid-line. Occasionally the child presents with haematuria (25% of children at diagnosis). Other symptoms are non-specific, such as abdominal pain mimicking appendicitis, abdominal fullness, acute abdominal pain (resulting from tumour rupture and haemorrhage), gastrointestinal upset, fever, weight loss, malaise and anaemia. Rarely, vascular extension of Wilms' tumour into the left renal vein results in left varicocele; occlusion of the hepatic vein may cause hepatomegaly and ascites. Hypertension may be present in 25–50% of patients and in part may be due to the renin production in response to ischaemia by tumour compression.

Investigations

Generally imaging studies cannot always reliably establish the correct preoperative diagnosis for a renal mass in children. However, ultrasonography is the first investigative tool for evaluation of a renal mass to determine if the mass is solid or cystic (e.g. multicystic kidney or hydronephrosis). Ultrasonography may also help to detect a tumour in the contralateral kidney, tumour thrombi in the renal vein or inferior vena cava and abdominal metastasis. Plain abdominal radiography usually reveals a soft tissue shadow without calcification. Abdominal CT scan with contrast can show an intrarenal neoplasm that displaces the collecting system medially and there is usually a sharp distinction between the tumour and normal renal parenchyma (Figure 51.2). CT scan can also indicate if there is tumour invasion of the perirenal fat, involvement of regional lymph nodes, tumour extension into the renal vein and vena cava and liver metastasis. In the absence of a CT scan, intravenous urography can be diagnostic and may reveal distortion of the renal contour with splaying of the calyceal system. A chest radiograph or CT should always be performed to detect possible pulmonary metastasis, which may be evident in 10–15% of patients at the time of diagnosis. Echocardiography is indicated if tumour extension into the right atrium is suspected.

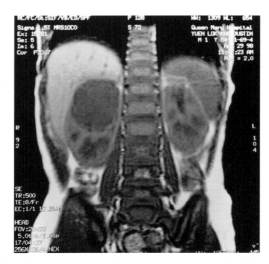

Figure 51.2 Contrast-enhanced CT scan (coronal section) of a Wilms' tumour (nephroblastoma) at right upper kidney. Normal renal parenchyma is still visible at the lower part.

Staging

The staging system designed by the National Wilms' Tumour Study (NWTS) mainly depends on the surgical findings at laparotomy and light-microscopic features. Factors determining the staging include the extension of disease, resectability of the primary tumour, the involvement of perirenal fat, capsule and lymph nodes, tumour histology, the presence of distant metastasis or contralateral involvement (Box 51.1).

Box 51.1	NWTS Wilms' tumour staging system
I	Tumour limited to kidney and completely excised
II	Tumour extends beyond the kidney but is completely excised
III	Residual non-haematogenous tumour confined to abdomen (lymph node involvement, diffuse tumour spillage, peritoneal implants, incomplete resection)
IV	Haematogenous metastasis
V	Bilateral renal involvement at diagnosis

Treatment

Treatment of Wilms' tumour is multimodal and is dependent on staging and histology. Box 51.2 lists the recommended treatment regimen of Wilms' tumour. Surgical removal of the involved kidney without spillage is still the mainstay of treatment even when pulmonary metastasis is present. The contralateral kidney, para-aortic lymph nodes, renal vein and inferior vena cava should be carefully inspected. The renal vein should be clamped before any manipulation of the affected kidney commences. Any suspicious para-aortic lymph node should be removed. If there is no gross involvement, at least one para-aortic lymph node should be sampled. The inferior vena cava should be controlled and opened if tumour thrombi extend from the renal vein to the inferior vena cava. Surgical excision of extensive neoplastic thrombus with cardiopulmonary bypass is suggested in the case of life-threatening thrombosis in the right atrium.

Box 51.2	Recommended treatment of Wilms' tumour
Favourable histology	
Stage I	Surgery and chemotherapy for 10 weeks to 6 months
Stage II	Surgery and chemotherapy for 18 months
Stage III	Surgery and radiotherapy (10–20 Gy) and chemotherapy for 15 months
Unfavourable histology (any stage) and all stage IV	
Surgery, radiotherapy (20 Gy) and chemotherapy for 18 months	

Wilms' tumour is sensitive to both radiotherapy and chemotherapy. Postoperative radiotherapy is usually effective but the delayed side effects on the growth of bones and soft tissues have limited its application. Instead, postoperative adjuvant chemotherapy including vincristine and actinomycin-D has become an integral part of treatment of Wilms' tumour.

Adriamycin has also been used on high-risk patients. In selected patients, preoperative chemotherapy could be used to reduce the size of the tumour, especially in patients with bilateral diseases.

Bilateral Wilms' tumour (stage V)

Bilateral disease occurs in 6% (synchonous, 5%; metachronous, 1%) of patients; the incidence increases to 20% in familial cases. Treatment has to be tailored for each patient. Primary resection of bilateral tumours has a survival rate comparable to that of resection after preoperative chemotherapy, but the latter approach increases the likelihood of sparing more normal renal tissues. Thus, preoperative chemotherapy followed by nephron-sparing surgery is indicated in patients with bilateral Wilms' tumour, while in those with diffuse anaplasia nephron-sparing surgery is contraindicated. The NWTS-5 suggests that for bilateral tumours initial biopsy should be performed followed by preoperative chemotherapy. Radical resection should not be performed in the first setting. At the completion of chemotherapy, a second-look laparotomy is performed for partial nephrectomies or wedge resections if negative margins can be obtained. In patients who require bilateral nephrectomies, haemodialysis should be performed. Renal transplantation should be delayed for at least two years after nephrectomy to ensure there is no evidence of recurrence.

Prognosis

Overall survival rate for Wilms' tumour is around 90%. The most important prognostic variables are histology, stage and age of onset. Onset before the age of two years is associated with a better prognosis. With favourable histology, four-year survival rate in stage I is 97%; stage II, 95%; stage III, 91%; stage IV, 87%. With unfavourable histology, four-year survival rate is: stage I–III, 68%; stage IV, 58%. Patients with stage V (bilateral tumours) have a survival rate similar to that of stage II disease. Any relapse or recurrence carries a poorer prognosis.

Mesoblastic nephroma

Congenital mesoblastic nephroma was initially regarded as a variant of Wilms' tumour, but now has been classified as a separate identity. It usually presents as a bulky, firm, solitary and infiltrative renal mass in the neonatal period and accounts for the majority of antenatally detected renal neoplasms. This tumour is benign in nature, therefore surgical removal represents adequate treatment. Ultrasonography and CT scan are useful in delineation but differentiation from Wilms' tumour is difficult from image studies (Figure 51.3). Prognosis of mesoblastic nephroma is excellent (virtually 100% survival). Chemotherapy or radiotherapy is usually not required.

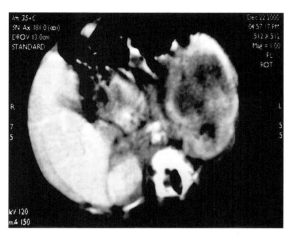

Figure 51.3 Contrast-enhanced CT scan of a newborn baby with a congenital mesoblastic nephroma of the left kidney. Heterogenous contrast enhancement and central hypodense areas are noted within the tumour.

NEUROBLASTOMA

Pathology

Neuroblastoma is the second most common solid malignant tumour of infancy and childhood after brain tumours, representing about 10% of all childhood tumours. It arises from the neural crest and therefore may occur in the adrenal medulla or in any part of the sympathetic chain from brain, neck, mediastinum, para-aortic sympathetic ganglion to the pelvis. The majority of neuroblastomas arise in the abdomen (75%), followed by the chest (15–20%) and the neck and pelvis (5–10%).

Grossly most neuroblastomas are usually big in size, with a lobulated appearance and an uneven surface. Tumours that are composed mainly of immature cells appear purple red or dark brown in colour, are fragile with high vascularity and are vulnerable to haemorrhage and cystic changes internally. In contrast, tumours consisting mainly of mature cells look greyish white or light yellow and appear in a more solid form. Internal calcification of the mature neuroblastoma cells also contributes to the hard-core consistency of the tumours. Microscopically, neuroblastoma is composed of small round blue cells with scanty cytoplasm and neurofibrillary matrix (Figure 51.4). Cells are usually arranged in rosettes (Homer–Wright pseudorosettes) with fine nerve fibres in the centres. The degree of differentiation varies widely among different neural crest tumours. At the mature end of such a spectrum is the benign ganglioneuroma, which is composed primarily of mature ganglion cells, Schwann's cells and neuropils. At the other end is the immature, anaplastic neuroblastoma.

Virtually all foetal adrenal tissues studied at the 17th to 20th weeks of gestational age contain neuroblastoma *in situ* but only 0.4–3% of the adrenal glands from infants less than three months old show the presence of neuroblastoma cells. Neuroblastomas *in situ*, therefore, may undergo spontaneous regression with differentiation.

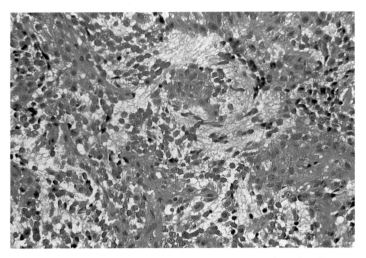

Figure 51.4 A neuroblastoma in which there is an intermingling of small hyperchromatic cells with a pale neurofibrillary matrix. Rosette formation is noted in the centre and ganglion cells are not identified in this area.

Clinical tumour development may be due to defective regression or malignant differentiation.

Neuroblastomas can produce and secrete hormones such as vasoactive intestinal polypeptide (VIP) and vasoactive substances including the catecholamines and their byproducts (vanillylmandelic acid, VMA; homovanillic acid, HVA; metanephrines and dopamine). VMA and HVA have been used as tumour markers for neuroblastomas. VMA is derived from norepinephrine that is secreted by more differentiated neuroblastomas and it indicates a better prognosis if the ratio of VMA to HVA is greater than 1. Neurone-specific enolase (NSE) has also been used as a tumour marker and can be identified immunohistochemically by special staining (Figure 51.5). Distant metastasis of neuroblastoma usually is accompanied by an increased level of serum ferritin and lactate dehydrogenase (LDH). Ten percent of the neuroblastomas secrete acetylcholine (ACh) instead of HVA or VMA and behave in a more malignant manner with a poorer prognosis.

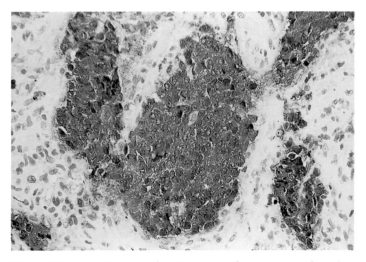

Figure 51.5 A neuroblastoma with positive staining for neurone-specific enolase.

Incidence

Neuroblastomas occur more frequently in boys (2:1) and the incidence is reported as 8.5–9.6 in a million. Ninety percent of the patients are under eight years old and over half are under two years of age. Neuroblastoma is also the most common intra-abdominal malignancy in neonates. Familial occurrence has been reported.

Associated anomalies

Neuroblastomas have been associated with other genetic diseases: Beckwith–Wiedemann syndrome, Hirschsprung's disease, Klippel–Feil syndrome (short, immobile neck due to cervical vertebral fusion), di George syndrome, Ondine's curse and trisomy 18.

Clinical picture

Clinical presentation of neuroblastoma is mainly determined by the location of the primary lesion and the presence of metastasis. A palpable abdominal mass is noted in over 50% of the patients from a primary adrenal or paraspinal tumour and may be accompanied by non-specific symptoms such as weight loss, failure to thrive, nausea, vomiting, fever, anorexia, abdominal fullness or pain. Gastrointestinal obstruction is uncommon. A paraspinal tumour may extend through the vertebral foramen (dumb-bell tumour) and cause neurological deficits ranging from radiculopathy to paraplegia. Cervical neuroblastoma usually presents as a neck mass and may result in Horner's syndrome if the stellate ganglion is involved. Intrathoracic neuroblastoma may cause respiratory symptoms but more frequently is diagnosed from a chest radiograph for unrelated reasons. Pelvic tumours may cause disturbances of urinary function and defaecation. Rarely, intractable diarrhoea or hypertension due to the secretion of VIP and catecholamine, respectively, may be present.

At the time of diagnosis, about one-third of patients have lymphatic metastasis and more than half have haematogenous spread, which gives rise to symptoms such as bone pain, subcutaneous nodules, jaundice, lymphadenopathy and limping. Rarely, the patient may develop acute cerebellar encephalopathy, a paraneoplastic syndrome associated with neuroblastoma, manifested as opsomyoclonus (the 'dancing eye', cerebellar ataxia and dementia).

Investigations

Up to 95% of neuroblastomas produce detectable urinary levels of the catecholamine metabolites HVA and VMA. Analysis of these two chemicals in a 24-hour urine collection aids in the diagnosis and the detection of recurrence. Elevated serum levels of NSE have been found in neuroblastomas and are directly proportional to the staging.

Plain radiography can reveal stippled calcification in a posterior mediastinal mass, an abdominal mass or a cortical bone lesion. Bone scan is an important tool in detecting cortical bone metastasis (Figure 51.6). Ultrasonography can distinguish neuroblastomas, solid and extrarenal, from cystic lesions and renal tumours. CT

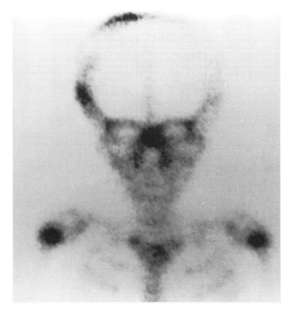

Figure 51.6 99mTc-MDP bone scan of a neuroblastoma patient showing increased uptake at right parietal and right occipital skull, indicating bony metastasis.

scan and MRI can disclose the extent of the primary tumour and lymph node (Figure 51.7) or vessel involvement (Figure 51.8), and the presence of metastasis on either side of the diaphragm or within the head and neck. Meta-iodobenzylguanindine (MIBG) has a molecular structure similar to that of adrenaline and is specifically taken up by neurodermal tumours. [I131]-MIBG scan can identify primary disease and differentiate cortical disease from

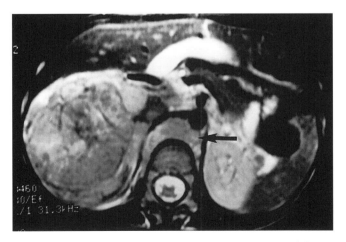

Figure 51.7 Axial T2-weighted MRI of the right neuroblastoma with heterogenously hyperintense signals. The normal kidney is compressed posteriorly and the pancreas is displaced anteriorly. Note the hyperintense enlarged retrocrural lymph node (arrow).

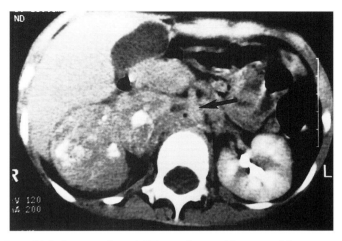

Figure 51.8 Contrast-enhanced CT scan of a neuroblastoma at right suprarenal region with central calcification, crossing the mid-line and encasing the origin of the superior mesenteric artery (arrow).

normal bone (Figure 51.9), and therefore is a sensitive and specific method of assessing primary, residual, metastatic or recurrent neuroblastoma. Radiolabelled monoclonal antibody scanning has been used for the detection of marrow metastasis and seems to be more specific than CT and MRI. Surgical biopsy of the primary tumour or occasionally of the skin nodules or lymph nodes is usually required for histological diagnosis and evaluation of tumour biology. Bone marrow aspiration from both the anterior or posterior iliac crests is also helpful for determination of staging.

Staging

Currently the Shimada pathologic classification divides neuroblastomas into stroma-rich and stroma-poor categories, with

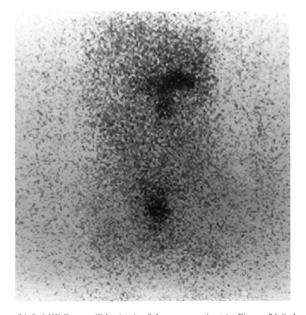

Figure 51.9 MIBG scan (PA view) of the same patient in Figure 51.8 showing uptake in the neuroblastoma at right adrenal region.

prognostic value (Table 51.1). Stroma-rich tumours contain Schwann-like spindle cell stroma with the appearance of a ganglioneuroblastoma and have a favourable prognosis. Unfavourable stroma-rich tumours usually have a nodular appearance. The prognosis of stroma-poor tumours depends on three parameters: age at diagnosis, differentiation of neuroblast cells and the mitosis-karyorrhexis index (MKI). The MKI refers to the sum of a variety of nuclear abnormalities including the

number of necrotic tumour cells, the number of cells with mitotic activities and the number of cells with malformed, lobulated or pyknotic nuclei.

Staging of neuroblastomas is determined by preoperative clinical and operative criteria, which includes the Evans, St Jude, Paediatric Oncology Group, and International neuroblastoma staging systems. Among these, the Evans and the International neuroblastoma staging systems (Table 51.2) have been long used. All these systems are in basic agreement regarding the categorisation of a localised completely resected tumour, distant metastasis to bony cortex and infants less than one year of age with subcutaneous nodules, involvement of liver and bone marrow but no bony cortex metastasis.

Treatment

Treatment of neuroblastoma is based on the stage of the tumour. The present recommended treatment regimen is listed in Table 51.3. Generally, the mainstay of treatment for stages I and II is complete surgical resection. Stages III and IV are treated with

Table 51.1 Shimada pathologic classification system of neuroblastoma

	Favourable histology	Unfavourable histology
Stroma rich	Well differentiated all ages, no nodular pattern	All ages, nodular pattern (+)
Stroma poor		
Age <18 mo	MKI*<200	MKI<100
Age 18 mo–5 yr	MKI>100	MKI<100
	Differentiated	Undifferentiated
Age >5 yr	None	All

*MKI, mitosis-karyorrhexis index (number of mitoses and karyorrhexis /5000 cells)

Table 51.2 Evans and International neuroblastoma staging systems

Stage	Evans staging system	International staging system
I	Tumour confined to the organ or structure of origin	Localised tumour with complete gross excision, with or without microscopic residual disease; representative ipsilateral lymph nodes negative for tumour microscopically (nodes attached to and removed with the primary tumour may be positive)
II	Tumour extending in continuity beyond the organ or structure of origin but not crossing the mid-line. Regional lymph nodes on the homolateral side may be involved	Stage IIA: localised tumour with incomplete gross excision; representative ipsilateral non-adherent lymph nodes negative for tumour microscopically

Stage IIB: localised tumour with or without complete gross excision, with ipsilateral non-adherent lymph nodes positive for tumour. Enlarged contralateral lymph nodes must be negative microscopically |
III	Tumor invasively extending in continuity beyond the mid-line. Regional lymph nodes may be involved bilaterally	Unresectable unilateral tumour infiltrating across the mid-line, with or without regional lymph node involvement; or localised unilateral tumour with contralateral regional lymph node involvement; or mid-line tumour with bilateral extension by infiltration (unresectable) or by lymph node involvement. The mid-line is defined as the vertebral column. Tumours originating on one side and crossing the mid-line must infiltrate to or beyond the opposite side of the vertebral column
IV	Remote disease involving skeleton, parenchymatous organs, soft tissues, distant lymph node groups, etc.	Any primary tumour with dissemination to distant lymph nodes, bone, bone marrow, liver, skin and/or other organs (except as defined for stage IVs)
IVs	Patients who would otherwise be stage I or II but have remote disease confined to one or more of the following sites only: liver, skin or bone marrow (without radiographic evidence of bone metastases on complete skeletal survey)	Localised primary tumour (as defined for stage I, IIA or IIB), with dissemination limited to skin, liver and/or bone marrow (limited to infants less than 1 year of age). Marrow involvement should be minimal (i.e. <10% of total nucleated cells identified as malignant by bone biopsy or bone marrow aspirate). More extensive bone marrow involvement would be considered to be stage IV disease. The results of the MIBG scan (if performed) should be negative for disease in the bone marrow

Table 51.3 Recommended treatment regimens for neuroblastoma

Stage	Treatment regimens
I	Total excision alone
II	Total excision ± postoperative radiotherapy and/or chemotherapy
III	Resectable tumours: excision + chemotherapy + radiotherapy Unresectable tumours: cytoreduction with chemo- and radiotherapy, followed by excision of shrunken tumour
IV	Combination chemotherapy, and may be followed by surgical excision for those responding to chemotherapy (delayed primary excision)
IVs	Excision of primary tumour. Occasionally respiratory distress may develop from a rapidly enlarging liver, which can be treated by low-dose irradiation or enlarging the abdominal cavity temporarily by placing a Silastic patch in the abdominal wall as in the treatment of gastroschisis/giant exomphalos

combination therapy, i.e. chemotherapy and radiotherapy followed by surgical excision of shrunken tumour. Treatment for stage IVs is controversial but if detectable, excision of the primary tumour is preferable.

Prognosis

For the last two decades neuroblastoma has been one of the paediatric malignancies with the poorest prognosis. The overall three-year survival rate for all stages is 30–50%. Two key determinants of survival are the age of patient and the stage of disease at diagnosis. Patients younger than two years old have a survival rate of 70–80%, in contrast to 30–40% for patients older than two years. Survival is inversely proportional to the stage of disease, except for stage IVs: stage I, 100%; stage II, 80–85%; stage III, 40%; stage IV, 20–40%; stage IVs, over 90%. Other poor prognostic factors include unfavourable histology, high serum NSE level, high serum ferritin level, 1p36 chromosome deletion, diploidy and high number of N-myc protooncogene copies. Amplification of the N-myc gene may lead to the prevention of tumour apoptosis by inhibiting the caspase activities and is associated with poor outcome.

New strategies for treatment of advanced diseases include high-dose chemotherapy, total body irradiation and allogeneic or autologous bone marrow transplantation. Autologous bone marrow transplantation requires complete removal of the tumour cells by treatment with cytotoxic agents coupled with monoclonal antibodies against neuroblastoma cells, before reinfusion back into the patient. Several clinical trials of immunotherapy have been undertaken, including the use of monoclonal antibody antiganglioside G(D2) to induce lysis of neuroblastoma cells by antibody-dependent cellular cytotoxicity and complement-dependent cytotoxicity, and the use of retinoid acid to induce differentiation and apoptosis of neuroblastoma cells. Initial results show some promises but long-term follow-up is required for confirmation of their efficacy.

RHABDOMYOSARCOMA

Pathology

Rhabdomyosarcomas are highly malignant and tend to have early local invasion and eventual metastasis to distant sites. Rhabdomyosarcoma arises from the same embryonic mesenchyme as the striated muscle, so it can occur anywhere in the body. Because of the similar morphologic features, rhabdomyosarcoma and other soft tissue sarcomas, such as Ewing's sarcoma, neuroblastoma and lymphoma, are grouped as 'small round cell tumours'. Differentiation of rhabdomyosarcoma from other soft tissue sarcomas depends on the positive staining with antibodies against actin, myosin and myoglobulin and with the periodic acid-Schiff (PAS) technique. Characteristic features on electron microscopy include intracytoplasmic filaments and Z-band materials.

The Intergroup Rhabdomyosarcoma Study (IRS) has divided rhabdomyosarcoma into five histologic subtypes: the embryonal type (60%), the botryoid type (6%), the alveolar type (20%), the undifferentiated type (20%) and the pleomorphic type (1%). The botryoid type is an embryonal variant and is so named because the tumour cells with their oedematous stroma may project like a bunch of grapes into hollow organ cavities, such as vagina, uterus, bladder, nasopharynx and the middle ear. The tissue typing affects the survival: the embryonal type has a favourable prognosis whereas the alveolar type has an unfavourable outcome. If there is more than one tissue in the tumour, the predominant cells determine the category and prognosis.

Incidence

Rhabdomyosarcoma is the most common soft tissue tumour in childhood and represents the fifth most common paediatric malignancy, after leukaemia, central nervous system tumours, neuroblastoma and Wilms' tumour. It represents 10–15% of all the solid tumours and 6–8% of all paediatric malignancies. There are two peak incidences for the onset of rhabdomyosarcoma: an early peak before the age of five years and a second peak at the age of 12–18 years. About 70% of the patients are under the age of 10 years. Younger children have tumours more frequently occurring in the head, neck and distal urogenital tract. Trunk and paratesticular tumours occur mostly in adolescence. Rhabdomyosarcoma is more common in boys than girls, at a ratio of 3:2.

Associated anomalies

A familial aggregation of rhabdomyosarcoma with other sarcomas and tumours of central nervous system has been documented. Rhabdomyosarcoma may be associated with neurofibromatosis, Li Fraumeni syndrome and p53 suppression gene mutation. The female family members of children with rhabdomyosarcoma may have a higher incidence of breast cancer.

Clinical features

The clinical presentation of rhabdomyosarcoma relates to the site of origin. Tumours at the distal urogenital tract may present as a mass on abdominal or rectal examination, urinary symptoms due to obstruction, recurrent urinary infection, haematuria, incontinence or vaginal discharge. Vaginal rhadomyosarcoma may present as a grape-like mass projecting through the vaginal orifice and may be associated with vaginal bleeding, obstruction of the urethra or rectum. Head and neck rhadomyosarcoma may present as a mass at the orbit, parameningeal (middle ear, nasal cavity, nasopharynx, paranasal sinus and infratemporal fossa) or non-parameningeal region. Tumours at the nasopharynx may cause nasal obstruction, epistaxis, dysphagia and possibly intracranial invasion. Proptosis, ptosis, periorbital oedema and change of visual acuity may occur if the orbit is involved. Involvement of the middle ear may cause pain, otorrhoea and loss of hearing. Tumours at the face or cheek may be associated with pain, swelling, trismus and cranial nerve palsy if tumour extension occurs. Rhabdomyosarcomas at the trunk and extremities present as detectable masses and sometimes may be mistaken for haematomas. Involvement of the paratesticular tissue leads to a rapid enlargement of the scrotum due to progressive tumour growth. Lungs, bone marrow and bone cortex are the common sites of metastasis and their involvement may result in respiratory distress, bone pain and symptomatic hypercalcaemia.

Investigations

Early diagnosis of rhabdomyosarcoma depends on the physician's alertness. The area of involvement determines the diagnostic procedures and the extent of the tumour directs therapy. For tumours at the head and neck, plain roentgenograms are helpful in determining the location, bony erosion and intracranial extension. Ultrasonography and CT scan with contrast may help delineate the extent of the tumour in the abdomen. In selected patients, MRI may provide more precise delineation of tumour margins. Before surgery, evidence of metastasis should be sought for carefully by bone scan, bone marrow biopsy and chest radiograph or CT. Definite diagnosis, however, is established on incisional or excisional biopsy. If incisional biopsy is performed initially, the incision should be planned so that the incision scar will be included in subsequent excision, e.g. axial incision for rhabdomyosarcoma of extremities.

Treatment

Treatment is adjusted according to the location and grouping. The IRS clinical group system is based upon pretreatment and operative outcome and is shown in Box 51.3.

Treatment for rhabdomyosarcoma is multimodal, consisting of surgery, chemotherapy and radiotherapy. The general principle for surgery is complete, wide excision of the primary tumour and

---

Box 51.3 Intergroup Rhabdomyosarcoma Study (IRS-III) grouping system

I   Localised disease, completely resected, no regional lymph node involvement
   (a) Confined to muscle or organ of origin
   (b) Infiltration outside origin but nodes negative

II Localised or regional disease with grossly total resection
   (a) Grossly resected tumour with microscopic residual disease but nodes negative
   (b) Regional disease, completely resected without microscopic residual, nodes positive
   (c) Regional disease with involved nodes resected, but with microscopic residual disease

III Incomplete resection or biopsy with gross residual disease
   (a) Only biopsy or less than 50% tumour resected
   (b) More than 50% but less than 100% tumour resected

IV Distant metastasis at the time of diagnosis

---

surrounding tissues without affecting the cosmesis and function. However, complete excision of rhabdomyosarcomas is not always feasible; in such cases, incisional biopsy for tissue diagnosis only is justifiable. Chemotherapy and/or radiotherapy may reduce the size of a massive tumour to an extent that allows a delayed complete resection. Second excision after initial biopsy and adjuvant chemoradiotherapy offers a better outcome than incomplete excision in the first setting. Postoperative chemotherapy is helpful in eradicating microscopic residual disease and micrometastasis. For group I patients, chemotherapy is given after complete local excision to reduce the likelihood of subsequent metastasis. For group II and III patients, local radiation and systemic chemotherapy should be given after initial surgery. Group IV patients are usually treated with systemic chemotherapy.

Prognosis

The survival rate depends upon the site of the primary tumour, clinical grouping and staging. Tumours of the orbit, vagina, vulva and paratesticular region have a favourable prognosis. Tumours of the limbs, prostate, bladder, uterus and non-parameningeal areas of the head and neck have an intermediate prognosis. A poorer prognosis is noted for tumours at the biliary trees, retroperitoneum, chest wall, trunk, perineum, buttock and metastatic tumours to bone marrow and lymph nodes. In general, the overall two-year survival rate has increased from 20% to 65% or so in the past two decades. The overall survival rate in the IRS-III is about 70%: it is about 90% in clinical group I, 80–85% in group II, 65–70% in group III and only 30% in group IV.

OTHER SOFT TISSUE SARCOMAS

Other frequently seen soft tissue sarcomas in the paediatric population include fibrosarcoma, liposarcoma, leiomyosarcoma, neurofibrosarcoma, synovial sarcoma, extraosseous Ewing's sarcoma, small cell soft tissue sarcomas and primitive neuroectodermal tumours. The site of occurrence is as the nomenclature indicates. The management of these tumours is similar to that of rhabdomyosarcoma.

MALIGNANT LIVER TUMOURS

Malignant liver tumours are relatively rare and constitute about 2% of all malignant tumours in childhood. Two types of primary liver malignancies may occur in children: hepatoblastoma and hepatocellular carcinoma (HCC or hepatoma).

Hepatoblastoma

Hepatoblastoma (Figure 51.10) is more common than HCC and is seen almost exclusively in infancy and early childhood with a male predominance in a ratio of 1.5:1. The incidence of paediatric HCC has two peaks: before the age of four years and at 12–15 years. HCC predominates in males by a ratio of 1.3:1. Hepatoblastoma may consist of cells with an epithelial appearance or a mixture of mesenchymal components. The histology of paediatric HCC is similar to that in adults. HCC often arises in a previously abnormal liver, e.g. history of hepatitis, cirrhosis due to biliary atresia, total parenteral nutrition-associated cholestasis, metabolic disease, etc. In both forms of liver malignancies, the right lobe is more commonly involved than the left. However, multicentricity of the tumour or bilateral lobal involvement can be seen in about half of patients.

The clinical presentation is usually an abdominal mass with abdominal distension. Pain is present in one-fifth of patients at the time of diagnosis. Other non-specific symptoms include anorexia, body weight loss, vomiting and jaundice. Diagnosis is mainly dependent on image studies such as ultrasonography, CT scan (Figure 51.11) or MRI. The major diagnostic difficulty is to

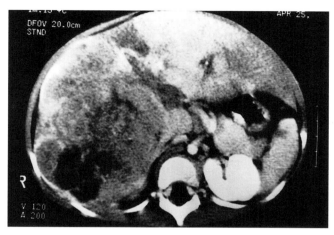

Figure 51.11 Contrast-enhanced CT scan of a hepatoblastoma replacing the right lobe of the liver. Central hypodense area consistent with tumour necrosis or haemorrhage is not uncommonly seen.

differentiate the primary tumour from those caused by other diseases such as metastatic neuroblastoma, infantile haemangioendothelioma, cavernous haemangioma or metabolic storage diseases. Most of the laboratory results are normal. However, most patients have an increased serum alpha-fetoprotein (AFP) level, which is a useful marker for postoperative monitoring. Pulmonary metastasis can be detected in 10% of the patients at the time of diagnosis. Therefore, abdominal and chest CT scan should be performed for the staging. Angiography may provide delineation of blood supply of the tumour by which the resectability can be determined.

Tumour resection is the main form of treatment. In about one-third of patients complete resection is possible at the time of diagnosis. Generally children have a better capacity for hepatic regeneration than adults and can tolerate liver resection of up to 80% of the liver volume. Hepatoblastoma is chemosensitive; the chemotherapeutic agents used include adriamycin, vincristine, cisplastin and cyclophosphamide. Chemotherapy is given as adjuvant therapy after hepatectomy or preoperatively to render a non-resectable heptoblastoma resectable. Radiotherapy may be used in selected patients with limited effects. Inoperable HCC may be treated by transarterial oily chemoembolisation (TOCE).

Overall survival for hepatoblastoma is 70% and for HCC 13% only. Patients who have had complete surgical excision have a survival rate of 80% at two years. Incomplete resection always results in recurrence and eventual mortality. Liver transplantation may give good results in selected patients.

GERM CELL TUMOURS AND TERATOMA

Germ cell tumour is uncommon in children. Malignant germ cell tumours account for about 3–4% of childhood malignancies, in which sacrococcygeal teratoma (a type of germ cell tumour; see below) remains the most common solid tumour in the newborn.

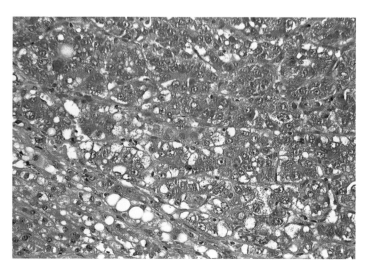

Figure 51.10 A malignant liver tumour (hepatoblastoma) composed of pleomorphic small to medium-sized liver cells without bile production. Normal liver is present in the left lower quadrant.

Germ cell tumours may occur in both gonadal and extragonadal sites as a result of aberrant migration of primitive germ cells (Figure 51.12). Extragonadal and testicular tumours are mostly seen in children younger than three years of age. Gonadal tumours are more frequently seen in late adolescence or young adults. Germ cell tumours may arise from primitive germ cells that lack the ability for further differentiation, such as seminoma and dysgerminoma, or from totipotential stem cells capable of differentiating into embryonal (teratoma) or extraembryonal tumours (choriocarcinoma or yolk sac tumour).

Most of the germ cell tumours secrete hormonal markers that allow post-excisional disease progression to be monitored biochemically. For example, AFP is a sensitive marker for teratoma and yolk sac tumour (or called endodermal sinus tumour). Human chorionic gonadotropin (hCG) is elevated in choriocarcinoma.

Ultrasound, CT or MRI is useful for evaluating the extent of disease. For resectable tumours, surgical excision should be undertaken. Ovarian tumours are often excised by salpingo-oophorectomy. Testicular tumours require radical orchidectomy via a groin incision with or without and dissection of the retroperitoneal lymph node sampling/debulking in advanced cases. The introduction of cisplastin-based chemotherapy has improved the survival rate. Although some of the germ cell tumours are radiosensitive, the success of the combination of surgery and chemotherapy has diminished the need for radiotherapy.

Teratoma

Teratoma represents the most common form of paediatric germ cell tumour. Histologically teratomas are composed of tissues from all three embryonal germ layers (Figure 51.13). Teratomas

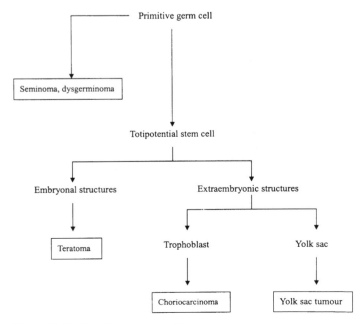

Figure 51.12 The origins of germ cell tumours.

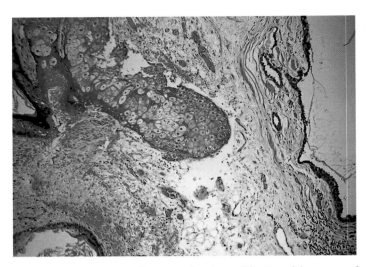

Figure 51.13 Sacrococcygeal teratoma showing proliferation of three types of cells. There is squamous and metaplastic epithelium present with the epithelia separated by a stroma that contains muscle, vessels and fat.

may arise from any part but usually occur in the mid-line or paraaxis of body. By location, the sacrococcygeal region is the most common site for teratoma (40%), followed by the ovary (one-third of all cases), head and neck, mediastinum, retroperitoneum and abdomen, brain and spinal cord and testes. Ovarian teratoma (Figure 51.14) usually presents with an abdominal mass and may be associated with bleeding, torsion or rupture. Thoracic teratoma may present as a mediastinal mass on imaging studies. Other retroperitoneal teratomas often present as abdominal or flank masses. Unlike other paediatric tumours, teratoma is not sensitive to chemotherapy or radiotherapy so the goal of treatment is complete excision.

Sacrococcygeal teratoma

Sacrococcygeal teratoma is the most common type of teratoma and also represents the most common neoplasm of the newborn, with an incidence of about 1:35 000. It has a strong female predominance with a girl:boy ratio of 3–4:1. Sacrococcygeal teratoma usually presents as a protruding mass between the anus and the coccyx and nowadays can be diagnosed by antenatal ultrasonography. However, the mass may be as small as several centimeters in diameter or as large as the size of the infant. There is a unique form of sacrococcygeal teratoma which does not present externally but grows into the presacral space as a primary pelvic lesion and usually is undetectable until late childhood. The late-detected pelvic sacrococcygeal teratoma is usually malignant.

Most sacrococcygeal teratomas (>80%) are benign and can be identified at birth, but there is a malignant potential if the tumours are not completely excised. The incidence of malignant change increases as age advances: 7% at birth, 37% at one year and 50% at two years. Early complete excision of the tumour is the only definite cure for sacrococcygeal teratoma, as delay in surgery and retention of the coccyx increase the risk of malig-

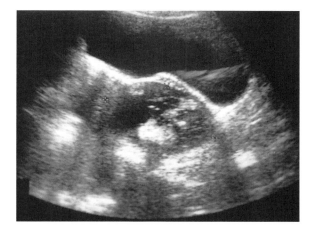

A

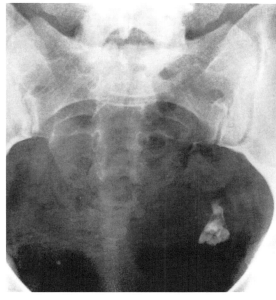

B

Figure 51.14 A. Ultrasound examination of an ovary showing a well-circumscribed mass with mixed echogenicity. It is predominantly cystic with a central echogenic area, which demonstrates posterior acoustic shadowing, compatible with a focus of calcification. Features are characteristic of a mature teratoma. **B.** Plain abdominal X-ray of a patient with a mature teratoma of the left ovary showing a calcified 'molar tooth'.

nant transformation. The urogenital organs or the rectum may be distorted but should be preservable during dissection. Postoperative follow-up should include rectal examination for detection of presacral recurrence and serial measurements of serum AFP.

The prognosis of benign sacrococcygeal teratoma after complete excision is excellent. Perioperative haemorrhage and hypothermia, however, are possible lethal complications of the excision of a massive benign tumour. Some patients may have bowel or urinary incontinence on long-term follow-up. Malignant sacrococcygeal teratoma, in contrast, requires aggressive multimodal therapy, including surgery, chemotherapy and radiotherapy. Prognosis for malignant sacrococcygeal teratoma is poor, with an overall mortality rate of more than 80%.

LYMPHOMA

Lymphoma is a common malignancy in childhood. Childhood lymphomas can be either Hodgkin's disease (HD) or non-Hodgkin's lymphoma (NHL), which have a similar histology but a remarkable difference in tumour behaviour, treatment and prognosis. HD and NHL represent 5% and 10% of all childhood malignancies respectively and predominate in males.

Prognosis of lymphomas in childhood after treatment with systemic chemotherapy is excellent, with or without radiotherapy. The overall survival rate for children with HD is over 90% and 70–85% for NHL.

Hodgkin's lymphoma

HD has a peak age of onset at 11–15 years and is more common than NHL in teenagers and young adults. The malignant cells in HD are the Reed–Sternberg cells. There is increasing evidence that HD is derived from malignant transformation of B cells and may be associated with Epstein–Barr virus infection. Most of the patients have no systemic complaints except enlarged lymph nodes. The sites of involvement, in order of frequency, are cervical, supraclavicular, mediastinal, abdominal, axillary and inguinal areas. Four major histologic types of HD have been suggested in Rye's classification:

- lymphocyte predominant (3%)
- lymphocyte depleted (5%)
- mixed cellularity (25%)
- nodular sclerosis (67%).

Nodular sclerosis is the most common histologic type and also accounts for the increase in the incidence of HD in childhood in recent years.

The surgeon's role is to obtain tissue diagnosis and to perform staging laparotomy, including liver biopsy, splenectomy, bone marrow biopsy, sampling of iliac, mesenteric, para-aortic, periportal, splenic and coeliac lymph nodes. The information obtained from staging laparotomy is sometimes significant and may not be revealed by CT/MRI, gallium scan or lymphangiography. A change in the clinical staging of HD as a result of laparotomy has been reported in 25–53%. However, as low-stage patients respond to combination chemotherapy as well as radiotherapy, the significance of precise staging, and consequently the need for staging laparotomy, has decreased.

Non-Hodgkin's lymphoma

NHL is far less common than HD in total case incidence but in the infant and toddler age group, it is more common than HD. NHL may occur throughout the body and the sites of involvement may be diffuse and disseminated. The common primary sites are the abdomen, mediastinum, peripheral nodes and head and neck. NHL can be subcategorised into three types:

- undifferentiated (also called small non-cleaved cell lymphoma, 40–50%)

- lymphoblastic (30–40%)

- large cell (15%).

Based on the histology under light microscopy, the undifferentiated NHL can be divided into Burkitt's and non-Burkitt's lymphoma, both of which are believed to differentiate from B cell precursors. More than 90% of undifferentiated NHL present with a palpable abdominal mass, which can cause abdominal pain, distension, obstruction, intestinal bleeding, intussusception or bowel perforation. Occasionally the tumour at the right iliac fossa may be mistakenly diagnosed as appendicitis or appendiceal abscess.

Laparotomy is not indicated in NHL for staging because all patients require systemic chemotherapy. However, laparotomy may still have to be performed on NHL patients because of abdominal complications such as intussusception, intestinal bleeding or simulated appendicitis. Intussusception in patients above two years of age should raise the suspicion of an uncommon pathology, such as Meckel's diverticulum or lymphoma.

FURTHER READING

Andrassy RJ, ed., *Pediatric Surgical Oncology*. Philadelphia: WB Saunders, 1998

Carachi R, Azmy A, Grosfeld JL, ed. *The Surgery of Childhood Tumours*. London: Arnold, 1999

Cooper CS, Jaffe WI, Huff DS et al. The role of renal salvage procedures for bilateral Wilms tumor: a 15-year review. *J Urol* 2000; **163**:265–268

Coppes MJ, Pritchard-Jones K. Principles of Wilms tumor biology. *Urologic Clin North Am* 2000; **27**:423–433

Cotterill SJ, Pearson AD, Pritchard J et al. Clinical prognostic factors in 1277 patients with neuroblastoma: results of the European Neuroblastoma Study Group 'Survey' 1982–1992. *Eur J Cancer* 2000; **36**:901–908

Fiore NF Jr, Grosfeld JL. Solid tumors of childhood. *Asian J Surg* 1999; **22**:102–119

Greenlee RT, Murray T, Bolden S, Wingo PA. Cancer statistics 2000. *Ca Cancer J Clin* 2000; **50**:7–11

Giannoulia-Karadana A, Moschovi M, Koutsovitis P, Tolis G, Tzortzatou-Stathopoulou F. Inferior vena cava and right atrial thrombosis in children with nephroblastoma: diagnostic and therapeutic problems. *J Pediatr Surg* 2000; **35**:1459–1461

Hays DM, Fryer CJ, Pringle KC et al. An evaluation of abdominal staging procedures performed in pediatric patients with advanced Hodgkin's disease: a report from the Children's Cancer Study Group. *J Pediatr Surg* 1992; **27**:1175–1180

Matz LR, Finlay-Jones LR, Waters ED et al. The Rye classification of a population based series of Hodgkin's disease patients in Western Australia. *Pathology* 1981; **13**:263–276

Ozkaynak MF, Sondel PM, Krailo MD et al. Phase I study of chimeric human/murine anti-ganglioside G(D2) monoclonal antibody (ch14.18) with granulocyte-macrophage colony-stimulating factor in children with neuroblastoma immediately after hematopoietic stem-cell transplantation: a Children's Cancer Group Study. *J Clin Oncol* 2000; **18**:4077–4085

Suc A, Lumbroso J, Rubie H et al. Metastatic neuroblastoma in children older than one year: prognostic significance of the initial metaiodobenzylguanidine scan and proposal for a scoring system. *Cancer* 1996; **77**:805-811

Spinal dysraphism

Paul K.H. Tam, Gilbert K.K. Leung

INTRODUCTION

Development of the central nervous system begins in the second week of gestation when the neural plate, consisting of neuroectoderm, folds to form the neural tube in a process termed neurulation. The surrounding mesoderm and somatic ectoderm subsequently migrate dorsally to form the vertebral column and myocutaneous coverings over the future brain and spinal cord (Figure 52.1). Failure of this mid-line closure results in neural tube defect, which may affect any part of the craniospinal axis. The term spinal dysraphism encompasses several distinct spinal neural tube defects. In spina bifida occulta, defects of the posterior vertebral arch are masked by normal skin, i.e. closed, whereas in spina bifida cystica, the underlying malformed neural elements are exposed through a skin defect, i.e. open (Figure 52.2).

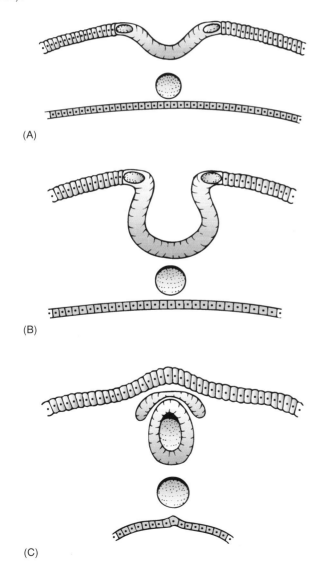

Figure 52.1 Normal neural tube development. **A**. Neuroectoderm forms a neural plate. **B**. A neural groove. **C**. A neural tube with mesodermal and ecto-dermal coverings.

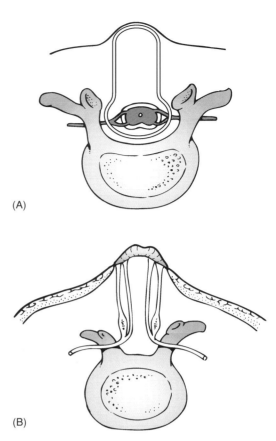

Figure 52.2 Spina bifida. **A**. Meningocoele. **B**. Myelomeningocoele.

SPINA BIFIDA OCCULTA

This condition is usually an incidental and asymptomatic radio-logical finding. The primary defect is the absence of spinous processes and variable amounts of laminae over one or two levels. There may be overlying cutaneous stigmata such as a tuft of hair, port wine stain or skin dimple. The infant is otherwise normal. In some cases, however, other associated conditions in the region may present later in life with pain, sensorimotor deficits, gait disturbance and urological dysfunction. There may be progressive spinal and foot deformities such as scoliosis, high-arch feet and claw toes. These symptoms may appear in different chronological orders and combinations.

The pathogenesis of these separate, yet frequently co-existing conditions is incompletely understood but most probably involves failed regression of embryonic caudal structures. Examples include tethered cord syndrome, lipomyelomeningocoele, split cord condition and dermal sinus.

Tethered cord syndrome

This is characterised by a low-lying conus medullaris (below L2) associated with an abnormally short and thickened filum terminale.

Since the spinal cord is effectively 'tethered' within the vertebral canal, traction and cord ischaemia may result, especially during growth spurts, giving rise to neurological symptoms. Although the condition is more often a late complication of myelomeningocoele (see below), in occult cases, it may present late in previously healthy children or even in adults. Treatment with laminectomy and division of the filum terminale is indicated in symptomatic cases or as a prophylactic measure, although the effectiveness of the latter is difficult to confirm. Re-tethering may occur and vigilant follow-up is mandatory.

Lipomyelomeningocoele

This usually presents as a palpable subcutaneous lipomatous mass, which passes through a mid-line defect of the lumbosacral fascia, vertebral arch and dura, and merges with a low-lying conus medullaris. Direct spinal cord compression or tethering may cause neurological symptoms. The condition must be distinguished from a subcutaneous lipoma. Whenever clinical or intraoperative findings suggest involvement of deep structures, exploration must be deferred and further imaging studies performed. Patient weight reduction may result in shrinkage of the lipoma and improvement in symptoms. Definitive treatment aims at removal of the lipoma, untethering of the cord and reconstruction of the dural tube.

Split cord malformation

This rare condition is characterised by splitting or duplication of the caudal spinal cord. The two hemicords may lie in separate dural tubes (diastematomyelia) or within a single dural tube (diplomyelia). The hemicords are usually separated by a fibrous or osseocartilaginous median septum, with associated malformations such as hemivertebrae or kyphoscoliosis. Surgical untethering of the cord may be required prior to correction of the spinal deformities which may otherwise cause neurological deterioration.

Dermal sinus

This appears as a mid-line dimple in the lumbosacral area. The sinus may extend as far down as the intradural compartment and may act as a pathway for repeated bouts of meningitis. Formation of epidermoid or dermoid cysts is not uncommon as it is lined with cutaneous squamous epithelium. Clinically it must be distinguished from a pilonidal sinus or from a sacrococcygeal dimple. A pilonidal sinus or a sacrococcygeal dimple which is situated in a very low position (overlying the tip of the coccyx), is not associated with a tethered cord and does not require surgical intervention. The tract of a lumbosacral sinus should not be probed or injected with contrast. Plain radiographs or magnetic resonance imaging may demonstrate underlying spina bifida. Surgical excision is indicated for cord tethering and prevention of infection. Cranial dermal sinus may sometimes occur in the occipital region.

SPINA BIFIDA CYSTICA

Meningocoele

This protrusion of the meningeal coverings through a defect in the spinal column is relatively uncommon. The condition affects primarily the posterior lumbosacral spine but may sometimes involve other regions, including the skull. Clinically, it presents at birth as a soft, reducible and pedunculated mass that trans-illuminates well. The surface may be covered by very attenuated skin and CSF may be visible. The underlying spinal cord is normal. In contrast to myelomeningocoele, there is no neurological dysfunction or lower limb deformity. Hydrocephalus is uncommon.

The condition should be distinguished from other dorsal mid-line masses. A lipomatous mass is clinically not reducible and usually broad based. A sacrococcygeal teratoma is covered by normal skin and located at the tip of the coccyx. A meningocoele may very occasionally herniate anteriorly through a sacral defect and present as a laparotomy finding or a pelvic mass with obstructive symptoms. Treatment of meningocoele aims at decompression, obliteration of the CSF fistula and release of spinal cord tethering.

Myelomeningocoele

Epidemiology

Myelomeningocoele is the most important spinal dysraphic disorder with an incidence of 1–2 per 1000 live births. It is a major cause of fetal and infant mortality and survivors suffer from multiple long-term problems with medical, economic and social implications. There has been a worldwide decline in prevalence recently, probably due to effective prenatal screening and increasing therapeutic abortion. However, the prevalence is higher in the British Isles and populations of Celtic origin and lower in Asians. The risk of a first-born child being affected is around 1 in 250 and increases to 1 in 25 in the next pregnancy.

Aetiology

The aetiology is multifactorial and heterogeneous. Additional congenital abnormalities are found in 20% of affected infants. Chromosomal abnormalities and mutations of genes, including those that encode folate receptors (e.g. 5, 10-methylene-terahydrofolate reductase – MTHFR) have been identified in some cases but the genetic control of neural tube closure is yet to be determined. Environmental factors, such as poverty and famine, and drug use, e.g. carbamazepine and valproic acid, seem to play a role. Furthermore, there is conclusive evidence showing that maternal folate insufficiency constitutes additional risk. Population-based intervention studies have demonstrated that folic acid supplement around the time of conception may prevent 72% of occurrences. The current recommendation is that women of child-bearing age should take 0.4 mg of folic acid per day.

Associated anomalies

Primary anomalies

Myelomeningocoele is nearly always associated with the Arnold–Chiari malformation (prolongation of the medulla and the tonsils and vermis of the cerebellum through the foramen magnum) which results in hydrocephalus. Vertebral anomalies are common and result in kyphosis and kyphoscoliosis.

Secondary anomalies due to neurological deficit

Lower limbs may be affected by paralysis and sensory loss. Autonomic dysfunction leads to neurogenic bladder and bowel incontinence.

Prenatal screening

Prenatal diagnosis of an affected pregnancy provides an opportunity for parent counselling and planning of termination as well as perinatal management. Maternal serum alpha-fetoprotein (AFP) measured between 14 and 21 weeks is an effective screening tool. Almost all maternal serum AFP is fetal in origin. It is normally raised in pregnancy but a level twice that of the median (adjusted to gestation week) is highly suggestive of an open neural tube defect. The sensitivity is around 90%. However, a false positive may occur if other abnormalities, such as congenital nephrosis, abdominal wall defect and duodenal atresia, are present. The diagnosis can be confirmed on high-resolution ultrasonography which detects up to 95% of cases. Amniocentesis, with subsequent measurement of amniotic fluid AFP and acetyl cholinesterase (AChE), is a useful adjunct but carries additional procedure-related risks.

If the decision is to continue with the pregnancy, regular assessment with ultrasonography is required to monitor the development of such conditions as congenital hydrocephalus. *In utero* shunting for the hydrocephalus carries high risks without showing any proven benefit. Intrauterine exposure of the spinal cord to neurotoxic substances within the amniotic fluid, e.g. glutamine, and trauma induced during labour have been shown to increase neurological injury. The controversy remains whether delivery before term by elective caesarean section may improve outcome. *In utero* repair of spina bifida in mid trimester to reduce neurological damage has been attempted but the long-term outcome remains unknown.

Initial assessment

Myelomeningocoele varies in severity. The neural plate may remain entirely open (myeloschisis) or be fused, with varying degrees of herniation of neural elements through the skin defect. The lesion is commonly oval, lying longitudinally in the lumbo-sacral or thoracolumbar region. The caudal neural 'placode' is usually covered by a membranous sac and surrounded by a pearly 'zona epitheliosa' (see Figure 52.2). There may be signs of congenital hydrocephalus, which occurs in 60–80% of cases. The size and level of the spinal lesion and the head circumference should be carefully documented at birth.

When assessing motor function, it is important to distinguish spontaneous from reflex movements. The latter are often stereo-typed and disappear on cessation of painful stimuli. Motor deficits may be asymmetrical and of mixed upper and lower motor neurone types. On inspection there may be fixed lower limb deformity (e.g. hip flexion) secondary to intrauterine onset of paralysis.

Neurological examination aimed at detecting the level of functional loss correlates well with the level of spinal defect. As a general guideline, lesions below T12 are associated with complete paraplegia. Below L2, there is retained hip flexion. Knee extension and ankle dorsiflexion and inversion are preserved for lesions below L4. Lesions below S1 may only exhibit weakness of the intrinsic foot muscles. Urine dripping suggests bladder dysfunction and a patulous anus lacking sensation implies sacral denervation.

Imaging studies with plain radiographs and MRI may serve as a useful baseline but rarely affect immediate management. Cranial ultrasonography should be performed to detect hydrocephalus and other malformations.

Management

The complexity of congenital maldevelopment calls for a multi-disciplinary approach involving neonatologists, neurosurgeons, physiotherapists and paediatric and orthopaedic surgeons at an early stage. Cardiac and lung functions must be stabilised and assessed for prognostication and anaesthetic risks. The patient is nursed prone to avoid pressure on the spinal defect, which is loosely covered with sterile saline-soaked gauze to prevent desiccation and bacterial colonisation. Neurotoxic iodine-containing solution must be avoided. Antibiotics are indicated if there is rupture of the sac or CSF leakage. Oral feeding is with-held to ensure an aseptic bowel. The urinary bladder is catheterised to avoid contamination of the field. Susceptibility to latex allergy is associated with this condition and should be documented.

Surgical repair of myelomeningocoele aims at preservation of existing neurological function and prevention of CSF leakage, infection and death. Surgery cannot restore lost function but may prevent further deterioration. A policy of selective treatment based on the chance and quality of survival was adopted in the past but since not all untreated patients die, the current practice is that surgery should be performed unless it carries unacceptable risks or when death is inevitable. There is no conclusive evidence that the timing of surgery affects outcome in terms of infection, motor or mental function. Generally, closure is performed within 48–72 hours.

The operation is performed under general anaesthesia with the patient in the prone position. The exposed neural placode is first dissected from any adjoined dura and herniating nerve roots are preserved and replaced within the canal. The dura is then dissected free from the skin, followed by reconstitution of a dural tube and meticulous closure of the fascia and skin (Figure 52.3). Complex plastic surgery is rarely needed. Occasionally, closure may exacerbate previously subclinical hydrocephalus. Progressive hydrocephalus occurs regardless in about 80% of patients with spina bifida and is treated by insertion of a ventriculo-peritoneal shunt.

Outcomes

With modern treatment, 85% of patients survive with varying degrees of disability. Mortality, however, is higher with thoraco-lumbar lesions. Furthermore, myelomeningocoele is almost always associated with the Arnold–Chiari malformation, which may cause severe brain dysfunction. Untreated patients most often die of meningitis, hydrocephalus and its associated Chiari malformation.

Many long-term problems affect the survivor's quality of life and are a significant burden on the family and the community. For instance, although around two-thirds of patients have an intelligence quotient (IQ) above 80, many suffer from significant psychosocial and learning difficulties. Approximately three-quarters of patients are able to walk independently or with aids. However, progressive spinal and lower limb deformities may cause secondary deterioration and hamper rehabilitation. Constipation is common and most patients are incontinent of urine. Neurogenic bladder and vesicoureteric reflux may result in hydronephrosis and renal failure leading to death, although many patients are successfully managed with intermittent self-catheterisation. Delayed neurological problems include syringomyelia, tethered cord syndrome and symptomatic Chiari malformation, while shunt complications may require repeated operations.

FURTHER READING

Banta JV, Bonanni C, Prebluda J. Latex anaphylaxis during spinal surgery in children with myelomeningocele. *Dev Med Child Neurol* 1993; **35**:543–548

Brown S, Bailie A. Early management of meningomyelocele. *Eur J Pediatr Surg* 2000; **10** (suppl 1):40–41

Choi S, McComb JG. Long-term outcome of terminal myelocystocele patients. *Pediatr Neurosurg* 2000; **32**(2):86–91

Kanev PM, Bierbrauer KS. Reflections on the natural history of lipomyelomeningocele. *Pediatr Neurosurg* 1995; **22**:137–140

Lemire RJ. Neural tube defects. *JAMA* 1988; **259**:558-562

Lindhout D, Omtzigt JG. Teratogenic effects of antiepileptic drugs: implications for the management of epilepsy in women of childbearing age. *Epilepsia* 1994; **35**:S19–28

McComb JG. Congenital dermal sinus. In: Wilkins RH, Rengachary SS, eds. *Neurosurgery*, 2nd edn. New York: McGraw-Hill, 1996: 3561–3564

McCullough DC, Johnson DL. Myelomeningocele repair: technical considerations and complications. *Pediatr Neurosurg* 1994; **21**:83–89

Pang D, Dias MS. Cervical myelomeningoceles. *Neurosurgery* 1993; **33**:363–373

Pang D, Dias MS, Ahab-Barmada M. Split cord malformation: Part 1: a unified theory of embryogenesis for double spinal cord malformations. *Neurosurgery* 1992; **31**:451–480

Parent AD, McMillan T. Contemporaneous shunting with repair of myelomeningocoele. *Pediatr Neurosurg* 1995; **22**:132–136

Perez LM, Wilbanks JT, Joseph DB, Oakes WJ. Urological outcome of patients with cervical and upper thoracic myelomeningocele. *J Urol* 2000; **164**(3 pt 2):962–964

Rosengerg IH. Folic acid and neural-tube defects – time for action? *N Engl J Med* 1992; **327**:1875–1877

Sathi S, Madsen JR, Bauer S, Scott RM. Effects of surgical repair on the neurologic function in infants with lipomeningocele. *Pediatr Neurosurg* 1993; **19**:256–259

Shurtleff DB, Lemire RJ. Epidemiology, etiologic factors, and prenatal diagnosis of open spinal dysraphism. *Neurosurg Clin North Am* 1995; **6**:183–193

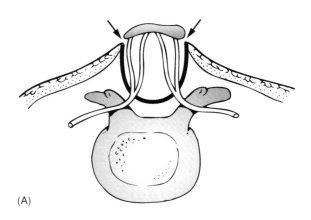

(A)

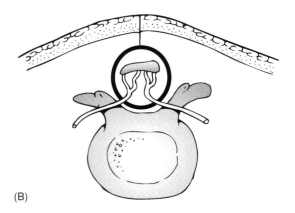

(B)

Figure 52.3 Surgical repair of a myelomeningocoele. **A**. The neural placode is dissected free from the attached skin and dura. **B**. Reconstitution of the dural tube, fascia and skin.

Swank M, Dias L. Myelomeningocele: a review of the orthopedic aspects of 206 patients treated from birth with no selection criteria. *Dev Med Child Neurol* 1992; **34**:1047–1052

Tortori-Donati P, Rossi A, Cama A. Spinal dysraphism: a review of neuro-radiological features with embryological correlations and proposal for a new classification. *Neuroradiology* 2000; **42**(7):471–491

Warder DE, Oakes WJ. Tethered cord syndrome: the low-lying and normally positioned conus. *Neurosurgery* 1994; **34**:597–600

White BD, Firth JL. Anterior spinal hernia: an increasingly recognised cause of thoracic cord dysfunction. *J Neurol Neurosurg Pyschiatr* 1994; **57**:1433–1435

Epilogue

53

Clinical governance

J. Adrian Copplestone

CLINICAL GOVERNANCE

The term 'clinical governance' first came into use after the publication of *The New NHS – Modern and Dependable*, in 1997. It was said to be a new initiative to assure and improve clinical standards at a local level throughout the NHS. Detailed proposals appeared the following year in *A First Class Service*, where clinical governance was defined as a framework through which NHS organisations are accountable for continuously improving the quality of their services and safeguarding high standards of care by creating an environment in which excellence in clinical care will flourish.

From a clinician's point of view, clinical governance can be summarised as:

- demonstrating that we are doing things correctly
- demonstrating that we are up-to-date and fit to practise
- demonstrating continuous improvement in the quality of clinical services.

From an organisational perspective, this represents a major change in policy – rather than the consultant being the sole person responsible for a patient, the Chief Executive, a manager, now has personal, statutory responsibility for clinical outcomes within the hospital. This responsibility is often delegated to the Medical Director or Director of Clinical Governance, but serves to bring the 'system' to account when things go wrong. It should lead to resources being allocated on the basis of relative clinical risk a clinical need.

Within a Trust, arrangements for clinical governance will include:

- Trust Board subcommittee similar to the Audit subcommittee, which monitors financial probity
- Lead Clinician with day-to-day responsibility for the implementation of clinical governance
- Clinical Governance Steering Group bringing together all the elements
- Clinical effectiveness
  - clinical audit
  - evidence-based practice
  - implementation of NICE guidelines and National Service Frameworks
- Clinical risk management
  - risk management policies, e.g. blood transfusion, infection control
  - Critical incident reporting
- Professional performance
  - detecting poor performance and reporting concerns
  - continuing professional development and training
  - support mechanisms for staff
  - workforce planning to ensure the right staff are available
- Systems for performance management and reporting.

The other major change in the medical environment is the impact of increasing numbers of external bodies which set standards or guidelines to determine 'best clinical practice'. These include:

- Royal Colleges
- National Institute for Clinical Excellence (NICE)
- Scottish Intercollegiate Guidelines Network (SIGN)
- Clinical Oncology Guidelines (COG), now taken over by NICE
- Medical Devices Agency (MDA)
- National Patient Safety Agency (NPSA)
- Specialist societies
- Consensus conferences.

External agencies to check that hospitals are complying with this profusion of advice include:

- Commission for Health Improvement (CHI)
- Audit Commission
- Ombudsman (complaints)
- Legal system.

Clinical governance is thus the system by which a Trust can monitor the quality of its services and is the meat in the quality sandwich (see Figure 53.1).

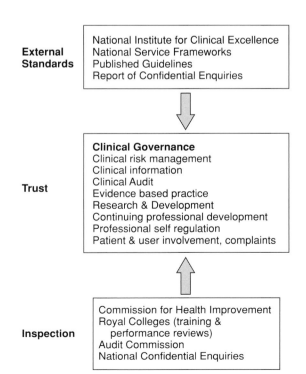

Figure 53.1 Clinical governance – the meat in the sandwich.

Clinical audit

Audit is a tool to assess whether the quality and outcome of patient care achieves a defined standard, through a process of structured peer review. Many different facets of care can be audited but often the most useful audits have a simple question and defined, measurable endpoints. There is no point in doing an audit unless it leads to improvements in practice.

Audits are often divided into audits of outcome or process. They can be viewed in other ways:

- Horizontal audit – a look across a clinical unit, e.g. do all members have sufficient training and up-to-date logs/CPD books?

- Vertical audit – if a patient is followed through a clinical pathway, are there defined policies for the different outcomes?

- Real-time audit – the hardest of all audits, but often the most useful – if a patient is followed through a pathway, are the policies followed correctly?

If the question is phrased correctly, the data can be collected prospectively and be presented in an audit meeting, often in an anonymous form. From the discussion of the data provided, benchmarking (comparison with other similar groups) and recent literature, a plan can be made for improvements in clinical practice. It is important that changes have the support of all the clinical team members and that a subsequent audit takes place to ensure that the expected improvement has occurred. This process is termed the 'audit cycle' (see Figure 53.2).

Ideally audits should be planned throughout the year to make the best use of clerical and computing help available, but there will be urgent problems arising from clinical risk management, complaints or external pressures that require immediate attention. Audit activity does tend to merge into research when the 'optimum treatment' is not well defined, but limited resources mean

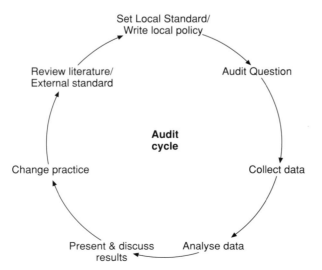

Figure 53.2 The audit cycle.

that projects have to be prioritised and an annual programme is a good way of achieving this.

Complaints

In most societies, people are much less accepting and complain more often than they did a decade ago. Most patients who complain want an explanation, an apology and the organisation to put things right so problems do not recur. Under the Patients Charter complaints need to be answered within 21 days. Usually an investigation of the complaint follows and a letter is drafted for the Chief Executive to reply to the patient. Although some staff are worried about the risk of subsequent litigation, an early explanation and full apology to patients at an early stage can often prevent later problems. Investigations can take time, especially when many different clinicians are involved.

A recent initiative is the Patient Advisory Liaison Service (PALS). This service's staff receive complaints, look into matters and aim to give an on-the-spot explanation. For simple administrative problems, PALS can resolve problems rapidly and stop the escalation that results when delays occur.

If a complainant is not satisfied, they may request an independent review. The convenor of this review is usually a non-executive director of the Trust or Health Authority and works with an independent lay-chairman to decide if an independent panel is able to resolve complaints. These may be of a complex nature and independent clinical advice may be sought.

At any stage in the process, a complainant may wish to refer their complaint to the Ombudsman (Health Service Commissioner) who has the jurisdiction of the whole range of NHS complaints, except of personnel and contractual matters.

Critical incidents

Recording adverse clinical incidents is a very useful way of improving clinical practice and surgical teams have done this for many years in Mortality and Morbidity Review Meetings. It is a process that can monitor equipment failure, lack of facilities or manpower on a prospective basis. It is useful if near-misses are also recorded, as these are informative events. Reporting needs to be made within a no-blame culture, where the whole team can benefit from discussing the event – often other system errors are identified.

An example of such an incident is given in Box 53.1.

Sometimes staff are unsure about whether to report events. This is a difficult area when clinical teams use this reporting system to highlight differences in clinical practice. In this situation the team should complete the form together following discussion.

There needs to be adequate monitoring of these reports at Directorate and Trust level so appropriate action can be taken and lessons learnt can be applied in other clinical areas.

Box 53.1

Critical Incident: Patient was transfused with the wrong blood.

Clinical Scenario: A patient with multiple injuries, including four limb fractures, was admitted through the Accident and Emergency (A&E) department. He had a cardiac arrest on arrival and was resuscitated. Group O RhD-negative blood was transfused. There were problems obtaining venous access due to the nature of his injuries. His identity was known. A correctly labelled cross-matched sample was sent to the transfusion laboratory. He was transferred urgently to the emergency theatre with such speed that the casenotes followed after.

At the same time, Blood Bank had been asked for an urgent cross-match for a patient undergoing neurosurgery in the emergency theatre later that day. When this blood was ready, theatre received a call, which was taken by a new member of staff. A porter collected the blood (for the neurosurgery patient) and this was given to the anaesthetist.

In the absence of a patient identity bracelet and notes, the theatre staff asked for the patient's name and were incorrectly given the name on the blood pertaining to the second patient and this was placed on the operating theatre board. The patient was bleeding extensively and more blood was requested. Pretransfusion identity checks used the name on the theatre board. Once the notes arrived, it was realised that this was a different patient and the transfusion was stopped. Fortunately there had been no ABO incompatibility.

Critical Incident Review: A no-blame multidisciplinary meeting was convened and a number of problems were identified leading to the final error:

- No patient identification bracelet was attached
- Problems with the verbal handover of the patient from A&E staff to theatre staff
- The notes did not come with the patient
- The patient identification on the theatre board was inaccurate
- The porter brought the blood directly to theatre (it would normally be delivered to the theatre co-ordinator or put in theatre blood fridge)
- Inadequate checking of the blood prior to the transfusion as the location and age/date of birth details would have identified the error

Changes to policies and procedures: As a result of this review, changes were made in both A&E and theatres including patient identification, handover, and delivery of blood to theatres.

An *Organisation with a Memory* (DOH, 2001) set up a reporting system, the National Patient Safety Agency, to try to learn from adverse events and near-misses.

Clinical risk management

This is an important element of clinical governance and not least because of the increase in litigation and the fact that the NHS has lost Crown Immunity against prosecution since 1990. Health Authorities and Trusts insure themselves against the costs of litigation under the Clinical Negligence Scheme for Trusts (CNST) run by the NHS Litigation Authority. Trusts are able to earn large discounts in the premiums if they can demonstrate high standards of risk management. So far these have been related to

organisational policies and documentation, but in future it is likely that standards will cover specific clinical issues and non-clinical risk areas.

Professional performance

This area of clinical governance is often seen as the most personally threatening, but should not be so provided clinicians take other aspects of clinical governance seriously. Recent medical and surgical scandals have eroded public confidence in the profession. The General Medical Council has produced new fitness to practice procedures, which are different to their disciplinary procedures. Continuing registration will be subject to regular revalidation, based on evidence obtained in annual appraisals.

Trusts need to have processes for dealing sensitively with concerns for medical performance. This is usually conducted through the office of Medical Director. All doctors have a duty to protect patients if they may come to harm. The doctors need to be able to raise concerns freely, without criticism and know that they will be dealt with appropriately. At the same time the staff that are the subject of the concern, need to be treated fairly and supported, as often there are many contributory factors.

Continuing professional development

One way of ensuring professional performance is maintained is by a structured approach to continuing professional development (CPD). Most Royal Colleges have CPD schemes to accredit continuing training and all contracted staff will have access to study leave. Arrangements vary from hospital to hospital but are typically 10 days per annum, with partial costs reimbursed. However CPD can come from a variety of sources:

- Courses
- Specialist conferences
- Reading and writing for textbooks, journals, Internet
- Case presentations
- Visiting other centres (especially where transfer of skills is involved).

In many cases, the CPD is haphazard and choices depend on the location of the conference rather than its content. It is better to have a long-term, structured plan, taking into account the development needs of the clinical team in which a surgeon works.

Performance management

Performance management involves systematic review of performance with the aim of continuous improvement. The measures and targets of performance should be defined and ideally agreed beforehand. For surgical specialties, an increasing number of clinical indicators are being used (and published) by the NHS and Dr Foster (a private organisation). Examples include:

- Deaths in hospital and after discharge within 30 days of surgery
- Deaths in hospital and after discharge within 30 days following emergency admission for fracture of neck of femur
- Emergency re-admissions within 28 days.

Much of the data for these indicators are derived from coding of hospital discharges, so it pays to make sure that the level of coding is accurate and complete. Good coding is time-consuming but if the data is accurate it makes regular audit much easier to achieve.

Achieving change

The whole point of clinical governance is to improve clinical services. Some changes are obvious and easy to achieve; others are harder and often the system seems to be resistant to change. The first step is to try to define what needs to be changed and why. If there is evidence of a problem, this is a good start to opening discussions with other members of your team.

The next step is to think about other people who would be affected by your proposals. Very often in hospitals, clinical teams or departments have systems set up to optimise their work flow, but in the overall system this can cause blocks or problems elsewhere. There are often duplications of processes as patients move through the hospital. Occasionally the requirements are contradictory. If you can work with others in the clinical pathway and meet their needs, benefits grow and change is likely to be maintained.

After discussion, it is necessary to document the changes. Depending on the degree of change, it may be a simple update of a policy that is required. For larger projects *a case of need* and *an option appraisal* will be required. Often termed a 'business plan', this sets out the problem, options considered including 'do nothing/present system', and the likely costs involved. The Directorate business manager should be able to help you with this. These proposals will need to be discussed at a clinical team or Directorate meeting and it is good idea if you can have discussed them already and have supporters present to carry the day.

Many of the changes in hospital require money in one form or another. Capital refers to equipment or estate over the value of £5000. It is allocated usually a year ahead in a competitive bidding process. There is an annual cycle so choosing your timing is important. Alternative sources of money include sums allocated for specific projects (e.g. NSFs), capital retained for special areas (e.g. equipment for new consultants), charitable sources and leasing. It is important to realise that equipment often has running expenses (e.g. disposables, maintenance and capital charges) and money will have to be identified for this as well.

The other source of money is termed 'revenue' which is broadly divided into pay and non-pay. The budget is the financial plan for a department. Much of the money will be allocated but managers are always interested in schemes that will identify savings in the long-term. New money for developments is available but usually goes through an intense competitive process so your plans must be sound and well documented. It is also important to bear the annual financial cycle in mind:

April	New financial year
May	Budget usually meaning less
June	Budgets have changes with agreed funding
September	Plans needed for next year
October	Trust sorting priorities internally
December	Negotiations start with commissioners
January	Negotiations continue
February	Starts to get difficult to make changes to budget
March	Service and Financial Framework (SAFF) Agreement made; impossible to get changes to budget. Opportunity for savings or sudden release of capital to be spent by year-end.
April	A new financial year – time to update that plan.

Once a plan has been approved, all parties need to be informed of the change and the date it is to be introduced. Since it may be months since you spoke to other teams and some staff (e.g. junior medical staff) will have moved on, you will have to explain to all why the changes are being made. Purchases need chasing through the system otherwise the paperwork gets 'lost'. When it all comes together, don't forget to celebrate your success with the team, and re-audit the changes to see if they have brought the benefits you envisaged.

SUMMARY

Clinical governance is a multifaceted process, which should lead to improved patient care. The steps taken are not new and were utilised by good clinicians in the past. The new feature is the institutional structures to support and demonstrate that clinical practice is up to date. Surgeons should embrace the culture in the knowledge that they will be able to prove competence and obtain resources for improvements in future.

FURTHER READING AND WEBSITES

Department of Health (1997) *The New NHS – Modern and Dependable.* The Stationery Office, London

Department of Health (1998) *A First Class Service; Quality in the new NHS.* The Stationery Office, London

Department of Health (2001) *An Organisation with a Memory.* The Stationery Office, London

General Medical Council (1998) *Good Medical Practice.* General Medical Council, London

www.clinicalevidence.nhs.uk

www.nice.org.uk [National Institute for Clinical Excellence]

www.chi.nhs.uk [commission for Health improvement]

www.nelh-pc.nhs.uk [National electronic library for health]

www.cgsupport.org [clinical governance support]

www.medical-devices.gov.uk

www.sign.ac.uk [Scottish intercollegiate guidelines network]

www.gmc-uk.org

Index